Medical Microbiology

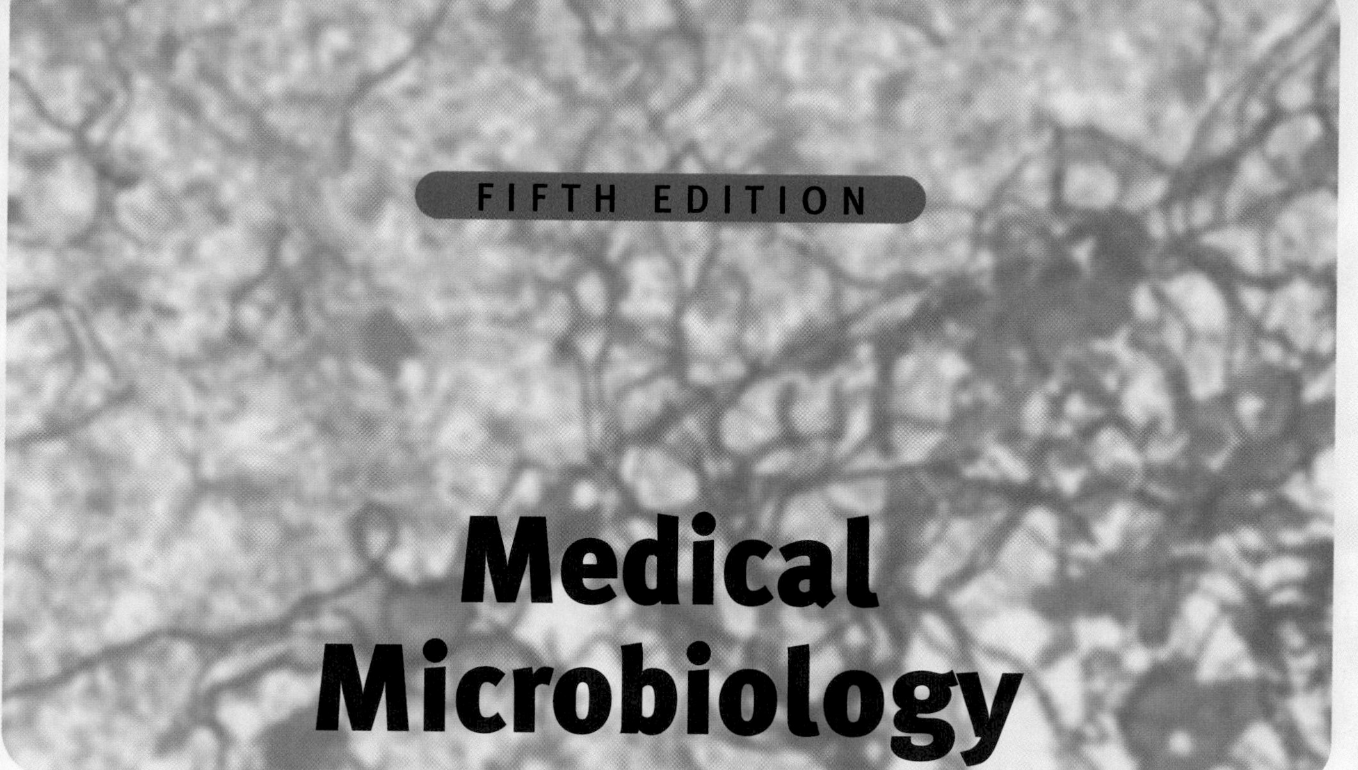

FIFTH EDITION

Medical Microbiology

Patrick R. Murray, PhD

Chief, Microbiology Service
Department of Laboratory Medicine
National Institutes of Health
Bethesda, Maryland

Ken S. Rosenthal, PhD

Professor
Department of Microbiology and Immunology
Northeastern Ohio Universities College of Medicine
Rootstown, Ohio

Michael A. Pfaller, MD

Professor, Pathology and Epidemiology
Director, Molecular Epidemiology and Fungus Testing Laboratory
Department of Pathology, Carver College of Medicine
University of Iowa College of Medicine
Iowa City, Iowa

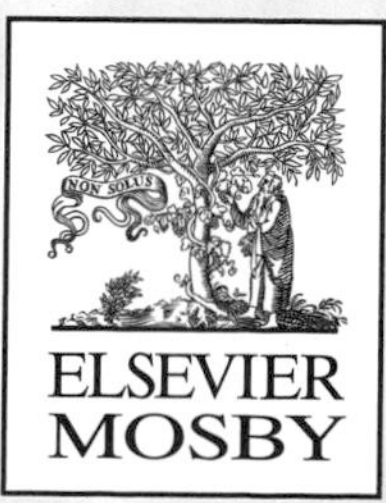

ELSEVIER
MOSBY

ELSEVIER
MOSBY

1600 John F. Kennedy Boulevard, Suite 1800
Philadelphia, Pennsylvania 19103-2899

Medical Microbiology
Fifth Edition

Copyright © 2005, 2002, 1998, 1994, and 1990 by Elsevier Inc. All rights reserved.

No part of this publication may be reproduced or transmitted in any form or by any means, electronic or mechanical, including photocopying, recording, or any information storage and retrieval system, without permission in writing from the publisher. Permissions may be sought directly from Elsevier's Health Sciences Rights Department in Philadelphia, PA, USA: phone: (+1) 215 239 3804, fax: (+1) 215 239 3805, e-mail: healthpermissions@elsevier.com. You may also complete your request on-line via the Elsevier homepage (http://www.elsevier.com), by selecting "Customer Support" and then "Obtaining Permissions."

NOTICE

Knowledge and best practice in this field are constantly changing. As new research and experience broaden our knowledge, changes in practice, treatment, and drug therapy may become necessary or appropriate. Readers are advised to check the most current information provided (i) on procedures featured or (ii) by the manufacturer of each product to be administered, to verify the recommended dose or formula, the method and duration of administration, and contraindications. It is the responsibility of the practitioner, relying on his or her own experience and knowledge of the patient, to make diagnoses, to determine dosages and the best treatment for each individual patient, and to take all appropriate safety precautions. To the fullest extent of the law, neither the Publisher nor the Authors assume any liability for any injury and/or damage to persons or property arising out or related to any use of the material contained in this book.

Patrick R. Murray's role as author of this book was carried out in his private capacity, and his contribution does not reflect official support or endorsement by the National Institutes of Health or the Department of Health and Human Services.

Previous editions copyrighted 2002, 1998, 1994, and 1990.

Library of Congress Cataloging-in-Publication Data
Murray, Patrick R.
Medical microbiology / Patrick R. Murray, Kenneth S. Rosenthal, Michael A. Pfaller.—5th ed.
p. ; cm.
Rev. ed. of: Medical microbiology / Patrick R. Murray . . . [et al.]. 4th ed. c2002.
Includes bibliographical references and index.
ISBN-10: 0-323-03303-2 ISBN-13: 978-0-323-03303-9
1. Medical microbiology. I. Rosenthal, Ken S. II. Pfaller, Michael A. III. Title.
[DNLM: 1. Microbiology. 2. Microbiological Techniques. 3. Parasitology. QW4 M983m 2005]
QR46.M4683 2005
616.9'041—dc22 2005047941

Acquisitions Editor: William Schmitt
Developmental Editor: Katie Miller
Publishing Services Manager: Joan Sinclair
Project Manager: Cecelia Bayruns
Illustrator: Lisa Lambert

Printed in the United States of America.

Last digit is the print number: 9 8 7 6 5 4 3 2

Working together to grow
libraries in developing countries
www.elsevier.com | www.bookaid.org | www.sabre.org
ELSEVIER BOOK AID International Sabre Foundation

To all who use
this textbook,
that they may benefit
from its use
as much as we did
in its preparation.

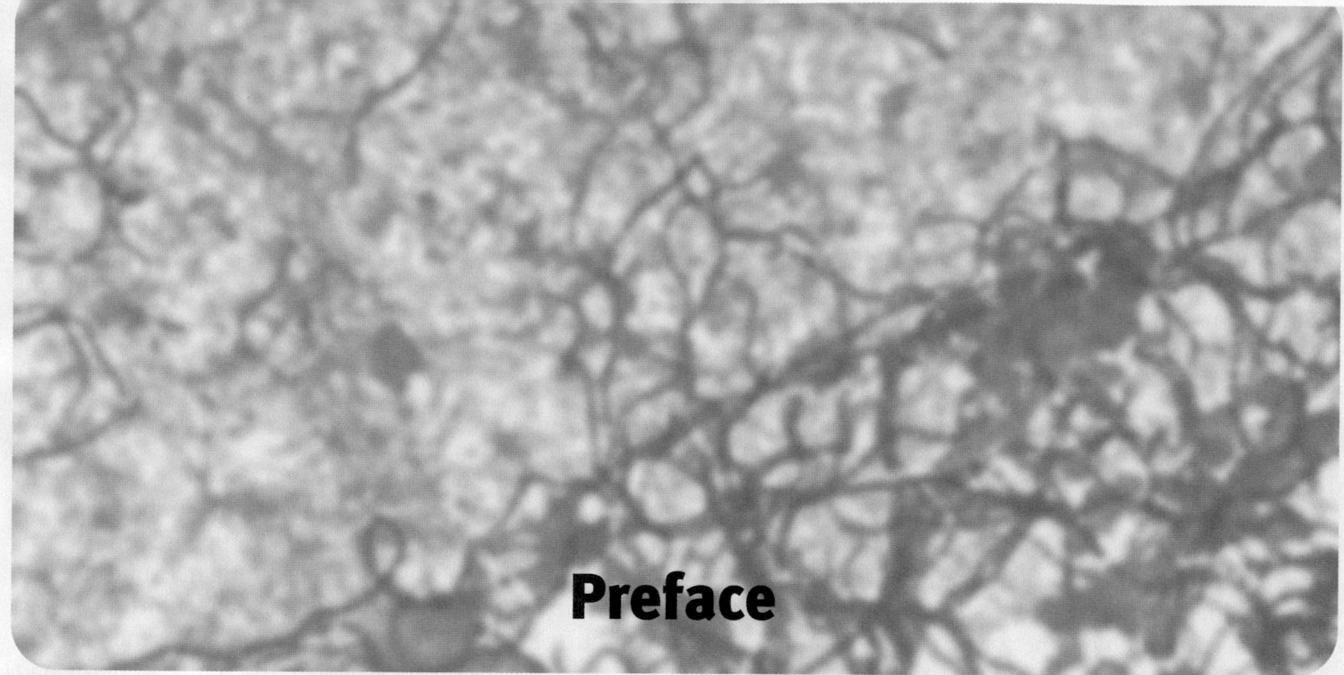

Preface

Medical microbiology can be a bewildering field to the novice. The student is faced with many questions when learning microbiology. How do I learn all the names? Which infectious agents cause which diseases? Why? When? Who is at risk? Is there a treatment? However, all these concerns can be reduced to one essential question: What information do I need to know that will help me understand how to diagnose and treat an infected patient?

Certainly, there are a number of theories about what a student needs to know and how to teach it, which supposedly validates the plethora of microbiology textbooks that have flooded the bookstores in recent years. Although we do not claim to have the one right approach to teaching medical microbiology (there is truly no one perfect approach to medical education), we have founded the revisions of this textbook on our experience gained through years of teaching medical students, residents, and infectious disease fellows as well as on the work devoted to the four previous editions. We have tried to present the basic concepts of medical microbiology clearly and succinctly in a manner that addresses different types of learners. The text is written in a straightforward manner with, it is hoped, uncomplicated explanations of difficult concepts. **Details** are summarized in tabular format rather than in lengthy text, and there are colorful illustrations for the visual learner. **Important points** are emphasized in **boxes** to aid the student, especially in their **review;** and the **study questions** address relevant aspects of each chapter, including **clinical cases.**

The material included in this text—and maybe more importantly, the material excluded—can be a subject for debate, but we have used our perception of the practical needs of the student as our guide. We are faced with the dilemma that new and exciting discoveries add not only to our foundation of knowledge but can also add to the length of the book. We used our experience as authors and teachers to choose the most important information and explanations for inclusion in this textbook. Each chapter has been carefully updated and expanded to include new, medically relevant discoveries. In each of these chapters, we have attempted to present the material that we feel will help the student gain a clear understanding of the significance of the individual microbes and their diseases.

With each edition of *Medical Microbiology* we refine and update our presentation. The obvious changes with this fifth edition include the addition of many new summary boxes, tables, and clinical photographs. We feel these are useful teaching aids for the students and the most efficient way to present this complex subject. We have reorganized and expanded the mycology section, consistent with the increased role of fungi in infectious diseases, particularly in the immunocompromised host. The student will also find discussions of newly discovered pathogens (e.g., SARS coronavirus, avian influenza virus) and old pathogens associated with new diseases (e.g., *Staphylococcus aureus* responsible for community-acquired necrotizing pneumonia). Finally, the student is provided with access to the Student Consult website, which provides links to additional reference materials, clinical photographs, and practice exam questions.

To the Student

How can the student digest what appear to be innumerable facts? On first impression, success in medical microbiology would seem to depend on memorization. Although memorization is an important part of any medical discipline, understanding the basic principles and developing a system for storing this information plays an important role in mastering this science. We suggest that the student concentrate on learning what is important by

thinking like a physician. Continue to ask seven basic questions as you approach this material: Who? Where? When? Why? Which? What? and How? For example: Who is at risk for disease? Where does this organism cause infections (both body site and geographic area)? When is isolation of this organism important? Why is this organism able to cause disease? Which species and genera are medically important? What diagnostic tests should be performed? How is this infection managed? Each organism that is encountered can be systematically examined. Know the specifics about how the organism grows, the virulence properties of the organism, and the diseases it causes; understand the epidemiology of infections; know what specimens should be collected and the basic identification tests that should be performed; and be familiar with preventive and therapeutic strategies. Learn three to five words or phrases that are associated with the microbe—words that will stimulate your memory **(trigger words)** and organize the diverse facts into a logical picture. Develop **alternative associations.** For example, this textbook presents organisms in the systematic taxonomic structure (frequently called a "bug parade," but which the authors think is the easiest way to introduce the organisms). Take a given virulence property (e.g., toxin production) or type of disease (e.g., meningitis) and list the organisms that share this property. Pretend that an imaginary patient is infected with a specific agent and create the case history. Explain the diagnosis to the imaginary patient and also to your future professional colleagues. In other words, do not simply attempt to memorize page after page of facts; rather, use techniques that stimulate your mind and challenge your understanding of the facts presented throughout the text.

No textbook of this magnitude would be successful without the contributions of numerous individuals. We thank Roberta Kamin-Lewis, Ph.D. for updates on HIV. We are grateful for the valuable professional help and support provided by the staff at Elsevier, particularly William Schmitt, Katie Miller, Jamey Stegmaier, and Cecelia Bayruns. We also want to thank the many students and professional colleagues who have offered their advice and constructive criticism throughout the development of this fifth edition of *Medical Microbiology*.

Patrick R. Murray, PhD
Ken S. Rosenthal, PhD
Michael A. Pfaller, MD

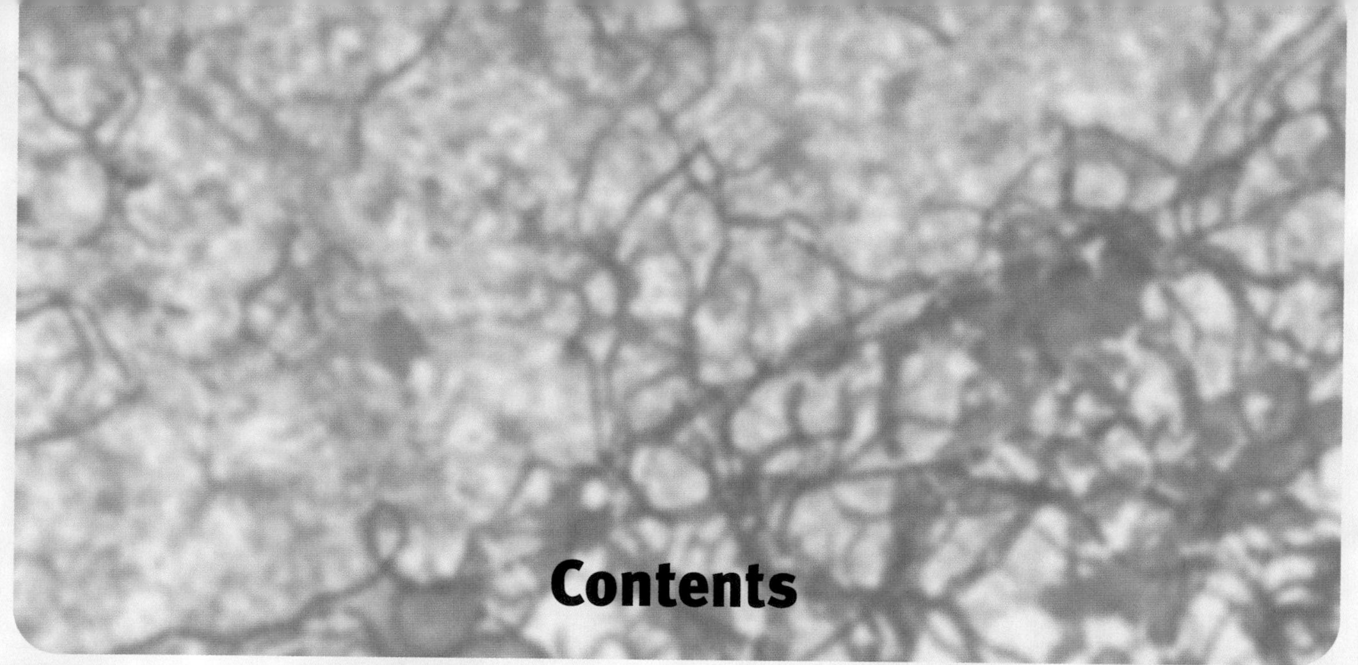

Contents

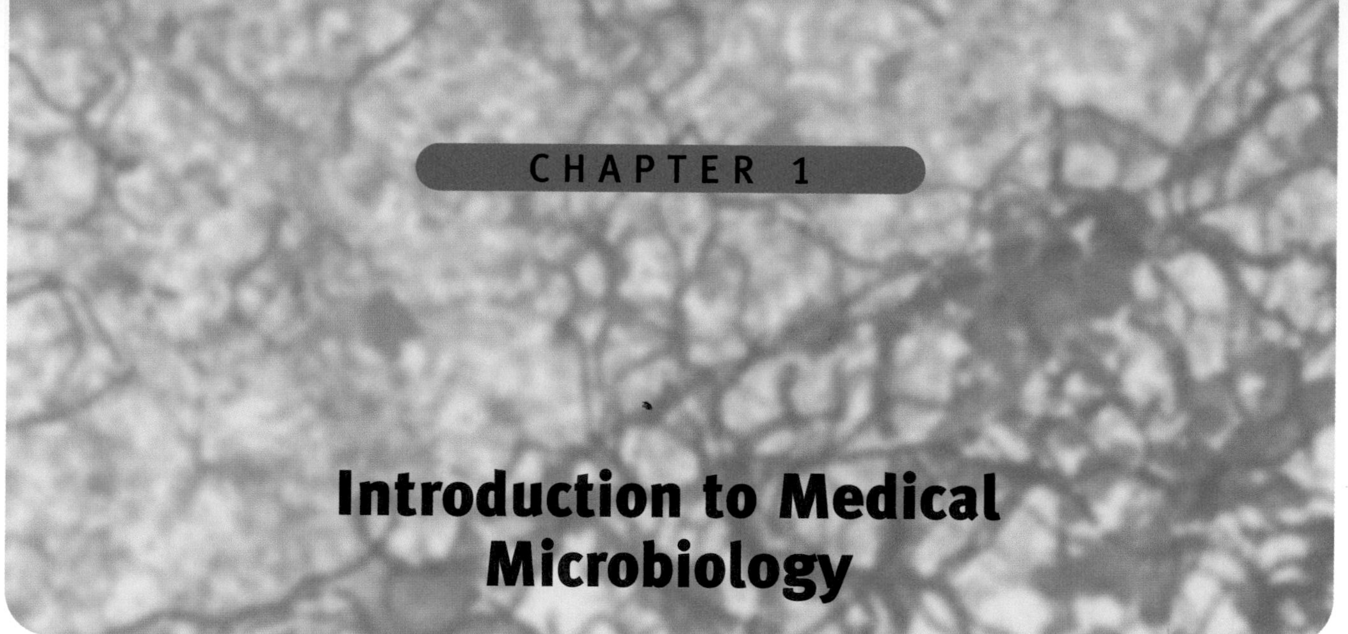

Introduction to Medical Microbiology

Since the last edition of this textbook, we have discovered new pathogens and their diseases (e.g., severe acute respiratory syndrome coronavirus [SARS-CoV] and H5N1 avian influenza A virus), old pathogens causing old diseases (e.g., vaccinia-associated vaccine complications), old pathogens causing new diseases (e.g., monkeypox virus), and bioterrorism (e.g., anthrax). We have also had to learn many new names for old organisms as the technology for microbial classification has become more sophisticated and discriminating. Some would challenge the wisdom or saneness of this development. Finally, the antibiotics that were so effective in the past are now impotent against some very common and important pathogens, because these drugs have been freely prescribed to humans and farm animals alike. Thus we find that the science of microbiology is in dynamic flux—an intellectually satisfying, but for the student, frustrating, development.

The Microbial World

Imagine the excitement felt by the Dutch biologist Anton van Leeuwenhoek in 1674 as he peered through his carefully ground microscopic lenses at a drop of water and discovered a world of millions of tiny "animalcules." Almost 100 years later, the Danish biologist Otto Müller extended van Leeuwenhoek's studies and organized bacteria into genera and species according to the classification methods of Carolus Linnaeus. This was the beginning of the taxonomic classification of microbes. In 1840 the German pathologist Friedrich Henle proposed criteria for proving that microorganisms were responsible for causing human disease (the "germ theory" of disease). Robert Koch and Louis Pasteur confirmed this theory in the 1870s and 1880s with a series of elegant experiments proving that microorganisms were responsible for causing anthrax, rabies, plague, cholera, and tuberculosis. Other brilliant scientists went on to prove that a diverse collection of microbes was responsible for causing human disease. The era of chemotherapy began in 1910, when the German chemist Paul Ehrlich discovered the first antibacterial agent, a compound effective against the spirochete that causes syphilis. This was followed by Alexander Fleming's discovery of penicillin in 1928, Gerhard Domagk's discovery of sulfanilamide in 1935, and Selman Waksman's discovery of streptomycin in 1943. In 1946, the American microbiologist John Enders was the first to cultivate viruses in cell cultures, leading the way to the large-scale production of virus cultures for vaccine development. Thousands of scientists have followed these pioneers, each building on the foundation established by his or her predecessors, and each adding an observation that expanded our understanding of microbes and their role in disease.

The world that van Leeuwenhoek discovered was complex, consisting of protozoa and bacteria of all shapes and sizes. However, the complexity of medical microbiology we know today rivals the limits of the imagination. We now know that there are thousands of different types of microbes that live in, on, and around us—and hundreds that cause serious human diseases. To understand this information and organize it in a useful manner, it is important to understand some of the basic aspects of medical microbiology. To start, the microbes can be subdivided into the following four groups: viruses, bacteria, fungi, and parasites, each having its own level of complexity.

VIRUSES

Viruses are the smallest infectious particles, ranging in diameter from 18 to nearly 300 nanometers (most viruses are less than 200 nm and cannot be seen with a light microscope). Twenty-five families with more than 1550 species of viruses have been described, and many are associated with human disease. Viruses consist of either deoxyribonucleic acid (DNA) or ribonucleic acid (RNA) (but not both) and may also contain proteins required for replication and pathogenesis. These components are then enclosed in a protein coat with or without a lipid membrane coat. Viruses are true parasites, requiring host cells for replication. The cells they infect and the host response to the infection dictate the nature of the clinical manifestation. Infection can lead either to rapid replication and destruction of the cell or to a long-term chronic relationship with possible integration of the viral genetic information into the host genome. The factors that determine which of these takes place are only partially understood. For example, infection with the human immunodeficiency virus, the etiologic agent of the acquired immunodeficiency syndrome (AIDS), can result in the latent infection of CD4 lymphocytes or the active replication and destruction of these immunologically important cells. Likewise, infection can spread to other susceptible cells, such as the microglial cells of the brain, resulting in the neurologic manifestations of AIDS. Thus the diseases caused by viruses can range from the common cold to gastroenteritis to fatal catastrophes such as rabies, ebola, smallpox, or AIDS.

BACTERIA

Bacteria are relatively simple in structure. They are **prokaryotic** organisms—simple unicellular organisms with no nuclear membrane, mitochondria, Golgi bodies, or endoplasmic reticulum—that reproduce by asexual division. The bacterial cell wall is complex, consisting of one of two basic forms: a gram-positive cell wall with a thick peptidoglycan layer, and a gram-negative cell wall with a thin peptidoglycan layer and an overlying outer membrane (additional information about this structure is presented in Chapter 3). Some bacteria lack this cell wall structure and compensate by surviving only inside host cells or in a hypertonic environment. The size (1 to 20 μm or larger), shape (spheres, rods, spirals), and spatial arrangement (single cells, chains, clusters) of the cells are used for the preliminary classification of bacteria, and the phenotypic and genotypic properties of the bacteria form the basis for the definitive classification. The human body is inhabited by thousands of different bacterial species—some living transiently, others in a permanent parasitic relationship. Likewise, the environment that surrounds us, including the air we breathe, water we drink, and food we eat, is inhabited by bacteria, many of which are relatively avirulent and some of which are capable of producing life-threatening disease. Disease can result from the toxic effects of bacterial products (toxins) or when bacteria inhabit normally sterile body sites.

FUNGI

In contrast to bacteria, the cellular structure of fungi is more complex. These are **eukaryotic** organisms that contain a well-defined nucleus, mitochondria, Golgi bodies, and endoplasmic reticulum. Fungi can exist either in a unicellular form **(yeast)** that can replicate asexually or in a filamentous form **(mold)** that can replicate asexually and sexually. Most fungi exist as either yeasts or molds; however, some fungi can assume either morphology. These are known as **dimorphic** fungi and consist of such organisms as *Histoplasma*, *Blastomyces*, and *Coccidioides*.

PARASITES

Parasites are the most complex microbes. Although all parasites are classified as eukaryotic, some are unicellular and others are multicellular. They range in size from tiny protozoa as small as 1 to 2 μm in diameter (the size of many bacteria) to arthropods and tapeworms that can measure up to 10 meters in length. Indeed, considering the size of some of these parasites, it is hard to imagine how these organisms came to be classified as microbes. Their life cycles are equally complex, with some parasites establishing a permanent relationship with humans and others going through a series of developmental stages in a progression of animal hosts. One of the difficulties confronting students is not only an understanding of the spectrum of diseases caused by parasites, but also an appreciation of the epidemiology of these infections, which is vital for understanding the diagnosis, control, and prevention of these infections.

Microbial Disease

One of the most important reasons for studying microbes is to understand the diseases they cause and the ways to control them. Unfortunately, the relationship between many organisms and their diseases is not simple. Specifically, most organisms do not cause a single, well-defined disease, although there are certainly ones that do (e.g., *Treponema pallidum*, syphilis; poliovirus, polio; *Plasmodium* species, malaria). Instead, it is more common for a particular organism to produce many manifestations of disease (e.g., *Staphylococcus aureus*—endocarditis, pneumonia, wound infections, food poisoning) or for many organisms to produce the same disease (e.g., meningitis caused by viruses, bacteria, fungi, and parasites). In addition, relatively few organisms can be classified as always pathogenic, although some do belong in this category (e.g., rabies virus, *Bacillus anthracis*, *Sporothrix schenckii*, *Plasmodium* species). Instead, most organisms are able to establish disease only under well-defined circumstances (e.g., the introduction of an organism with a potential for causing disease into a normally sterile site, such as the brain, lungs, and peritoneal cavity). Some diseases arise when a person is exposed to organisms from external sources. These are known as **exogenous infections** and examples include diseases caused by influenza virus, *Clostridium tetani, Neisseria gonorrhoeae, Coccidioides immitis,* and *Entamoeba histolytica.* Most human diseases, however, are produced by organisms in the person's own microbial flora that spread to inappropriate body sites where disease can ensue **(endogenous infections).**

The interaction between an organism and the human host is complex. The interaction can result in transient colonization, a long-term symbiotic relationship, or disease. The virulence of the organism, the site of exposure, and the host's ability to respond to the organism determine the outcome of this interaction. Thus the manifestations of disease can range from mild symptoms to organ failure and death. The role of microbial virulence and the host's immunologic response is discussed in depth in subsequent chapters.

The human body is remarkably adapted to controlling exposure to pathogenic microbes. Physical barriers prevent invasion by the microbe; innate responses recognize molecular patterns on the microbial components and activate local defenses and specific immune responses that target the microbe for elimination. Unfortunately, the immune response is often too late or too slow. To improve the human body's ability to prevent infection, the immune system can be augmented either through the passive transfer of antibodies present in immune globulin preparations or through active immunization with components of the microbes (antigens). Infections can also be controlled with a variety of chemotherapeutic agents. Unfortunately, many microbes can alter their antigenic complexion **(antigenic variation)** or develop resistance to even the most potent antibiotics. Thus the battle for control between microbe and host continues, with neither side yet able to claim victory (although the microbes have demonstrated remarkable ingenuity).

Diagnostic Microbiology

The clinical microbiology laboratory plays an important role in the diagnosis and control of infectious diseases. However, the ability of the laboratory to perform these functions is limited by the quality of the specimen collected from the patient, the means by which it is transported from the patient to the laboratory, and the techniques used to demonstrate the microbe in the sample. Because most diagnostic tests are based on the ability of the organism to grow, transport conditions must ensure the viability of the pathogen. In addition, the most sophisticated testing protocols are of little value if the collected specimen is not representative of the site of infection. This seems obvious, but many specimens sent to laboratories for analysis are contaminated during collection with the organisms that colonize the mucosal surfaces. It is virtually impossible to interpret the testing results with contaminated specimens because most infections are caused by endogenous organisms.

The laboratory is also able to determine the antimicrobial activity of selected chemotherapeutic agents, although the value of these tests is limited. The laboratory must test only organisms capable of producing disease and only medically relevant antimicrobials. To test all isolated organisms or an indiscriminate selection of drugs can yield misleading results with potentially dangerous consequences. Not only can a patient be treated inappropriately with unnecessary antibiotics, but also the true pathogenic organism may not be recognized among the plethora of organisms isolated and tested. Finally, the in vitro determination of an organism's susceptibility to a variety of antibiotics is only one aspect of a complex picture. The virulence of the organism, site of infection, and patient's ability to respond to the infection influence the host-parasite interaction and must also be considered when planning treatment.

Summary

It is important to realize that, as was stated at the beginning of this chapter, our knowledge of the microbial world is evolving continually. Just as the early microbiologists built their discoveries on the foundations established by their predecessors, so, too, will we (and future generations) continue to discover new microbes, new diseases, and new therapies. The following chapters are intended as a foundation of knowledge that can be used to enrich your understanding of microbes and their diseases.

SECTION I

Basic Principles of Medical Microbiology

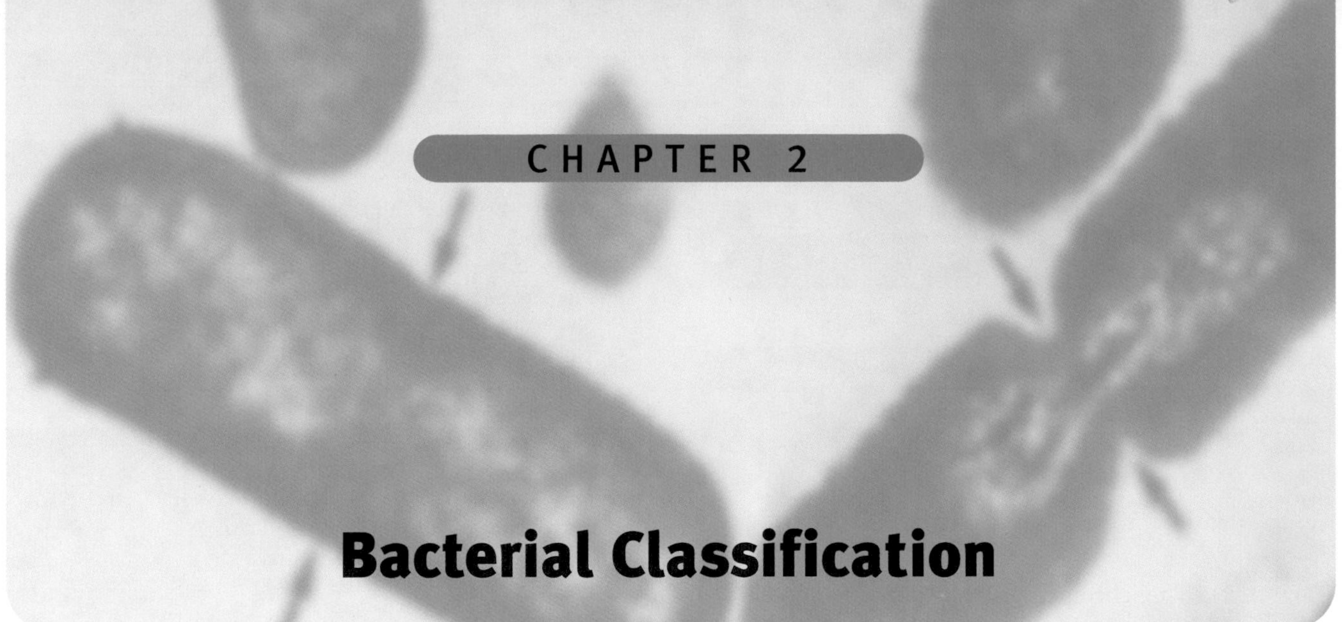

CHAPTER 2

Bacterial Classification

Understanding the relevance and complex nomenclature of literally hundreds of "important" bacteria can be challenging. The mastery of this exercise depends on the systematic organization of the bewildering array of different organisms into logical relationships (i.e., the taxonomic classification of the organisms).

Phenotypic Classification

The **microscopic** and **macroscopic morphologies** of bacteria were the first characteristics used to identify bacteria and form the cornerstones for most identification algorithms used today (Box 2–1). For example, bacteria can be classified by their ability to retain the Gram stain (gram-positive or gram-negative) and by the shape of the individual organisms (cocci, rods, curved, or spiral). The macroscopic appearance of colonies of bacteria (e.g., hemolytic properties on agar containing blood, pigmentation of the colonies, size and shape of the colonies, odor of the colonies) can also be used to identify bacteria. Thus, *Streptococcus pyogenes* is a gram-positive bacterium that forms long chains of cocci and appears as small, white, hemolytic colonies on blood agar plates. Because many organisms can appear very similar on microscopic and macroscopic examination, morphologic characteristics are used to provide a tentative identification of the organism and to select more discriminating classification methods.

The most common methods that are still used to identify bacteria consist of measuring the presence or absence of specific biochemical markers (e.g., ability to ferment specific carbohydrates or use different compounds as a source of carbon for growth; presence of specific proteases, lipases, or nucleases; presence of specific hydrolytic enzymes such as lipases and nucleases). With the use of carefully selected biochemical tests, most clinically significant isolates can be identified with a high degree of precision. These methods have also been used for subdividing groups of organisms beyond the species level, primarily for epidemiologic purposes (e.g., to determine whether a group of organisms from the same genus and species is from a common source or from distinct sources). This epidemiologic method is referred to as **biotyping.**

Many bacteria possess antigens that are unique, and antibodies used to detect these antigens are powerful tools for their identification **(serotyping)**. These serologic tests can be used to identify organisms that are inert in biochemical testing (e.g., *Francisella,* the organism that causes tularemia), are difficult or impossible to grow (e.g., *Treponema pallidum*, the organism responsible for syphilis), are associated with specific disease syndromes (e.g., *Escherichia coli* serotype O157, responsible for hemorrhagic colitis), or need to be identified rapidly (e.g., *S. pyogenes*, responsible for streptococcal pharyngitis). Serotyping is also used to subdivide bacteria below the species level for epidemiologic purposes.

Other examples of phenotypic methods used to classify bacteria include analysis of **antibiogram patterns** (patterns of susceptibility to various antibiotics) and **phage typing** (susceptibility to viruses that infect bacteria—bacteriophages). Assessment of antibiotic susceptibility patterns is commonly performed but has limited discriminatory power. Phage typing is technically cumbersome and has been replaced by more sensitive genetic techniques.

Analytic Classification

The analytic characteristics of bacteria have been used to classify bacteria at the genus, species, or subspecies level

BOX 2–1. Phenotypic Classification of Bacteria

Microscopic morphology	Serotyping
Macroscopic morphology	Antibiogram patterns
Biotyping	Phage typing

BOX 2–2. Analytic Classification of Bacteria

Cell wall fatty-acid analysis
Whole cell lipid analysis
Whole cell protein analysis
Multifocus locus enzyme electrophoresis

(Box 2–2). The chromatographic pattern of cell wall mycolic acids is unique for many of the individual species of mycobacteria and has been used for many years to identify the most commonly isolated species. Analysis of the lipids in the entire cell has also proved to be a useful method for characterizing many bacterial species and yeasts. Analyses of the whole cell proteins (proteomic analysis by **mass spectroscopy**) and cellular enzymes **(multilocus enzyme electrophoresis)** are also techniques that have been used to characterize bacteria, most typically at the subspecies level for epidemiologic investigations. Although these analytic methods are accurate and reproducible, they are labor intensive and the instrumentation is expensive. For these reasons the analyses are used primarily in reference laboratories.

Genotypic Classification

The most precise method for classifying bacteria is by analysis of their genetic material (Box 2–3). Organisms were initially classified by the **ratio of guanine to cytosine;** however, this procedure has largely been forsaken for more discriminating methods. **DNA** (deoxyribonucleic acid) **hybridization** was used initially to determine the relationship among bacterial isolates (i.e., to determine whether two isolates were in the same genus or species). More recently this technique has been exploited for the rapid identification of organisms by use of molecular probes. That is, DNA from an organism to be identified is extracted and exposed to species-specific molecular probes. If the probe binds to the DNA, then the organism's identity is confirmed. This technique has also been used to detect organisms directly in clinical specimens, thus avoiding the need to grow the organisms. DNA hybridization has proved to be a valuable tool for the rapid detection and identification of slow-growing organisms such as mycobacteria and fungi.

An extension of the hybridization method is **nucleic acid sequence analysis.** Probes are used to localize specific nucleic acid sequences that are unique to a genus, species, or subspecies. These sequences are amplified so that millions of copies are produced, and then the amplified genetic material is sequenced to define the precise identity of the isolate. The most common application of this technique is analysis of sequences of ribosomal DNA (because highly conserved [family- or genus-specific] sequences and highly variable [species- or subspecies-specific] sequences are present). It has also been used to define the evolutionary relationship among organisms and to identify organisms that are difficult or impossible to grow. Most of the recent changes in taxonomic nomenclature were determined by nucleic acid sequence analysis. An extension of this work is the complete sequencing of a bacterium's entire genome, a technique that has become technically feasible, although not yet used in for diagnostic purposes.

BOX 2–3. Genotypic Classification of Bacteria

Guanine plus cytosine ratio
DNA hybridization
Nucleic acid sequence analysis
Plasmid analysis
Ribotyping
Chromosomal DNA fragment analysis

BOX 2–4. Aerobic, Gram-Positive Cocci

Catalase-Positive Cocci	Catalase-Negative Cocci
Micrococcus	*Aerococcus*
Staphylococcus	*Alloiococcus*
	Enterococcus
	Lactococcus
	Leuconostoc
	Pediococcus
	Streptococcus

Various other methods that have been used, primarily to classify organisms at the subspecies level for epidemiologic investigations, include the following: **plasmid analysis, ribotyping,** and **analysis of chromosomal DNA fragments.** In recent years the technical aspects of these methods have been simplified to the point that most clinical laboratories use variations of these methods in their day-to-day practice.

Boxes 2–4 through 2–8 provide a useful classification scheme for organizing the many bacteria that are discussed in subsequent chapters. It should be noted that the list of organisms is not exhaustive. Many genera that are recovered in clinical specimens are omitted for the sake of simplifying this presentation. The organisms included in these summary boxes are only those that are discussed in subsequent chapters. In addition, the precise arrangement of bacteria in families, genera, and species continues to change.

BOX 2–5. Aerobic, Gram-Positive Rods

Actinomycetes with Cell Wall Mycolic Acids
Corynebacterium
Gordonia
Nocardia
Rhodococcus
Tsukamurella
Mycobacterium

Actinomycetes with No Cell Wall Mycolic Acids
Actinomadura
Dermatophilus
Nocardiopsis
Oerskovia
Rothia
Streptomyces
Thermophilic actinomycetes
  Saccharomonospora
  Saccharopolyspora
  Thermoactinomyces
Tropheryma

Miscellaneous Gram-Positive Rods
Arcanobacterium
Bacillus
Brevibacterium
Erysipelothrix
Gardnerella
Listeria
Turicella

BOX 2–6. Aerobic, Gram-Negative Cocci, Coccobacilli, and Rods

Cocci and Coccobacilli
Branhamella
Moraxella
Neisseria

Rods
Enterobacteriaceae
  Citrobacter
  Enterobacter
  Escherichia
  Klebsiella
  Morganella
  Plesiomonas
  Proteus
  Salmonella
  Serratia
  Shigella
  Yersinia
Vibrionaceae
  Vibrio
Aeromonadaceae
  Aeromonas
Campylobacteriaceae
  Arcobacter
  Campylobacter
Helicobacteriaceae
  Helicobacter
Pseudomonadaceae
  Pseudomonas
Pasteurellaceae
  Actinobacillus
  Haemophilus
  Pasteurella

Miscellaneous Genera
Acinetobacter
Bartonella
Bordetella
Brucella
Burkholderia
Capnocytophaga
Cardiobacterium
Eikenella
Francisella
Kingella
Legionella
Stenotrophomonas
Streptobacillus

BOX 2–7. Anaerobic Gram-Positive and Gram-Negative Bacteria

Gram-Positive Cocci
Anaerococcus
Finegoldia
Micromonas
Peptostreptococcus
Schleiferella

Gram-Negative Cocci
Veillonella

Gram-Positive Rods
Actinomyces
Bifidobacterium
Clostridium
Eubacterium
Lactobacillus
Mobiluncus
Propionibacterium

Gram-Negative Rods
Bacteroides
Fusobacterium
Porphyromonas
Prevotella

BOX 2–8. Miscellaneous, Medically Important Bacteria

Mycoplasmataceae
  Mycoplasma
  Ureaplasma
Spirochaetaceae
  Borrelia
  Treponema
Leptospiraceae
  Leptospira
Chlamydiaceae
  Chlamydia
  Chlamydophila
Other bacteria
  Coxiella
  Ehrlichia
  Orientia
  Rickettsia

QUESTIONS

1. Name three examples each of phenotypic, analytic, and genotypic characteristics used to classify bacteria.
2. Describe the microscopic morphology (e.g., Gram-stain characteristic, shape of organism) of the following bacteria: *Staphylococcus, Escherichia, Neisseria, Clostridium, Enterococcus,* and *Pseudomonas.*
3. Which of the following organisms have mycolic acids in their cell walls: *Staphylococcus, Nocardia, Mycobacterium,* and *Klebsiella?*

Bibliography

Balows A et al, editors: *The prokaryotes,* ed 2, New York, 1992, Springer-Verlag.

Murray PR et al, editors: *Manual of clinical microbiology,* ed 8, Washington, 2003, American Society for Microbiology.

Murray PR, Shea Y: *Pocket guide to clinical microbiology,* ed 3, Washington, 2004, American Society for Microbiology.

CHAPTER 3

Bacterial Morphology and Cell Wall Structure and Synthesis

Cells are the fundamental units of living things, from the smallest bacterium to the largest of the plants and animals. Bacteria, the smallest cells, are visible only with the aid of a microscope. The smallest bacteria (*Chlamydia* and *Rickettsia*) are just 0.1 to 0.2 μm in diameter, whereas larger bacteria may be many microns in length. A newly described species is hundreds of times larger than the average bacterial cell and is visible to the naked eye. Most species, however, are approximately 1 μm in diameter and are therefore visible with the use of the light microscope, which has a resolution of 0.2 μm. In comparison, animal and plant cells are much larger, ranging from 7 μm (the diameter of a red blood cell) to several feet (the length of certain nerve cells).

Each cell contains the genetic basis for reproduction in its deoxyribonucleic acid (DNA) genome, the biochemical machinery for transcribing genetic information into messenger ribonucleic acid (mRNA) and translating the mRNA into proteins, and the machinery for energy production and biosynthesis, which is all packaged by a membrane. In addition, each cell replicates by cell division. The mechanisms and machinery for accomplishing these functions are basically similar, but the specifics may be different for bacteria and for the higher-order organisms. These differences are influenced by the structure of the cell, the environment in which the cell lives, the source and means of the cell's energy production, and the nature of and requirement for cell interaction (or lack thereof).

Differences Between Eukaryotes and Prokaryotes

Cells from animals, plants, and fungi are **eukaryotes** (Greek for "true nucleus"), whereas bacteria and blue-green algae belong to the **prokaryotes** (Greek for "primitive nucleus"). In addition to lacking a nucleus and other organelles, prokaryotes use a smaller ribosome, the 70S ribosome, and in most bacteria a meshlike peptidoglycan cell wall surrounds the membranes to protect them against the environment. Bacteria can survive and, in some cases, grow in hostile environments in which the osmotic pressure outside the cell is so low that most eukaryotic cells would lyse at temperature extremes (both hot and cold), with dryness, and with very dilute and diverse energy sources. Bacteria have evolved their structures and functions to adapt to these conditions. These and other distinguishing features are depicted in Figure 3–1 and outlined in Table 3–1. Several of these distinctions provide the basis for antimicrobial action.

Differences Among Prokaryotes

Bacteria can be distinguished from one another by their morphology (size, shape, and staining characteristics) and metabolic, antigenic, and genetic characteristics. Although bacteria are difficult to differentiate by size, they do have different shapes. A spherical bacterium, such as *Staphylococcus*, is a **coccus;** a rod-shaped bacterium, such as *Escherichia coli*, is a **bacillus;** and the snakelike treponeme is a **spirillum.** In addition, *Nocardia* and *Actinomyces* species have **branched filamentous** appearances similar to those of fungi. Some bacteria form aggregates such as the grapelike clusters of *Staphylococcus aureus* or the **diplococcus** (two cells together) observed in *Streptococcus* or *Neisseria* species.

Gram stain is a powerful, easy test that allows clinicians to distinguish between the two major classes of bacteria and to initiate therapy (Figure 3–2). Bacteria that are heat fixed or otherwise dried onto a slide are stained with **crystal violet** (Figure 3–3), a stain that is precipitated

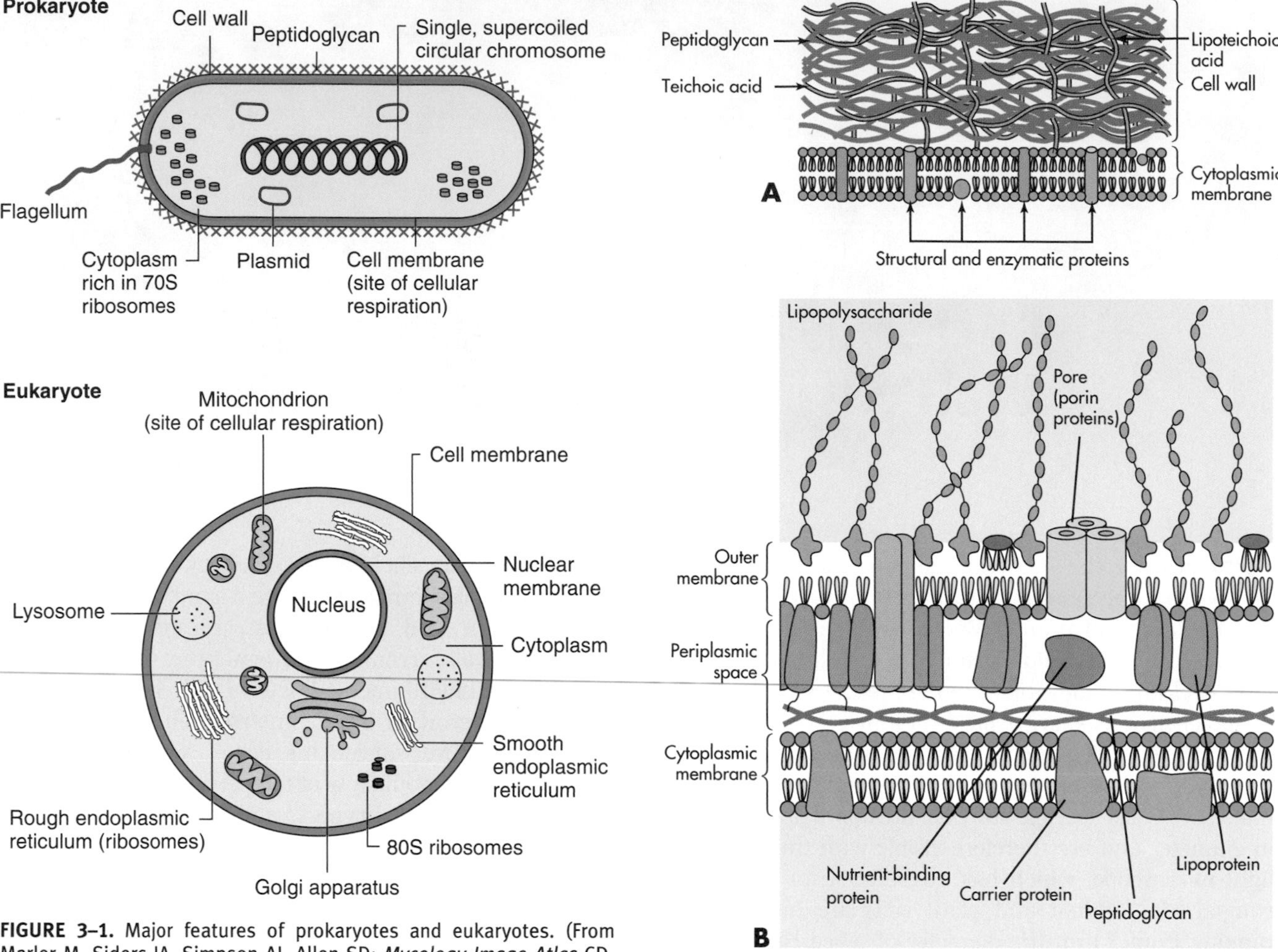

FIGURE 3–1. Major features of prokaryotes and eukaryotes. (From Marler M, Siders JA, Simpson AI, Allen SD: *Mycology Image Atlas* CD-Rom, Indiana Pathology Images, 2004.)

FIGURE 3–2. Comparison of the gram-positive and gram-negative bacterial cell walls. **A,** A gram-positive bacterium has a thick peptidoglycan layer that contains teichoic and lipoteichoic acids. **B,** A gram-negative bacterium has a thin peptidoglycan layer and an outer membrane that contains lipopolysaccharide, phospholipids, and proteins. The periplasmic space between the cytoplasmic and outer membranes contains transport, degradative, and cell wall synthetic proteins. The outer membrane is joined to the cytoplasmic membrane at adhesion points and is attached to the peptidoglycan by lipoprotein links. (From Marler M, Siders JA, Simpson AI, Allen SD: *Mycology Image Atlas* CD-Rom, Indiana Pathology Images, 2004.)

with **iodine,** and then the unbound and excess stain is removed by washing with the acetone-based **decolorizer** and water. A red counterstain, **safranin,** is added to stain any decolorized cells. This process takes less than 10 minutes.

For **gram-positive bacteria,** which turn **purple,** the stain gets trapped in a thick, cross-linked, meshlike structure, the peptidoglycan layer, which surrounds the cell. **Gram-negative bacteria** have a thin peptidoglycan layer that does not retain crystal violet stain, so the cells must be counterstained with safranin and turned red (Figure 3–4). A mnemonic device that may help is **"P-PURPLE-POSITIVE."** Gram stain is not a dependable test for bacteria that are starved (e.g., old or stationary phase cultures) or treated with antibiotics due to degradation of the peptidoglycan.

Bacteria that cannot be classified by Gram stain include mycobacteria, which have a waxy outer shell and are distinguished with the acid-fast stain, and mycoplasmas, which have no peptidoglycan.

Bacterial Ultrastructure

CYTOPLASMIC STRUCTURES

Gram-positive and gram-negative bacteria have similar internal structures, but their external structures are quite different. The cytoplasm of the bacterial cell contains the DNA chromosome, mRNA, ribosomes, proteins, and metabolites (see Figure 3–4). Unlike eukaryotes, the **bacterial chromosome** is a single, double-stranded circle that is contained not in a nucleus, but in a discrete area known as the **nucleoid.** Histones are not present to

TABLE 3–1. Major Characteristics of Eukaryotes and Prokaryotes

Characteristic	Eukaryote	Prokaryote
Major groups	Algae, fungi, protozoa, plants, animals	Bacteria
Size (approximate)	>5 μm	0.5-3.0 μm
Nuclear Structures		
Nucleus	Classic membrane	No nuclear membrane
Chromosomes	Strands of DNA Diploid genome	Single, circular DNA Haploid genome
Cytoplasmic Structures		
Mitochondria	Present	Absent
Golgi bodies	Present	Absent
Endoplasmic reticulum	Present	Absent
Ribosomes (sedimentation coefficient)	80S (60S + 40S)	70S (50S + 30S)
Cytoplasmic membrane	Contains sterols	Does not contain sterols
Cell wall	Present for fungi; otherwise absent	Is a complex structure containing protein, lipids, and peptidoglycans
Reproduction	Sexual and asexual	Asexual (binary fission)
Movement	Complex flagellum, if present	Simple flagellum, if present
Respiration	Via mitochondria	Via cytoplasmic membrane

Modified from Holt S: In Slots J, Taubman M, editors: *Contemporary oral microbiology and immunology,* St Louis, 1992, Mosby.

maintain the conformation of the DNA, and the DNA does not form nucleosomes. **Plasmids,** which are smaller, circular, extrachromosomal DNAs, may also be present. Plasmids are most commonly found in gram-negative bacteria, and although not usually essential for cellular survival, they often provide a selective advantage: many confer resistance to one or more antibiotics.

The lack of a nuclear membrane simplifies the requirements and control mechanisms for the synthesis of proteins. Without a nuclear membrane, transcription and translation are coupled; in other words, ribosomes can bind to the mRNA, and protein can be made as the mRNA is being synthesized and still attached to the DNA.

The **bacterial ribosome** consists of 30S + 50S subunits, forming a 70S ribosome. This is unlike the eukaryotic 80S (40S + 60S) ribosome. The proteins and RNA of the bacterial ribosome are significantly different from those of eukaryotic ribosomes and are major targets for antibacterial drugs.

The **cytoplasmic membrane** has a lipid bilayer structure similar to the structure of the eukaryotic membranes, but it contains no steroids (e.g., cholesterol); mycoplasmas are the exception to this rule. The cytoplasmic membrane is responsible for many of the functions attributable to organelles in eukaryotes. These tasks include electron transport and energy production, which are normally achieved in the mitochondria (Figure 3–5). In addition, the membrane contains transport proteins that allow the uptake of metabolites and the release of other substances, ion pumps to maintain a membrane potential, and enzymes. A coiled cytoplasmic membrane, the **mesosome,** acts as an anchor to bind and pull apart daughter chromosomes during cell division. The inside of the membrane is lined with actinlike protein filaments, which help determine the shape of the bacteria and the site of septum formation for cell division. Although recently described for other bacteria, the filaments are a characteristic of the treponemes, a spirilla-shaped bacteria.

CELL WALL

The structure (Table 3–2), components, and functions (Table 3–3) of the cell wall distinguish gram-positive from gram-negative bacteria. Cell wall components are also unique to bacteria, and their repetitive structure elicits innate protective immune responses in humans. The important differences in membrane characteristics are outlined in Table 3–4. Rigid **peptidoglycan (murein)** layers surround the cytoplasmic membrances of most prokaryotes. The exceptions are *Archaeobacteria* organisms

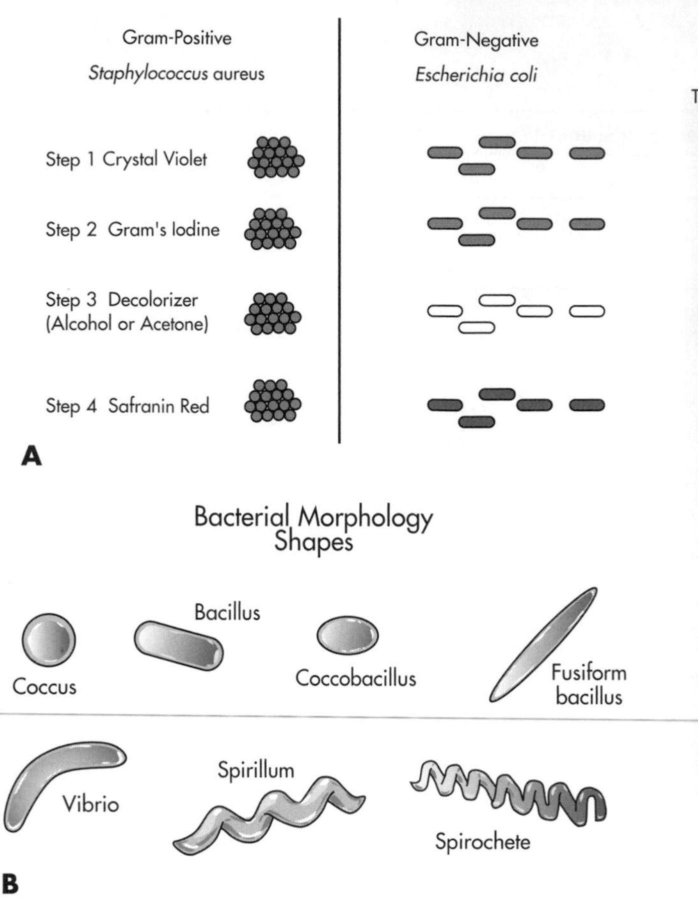

FIGURE 3–3. Gram-stain morphology of bacteria. **A,** The crystal violet of Gram stain is precipitated by Gram iodine and is trapped in the thick peptidoglycan layer in gram-positive bacteria. The decolorizer disperses the gram-negative outer membrane and washes the crystal violet from the thin layer of peptidoglycan. Gram-negative bacteria are visualized by the red counterstain. **B,** Bacterial morphologies.

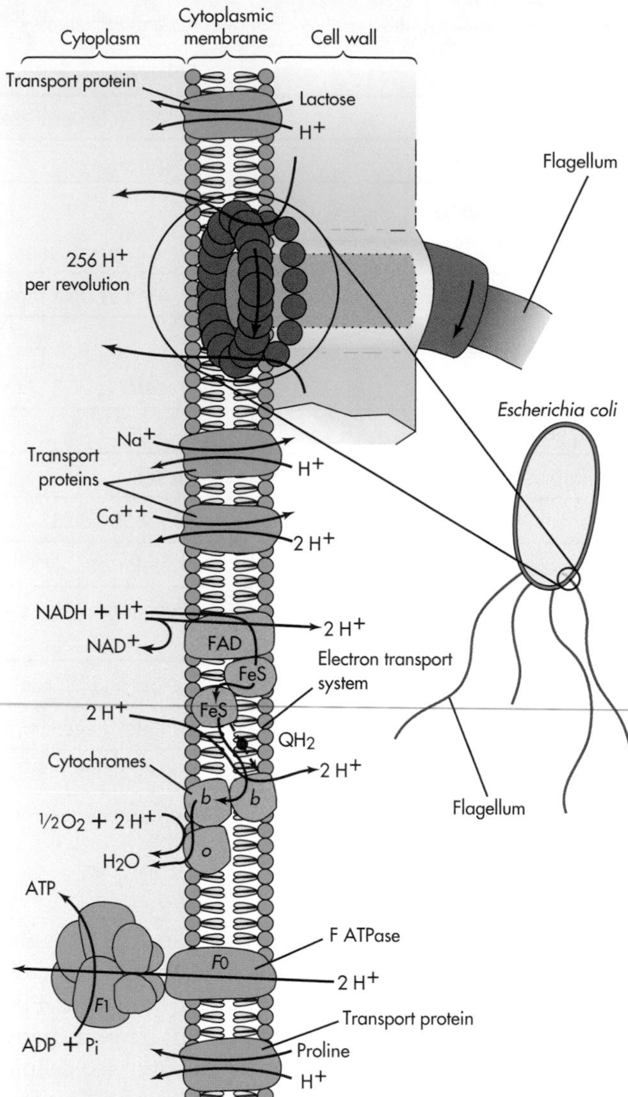

FIGURE 3–5. The cytoplasmic membrane contains the machinery for the production of adenosine triphosphate (ATP) (electron transport system, cytochromes, F1-adenosine triphosphatase [F1-ATPase]) and membrane potential. The membrane potential provides electrochemical energy for transport proteins and the flagellum 'motor.' ADP, adenosine diphosphate; FAD, flavin adenine dinucleotide; NAD, nicotine adenine dinucleotide; NADH, reduced form of nicotine adenine dinucleotide; Pi, phosphate. (From Marler M, Siders JA, Simpson AI, Allen SD: *Mycology Image Atlas* CD-Rom, Indiana Pathology Images, 2004.)

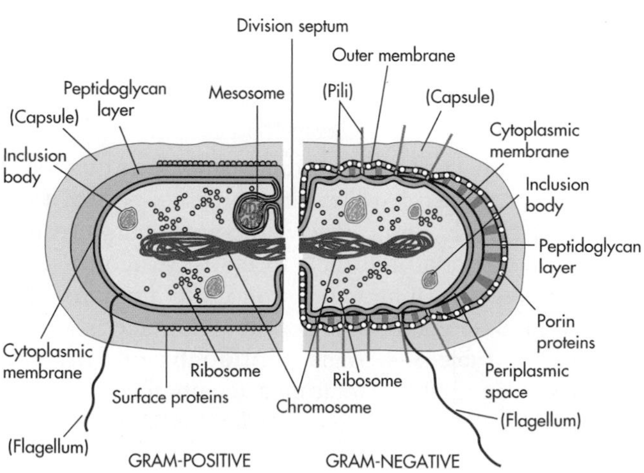

FIGURE 3–4. Gram-positive and gram-negative bacteria. A gram-positive bacterium has a thick layer of peptidoglycan (filling the purple space) *(left)*. A gram-negative bacterium has a thin peptidoglycan layer (single black line) and an outer membrane *(right)*. Structures in listed in parentheses are not found in all bacteria. Upon cell division the membrane and peptidoglycan grow toward each other to form a division septum to separate the daughter cells. (From Marler M, Siders JA, Simpson AI, Allen SD: *Mycology Image Atlas* CD-Rom, Indiana Pathology Images, 2004.)

TABLE 3–2. Bacterial Membrane Structures

Structure	Chemical Constituents
Plasma membrane	Phospholipids, proteins, and enzymes involved in generation of energy, membrane potential, and transport
Cell Wall	
Gram-positive bacteria	
Peptidoglycan	Glycan chains of GlcNAc and MurNAc cross-linked by peptide bridge
Teichoic acid	Polyribitol phosphate or glycerol phosphate cross-linked to peptidoglycan
Lipoteichoic acid	Lipid-linked teichoic acid
Gram-negative bacteria	
Peptidoglycan	Thinner version of that found in gram-positive bacteria
Periplasmic space	Enzymes involved in transport, degradation, and synthesis
Outer membrane	Phospholipids with saturated fatty acids
Proteins	Porins, lipoprotein, transport proteins
LPS	Lipid A, core polysaccharide, O antigen
Other structures	
Capsule	Polysaccharides (disaccharides and trisaccharides) and polypeptides
Pili	Pilin, adhesins
Flagellum	Motor proteins, flagellin
Proteins	M protein of streptococci (as an example)

GlcNAc, *N*-Acetylglucosamine; LPS, lipopolysaccharide; MurNAc, *N*-acetylmuramic acid.

(which contain pseudoglycans or pseudomureins related to peptidoglycan) and mycoplasmas (which have no cell walls). Because the peptidoglycan provides rigidity, it also helps to determine the shape of the particular bacterial cell. Gram-negative bacteria are also surrounded by outer membranes.

GRAM-POSITIVE BACTERIA

A gram-positive bacterium has a *thick, multilayered cell wall consisting mainly of peptidoglycan* (150 to 500 Å) surrounding the cytoplasmic membrane (see Figure 3–6). The peptidoglycan is a meshlike exoskeleton similar in function to the exoskeleton of an insect. Unlike the exoskeleton of the insect, however, the peptidoglycan of

TABLE 3–3. Functions of the Bacterial Envelope

Function	Component
Structure	
Rigidity	All
Packaging of internal contents	All
Bacterial Functions	
Permeability barrier	Outer membrane or plasma membrane
Metabolic uptake	Membranes and periplasmic transport proteins, porins, permeases
Energy production	Plasma membrane
Motility	Flagella
Mating	Pili
Host Interaction	
Adhesion to host cells	Pili, proteins, teichoic acid
Immune recognition by host	All outer structures
Escape from host immune recognition	Capsule, M protein
Medical Relevance	
Antibiotic sensitivity	Peptidoglycan synthetic enzymes
Antibiotic resistance	Outer membrane

TABLE 3–4. Membrane Characteristics of Gram-Positive and Gram-Negative Bacteria

Characteristic	Gram-Positive	Gram-Negative
Outer membrane	–	+
Cell wall	Thicker	Thinner
LPS	–	+
Endotoxin	–	+
Teichoic acid	Often present	–
Sporulation	Some strains	–
Capsule	Sometimes present	Sometimes present
Lysozyme	Sensitive	Resistant
Antibacterial activity of penicillin	More susceptible	More resistant
Exotoxin production	Some strains	Some strains

LPS, Lipopolysaccharide.

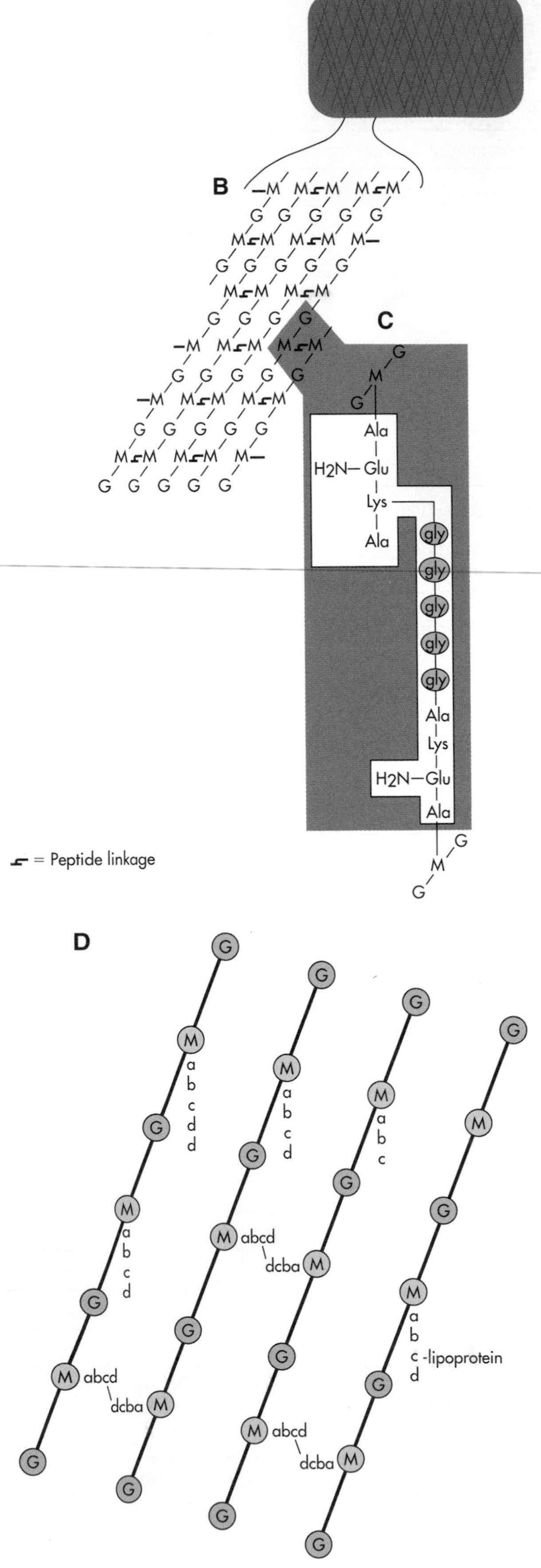

the cell is sufficiently porous to allow diffusion of metabolites to the plasma membrane. The *peptidoglycan is essential* for the structure, for replication, and for survival in the normally hostile conditions in which bacteria grow. During infection the peptidoglycan can interfere with phagocytosis and stimulate innate responses, including pyrogenic activity (i.e., induce fever).

The peptidoglycan can be degraded by treatment with **lysozyme.** Lysozyme is an enzyme in human tears and mucus, but is also produced by bacteria and other organisms. Lysozyme degrades the glycan backbone of the peptidoglycan. Without the peptidoglycan, the bacteria succumb to the large osmotic pressure differences across the cytoplasmic membrane and lyse. Removal of the cell wall produces a **protoplast** that lyses unless it is osmotically stabilized.

The gram-positive cell wall may also include other components such as teichoic and lipoteichoic acids and complex polysaccharides (usually called C polysaccharides). The M protein of streptococci and R protein of staphylococci also associate with the peptidoglycan. **Teichoic acids** are water-soluble, anionic polymers of polyol phosphates, which are covalently linked to the peptidoglycan and essential to cell viability. **Lipoteichoic acids** have a fatty acid and are anchored in the cytoplasmic membrane. These molecules are common surface antigens that distinguish bacterial serotypes and promote attachment to other bacteria and to specific receptors on mammalian cell surfaces (adherence). Teichoic acids are important factors in virulence. Lipoteichoic acids are shed into the media and host and, although weaker, can initiate host responses similar to endotoxin.

GRAM-NEGATIVE BACTERIA

Gram-negative cell walls are more complex than gram-positive cell walls, both structurally and chemically (see Figure 3–2). Structurally, a gram-negative cell wall contains two layers external to the cytoplasmic membrane.

FIGURE 3–6. General structure of the peptidoglycan component of the cell wall. **A,** The peptidoglycan forms a meshlike layer around the cell. **B,** The peptidoglycan mesh consists of a polysaccharide polymer that is cross-linked by peptide bonds. **C,** Peptides are cross-linked through a peptide bond between the terminal D-alanine (D-ala) from one chain and a lysine (lys) (or another diamino amino acid) from the other chain. A pentaglycine bridge (gly_5) expands the cross-link in *Staphylococcus aureus* (as shown). **D,** Representation of the *Escherichia coli* peptidoglycan structure. Diaminopimelic acid, the diamino amino acid in the third position of the peptide, is *directly linked* to the terminal alanine of another chain to cross-link the peptidoglycan. Lipoprotein anchors the outer membrane to the peptidoglycan. G, *N*-acetylglucosamine; Glu, glucosamine; gly, glycine; M, *N*-acetylmuramic acid. (From Marler M, Siders JA, Simpson AI, Allen SD: *Mycology Image Atlas* CD-Rom, Indiana Pathology Images, 2004.)

Immediately external to the cytoplasmic membrane is a *thin peptidoglycan layer,* which accounts for only 5% to 10% of the gram-negative cell wall by weight. There are *no teichoic or lipoteichoic acids* in the gram-negative cell wall. External to the peptidoglycan layer is the **outer membrane,** which is unique to gram-negative bacteria. The area between the external surface of the cytoplasmic membrane and the internal surface of the outer membrane is referred to as the **periplasmic space.** This space is actually a compartment containing a variety of hydrolytic enzymes that are important to the cell for the breakdown of large macromolecules for metabolism. These enzymes typically include proteases, phosphatases, lipases, nucleases, and carbohydrate-degrading enzymes. In the case of pathogenic gram-negative species, many of the lytic virulence factors, such as collagenases, hyaluronidases, proteases, and β-lactamase, are in the periplasmic space. This space also contains components of the sugar transport systems and other binding proteins to facilitate the uptake of different metabolites and other compounds. Some binding proteins can be components of a chemotaxis system, which senses the external environment of the cell.

As mentioned previously, outer membranes (see Figure 3–2) are unique to gram-negative prokaryotes. The outer membrane is like a stiff canvas sack around the bacteria. *The outer membrane maintains the bacterial structure and is a permeability barrier to large molecules* (e.g., proteins such as lysozyme) *and hydrophobic molecules.* It also provides protection from adverse environmental conditions such as the digestive system of the host (important for Enterobacteriaceae organisms). The outer membrane has an asymmetric bilayer structure that differs from any other biologic membrane in the structure of the outer leaflet of the membrane. The inner leaflet contains phospholipids normally found in bacterial membranes. However, the outer leaflet is composed primarily of an amphipathic molecule (meaning that it has both hydrophobic and hydrophilic ends) called **lipopolysaccharide (LPS).** Except for those LPS molecules in the process of synthesis, the outer leaflet of the outer membrane is the only location where LPS molecules are found.

LPS is also called **endotoxin,** a powerful stimulator of innate and immune responses. LPS activates B cells and induces macrophage, dendritic, and other cells to release interleukin-1 and interleukin-6, tumor necrosis factor, and other factors. LPS causes fever and can cause shock. The **Shwartzman reaction** (disseminated intravascular coagulation) follows the release of large amounts of endotoxin into the bloodstream. LPS is shed from the bacteria into the media and host. *Neisseria* bacteria shed large amounts of a related compound, lipooligosaccharide **(LOS),** resulting in fever and severe symptoms.

The variety of proteins found in gram-negative outer membranes is limited, but several of the proteins are present in high concentration, resulting in a total protein content that is higher than that of the cytoplasmic membrane. Many of the proteins traverse the entire lipid bilayer and are thus transmembrane proteins. A group of these proteins is known as **porins** because they form pores **that allow the diffusion of hydrophilic molecules less than 700 Da in mass through the membrane.** *The porin channel allows passage of metabolites and small hydrophilic antibiotics, but the outer membrane is a barrier for large or hydrophobic antibiotics and proteins such as lysozyme.*

The outer membrane also contains structural proteins and receptor molecules for bacteriophages and other ligands. The outer membrane is connected to the cytoplasmic membrane at **adhesion sites** and is tied to the peptidoglycan by **lipoprotein.** The lipoprotein is covalently attached to the peptidoglycan and is anchored in the outer membrane. The adhesion sites provide a membranous route for the delivery of newly synthesized outer membrane components to the outer membrane.

The outer membrane is held together by divalent cation (Mg^{+2} and Ca^{+2}) linkages between phosphates on LPS molecules and hydrophobic interactions between the LPS and proteins. These interactions produce a stiff, strong membrane that can be disrupted by antibiotics (e.g., polymyxin) or by the removal of Mg and Ca ions (chelation with ethylenediaminetetraacetic acid [EDTA] or tetracycline). Disruption of the outer membrane weakens the bacteria and allows the permeability of large, hydrophobic molecules. The addition of lysozyme to cells with a disrupted outer membrane produces **spheroplasts,** which, like protoplasts, are osmotically sensitive.

EXTERNAL STRUCTURES

Some bacteria (gram-positive or gram-negative) are closely surrounded by loose polysaccharide or protein layers called **capsules.** In cases in which it is loosely adherent and nonuniform in density or thickness, the material is referred to as a **slime layer.** The capsules and slime layers are also called the **glycocalyx.** *Bacillus anthracis,* the exception to this rule, produces a polypeptide capsule. The capsule is hard to see in a microscope but can be visualized by the exclusion of India ink particles.

Capsules and slimes are unnecessary for the growth of bacteria but are very important for survival in the host. *The capsule is poorly antigenic and antiphagocytic and is a major virulence factor* (e.g., *Streptococcus pneumoniae*). The capsule can also act as a barrier to toxic hydrophobic molecules, such as detergents, and can promote **adherence** to other bacteria or to host tissue surfaces. For *Streptococcus mutans,* the dextran and levan capsules are the means by which the bacteria attach and stick to the tooth enamel. Bacterial strains lacking a capsule may arise during growth under laboratory conditions, away from the selective pressures of the host, and are therefore less virulent. Some bacteria (e.g. *Pseudomonas aeroginosa*) will produce a polysaccharide **biofilm** under certain conditions, which establishes a bacterial community and protects them from antibiotics and host defenses. Another example of a biofilm is tooth plaque produced by *Streptococcus mutans*.

Flagella are ropelike propellers composed of helically coiled protein subunits **(flagellin)** that are anchored in the bacterial membranes through hook and basal body structures and are driven by membrane potential (see Figure 3–5). Bacterial species may have one or several flagella on their surfaces, and they may be anchored at different parts of the cell. Flagella provide motility for bacteria, allowing the cell to swim **(chemotaxis)** toward food and away from poisons. Bacteria approach food by swimming straight and then tumbling in a new direction. The swimming period becomes longer as the concentration of chemoattractant increases. The direction of flagellar spinning determines whether the bacteria swim or tumble. Flagella also express antigenic and strain determinants.

Fimbriae (pili) (Latin for "fringe") are hairlike structures on the outside of bacteria; they are composed of protein subunits **(pilin).** Fimbriae can be morphologically distinguished from flagella because they are smaller in diameter (3 to 8 nm versus 15 to 20 nm) and usually are not coiled in structure. Generally, several hundred fimbriae are arranged peritrichously (uniformly) over the entire surface of the bacterial cell. They may be as long as 15 to 20 μm, or many times the length of the cell.

Fimbriae promote adherence to other bacteria or to the host (alternative names are adhesins, lectins, evasins, and aggressins). As an adherence factor **(adhesin),** fimbriae are an important virulence factor for *E. coli* colonization and infection of the urinary tract, *Neisseria gonorrhoeae*, and other bacteria. The tips of the fimbriae may contain proteins (lectins) that bind to specific sugars (e.g., mannose). **F pili (sex pili)** bind to other bacteria and are a tube for transfer of large segments of bacterial chromosomes between bacteria. These pili are encoded by a plasmid (F).

BACTERIAL EXCEPTIONS

Mycobacteria have a peptidoglycan layer (slightly different structure), which is intertwined with and covalently attached to an arabinogalactan polymer and surrounded by a waxlike lipid coat of mycolic acid (large α-branched β-hydroxy fatty acids), cord factor (glycolipid of trehalose and two mycolic acids), waxD (glycolipid of 15 to 20 mycolic acids and sugar), and sulfolipids. These bacteria are described as **acid-fast staining.** The coat is responsible for virulence and is antiphagocytic. *Corynebacterium* and *Nocardia* organisms also produce mycolic acid lipids. The **mycoplasmas** are also exceptions in that they have no peptidoglycan cell wall and they incorporate steroids from the host into their membranes.

Structure and Biosynthesis of the Major Components of the Bacterial Cell Wall

The cell wall components are large structures made up of polymers of subunits. This type of structure facilitates their synthesis. Like astronauts building a space station, bacteria face problems assembling their cell walls. Synthesis of the peptidoglycan, LPS, teichoic acid, and capsule occurs on the outside of the bacteria, away from the synthetic machinery and energy sources of the cytoplasm and in an inhospitable environment. For both the space station and the bacteria, prefabricated precursors and subunits of the final structure are assembled in a factory-like setting on the inside, attached to a structure similar to a conveyor belt, brought to the surface, and then attached to the preexisting structure. For bacteria, the molecular conveyor belt–like structure is a large hydrophobic phospholipid called **bactoprenol (undecaprenol, [C_{55} isoprenoid]).** The prefabricated precursors must also be activated with high-energy bonds (e.g., phosphates) or other means to power the attachment reactions occurring outside the cell. For gram-negative bacteria, the outer membrane components are delivered through adhesion sites.

PEPTIDOGLYCAN (MUCOPEPTIDE, MUREIN)

The peptidoglycan is a rigid mesh made up of ropelike linear polysaccharide chains cross-linked by peptides. The polysaccharide is made up of repeating disaccharides of **N-acetylglucosamine (GlcNAc, NAG, G)** and **N-acetylmuramic acid (MurNAc, NAM, M)** (Figures 3-6 and 3-7).

A tetrapeptide is attached to the MurNAc. The peptide is unusual because it contains both D and L amino acids (D amino acids are not normally used in nature), and the peptide is produced enzymatically rather than by a ribosome. The first two amino acids attached to the MurNAc may vary for different organisms.

The diamino amino acids in the third position are essential for the cross-linking of the peptidoglycan chain. Examples of diamino amino acids include lysine and diaminopimelic and diaminobutyric acids. The peptide cross-link is formed between the free amine of the diamino amino acid and the D-alanine in the fourth position of

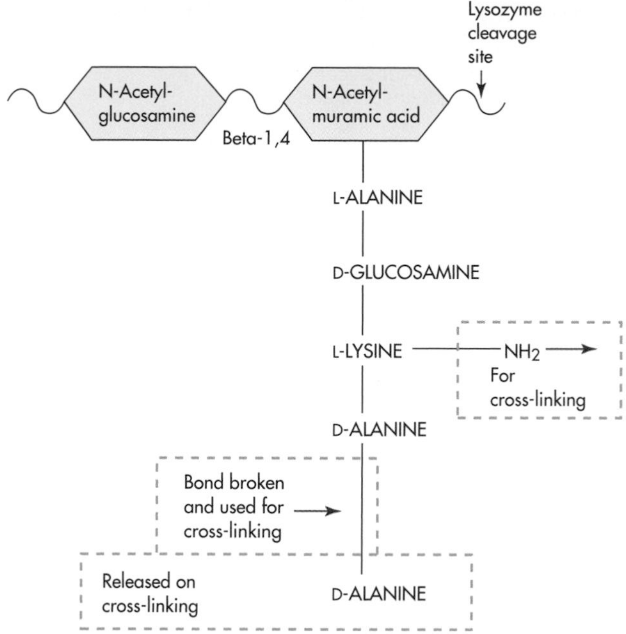

FIGURE 3–7. Precursor of peptidoglycan. The peptidoglycan is built from prefabricated units that contain a pentapeptide attached to the MurNAc. The pentapeptide contains a terminal D-alanine-D-alanine unit. This dipeptide is required for cross-linking the peptidoglycan and is the basis for the action of β-lactam and vancomycin antibiotics.

another chain. The bacteria *S. aureus* and other gram-positive bacteria use an amino acid bridge (e.g., a $glycine_5$ peptide) between these amino acids to lengthen the cross-link. The precursor form of the peptide has an extra D-alanine, which is released during the cross-linking step.

The peptidoglycan in gram-positive bacteria forms multiple layers and is often cross-linked in three dimensions, providing a very strong, rigid cell wall. In contrast, the peptidoglycan in gram-negative cell walls is usually only one molecule (layer) thick. The number of cross-links and the length of the cross-link determine the rigidity of the peptidoglycan mesh. The site where **lysozyme** cleaves the glycan of the peptidoglycan is shown in Figure 3–7.

PEPTIDOGLYCAN SYNTHESIS

Peptidoglycan synthesis occurs in four steps (see Figure 3–8). First, inside the cell, glucosamine is enzymatically converted into MurNAc and then energetically activated by a reaction with uridine triphosphate (UTP) to produce uridine diphosphate-*N*-acetylmuramic acid (UDP-MurNAc). Next, the UDP-MurNAc-pentapeptide precursor is assembled in a series of enzymatic steps.

Second, the UDP-MurNAc pentapeptide is attached to the **bactoprenol** "conveyor belt" in the cytoplasmic membrane through a pyrophosphate link, with the release of uridine monophosphate (UMP). GlcNAc is added to make the disaccharide building block of the peptidoglycan. Some bacteria (e.g., *S. aureus*) add a pentaglycine or another chain to the diamino amino acid at the third position of the peptide chain to lengthen the cross-link. Third, the bactoprenol molecule translocates the disaccharide:peptide precursor to the outside of the cell. The GlcNAc-MurNAc disaccharide is then attached to a peptidoglycan chain, using the pyrophosphate link between itself and the bactoprenol as energy to drive the reaction by enzymes called **transglycosylases.** The pyrophosphobactoprenol is converted back to a phosphobactoprenol and recycled. Fourth, outside the cell but near the membrane surface, peptide chains from adjacent glycan chains are cross-linked to each other by a peptide bond exchange **(transpeptidation)** between the free amine of the amino acid in the third position of the pentapeptide (e.g., lysine), or the *N*-terminus of the attached pentaglycine chain, and the D-alanine at the fourth position of the other peptide chain, releasing the terminal D-alanine of the precursor. This step requires no additional energy because peptide bonds are "traded."

The cross-linking reaction is catalyzed by membrane-bound **transpeptidases.** Related enzymes, **DD-carboxypeptidases,** remove unreacted terminal D-alanines to limit the extent of cross-linking. The transpeptidases and carboxypeptidases are called **penicillin-binding proteins (PBPs)** because they are targets for penicillin and other β-lactam antibiotics. Penicillin and related β-lactam antibiotics resemble the "transition state" conformation of the D-ALA-D-ALA substrate when bound to these enzymes. Different PBPs are used for extending the peptidoglycan, creating a septum for cell division, and curving the peptidoglycan mesh (cell shape).

The peptidoglycan is constantly being synthesized and degraded. **Autolysins** such as lysozyme are important for determining bacterial shape. Inhibition of synthesis or the cross-linking of the peptidoglycan does not stop the autolysins, and their action weakens the mesh and the bacterial structure and leads to lysis and cell death. New peptidoglycan synthesis does not occur during starvation, which leads to a weakening of the peptidoglycan and a loss in the dependability of the Gram stain.

An understanding of the biosynthesis of peptidoglycan is essential in medicine, because these reactions are unique to bacterial cells and hence can be inhibited with little or no adverse effect on host (human) cells. A number of antibiotics target one or more steps in this pathway (see Chapter 20).

TEICHOIC ACID

Teichoic and **lipoteichoic acid** are polymers of chemically modified ribose or glycerol connected by phosphates

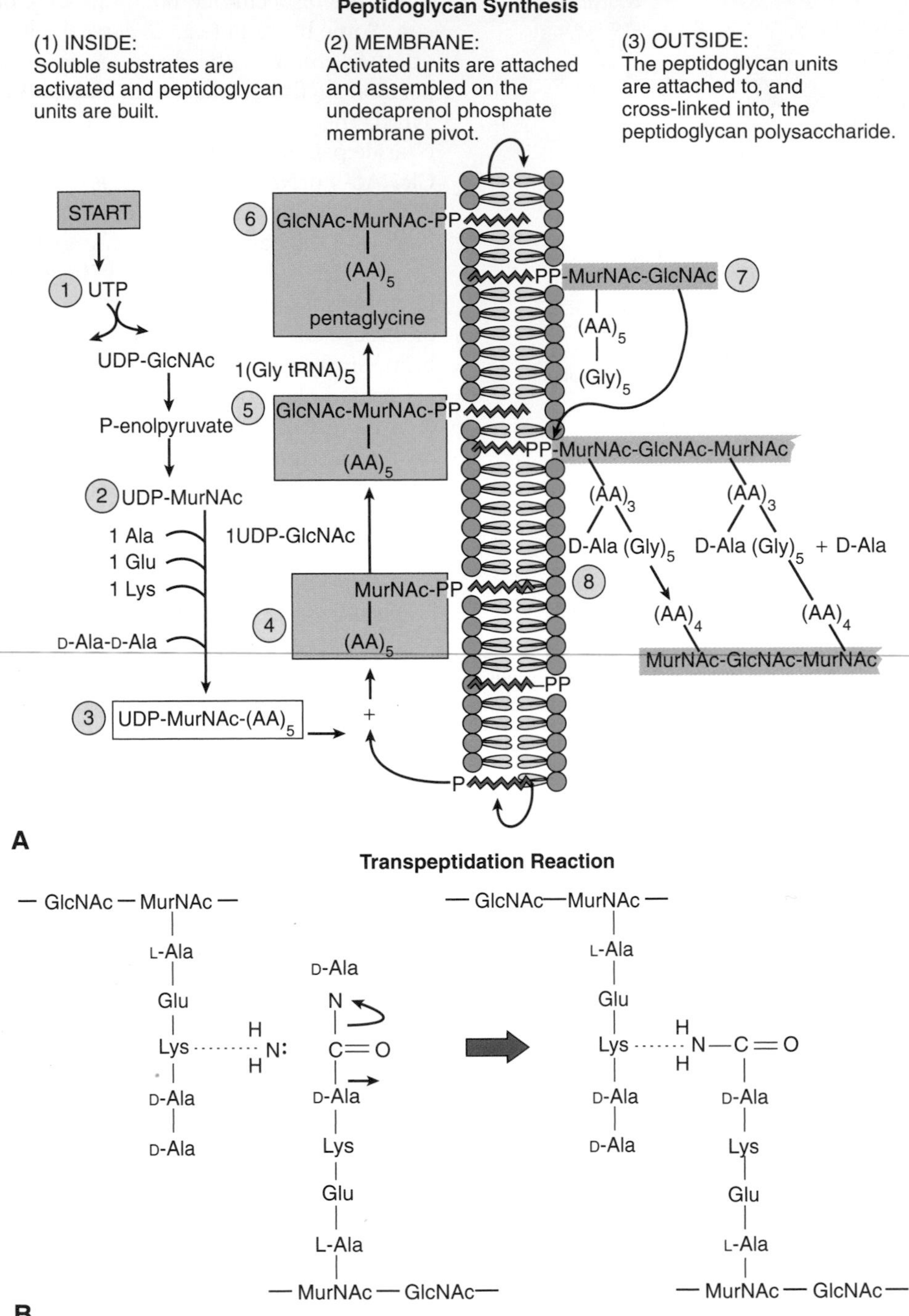

FIGURE 3–8. Peptidoglycan synthesis. **A,** Peptidoglycan synthesis occurs in the following three phases: (1) Peptidoglycan is synthesized from prefabricated units constructed and activated for assembly and transport inside the cell. (2) At the membrane the units are assembled onto the undecaprenol phosphate conveyor belt, and fabrication is completed. (3) The unit is translocated to the outside of the cell, where it is attached to the polysaccharide chain, and the peptide is cross-linked to finish the construction. Such a construction can be compared with the assembly of a space station. **B,** The cross-linking reaction is a transpeptidation. One peptide bond (produced inside the cell) is traded for another (outside the cell) with the release of D-alanine. The enzymes that catalyze the reaction are called D*-alanine,* D*-alanine transpeptidase-carboxypeptidases.* These enzymes are the targets of β-lactam antibiotics and are called *penicillin-binding proteins.* (© American Society of Clinical Pathologists. Reprinted with permission.)

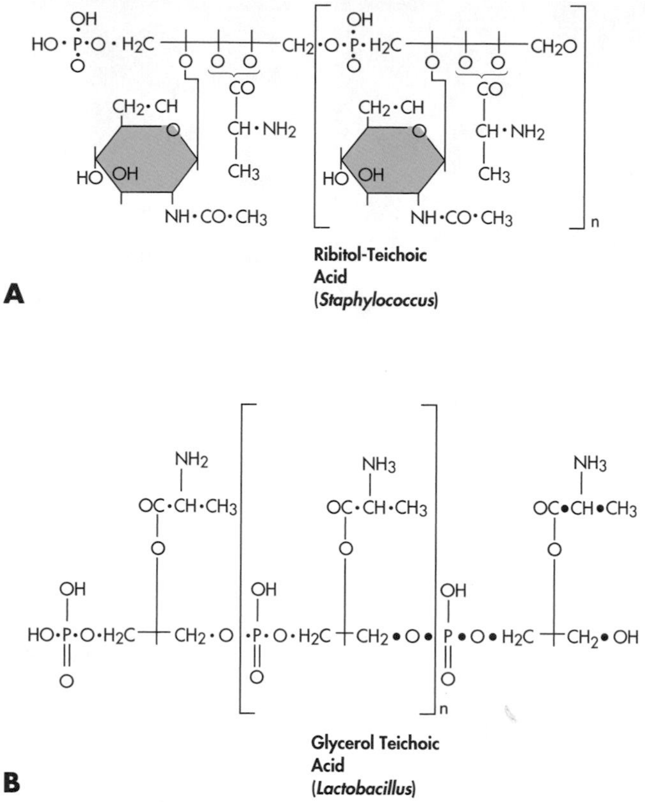

A

Ribitol-Teichoic Acid
(*Staphylococcus*)

B

Glycerol Teichoic Acid
(*Lactobacillus*)

FIGURE 3–9. Teichoic acid. Teichoic acid is a polymer of chemically modified ribitol **(A)** or glycerol phosphate **(B)**. The nature of the modification (e.g., sugars, amino acids) can define the serotype of the bacteria. Teichoic acid may be covalently attached to the peptidoglycan. Lipoteichoic acid is anchored in the cytoplasmic membrane by a covalently attached fatty acid.

(Figure 3–9). Sugars, choline, or D-alanine may be attached to the hydroxyls of the ribose or glycerol, providing antigenic determinants. These can be distinguished by antibodies and may determine the bacterial serotype. Lipoteichoic acid has a fatty acid and is anchored in the membrane. Teichoic acid is synthesized from building blocks using the bactoprenol in a manner similar to that of peptidoglycan. Teichoic acid and some **surface proteins** (e.g., protein A from *S. aureus*) are secreted from the cells and then enzymatically attached to the *N*-terminus of the peptide of peptidoglycan.

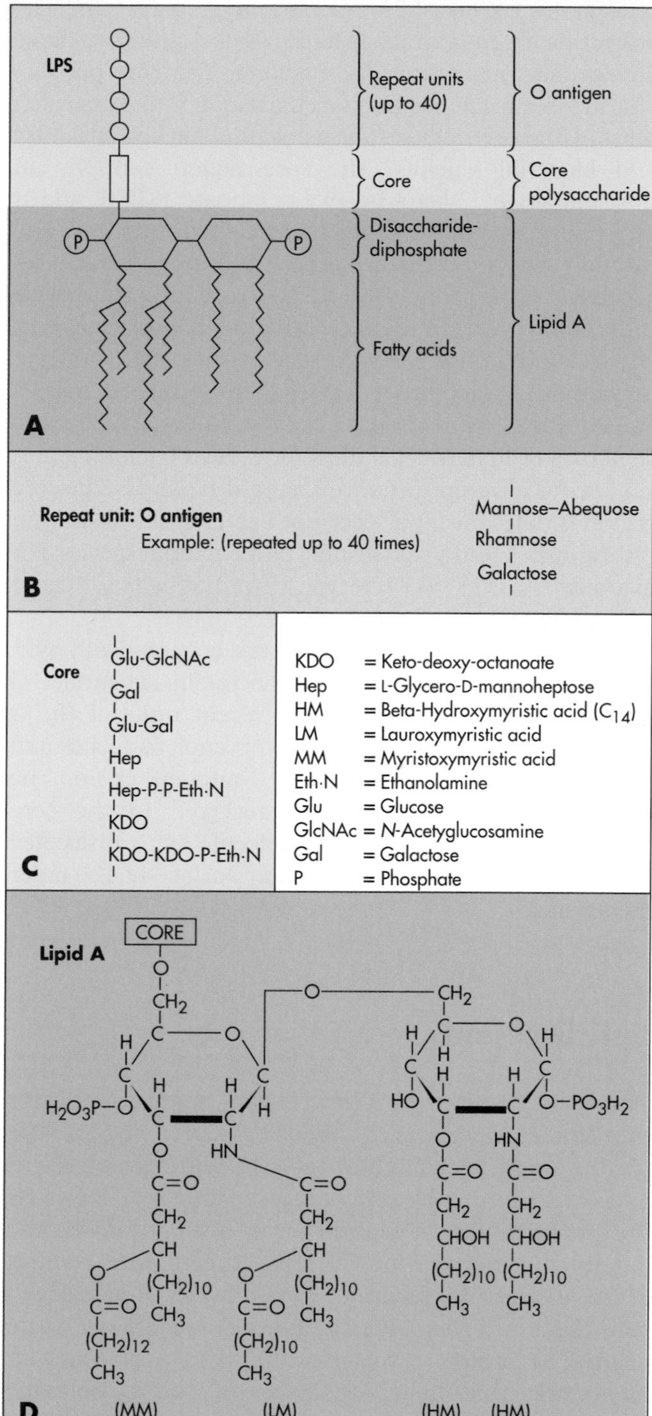

FIGURE 3–10. The lipopolysaccharide of the gram-negative cell envelope. **A,** Segment of the polymer showing the arrangements of the major constituents. Each LPS molecule has one Lipid A and one polysaccharide core unit but many repeats of O antigen. **B,** Structure of lipid A of *Salmonella typhimurium*. **C,** Polysaccharide core. **D,** Typical O antigen repeat unit *(S. typhimurium)*. (Redrawn from Brooks GF, Butel JS, Ornston LN, editors: *Jawetz, Melnick and Aldenberg's medical microbiology,* ed 19, Norwalk, Conn, 1991, Appleton & Lange.)

LIPOPOLYSACCHARIDE

LPS (endotoxin) *consists of three structural sections: Lipid A, core polysaccharide (rough core), and O antigen* (Figure 3–10). Lipid A is a basic component of LPS and is essential for bacterial viability. *Lipid A is responsible for the endotoxin activity of LPS.* It has a phosphorylated glucosamine disaccharide backbone with fatty acids attached to anchor the structure in the outer membrane. The phosphates connect LPS units into aggregates. One carbohydrate chain is attached to the disaccharide backbone and extends away from the bacteria. The core polysaccharide is a branched polysaccharide of 9 to 12 sugars. Most of the core region is also essential for LPS structure and bacterial viability. The core region contains an unusual sugar, 2-keto-3-deoxy-octanoate (KDO), and is phosphorylated. The O antigen is attached to the core and extends away from the bacteria. It is a long, linear polysaccharide consisting of 50 to 100 repeating saccharide units of four to seven sugars per unit. Lipooligosaccharide, which is present in *Neisseria* species, lack the O-antigen portion of LPS and are readily shed from the bacteria.

LPS structure is used to classify bacteria. The basic structure of lipid A is identical for related bacteria and is similar for all gram-negative *Enterobacteriaceae.* The core region is the same for a species of bacteria. The O antigen distinguishes serotypes (strains) of a bacterial species. For example, the O157:H7 serotype identifies the *E. coli* agent of hemolytic-uremic syndrome.

The lipid A and core portions are enzymatically synthesized in a sequential manner on the inside surface of the cytoplasmic membrane. The repeat units of the O antigen are assembled on a bactoprenol molecule and then transferred to a growing O-antigen chain. The finished O-antigen chain is transferred to the core lipid A structure. The LPS molecule is translocated through adhesion sites to the outer surface of the outer membrane.

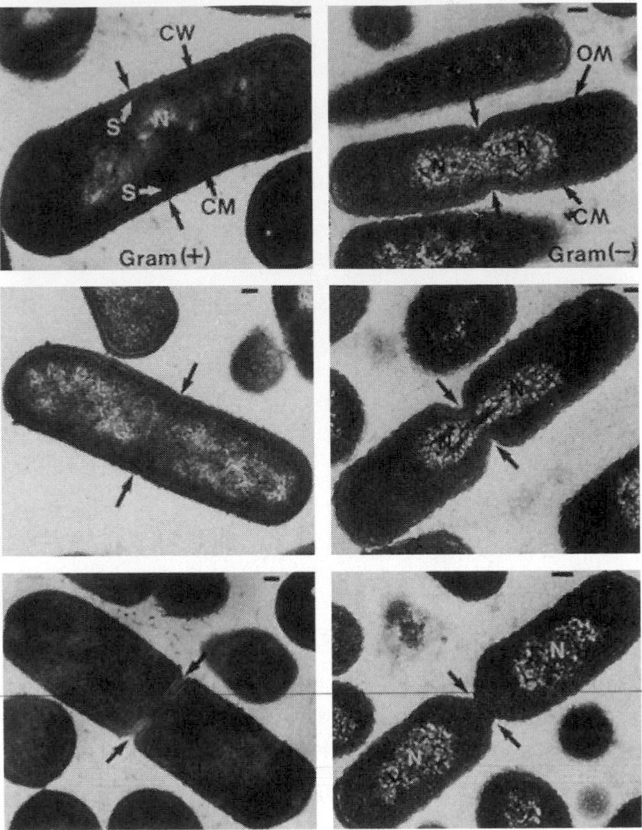

FIGURE 3–11. Electron photomicrographs of gram-positive cell division *(Bacillus subtilis) (left)* and gram-negative cell division *(Escherichia coli) (right)*. Progression in cell division from top to bottom. CM, cytoplasmic membrane; CW, cell wall; N, nucleoid; OM, outer membrane; S, septum. Bar = 0.2 μm. (From Slots J, Taubman MA, editors: *Contemporary oral biology and immunology,* St Louis, 1992, Mosby.)

Cell Division

The replication of the bacterial chromosome also triggers the initiation of cell division (Figure 3–11). The production of two daughter bacteria requires the growth and extension of the cell wall components, followed by the production of a septum (cross wall) to divide the daughter bacteria into two cells. The septum consists of two membranes separated by two layers of peptidoglycan. Septum formation is initiated at midcell, at a site defined by protein complexes affixed to a protein filament ring that lines the inside of the cytoplasmic membrane. The septum grows from opposite sides toward the center of the cell, causing cleavage of the daughter cells. This process requires special transpeptidases (PBPs) and other enzymes. For streptococci, the growth zone is located at 180 degrees from each other, producing linear chains of bacteria. In contrast, the growth zone of staphylococci is at 90 degrees. Incomplete cleavage of the septum can cause the bacteria to remain linked, forming chains (e.g., streptococci) or clusters (e.g., staphylococci).

Spores

Some gram-positive, but never gram-negative, bacteria, such as members of the genera *Bacillus* (e.g., *Bacillus anthracis*) and *Clostridium* (e.g., *Clostridium tetanii* or *botulinum*) (soil bacteria), are spore formers. Under harsh environmental conditions, such as the loss of a nutritional requirement, these bacteria can convert from a **vegetative state** to a **dormant state,** or **spore.** The location of the spore within a cell is a characteristic of the bacteria and can assist in identification of the bacterium.

The spore is a dehydrated, multishelled structure that protects and allows the bacteria to exist in "suspended animation" (Figure 3–12). It contains a complete copy of the chromosome, the bare minimum concentrations of essential proteins and ribosomes, and a high concentration of **calcium bound to dipicolinic acid.** The spore has an inner membrane, two peptidoglycan layers, and an outer keratin-like protein coat. The spore looks refractile (bright) in the microscope. The structure of the spore protects the

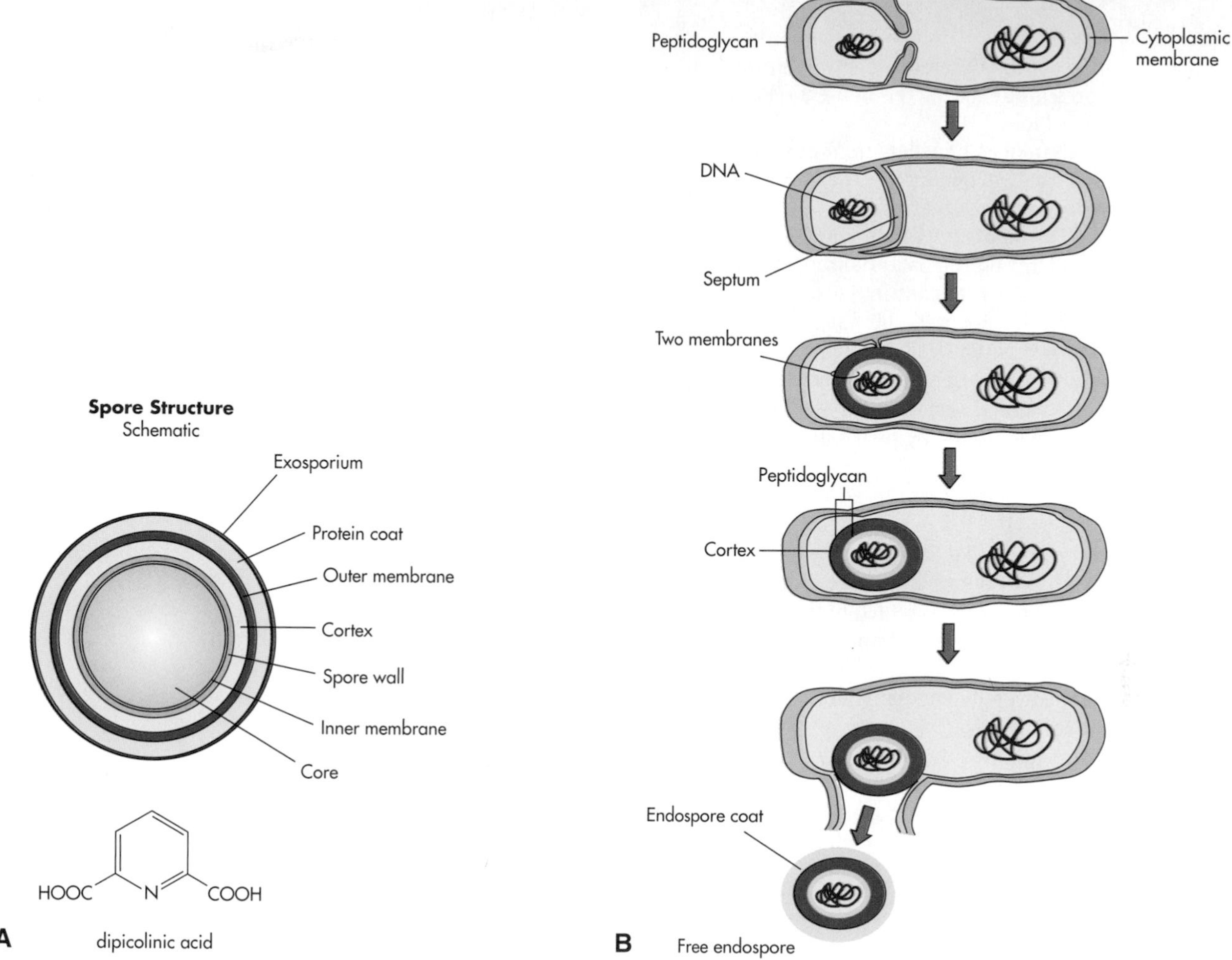

FIGURE 3–12. Endospores. **A,** Structure of a spore. **B,** Sporogenesis, the process of endospore formation.

genomic DNA from intense heat, radiation, and attack by most enzymes and chemical agents. In fact, bacterial spores are so resistant to environmental factors that they can exist for centuries as viable spores. Spores are also difficult to decontaminate with standard disinfectants.

Depletion of specific nutrients (e.g., alanine) from the growth medium triggers a cascade of genetic events (comparable to differentiation) leading to the production of a spore. Spore mRNA are transcribed, and other mRNA are turned off. Dipicolinic acid is produced, and antibiotics and toxins are often excreted. After duplication of the chromosome, one copy of the DNA and cytoplasmic contents **(core)** are surrounded by the cytoplasmic membrane, the peptidoglycan, and the membrane of the septum. This wraps the DNA in the two layers of membrane and peptidoglycan that would normally divide the cell. These two layers are surrounded by the **cortex,** which is made up of a thin inner layer of tightly cross-linked peptidoglycan surrounding a membrane (which used to be the cytoplasmic membrane) and a loose outer peptidoglycan layer. The cortex is surrounded by the tough, **keratin-like protein coat,** which protects the spore. The process requires 6 to 8 hours for completion.

The germination of spores into the vegetative state is stimulated by disruption of the outer coat by mechanical stress, pH, heat, or another stressor and requires water and a triggering nutrient (e.g., alanine). The process takes approximately 90 minutes. After the germination process begins, the spore will take up water, swell, shed its coats, and produce one new vegetative cell identical to the original vegetative cell, thus completing the entire cycle. Once germination has begun and the spore coat has been compromised, the spore is weakened, vulnerable, and can be inactivated like other bacteria.

QUESTIONS

1. How does each of the differences between prokaryotes and eukaryotes influence bacterial infection and treatment (see Table 3–1)?
2. How do the differences between gram-positive and gram-negative cell walls influence the cells' clinical behavior, detection, and treatment?
3. List the cell wall components that contribute to virulence by protecting the bacteria from immune responses. List those that contribute to virulence by eliciting toxic responses in the human host.
4. When peptidoglycan synthesis is inhibited, what processes kill the bacteria? List the precursors that would build up within the bacteria if recycling of bactoprenol were inhibited by penicillin, vancomycin, or bacitracin.
5. Why are spores more resistant to environmental stresses?
6. The laboratory would like to selectively eliminate gram-positive bacteria from a mixture of gram-positive and gram-negative bacteria. Which of the following procedures would be more appropriate and why or why not?
   a. Treatment with ethylenediaminetetraacetic acid (a divalent cation chelator)
   b. Treatment with mild detergent
   c. Treatment with lysozyme
   d. Treatment with transpeptidase
   e. Treatment with ampicillin (a hydrophilic β-lactam antibiotic)

Bibliography

Daniel RA, Errington J: Control of cell morphogenesis in bacteria: two distinct ways to make a rod-shaped cell, *Cell* 113:767-776, 2003.

Davis BD et al, editors: *Microbiology*, ed 4, Philadelphia, 1990, Lippincott.

Lutkenhaus J: The regulation of bacterial cell division: a time and place for it, *Curr Opin Microbiol* 1: 210-215, 1998.

Nanninga N: Morphogenesis of Escherichia coli, *Microbiol Mol Biol Rev* 62:110-129, 1998.

Strauss JM, Strauss EG: *Viruses and human disease*, San Diego, Academic Press, 2002.

Talaro K, Talaro A, editors: *Foundations in microbiology*, ed 4, New York, 2002, McGraw Hill.

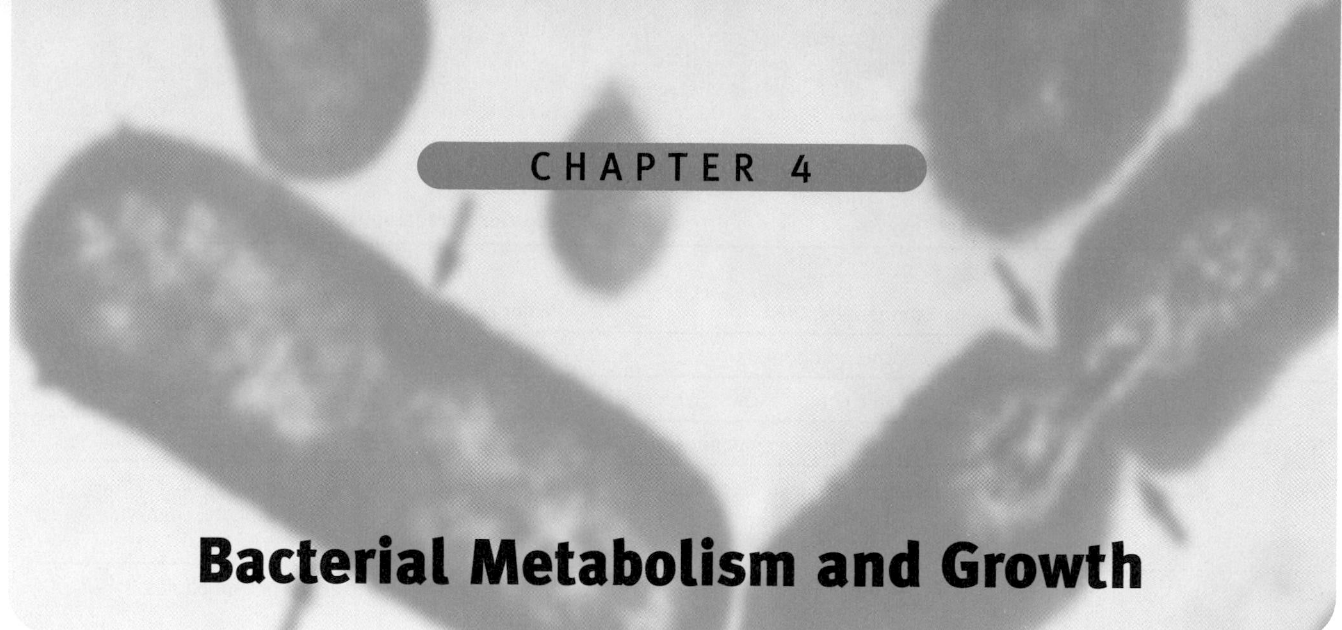

Bacterial Metabolism and Growth

Metabolic Requirements

Bacterial growth requires a source of energy and the raw materials to build the proteins, structures, and membranes that make up the structure and biochemical machines of the cell. Bacteria must obtain or synthesize the amino acids, carbohydrates, and lipids used as building blocks of the cell.

The minimum requirement for growth is a source of carbon and nitrogen, an energy source, water, and various ions. The essential elements and their functions are listed in Table 4–1. **Iron** is so important that many bacteria secrete special proteins (siderophores) to sequester iron from dilute solutions.

Oxygen (O_2 gas), although essential for the human host, is actually a poison for many bacteria. Some organisms, such as *Clostridium perfringens*, which causes gas gangrene, cannot grow in the presence of oxygen. Such bacteria are referred to as **obligate anaerobes.** Other organisms, such as *Mycobacterium tuberculosis*, which causes tuberculosis, require the presence of molecular oxygen for growth and are therefore referred to as **obligate aerobes.** Most bacteria, however, grow in either the presence or the absence of oxygen. These bacteria are referred to as **facultative anaerobes.**

Although some bacteria (e.g., chemotrophs) can derive energy directly from the oxidation of metal ions, such as iron, and other bacteria (e.g., blue-green algae) are capable of photosynthesis, pathogenic bacteria derive their energy by metabolizing sugars, fats, and proteins. Some bacteria, such as certain strains of *Escherichia coli* (a member of the intestinal flora), can synthesize all the amino acids, nucleotides, lipids, and carbohydrates necessary for growth and division when provided with the inorganic nutrients listed in Table 4–1 plus a simple source of carbon, such as glucose. At the other extreme are bacteria, such as the causative agent of syphilis, *Treponema pallidum*, whose growth requirements are so complex that a defined laboratory medium capable of supporting its growth has yet to be developed.

Growth requirements and metabolic by-products may be used as a convenient means of classifying different bacteria. Those that can rely entirely on inorganic chemicals for their energy and source of carbon (CO_2) are referred to as autotrophs (lithotrophs), whereas many bacteria and animal cells that require organic carbon sources are known as heterotrophs (organotrophs). Clinical microbiology laboratories distinguish bacteria by their ability to grow on specific carbon sources (e.g., lactose) and the end products of metabolism (e.g., ethanol, lactic acid, succinic acid).

Metabolism and the Conversion of Energy

All cells require a constant supply of energy to survive. This energy, typically in the form of adenosine triphosphate (ATP), is derived from the controlled breakdown of various organic substrates (carbohydrates, lipids, and proteins). This process of substrate breakdown and conversion into usable energy is known as **catabolism.** The energy produced may then be used in the synthesis of cellular constituents (cell walls, proteins, fatty acids, and nucleic acids), a process known as **anabolism.** Together these two processes, which are interrelated and tightly integrated, are referred to as **intermediary metabolism.**

The metabolic process generally begins with hydrolysis of large macromolecules in the external cellular environment by specific enzymes (Figure 4–1). The smaller molecules that are produced (e.g., monosaccharides, short

TABLE 4–1. Essential Elements, Their Sources, and Functions in Prokaryotes

Element	Source	Function in Metabolism
Major Essential Elements		
C	Organic compounds, CO_2	Major components of cellular material
O	O_2, H_2O, organic compounds	
H	H_2, H_2O, organic compounds	
N	NH_4^+, NO_3^-, N_2, organic compounds	
S	SO_4^{2-}, HS^-, S^0, organic sulfur compounds	Constituent of S-containing amino acids, cysteine, methionine, thiamine pyrophosphate, coenzyme A, biotin, and α-lipoic acid
P	HPO_4^{2-}	Constituent of nucleic acids, phospholipids, nucleotides
K	K^+	Major inorganic cation, co-factor (e.g., pyruvate kinase)
Mg	Mg^{2+}	Cofactor of many enzymes (e.g., kinases); component of cell walls, membranes, ribosomes
Ca	Ca^{2+}	Component of exoenzymes (amylases, proteases) and cell walls; major component of endospores as Ca-dipicolinate
Fe	Fe^{2+}, Fe^{3+}	Present in cytochromes, ferredoxins, and other iron-sulfur proteins; cofactor (dehydratases)
Na	Na^+	Transport
Cl	Cl^-	Important inorganic anion
Minor Essential Elements		
Zn	Zn^{2+}	Component of the enzymes alcohol dehydrogenase, alkaline phosphatase, aldolase, RNA and DNA polymerase
Mn	Mn^{2+}	Present in superoxide dismutase; cofactor of the enzymes PEP carboxykinase, isocitrate synthase
Mo	MoO_4^{2-}	Present in nitrate reductase, nitrogenase, xanthine dehydrogenase, formate dehydrogenase
Se	SeO_3^{2-}	Component of glycine reductase and formate dehydrogenase
Co	Co^{2+}	Required element in coenzyme B_{12}–containing enzymes (glutamate mutase, methylmalonyl coenzyme A mutase)
Cu	Cu^{2+}	Present in cytochrome oxidase and nitrite reductase
Ni	Ni^{2+}	Present in urease, hydrogenase, and factor F_{430}
W	WO_4^{2-}	Present in some formate dehydrogenases

Modified from Gottschalk E: *Bacterial metabolism*, ed 2, New York, 1985, Springer-Verlag.

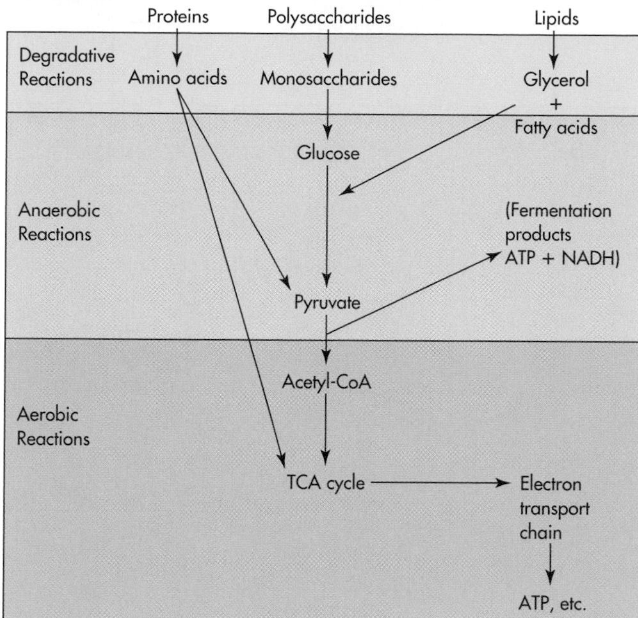

FIGURE 4–1. Catabolism of proteins, polysaccharides, and lipids produces glucose, pyruvate, or intermediates of the tricarboxylic acid (TCA) cycle and, ultimately, energy in the form of adenosine triphosphate (ATP) or the reduced form of nicotinamide-adenine dinucleotide (NADH).

peptides, and fatty acids) are transported across the cell membranes into the cytoplasm by active or passive transport mechanisms specific for the metabolite. These mechanisms may use specific carrier or membrane transport proteins to help concentrate metabolites from the medium. The metabolites are converted via one or more pathways to one common, universal intermediate, **pyruvic acid.** From pyruvic acid the carbons may be channeled toward energy production or the synthesis of new carbohydrates, amino acids, lipids, and nucleic acids.

METABOLISM OF GLUCOSE

For the sake of simplicity, this section presents an overview of the pathways by which the model carbohydrate glucose is metabolized to produce energy or other usable substrates. Instead of releasing all the molecule's energy as heat (as for burning), the bacteria break down the glucose in discrete steps to allow the energy to be captured in usable forms. *Bacteria can produce energy from* glucose by—in order of increasing efficiency—fermentation, anaerobic respiration (both of which occur in the absence of oxygen), or aerobic respiration. Aerobic respiration can completely convert the six carbons of glucose to CO_2 and H_2O plus energy, whereas two- and three-carbon compounds are the end products of fermentation. For a discussion of the metabolism of other organic compounds, including proteins and lipids, refer to a textbook on biochemistry.

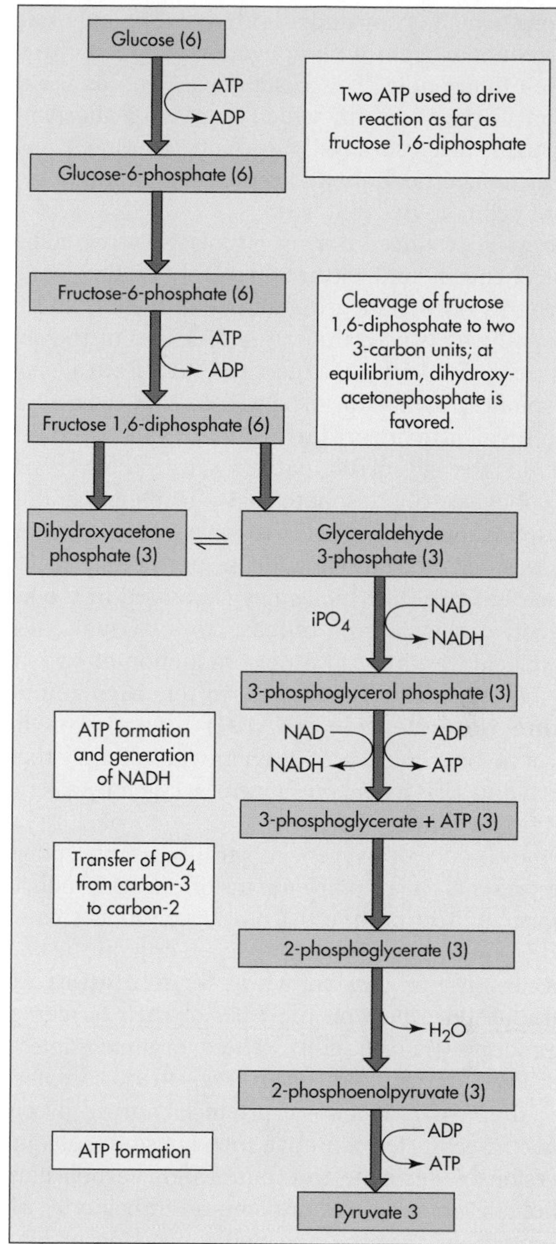

FIGURE 4–2. Embden-Meyerhof-Parnas (EMP) glycolytic pathway results in conversion of glucose to pyruvate. The sum of glucose + 2 ADP + 2 Pi + 2 NAD → 2 pyruvate + 4 ATP + 2 NADH + 2 H^+. Double arrows denote 2 moles reacting per mole of glucose. ADP, adenosine diphosphate; ATP, adenosine triphosphate; iPO_4, inorganic phosphate; NAD, nicotinamide adenine dinucleotide; NADH, reduced form of NAD.

EMBDEN-MEYERHOF-PARNAS PATHWAY

Bacteria use three major metabolic pathways in the catabolism of glucose. Most common among these is the **glycolytic**, or Embden-Meyerhof-Parnas (EMP), pathway (Figure 4–2). This pathway represents the primary means in both bacteria and eukaryotic cells for the conversion of glucose to pyruvate, which, as noted previously, is central to various other cellular metabolic pathways. These reactions, which occur under both **aerobic** and **anaerobic** conditions, begin with activation of glucose to form glucose-6-phosphate. This reaction, as well as the third reaction in the series, in which fructose-6-phosphate is converted to fructose-1,6-diphosphate, requires 1 mole of ATP per mole of glucose and represents an initial investment of cellular energy stores.

Energy is produced during glycolysis in two different forms, chemical and electrochemical. In the first, the high-energy phosphate group of one of the intermediates in the pathway is used under the direction of the appropriate enzyme (a **kinase**) to generate **ATP** from adenosine diphosphate (ADP). This type of reaction, termed **substrate-level phosphorylation,** occurs at two different points in the glycolytic pathway (i.e., conversion of 3-phosphoglycerol phosphate to 3-phosphoglycerate and 2-phosphoenolpyruvic acid to pyruvate). Four ATP molecules per molecule of glucose are produced in this manner, but two ATP molecules were used in the initial glycolytic conversion of glucose to two molecules of pyruvic acid, resulting in a net production of two molecules of ATP. The reduced form of **nicotinamide-adenine dinucleotide (NADH)** that is produced represents the second form of energy, which may then be converted to ATP in the presence of oxygen by a series of oxidation reactions.

In the absence of oxygen, substrate-level phosphorylation represents the primary means of energy production. The pyruvic acid produced from glycolysis is then converted to various end products, depending on the bacterial species, in a process known as **fermentation.** Many bacteria are identified on the basis of their fermentative end products (Figure 4–3). These organic molecules, rather than oxygen, are used as electron acceptors to recycle the NADH, which was produced during glycolysis, to NAD. In yeast, fermentative metabolism results in the conversion of pyruvate to ethanol plus carbon dioxide. Alcoholic fermentation is uncommon in bacteria, which most commonly use the one-step conversion of pyruvic acid to lactic acid. This process is responsible for making milk into yogurt and cabbage into sauerkraut. Other bacteria use more complex fermentative pathways, producing various acids, alcohols, and often gases (many of which have vile odors). These products lend flavors to various cheeses and wines.

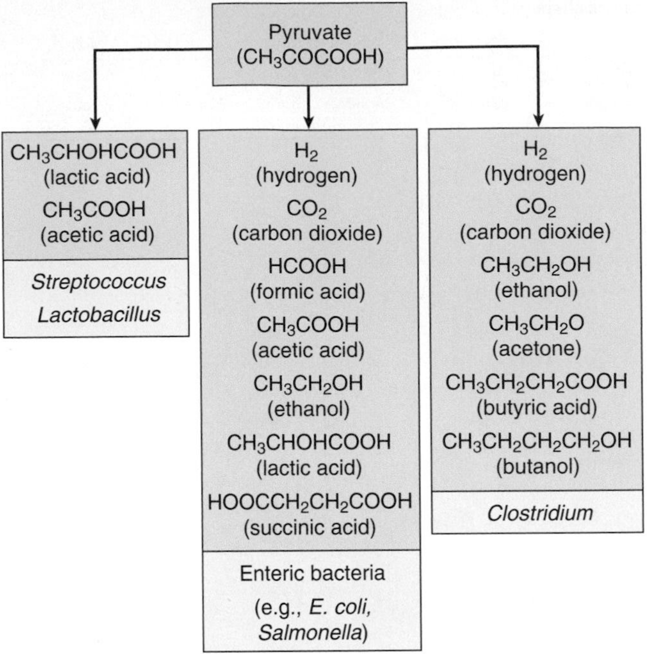

FIGURE 4–3. Fermentation of pyruvate by different microorganisms results in different end products. The clinical laboratory uses these pathways and end products as a means of distinguishing different bacteria.

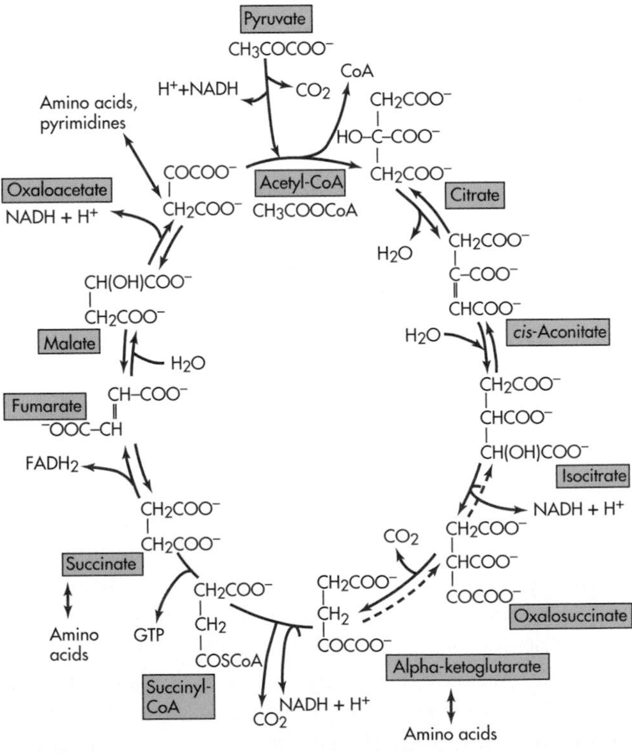

FIGURE 4–4. Tricarboxylic acid cycle occurs in aerobic conditions and is an amphibolic cycle. Precursors for the synthesis of amino acids and nucleotides are also shown. CoA, coenzyme A; $FADH_2$, flavin adenine dinucleotide; GTP, guanosine triphosphate.

TRICARBOXYLIC ACID CYCLE

In the presence of oxygen, the pyruvic acid produced from glycolysis and from the metabolism of other substrates may be completely oxidized (controlled burning) to water and CO_2 using the tricarboxylic acid (TCA) cycle (Figure 4–4), which results in production of additional energy. The process begins with the oxidative decarboxylation (release of CO_2) of pyruvate to the high-energy intermediate, acetyl coenzyme A (acetyl CoA); this reaction also produces NADH. The two remaining carbons derived from pyruvate then enter the TCA cycle in the form of acetyl CoA by condensation with oxaloacetate, with the formation of the six-carbon citrate molecule. In a stepwise series of oxidative reactions the citrate is converted back to oxaloacetate, with the net production of 2 moles of CO_2, 3 moles of NADH, 1 mole of flavin adenine dinucleotide ($FADH_2$), and 1 mole of guanosine triphosphate (GTP). GTP is produced via substrate-level phosphorylation in a reaction in which succinyl CoA is converted to succinate.

The TCA cycle allows the organism to generate substantially more energy per mole of glucose than is possible from glycolysis alone. In addition to the GTP (an ATP equivalent) produced by substrate-level phosphorylation, the NADH and $FADH_2$ yield ATP from the electron transport chain. In this chain the electrons carried by NADH (or $FADH_2$) are passed in a stepwise fashion through a series of donor-acceptor pairs and, ultimately, to oxygen (Figure 4–5). This process, known as **aerobic respiration,** results in the generation of 3 moles of ATP per mole of NADH and 2 moles of ATP per mole of $FADH_2$. The energetics of aerobic glucose metabolism are depicted in Figure 4–5.

Some bacteria can use compounds other than oxygen (e.g., NO_3^-, SO_4^{-2}, CO_2) as terminal electron acceptors during **anaerobic respiration.** Although this approach is more efficient than fermentation, which uses organic molecules as electron acceptors, it is less efficient than aerobic respiration because it produces less ATP.

Anaerobic organisms are less efficient at energy production than aerobic organisms. Fermentation, without aerobic electron transport and a complete TCA cycle, produces only 2 ATP molecules per glucose, whereas aerobic metabolism can generate 19 times more energy (38 ATP molecules) from the same starting material (and it is much less smelly) (Figure 4–6).

In addition to the efficient generation of ATP from glucose (and other carbohydrates), the TCA cycle provides a means by which carbons derived from **lipids** (in the form of acetyl CoA) may be shunted toward either energy production or the generation of biosynthetic precursors. Similarly, the cycle includes several points at which **deaminated amino acids** may enter (see Figure 4–4). For example, deamination of glutamic acid yields α-ketoglutarate, whereas deamination of aspartic acid yields oxaloacetate, both of which are TCA cycle intermediates. The TCA cycle therefore serves the following functions:

1. It is the major mechanism for the generation of ATP.
2. It serves as the final common pathway for the complete oxidation of amino acids, fatty acids, and carbohydrates.
3. It supplies key intermediates (i.e., α-ketoglutarate, pyruvate, oxaloacetate) for the ultimate synthesis of amino acids (Figure 4–7), lipids, purines, and pyrimidines.

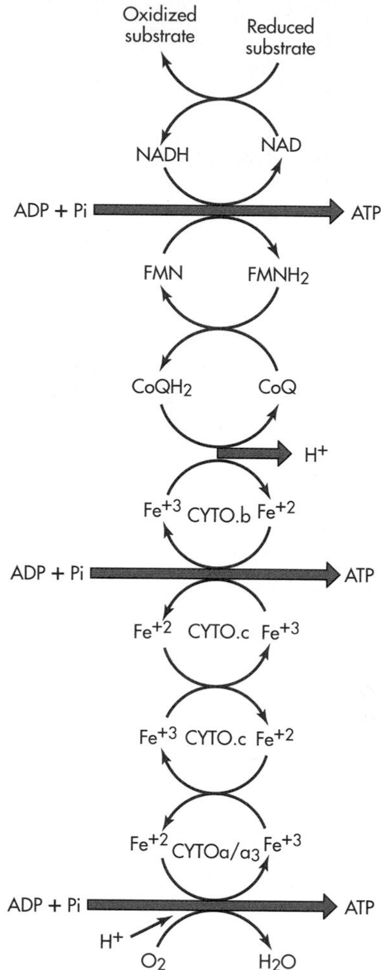

FIGURE 4–5. Electron transport chain, showing sequential oxidation and energy-generating steps. Electron transfer is accompanied by the flow of protons (H^+) from NADH, through coenzyme Q (CoQ), and electrons through the cytochromes (CYTO). Three ATPs are formed per molecule of NADH reoxidized, but only two ATPs are formed per molecule of $FADH_2$ reoxidized. FMN, flavin mononucleotide. (Modified from Slots J, Taubman MA, editors: *Contemporary oral microbiology and immunology,* St Louis, 1992, Mosby.)

The last two functions make the TCA cycle a so-called **amphibolic cycle** (i.e., it may function in the anabolic and the catabolic functions of the cell).

PENTOSE PHOSPHATE PATHWAY

The final pathway of glucose metabolism considered here is known as the **pentose phosphate pathway,** or the **hexose monophosphate shunt** (Figure 4–8). The function of this pathway is to provide precursors and reducing power in the form of nicotinamide-adenine dinucleotide phosphate (reduced form) **(NADPH)** for use in biosynthesis. In the first half of the pathway, glucose is converted to ribulose-5-phosphate, with consumption of 1 mole of

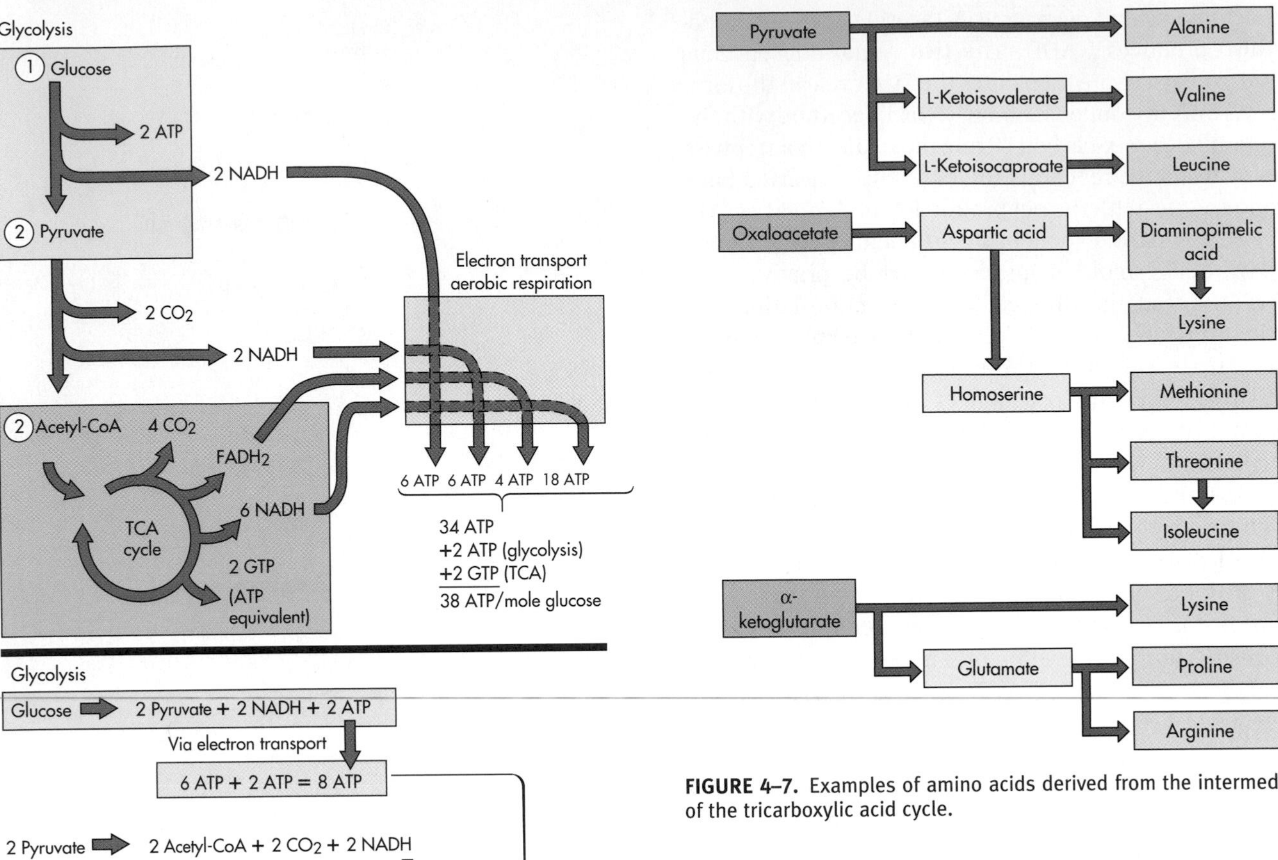

FIGURE 4–6. Aerobic glucose metabolism.

FIGURE 4–7. Examples of amino acids derived from the intermediates of the tricarboxylic acid cycle.

ATP and generation of 2 moles of NADPH per mole of glucose. The ribulose-5-phosphate may then be converted to ribose-5-phosphate (a precursor in nucleotide biosynthesis), or alternatively to xylulose-5-phosphate. The remaining reactions in the pathway use enzymes known as **transketolases** and **transaldolases** to generate various sugars, which may function as biosynthetic precursors or may be shunted back to the glycolytic pathway for use in energy generation.

Biosynthesis

We have thus far discussed primarily the catabolic pathways of the bacterial cell, pathways that result in the generation of ATP, NADH, NADPH, and various chemical intermediates. These products may be used for synthesizing major cellular constituents (i.e., peptidoglycan, lipopolysaccharide, proteins, nucleic acids). The following sections describe the important points of the synthesis of each macromolecule from component subunits. Deoxyribonucleic acid (DNA) and Ribonucleic acid (RNA) are discussed more fully in Chapter 5.

NUCLEIC ACID SYNTHESIS

The synthesis of the purine nucleotides (e.g., adenosine monophosphate and guanosine monophosphate) begins with ribose-5-phosphate formed as a product of the pentose phosphate pathway. The bicyclic purine ring system is constructed in a stepwise fashion on the sugar phosphate moiety. The product of this series of reactions is the purine nucleotide, inosine monophosphate, which may then be converted to guanosine or adenosine monophosphate. In contrast, the pyrimidine nucleotides are produced by the synthesis of the pyrimidine, orotate, which is then attached to the ribose phosphate, forming orotidine monophosphate. This nucleotide may then be converted to cytidine monophosphate or uridine monophosphate. The corresponding deoxyribonucleotides for use in DNA are obtained by removal of the hydroxyl at the 2′ carbon atom of the sugar portion of the ribonucleotide. Production of thymine, a unique and

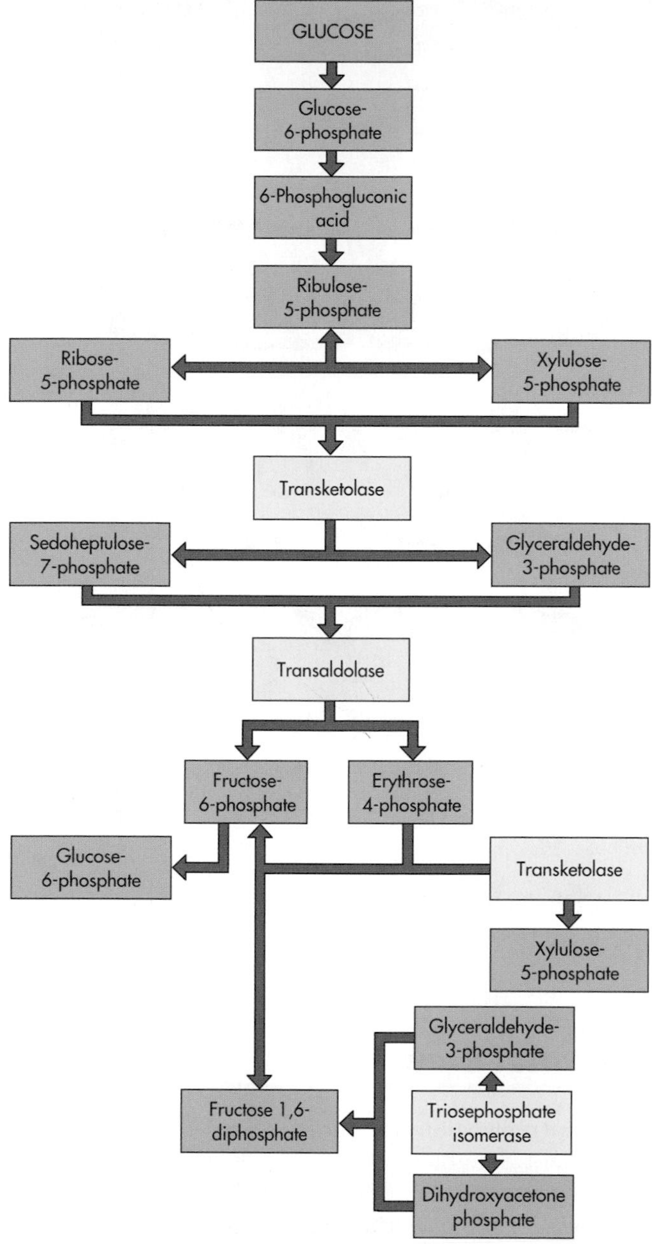

FIGURE 4–8. Pentose phosphate cycle or hexose monophosphate pathway. The enzymes transketolase and transaldolase are central to the cycle's activity.

required nucleotide for DNA, requires the tetrahydrofolate pathway, which makes this pathway a target for antibiotic action.

TRANSCRIPTION

The information carried in the genetic memory of the DNA is transcribed into a useful messenger RNA (mRNA) for subsequent translation into protein. RNA synthesis occurs in a manner similar to that of DNA replication, using a specific **DNA-dependent RNA polymerase.**

The process begins when **sigma factor** recognizes a particular sequence of nucleotides in the DNA (the **promoter;** see Chapter 5) and binds tightly to this site. Promoter sequences occur just before the start of the DNA that actually encodes a protein. Sigma factors bind to these promoters to provide a docking site for the RNA polymerase. Some bacteria encode several sigma factors to allow transcription of a group of genes under special conditions, such as heat shock, starvation, special nitrogen metabolism, or sporulation. Once the polymerase has bound to the appropriate site on the DNA, RNA synthesis proceeds with the sequential addition of ribonucleotides complementary to the sequence in the DNA. Once an entire gene or group of genes (**operon;** see Chapter 5) has been transcribed, the RNA polymerase dissociates from the DNA, a process mediated by signals within the DNA. The bacterial, DNA-dependent RNA polymerase is inhibited by rifampin, an antibiotic often used in the treatment of tuberculosis. The transfer RNA (tRNA), which is used in protein synthesis, and ribosomal RNA (rRNA), a component of the ribosomes, are also transcribed from the DNA.

TRANSLATION

Translation is the process by which the language of the **genetic code,** in the form of mRNA, is converted (translated) into a sequence of amino acids, the protein product. For the purposes of translation, the nucleotide sequence of the mRNA is divided into groups of three consecutive nucleotides. Each set of three nucleotides is known as a **codon** and encodes a particular amino acid. Because there are four different nucleotides, 4^3, 64 combinations of 3 are possible, each codon coding for only a single amino acid (or termination signal). However, because there are only 20 amino acids, each may be encoded by more than one triplet codon. This feature is known as the *degeneracy of the genetic code* and may function in protecting the cell from the effects of minor mutations in the DNA or mRNA. Each tRNA molecule contains a three-nucleotide sequence complementary to one of the codon sequences. This tRNA sequence is known as the **anticodon;** it allows base pairing and binds to the codon sequence on the mRNA. Attached to the opposite end of the tRNA is the amino acid that corresponds to the particular codon–anticodon pair.

The process of protein synthesis (Figure 4–9) begins with the binding of the 30S ribosomal subunit and a special initiator tRNA for formyl methionine (fmet) at the methionine codon (AUG) start codon to form the so-called **initiation complex.** The 50S ribosomal subunit binds to the complex to initiate mRNA synthesis. The ribosome contains two tRNA binding sites, the **A (aminoacyl) site** and the **P (peptidyl) site,** each of which allows base pairing between the bound tRNA and the codon sequence

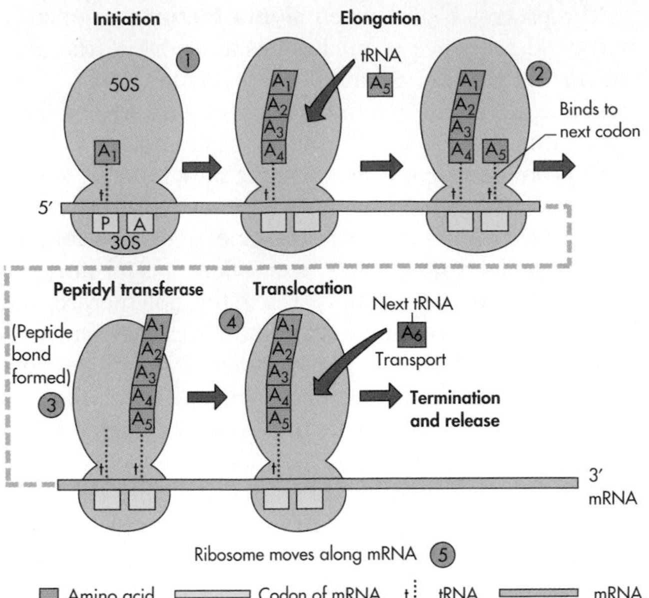

FIGURE 4–9. Bacterial protein synthesis. *1*, Binding of the 30S subunit to the messenger RNA (mRNA) with the formylmethionine transfer RNA (fmet-tRNA) at the AUG start codon allows assembly of the 70S ribosome. The fmet-tRNA binds to the peptidyl site (P). *2*, The next tRNA binds to its codon at the A site and 'accepts' the growing peptide chain *3*, *4*, Before translocation to the peptidyl site. *5*, The process is repeated until a stop codon and the protein are released.

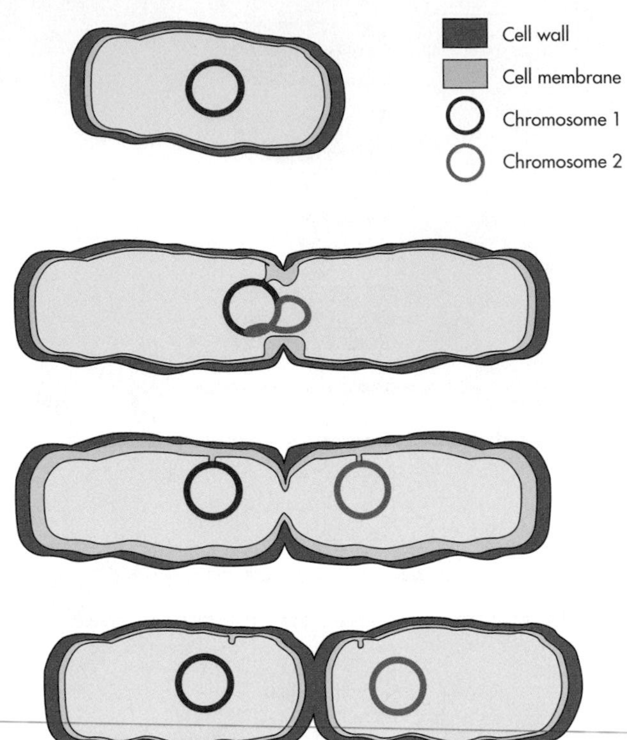

FIGURE 4–10. Bacterial cell division. Replication requires extension of the cell wall and replication of the chromosome and septum formation. Membrane attachment of the DNA pulls each daughter strand into a new cell.

in the mRNA. The tRNA corresponding to the second codon occupies the A site. The amino group of the amino acid attached to the A site forms a peptide bond with the carboxyl group of the amino acid in the P site in a reaction known as **transpeptidation.** This process leaves the tRNA in the P site uncharged (i.e., without an attached amino acid), allowing it to be released from the ribosome. The ribosome then moves down the mRNA exactly three nucleotides, thereby transferring the tRNA with attached nascent peptide to the P site and bringing the next codon into the A site. The appropriate charged tRNA is brought into the A site, and the process is then repeated. Translation continues until the new codon in the A site is one of the three termination codons, for which there is no corresponding tRNA. At that point the new protein is released to the cytoplasm and the translation complex may be disassembled, or the ribosome shuffles to the next start codon and initiates a new protein. The ability to shuffle along the mRNA to start a new protein is a characteristic of the 70S bacterial but not of the 80S eukaryotic ribosome. This has implications for the synthesis of proteins for some viruses.

The process of protein synthesis by the 70S ribosome represents an important target of antimicrobial action. The aminoglycosides (e.g., streptomycin and gentamicin) and the tetracyclines act by binding to the small ribosomal subunit and inhibiting normal ribosomal function. Similarly, the macrolide (e.g., erythromycin) and lincosamide (e.g., clindamycin) groups of antibiotics act by binding to the large ribosomal subunit.

Bacterial Growth

Bacterial replication is a coordinated process in which two equivalent daughter cells are produced. For growth to occur, there must be sufficient metabolites to support the synthesis of the bacterial components and especially the nucleotides for DNA synthesis. A cascade of regulatory events (synthesis of key proteins and RNA), much like a countdown at the Kennedy Space Center, must occur on schedule to initiate a replication cycle. *However, once it is initiated, DNA synthesis must run to completion, even if all nutrients have been removed from the medium.*

Chromosome replication is initiated at the membrane, and each daughter chromosome is anchored to a different portion of membrane. In some cells the DNA associates with mesosomes. Bacterial membrane, peptidoglycan synthesis, and cell division are linked together. As the bacterial membrane grows, the daughter chromosomes are pulled apart. Commencement of chromosome replication also initiates the process of cell division, which can be visualized by the start of septum formation between the two daughter cells (Figure 4–10; see also Chapter 3). New

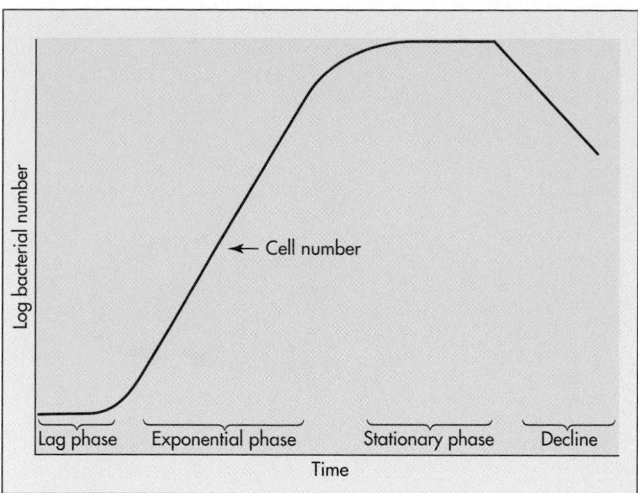

FIGURE 4–11. Phases of bacterial growth, starting with an inoculum of stationary-phase cells.

initiation events may occur even before completion of chromosome replication and cell division.

Depletion of metabolites (starvation) or a buildup of toxic by-products (e.g., ethanol) triggers the production of chemical **alarmones,** which causes synthesis to stop, but degradative processes continue. DNA synthesis continues until all initiated chromosomes are completed, despite the detrimental effect on the cell. Ribosomes are cannibalized for deoxyribonucleotide precursors, peptidoglycan and proteins are degraded for metabolites, and the cell shrinks. Septum formation may be initiated, but cell division may not occur. Many cells die. Similar signals may initiate **sporulation** in species capable of this process (see Chapter 3).

POPULATION DYNAMICS

When bacteria are added to a medium, they require time to adapt to the new environment before they begin dividing (Figure 4–11). This hiatus is known as the **lag phase** of growth. During the **log or exponential phase,** the bacteria will grow and divide with a **doubling time** characteristic of the strain and determined by the conditions. The number of bacteria will increase to 2^n, in which n is the number of generations (doublings). The culture eventually runs out of metabolites, or a toxic substance builds up in the medium; the bacteria then stop growing and enter the **stationary phase.**

QUESTIONS

1. How many moles of ATP are generated per mole of glucose in glycolysis, the TCA cycle, and electron transport? Which of these occur in anaerobic conditions and in aerobic conditions? Which is most efficient?
2. What products of anaerobic fermentation would be detrimental to host (human) tissue (e.g., *C. perfringens*)?
3. If the number of bacteria during log phase growth can be calculated by the following equation:

$$N_t = N_0 \times 2^{t/d}$$

in which N_t is the number of bacteria after time (t), t/d is the amount of time divided by the doubling time, and N_0 is the initial number of bacteria, how many bacteria will be in the culture after 4 hours if the doubling time is 20 minutes and the initial bacterial inoculum contained 1000 bacteria?

Bibliography

Davis BD et al, editors: *Microbiology,* ed 4, Philadelphia, 1990, JB Lippincott.

Jawetz E et al: *Review of medical microbiology,* ed 16, Los Altos, Calif, 1984, Lange.

Lehninger AL: *Principles of biochemistry,* New York, 1982, Worth.

Mandell GL, Bennet JE, Dolin R, editors: *Principles and practice of infectious diseases,* ed 6. Philadelphia, 2005, Churchill Livingstone.

Slots J, Taubman MA, editors: *Contemporary oral microbiology and immunology,* St Louis, 1992, Mosby.

Strauss JM, Strauss EG: *Virues and human disease,* San Diego, 2002, Academic Press.

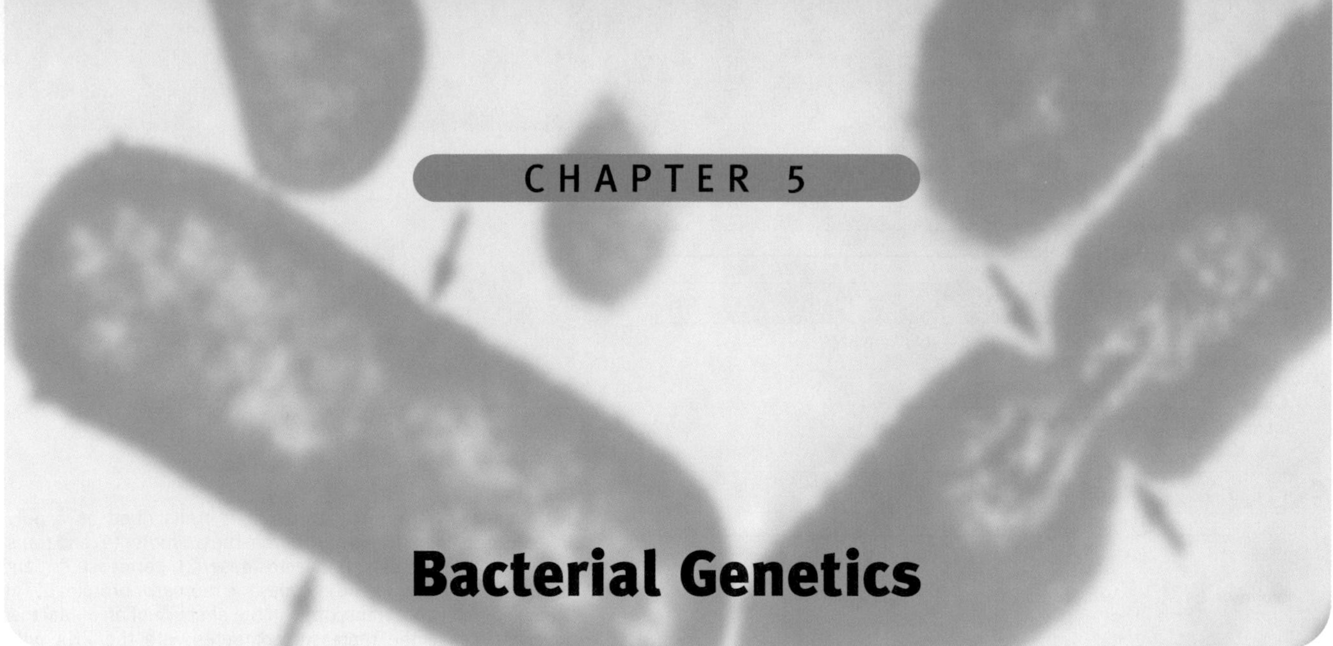

Bacterial Genetics

DNA: The Genetic Material

The bacterial genome is the total collection of genes carried by a bacterium, both on its chromosome and on its extrachromosomal genetic elements, if any. The bacterial chromosome differs from the human chromosome in several ways. The chromosome of a typical bacterium such as *Escherichia coli* is a single, double-stranded, circular molecule of deoxyribonucleic acid (DNA) containing approximately 5 million base pairs (or 5000 kilobase [kb] pairs), an approximate length of 1.3 mm (i.e., nearly 1000 times the diameter of the cell). The smallest bacterial chromosomes (from mycoplasmas) are approximately a fourth of this size. In comparison, humans have two copies of 23 chromosomes, which represent 2.9×10^9 base pairs 990 mm in length. Each genome contains many **operons,** which are made up of **genes.** Eukaryotes usually have two distinct copies of each chromosome (they are therefore diploid). Bacteria usually have only one copy of their chromosomes (they are therefore **haploid**). Because bacteria have only one chromosome, alteration of a gene (mutation) will have a more obvious effect on the cell. In addition, the structure of the bacterial chromosome is maintained by polyamines, such as spermine and spermidine, rather than by histones.

Bacteria may also contain **extrachromosomal genetic elements** such as **plasmids** or **bacteriophages** (bacterial viruses). These elements are independent of the bacterial chromosome and in most cases can be transmitted from one cell to another.

Genes are sequences of nucleotides that have a biologic function; examples are protein-structural genes (**cistrons,** which are coding genes), ribosomal ribonucleic acid (RNA) genes, and recognition and binding sites for other molecules (promoters and operators). **Promoters and operators** are nucleotide sequences that control the expression of a gene by influencing which sequences will be transcribed into messenger RNA (mRNA).

Operons are groups of one or more structural genes expressed from a particular promoter and ending at a transcriptional terminator. Thus all the genes coding for the enzymes of a particular pathway can be coordinately regulated. Operons with many structural genes are **polycistronic.** The *E. coli lac* operon includes all the genes necessary for lactose metabolism, as well as the control mechanisms for turning off (in the presence of glucose) or turning on (in the presence of galactose or an inducer) these genes only when they are needed. The *lac* operon includes a repressor sequence, a promoter sequence and structural genes for the β-galactosidase enzyme, a permease, and an acetylase (Figure 5–1). The *lac* operon is discussed later in this chapter.

Replication of DNA

The bacterial chromosome is a storehouse of information by which the characteristics of the cell are defined and all cellular processes are carried out. It is therefore essential that this molecule be duplicated without errors. Replication of the bacterial genome is triggered by a cascade of events linked to the growth rate of the cell. Replication of bacterial DNA is initiated at a specific sequence in the chromosome, called OriC. The replication process requires many enzymes, including an enzyme **(helicase)** to unwind the DNA at the origin to expose the DNA, an enzyme **(primase)** to synthesize primers to start the process, and the enzyme or enzymes **(DNA-dependent DNA polymerases)** that synthesize a copy of the DNA, but only if there is a primer sequence to add to and only in the 5′ to 3′ direction.

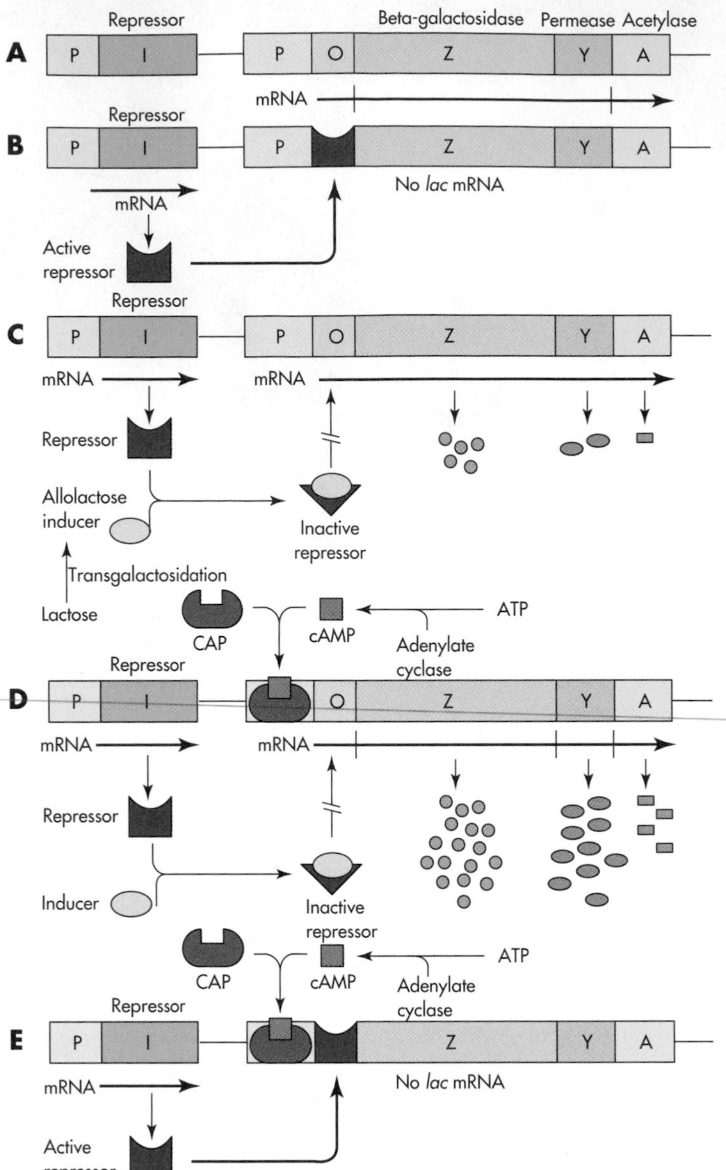

FIGURE 5–1. A, The lactose operon is transcribed as a polycistronic messenger RNA (mRNA) from the promoter (P) and translated into three proteins: β-galactosidase (Z), permease (Y), and acetylase (A). The *lac I* gene encodes the repressor protein. **B,** The lactose operon is not transcribed in the absence of an allolactose inducer, because the repressor competes with the RNA polymerase at the operator site (O). **C,** The repressor, complexed with the inducer, does not recognize the operator because of a conformation change in the repressor. The *lac* operon is thus transcribed at a low level. **D,** *Escherichia coli* is grown in a poor medium in the presence of lactose as the carbon source. Both the inducer and the CAP-cAMP complex are bound to the promoter, which is fully 'turned on,' and a high level of *lac* mRNA is transcribed and translated. **E,** Growth of *E. coli* in a poor medium without lactose results in the binding of the CAP-cAMP complex to the promoter region and binding of the active repressor to the operator sequence, because no inducer is available. The result will be that the *lac* operon will not be transcribed. ATP, adenosine triphosphate; CAP, catabolite gene-activator protein; cAMP, cyclic adenosine monophosphate.

New DNA is synthesized **semiconservatively,** using both strands of the parental DNA as templates. New DNA synthesis occurs at **growing forks** and proceeds **bidirectionally.** One strand (the leading strand) is copied continuously in the 5′ to 3′ direction, whereas the other strand (the lagging strand) must be synthesized as many pieces of DNA using RNA primers (Okazaki's fragments). The lagging-strand DNA must be extended in the 5′ to 3′ direction as its template becomes available. Then the pieces are ligated together by the enzyme DNA ligase (Figure 5–2). To maintain the high degree of accuracy required for replication, the DNA polymerases possess "proofreading" functions, which allow the enzyme to confirm that the appropriate nucleotide was inserted and to correct any errors that were made. During log-phase growth in rich medium, many initiations of chromosomal replication may occur before cell division. This process produces a series of nested bubbles of new daughter chromosomes, each with its pair of growth forks of new DNA synthesis. The polymerase moves down the DNA strand, incorporating the appropriate (complementary) nucleotide at each position. Replication is complete when the two replication forks meet 180 degrees from the origin. The process of DNA replication puts great torsional strain on the chromosomal circle of DNA; this strain is relieved by **topoisomerases** (e.g., gyrase), which supercoil the DNA. Topoisomerases are essential to the bacteria and are targets for the quinolone antibiotics.

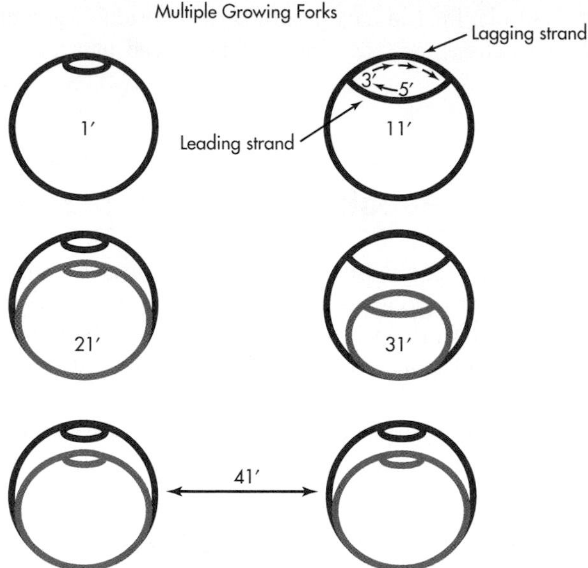

FIGURE 5–2. Bacterial DNA replication. New DNA synthesis occurs at growing forks and proceeds bidirectionally. DNA synthesis progresses in the 5′ to 3′ direction continuosly (leading strand) or in pieces (lagging strand). Assuming it takes 40 minutes to complete one round of replication and assuming new initiation every 20 minutes, initiation of DNA synthesis precedes cell division. Multiple growing forks may be initiated in a cell before complete septum formation and cell division. The daughter cells are "born pregnant."

Transcriptional Control

REGULATION OF GENE EXPRESSION

Bacteria have developed mechanisms to adapt quickly and efficiently to changes in concentrations of nutrients in their environment. The bacteria turn on a complete set of enzymes when necessary and avoid making the enzyme or enzymes of a pathway when the substrate is absent.

First, the organization of the genes of a biochemical pathway into an **operon,** with appropriate genetic control mechanisms, allows coordinated production of the necessary enzymes in response to a nutritional stimulus. Second, the transcription of the gene is regulated directly by repressor proteins (which bind to operators) in response to nutritional signals within the cell. Third, the rate of protein synthesis by the ribosome can regulate transcription in prokaryotes. The absence of a nuclear membrane in prokaryotes allows the ribosome to bind to the mRNA as it is being transcribed from the DNA.

TRANSCRIPTIONAL REGULATION

Initiation of transcription may be under positive or negative control. Genes under **negative control** are expressed unless they are switched off by a **repressor protein.** This repressor protein prevents gene expression by binding to a specific DNA sequence called the **operator,** making it impossible for the RNA polymerase to initiate transcription at the promoter. Inversely, genes whose expression is under **positive control** are not transcribed unless an active regulator protein, called an **apoinducer,** is present. The apoinducer binds to a specific DNA sequence and assists the RNA polymerase in the initiation steps by an unknown mechanism.

Operons can be **inducible or repressible.** Introduction of a substrate **(inducer)** into the growth medium may induce an operon to increase the expression of the enzymes necessary for its metabolism. An abundance of the end products **(co-repressors)** of a pathway may signal that a pathway should be shut down or repressed by reducing the synthesis of its enzymes.

The lactose *(lac)* operon responsible for the degradation of the sugar lactose is an inducible operon under positive and negative regulation (see Figure 5–1). Normally the bacteria use glucose and not lactose. In the absence of lactose the operon is repressed by the binding of the repressor protein to the operator sequence, thus impeding the RNA polymerase function. In the absence of glucose, however, the addition of lactose reverses this repression. Full expression of the *lac* operon also requires a protein-mediated, positive-control mechanism. In *E. coli,* a protein called the catabolite gene-activator protein (CAP) forms a complex with cyclic adenosine monophosphate (cAMP), acquiring the ability to bind to a specific DNA sequence present in the promoter. The CAP-cAMP complex enhances binding of the RNA polymerase to the promoter, thus allowing an increase in the frequency of transcription initiation. The CAP-cAMP complex may increase the operon transcription by protein-protein interaction with the RNA polymerase or by protein-DNA interaction.

The tryptophan operon **(trp operon)** contains the structural genes necessary for tryptophan biosynthesis and is under dual transcriptional control mechanisms (Figure 5–3). Although tryptophan is essential for protein synthesis, too much tryptophan in the cell can be toxic; therefore its synthesis must be regulated. At the DNA level the repressor protein is activated by an increased intracellular concentration of tryptophan to prevent transcription. At the protein synthesis level, rapid translation of a "test peptide" at the beginning of the mRNA in the presence of tryptophan promotes the formation of a double-stranded loop in the RNA, which terminates transcription. The same loop is formed if no protein synthesis is occurring, a situation in which tryptophan synthesis would similarly not be required. This regulates tryptophan synthesis at the mRNA level in a process termed **attenuation,** in which mRNA synthesis is prematurely terminated.

POST-TRANSCRIPTIONAL OR TRANSLATIONAL REGULATION

The rate and efficiency of protein synthesis can be controlled by other factors. These may include the structure of the mRNA or the concentrations of transfer RNA (tRNA) and amino acids in the cell. With polycistronic mRNAs, translational control may result in differences in the quantity of each protein expressed from each gene. For example, for the *lac* operon, β-galactosidase, galactoside permease, and acetylase are produced at a ratio of 10 : 5 : 2.

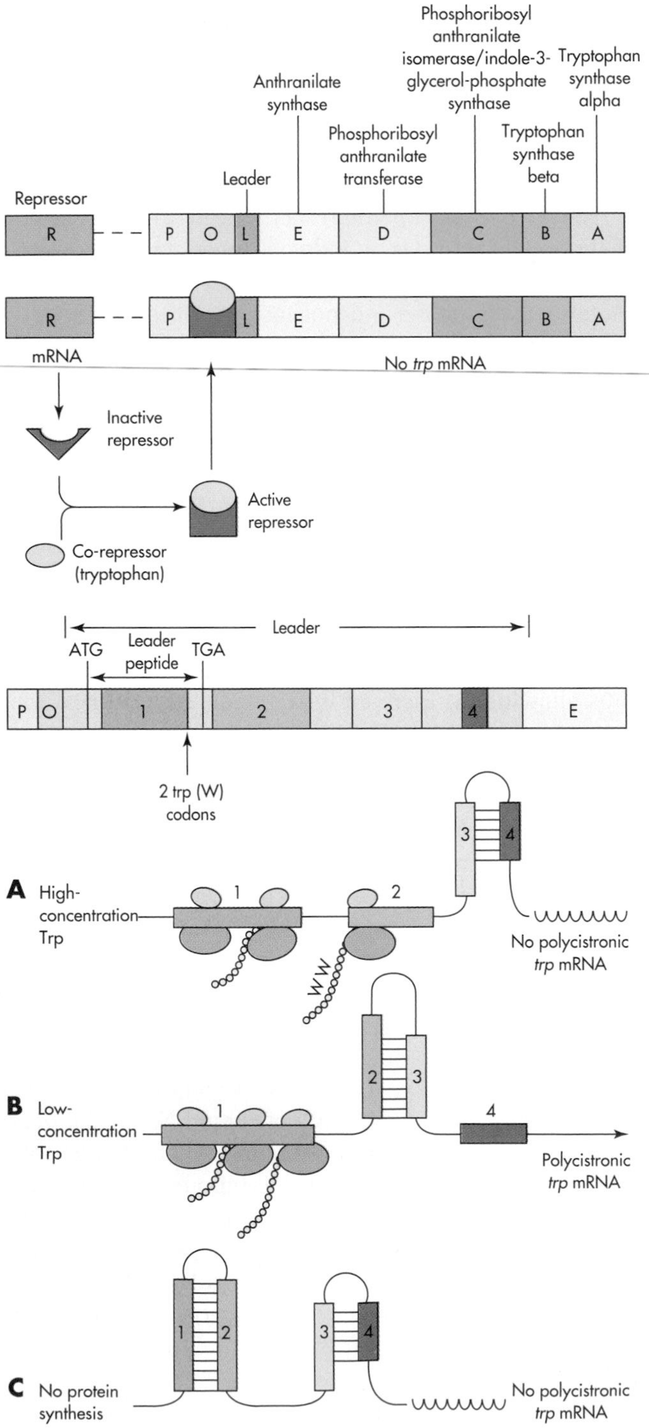

Mutation, Repair, and Recombination

DNA conveys genetic information; therefore cells must be able to replicate DNA accurately. Furthermore, accidental damage to DNA must be minimized by the elaboration of efficient DNA repair systems. These damage-containment systems are so important for the life of a cell that the bacterium devotes a large percentage of its genome to specify and control the enzymes involved.

MUTATIONS AND THEIR CONSEQUENCES

A mutation is any change in the base sequence of the DNA. A single base change can result in a **transition** in which one purine is replaced by another purine, or in which a pyrimidine is replaced by another pyrimidine. A **transversion,** in which, for example, a purine is replaced by a pyrimidine and vice versa, may also result. A **silent mutation** is a change at the DNA level that does not result in any change of amino acid in the encoded protein. This type of mutation occurs because more than one codon may encode an amino acid. A **missense mutation** results in a different amino acid being inserted in the protein, but this may be a **conservative mutation** if the new amino acid has similar properties (e.g., valine replacing alanine). A **nonsense mutation** changes a codon encoding an amino acid to a stop codon (e.g., TAG [thymidine-adenine-guanine]), which will cause the ribosome to fall off the mRNA and end the protein prematurely.

FIGURE 5–3. Regulation of the tryptophan *(trp)* operon. **A,** The *trp* operon encodes the five enzymes necessary for tryptophan biosynthesis. This *trp* operon is under dual control. **B,** The conformation of the inactive repressor protein is changed after its binding by the corepressor tryptophan. The resulting active repressor (R) binds to the operator (O), blocking any transcription of the *trp* mRNA by the RNA polymerase. **C,** The *trp* operon is also under the control of an attenuation-antitermination mechanism. Upstream of the structural genes are the promoter (P), the operator, and a leader (L), which can be transcribed into a short peptide containing two tryptophans (W), near its distal end. The leader mRNA possesses four repeats (1, 2, 3, and 4), which can pair differently according to the tryptophan availability, leading to an early termination of transcription of the *trp* operon or its full transcription. In the presence of a high concentration of tryptophan, regions 3 and 4 of the leader mRNA can pair, forming a terminator hairpin, and no transcription of the *trp* operon occurs. However, in the presence of little or no tryptophan the ribosomes stall in region 1 when translating the leader peptide, because of the tandem of tryptophan codons. Then regions 2 and 3 can pair, forming the antiterminator hairpin and leading to transcription of the *trp* genes. Finally, the regions 1:2 and 3:4 of the free leader mRNA can pair, also leading to cessation of transcription before the first structural gene *trpE*. A, adenine; G, guanine; T, thymine.

More drastic changes can occur when numerous bases are involved. A small deletion or insertion that *is not in multiples of three* produces a **frameshift mutation.** This results in a change in the reading frame, usually leading to a useless peptide and premature truncation of the protein. **Null mutations,** which completely destroy gene function, arise when there is an extensive insertion, deletion, or gross rearrangement of the chromosome structure. Insertion of long sequences of DNA (many thousands of base pairs) by recombination, by transposition, or during genetic engineering can produce **null mutations** by separating the parts of a gene and inactivating the gene.

Many mutations occur spontaneously in nature (e.g., by polymerase mistakes); however, physical or chemical agents can also induce mutations. Among the physical agents used to induce mutations in bacteria are heat, which results in deamination of nucleotides; ultraviolet light, which causes pyrimidine dimer formation; and ionizing radiation, such as x-rays, which produce very reactive hydroxyl radicals that may be responsible for opening a ring of a base or causing single- or double-stranded breaks in the DNA. Chemical mutagens can be grouped into three classes. **Nucleotide-base analogues** lead to mispairing and frequent DNA replication mistakes. For example, incorporation of 5-bromouracil into DNA instead of thymidine allows base pairing with guanine instead of adenine, changing a T-A base pair to a G-C base pair. **Frameshift mutagens,** such as polycyclic, flat, molecules, like ethidium bromide or acridine derivatives, insert (or intercalate) between the bases as they stack with each other in the double helix. These intercalating agents increase the spacing of successive base pairs, destroying the regular sugar-phosphate backbone and decreasing the pitch of the helix. These changes cause the addition or deletion of a single base and lead to frequent mistakes during DNA replication. **DNA-reactive chemicals** act directly on the DNA to change the chemical structure of the base. These include nitrous acid (HNO_2) and alkylating agents, including nitrosoguanidine and ethyl methane sulfonate, which are known to add methyl or ethyl groups to the rings of the DNA bases. The modified bases may pair abnormally or not at all. The damage may cause the removal of the base from the DNA backbone.

REPAIR MECHANISMS OF DNA

A number of repair mechanisms have evolved in bacterial cells to minimize damage to DNA. These repair mechanisms can be divided into the following five groups:

1. **Direct DNA repair** is the enzymatic removal of damage, such as pyrimidine dimers and alkylated bases.

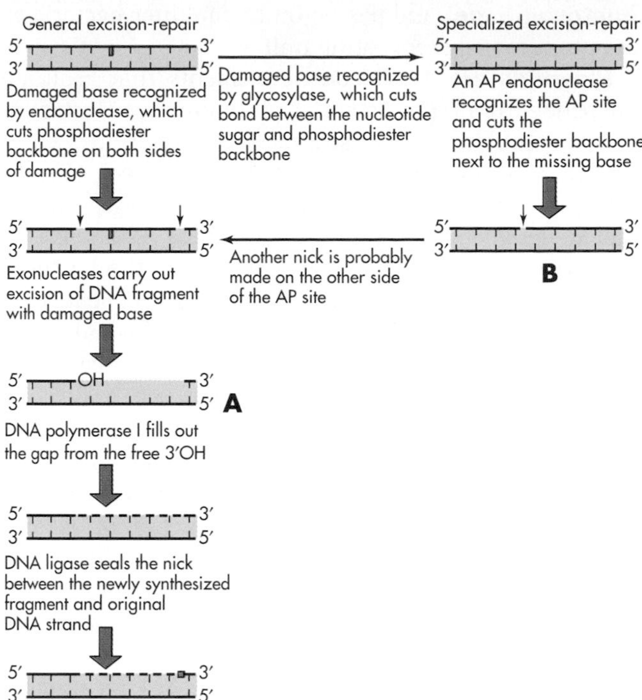

FIGURE 5–4. A, Generalized excision repair mechanism. **B,** Specialized excision repair mechanism. AP, apurinic (endonuclease).

2. **Excision repair** is the excision of a DNA segment containing the damage, followed by synthesis of a new DNA strand (Figure 5–4). Two types of excision-repair mechanisms, generalized and specialized, exist.
3. Recombinational or **postreplication repair** is the retrieval of missing information by genetic recombination when both DNA strands are damaged.
4. The **SOS response** is the induction of many genes (approximately 15) after DNA damage or interruption of DNA replication.
5. **Error-prone repair** is the last resort of a bacterial cell before it dies. It is used to fill in gaps with a random sequence when a DNA template is not available for directing an accurate repair.

Gene Exchange in Prokaryotic Cells

Many bacteria, especially many pathogenic bacterial species, are promiscuous with their DNA. The exchange of DNA between cells allows the exchange of genes and characteristics between cells, thus producing new strains of bacteria. This exchange may be advantageous for the recipient, especially if the exchanged DNA encodes antibiotic resistance. The transferred DNA can be integrated into the recipient chromosome or stably maintained as an extrachromosomal element **(plasmid)** or a bacterial virus

(bacteriophage) and passed on to daughter bacteria as an autonomously replicating unit.

Plasmids are small genetic elements that replicate independently of the bacterial chromosome. Most plasmids are circular, double-stranded DNA molecules varying from 1500 to 400,000 base pairs. However, *Borrelia burgdorferi*, the causative agent of Lyme disease, and the related *Borrelia hermsii* are unique among all eubacteria because they possess linear plasmids. Like the bacterial chromosomal DNA, they can autonomously replicate and, as such, are referred to as **replicons.** Some plasmids, such as the *E. coli* F plasmid, are **episomes,** which means that they can integrate into the host chromosome.

Plasmids carry genetic information, which may not be essential but can provide a selective advantage to the bacteria. For example, plasmids may confer high levels of antibiotic resistance, encoding the production of bacteriocins, toxins, virulence determinants, and other genes that may provide the bacteria with a unique growth advantage over other microbes or within the host (Figure 5–5). The number of copies of plasmid produced by a cell is determined by the particular plasmid. The copy number is the ratio of copies of the plasmid to the number of copies of the chromosome. This may be as few as one in the case of large plasmids or as many as 50 in smaller plasmids.

Large plasmids (20 to 120 kb), such as the **fertility factor F** found in *E. coli* or the resistance transfer factor (80 kb), can often mediate their own transfer from one cell to another by a process called **conjugation** (see the section on conjugation, later in this chapter). These conjugative plasmids encode all the necessary factors for their transfer. Other plasmids can be transferred into a bacterial cell by means other than conjugation, such as transformation or transduction. These terms are discussed later in the chapter.

Bacteriophages are bacterial viruses. These extrachromosomal genetic elements can survive outside of a host cell because a protein coat protects the nucleic acid genome (which may be DNA or RNA) (Figure 5–6).

Bacteriophages infect bacterial cells and either replicate to large numbers and cause the cell to lyse **(lytic infection)**, or in some cases **integrate** into the host genome without killing the host (the **lysogenic state**), such as the *E. coli* bacteriophage lambda (Figure 5–7). Some lysogenic bacteriophages carry toxin genes (e.g., corynephage beta carries the gene for the diphtheria toxin). Bacteriophage lambda remains lysogenic as long as a repressor protein is synthesized and prevents the phage from becoming unintegrated and replicating independently of the host chromosome. This reaction can be triggered if the host cell DNA is damaged by radiation or by another means or if the cell can no longer make the repressor protein, a signal that the host cell is unhealthy and is no longer a good place for "freeloading."

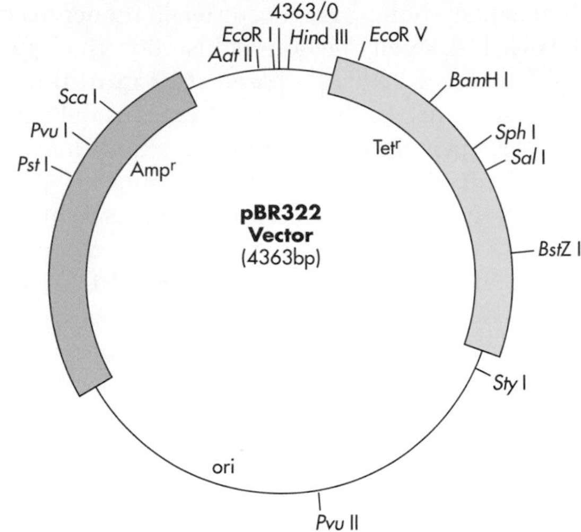

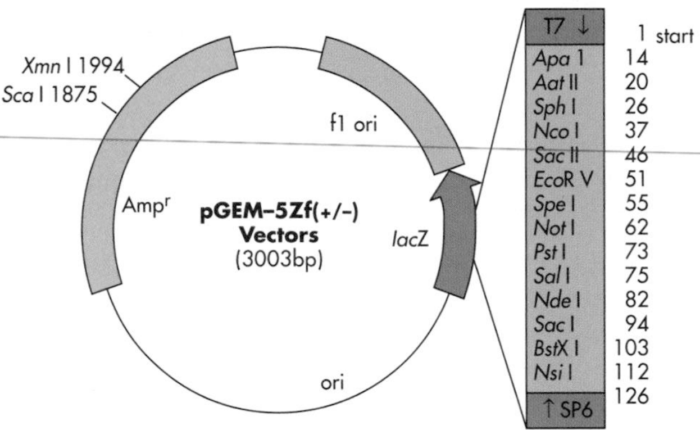

FIGURE 5–5. Plasmids. The pBR322 plasmid is one of the plasmids used for cloning DNA. This plasmid encodes resistance to ampicillin (Amp) and tetracycline (Tet) and an origin of replication (ori). The multiple cloning site in the pGEM plasmid provides different restriction enzyme cleavage sites for insertion of DNA within the β-galactosidase gene *(lacZ)*. The insert is flanked by bacteriophage promoters to allow directional messenger RNA expression of the cloned sequence.

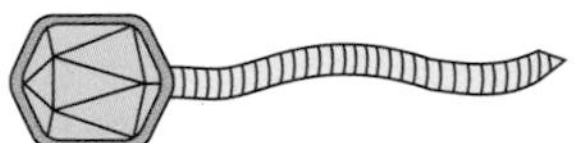

FIGURE 5–6. Bacteriophage lambda.

Transposons (jumping genes) are mobile genetic elements (Figure 5–8) that can transfer DNA within a cell, from one position to another in the genome or between different molecules of DNA (e.g., plasmid to plasmid or plasmid to chromosome). Transposons are present in prokaryotes and eukaryotes. The simplest transposons are called insertion sequences and range in length from 150 to 1500 base pairs with inverted repeats of 15 to 40 base pairs at their ends and the minimal genetic information

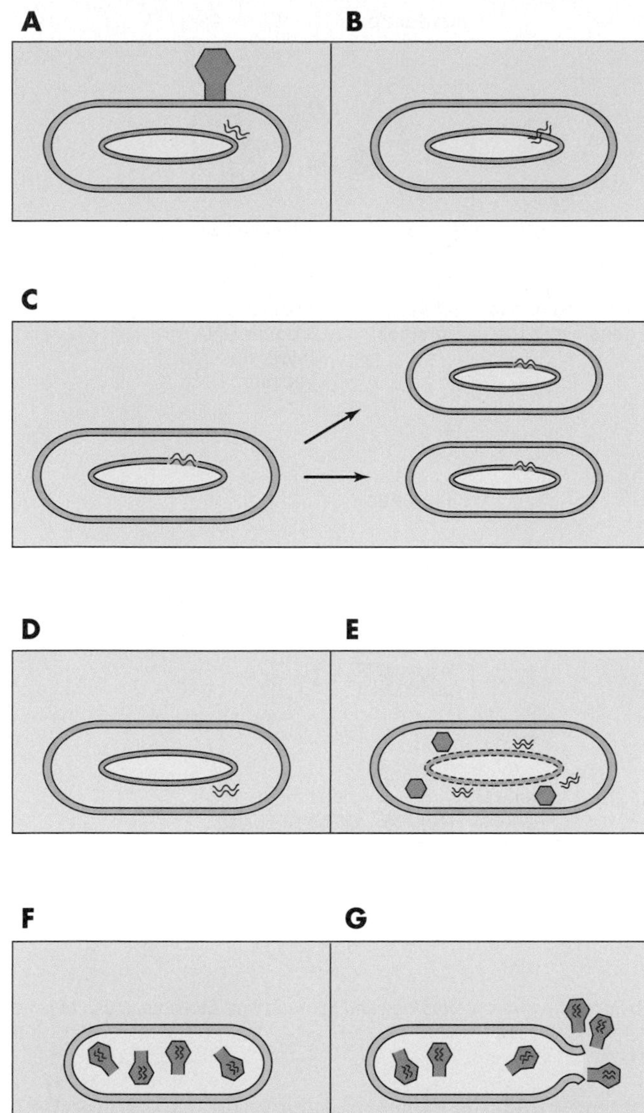

FIGURE 5–7. Lysogenic infection of bacterium with temperate bacteriophage. **A,** The phage infects a sensitive bacterium, and the phage DNA is injected. **B,** The phage DNA becomes integrated into the bacterial chromosome. **C,** The bacterium multiplies, apparently unaffected by the infection. It has been lysogenized. **D,** Occasionally the phage DNA is excised from the bacterial chromosome, takes control of the cell, and replicates. **E,** An individual cell (or, by induction, all the cells) produces phage components. **F,** The components are later assembled into phage particles. **G,** Ultimately, the cell lyses and releases mature phage particles.

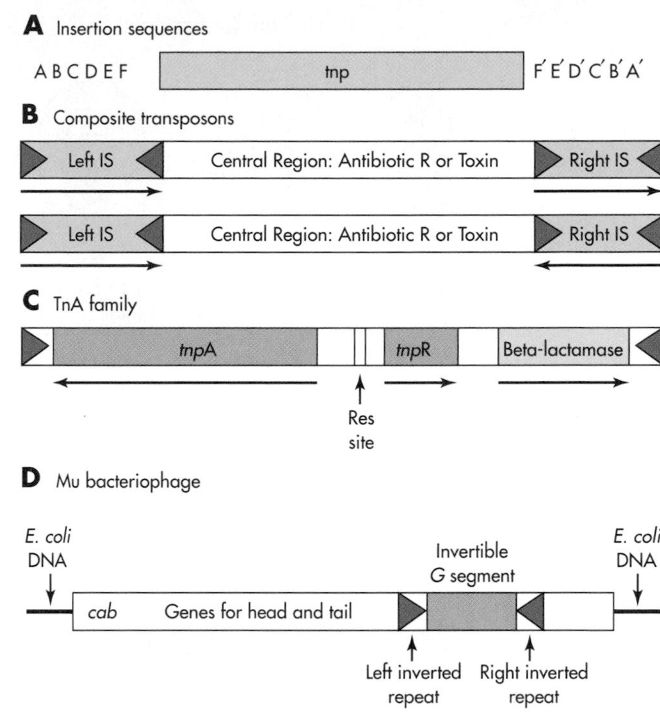

FIGURE 5–8. Transposons. **A,** The insertion sequences code only for a transposase *(tnp)* and possess inverted repeats (15 to 40 base pairs) at each end. **B,** The composite transposons contain a central-region coding for antibiotic resistances or toxins, flanked by two insertion sequences (IS), which can be either directly repeated or reversed. **C,** Tn3, a member of the TnA transposon family. The central region encodes three genes—a transposase (tnpA), a resolvase (tnpR), and a β-lactamase—conferring resistance to ampicillin. A resolution site (Res site) is used during the replicative transposition process. This central region is flanked on both ends by direct repeats of 38 base pairs. **D,** Phage-associated transposon is exemplified by the bacteriophage mu.

necessary for their own transfer (i.e., the gene coding for the transposase). Complex transposons carry other genes, such as genes that provide resistance against antibiotics. Transposons sometimes insert into genes and inactivate those genes. If insertion and inactivation occur in a gene that encodes an essential protein, the cell dies.

Some pathogenic bacteria use a transposon-like mechanism to coordinate the expression of a system of virulence factors. The genes for the activity may be grouped together in a **pathogenicity or virulence island,** which is surrounded by transposon-like mobile elements, allowing them to move within the chromosome and to other bacteria. The entire genetic unit can be triggered by an environmental stimulus (e.g., pH, heat, contact with the host cell surface) as a way to coordinate the expression of a complex process. For example, the SPI-1 island of *Salmonella* encodes 25 genes that allow the bacteria to enter nonphagocytic cells.

Mechanisms of Genetic Transfer Between Cells

The exchange of genetic material between bacterial cells may occur by one of three mechanisms (Figure 5–9): (1) **conjugation,** which is the mating or quasisexual exchange of genetic information from one bacterium (the donor) to another bacterium (the recipient); (2)

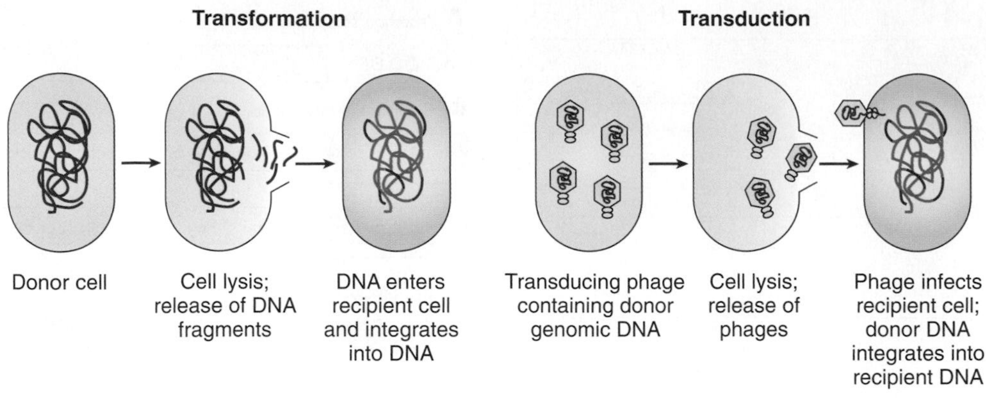

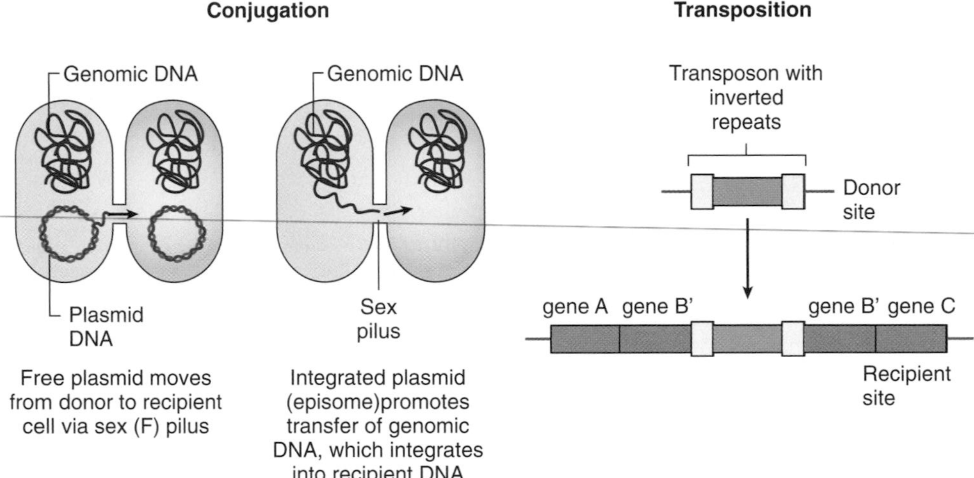

FIGURE 5–9. Mechanisms of bacterial gene transfer. (From Rosenthal KS, Tan J: *Rapid reviews microbiology and immunology,* St. Louis, 2002, Mosby.)

transformation, which results in acquisition of new genetic markers by the incorporation of exogenous or foreign DNA; or (3) **transduction,** which is the transfer of genetic information from one bacterium to another by a bacteriophage. Once inside a cell, a **transposon** can jump between different DNA molecules (e.g., plasmid to plasmid or plasmid to chromosome).

Transformation is the process by which bacteria take up fragments of naked DNA and incorporate them into their genomes. Transformation was the first mechanism of genetic transfer to be discovered in bacteria. In 1928, Griffith observed that pneumococcus virulence was related to the presence of a surrounding polysaccharide capsule and that extracts of encapsulated bacteria producing smooth colonies could transmit this trait to nonencapsulated bacteria, normally appearing with rough edges. Griffith's studies led to Avery, MacLeod, and McCarty's identification of DNA as the transforming principle some 15 years later.

Gram-positive and gram-negative bacteria can take up and stably maintain exogenous DNA. Certain species are naturally capable of taking up exogenous DNA (such species are then said to be competent), including *Haemophilus influenzae, Streptococcus pneumoniae, Bacillus* species, and *Neisseria* species. Competence develops toward the end of logarithmic growth, some time before a population enters the stationary phase. Most bacteria do not exhibit a natural ability for DNA uptake. Chemical methods or electroporation (the use of high-voltage pulses) can be used to introduce plasmid and other DNA into *E. coli* and other bacteria.

CONJUGATION

Conjugation occurs with most, if not all, eubacteria. Conjugation usually occurs between members of the same or related species but has also been demonstrated to occur between prokaryotes and cells from plants, animals, and fungi. Conjugation occurs for *E. coli,* bacteroides, enterococci, streptococci, streptomyces, and clostridia. Many of the large conjugative plasmids specify colicins or antibiotic resistance.

Genetic transfer in *E. coli* was first reported by Lederberg and Tatum in 1946, when they observed sexlike exchange between two mutant strains of *E. coli* K12. Conjugation is the process by which DNA is passed directly by cell-to-cell contact during the mating of the bacteria. Conjugation results in one-way transfer of DNA from a donor (or male) cell to a recipient (or female) cell through the **sex pilus.** Conjugative R (antibiotic resistance) for gram-positive bacteria, such as streptococci, streptomyces, and clostridia, are brought together by the presence of an adhesin molecule on the surface of the donor cell instead of pili.

The mating type (sex) of the cell depends on the presence (male) or absence (female) of a conjugative plasmid, such as the **F plasmid** of *E. coli.* The F plasmid is defined as conjugative because it carries all the genes necessary for its own transfer, including the ability to make sex pili and to initiate DNA synthesis at the transfer origin (OriT) of the plasmid. The F plasmid transfers itself, converting recipients into F^+ male cells (Figure 5–10). If a fragment of chromosomal DNA has been incorporated into the plasmid, it is designated an F prime (F′) plasmid. When it transfers into the recipient cell, it carries that fragment with it and converts it into an F′ male. If the F plasmid sequence is integrated into the bacterial chromosome, the cell is designated an Hfr (high frequency recombination) cell.

The DNA that is transferred by conjugation is not a double helix but a single-stranded molecule. Mobilization begins when a plasmid-encoded protein makes a single-stranded, site-specific cleavage at the OriT. The nick initiates rolling circle replication, and the displaced linear strand is directed to the recipient cell. The transferred, single-stranded DNA is recircularized and its complementary strand synthesized. Integration of an F plasmid into the bacterial chromosome generates an Hfr cell. Conjugation results in transfer of a part of the plasmid sequence and some portion of the bacterial chromosomal DNA. Because of the fragile connection between the mating pairs, the transfer is usually aborted before being completed such that only the chromosomal sequences adjacent to the integrated F are transferred. Artificial interruption of a mating between an Hfr and an F^- pair has been helpful in constructing a consistent map of the *E. coli* chromosomal DNA. In such maps the position of each gene is given in minutes (based on 100 minutes for

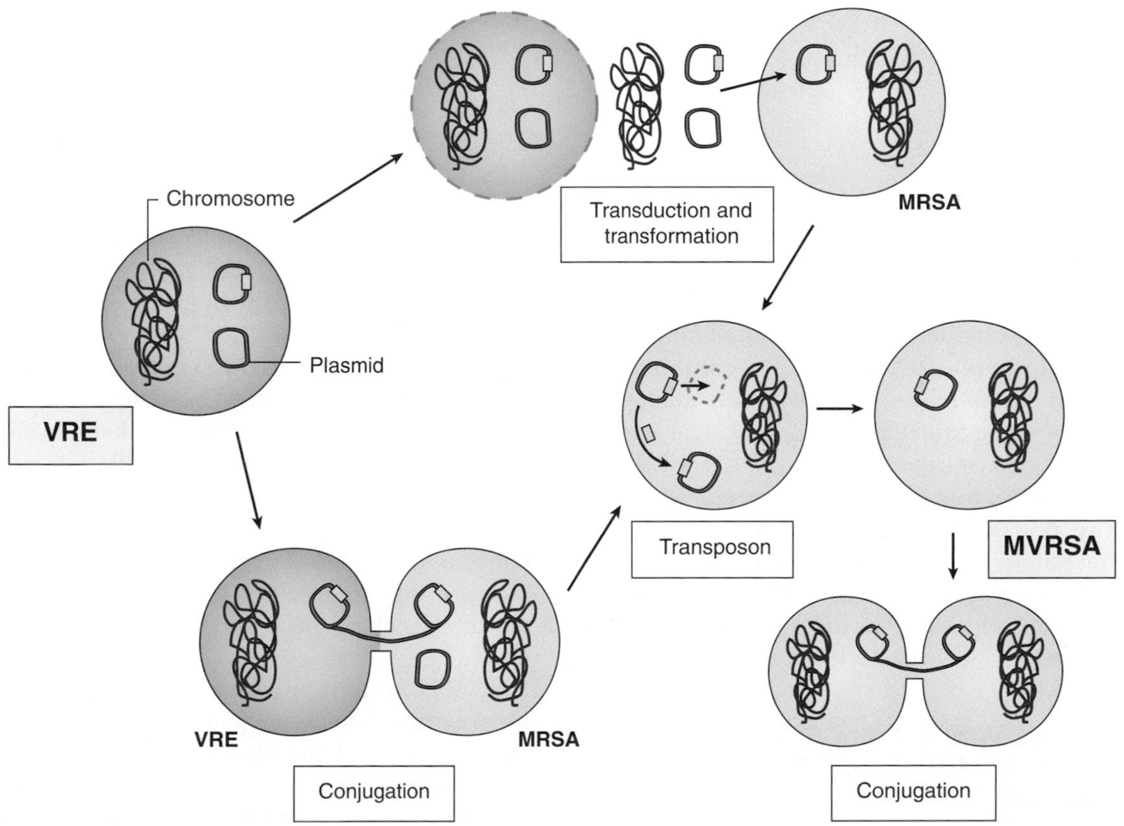

FIGURE 5–10. Genetic mechanisms of evolution of methicillin and vancomycin resistant *Staphylococcus aureus.* Vancomycin resistant enterococcus (VRE) *(in blue)* contains plasmids with multiple antibiotic resistance and virulence factors. During coinfection, a methicillin resistant *Staphylococcus aureus* (MRSA) may have acquired the enterococcal resistance plasmid (e-plasmid) by transformation (after lysis of the enterococcal cell and release of its DNA) or more likely, by conjugation. A transposon in the e-plasmid containing the vancomycin resistance gene jumped out and inserted into the multiple antibiotic resistance plasmid of the MRSA. The new plasmid is readily spread to other *S. aureus* bacteria by conjugation.

complete transfer at 37°C), according to its time of entry into a recipient cell in relation to a fixed origin.

TRANSDUCTION

Genetic transfer by transduction is mediated by bacterial viruses (bacteriophages), which pick up fragments of DNA and package them into bacteriophage particles. The DNA is delivered to infected cells and becomes incorporated into the bacterial genomes. Transduction can be classified as **specialized** if the phages in question transfer particular genes (usually those adjacent to their integration sites in the genome) or **generalized** if the selection of the sequences is random because of accidental packaging of host DNA into the phage capsid.

Generalized transducing particles should contain primarily bacterial DNA and little or no phage DNA. For example, the P1 phage of *E. coli* encodes a nuclease that degrades the host *E. coli* chromosomal DNA. A small percentage of the resultant phage particles package the DNA fragments into their capsids. The encapsulated DNA, instead of phage DNA, is injected into a new host cell, where it can recombine with the homologous host DNA. Generalized transducing particles are valuable in the **genetic mapping** of bacterial chromosomes. The closer two genes are within the bacterial chromosome, the more likely it is that they will be co-transduced in the same fragment of DNA.

Recombination

Incorporation of extrachromosomal (foreign) DNA into the chromosome occurs by recombination. There are two types of recombination: homologous and nonhomologous. **Homologous (legitimate) recombination** occurs between closely related DNA sequences and generally substitutes one sequence for another. The process requires a set of enzymes produced (in *E. coli*) by the *rec* genes. **Nonhomologous (illegitimate) recombination** occurs between dissimilar DNA sequences and generally produces insertions or deletions, or both. This process usually requires specialized (sometimes site-specific) recombination enzymes, such as those produced by many transposons and lysogenic bacteriophages.

GENERATION OF VANCOMYCIN-RESISTANT *STAPHYLOCOCCUS AUREUS* BY MULTIPLE GENETIC MANIPULATIONS

Until recently, vancomycin was the last-resort drug for *S. aureus* strains resistant to beta lactam (penicillin-related) antibiotics (e.g., methicillinresistant *S. aureus* [MRSA]). *S. aureus* acquired the vancomycin resistance gene during a mixed infection with *Enterococcus faecalis* (see Figure 5–10). The gene for the vancomycin resistance gene was contained within a **transposon** (TN1546) on a multiresistance conjugative plasmid. The plasmid was probably transferred by **conjugation** between *E. faecalis* and *S. aureus*. Alternatively, after lysis of the *E. faecalis*, *S. aureus* acquired the DNA by **transduction** and became **transformed** by the new DNA. The transposon then jumped from the *E. faecalis* plasmid, **recombined** and **integrated** into the *S. aureus* multiresistance plasmid, and the *E. faecalis* DNA was degraded. The resulting *S. aureus* plasmid encodes resistance to beta lactams, vancomycin, trimethoprim, and gentamycin/kanamycin/tobramycin antibiotics and to quaternary ammonium disinfectants and can transfer to other *S. aureus* strains by **conjugation.** (For more information, refer to Weigel in the bibliography at the end of the chapter.)

Genetic Engineering

Genetic engineering, also known as recombinant DNA technology, uses the techniques and tools developed by the bacterial geneticists to purify, amplify, modify, and express specific gene sequences. The use of genetic engineering and "cloning" has revolutionized biology and medicine. The basic components of genetic engineering are: (1) **cloning and expression vectors,** which can be used to deliver the DNA sequences into receptive bacteria and amplify the desired sequence; (2) the **DNA sequence** to be amplified and expressed; (3) **enzymes,** such as **restriction enzymes,** which are used to cleave DNA reproducibly at defined sequences (Table 5–1) and **DNA ligase,** the enzyme that links the fragment to the cloning vector.

Cloning and expression vectors must allow foreign DNA to be inserted into them but still must be able to replicate normally in a bacterial or eukaryotic host. Many types of vectors are currently used. Plasmid vectors, such as pUC, pBR322, and pGEM (see Figure 5–5), are used for DNA fragments up to 20 kb. Bacteriophages, such as lambda, are used for larger fragments up to 25 kb. More recently, **cosmid** vectors have combined some of the advantages of plasmids and phages for fragments up to 45 kb.

Most **cloning vectors** have been "engineered" to have a site for insertion of foreign DNA; a means of selection of the bacteria that have incorporated any plasmid (e.g., antibiotic resistance); and a means of distinguishing the bacteria that have incorporated those plasmids which contain inserted DNA. **Expression vectors** have DNA sequences to facilitate their replication in bacteria and eukaryotic cells and also the transcription of the gene into mRNA.

TABLE 5–1. Common Restriction Enzymes Used in Molecular Biology

Microorganism	Enzyme	Recognition Site
Acinetobacter calcoaceticus	AccI	5′ G T|(A/C) (G/T) A C C A (T/G) (C/A)|T G
Bacillus amyloliquefaciens H	BamHI	5′ G|G A T C C C C T A G|G
Escherichia coli RY13	EcoRI	5′ G|A A T T C C T T A A|G
Haemophilus influenzae Rd	HindIII	5′ A|A G C T T T T C G A|A
H. influenzae serotype c, 1160	HincII	5′ G T (C/T)|(G/A) A C C A (G/A)|(C/T) T G
Providencia stuartii 164	PstI	5′ C T G C A|G G|A C G T C
Serratia marcescens	SmaI	5′ C C C|G G G G G G|C C C
Staphylococcus aureus 3A	Sau3AI	5′|G A T C C T A G|
Xanthomonas malvacearum	XmaI	5′ C|C C G G G G G G C C|C

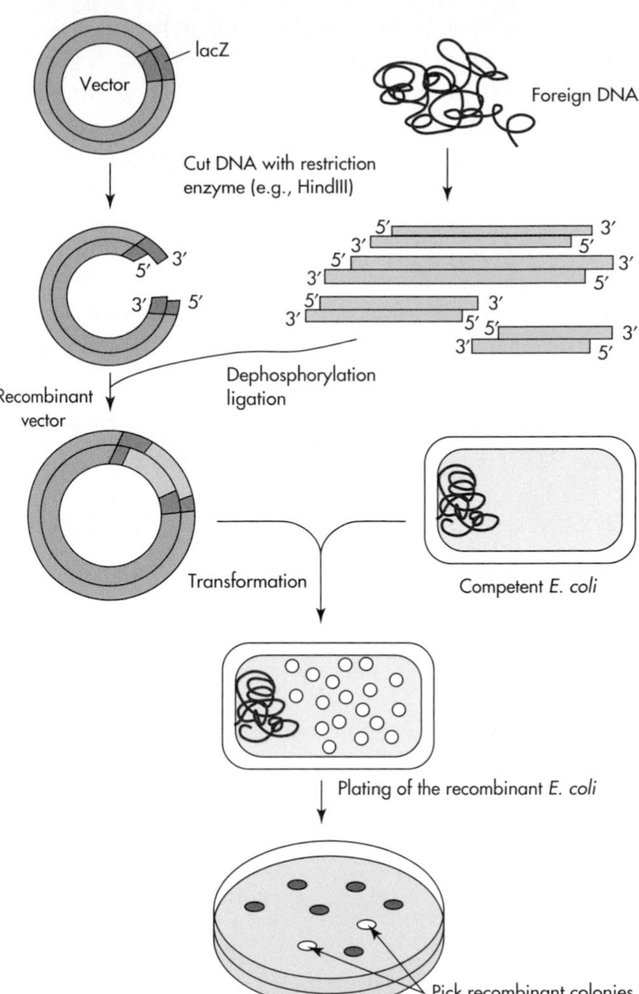

FIGURE 5–11. Cloning of foreign DNA in vectors. The vector and the foreign DNA are first digested by a restriction enzyme. Insertion of foreign DNA into the *lacZ* gene inactivates the β-galactosidase gene, allowing subsequent selection. The vector is then ligated to the foreign DNA, using bacteriophage T4 DNA ligase. The recombinant vectors are transformed into competent *Escherichia coli* cells. The recombinant *E. coli* cells are plated onto agar containing antibiotic, an inducer of the *lac* operon, and a chromophoric substrate that turns blue in cells having plasmid but not insert; those cells with plasmid containing the insert remain white.

The DNA to be cloned can be obtained by purification of chromosomal DNA from cells, viruses, or other plasmids or by selective amplification of DNA sequences by a technique known as polymerase chain reaction (PCR). (PCR is explained further in Chapter 17.) Both the vector and the foreign DNA are cleaved with restriction enzymes (Figure 5–11). Restriction enzymes recognize a specific palindromic sequence and make a staggered cut, which generates sticky ends, or a blunt cut, which generates blunt ends (see Table 5–1). Most cloning vectors have a sequence that can be cleaved by many restriction enzymes, called the **multiple cloning site.** Ligation of the vector with the DNA fragments generates a molecule capable of replicating the inserted sequence called **recombinant DNA** (see Figure 5–9). The total number of recombinant vectors obtained when cloning all the fragments that result from cleavage of chromosomal DNA is known as a **genomic library** because there should be at least one representative of each gene in the library. An alternative approach to cloning the gene for a protein is to convert the mRNA for the protein into DNA using a retrovirus enzyme called reverse transcriptase (RNA-dependent DNA polymerase) to produce a complementary DNA (cDNA). A **cDNA library** represents the genes that are expressed as mRNA in a particular cell.

The recombinant DNA is then transformed into a bacterial host, usually *E. coli,* and the plasmid-containing bacteria are selected for antibiotic resistance (e.g., ampicillin resistance). The library can then be screened to find an *E. coli* clone possessing the desired DNA fragment. Various screening techniques can be used to identify the bacteria containing the appropriate recombinant DNA. The multiple cloning site used for inserting the foreign DNA is often part of the *lacZ* gene of the *lac* operon. Insertion of the foreign DNA into the *lacZ* gene inactivates the gene (acting almost like a transposon) and prevents the plasmid-directed synthesis of β-galactosidase in the recipient cell, which results in white bacterial colonies instead of blue colonies if β-galactosidase were able to cleave an appropriate chromophore.

Genetic engineering has been used to isolate and express the genes for useful proteins in bacteria, yeast, or even insect cells such as insulin, interferon, growth hormones, and interleukin. Large amounts of pure immunogen for a vaccine can be prepared without the need to work with the intact disease organisms.

The development of a vaccine against hepatitis B virus represents the first success of recombinant DNA vaccines approved for human use by the U.S. Food and Drug Administration. The hepatitis B surface antigen is produced by the yeast *Saccharomyces cerevisiae.* In the future it may be sufficient to inject plasmid DNA capable of expressing the desired immunogen (DNA vaccine) into an individual to let the host cells express the immunogen and generate the immune response. Recombinant DNA technology has also become essential to laboratory diagnosis, forensic science, agriculture, and many other disciplines.

QUESTIONS

1. What are the principal properties of a plasmid?
2. Give two mechanisms of regulation of bacterial gene expression. Use specific examples.
3. What types of mutations affect DNA, and what agents are responsible for such mutations?
4. Which mechanisms may be used by a bacterial cell for the exchange of genetic material? Briefly explain each mechanism.
5. Discuss the applications of molecular biotechnology to medicine, including contributions and uses in diagnoses.

Bibliography

Alberts B et al: *Molecular biology of the cell,* ed 3, New York, 1994, Garland.

Cooper GM: *The cell: a molecular approach,* Washington, 1997, American Society for Microbiology.

Lehninger AL, Nelson DL, Fox MM: *Principles of biochemistry,* ed 2, New York, 1993, Worth.

Lewin B: *Genes VI,* Oxford, England, 1997, Oxford University.

Lodish H et al: *Molecular cell biology,* ed 4, New York, 2000, WH Freeman.

Stryer L: *Biochemistry,* ed 4, New York, 1995, Freeman.

Voet D, Voet JG: *Biochemistry,* ed 2, New York, 1995, Wiley.

Watson JD et al: *Molecular biology of the gene,* ed 4, Menlo Park, Calif, 1987, Benjamin-Cummings.

Weigel LM et al: Genetic analysis of a high-level vancomycin-resistant isolate of Staphylococcus aureus, *Science* 302:1569-1571, 2003.

CHAPTER 6

Viral Classification, Structure, and Replication

Viruses were first described as "filterable agents." Their small size allows them to pass through filters designed to retain bacteria. Unlike most bacteria, fungi, and parasites, **viruses are obligate intracellular parasites** that depend on the biochemical machinery of the host cell for replication. In addition, *reproduction of viruses occurs by assembly of the individual components rather than by binary fission* (Boxes 6–1 and 6–2).

The simplest viruses consist of a genome of deoxyribonucleic acid (DNA) or ribonucleic acid (RNA) packaged in a protective shell of protein and, for some viruses, a membrane (Figure 6–1). Viruses lack the capacity to make energy or substrates, cannot make their own proteins, and cannot replicate their genome independently of the host cell. To use the cell's biosynthetic machinery, the virus must be adapted to the biochemical rules of the cell.

The physical structure and genetics of viruses have been optimized by mutation and selection to infect humans and other hosts. To do this, the virus must be capable of transmission through potentially harsh environmental conditions, must traverse the skin or other protective barriers of the host, must be adapted to the biochemical machinery of the host cell for replication, and must escape elimination by the host immune response.

Knowledge of the structural (size and morphology) and genetic (type and structure of nucleic acid) features of a virus provides insight into how the virus replicates, spreads, and causes disease. The concepts presented in this chapter are repeated in greater detail in the discussions of specific viruses in later chapters.

Classification

Viruses range from the structurally simple and small parvoviruses and picornaviruses to the large and complex poxviruses and herpesviruses. Their names may describe viral characteristics, the diseases they are associated with, or even the tissue or geographic locale where they were first identified. Names such as *picornavirus* (*pico,* "small"; *rna,* "ribonucleic acid") or *togavirus* (*toga,* Greek for "mantle," referring to a membrane envelope surrounding the virus) describe the structure of the virus, whereas the name *papovavirus* describes the members of its family (*pa*pilloma, *po*lyoma, and *va*cuolating viruses). The name *retrovirus* (*retro,* "reverse") refers to the virus-directed synthesis of DNA from an RNA template, whereas the *poxviruses* are named for the disease smallpox, caused by one of its members. The *adenoviruses* (*adeno*ids) and the *reoviruses* (*r*espiratory, *e*nteric, *o*rphan) are named for the body site from which they were first isolated. Reovirus was discovered before it was associated with a specific disease, and thus it was designated an "orphan" virus. Norwalk virus is named for Norwalk, Ohio; coxsackievirus is named for Coxsackie, N.Y.; and many of the togaviruses, arenaviruses, and bunyaviruses are named after African places where they were first isolated.

Viruses can be grouped by characteristics such as disease (e.g., hepatitis), target tissue, means of transmission (e.g., enteric, respiratory), or vector (e.g., arboviruses; arthropod-borne virus) (Box 6–3). *The most consistent and current means of classification is by physical and biochemical characteristics, such as size, morphology (e.g., presence or absence of a membrane envelope), type of genome, and means of replication* (Figures 6–2 and 6–3). DNA viruses associated with human disease are divided into seven families (Tables 6–1 and 6–2). The RNA viruses may be divided into at least 14 families (Tables 6–3 and 6–4).

Virion Structure

The units for measurement of virion size are nanometers (nm). The clinically important viruses range from 18 nm

BOX 6–1. Definition and Properties of a Virus

Viruses are filterable agents.
Viruses are obligate intracellular parasites.
Viruses cannot make energy or proteins independently of a host cell.
Viral genomes may be RNA or DNA but not both.
Viruses have a naked capsid or an envelope morphology.
Viral components are assembled and do not replicate by "division."

BOX 6–2. Consequences of Viral Properties

Viruses are not living.
Viruses must be infectious to endure in nature.
Viruses must be able to use host cell processes to produce their components (viral messenger RNA, protein, and identical copies of the genome).
Viruses must encode any required processes not provided by the cell.
Viral components must self-assemble.

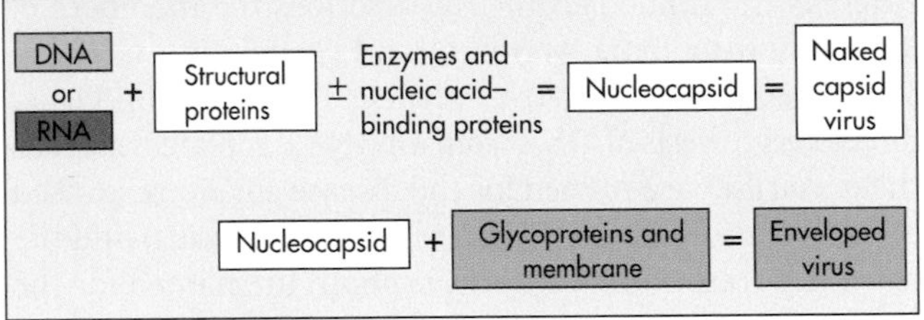

FIGURE 6–1. Components of the basic virion.

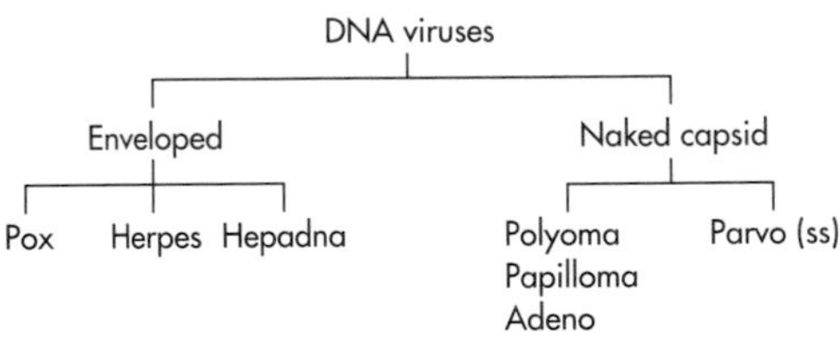

FIGURE 6–2. The DNA viruses and their morphology. The viral families are determined by the structure of the genome and the morphology of the virion.

(parvoviruses) to 300 nm (poxviruses) (Figure 6–4). The latter are almost visible with a light microscope and are approximately one fourth the size of *Staphylococcus* bacteria. *Larger virions can hold a larger genome that can encode more proteins, and they are generally more complex.*

The **virion** (the virus particle) consists of a nucleic acid **genome** packaged into a protein coat **(capsid)** or a membrane **(envelope)** (Figure 6–5). The virion may also contain certain essential or accessory enzymes or other proteins. Capsid or nucleic acid–binding proteins may associate with the genome to form a **nucleocapsid,**

BOX 6–3. Means of Classification and Naming of Viruses

Structure: size, morphology, and nucleic acid (e.g., picornavirus [small RNA], togavirus)
Biochemical characteristics: structure and mode of replication*
Disease: encephalitis and hepatitis viruses, for example
Means of transmission: arbovirus spread by insects, for example
Host cell (host range): animal (human, mouse, bird), plant, bacteria
Tissue or organ (tropism): adenovirus and enterovirus, for example

*This is the current means of taxonomic classification of viruses.

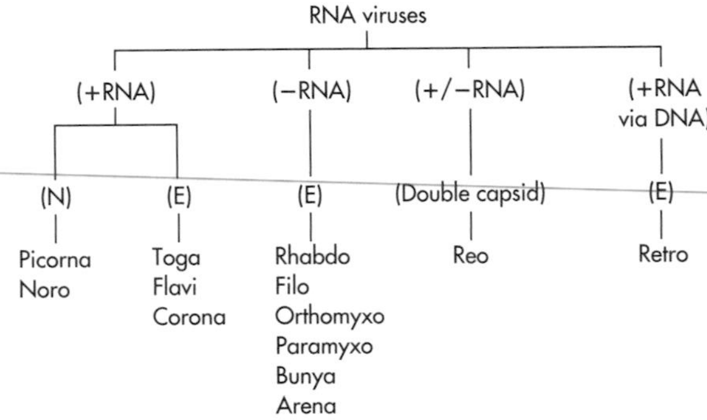

FIGURE 6–3. The RNA viruses, their genome structure, and their morphology. The viral families are determined by the structure of the genome and the morphology of the virion.

TABLE 6–1. Families of DNA Viruses and Some Important Members

Family	Members*
POXVIRIDAE[†]	*Smallpox virus,* vaccinia virus, monkeypox, molluscum contagiosum
Herpesviridae	*Herpes simplex virus* types 1 and 2, varicella-zoster virus, Epstein-Barr virus, cytomegalovirus, human herpesviruses 6, 7, and 8
Adenoviridae	*Adenovirus*
Hepadnaviridae	*Hepatitis B virus*
Polyoma viridae	*JC virus,* BK virus, SV40
Papilloma viridae	*Papilloma virus*
Parvoviridae	*Parvovirus B19,* adeno-associated virus

*The italicized virus is the important, or prototype, virus for the family.
[†]The size of type is indicative of the relative size of the virus.

TABLE 6–2. Properties of Virions of Human DNA Viruses

Family	Genome*		Viron		
	Molecular Mass × 10^6 Daltons	Nature	Shape	Size (nm)	DNA Polymerase[†]
Poxviridae	85-140	ds, linear	Brick-shaped, enveloped	300 by 240 by 100	+[‡]
Herpesviridae	100-150	ds, linear	Icosahedral, enveloped	Capsid, 100-110 Envelope, 120-200	+
Adenoviridae	20-25	ds, linear	Icosahedral	70-90	+
Hepadnaviridae	1.8	ds, circular[§]	Spherical, enveloped	42	+[‡‖]
Polyoma and papilloma viridae	3-5	ds, circular	Icosahedral	45-55	—
Parvoviridae	1.5-2.0	ss, linear	Icosahedral	18-26	—

ds, Double-stranded; ss, single-stranded.
*Genome invariably a single molecule.
[†]Polymerase encoded by virus.
[‡]Polymerase carried in the virion.
[§]Circular molecule is double-stranded for most of its length but contains a single-stranded region.
[‖]Reverse transcriptase.

TABLE 6–3. Families of RNA Viruses and Some Important Members

Family	Members*
Paramyxoviridae[†]	Parainfluenza virus, Sendai virus, *measles virus,* mumps virus, respiratory syncytial virus, metapneumovirus
Orthomyxoviridae	*Influenza virus* types A, B, and C
Coronaviridae	*Coronavirus,* SARS (severe acute respiratory syndrome)
Arenaviridae	*Lassa fever virus,* Tacaribe virus complex (Junin and Machupo viruses), lymphocytic choriomeningitis virus
Rhabdoviridae	*Rabies virus,* vesicular stomatitis virus
Filoviridae	*Ebola virus,* Marburg virus
Bunyaviridae	*California encephalitis virus,* LaCrosse virus, sandfly fever virus, hemorrhagic fever virus, Hanta virus
Retroviridae	Human T-cell leukemia virus types I and II, *human immunodeficiency virus,* animal oncoviruses
Reoviridae	*Rotavirus,* Colorado tick fever virus
Picornaviridae	Rhinoviruses, *poliovirus,* echoviruses, coxsackievirus, hepatitis A virus
Togaviridae	*Rubella virus;* western, eastern, and Venezuelan equine encephalitis virus; Ross River virus; Sindbis virus; Semliki Forest virus
Flaviviridae	*Yellow fever virus,* dengue virus, St. Louis encephalitis virus, West Nile virus, hepatitis C virus
Noroviridae	*Norwalk virus,* calicivirus
Delta	Delta agent

*The italicized virus is the important or prototype virus for the family.
[†]The size of the type is indicative of the relative size of the virus.

TABLE 6–4. Properties of Virions of Human RNA Viruses

Family	Genome*		Virion			
	Molecular Mass × 106 *Daltons*	Nature	Shape*	Size (nm)	Polymerase in Virion	Envelope
Paramyxoviridae	5-7	ss, –	Spherical	150-300	+	+
Orthomyxoviridae	5-7	ss, –, seg	Spherical	80-120	+	+
Coronaviridae	6-7	ss, +	Spherical	80-130	–	+†
Arenaviridae	3-5	ss, –, seg	Spherical	50-300	+	+†
Rhabdoviridae	4-7	ss, –	Bullet-shaped	180 by 75	+	+
Filoviridae	4-7	ss, –	Filamentous	800 by 80	+	+
Bunyaviridae	4-7	ss, –	Spherical	90-100	+	+†
Retroviridae	2 × (2-3)‡	ss, +	Spherical	80-110	+§	+
Reoviridae	11-15	ds, seg	Icosahedral	60-80	+	–
Picornaviridae	2.5	ss, +	Icosahedral	25-30	–	–
Togaviridae	4-5	ss, +	Icosahedral	60-70	–	+
Flaviviridae	4-7	ss, +	Spherical	40-50	–	+
Noroviridae	2.6	ss, +	Icosahedral	35-40	–	–

ds, Double-stranded; seg, segmented; ss, single-stranded; + or –, polarity of single-stranded nucleic acid.
*Some enveloped viruses are very pleomorphic (sometimes filamentous).
†No matrix protein.
‡Genome has two identical single-stranded RNA molecules.
§Reverse transcriptase.

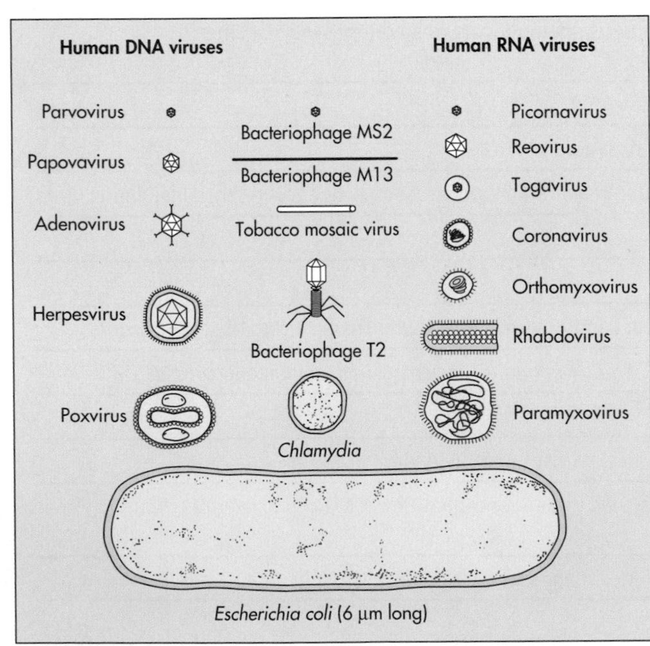

FIGURE 6–4. Relative sizes of viruses and bacteria. (Courtesy the Upjohn Company, Kalamazoo, Mich.)

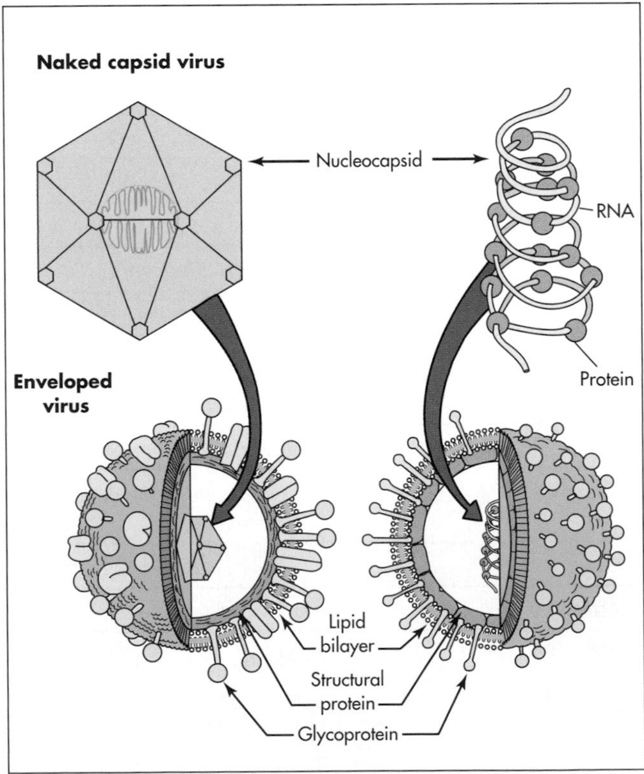

FIGURE 6–5. The structures of a naked capsid virus *(top left)* and enveloped viruses with an icosahedral *(left)* nucleocapsid or a helical *(right)* ribonucleocapsid. The helical ribonucleocapsid is formed by viral proteins associated with an RNA genome.

which may be the same as the virion or surrounded by an envelope.

The genome of the virus consists either of DNA or RNA. *The DNA can be single or double stranded, linear or circular. The RNA can be either positive sense (+) (like messenger RNA [mRNA]) or negative sense (−) (analogous to a photographic negative), double stranded (+/−) or ambisense (containing + and − regions of RNA attached end to end).* The RNA genome may also be *segmented* into pieces, with each piece encoding an individual gene. Just as there are many different types of computer memory devices, all of these forms of nucleic acid can maintain and transmit the genetic information of the virus. Similarly, the larger the genome, the more information (genes) it can carry and the larger the capsid or envelope structure required to contain the genome.

The outer layer of the virion is the **capsid** or **envelope.** These structures are the package, protection, and delivery vehicle during transmission of the virus from one host to another and for spread within the host to the target cell. The surface structures of the capsid and envelope mediate the interaction of the virus with the target cell. Removal or disruption of the outer package inactivates the virus. Antibodies generated against the components of these structures prevent virus infection.

The **capsid** is a rigid structure able to withstand harsh environmental conditions. Viruses with naked capsids are generally resistant to drying, acid, and detergents, including the acid and bile of the enteric tract. Many of these viruses are transmitted by the fecal-oral route and can endure transmission even in sewage.

The **envelope** is a membrane composed of lipids, proteins, and glycoproteins. The membranous structure of the envelope can be maintained only in aqueous solutions. It is readily disrupted by drying, acidic conditions, detergents, and solvents such as ether, which results in inactivation of the virus. As a result, enveloped viruses must remain wet and are generally transmitted in fluids, respiratory droplets, blood, and tissue. Most cannot survive the harsh conditions of the gastrointestinal tract. The influence of virion structure on viral properties is summarized in Boxes 6–4 and 6–5.

BOX 6–4. Viral Structure: Naked Capsid

Component
Protein

Properties
Is environmentally stable to the following:
- Temperature
- Acid
- Proteases
- Detergents
- Drying

Is released from cell by lysis

Consequences
Can be spread easily (on fomites, from hand to hand, by dust, by small droplets)
Can dry out and retain infectivity
Can survive the adverse conditions of the gut
Can be resistant to detergents and poor sewage treatment
Antibody may be sufficient for immunoprotection

BOX 6–5. Virus Structure: Envelope

Components
- Membrane
- Lipids
- Proteins
- Glycoproteins

Properties
Is environmentally labile—is disrupted by the following:
- Acid
- Detergents
- Drying
- Heat

Modifies cell membrane during replication
Is released by budding and cell lysis

Consequences
Must stay wet
Cannot survive the gastrointestinal tract
Spreads in large droplets, secretions, organ transplants, and blood transfusions
Does not need to kill the cell to spread
May need antibody and cell-mediated immune response for protection and control
Elicits hypersensitivity and inflammation to cause immunopathogenesis

CAPSID VIRUSES

The viral capsid is assembled from individual proteins associated into progressively larger units. All of the components of the capsid have chemical features that allow them to fit together and to assemble into a larger unit. Individual structural proteins associate into **subunits,** which associate into **protomers, capsomeres** (distinguishable in electron micrographs), and, finally, a recognizable **procapsid** or **capsid** (Figure 6–6). A procapsid requires further processing to the final, transmissible capsid. For some viruses the capsid forms around the genome; for others the capsid forms as an empty shell (procapsid) to be filled by the genome.

The simplest viral structures that can be built stepwise are symmetrical and include **helical** and **icosahedral** structures. Helical structures appear as rods, whereas the icosahedron is an approximation of a sphere assembled from symmetrical subunits (Figure 6–7). Nonsymmetrical capsids are complex forms and are associated with certain bacterial viruses (phages).

The classic example of a virus with helical symmetry is the tobacco mosaic plant virus. Its capsomeres self-

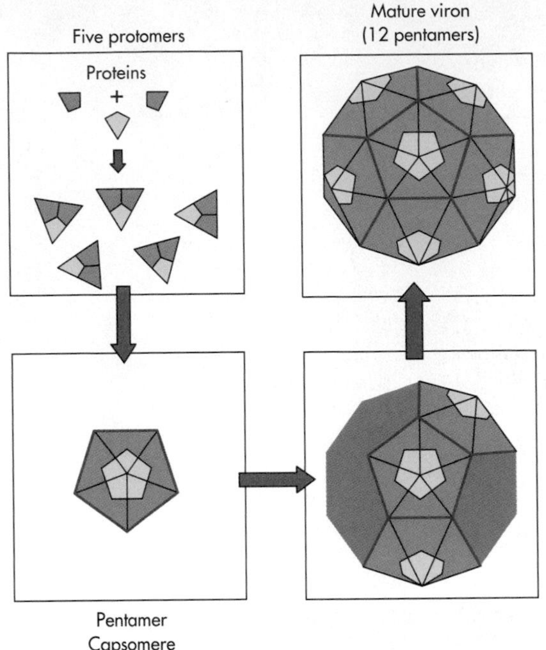

FIGURE 6–6. Capsid assembly of the icosahedral capsid of a picornavirus. Individual proteins associate into subunits, which associate into protomers, capsomeres, and an empty procapsid. Inclusion of the (+) RNA genome triggers its conversion to the final capsid form.

assemble on the RNA genome into rods that extend the length of the genome. The capsomeres cover and protect the RNA. Helical nucleocapsids are observed within the envelope of most negative-strand RNA viruses (see Figure 59–1).

Simple **icosahedrons** are used by small, simple viruses such as the picornaviruses and parvoviruses. The icosahedron is made of 12 capsomeres, each with fivefold symmetry **(pentamer** or **penton).** For the picornaviruses, every pentamer is made up of five protomers, each of which is composed of three subunits of four separate proteins (see Figure 6–6). X-ray crystallography and image analysis of cryoelectron microscopy have defined the structure of the picornavirus capsid to the molecular level. These studies have depicted a canyonlike cleft, which is a "docking site" to bind to the receptor on the surface of the target cell (see Figure 57–2).

Larger capsid virions are constructed by inserting structurally distinct capsomeres between the pentons at the vertices. These capsomeres have six nearest neighbors **(hexons).** This extends the icosahedron and is called an **icosadeltahedron,** and its size is determined by the number of hexons inserted along the edges and within the surfaces between the pentons. *A soccer ball is an icosadeltahedron.* For example, the herpesvirus nucleocapsid has 12

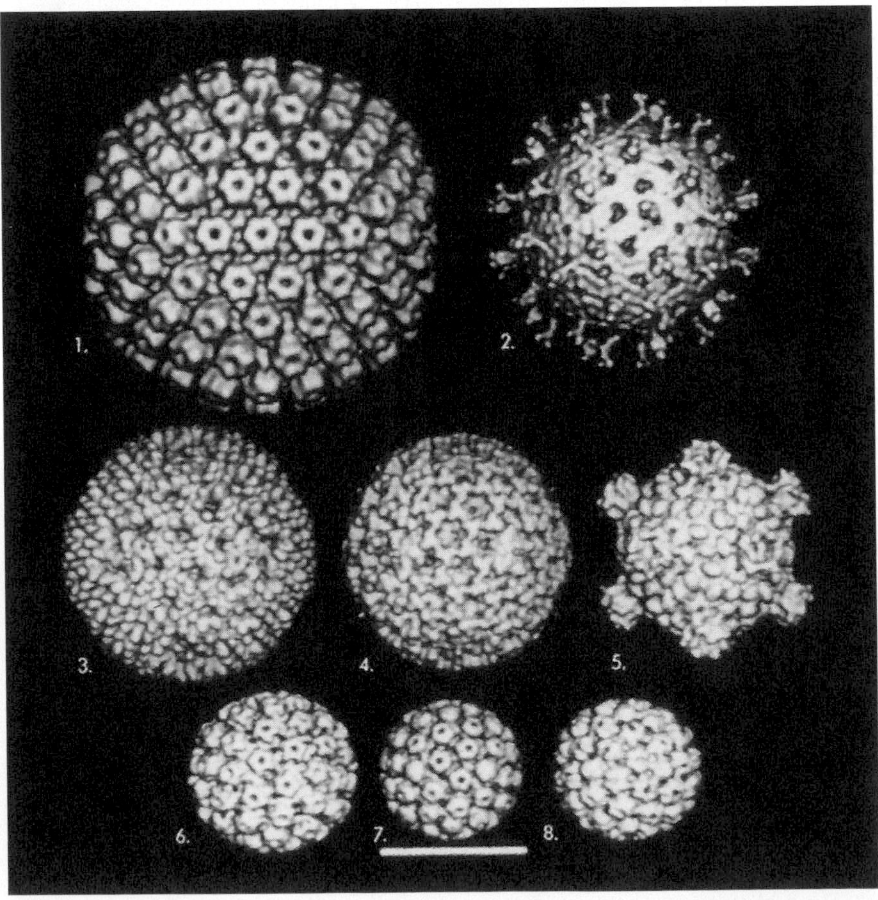

FIGURE 6–7. Cryoelectron microscopy and computer-generated three-dimensional image reconstructions of several icosahedral capsids. These images show the symmetry of capsids and the individual capsomeres. During assembly, the genome may fill the capsid through the holes in the herpesvirus and papovavirus capsomeres. *1,* Equine herpesvirus nucleocapsid; *2,* simian rotavirus; *3,* reovirus type 1 (Lang) virion; *4,* intermediate subviral particle (reovirus); *5,* core (inner capsid) particle (reovirus); *6,* human papillomavirus type 19; *7,* mouse polyomavirus; *8,* cauliflower mosaic virus. Bar = 50 nm. (Courtesy Dr. Tim Baker, Purdue University, West Lafayette, IN.)

pentons and 150 hexons. The herpesvirus nucleocapsid is also surrounded by an envelope. The adenovirus capsid is composed of 252 capsomeres, with 12 pentons and 240 hexons. A long fiber is attached to each penton of adenovirus to serve as the **viral attachment protein (VAP)** to bind to target cells, and it also contains the type-specific antigen (see Figure 53–1). The reoviruses have an icosahedral double capsid with fiberlike proteins partially extended from each vertex. The outer capsid protects the virus and promotes its uptake across the gastrointestinal tract and into target cells, whereas the inner capsid contains enzymes for the synthesis of RNA (see Figure 6–7 and Figure 62–2).

ENVELOPED VIRUSES

The virion envelope is composed of lipids, proteins, and glycoproteins (see Figure 6–5 and Box 6–5). It has a membrane structure similar to cellular membranes. Cellular proteins are rarely found in the viral envelope, even though the envelope is obtained from cellular membranes. Most enveloped viruses are round or pleomorphic. (See Figures 6–2 and 6–3 for the complete listing of enveloped viruses.) Two exceptions are the poxvirus, which has a complex internal and a bricklike external structure, and the rhabdovirus, which is bullet shaped.

Most viral glycoproteins have asparagine-linked (N-linked) carbohydrate and extend through the envelope and away from the surface of the virion. For many viruses, these can be observed as spikes (Figure 6–8). Most glycoproteins act as **VAPs,** capable of binding to structures on target cells. VAPs that also bind to erythrocytes are termed ***hemagglutinins (HAs).*** Some glycoproteins have other functions, such as the neuraminidase of orthomyxoviruses (influenza) and the Fc receptor and the C3b receptor associated with herpes simplex virus glycoproteins, or the fusion glycoproteins of paramyxoviruses. Glycoproteins are also major antigens that elicit protective immunity.

The envelope of the togaviruses surrounds an icosahedral nucleocapsid containing a positive-strand RNA genome. The envelope contains spikes consisting of two or three glycoprotein subunits anchored to the virion's icosahedral capsid. This causes the envelope to adhere tightly and conform (shrink-wrap) to an icosahedral structure discernible by cryoelectron microscopy.

All of the negative-strand RNA viruses are enveloped. Components of the viral RNA-dependent RNA polymerase associate with the (–) RNA genome of the orthomyxoviruses, paramyxoviruses, and rhabdoviruses to form helical nucleocapsids (see Figure 6–5). These enzymes are required to initiate virus replication, and their association with the genome ensures their delivery into the cell. Matrix proteins lining the inside of the envelope facilitate the assembly of the ribonucleocapsid into the virion.

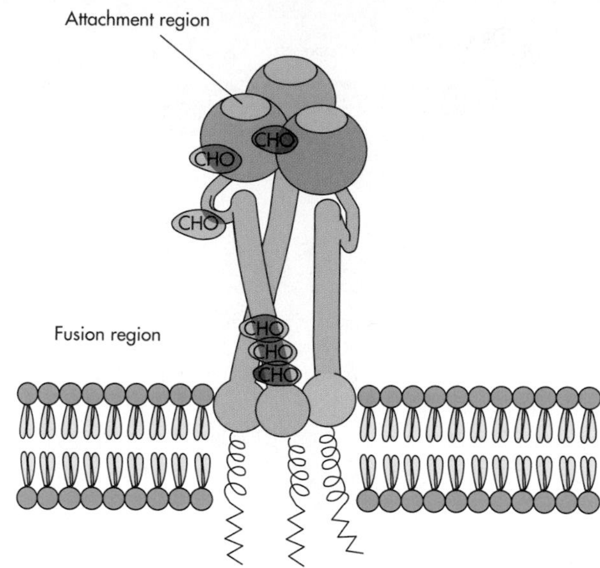

FIGURE 6–8. Diagram of the hemagglutinin glycoprotein trimer of influenza A virus, a representative spike protein. The region for attachment to the cellular receptor is exposed on the spike protein's surface. Under mild acidic conditions, the hemagglutinin changes conformation to expose a hydrophobic sequence at the "fusion region." CHO, *N*-linked carbohydrate attachment sites. (Modified from Schlesinger MJ, Schlesinger S: Domains of virus glycoproteins, *Adv Virus Res* 33:1-44, 1987.)

Influenza A (orthomyxovirus) is an example of a (–) RNA virus with a segmented genome. Its envelope is lined with matrix proteins and has two glycoproteins: the hemagglutinin, which is the VAP, and a neuraminidase (NA) (see Figure 60–1). Bunyaviruses do not have matrix proteins.

The herpesvirus envelope is a baglike structure that encloses the icosadeltahedral nucleocapsid (see Figure 54–1). Depending on the specific herpesvirus, the envelope may contain as many as 11 glycoproteins. The interstitial space between the nucleocapsid and the envelope is called the *tegument,* and it contains enzymes, other proteins, and even mRNA that facilitate the viral infection.

The poxviruses are enveloped viruses with large, complex, bricklike shapes (see Figure 55–1). The envelope encloses a dumbbell-shaped, DNA-containing nucleoid structure; lateral bodies; fibrils; and many enzymes and proteins, including the enzymes and transcriptional factors required for mRNA synthesis.

Viral Replication

The major steps in viral replication are the same for all viruses (Figure 6–9 and Box 6–6). The cell acts as a factory, providing the substrates, energy, and machinery necessary for the synthesis of viral proteins and replication of the genome. Processes not provided by the cell must be encoded in the genome of the virus. The manner

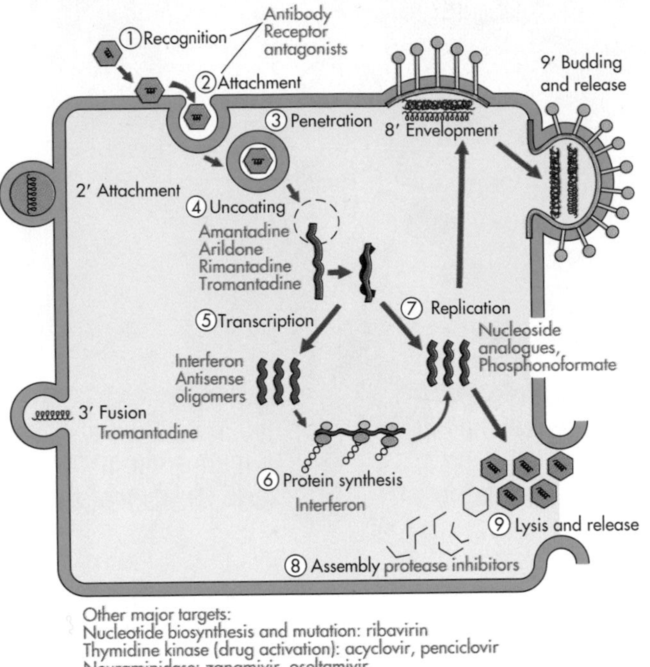

FIGURE 6–9. A general scheme of viral replication. Enveloped viruses have alternative means of entry (3) assembly, and exit from the cell (8′ and 9′). The antiviral drugs for susceptible steps in viral replication susceptible to antiviral drugs are listed in magenta.

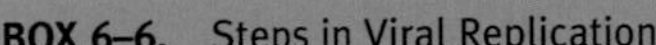

BOX 6–6. Steps in Viral Replication

1. Recognition of the target cell
2. Attachment
3. Penetration
4. Uncoating
5. Macromolecular synthesis
   a. Early messenger RNA (mRNA) and nonstructural protein synthesis: genes for enzymes and nucleic acid–binding proteins
   b. Replication of genome
   c. Late mRNA and structural protein synthesis
   d. Post-translational modification of protein
6. Assembly of virus
7. Budding of enveloped viruses
8. Release of virus

in which each virus accomplishes these steps and overcomes the cell's biochemical limitations is determined by the structure of the genome and of the virion (whether it is enveloped or has a naked capsid). This is illustrated in the examples in Figures 6–12 to 6–14.

A single round of the viral replication cycle can be separated into several phases. During the **early phase** of infection, the virus must recognize an appropriate target cell, attach to the cell, penetrate the plasma membrane and be taken up by the cell, release (uncoat) its genome into the cytoplasm, and, if necessary, deliver the genome

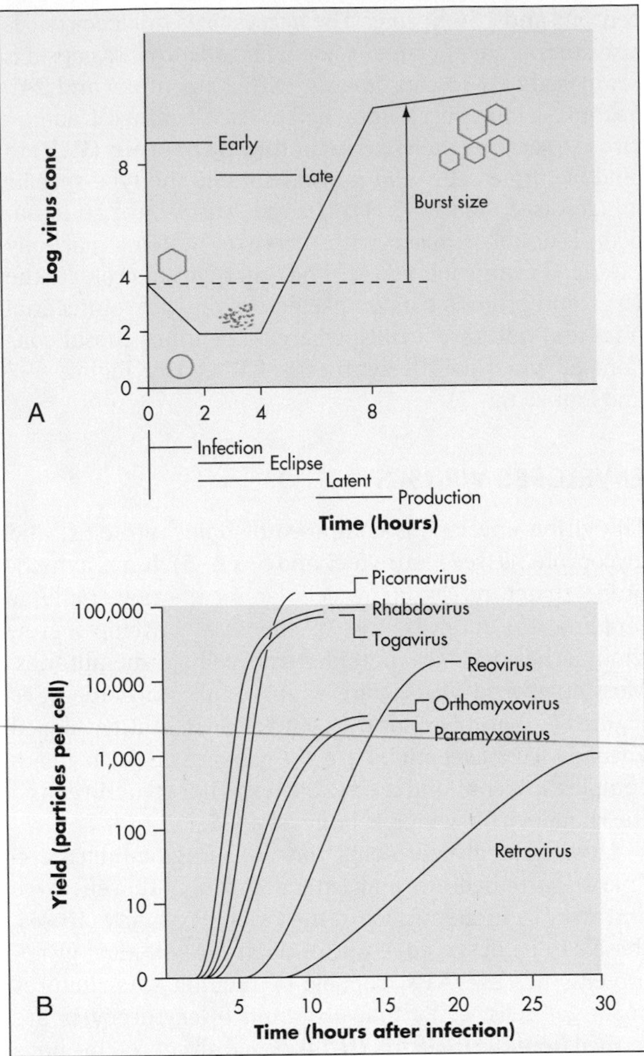

FIGURE 6–10. A, Single-cycle growth curve of a virus that is released on cell lysis. The different stages are defined by the presence or absence of visible viral components (eclipse period), infectious virus in the media (latent period), or macromolecular synthesis (early/late phases). **B,** Growth curve and burst size of representative viruses. (**A** modified from Davis BD et al: *Microbiology,* ed 4, Philadelphia, 1990, JB Lippincott; **B** modified from White DO, Fenner F: *Medical virology,* ed 3, New York, 1986, Academic Press.)

to the nucleus. The **late phase** begins with the start of genome replication and viral macromolecular synthesis and proceeds through viral assembly and release. Uncoating of the genome from the capsid or envelope during the early phase abolishes its infectivity and identifiable structure, thus initiating the eclipse period. The **eclipse period,** like a solar eclipse, ends with the appearance of new virions after virus assembly. The **latent period,** during which extracellular infectious virus is not detected, includes the eclipse period and ends with the release of new viruses (Figure 6–10). Each infected cell may produce as many as 100,000 particles; however, only 1% to 10% of these particles may be infectious. The noninfectious particles **(defective particles)** result from mutations and errors in the manufacture and assembly of the virion. The yield of infectious virus per cell, or **burst size,** and the time required for a single cycle of virus reproduction are determined by the properties of the virus and the target cell.

RECOGNITION OF AND ATTACHMENT TO THE TARGET CELL

The binding of the **VAPs** or structures on the surface of the virion capsid (Table 6–5) to **receptors on the cell** (Table 6–6) initially determines which cells can be infected by a virus. *The receptors for the virus on the cell may be proteins or carbohydrates on glycoproteins or glycolipids.* Viruses that bind to receptors expressed on specific cell types may be restricted to certain species **(host range)** (e.g., human, mouse) or specific cell types. The susceptible target cell defines the **tissue tropism** (e.g., neurotropic, lymphotropic). Epstein-Barr virus, a herpesvirus, has a very limited host range and tropism because it binds to the C3d receptor (CR2) expressed on human B cells. The B19 parvovirus binds to globoside (blood group P antigen) expressed on erythroid precursor cells.

The viral attachment structure for a capsid virus may be part of the capsid or a protein that extends from the capsid. A canyon on the surface of picornaviruses, such as the rhinovirus 14, serves as a "keyhole" for the insertion of a portion of the intercellular adhesion molecule (ICAM-1) from the cell surface. The fibers of the adenoviruses and the σ-1 proteins of the reoviruses at the vertices of the capsid interact with receptors expressed on specific target cells.

VAPs are specific glycoproteins of enveloped viruses. The HA of influenza A virus binds to sialic acid expressed on many different cells and has a broad host range and tissue tropism. Similarly, the α-togaviruses and the flaviviruses are able to bind to receptors expressed on cells of many animal species, including arthropods, reptiles, amphibians, birds, and mammals. This allows them to infect animals, mosquitoes, and other insects and to be spread by them.

TABLE 6–5. Examples of Viral Attachment Proteins

Virus Family	Virus	VAP
Picornaviridae	Rhinovirus	VP1-VP2-VP3 complex
Adenoviridae	Adenovirus	Fiber protein
Reoviridae	Reovirus Rotavirus	σ-1 VP7
Togaviridae	Semliki Forest virus	E1-E2-E3 complex gp
Rhabdoviridae	Rabies virus	G protein gp
Orthomyxoviridae	Influenza A virus	HA gp
Paramyxoviridae	Measles virus	HA gp
Herpesviridae	Epstein-Barr virus	gp350 and gp220
Retroviridae	Murine leukemia virus Human immunodeficiency virus	gp70 gp120

gp, Glycoprotein; VAP, viral attachment protein.

PENETRATION

Many interactions between the VAPs and the cellular receptors initiate the internalization of the virus into the cell. The mechanism of internalization depends on the virion structure and cell type. Most nonenveloped viruses enter the cell by receptor-mediated endocytosis or by viropexis. **Endocytosis** is a normal process used by the

TABLE 6–6. Examples of Viral Receptors

Virus	Target Cell	Receptor*
Epstein-Barr virus	B cell	C3d complement receptor CR2 (CD21)
Human immunodeficiency virus	Helper T cell	CD4 molecule and chemokine coreceptor
Rhinovirus	Epithelial cells	ICAM-1 (immunoglobulin superfamily protein)
Poliovirus	Epithelial cells	Immunoglobulin superfamily protein
Herpes simplex virus	Many cells	Immunoglobulin superfamily protein
Rabies virus	Neuron	Acetylcholine receptor
Influenza A virus	Epithelial cells	Sialic acid
B19 parvovirus	Erythroid precursors	Erythrocyte P antigen (globoside)

ICAM-1, Intercellular adhesion molecule.
*Other receptors for these viruses may also exist.

cell for the uptake of receptor-bound molecules such as hormones, low-density lipoproteins, and transferrin. Picornaviruses and papovaviruses may enter by **viropexis.** Hydrophobic structures of capsid proteins may be exposed after viral binding to the cells, and these structures help the virus or the viral genome slip through (direct penetration) the membrane.

Enveloped viruses fuse their membranes with cellular membranes to deliver the nucleocapsid or genome directly into the cytoplasm. The optimum pH for fusion determines whether penetration occurs at the cell surface at neutral pH or whether the virus must be internalized by endocytosis and fusion occurs in an endosome at acidic pH. The fusion activity may be provided by the VAP or another protein. The HA of influenza A (see Figure 6–8) binds to sialic acid receptors on the target cell. Under the mild acidic conditions of the endosome, the HA undergoes a dramatic conformational change to expose hydrophobic portions capable of promoting membrane fusion. Paramyxoviruses have a fusion protein that is active at neutral pH to promote virus-cell fusion. Paramyxoviruses can also promote cell-cell fusion to form multinucleated giant cells **(syncytia).** Some herpesviruses and retroviruses fuse with cells at a neutral pH and induce syncytia after replication.

UNCOATING

Once internalized, the nucleocapsid must be delivered to the site of replication within the cell and the capsid or envelope removed. The genome of DNA viruses, except for poxviruses, must be delivered to the nucleus, whereas most RNA viruses remain in the cytoplasm. The uncoating process may be initiated by attachment to the receptor or promoted by the acidic environment or proteases found in an endosome or lysosome. Picornavirus capsids are weakened by the release of the VP4 capsid protein to allow uncoating. VP4 is released by insertion of the receptor into the keyhole-like canyon attachment site of the capsid. Enveloped viruses are uncoated on fusion with cell membranes. Fusion of the herpesvirus envelope with the plasma membrane releases its nucleocapsid, which then "docks" with the nuclear membrane to deliver its DNA genome directly to the site of replication. The release of the influenza nucleocapsid from its matrix and envelope is facilitated by the passage of protons from inside the endosome through the ion pore formed by the influenza M2 matrix protein to acidify the environment.

The reovirus and poxvirus are only partially uncoated on entry. The outer capsid of reovirus is removed, but the genome remains in an inner capsid, which contains the polymerases necessary for RNA synthesis. The initial uncoating of the poxviruses exposes a subviral particle to the cytoplasm, allowing synthesis of mRNA by virion-contained enzymes. An uncoating enzyme can then be synthesized to release the DNA-containing core into the cytoplasm.

MACROMOLECULAR SYNTHESIS

Once inside the cell the genome must direct the synthesis of viral mRNA, protein, and generate identical copies of itself. *Transcription, translation, and replication of the genome are therefore probably the most important steps in viral multiplication.* The genome is useless unless it can be transcribed into functional mRNAs capable of binding to ribosomes and being translated into proteins. The means by which each virus accomplishes these steps depends on the structure of the genome (Figure 6–11) and the site of replication.

The cell's machinery for transcription and mRNA processing is found in the nucleus. *Most DNA viruses use the cell's DNA-dependent RNA polymerase* II *and other enzymes to make mRNA.* For example, eukaryotic mRNAs acquire a 3′ polyadenylated (poly A) tail and a 5′ methylated cap (for binding to the ribosome) and are processed to remove introns before being exported to the cytoplasm. Viruses that replicate in the cytoplasm must provide these functions or an alternative. Although poxviruses are DNA viruses, they replicate in the cytoplasm and therefore must encode enzymes for all these functions. *Most RNA viruses replicate and produce mRNA in the cytoplasm,* except for orthomyxoviruses and retroviruses. *RNA viruses must encode the necessary enzymes for transcription and replication because the cell has no means of replicating RNA.* The mRNAs for RNA viruses may or may not acquire a 5′ cap or poly A tail.

The naked genome of DNA viruses (except poxviruses) and the positive-sense RNA viruses (except retroviruses) are sometimes referred to as **infectious nucleic acids** because they are sufficient for initiating replication on injection into a cell. These genomes can interact directly with host machinery to promote mRNA or protein synthesis, or both.

In general, mRNA for nonstructural proteins is transcribed first (Figure 6–12). **Early gene products** (nonstructural proteins) are often DNA-binding proteins and enzymes, including virus-encoded polymerases. These proteins are catalytic, and only a few are required. *Replication of the genome usually initiates the transition to transcription of late gene products.* **Late viral genes** encode structural proteins. Many copies of these proteins are required to package the virus but are generally not required before the genome is replicated. Newly replicated genomes also provide new templates for more late gene mRNA synthesis. Different DNA and RNA viruses control the time and amount of viral gene and protein synthesis in different ways.

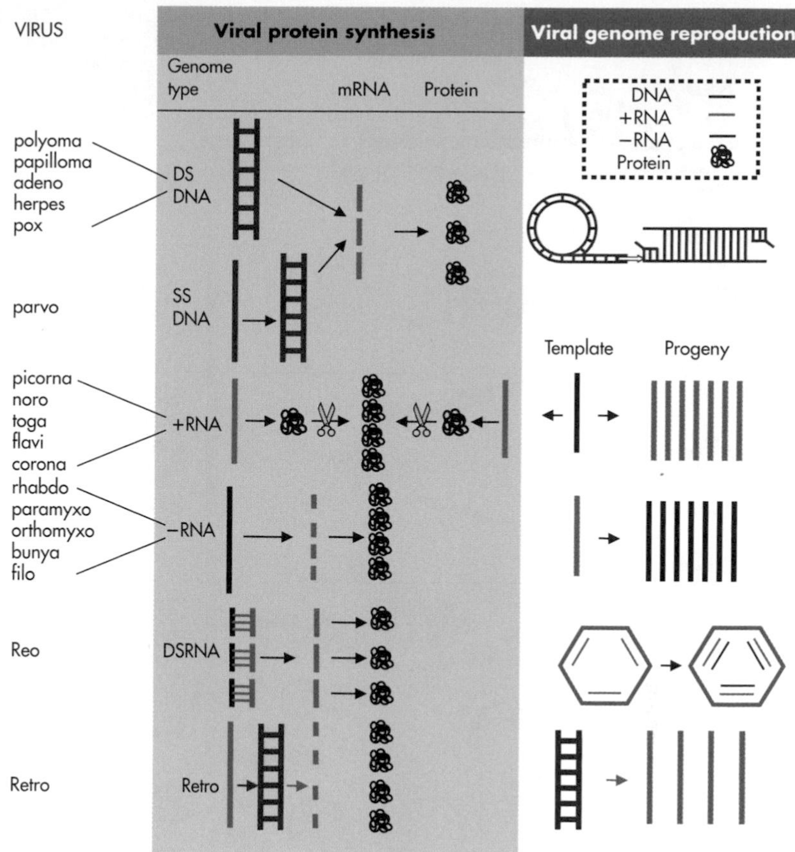

FIGURE 6–11. Viral macromolecular synthesis steps: The mechanism of viral mRNA and protein synthesis and genome replication are determined by the structure of the genome. 1. Double-stranded DNA (DS DNA) uses host machinery in the nucleus (except poxviruses) to make mRNA, which is translated by host cell ribosomes into proteins. Replication of viral DNA occurs by semiconservative means, by rolling circle, linear, and in other ways. 2. Single-stranded DNA (SS DNA) is converted into DS DNA and replicates like DS DNA. 3. (+) RNA resembles an mRNA that binds to ribosomes to make a polyprotein that is cleaved into individual proteins. One of the viral proteins is an RNA polymerase that makes a (–) RNA template and then more (+) RNA genome progeny and mRNAs. 4. (–) RNA is transcribed into mRNAs and a full-length (+) RNA template by an RNA polymerase carried in the virion. The (+) RNA template is used to make (–) RNA genome progeny. 5. DS RNA acts like (–) RNA. The (–) strands are transcribed into mRNAs by an RNA polymerase in the capsid. (+) RNAs get encapsidated and (–) RNAs are made in the capsid. 6. Retroviruses are (+) RNA that are converted to complementary DNA (cDNA) by reverse transcriptase carried in the virion. cDNA integrates into the host chromosome, and the host makes mRNAs, proteins, and full-length RNA genome copies.

DNA VIRUSES

Replication of the DNA genome requires a DNA-dependent DNA polymerase, other enzymes, and deoxyribonucleotide triphosphates, especially thymidine (Box 6-7). Transcription of the DNA virus genome (except for poxviruses) occurs in the nucleus, using host cell polymerases and other enzymes for viral mRNA synthesis. Transcription of the viral genes is regulated by the interaction of specific DNA-binding proteins with promoter and enhancer elements in the viral genome. The viral promoter and enhancer elements are similar in sequence to those of the host cell to allow binding of the cell's transcriptional activation factors and DNA-dependent RNA polymerase. Cells from some tissues do not express the DNA-binding proteins necessary for activating the transcription of viral genes, and replication of the virus in that cell is thus prevented or limited. For example, neurons transcribe only one gene for herpes simplex virus unless activated by stress, and as a result, the virus remains in latency in the cell. Transcription is therefore a factor in determining the tissue tropism and host range of the virus.

Different DNA viruses control the duration, timing, and quantity of viral gene and protein synthesis in different ways. The more complex viruses encode their own transcriptional activators, which enhance or regulate the expression of viral genes. For example, the herpes simplex virus encodes many proteins that regulate the kinetics of viral gene expression, including the VMW 65 (α-TIF protein, VP16). VMW 65 is carried in the virion, binds to the host cell transcription-activating complex (Oct-1), and enhances its ability to stimulate transcription of the immediate early genes of the virus.

Genes may be transcribed from either DNA strand of the genome and in opposite directions. For example, the early and late genes of the SV40 papovavirus are on opposite, nonoverlapping DNA strands. Viral genes may have introns requiring post-transcriptional processing of the mRNA by the cell's nuclear machinery (splicing). The late genes of papovaviruses and adenoviruses are initially transcribed as a large RNA from a single promoter and then processed to produce several different mRNAs after removal of different intervening sequences (introns).

Replication of viral DNA follows the same biochemical rules as for cellular DNA. Replication is initiated at a unique DNA sequence of the genome, called the **origin (ori).** This is a site recognized by cellular or viral nuclear factors and the **DNA-dependent DNA polymerase.** Viral DNA synthesis is semiconservative, and viral and

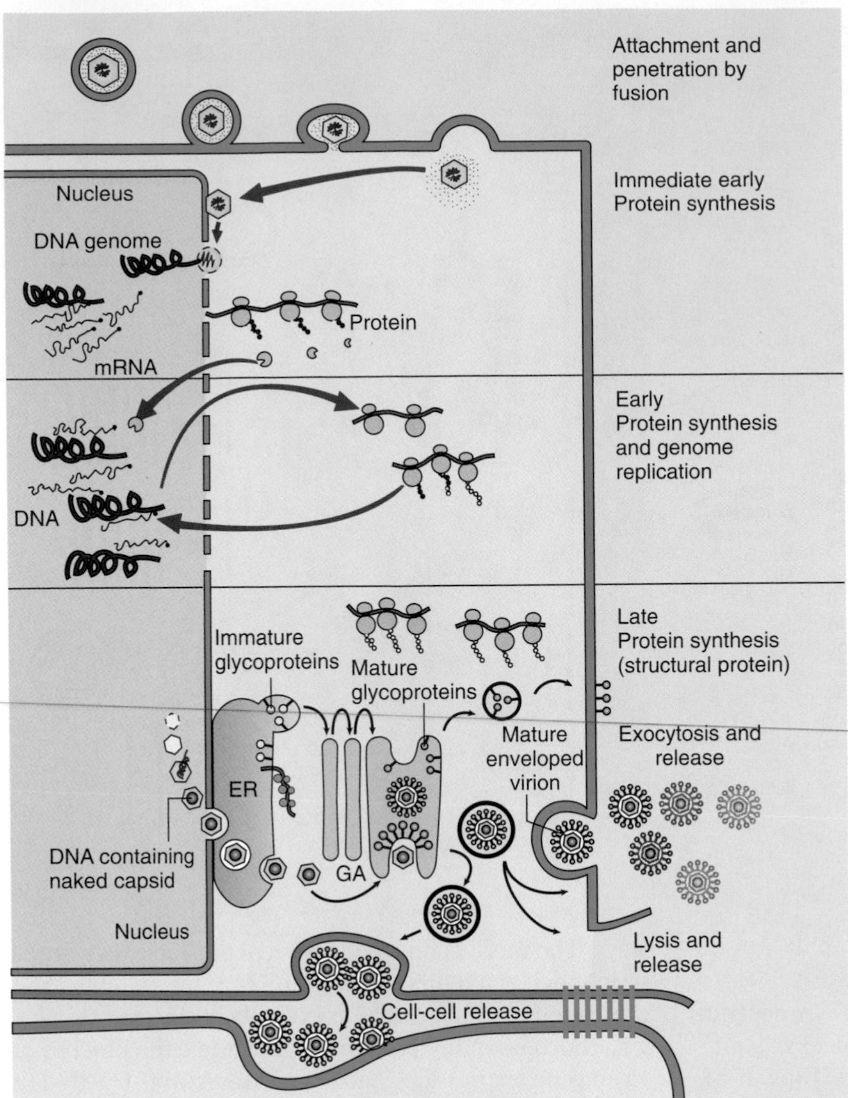

FIGURE 6–12. Replication of herpes simplex virus, a complex enveloped DNA virus. The virus binds to specific receptors and fuses with the plasma membrane. The nucleocapsid then delivers the DNA genome to the nucleus. Transcription and translation occur in three phases: immediate early, early, and late. Immediate early proteins promote the takeover of the cell; early proteins consist of enzymes, including the DNA-dependent DNA polymerase; and the late proteins are structural proteins, including the viral capsid and glycoproteins. The genome is replicated before transcription of the late genes. Capsid proteins migrate into the nucleus, assemble into icosadeltahedral capsids, and are filled with the DNA genome. The capsids filled with genomes bud through the nuclear and endoplasmic reticulum membranes into the cytoplasm, acquire tegument proteins, and then bud through the viral glycoprotein modified membranes of the trans Golgi network. The virus is released by exocytosis or cell lysis.

cellular *DNA polymerases require a primer* to initiate synthesis of the DNA chain. The parvoviruses have DNA sequences that are inverted and repeated to allow the DNA to fold back and hybridize with itself to provide a primer. Replication of the adenovirus genome is primed by deoxycytidine monophosphate attached to a terminal protein. A cellular enzyme (primase) synthesizes an RNA primer to start the replication of the papovavirus genome while the herpesviruses encode a primase.

Replication of the genome of the simple DNA viruses (e.g., parvoviruses, papovaviruses) uses the host DNA-dependent DNA polymerases, whereas the larger, more complex viruses (e.g., adenoviruses, herpesviruses, poxviruses) encode their own polymerases. Viral polymerases are usually faster but less precise than host cell polymerases, causing a higher mutation rate in viruses and providing a target for nucleotide analogues as antiviral drugs.

Hepadnavirus replication is unique in that a circular, positive-strand RNA intermediate is first synthesized by the cell's DNA-dependent RNA polymerase. Viral proteins surround the RNA, an RNA-dependent DNA polymerase (reverse transcriptase) in this virion core makes a negative-strand DNA, and then the RNA is degraded. Positive-strand DNA synthesis is initiated but stops when the genome and core are enveloped, yielding a partially double-stranded circular DNA genome.

Major limitations for replication of a DNA virus include availability of the DNA polymerase and deoxyribonucleotide substrates. Most cells in the resting phase of growth are not undergoing DNA synthesis because the necessary enzymes are not present and deoxythymidine pools are limited. *The smaller the DNA virus, the more dependent the virus is on the host cell* to provide these functions (see Box 6–7). The parvoviruses are the smallest DNA viruses and replicate only in growing cells, such as

BOX 6–7. Properties of DNA Viruses

DNA is not transient or labile.
Viral genomes remain in the infected cell.
Many DNA viruses establish persistent infections (e.g., latent, immortalizing).
DNA genomes reside in the nucleus (except for poxviruses).
Viral DNA resembles host DNA for transcription and replication.
Viral genes must interact with host transcriptional machinery (except for poxviruses).
Viral gene transcription is temporally regulated.
 Early genes encode DNA-binding proteins and enzymes.
 Late genes encode structural proteins.
DNA polymerases require a primer to replicate the viral genome.
The larger DNA viruses encode means to promote efficient replication of their genome.
Parvovirus: requires cells undergoing DNA synthesis to replicate.
Papovavirus: stimulates cell growth and DNA synthesis.
Hepadnavirus: stimulates cell growth (?) and encodes its own polymerase.
Adenovirus: stimulates cellular DNA synthesis and encodes its own polymerase.
Herpesvirus: stimulates cell growth, encodes its own polymerase and enzymes to provide deoxyribonucleotides for DNA synthesis, establishes latent infection in host.
Poxvirus: encodes its own polymerase and enzymes to provide deoxyribonucleotides for DNA synthesis, replication machinery, and transcription machinery in the cytoplasm.

erythroid precursor cells or fetal tissue. Speeding up the growth of the cell can enhance viral DNA and mRNA synthesis. The T antigen of SV40, the E6 and E7 of papillomavirus, and the E1a protein of adenovirus bind to and prevent the function of growth-inhibitory proteins (p53 and the retinoblastoma gene product), resulting in cell growth, which also promotes virus replication. The larger DNA viruses may encode a DNA polymerase and other proteins to facilitate DNA synthesis and are more independent. Herpes simplex virus encodes a DNA polymerase and scavenging enzymes, such as deoxyribonuclease, ribonucleotide reductase, and thymidine kinase, to generate the necessary deoxyribonucleotide substrates for replication of its genome.

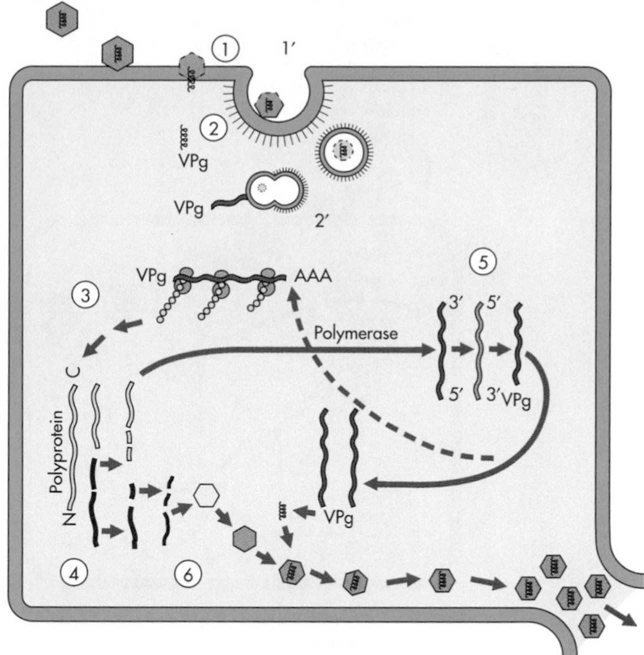

FIGURE 6–13. Replication of picornaviruses: a simple (+) RNA virus. *1,* Interaction of the picornaviruses with receptors on the cell surface defines the target cell and weakens the capsid. *2,* The genome is injected through the virion and across the cell membrane. *2′,* The virion is endocytosed, and then the genome is released. *3,* Alternatively, the genome is used as mRNA for protein synthesis. One large polyprotein is translated from the virion genome. *4,* Then the polyprotein is proteolytically cleaved into individual proteins, including an RNA-dependent RNA polymerase. *5,* The polymerase makes a (–) strand template from the genome and replicates the genome. A protein (VPg) is covalently attached to the 5′ end of the viral genome. *6,* The structural proteins associate into the capsid structure, the genome is inserted, and the virions are released on cell lysis.

RNA VIRUSES

Replication and transcription of RNA viruses are similar processes because the viral genomes are usually either an mRNA (positive-strand RNA) (Figure 6–13) or a template for mRNA (negative-strand RNA) (Box 6–8; Figure 6–14). During replication and transcription, a double-stranded RNA replicative intermediate, a structure not normally found in uninfected cells, is formed.

The RNA virus genome must code for **RNA-dependent RNA polymerases (replicases and transcriptases)** because the cell has no means of replicating RNA. Because RNA is degraded relatively quickly, the RNA-dependent RNA polymerase must be provided or synthesized soon after uncoating, to generate more viral RNA, or the infection will be aborted. Most viral RNA polymerases work at a fast pace but are also error prone, causing mutations. Replication of the genome provides new templates for production of more mRNA, which amplifies and accelerates virus replication.

The **positive-strand RNA viral genomes** of the picornaviruses, noroviruses, coronaviruses, flaviviruses, and togaviruses act as mRNA, bind to ribosomes, and direct protein synthesis. *The naked positive-strand RNA viral genome is sufficient to initiate infection by itself.* After the virus-encoded, RNA-dependent RNA polymerase is produced, a negative-strand RNA template is synthesized. The template can then be used to generate more mRNA and to replicate the genome. For the togaviruses and noroviruses, the negative-sense RNA template is also used to produce a smaller RNA for the structural proteins (late genes). The mRNAs for these viruses are not capped at the 5′ end, but the genome encodes a short poly A sequence.

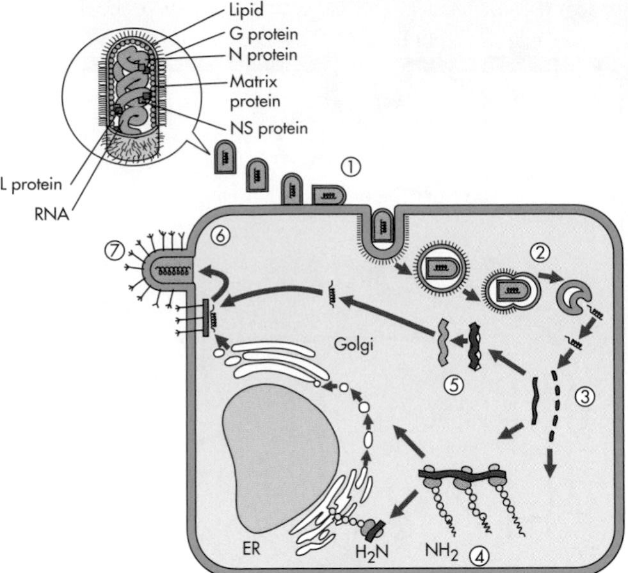

FIGURE 6–14. Replication of rhabdoviruses: a simple enveloped (–) RNA virus. *1,* Rhabdoviruses bind to the cell surface and are (*2*) endocytosed. The envelope fuses with the endosome vesicle membrane to deliver the nucleocapsid to the cytoplasm. The virion must carry a polymerase, which (*3*) produces five individual messenger RNAs (mRNAs) and a full-length (+) RNA template. *4,* Proteins are translated from the mRNAs, including one glycoprotein (G), which is co-translationally glycosylated in the endoplasmic reticulum (ER), processed in the Golgi apparatus, and delivered to the cell membrane. *5,* The genome is replicated from the (+) RNA template, and N, L, and NS proteins associate with the genome to form the nucleocapsid. *6,* The matrix protein associates with the G protein–modified membrane, which is followed by assembly of the nucleocapsid. *7,* The virus buds from the cell in a bullet-shaped virion.

BOX 6–8. Properties of RNA Viruses

RNA is labile and transient.
Most RNA viruses replicate in the cytoplasm.
Cells cannot replicate RNA. RNA viruses must encode an RNA-dependent RNA polymerase.
The genome structure determines the mechanism of transcription and replication.
RNA viruses are prone to mutation.
The genome structure and polarity determine how viral messenger RNA (mRNA) is generated and proteins are processed.
RNA viruses, except (+) RNA genome, must carry polymerases.
All (–) RNA viruses are enveloped.
Picornaviruses, togaviruses, flaviviruses, noroviruses, and coronaviruses
(+) RNA genome resembles mRNA and is translated into a polyprotein, which is proteolyzed. A (–) RNA template is used for replication. Togaviruses, coronaviruses, and noroviruses have early and late genes.
Orthomyxoviruses, paramyxoviruses, rhabdoviruses, filoviruses, and bunyaviruses
(–) RNA genome is a template for individual mRNAs, but full-length (+) RNA template is required for replication. Orthomyxoviruses replicate and transcribe in nucleus, and each segment of the genome encodes one mRNA and template.
Reoviruses
(+/–) Segmented RNA genome is a template for mRNA. (+) RNA may also be encapsulated to generate the (+/–) RNA and then more mRNA.
Retroviruses
(+) Retrovirus RNA genome is converted into DNA, which is integrated into the host chromatin and transcribed as a cellular gene.

Transcription and replication of coronaviruses share many of these aspects but are more complex.

The **negative-strand RNA virus genomes** of the rhabdoviruses, orthomyxoviruses, paramyxoviruses, filoviruses, and bunyaviruses are the templates for production of mRNA. The negative-strand RNA genome is not infectious by itself, and *a polymerase must be carried into the cell with the genome* (associated with the genome as part of the nucleocapsid) to make individual mRNA for the different viral proteins. As a result, a full-length positive-strand RNA must also be produced by the viral polymerase to act as a template to generate more copies of the genome. The (–) RNA genome is like the negatives from a roll of 35-mm film: Each frame encodes a photo/mRNA, but a full-length positive is required for replicating the roll. *Except for influenza viruses, transcription and replication of negative-strand RNA viruses occur in the cytoplasm.* The influenza transcriptase requires a primer to produce mRNA. It uses the 5′ ends of cellular mRNA in the nucleus as primers for its polymerase and, in the process, steals the 5′ cap from the cellular mRNA. The influenza genome is also replicated in the nucleus.

The reoviruses have a **segmented, double-stranded RNA genome** and undergo a more complex means of replication and transcription. The reovirus RNA polymerase is part of the inner capsid core. mRNA units are transcribed from each of the 10 or more segments of the genome while they are still in the core. The negative strands of the genome segments are used as templates for mRNA in a manner similar to that of the negative-strand RNA viruses. Reovirus-encoded enzymes contained in the inner capsid core add the 5′ cap to viral mRNA. The mRNA does not have poly A. The mRNAs are released into the cytoplasm, where they direct protein synthesis or are sequestered into new cores. The positive-strand RNA in the new cores acts as a template for negative-strand RNA, and the core polymerase produces the progeny double-stranded RNA.

The arenaviruses have an **ambisense circular genome** with (+) sequences adjacent to (–) sequences. The early genes of the virus are transcribed from the negative-sense portion of the genome, and the late genes of the virus are transcribed from the full-length replicative intermediate.

Although the **retroviruses** have a positive-strand RNA genome, the virus provides no means for replication of the RNA in the cytoplasm. Instead, the retroviruses carry two copies of the genome, two transfer RNA (tRNA) molecules, and an RNA-dependent DNA polymerase **(reverse transcriptase)** in the virion. The tRNA is used as a primer for synthesis of a circular complementary DNA copy **(cDNA)** of the genome. The cDNA is synthesized in the cytoplasm, travels to the nucleus, and is then integrated into the host chromatin. The viral genome becomes a cellular gene. Promoters at the end of the integrated viral genome enhance the transcription of the viral DNA sequences by the cell. Full-length RNA transcripts are used as new genomes, and individual mRNAs are generated by differential splicing of this RNA.

The most unusual mode of replication is reserved for the **deltavirus.** The deltavirus resembles a viroid. The genome is a circular, rod-shaped, single-stranded RNA, which is extensively hybridized to itself. As the exception, the deltavirus RNA genome is replicated by the host cell DNA-dependent RNA polymerase II in the nucleus. A portion of the genome forms an RNA structure called a ribozyme, which cleaves the RNA circle to produce an mRNA.

VIRAL PROTEIN SYNTHESIS

All viruses depend on the host cell ribosomes, tRNA, and mechanisms for post-translational modification to produce their proteins. The binding of mRNA to the ribosome is mediated by a 5′ cap structure of methylated guanosine or a special RNA loop structure (internal ribosome entry sequence [IRES]), which binds within the ribosome to initiate protein synthesis. The cap structure, if used, is attached to mRNA in different ways by different viruses. The IRES structure was discovered first in the picornavirus genome and then in selected cellular mRNAs. Most, but not all, viral mRNA have a polyadenosine (polyA) tail, like eukaryotic mRNAs.

Unlike bacterial ribosomes, which can bind to a polycistronic mRNA and translate several gene sequences into separate proteins, the eukaryotic ribosome binds to mRNA and can make only one continuous protein, and then it falls off the mRNA. Each virus deals with this limitation differently, depending on the structure of the genome. For example, the entire genome of a positive-strand RNA virus is read by the ribosome and translated into one giant **polyprotein.** The polyprotein is, subsequently, cleaved by cellular and viral proteases into functional proteins. DNA viruses, retroviruses, and most negative-strand RNA viruses transcribe separate mRNA for smaller polyproteins or individual proteins. The orthomyxovirus and reovirus genomes are segmented, and most of the segments code for single proteins for this reason.

Viruses use different tactics to promote preferential translation of their viral mRNA instead of cellular mRNA. In many cases, the concentration of viral mRNA in the cell is so large that it occupies most of the ribosomes, preventing translation of cellular mRNA. Adenovirus infection blocks the egress of cellular mRNA from the nucleus. Herpes simplex virus and other viruses inhibit cellular macromolecular synthesis and induce degradation of the cell's DNA and mRNA. To promote selective translation of its mRNA, poliovirus uses a virus-encoded protease to inactivate the 200,000-Da cap-binding protein of the ribosome to prevent binding and translation of 5′ capped cellular mRNA. Togaviruses and many other viruses increase the permeability of the cell's membrane; thus the ribosomal affinity for most cellular mRNA is decreased. All these actions also contribute to the cytopathology of the virus infection. The pathogenic consequences of these actions are discussed further in Chapter 49.

Some viral proteins require **post-translational modifications,** such as phosphorylation, glycosylation, acylation, or sulfation. Protein phosphorylation is accomplished by cellular or viral protein kinases and is a means of modulating, activating, or inactivating proteins. Several herpesviruses and other viruses encode their own protein kinase. *Viral glycoproteins are synthesized on membrane-bound ribosomes and have the amino acid sequences to allow insertion into the rough endoplasmic reticulum and N-linked glycosylation.* The high-mannose precursor form of the glycoproteins progresses from the endoplasmic reticulum through the vesicular transport system of the cell and is processed through the Golgi apparatus. The sialic acid–containing mature glycoprotein is expressed on the plasma membrane of the cell unless the glycoprotein expresses protein sequences for retention in an intracellular organelle. The presence of the glycoproteins determines where the virion will assemble. Other modifications, such as *O*-glycosylation, acylation, and sulfation of the proteins, can also occur during progression through the Golgi apparatus.

ASSEMBLY

Virion assembly is analogous to a three-dimensional interlocking puzzle that puts itself together in the box. The virion is built from small, easily manufactured parts that enclose the genome in a functional package. Each part of the virion has recognition structures that allow the virus to form the appropriate protein–protein, protein–nucleic acid, and (for enveloped viruses) protein–membrane interactions needed to assemble into the final structure. The assembly process begins when the necessary pieces are synthesized and the concentration of structural proteins in the cell is sufficient to drive the process thermodynamically, much like a crystallization reaction. The assembly process may be facilitated by scaffolding proteins or other proteins that are activated or release energy on proteolysis. For example, cleavage of the VP0 protein of poliovirus releases the VP4 peptide, which solidifies the capsid.

The site and mechanism of virion assembly in the cell depend on where genome replication occurs and whether the final structure is a naked capsid or an enveloped virus. Assembly of the DNA viruses, other than poxviruses, occurs in the nucleus and requires transport of the virion proteins into the nucleus. RNA virus and poxvirus assembly occurs in the cytoplasm.

Capsid viruses may be assembled as empty structures (procapsids) to be filled with the genome (e.g., picornaviruses), or they may be assembled around the genome. Nucleocapsids of the retroviruses, togaviruses, and the negative-strand RNA viruses assemble around the genome and are, subsequently, enclosed in an envelope. The helical nucleocapsid of negative-strand RNA viruses includes the RNA-dependent RNA polymerase necessary for mRNA synthesis in the target cell.

For enveloped viruses, newly synthesized and processed viral glycoproteins are delivered to cellular membranes by vesicular transport. Acquisition of an envelope occurs after association of the nucleocapsid with the viral glycoprotein-containing regions of host cell membranes in a process called **budding.** Matrix proteins for negative-strand RNA viruses line and promote the adhesion of nucleocapsids with the glycoprotein-modified membrane. As more interactions occur, the membrane surrounds the nucleocapsid and the virus buds from the membrane.

The type of genome and the protein sequence of the glycoproteins determine the site of budding. Most RNA viruses bud from the plasma membrane, and the virus is released from the cell at the same time. The flaviviruses, coronaviruses, and bunyaviruses acquire their envelope by budding into the endoplasmic reticulum and Golgi membranes and may remain cell-associated in these organelles. The herpes simplex virus nucleocapsid assembles in the nucleus and buds into and then out of the endoplasmic reticulum. The nucleocapsid is dumped into the cytoplasm, viral proteins associate with the capsid, and then the envelope is acquired by budding into a Golgi membrane decorated with the 10 viral glycoproteins. The virion is transported to the cell surface and released by exocytosis, on cell lysis, or transmitted through cell–cell bridges.

Viruses use different tricks to ensure that all the parts of the virus are assembled into complete virions. The RNA polymerase required for infection by negative-strand RNA viruses is carried on the genome as a helical nucleocapsid. The human immunodeficiency virus and other retrovirus genomes are packaged in a procapsid consisting of a polyprotein containing the protease, polymerase, integrase, and structural proteins. This procapsid binds to viral glycoprotein-modified membranes, and the virion buds from the membrane. The virus-encoded protease is activated within the virion and cleaves the polyprotein to produce the final, infectious nucleocapsid and the required proteins within the envelope.

Assembly of a complete, functional influenza or reovirus virion requires accumulation of at least one copy of each gene segment. Although the influenza virus requires eight unique genome segments, virions can randomly package 10 to 11 segments. Statistically, this yields approximately one complete set of genomes and functional virus per 20 defective viruses. Reovirus genomes are likely to assemble in a similar manner.

Errors are made during viral assembly. Empty virions and virions containing defective genomes are produced. As a result, the particle to infectious virus ratio, also called particle to plaque-forming unit ratio, is high, usually greater than 10, and during rapid viral replication can even be 10^4. Defective viruses can occupy the machinery required for normal virus replication to prevent (interfere with) virus production **(defective interfering particles).**

RELEASE

Viruses can be released from cells after lysis of the cell, by exocytosis, or by budding from the plasma membrane. Naked capsid viruses are generally released after lysis of the cell. Release of many enveloped viruses occurs after budding from the plasma membrane without killing the cell. Lysis and plasma membrane budding are efficient means of release. Viruses that bud or acquire their membrane in the cytoplasm (e.g., flaviviruses, poxviruses) remain cell-associated and are released by exocytosis or cell lysis. Viruses that bind to sialic acid receptors (e.g., orthomyxoviruses, certain paramyxoviruses) may also have a neuraminidase. The neuraminidase removes potential sialic acid receptors on the glycoproteins of the virion and the host cell to prevent clumping and facilitate release.

REINITIATION OF THE REPLICATION CYCLE

The virus released to the extracellular medium is usually responsible for initiating new infections; however, **traversal of cell–cell bridges, virus-induced cell–cell fusion, or vertical transmission** of the genome to daughter cells can also spread the infection. The latter means allow the virus to escape antibody detection. Some herpesviruses, retroviruses, and paramyxoviruses can induce cell–cell fusion to merge the cells into multinucleated giant cells **(syncytia),** which become huge virus factories. The retroviruses and some DNA viruses can transmit their integrated copy of the genome vertically to daughter cells on cell division.

Viral Genetics

Mutations spontaneously and readily occur in viral genomes, creating new virus strains with properties differing from the **parental,** or **wild-type, virus.** These variants can be identified by their nucleotide sequences, antigenic differences (serotypes), or differences in functional or structural properties. Most mutations have no effect or are detrimental to the virus. Mutations in essential genes inactivate the virus, but mutations in other genes can produce antiviral drug resistance or alter the antigenicity or pathogenicity of the virus.

Errors in copying the viral genome during virus replication produce many mutations. This is because of the *poor fidelity of the viral polymerase and the rapid rate of genome replication.* In addition, *RNA viruses do not have a genetic error-checking mechanism.* As a result, the rates of mutation for RNA viruses are usually greater than for DNA viruses.

Mutations in essential genes are termed **lethal mutations.** These mutants are difficult to isolate because the virus cannot replicate. A **deletion mutant** results from the loss or selective removal of a portion of the genome and the function that it encodes. Other mutations may produce **plaque mutants,** which differ from the wild type in the size or appearance of the infected cells; **host range mutants,** which differ in the tissue type or species of target cell that can be infected; or **attenuated mutants,** which are variants that cause less serious disease in animals or humans. **Conditional mutants**, such as **temperature-sensitive (ts)** or **cold-sensitive mutants,** have a mutation in a gene for an essential protein that allows virus production only at certain temperatures. ts mutants generally grow well or relatively better at 30° to 35°C, whereas the encoded protein is inactive at elevated temperatures of 38° to 40°C, preventing virus production.

New virus strains can also arise by genetic interactions between viruses or between the virus and the cell (Figure 6–15). Intramolecular genetic exchange between viruses or the virus and the host is termed **recombination.** Recombination can occur readily between two related DNA viruses. For example, coinfection of a cell with the two closely related herpesviruses (herpes simplex virus types 1 and 2) yields intertypic recombinant strains. These new hybrid strains have genes from types 1 and 2. Integration of retroviruses into host cell chromatin is a form of recombination. Recombination of two related RNA viruses, Sindbis and eastern equine encephalitis virus, resulted in creation of another togavirus, western equine encephalitis virus.

Viruses with segmented genomes (e.g., influenza viruses and reoviruses) form hybrid strains on infection of one cell with more than one virus strain. This process, termed **reassortment,** is analogous to picking 10 marbles out of a box containing 10 black and 10 white marbles. New strains of influenza A virus are created on coinfection with a virus from different species (see Figure 60–5).

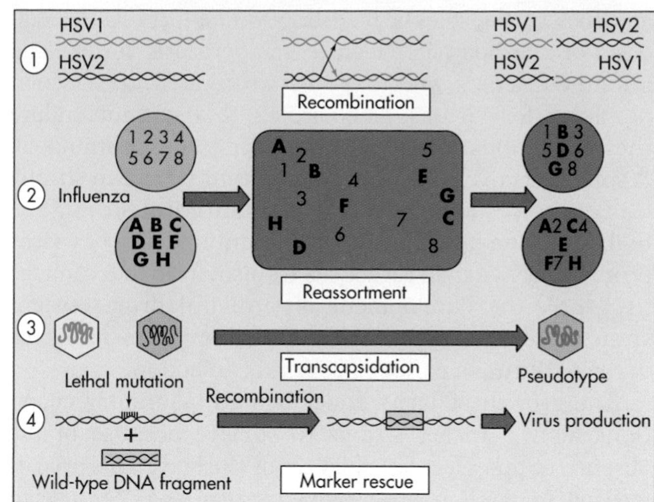

FIGURE 6–15. Genetic exchange between viral particles can give rise to new viral types, as illustrated. Representative viruses include the following: *1*, intertypic recombination of herpes simplex virus type 1 *(HSV1)* and type 2 *(HSV2)*; *2*, reassortment of two strains of influenza virus; *3*, rescue of a papovavirus defective in assembly by a complementary defective virus (transcapsidation); and *4*, marker rescue of a lethal or conditional mutation.

In some cases, a defective viral strain can be rescued by the replication of another mutant, by the wild-type virus, or by a cell line bearing a replacement viral gene. Replication of the other virus or expression of the gene in the cell provides the missing function required by the mutant **(complementation),** allowing replication to occur. A herpes simplex disabled infectious single cycle (DISC) vaccine virus lacks is an essential gene and grown in a cell line that expresses that gene product to "complement" the virus. The virus that is produced can infect the normal cells of the vaccinated individual, but the virions that are produced cannot replicate in the normal cells of a vaccinated individual. Rescue of a lethal or conditional-lethal mutant with a defined genetic sequence, such as a restriction endonuclease DNA fragment, is called **marker rescue.** Marker rescue is used to map the genomes of viruses such as herpes simplex virus. Virus produced from cells infected with different virus strains may be phenotypically mixed and have the proteins of one strain but the genome of the other **(transcapsidation). Pseudotypes** are generated when transcapsidation occurs between different types of virus, but this is rare.

Individual virus strains or mutants are **selected** by their ability to use the host cell machinery and to withstand the conditions of the body and the environment. Cellular properties that can act as selection pressures include the growth rate of the cell and tissue-specific expression of certain proteins required by the virus (e.g., enzymes, glycoproteins, transcription factors). The conditions of the body, its elevated temperature, innate and immune defenses, and tissue structure are also selection pressures for viruses. The viruses that cannot endure these conditions or evade the host defenses are eliminated. A small selective advantage in a mutant virus can shortly lead to its becoming the predominant viral strain. The high mutation rate of the human immunodeficiency virus promotes a switch in target cell tropism from macrophage to T cell, the development of antiviral drug-resistant strains after treatment, and the generation of antigenic variants during a patient's course of infection.

The growth of virus under benign laboratory conditions allows weaker strains to survive because of the absence of the selective pressures of the body. This process is used to develop attenuated virus strains for use in vaccines.

Viral Vectors for Therapy

Genetically manipulated viruses can be excellent delivery systems for foreign genes. Viruses can provide gene replacement therapy, can be used as vaccines to promote immunity to other agents or tumors, and can act as targeted killers of tumors. The advantages of using viruses are that they can be readily amplified by replication in appropriate cells and they target specific tissues and deliver the DNA or RNA into the cell. Viruses that are being developed as vectors include retroviruses, adenoviruses, herpes simplex virus, adeno-associated virus (parvovirus), poxviruses (e.g., vaccinia and canarypox) (see Figure 55–3), and even some togaviruses. The viral vectors are usually defective or attenuated viruses, in which the foreign DNA replaces a virulence or unessential gene. The foreign gene may be under the control of a viral promoter or even a tissue-specific promoter. Defective virus vectors are grown in cell lines that express the missing viral functions "complementing" the virus. The progeny can deliver their nucleic acid but not produce infectious virus. Retroviruses and adeno-associated viruses can integrate into cells and permanently deliver a gene into the cell's chromosome. Adenovirus and herpes simplex virus promote targeted delivery of the foreign gene to receptor-bearing cells. Genetically attenuated herpes simplex viruses are being developed to specifically kill the growing cells of glioblastomas while sparing the surrounding neurons. Vaccinia virus carrying a gene for the rabies glycoprotein is already being used successfully to immunize raccoons, foxes, and skunks in the wild. Some day, virus vectors may be routinely used to treat cystic fibrosis, Duchenne's muscular dystrophy, lysosomal storage diseases, and immunologic disorders.

QUESTIONS

1. Which features of these viruses are similar, and which are different?
   a. Poliovirus and rhinovirus
   b. Poliovirus and rotavirus
   c. Poliovirus and western equine encephalitis virus
   d. Yellow fever virus and dengue virus
   e. Epstein-Barr virus and cytomegalovirus
2. Match the characteristics from column A with the appropriate viral families in column B, based on your knowledge of their physical and genome structure and their implications.

A	B
1. Are resistant to detergents	Picornaviruses
2. Are resistant to drying	Togaviruses
3. Replication in the nucleus	Orthomyxoviruses
4. Replication in the cytoplasm	Paramyxoviruses
5. Can be released from the cell without cell lysis	Rhabdoviruses
	Reoviruses
6. Provide a good target for antiviral drug action	Retroviruses
	Herpesviruses
7. Undergo reassortment on coinfection with two strains	Papovaviruses
	Adenoviruses
8. Make DNA from an RNA template	Poxviruses
9. Use a (+) RNA template to replicate the genome	Hepadnaviruses
10. Genome translated into a polyprotein	

3. Based on structural considerations, which of the virus families listed in question 2 should be able to endure fecal-oral transmission?
4. List the essential enzymes encoded by the virus families listed in question 2.
5. A mutant defective in the herpes simplex virus type 1 DNA polymerase gene replicates in the presence of herpes simplex virus type 2. The progeny virus contains the herpes simplex virus type 1 genome but is recognized by antibodies to herpes simplex virus type 2. Which genetic mechanisms may be occurring?
6. How are the early and late genes of the togaviruses, papovaviruses, and herpesviruses distinguished, and how is the time of their expression regulated?
7. What are the consequences (no effect, decreased efficiency, or inhibition of replication) of a deletion mutation in the following viral enzymes?
   a. Epstein-Barr virus polymerase
   b. Herpes simplex virus thymidine kinase
   c. Human immunodeficiency virus reverse transcriptase
   d. Influenza B virus neuraminidase
   e. Rabies virus (rhabdovirus) G protein

Bibliography

Belshe RB, editor: *Textbook of human virology,* ed 2, St Louis, 1991, Mosby.

Cann AJ: *Principles of molecular virology,* San Diego, 2001, Academic Press.

Cohen J, Powderly WG, editors: *Infectious diseases,* ed 2, St Louis, 2004, Mosby.

Electron microscopic images of viruses, by Linda Stannard, University of Capetown, South Africa. Available at www.uct.ac.za/depts/mmi/stannard/linda.html.

Flint SJ et al: *Principles of virology: molecular biology, pathogenesis and control of animal viruses,* ed 2, Washington, 2003, American Society for Microbiology Press.

Knipe DM, Howley PM, editors: *Fields virology,* ed 4, New York, 2001, Lippincott-Williams and Wilkins.

Richman DD, Whitley RJ, Hayden FG: *Clinical virology,* New York, 1997, Churchill Livingstone.

Robbins PD, Ghivizzani SC: Viral vectors for gene therapy, *Pharmacol Ther* 80:35–47, 1998.

Specter S, Hodinka RL, Young SA: *Clinical virology manual,* ed 3, Washington, 2000, ASM Press.

Strauss JM, Strauss EG: *Viruses and human disease,* San Diego, 2002, Academic Press.

White DO, Fenner FJ: *Medical virology,* ed 4, Orlando, 1994, Academic Press.

Viruses in cell culture. Available at www.uct.ac.za/depts/mmi/stannard/linda.html

CHAPTER 7

Fungal Classification, Structure, and Replication

This chapter provides an overview of fungal classification, structure, and reproduction. The very basic aspects of fungal cell organization and morphology are discussed, as well as the broad categories of human mycoses. We have purposely simplified the fungal taxonomy and use it to highlight the following major classes of fungi causing disease in humans: the Zygomycetes, the Ascomycetes, the Archiascomycetes, the Basidiomycetes, and the Deuteromycetes.

Importance of Fungi

The fungi represent a ubiquitous and diverse group of organisms, the main purpose of which is to degrade organic matter. All fungi lead a heterotrophic existence as **saprobes** (organisms that live on dead or decaying matter), **symbionts** (organisms that live together and in which the association is of mutual advantage), **commensals** (organisms living in a close relationship in which one benefits from the relationship and the other neither benefits nor is harmed), or as **parasites** (organisms that live on or within a host, from which they derive benefits without making any useful contribution in return; in the case of pathogens the relationship is harmful to the host).

Fungi have emerged in the past two decades as major causes of human disease (Table 7–1), especially among those individuals who are immunocompromised or hospitalized with serious underlying diseases. Among these patient groups, fungi serve as opportunistic pathogens causing considerable morbidity and mortality. The overall incidence of specific invasive mycoses continues to increase with time (Table 7–2), and the list of opportunistic fungal pathogens likewise increases each year. In short, *there are no nonpathogenic fungi!* This increase in fungal infections can be attributed to the ever-growing number of immunocompromised patients, including transplant patients, individuals with acquired immune deficiency syndrome (AIDS), patients with cancer and who are undergoing chemotherapy, and those individuals who are hospitalized with other serious underlying conditions and who undergo a variety of invasive procedures.

Fungal Taxonomy, Structure, and Replication

The fungi are classified into their own separate kingdom, Kingdom Fungi (Myceteae). They are eukaryotic organisms that are distinguished from other eukaryotes by a rigid cell wall composed of chitin and glucan, and a cell membrane in which ergosterol is substituted for cholesterol as the major sterol component (Figure 7–1).

Classic fungal taxonomy relies heavily on morphology and mode of spore production; however, increasingly, ultrastructural features, biochemical and molecular characteristics, are brought to bear, often resulting in changes in the original taxonomic designation. Fungi may be unicellular or multicellular. The simplest grouping based on morphology lumps fungi into either **yeasts** or **moulds.** A yeast can be defined morphologically as a cell that reproduces by budding or by fission (Figure 7–2), in which a progenitor or "mother" cell pinches off a portion of itself to produce a progeny or "daughter" cell. The daughter cells may elongate to form sausagelike **pseudohyphae.** Yeasts are usually unicellular and produce round, pasty, or mucoid colonies on agar. Moulds, on the other hand, are multicellular organisms consisting of threadlike tubular structures called **hyphae** (see Figure 7–2) that elongate at their tips by a process known as apical extension. Hyphae are either **coenocytic** (hollow and

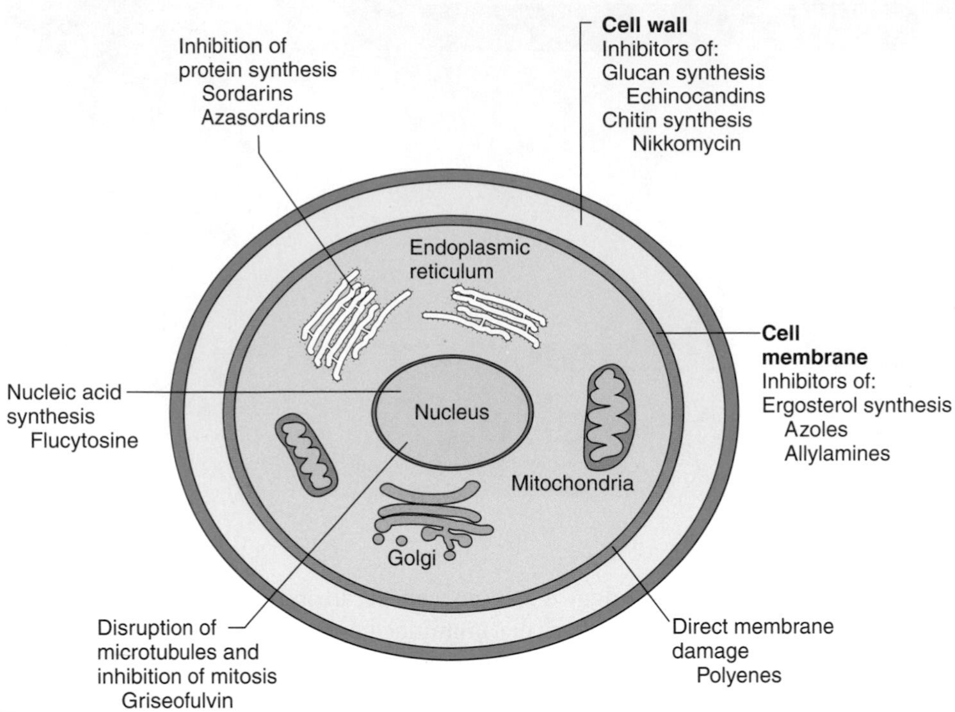

FIGURE 7–1. Diagram of a fungal cell.

TABLE 7–1. Incidence and Case-Fatality Ratios of Selected Invasive Fungal Infections

Pathogen	No. of Cases Per Million Per Year Incidence	Case-Fatality Ratio (%) for First Episode
Candida species	72.8	33.9
Cryptococcus neoformans	65.5	12.7
Coccidioides immitis	15.3	11.1
Aspergillus species	12.4	23.3
Histoplasma capsulatum	7.1	21.4
Agents of Zygomycosis	1.7	30.0
Agents of Hyalohyphomycosis	1.2	14.3
Agents of Phaeohyphomycosis	1.0	0
Sporothrix schenckii	<1	20.0
Malassezia furfur	<1	0
Total	178.3	22.4

Adapted from Rees et al (1998).

TABLE 7–2. Cumulative Incidences of Selected Invasive Mycoses

Mycosis	Incidence Per Million Per Year		
	CPHA* 1980-1982	CDC† 1992-1993	NHDS‡ 1996
Candidiasis	2.6	72.8	228.2
Histoplasmosis	13.9	7.1	13.6
Aspergillosis	8.4	12.4	34.3
Cryptococcosis	4.0	65.5	29.6

*CPHA, Commission on Hospital and Professional Activities (Reingold et al, 1986).
†CDC, Centers for Disease Control (Rees et al, 1998).
‡NHDS, National Hospital Discharge Survey (Wilson et al, 2002).

multinucleate) or **septate** (divided by partitions or cross-walls) (see Figure 7–2). The hyphae form together to produce a matlike structure called a **mycelium.** The colonies formed by moulds are often described as filamentous, hairy, or woolly. When growing on agar or other solid surfaces, moulds produce hyphae, termed **vegetative hyphae,** which grow on or beneath the surface of the culture medium, and also hyphae that project above the surface of the medium, so-called **aerial hyphae.** The aerial hyphae may produce specialized structures known as **conidia** (asexual reproductive elements) (Figure 7–3). The conidia are easily airborne and serve to disseminate the fungus. The size, shape, and certain developmental features of conidia are used as a means of identifying fungi to genus and species. Many fungi of medical importance are termed **dimorphic** because of the fact that they may exist in both a yeast form and a mould form.

Most fungi exhibit aerobic respiration, although some are facultatively anaerobic (fermentative) and others are strict anaerobes. Metabolically, fungi are heterotrophic

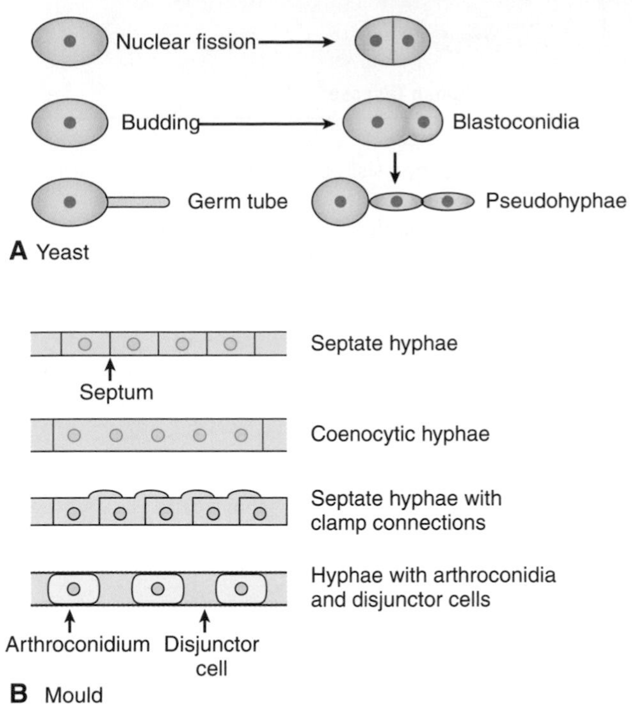

FIGURE 7–2. Fungal cell morphology. **A,** Yeast cells reproducing by nuclear fission and blastoconidia formation. The elongation of budding yeast cells to form pseudohyphae is shown, as is the formation of a germ tube. **B,** Types of hyphae seen with various moulds.

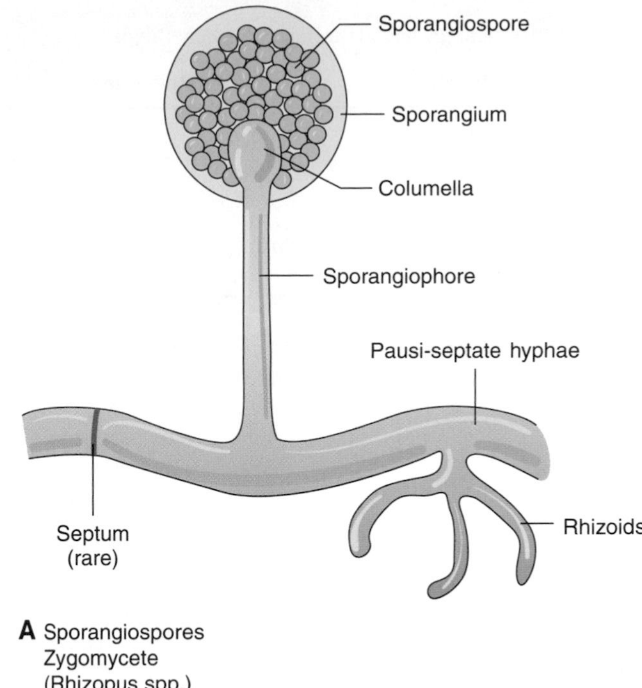

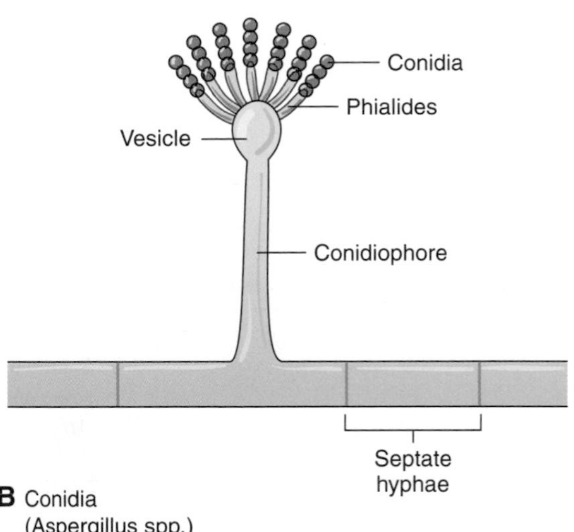

FIGURE 7–3. Examples of asexual spore formation and associated structures seen with a Zygomycete (**A**) and an *Aspergillus* spp. (**B**).

and biochemically versatile, producing both primary (e.g., citric acid, ethanol, glycerol) and secondary (e.g., antibiotics [penicillin], amanitens, aflatoxins) metabolites. Relative to the bacteria, fungi are slow growing with cell-doubling times in terms of hours rather than minutes.

A simplified taxonomic scheme listing the five major classes of fungi of medical importance is shown in Table 7–3. Of the estimated hundreds of thousands of different fungi, only approximately 200 are known to cause human disease, although this number appears to be increasing.

Fungi reproduce by the formation of spores, which may be sexual (involving meiosis, preceded by fusion of the protoplasm and nuclei of two compatible mating types) or asexual (involving mitosis only). The fungi in the classes Zygomycetes, Ascomycetes, Archiascomycetes, and Basidiomycetes produce both sexual and asexual spores (Table 7–4). The form of the fungus producing sexual spores is termed the **teleomorph,** and the form producing asexual spores is termed the **anamorph.** The fact that the teleomorph and anamorph of the same fungus have different names (e.g., *Ajellomyces capsulatum* [teleomorph] and *Histoplasma capsulatum* [anamorph]) is a source of confusion for nonmycologists.

The largest group of fungi causing infections in humans, the **Deuteromycetes** (see Table 7–4), does not produce known sexual spores. Irrespective of the ability of a given fungus to produce sexual spores, in clinical situations it is common to refer to the organisms by their asexual designations. This is because the anamorphic (asexual) state is isolated from clinical specimens and the sexual or teleomorphic phase occurs only under very specialized conditions in the laboratory.

Asexual spores consist of two general types: **sporangiospores** and **conidia.** Sporangiospores are asexual spores produced in a containing structure or **sporangium** (see Figure 7–3) and are characteristic of genera belonging to the class Zygomycetes, such as *Rhizopus* and *Mucor* spp. Conidia are asexual spores that are borne

TABLE 7–3. Medically Important Fungi (Kingdom Fungi)

Taxonomic Designation	Representative Genera	Human Disease
Class: Zygomycetes		
Order: Mucorales	*Rhizopus, Mucor, Absidia, Saksenaea*	Zygomycosis: Opportunistic in patients with diabetes, leukemia, severe burns, or malnutrition; rhinocerebral infections.
Order: Entomophthorales	*Basidiobolus, Conidiobolus*	Zygomycosis: Subcutaneous and gastrointestinal infections
Class: Ascomycetes		
Order: Endomycetales	*Saccharomyces, Pichia*	Numerous mycoses
Order: Onygenales	*Arthroderma* (teleomorphs of *Trichophyton* and *Microsporum*)	Dermatophytoses
	Ajellomyces (teleomorphs of *Histoplasma* and *Blastomyces*)	Systemic mycoses
Order: Eurotiales	Teleomorphs of some *Aspergillus* and *Penicillium* spp.	Aspergillosis; Hyalohyphomycosis
Class: Archiascomycetes	*Pneumocystis jiroveci* (*carinii*)	Pneumonia
Class: Basidiomycetes	*Amanita, Agaricus, Filobasidiella* (teleomorph of *Cryptococcus neoformans*)	Mushroom poisoning; Cryptococcosis
Class: Deuteromycetes		
Order: Cryptococcales	Imperfect yeasts: *Candida, Cryptococcus, Trichosporon, Malassezia*	Numerous mycoses
Order: Moniliales		
Family: Moniliaceae	*Epidermophyton, Coccidioides, Paracoccidioides, Sporothrix, Aspergillus*	Numerous mycoses
Family: Dematiaceae	*Phialophora, Fonsecaea, Exophiala, Wangiella, Bipolaris, Alternaria*	Chromoblastomycoses, mycetoma, and phaeohyphomycoses

Adapted from Fromtling et al (2003).

TABLE 7–4. Biologic, Morphologic, and Reproductive Characteristics of Pathogenic Fungi

Organism Class	Representative Genera	Morphology	Reproduction
Zygomycetes	*Rhizopus, Mucor, Absidia, Basidiobolus*	Broad, thin-walled, coenocytic hyphae, 6-25μm, with nonparallel sides; spores contained within sporangium; rootlike structures called rhizoids characteristic of some genera	Asexual: production of sporangiospores within sporangium Sexual: production of zygospores formed by fusion of compatible mating types
Ascomycetes	*Saccharomyces*, some *Aspergillus* spp., *Histoplasma, Trichophyton*	Budding yeasts, septate hyphae, spores (conidia) borne on conidiophores	Asexual: production of conidia Sexual: ascospores produced in specialized structure called an ascus
Archiascomycetes	*Pneumocystis*	Trophic forms and cystlike structures	Asexual: binary fission Sexual: fusion of compatible mating types to form zygote; compartmentalization of spores within cyst
Basidiomycetes	*Filobasidiella* (sexual form of *Cryptococcus neoformans*)	Hyphae that produce basidiospores (not seen in nature or in patients)	Sexual: fusion of compatible nuclei, followed by meiosis to form basidiospores
Deuteromycetes	*Candida, Cryptococcus, Coccidioides, Aspergillus, Bipolaris*	Budding yeasts, septate hyphae, pseudohyphae, asexual conidia borne on specialized structure or within the hyphae	Asexual: production of conidia by budding from a mother cell or within a hyphal fragment Sexual: not identified

naked on specialized structures, as seen in *Aspergillus* spp. (see Figure 7–3), *Penicillium* spp., and the dermatophytes.

ZYGOMYCETES

The Zygomycetes are moulds with broad, sparsely septate, coenocytic hyphae. The Zygomycetes produce sexual zygospores following the fusion of two compatible mating types. The asexual spores of the order Mucorales (see Table 7–3) are contained within a sporangium (sporangiospores). The sporangia are borne at the tips of stalklike **sporangiophores** that terminate in a bulbous swelling called the **columella** (see Figure 7–3). The presence of rootlike structures, called **rhizoids,** is helpful in identifying specific genera within the Mucorales. Most Zygomycetes encountered clinically belong to the order Mucorales. The other order, the Entomophthorales, are less common and include the genera, *Basidiobolus* and *Conidiobolus.* These organisms cause tropical subcutaneous zygomycosis. The asexual spores are borne singly on short sporophores and are forcibly ejected when mature.

ASCOMYCETES

Ascomycetes include both yeasts (e.g., **Saccharomycetes**) and moulds. The hyphae are septate, and asexual spores are produced from conidiogenous cells borne on conidiophores. The sexual spore of the Ascomycetes is the ascospore, characterized by its production within a sac or **ascus.**

ARCHIASCOMYCETES

Archiascomycetes is a new class that was recently described to include an organism, *Pneumocystis carinii,* that had formerly been considered a protozoan. The reclassification of *Pneumocystis* was based on molecular evidence that it was most closely related to the ascomycete *Schizosaccharomyces pombe.* Further molecular studies resulted in the naming of human-derived strains as *Pneumocystis jiroveci.* The organism exists in a vegetative, trophic form that reproduces asexually by binary fission. Fusion of compatible mating types results in a spherical cyst or spore case, which on maturity contains eight spores.

BASIDIOMYCETES

The Basidiomycetes are rarely encountered clinically. The only human pathogen is *Filobasidiella neoformans,* the sexual form of *Cryptococcus neoformans.* The sexual spore of the Basidiomycetes is the basidiospore, characterized by the extension from a club-shaped structure, the basidium.

DEUTEROMYCETES

Deuteromycetes includes both yeasts and moulds that share a common lack of a sexual phase. Many of the fungi pathogenic to humans are included in this class. In general, these organisms have septate hyphae and produce conidia from conidiophores and conidiogenous cells. The yeasts reproduce by budding, and the moulds produce conidia by either a blastic (budding) process or a thallic process, in which hyphal segments fragment into individual cells or **arthroconidia.** Identification of individual genus and species is based in part on microscopic evaluation of the mode of development of the conidium from the conidiogenous cell.

Classification of Human Mycoses

In addition to the formal taxonomic classification of fungi, fungal infections may be classified according to the tissues infected, as well as by specific characteristics of organism groups. These classifications include the superficial, cutaneous, and subcutaneous mycoses; the endemic mycoses; and the opportunistic mycoses (Table 7–5).

SUPERFICIAL MYCOSES

The superficial mycoses are those infections that are limited to the very superficial surfaces of the skin and hair. They are nondestructive and of cosmetic importance only. The clinical infection pityriasis versicolor is characterized by discoloration or depigmentation and scaling of the skin. Tinea nigra refers to brown- or black-pigmented, macular patches localized primarily to the palms. The clinical entities of black and white piedra involve the hair and are characterized by nodules composed of hyphae that encompass the hair shaft. The fungi associated with these superficial infections include *Malassezia furfur, Phaeoannelomyces (Exophiala) werneckii, Piedraia hortae,* and *Trichosporon* spp.

CUTANEOUS MYCOSES

Cutaneous mycoses are infections of the keratinized layer of skin, hair, and nails. These infections may elicit a host response and become symptomatic. Signs and symptoms include itching, scaling, broken hairs, ringlike patches of the skin, and thickened, discolored nails. The Dermatophytes are fungi classified in the genera *Trichophyton, Epidermophyton,* and *Microsporum.* Infections of the skin involving these organisms are called dermatophytoses. Tinea unguium refers to infections of the toes involving these agents. Onychomycoses includes infections of the nails caused by the dermatophytes, as well as nondermatophytic fungi such as *Candida* spp. and *Aspergillus* spp.

TABLE 7–5. Classification of Human Mycoses and Representative Etiologic Agents

Superficial Mycoses	Cutaneous and Subcutaneous Mycoses	Endemic Mycoses	Opportunistic Mycoses
Black piedra	Dermatophytoses	Blastomycosis	Aspergillosis
Piedraia hortae	*Microsporum* spp.	*Blastomyces*	*Aspergillus fumigatus*
Tinea nigra	*Trichophyton* spp.	*dermatitidis*	*A. flavus*
Phaeoannelomyces wernickii	*Epidermophyton floccosum*	Histoplasmosis	*A. niger*
Pityriasis versicolor	Tinea unguium	*Histoplasma*	*A. terreus*
Malassezia furfur	*Trichophyton* spp.	*capsulatum*	Candidiasis
White piedra	*E. floccosum.*	Coccidioidomycosis	*Candida albicans*
Trichosporon spp.	Onychomycosis	*Coccidioides immitis*	*C. glabrata*
	Candida spp.	Penicilliosis	*C. parapsilosis*
	Aspergillus spp.	*Penicillium marneffei*	*C. tropicalis*
	Trichosporon spp.	Paracoccidioidomycosis	Cryptococcosis
	Geotrichum spp.	*Paracoccidioides*	*Cryptococcus*
	Mycotic keratitis	*brasiliensis*	*neoformans*
	Fusarium spp.		Trichosporonosis
	Aspergillus spp.		*Trichosporon* spp.
	Candida spp.		Hyalohyphomycosis
	Chromoblastomycosis		*Acremonium* spp.
	Cladosporium spp.		*Fusarium* spp.
	Fonsicaea spp.		*Paecilomyces* spp.
	Phialophora spp.		*Scedosporium* spp.
			Zygomycosis
			Rhizopus spp.
			Mucor spp.
			Absidia spp.
			Phaeohyphomycosis
			Alternaria spp.
			Curvularia spp.
			Bipolaris spp.
			Wangiella spp.
			Pneumocystosis
			Pneumocystis jiroveci

SUBCUTANEOUS MYCOSES

Subcutaneous mycoses involve the deeper layers of the skin, including the cornea, muscle, and connective tissue, and are caused by a broad spectrum of taxonomically diverse fungi. The fungi gain access to the deeper tissues, usually by traumatic inoculation, and remain localized, causing abscess formation, nonhealing ulcers, and draining sinus tracts. The host immune system recognizes the fungi, resulting in variable tissue destruction and, often, epitheliomatous hyperplasia. Infections may be caused by hyaline moulds such as *Acremonium* spp. and *Fusarium* spp. and by pigmented or dematiaceous fungi such as *Alternaria* spp., *Cladosporium* spp., and *Exophiala* spp. (Phaeohyphomycoses, Chromoblastomycoses). Subcutaneous mycoses tend to remain localized and rarely disseminate systemically.

ENDEMIC MYCOSES

The endemic mycoses are fungal infections caused by the classic dimorphic fungal pathogens *Histoplasma capsulatum, Blastomyces dermatitidis, Coccidioides immitis,* and *Paracoccidioides brasiliensis*. These fungi exhibit thermal dimorphism (i.e., exist as yeast at 37°C and mould at 25°C) and are generally confined to specific geographic regions where they occupy specific environmental or ecologic niches. The endemic mycoses are often referred to as **systemic mycoses,** because these organisms are true pathogens and can cause infection in healthy individuals. Recently the dimorphic fungus *Penicillium marneffei* was added to the list of agents causing endemic mycoses. All of these agents produce a primary infection in the lung, with subsequent dissemination to other organs and tissues.

OPPORTUNISTIC MYCOSES

The opportunistic mycoses are infections caused by fungi that are normally found as human commensals or in the environment. With the exception of *Cryptococcus neoformans*, these organisms exhibit inherently low or limited virulence and cause infection in individuals who are debilitated, immunosuppressed, or who carry implanted prosthetic devices or vascular catheters. Virtually any fungus can serve as an opportunistic pathogen, and the list of those identified as such becomes longer each year. The most common opportunistic fungal pathogens are the yeasts *Candida* spp. and *Cryptococcus neoformans*, the mould *Aspergillus* spp., and *Pneumocystis jiroveci*. Because of its inherent virulence, *Cryptococcus neoformans* is often considered a "systemic" pathogen. Although this fungus may cause infection in immunologically normal individuals, it clearly is seen more often as an opportunistic pathogen in the immunocompromised population.

Summary

With the ever-increasing number of individuals at risk for fungal infection, it is imperative that physicians "think fungus" when confronting a suspected infection. The list of documented fungal pathogens is extensive, and one can no longer ignore or dismiss fungi as "contaminants" or clinically insignificant when isolated from clinical material. It is also apparent that the prognosis and response to therapy may vary with the type of fungus causing infection, as well as with the immunologic status of the host. Thus physicians must become familiar with the various fungi and their epidemiologic and pathogenic features, as well as the optimal approaches to diagnosis and therapy. These issues will be discussed in detail in subsequent chapters according to the classification scheme shown in Table 7–5.

QUESTIONS

1. How do fungi differ from bacteria (i.e., size, nucleus, cytosol, plasma membrane, cell wall, physiology, generation time)?
2. How do the plasma membranes of fungi differ from those of other eukaryotic (e.g., mammalian) cells?
3. What is the difference between a yeast and a mould?
4. What do the terms *anamorph* and *teleomorph* mean, and why are they important?

Bibliography

Fromtling RA, Rhodes JC, Dixon DM: Taxonomy, classification, and morphology of the fungi. In Murray PR et al, editors: *Manual of clinical microbiology*, ed 8, Washington, 2003, American Society for Microbiology.

Rees JR et al: The epidemiological features of invasive mycotic infections in the San Francisco Bay Area, 1992-1993: Results of population-based laboratory active surveillance, *Clin Infect Dis* 27:1138-1147, 1998.

Rheingold AL et al: Systemic mycoses in the United States, 1980-1982, *J Med Vet Mycol* 24:433-436, 1986.

Wilson LS et al: The direct cost and incidence of systemic fungal infections, *Value Health* 5:26-34, 2002.

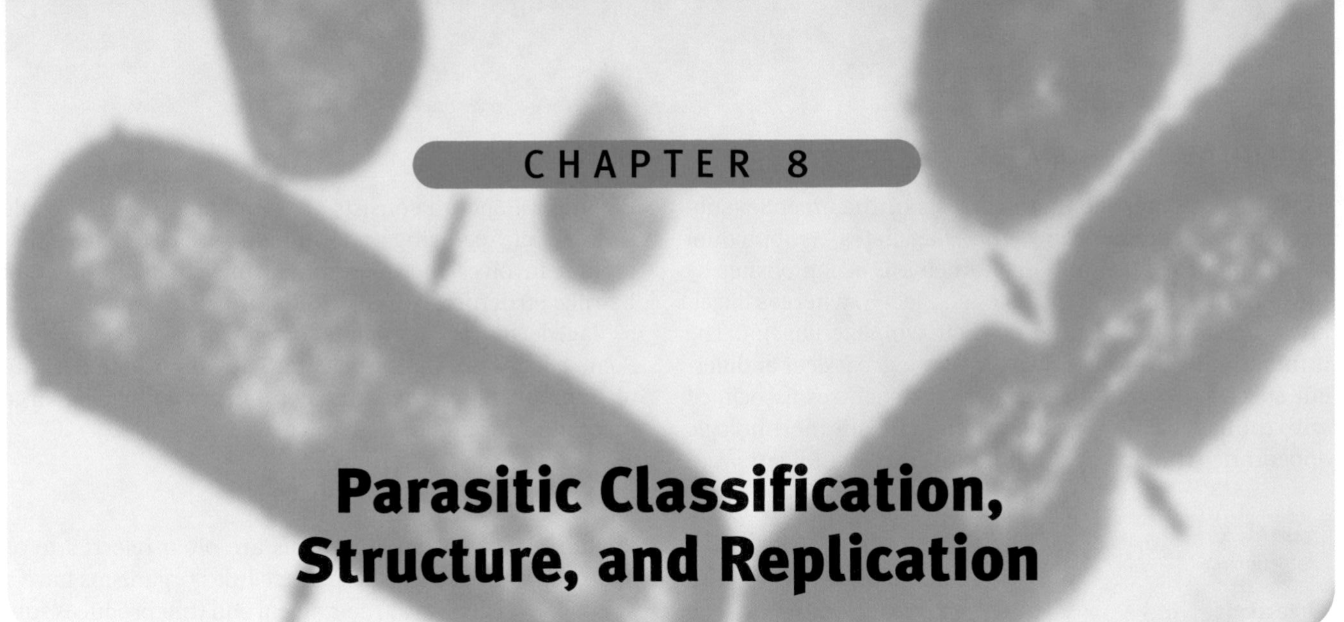

Parasitic Classification, Structure, and Replication

This chapter provides an introduction to parasite classification and physiology. This brief review is intended to enhance the reader's comprehension of the interrelationships among parasitic organisms, their epidemiology and transmission of disease, the specific disease processes involved, and the possibilities for prevention and control of maladies. We have deliberately attempted to simplify the taxonomy by using it to address the major divisions involved in medical parasitology—specifically, intestinal and urogenital protozoa, blood and tissue protozoa, nematodes, trematodes, and cestodes.

Importance of Parasites

Medical parasitology is the study of invertebrate animals capable of causing disease in humans and other animals. Although parasitic diseases are often considered "tropical," and thus of little importance to physicians practicing in the more temperate, developed countries of the world, it is clear that the world has become a very small place and that physicians' knowledge of parasitic diseases is essential. The global impact of parasitic infections and the number of parasite-associated deaths is staggering and must be of concern to all health care workers (Table 8–1). Increasingly, tourists, missionaries, Peace Corps volunteers, and others are visiting and working for extended periods in exotic, remote parts of the world. Thus they are at risk for parasitic and other infections that are rare in the United States and other more developed countries. Another source of infected patients is the ever-increasing number of refugees from developing countries. Finally, the profound immunosuppression problems that accompany advances in medical therapy (e.g., organ transplantation), as well as those associated with persons infected with human immunodeficiency virus (HIV), place a growing number of individuals at risk for developing infections caused by certain parasites. Given these considerations, clinicians and laboratory workers should be aware of the possibility of parasitic disease and should be trained in ordering, performing, and interpreting the appropriate laboratory tests to aid in the diagnosis and therapy.

Classification and Structure

The parasites of humans are classified within the kingdom Animalia and are separated into two subkingdoms, Protozoa and Metazoa (Table 8–2). Parasite classification takes into account the morphology of intracytoplasmic structures, such as the nucleus, the type of locomotive organelles, and the mode of reproduction (Table 8–3). The Protozoa are animals whose life functions occur in a single cell. The Metazoa are multicellular animals in which life functions occur in cellular structures organized as tissue and organ systems.

Protozoa

Protozoa are simple microorganisms that range in size from 2 to 100 μm. Their protoplasm is enclosed by a cell membrane and contains numerous organelles, including a membrane-bound nucleus, an endoplasmic reticulum, food-storage granules, and contractile and digestive vacuoles. The nucleus contains clumped or dispersed chromatin and a central karyosome. Organs of motility vary from simple cytoplasmic extrusions or pseudopods to more complex structures, such as flagella and cilia. The subkingdom Protozoa comprises seven major subgroups, or phyla, four of which are the concern of medical parasitology.

SARCOMASTIGOPHORA

Phylum Sarcomastigophora consists of the amebae (subphylum Sarcodina) and the flagellates (subphylum Mastigophora). Locomotion of amebae is accomplished by the extrusion of pseudopodia ("false feet"), whereas flagellates move by the lashing of their whiplike flagella. The number and position of flagella vary a great deal in different species. In addition, specialized structures associated with the flagella may produce a characteristic morphologic appearance that may be useful in species identification.

TABLE 8–1. Estimated Worldwide Disease Burden of Parasitic Infections

Infection	Disease Burden in DALYs (thousands)	Deaths (thousands)*
Malaria	42,280	1,124
Lymphatic filariasis	5,644	0
Leishmaniasis	2,357	59
Hookworm	1,825	—
Schistosomiasis	1,760	15
Trichuriasis	1,649	—
African trypanosomiasis	1,598	50
Ascariasis	1,181	—
Onchocerciasis	987	0
Chagas Disease	649	13

Adapted from Edwards G, Krishna S: Pharmacokinetic and pharmacodynamic issues in the treatment of parasite infections. *Eur J Clin Microbiol Infect Dis* 23:233-242, 2004.

DALYs, disability-adjusted life years (the number of healthy years of life lost because of premature death and disability).

*Mortality data included where available.

CILIOPHORA

Phylum Ciliophora consists of the ciliates, which include a variety of free-living and symbiotic species. Ciliate locomotion involves the coordinated movement of rows of hairlike structures, or cilia. Cilia are structurally similar to flagella but are usually shorter and more numerous. Some ciliates are multinucleate. The only ciliate parasite of humans, *Balantidium coli,* contains two nuclei: a large macronucleus and a small micronucleus.

APICOMPLEXA

Phylum Apicomplexa organisms are often referred to as Sporozoa or Coccidia. These unicellular organisms have a system of organelles at their apical end that produces substances to help the organism penetrate host cells and thus become an intracellular parasite.

MICROSPORA

Phylum Microspora organisms were formerly classified with the Sporozoa (Apicomplexa). The Microspora are small intracellular parasites that differ significantly in structure from the Apicomplexa organisms. These parasites are characterized by the structure of their spores, which have a complex, tubular extrusion mechanism (polar tubule) used to inject the infective material (sporoplasm) into host cells.

Metazoa

The subkingdom Metazoa includes all animals that are not Protozoa. This chapter discusses two groups of organisms of major importance: the helminths ("worms") and the arthropods (crabs, insects, ticks, and the like).

TABLE 8–2. Medically Important Parasites (Kingdom Animalia)

Subkingdom	Phylum	Organisms
Protozoa	Sarcomastigophora	Ameba, flagellates
	Ciliophora	Ciliates
	Apicomplexa	Sporozoa, Coccidia
	Microspora	Microsporidia
Metazoa	Nematoda	Roundworms
	Platyhelminthes	Flatworms
	Trematodes	Flukes
	Cestodes	Tapeworms
	Arthropoda	
	Chilopoda	Centipedes
	Pentastomida	Tongue worms
	Crustacea	Crabs, crayfish, shrimp, copepods
	Arachnida	Mites, ticks, spiders, scorpions
	Insecta	Mosquitoes, flies, lice, fleas, wasps, ants, beetles, moths, roaches, true bugs

TABLE 8–3. Biologic, Morphologic, and Physiologic Characteristics of Pathogenic Parasites

Organism Class	Morphology	Reproduction	Organelles of Locomotion	Respiration	Nutrition
Protozoa					
Ameba	Unicellular; cyst and trophozoite forms	Binary fission	Pseudopods	Facultative anaerobe	Assimilation by pinocytosis or phagocytosis
Flagellates	Unicellular; cyst and trophozoite forms; possibly intracellular	Binary fission	Flagella	Facultative anaerobe	Simple diffusion or ingestion via cytostome, pinocytosis, or phagocytosis
Ciliates	Unicellular; cysts and trophozoite	Binary fission or conjugation	Cilia	Facultative anaerobe	Ingestion via cytostome, food vacuole
Coccidia	Unicellular, frequently intracellular; multiple forms, including trophozoites, sporozoites, cysts (oocysts), gametes	Schizogony and sporogony	None	Facultative anaerobe	Simple diffusion
Microsporidia	Obligate intracellular forms; small, simple cells and spores	Binary fission, schizogony and sporogony	None	Facultative anaerobe	Simple diffusion
Helminths					
Nematodes	Multicellular; round, smooth, spindle shaped, tubular alimentary tract; possibility of teeth or plates for attachment	Separate sexes	No single organelle; active muscular motility	Adults: usually anaerobic; larvae: possibly aerobic	Ingestion or absorption of body fluids, tissue, or digestive contents
Trematodes	Multicellular; leaf shaped with oral and ventral suckers; blind alimentary tract	Hermaphroditic (Schistosoma group has separate sexes)	No single organelle; muscle-directed motility	Adults: usually anaerobic	Ingestion or absorption of body fluids, tissue, or digestive contents
Cestodes	Multicellular; head with segmented body (proglottids); lack of alimentary tract; head equipped with hooks and/or suckers for attachment	Hermaphroditic	No single organelle; usually, attachment to mucosa, possible muscular motility (proglottids)	Adults: usually anaerobic	Absorption of nutrients from intestine
Arthropods					
Chilopoda	Elongated; many legs; distinctive head and trunk; poisoning claws on first segment	Separate sexes	Legs	Aerobic	Carnivore

TABLE 8–3. Biologic, Morphologic, and Physiologic Characteristics of Pathogenic Parasites—*cont'd*

Organism Class	Morphology	Reproduction	Organelles of Locomotion	Respiration	Nutrition
Pentastomida	Wormlike; cylindrical, or flattened; two distinct body regions; digestive and reproductive organs; lack of circulatory and respiratory systems	Separate sexes	Muscle-directed motility	Aerobic	Ingestion of body fluids and tissue
Crustacea	Hard external carapace; one pair of maxillae; five pairs of biramous legs	Separate sexes	Legs	Aerobic	Ingestion of body fluids and tissue, carnivorous
Arachnida	Body divided into cephalothorax and abdomen; eight legs and poisoning fangs	Separate sexes	Legs	Aerobic	Carnivore
Insecta	Body: head, thorax, and abdomen; one pair of antennae; three pairs of appendages, up to two pairs of wings	Separate sexes	Legs, wings	Aerobic	Ingestion of fluids and tissues

HELMINTHS

The helminths are complex, multicellular organisms that are elongated and bilaterally symmetrical. They are considerably larger than the protozoan parasites and generally are macroscopic, ranging in size from less than 1 mm to 1 m or larger. The external surface of some worms is covered with a protective cuticle, which is acellular and may be smooth or possess ridges, spines, or tubercles. The protective covering of flatworms is known as a tegument. Often, helminths possess elaborate attachment structures such as hooks, suckers, teeth, or plates. These structures are usually located anteriorly and may be useful in classifying and identifying the organisms (see Table 8–3). Helminths typically have primitive nervous and excretory systems. Some have alimentary tracts; however, none have a circulatory system. The helminths are separated into two phyla, the Nematoda and the Platyhelminthes.

Nematoda

Phylum Nematoda consists of the roundworms, which have cylindrical bodies. The sexes of roundworm are separate, and these organisms have a complete digestive system. The nematodes may be intestinal parasites or may infect the blood and tissue.

Platyhelminthes

Phylum Platyhelminthes consists of the flatworms, which have flattened bodies that are leaflike or resemble ribbon segments. Platyhelminthes can be further separated into trematodes and cestodes.

Trematodes, or flukes, have leaf-shaped bodies. Most are hermaphroditic, with male and female sex organs in a single body. Their digestive systems are incomplete and only have saclike tubes. Their life cycle is complex; snails serve as first intermediate hosts, and other aquatic animals or plants serve as second intermediate hosts.

Cestodes, or tapeworms, have bodies composed of ribbons of proglottids, or segments. All are hermaphroditic, and all lack digestive systems, with nutrition being absorbed through the body walls. The life cycles of some cestodes are simple and direct, whereas those of others are complex and require one or more intermediate hosts.

ARTHROPODS

Phylum Arthropoda is the largest group of animals in the kingdom Animalia. Arthropods are complex, multicellular organisms that may be involved directly in causing invasive or superficial (infestation) disease processes or indirectly as intermediate hosts and vectors of many infectious agents, including protozoan and metazoan parasites (Table 8–4). In addition, envenomization by biting and stinging arthropods can result in adverse reactions in humans that range from local allergic and hypersensitivity reactions to severe anaphylactic shock and death. There are five major classes of arthropods (see Table 8–2).

Chilopoda

Class Chilopoda consists of terrestrial forms, such as centipedes. These organisms are of medical importance because of their poisoning claws, which may produce a painful "bite."

TABLE 8–4. Transmission and Distribution of Pathogenic Parasites

Organism	Infective Form	Mechanism of Spread	Distribution
Intestinal Protozoa			
Entamoeba histolytica	Cyst/trophozoite	Indirect (fecal-oral) Direct (venereal)	Worldwide
Giardia lamblia	Cyst	Fecal-oral route	Worldwide
Dientamoeba fragilis	Trophozoite	Fecal-oral route	Worldwide
Balantidium coli	Cyst	Fecal-oral route	Worldwide
Isospora belli	Oocyst	Fecal-oral route	Worldwide
Cryptosporidium species	Oocyst	Fecal-oral route	Worldwide
Enterocytozoon bieneusi	Spore	Fecal-oral route	North America, Europe
Urogenital Protozoa			
Trichomonas vaginalis	Trophozoite	Direct (venereal) route	Worldwide
Blood and Tissue Protozoa			
Naegleria and Acanthamoeba species	Cyst/trophozoite	Direct inoculation, inhalation	Worldwide
Plasmodium species	Sporozoite	Anopheles mosquito	Tropical and subtropical areas
Babesia species	Pyriform body	Ixodes tick	North America, Europe
Toxoplasma gondii	Oocysts and tissue cysts	Fecal-oral route, carnivorism	Worldwide
Leishmania species	Promastigote	Phlebotomus sandfly	Tropical and subtropical areas
Trypanosoma cruzi	Trypomastigote	Reduviid bug	North, Central, and South America
Trypanosom brucei	Trypomastigote	Tsetse fly	Africa
Nematodes			
Enterobius vermicularis	Egg	Fecal-oral route	Worldwide
Ascaris lumbricoides	Egg	Fecal-oral route	Areas of poor sanitation
Toxocara species	Egg	Fecal-oral route	Worldwide
Trichuris trichiura	Egg	Fecal-oral route	Worldwide
Ancylostoma duodenale	Filariform lava	Direct skin penetration from contaminated soil	Tropical and subtropical areas
Necator americanus	Filariform larva	Direct skin penetration, autoinfection	Tropical and subtropical areas
Strongyloides	Filariform larva	Direct skin penetration, autoinfection	Tropical and subtropical areas
Trichinella spiralis	Encysted larva in tissue	Carnivorism	Worldwide
Wuchereria bancrofti	Third-stage larva	Mosquito	Tropical and subtropical areas
Brugia malayi	Third-stage larva	Mosquito	Tropical and subtropical areas
Loa loa	Filariform larva	Chrysops fly	Africa
Mansonella species	Third-stage larva	Biting midges or black flies	Africa and Central and South America
Onchocerca volvulus	Third-stage larva	Simulium black fly	Africa and Central and South America
Dracunculus medinensis	Third-stage larva	Ingestion of infected cyclops	Africa, Asia
Dirofilaria immitis	Third-stage larva	Mosquito	Japan, Australia, United States

TABLE 8–4. Transmission and Distribution of Pathogenic Parasites—*cont'd*

Organism	Infective Form	Mechanism of Spread	Distribution
Trematodes			
Fasciolopsis buski	Metacercaria	Ingestion of metacercaria encysted on aquatic plants	China, Southeast Asia, India
Fasciola hepatica	Metacercaria	Metacercaria on water plants	Worldwide
Opisthorchis (Clonorchis) sinensis	Metacercaria	Metacercaria encysted in freshwater fish	China, Japan, Korea, Vietnam
Paragonimus westermani	Metacercaria	Metacercaria encysted in freshwater crustaceans	Asia, Africa, India, Latin America
Schistosoma species	Cercaria	Direct penetration of skin by free-swimming cercaria	Africa, Asia, India, Latin America
Cestodes			
Taenia solium	Cysticercus, embryonated egg or proglottid	Ingestion of infected pork; ingestion of egg (cysticercosis)	Pork-eating countries: Africa, Southeast Asia, China, Latin America
Taenia saginata	Cysticercus	Ingestion of cysticercus in meat	Worldwide
Diphyllobothrium latum	Sparganum	Ingestion of sparganum in fish	Worldwide
Echinococcus granulosus	Embryonated egg	Ingestion of eggs from infected canines	Sheep-raising countries: Europe, Asia, Africa, Australia, United States
Echinococcus multilocularis	Embryonated egg	Ingestion of eggs from infected animals, fecal-oral route	Canada, Northern United States, Central Europe
Hymenolepsis nana	Embryonated egg	Ingestion of eggs; fecal-oral route	Worldwide
Hymenolepsis diminuta	Cysticercus	Ingestion of infected beetle larvae in contaminated grain products	Worldwide
Dipylidium caninum	Cysticercus	Ingestion of infected fleas	Worldwide

Pentastomida

The pentastomids, or tongue worms, are bloodsucking endoparasites of reptiles, birds, and mammals. Adult pentastomids are white and cylindrical or flattened parasites that possess two distinct body regions: an anterior cephalothorax and an abdomen. Humans may serve as intermediate hosts for these parasites.

Crustacea

Class Crustacea consists of familiar aquatic forms, such as crabs, crayfish, shrimp, and copepods. Several are involved as intermediate hosts in life cycles of various intestinal or blood and tissue helminths.

Arachnida

Class Arachnida consists of familiar terrestrial forms, such as mites, ticks, spiders, and scorpions. Unlike insects, these animals have no wings or antennae, and adults have four pairs of legs, as opposed to three pairs for insects. Of medical importance are those serving as vectors for microbial diseases (mites and ticks) or as venomous animals that bite (spiders) or sting (scorpions).

Insecta

Class Insecta consists of familiar aquatic and terrestrial forms, such as mosquitoes, flies, midges, fleas, lice, bugs, wasps, and ants. Wings and antennae are present, and adult forms have three pairs of legs. Of medical importance are the many insects that serve as vectors for microbial diseases (mosquitoes, fleas, flies, lice, and bugs) or as venomous animals that sting (bees, wasps, and ants).

Physiology And Replication

PROTOZOA

The nutritional requirements of the parasitic protozoa are generally simple and require the assimilation of organic nutrients. The amebae, ameboflagellates, and certain other protozoa accomplish this assimilation by the rather primitive process of pinocytosis, or phagocytosis, of soluble or particulate matter (see Table 8–3). The engulfed material is enclosed in digestive vacuoles. The flagellates and ciliates generally ingest food at a definitive site or structure, the peristome or cytostome. Other protozoan parasites, such as the intracellular microsporidia, assimilate nutrients by simple diffusion. The ingested food material may be retained in intracytoplasmic granules or in vacuoles. The undigested particles and waste may be eliminated from the cell by extrusion of the material at the cell surface. Facultatively anaerobic processes accomplish respiration in most parasitic protozoa.

To ensure survival under harsh or unfavorable environmental conditions, many parasitic protozoa develop into a cyst form that is less metabolically active. This cyst is surrounded by a thick external cell wall capable of protecting the organism from otherwise lethal physical and chemical insults. The cyst form is an integral part of the life cycle of many protozoan parasites and facilitates the transmission of the organism from host to host in the external environment. Parasites that cannot form cysts must rely on direct transmission from host to host or require an arthropod vector to complete their life cycles (see Table 8–4).

In addition to cyst formation, many protozoan parasites have developed elaborate immunoevasive mechanisms that allow them to respond to attack by the host immune system by continuously changing their surface antigens, thus ensuring continued survival within the host. Reproduction among the protozoa is generally by simple binary fission (merogony), although the life cycle of some protozoa, such as the sporozoans, includes cycles of multiple fission (schizogony), alternating with a period of sexual reproduction (sporogony or gametogony).

METAZOA

Helminths

The nutritional requirements of helminthic parasites are met by active ingestion of host tissue, fluids, or both, with resultant tissue destruction, or by more passive absorption of nutrients from the surrounding fluids and intestinal contents (see Table 8–3). The muscular motility of many helminths expends considerable energy, and the worms rapidly metabolize carbohydrates. Nutrients are stored in the form of glycogen, the content of which is high in most helminths. Similar to respiration in protozoa, respiration in helminths is primarily anaerobic, although the larval forms may require oxygen.

A significant proportion of the energy requirement of helminths is dedicated to supporting the reproductive process. Many worms are quite prolific, producing as many as 200,000 offspring each day. In general, helminthic parasites lay eggs (oviparous), although a few species may bear live young (viviparous). The resulting larvae are always morphologically distinct from the adult parasites and must undergo several developmental stages or molts before attaining adulthood.

The major protective barrier for most helminths is the tough external layer (cuticle or tegument). Worms may also secrete enzymes that destroy host cells and neutralize immunologic and cellular defense mechanisms. Similar to protozoan parasites, some helminths possess the ability to alter the antigenic properties of their external surfaces and thus evade the host immune response. This is accomplished in part by incorporating host antigens into their external cuticular layer. In this way, the worm avoids immunologic recognition, and in some diseases (e.g., schistosomiasis) it allows the parasite to survive within the host for decades.

Arthropods

Arthropods have segmented bodies, paired jointed appendages, and well-developed digestive and nervous systems. Sexes are separate. Respiration by aquatic forms is via gills and by terrestrial forms is via tubular body structures. All have a hard chitin covering as an exoskeleton.

Summary

Physician awareness of parasitic diseases is undoubtedly more critical now than at any time in the history of medical practice. Physicians today must be prepared to answer questions from patients about protection from malaria and the risks of drinking water and eating fresh fruits and vegetables in remote areas where they may be traveling. With this knowledge of parasitic diseases, the physician can also evaluate signs, symptoms, and incubation periods in returning travelers and make a diagnosis and begin treatment for a patient with a possible parasitic disease. The risks of parasitic diseases in immunosuppressed individuals, and those with acquired immunodeficiency syndrome, must also be understood and taken into account.

Proper education regarding parasitic diseases in medical curricula cannot be overemphasized as a requirement for physicians whose practice includes travelers to foreign countries and refugee populations. Many of the important parasites responsible for human diseases are transmitted by arthropod vectors or are acquired by the consumption of contaminated food or water. The various modes of transmission and distribution of parasitic diseases are presented in appropriate detail in the following chapters; however, the data in Table 8–4 are provided as an outline.

QUESTIONS

1. How do protozoa adapt to harsh environmental conditions?
2. Which morphologic form is important in the transmission of protozoa from host to host?
3. How do helminths, such as schistosomes, avoid the host immune response?
4. How do arthropods cause human disease?

Bibliography

Cox FEC: History of human parasitology, *Clin Microbiol Rev* 15:595-612, 2002.

Edwards G, Krishna S: Pharmacokinetic and pharmacodynamic issues in the treatment of infections. *Eur J Clin Microbiol Infect Dis* 23:233-242, 2004.

Garcia LS, editor: *Diagnostic medical parasitology*, ed 4, Washington, 2001, American Society for Microbiology.

Markell EK, John DT, Krotoski WA, editors: *Markell and Voge's medical parasitology*, ed 8, Philadelphia, 1999, WB Saunders.

Murray PR et al, editors: *Manual of clinical microbiology*, ed 8, Washington, 2003, American Society for Microbiology.

Strickland GT, editors: Hunter's *Tropical medicine and emerging infectious disease*, ed 8, Philadelphia, 2000, WB Saunders.

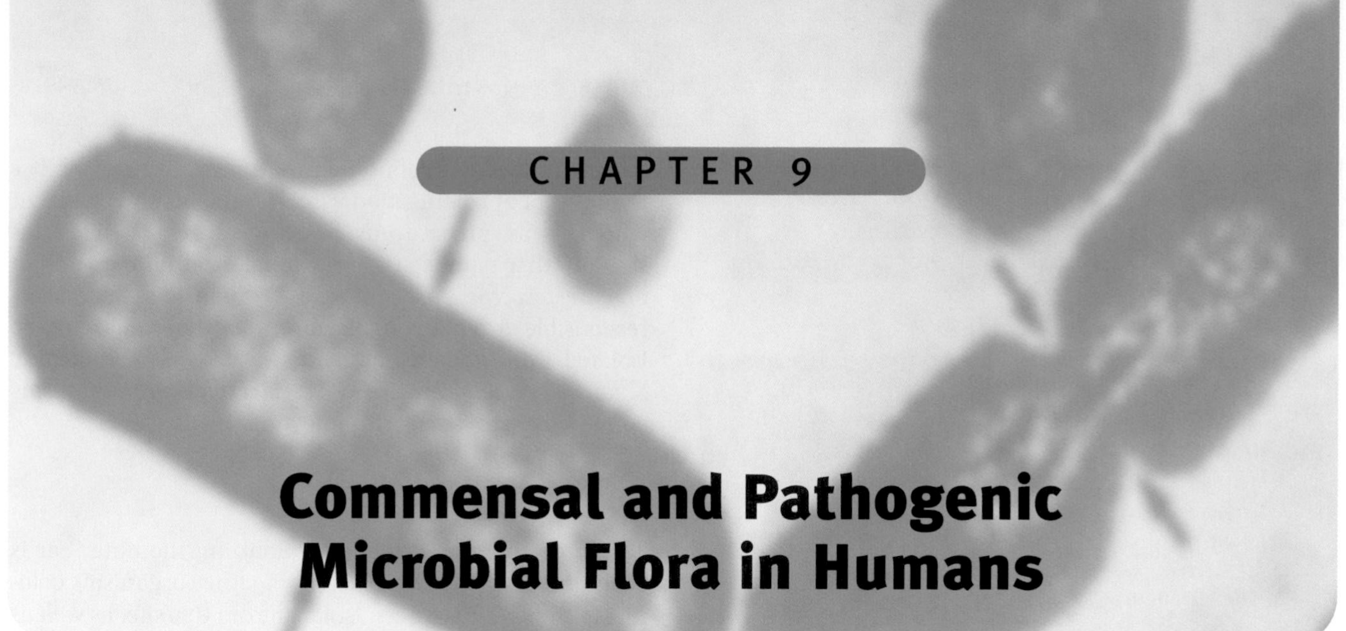

CHAPTER 9

Commensal and Pathogenic Microbial Flora in Humans

Medical microbiology is the study of the interactions between animals (primarily humans) and microorganisms, such as bacteria, viruses, fungi, and parasites. Although the primary interest is in diseases caused by these interactions, it must also be appreciated that microorganisms play a critical role in human survival. The normal commensal population of microbes participates in the metabolism of food products, provides essential growth factors, protects against infections with highly virulent microorganisms, and stimulates the immune response. In the absence of these organisms, life as we know it would be impossible.

The microbial flora in and on the human body is in a continual state of flux determined by a variety of factors, such as age, diet, hormonal state, health, and personal hygiene. Whereas the human fetus lives in a protected, sterile environment, the newborn human is exposed to microbes from the mother and the environment. The infant's skin is colonized first, followed by the oropharynx, gastrointestinal tract, and other mucosal surfaces. Throughout the life of an human being, this microbial population continues to change. Changes in health can drastically disrupt the delicate balance that is maintained among the heterogeneous organisms coexisting within us. For example, hospitalization can lead to the replacement of normally avirulent organisms in the oropharynx with gram-negative rods (e.g., *Klebsiella, Pseudomonas*) that can invade the lungs and cause pneumonia. Likewise, the indigenous bacteria present in the intestines restrict the growth of Clostridium difficile in the gastrointestinal tract. In the presence of antibiotics, however, this indigenous flora is eliminated, and *C. difficile* is able to proliferate and produce diarrheal disease and colitis.

Exposure of an individual to an organism can lead to one of three outcomes. The organism can: (1) transiently colonize the person, (2) permanently colonize the person, or (3) produce disease. It is important to understand the distinction between **colonization** and **disease** (Box 9–1). (Note: many people use the term *infection* inappropriately as a synonym for both terms.) Organisms that colonize humans (whether for a short period such as hours or days [transient] or permanently) do not interfere with normal body functions. In contrast, disease occurs when the interaction between microbe and human leads to a pathologic process characterized by damage to the human host. This process can result from microbial factors (e.g., damage to organs caused by the proliferation of the microbe or the production of toxins or cytotoxic enzymes) or the host's immune response to the organism (e.g., the pathology of several acute respiratory syndrome [SARS] coronavirus infections is primarily caused by the patient's immune response to the virus).

An understanding of medical microbiology requires knowledge not only of the different classes of microbes but also of their propensity for causing disease. A few infections are caused by **strict pathogens** (i.e., organisms always associated with human disease; see Box 9–1). A few examples of strict pathogens and the diseases they cause include *Mycobacterium tuberculosis* (tuberculosis), *Neisseria gonorrhoeae* (gonorrhea), *Francisella tularensis* (tularemia), *Plasmodium* spp. (malaria), and rabies virus (rabies). Most human infections are caused by **opportunistic pathogens** (see Box 9–1), organisms that are typically members of the patient's normal microbial flora (e.g., *Staphylococcus aureus, Escherichia coli, Candida albicans*). These organisms do not produce disease in their normal setting but establish disease when they are introduced into unprotected sites (e.g., blood, tissues). The specific factors responsible for the virulence of strict and opportunistic pathogens are discussed in later chapters. If a patient's immune system is defective, that patient is more susceptible to disease caused by opportunistic pathogens.

BOX 9–1. Key Terms

Colonization	Strict pathogen
Disease	Opportunistic pathogen

BOX 9–2. Most Common Microbes That Colonize the Upper Respiratory Tract

Bacteria	*Peptostreptococcus*
Acinetobacter	*Porphyromonas*
Actinobacillus	*Prevotella*
Actinomyces	*Propionibacterium*
Cardiobacterium	*Staphylococcus*
Corynebacterium	*Streptococcus*
Eikenella	*Stomatococcus*
Enterobacteriaceae	*Treponema*
Eubacterium	*Veillonella*
Fusobacterium	**Fungi**
Haemophilus	*Candida*
Kingella	**Parasites**
Moraxella	*Entamoeba*
Mycoplasma	*Trichomonas*
Neisseria	

The microbial population that colonizes the human body is numerous and diverse. The most common organisms that form the commensal flora and the organisms associated with disease are summarized in this chapter.

Respiratory Tract and Head

MOUTH, OROPHARYNX, AND NASOPHARYNX

The upper respiratory tract is colonized with numerous organisms, with 10 to 100 anaerobes for every aerobic bacterium (Box 9–2). The most common anaerobic bacteria are *Peptostreptococcus* and related anaerobic cocci, *Veillonella, Actinomyces,* and *Fusobacterium* spp. The most common aerobic bacteria are *Streptococcus, Haemophilus,* and *Neisseria* spp. The relative proportion of these organisms varies at different anatomic sites; for example, the microbial flora on the surface of a tooth is quite different from the flora in saliva or in the subgingival spaces. Most of the common organisms in the upper respiratory tract are relatively avirulent and are rarely associated with disease unless they are introduced into normally sterile sites (e.g., sinuses, middle ear, brain). Potentially pathogenic organisms, including *Streptococcus pyogenes, Streptococcus pneumoniae, S. aureus, Neisseria meningitidis, Haemophilus influenzae, Moraxella catarrhalis,* and *Enterobacteriaceae,* can also be found in the upper airways. Isolation of these organisms from an upper respiratory tract specimen does not define their pathogenicity (remember the concept of colonization vs. disease). Their involvement with a disease process must be demonstrated by the exclusion of other pathogens. For example, with the exception of *Streptococcus pyogenes,* these organisms are rarely responsible for pharyngitis, even though they can be isolated from patients with this disease. *S. pneumoniae, S. aureus, H. influenzae,* and *M. catarrhalis* are organisms commonly associated with infections of the sinuses.

EAR

The most common organism colonizing the outer ear is coagulase-negative *Staphylococcus.* Other organisms colonizing the skin have been isolated from this site, as well as potential pathogens such as *S. pneumoniae, Pseudomonas aeruginosa,* and members of the Enterobacteriaceae family.

EYE

The surface of the eye is colonized with coagulase-negative staphylococci, as well as rare numbers of organisms found in the nasopharynx (e.g., *Haemophilus* spp., *Neisseria* spp., viridans streptococci). Disease is typically associated with *S. pneumoniae, S. aureus, H. influenzae, N. gonorrhoeae, Chlamydia trachomatis, P. aeruginosa,* and *Bacillus cereus.*

LOWER RESPIRATORY TRACT

The larynx, trachea, bronchioles, and lower airways are generally sterile, although transient colonization with secretions of the upper respiratory tract may occur. More virulent bacteria present in the mouth (e.g., *S. pneumoniae, S. aureus,* members of the family Enterobacteriaceae such as *Klebsiella*) cause acute disease of the lower airway. Chronic aspiration may lead to a polymicrobial disease in which anaerobes are the predominant pathogens, particularly *Peptostreptococcus,* related anaerobic cocci, and anaerobic gram-negative rods. Fungi such as *Candida albicans* are a rare cause of disease in the lower airway, and invasion of these organisms into tissue must be demonstrated to exclude simple colonization. In contrast, the presence of the dimorphic fungi (e.g., *Histoplasma, Coccidioides,* and *Blastomyces* spp.) is diagnostic because asymptomatic colonization with these organisms never occurs.

Gastrointestinal Tract

The gastrointestinal tract is colonized with microbes at birth and remains the home for a diverse population of organisms throughout the life of the host (Box 9–3). Although the opportunity for colonization with new

BOX 9–3. Most Common Microbes That Colonize the Gastrointestinal Tract

Bacteria
- *Acinetobacter*
- *Actinomyces*
- *Bacteroides*
- *Bifidobacterium*
- *Campylobacter*
- *Clostridium*
- *Corynebacterium*
- *Eubacterium*
- Enterobacteriaceae
- *Enterococcus*
- *Fusobacterium*
- *Haemophilus*
- *Helicobacter*
- *Lactobacillus*
- *Mobiluncus*
- *Peptostreptococcus*
- *Porphyromonas*
- *Prevotella*
- *Propionibacterium*
- *Pseudomonas*
- *Staphylococcus*
- *Streptococcus*
- *Veillonella*

Fungi
- *Candida*

Parasites
- *Blastocystis*
- *Chilomastix*
- *Endolimax*
- *Entamoeba*
- *Iodamoeba*
- *Trichomonas*

organisms occurs daily with the ingestion of food and water, the population remains relatively constant, unless exogenous factors such as antibiotic treatment disrupt the balanced flora.

ESOPHAGUS

Oropharyngeal bacteria and yeast, as well as the bacteria that colonize the stomach, can be isolated from the esophagus; however, most organisms are believed to be transient colonizers that do not establish permanent residence. Bacteria rarely cause disease of the esophagus (esophagitis); *Candida* spp. and viruses such as herpes simplex virus and cytomegalovirus cause most infections.

STOMACH

Because the stomach contains hydrochloric acid and pepsinogen (secreted by the parietal and chief cells lining the gastric mucosa), the only organisms present are small numbers of acid-tolerant bacteria, such as the lactic acid–producing bacteria (*Lactobacillus* and *Streptococcus* spp.) and *Helicobacter pylori*. *H. pylori* is a cause of gastritis and ulcerative disease. The microbial population can dramatically change in numbers and diversity in patients receiving drugs that neutralize or reduce the production of gastric acids.

SMALL INTESTINE

In contrast with the anterior portion of the digestive tract, the small intestine is colonized with many different bacteria, fungi, and parasites. Most of these organisms are anaerobes, such as *Peptostreptococcus*, *Porphyromonas*, and *Prevotella*. Common causes of gastroenteritis (e.g., *Salmonella* and *Campylobacter* spp.) can be present in small numbers as asymptomatic residents; however, their detection in the clinical laboratory generally indicates disease. If the small intestine is obstructed, such as after abdominal surgery, then a condition called blind loop syndrome can occur. In this case, stasis of the intestinal contents leads to the colonization and proliferation of the organisms typically present in the large intestine, with a subsequent malabsorption syndrome.

LARGE INTESTINE

More microbes are present in the large intestine than anywhere else in the human body. It is estimated that more than 10^{11} bacteria per gram of feces can be found, with anaerobic bacteria in excess by more than 1000-fold. Various yeasts and nonpathogenic parasites can also establish residence in the large intestine. The most common bacteria include *Bifidobacterium*, *Eubacterium*, *Bacteroides*, *Enterococcus*, and the Enterobacteriaceae family. *E. coli* is present in virtually all humans from birth until death. Although this organism represents less than 1% of the intestinal population, it is the most common aerobic organism responsible for intraabdominal disease. Likewise, *Bacteroides fragilis* is a minor member of the intestinal flora, but it is the most common anaerobe responsible for intraabdominal disease. In contrast, *Eubacterium* and *Bifidobacterium* are the most common bacteria in the large intestine but are rarely responsible for disease. These organisms simply lack the diverse virulence factors found in *B. fragilis*.

Antibiotic treatment can rapidly alter the population, causing the proliferation of antibiotic-resistant organisms, such as *Enterococcus*, *Pseudomonas*, and fungi. *C. difficile* can also grow rapidly in this situation, leading to diseases ranging from diarrhea to pseudomembranous colitis. Exposure to other enteric pathogens, such as *Shigella*, enterohemorrhagic *E. coli*, and *Entamoeba histolytica*, can also disrupt the colonic flora and produce significant intestinal disease.

Genitourinary System

In general the anterior urethra and vagina are the only anatomic areas of the genitourinary system permanently colonized with microbes (Box 9–4). Although the urinary bladder can be transiently colonized with bacteria migrating upstream from the urethra, these should be cleared rapidly by the bactericidal activity of the uroepithelial cells and the flushing action of voided urine. The other structures of the urinary system should be sterile, except when disease or an anatomic abnormality is present. Likewise, the uterus should also remain free of organisms.

BOX 9–4. Most Common Microbes That Colonize the Genitourinary Tract

Bacteria
Actinomyces
Bacteroides
Bifidobacterium
Clostridium
Corynebacterium
Enterococcus
Enterobacteriaceae
Eubacterium
Fusobacterium
Gardnerella
Haemophilus
Lactobacillus
Mobiluncus
Mycoplasma
Peptostreptococcus
Porphyromonas
Prevotella
Propionibacterium
Staphylococcus
Streptococcus
Treponema
Ureaplasma

Fungi
Candida

ANTERIOR URETHRA

The commensal population of the urethra consists of a variety of organisms, with lactobacilli, streptococci, and coagulase-negative staphylococci the most numerous. These organisms are relatively avirulent and are rarely associated with human disease. In contrast, the urethra can be colonized transiently with fecal organisms such as *Enterococcus*, Enterobacteriaceae, and *Candida*—all of which can invade the urinary tract, multiply in urine, and lead to significant disease. Pathogens such as *N. gonorrhoeae* and *C. trachomatis* are common causes of urethritis and can persist as asymptomatic colonizers of the urethra. The isolation of these two organisms in clinical specimens should always be considered significant, regardless of the presence or absence of clinical symptoms.

VAGINA

The microbial population of the vagina is more diverse and is dramatically influenced by hormonal factors. Newborn girls are colonized with lactobacilli at birth, and these bacteria predominate for approximately 6 weeks. After that time, the levels of maternal estrogen have declined, and the vaginal flora changes to include staphylococci, streptococci, and Enterobacteriaceae. When estrogen production is initiated at puberty, the microbial flora again changes. Lactobacilli reemerge as the predominant organisms, and many other organisms are also isolated, including staphylococci (*S. aureus* less commonly than the coagulase-negative species), streptococci (including group B *Streptococcus*), *Enterococcus, Gardnerella, Mycoplasma, Ureaplasma,* Enterobacteriaceae, and a variety of anaerobic bacteria. *N. gonorrhoeae* is a common cause of vaginitis. In the absence of this organism, significant numbers of cases develop when the balance of vaginal bacteria is disrupted, resulting in decreases in the number of lactobacilli and increases in the number of *Mobiluncus* and *Gardnerella*. *Trichomonas vaginalis, C. albicans*, and *Candida glabrata* are also important causes of vaginitis. Although herpes simplex virus and papillomavirus would not be considered normal flora of the genitourinary tract, these viruses can establish persistent infections.

BOX 9–5. Most Common Microbes That Colonize the Skin

Bacteria
Acinetobacter
Aerococcus
Bacillus
Clostridium
Corynebacterium
Micrococcus
Peptostreptococcus
Propionibacterium
Staphylococcus
Streptococcus

Fungi
Candida
Malassezia

CERVIX

Although the cervix is not normally colonized with bacteria, *N. gonorrhoeae* and *C. trachomatis* are important causes of cervicitis. *Actinomyces* can also produce disease at this site.

Skin

Although many organisms come into contact with the skin surface, this relatively hostile environment does not support the survival of most organisms (Box 9–5). Gram-positive bacteria (e.g., coagulase-negative *Staphylococcus* and, less commonly, *S. aureus*, corynebacteria, and propionibacteria) are the most common organisms found on the skin surface. *Clostridium perfringens* is isolated on the skin of approximately 20% of healthy individuals, and the fungi *Candida* and *Malassezia* are also found on skin surfaces, particularly in moist sites. Streptococci can colonize the skin transiently, but the volatile fatty acids produced by the anaerobe propionibacteria are toxic for these organisms. Gram-negative rods do not permanently colonize the skin surface (with the exception of *Acinetobacter* and a few other less common genera) because the skin is too dry.

QUESTIONS

1. What is the distinction between *colonization* and *disease*?
2. Give examples of strict pathogens and opportunistic pathogens.
3. What factors regulate the microbial populations of organisms that colonize humans?

Bibliography

Balows A, Truper H: *The prokaryotes,* ed 2, New York, 1992, Springer-Verlag.

Granato P: Pathogenic and indigenous microorganisms of humans. In Murray P et al, editors: *Manual of clinical microbiology,* ed 8, Washington, 2003, American Society for Microbiology.

Murray P: Human microbiota. In Balows A et al: *Topley and Wilson's microbiology and microbial infections,* ed 10, London, 2005, Edward Arnold.

Murray P, Shea Y: *Pocket guide to clinical microbiology,* ed 3, Washington, 2004, American Society for Microbiology.

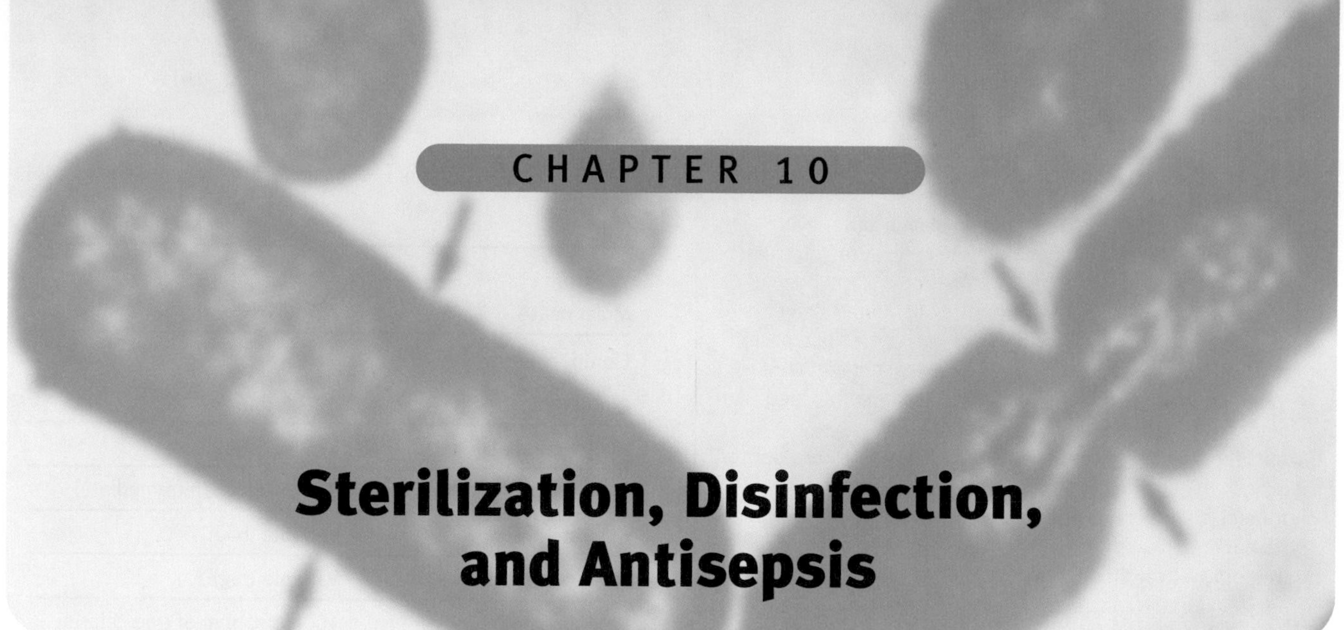

Sterilization, Disinfection, and Antisepsis

Medical microbiology involves the study of the pathogenesis and chemotherapy of infectious diseases, as well as the examination of how diseases can be prevented. An important aspect of the control of infections is an understanding of the principles of sterilization, disinfection, and antisepsis (Box 10–1).

Sterilization

Sterilization is the total destruction of all microbes, including the more resilient forms such as bacterial spores, mycobacteria, nonenveloped (nonlipid) viruses, and fungi. This can be accomplished using physical, gas vapor, or chemical sterilants (Table 10–1).

Physical sterilants such as **moist** and **dry heat** are the most common sterilizing methods used in hospitals and are indicated for most materials, except those that are heat sensitive or consist of toxic or volatile chemicals. **Filtration** is useful for removing bacteria and fungi from air (with high-efficiency particulate air [HEPA] filters) or from solutions. However, these filters are unable to remove viruses and some small bacteria. Sterilization by **ultraviolet** or **ionizing radiation** (e.g., microwave or gamma rays) is also commonly used. The limitation of ultraviolet radiation is that direct exposure is required.

Ethylene oxide is the most commonly used gas vapor sterilant. Although it is highly efficient, strict regulations limit its use because ethylene oxide is flammable, explosive, and carcinogenic to lab animals. Sterilization with **formaldehyde gas** is also limited because the chemical is carcinogenic. Its use is restricted primarily to sterilization of HEPA filters. **Hydrogen peroxide** vapors are effective sterilants because of the oxidizing nature of the gas. This sterilant is used for the sterilization of instruments. A variation is **plasma gas sterilization**, in which hydrogen peroxide is vaporized, and then reactive free radicals are produced with either microwave-frequency or radiofrequency energy. Because this is an efficient sterilizing method that does not produce toxic by-products, it is anticipated that plasma gas sterilization will replace many of the applications for ethylene oxide. However, it cannot be used with materials that absorb hydrogen peroxide or react with it.

Two chemical sterilants have also been used: **peracetic acid** and **glutaraldehyde**. Peracetic acid, an oxidizing agent, has excellent activity, and the end products (i.e., acetic acid and oxygen) are nontoxic. In contrast, safety is a concern with glutaraldehyde, and care must be used when handling this chemical.

Disinfection

Microbes are also destroyed by disinfection procedures, although more resilient organisms can survive. Unfortunately, the terms *disinfection* and *sterilization* are casually interchanged, which can result in some confusion. This occurs because disinfection processes have been categorized as high level, intermediate level, and low level. High-level disinfection can generally approach sterilization in effectiveness, whereas spore forms can survive intermediate-level disinfection, and many microbes can remain viable when exposed to low-level disinfection.

Even the classification of disinfectants (Table 10–2) by their level of activity is misleading. The effectiveness of these procedures is influenced by the nature of the item to be disinfected, number and resilience of the contaminating organisms, amount of organic material present (which can inactivate the disinfectant), type and concentration of disinfectant, and duration and temperature of exposure.

BOX 10–1. Definitions

Antisepsis: Use of chemical agents on skin or other living tissue to inhibit or eliminate microbes; no sporicidal action is implied

Disinfection: Use of physical procedures or chemical agents to destroy most microbial forms; bacterial spores and other relatively resistant organisms (e.g., mycobacteria, viruses, fungi) may remain viable; disinfectants are subdivided into high-, intermediate-, and low-level agents

Germicide: Chemical agent capable of killing microbes; spores may survive

High-level disinfectant: A germicide that kills all microbial pathogens except large numbers of bacterial spores

Intermediate-level disinfectant: A germicide that kills all microbial pathogens except bacterial endospores

Low-level disinfectant: A germicide that kills most vegetative bacteria and lipid-enveloped or medium-size viruses

Sporicide: Germicide capable of killing bacterial spores

Sterilization: Use of physical procedures or chemical agents to destroy all microbial forms, including bacterial spores

TABLE 10–1. Methods of Sterilization

Method	Concentration or Level
Physical Sterilants	
Steam under pressure	121°C or 132°C for various time intervals
Dry heat	1 hr at 171°C; 2 hr at 160°C; 16 hr at 121°C
Filtration	0.22- to 0.45-µm pore size; HEPA filters
Ultraviolet radiation	Variable exposure to 254-nm wavelength
Ionizing radiation	Variable exposure to microwave or gamma radiation
Gas Vapor Sterilants	
Ethylene oxide	450-1200 mg/L at 29° to 65°C for 2–5 hr
Formaldehyde vapor	2%–5% at 60° to 80°C
Hydrogen peroxide vapor	30% at 55° to 60°C
Plasma gas	Highly ionized hydrogen peroxide gas
Chemical Sterilants	
Peracetic acid	0.2%
Glutaraldehyde	2%

HEPA, High-efficiency particulate air.

TABLE 10–2. Methods of Disinfection

Method	Concentration (Level of Activity)
Heat	
Moist heat	75° to 100°C for 30 min (high)
Liquid	
Glutaraldehyde	2% (high)
Hydrogen peroxide	3%–25% (high)
Formaldehyde	3%–8% (high/intermediate)
Chlorine dioxide	Variable (high)
Peracetic acid	Variable (high)
Chlorine compounds	100-1000 ppm of free chlorine (high)
Alcohol (ethyl, isopropyl)	70%–95% (intermediate)
Phenolic compounds	0.4%–5.0% (intermediate/low)
Iodophor compounds	30–50 ppm of free iodine/L (intermediate)
Quaternary ammonium compounds	0.4%–1.6% (low)

High-level disinfectants are used for items involved with invasive procedures that cannot withstand sterilization procedures (e.g., certain types of endoscopes, surgical instruments with plastic or other components that cannot be autoclaved). Disinfection of these and other items is most effective if cleaning the surface to remove organic matter precedes treatment. Examples of high-level disinfectants include treatment with moist heat and use of liquids such as glutaraldehyde, hydrogen peroxide, peracetic acid, and chlorine compounds.

Intermediate-level disinfectants (i.e., alcohols, iodophor compounds, phenolic compounds) are used to clean surfaces or instruments in which contamination with bacterial spores and other highly resilient organisms is unlikely. These have been referred to as semicritical instruments and devices and include flexible fiberoptic endoscopes, laryngoscopes, vaginal specula, anesthesia breathing circuits, and other items.

Low-level disinfectants (i.e., quaternary ammonium compounds) are used to treat noncritical instruments and devices, such as blood pressure cuffs, electrocardiogram electrodes, and stethoscopes. Although these items come into contact with patients, they do not penetrate through mucosal surfaces or into sterile tissues.

The level of disinfectants used for environmental surfaces is determined by the relative risk these surfaces pose as a reservoir for pathogenic organisms. For example, a higher level of disinfectant should be used to clean the surface of instruments contaminated with blood than that used to clean surfaces that are "dirty," such as floors, sinks, and countertops. The exception to this rule is if a particular surface has been implicated in a nosocomial infection, such as a bathroom contaminated with *Clostridium difficile* (spore-forming anaerobic bacterium) or a sink contaminated with *Pseudomonas aeruginosa*. In these cases a disinfectant with appropriate activity against the implicated pathogen should be selected.

Antisepsis

Antiseptic agents (Table 10–3) are used to reduce the number of microbes on skin surfaces. These compounds are selected for their safety and efficacy. A summary of their germicidal properties is presented in Table 10–4. **Alcohols** have excellent activity against all groups of organisms, except spores, and are nontoxic, although they tend to dry the skin surface because they remove lipids. They also do not have residual activity and are inactivated by organic matter. Thus the surface of the skin should be cleaned before alcohol is applied. **Iodophors** are also excellent skin antiseptic agents, having a range of activity similar to that of alcohols. They are slightly more toxic to the skin than is alcohol, have limited residual activity, and are inactivated by organic matter. Iodophors and iodine preparations are frequently used with alcohols for disinfecting the skin surface. **Chlorhexidine** has broad antimicrobial activity, although it kills organisms at a much slower rate than does alcohol. Its activity persists, although organic material and high pH levels decrease its effectiveness. The activity of **parachlorometaxylenol** (PCMX) is limited primarily to gram-positive bacteria. Because it is nontoxic and has residual activity, it has been used in handwashing products. **Triclosan** is active against bacteria but not against many other organisms. It is a common antiseptic agent in deodorant soaps and some toothpaste products.

TABLE 10–3. Antiseptic Agents

Antiseptic Agent	Concentration
Alcohol (ethyl, isopropyl)	70%-90%
Iodophors	1-2 mg of free iodine/L; 1%-2% available iodine
Chlorhexidine	0.5%-4.0%
Parachlorometaxylenol	0.50%-3.75%
Triclosan	0.3%-2.0%

Mechanisms of Action

The following section briefly reviews the mechanisms by which the most common sterilants, disinfectants, and antiseptics work.

TABLE 10–4. Germicidal Properties of Disinfectants and Antiseptic Agents

Agents	Bacteria	Mycobacteria	Bacterial Spores	Fungi	Viruses
Disinfectants					
Alcohol	+	+	–	+	+/–
Hydrogen peroxide	+	+	+/–	+	+
Formaldehyde	+	+	+	+	+
Phenolics	+	+	–	+	+/–
Chlorine	+	+	+/–	+	+
Iodophors	+	+/–	–	+	+
Glutaraldehyde	+	+	+	+	+
Quaternary ammonium compounds	+/–	–	–	+/–	+/–
Antiseptic Agents					
Alcohol	+	+	–	+	+
Iodophors	+	+	–	+	+
Chlorhexidine	+	+	–	+	+
Parachlorometaxylenol	+/–	+/–	–	+	+/–
Triclosan	+	+/–	–	+/–	+

MOIST HEAT

Attempts to sterilize items using boiling water are inefficient because only a relatively low temperature (100°C) can be maintained. Indeed, spore formation by a bacterium is commonly demonstrated by boiling a solution of organisms and then subculturing the solution. Boiling vegetative organisms kills them, but the spores remain viable. If organisms grow on the subculture plate, the bacteria are capable of sporulating. In contrast, steam under pressure in an autoclave is a very effective form of sterilization; the higher temperature causes denaturation of microbial proteins. The rate of killing organisms during the autoclave process is rapid but is influenced by the temperature and duration of autoclaving, size of the autoclave, flow rate of the steam, density and size of the load, and placement of the load in the chamber. Care must be taken to avoid creating air pockets, which inhibit penetration of the steam into the load. In general, most autoclaves are operated at 121°C to 132 °C for 15 minutes or longer. Including commercial preparations of *Bacillus stearothermophilus* spores can help monitor the effectiveness of sterilization. An ampule of these spores is placed in the center of the load, removed at the end of the autoclave process, and incubated at 37°C. If the sterilization process is successful, the organisms fail to sporulate and do not grow.

DRY HEAT

Hot air can also be used to sterilize items such as glassware. This method is not as efficient as the moist air method because diffusion and penetration of heat is slow, long sterilization periods and high temperatures are required, materials can be damaged by the oxidation process of this prolonged heating, and dry heat tends to stratify in the processing chamber. Sterilization requires processing for 1 hour at 171°C, 2 hours at 160°C, or 16 hours at 121°C. The effectiveness is monitored with spore tests, using *Bacillus subtilis*, which is relatively resistant to killing by dry air (in contrast with *B. stearothermophilus*).

ETHYLENE OXIDE

Ethylene oxide is a colorless gas, soluble in water and common organic solvents, that is used to sterilize heat-sensitive items. The sterilization process is relatively slow and is influenced by the concentration of gas, relative humidity and moisture content of the item to be sterilized, exposure time, and temperature. The exposure time is reduced by 50% for each doubling of ethylene oxide concentration. Likewise, the activity of ethylene oxide approximately doubles with each temperature increase of 10°C. Sterilization with ethylene oxide is optimal in a relative humidity of approximately 30%, with decreased activity at higher or lower humidity. This is particularly problematic if the contaminated organisms are dried onto a surface or lyophilized. Ethylene oxide exerts its sporicidal activity through the alkylation of terminal hydroxyl, carboxyl, amino, and sulfhydryl groups. This process blocks the reactive groups required for many essential metabolic processes. Examples of other strong alkylating gases used as sterilants are formaldehyde and β-propiolactone. Because ethylene oxide can damage viable tissues, the gas must be dissipated before the item can be used. This aeration period is generally 16 hours or longer. The effectiveness of sterilization is monitored with the *B. subtilis* spore test.

ALDEHYDES

As with ethylene oxide, aldehydes exert their effect through alkylation. The two best-known aldehydes are **formaldehyde** and **glutaraldehyde**, both of which can be used as sterilants or high-level disinfectants. Formaldehyde gas can be dissolved in water (creating a solution called *formalin*) at a final concentration of 37%. Stabilizers such as methanol are added to formalin. Low concentrations of formalin are bacteriostatic (i.e., they inhibit but do not kill organisms), whereas higher concentrations (e.g., 20%) can kill all organisms. Combining formaldehyde with alcohol (e.g., 20% formalin in 70% alcohol) can enhance this microbicidal activity. Exposure of skin or mucous membranes to formaldehyde can be toxic. Glutaraldehyde is less toxic for viable tissues, but it can still cause burns on the skin or mucous membranes. Glutaraldehyde is more active at alkaline pH levels ("activated" by sodium hydroxide) but is less stable. Glutaraldehyde is also inactivated by organic material, so items to be treated must first be cleaned.

OXIDIZING AGENTS

Examples of oxidants include ozone, peracetic acid, and hydrogen peroxide, the last used most commonly. **Hydrogen peroxide** effectively kills most bacteria at a concentration of 3% to 6% and kills all organisms, including spores, at higher concentrations (10% to 25%). The active oxidant form is not hydrogen peroxide but rather the free hydroxyl radical formed by the decomposition of hydrogen peroxide. Hydrogen peroxide is used to disinfect plastic implants, contact lenses, and surgical prostheses.

HALOGENS

Halogens, such as compounds containing iodine or chlorine, are used extensively as disinfectants. **Iodine compounds** are the most effective halogens available for disinfection. Iodine is a highly reactive element that precipitates proteins and oxidizes essential enzymes. It is microbicidal against virtually all organisms, including spore-forming bacteria and mycobacteria. Neither the concentration nor the pH of the iodine solution affects the microbicidal activity, although the efficiency of iodine solutions is increased in acid solutions because more free iodine is liberated. Iodine acts more rapidly than do other halogen compounds or quaternary ammonium compounds. However, the activity of iodine can be reduced in the presence of some organic and inorganic compounds, including serum, feces, ascitic fluid, sputum, urine, sodium thiosulfate, and ammonia. Elemental iodine can be dissolved in aqueous potassium iodide or alcohol, or it can be complexed with a carrier. The latter compound is referred to as an *iodophor* (iodo, "iodine"; phor, "carrier"). Povidone iodine (iodine complexed with polyvinylpyrrolidone) is used most commonly and is relatively stable and nontoxic to tissues and metal surfaces, but it is expensive compared with other iodine solutions.

Chlorine compounds are also used extensively as disinfectants. Aqueous solutions of chlorine are rapidly bactericidal, although their mechanisms of action are not defined. Three forms of chlorine may be present in water: elemental chlorine (Cl_2), which is a very strong oxidizing agent; hypochlorous acid (HOCl); and hypochlorite ion (OCl_2). Chlorine also combines with ammonia and other nitrogenous compounds to form chloramines, or *N*-chloro compounds. Chlorine can exert its effect by the irreversible oxidation of sulfhydryl (SH) groups of essential enzymes. Hypochlorites are believed to interact with cytoplasmic components to form toxic *N*-chloro compounds, which interfere with cellular metabolism. The efficacy of chlorine is inversely proportional to the pH, with greater activity observed at acid pH levels. This is consistent with greater activity associated with hypochlorous acid rather than with hypochlorite ion concentration. The activity of chlorine compounds also increases with concentration (e.g., a twofold increase in concentration results in a 30% decrease in time required for killing) and temperature (e.g., a 50% to 65% reduction in killing time with a 10°C increase in temperature). Organic matter and alkaline detergents can reduce the effectiveness of chlorine compounds. These compounds demonstrate good germicidal activity, although spore-forming organisms are tenfold to 1000-fold more resistant to chlorine than are vegetative bacteria.

PHENOLIC COMPOUNDS

Phenolic compounds (germicides) are rarely used as disinfectants. However, they are of historical interest because they were used as a comparative standard for assessing the activity of other germicidal compounds. The ratio of germicidal activity by a test compound to that by a specified concentration of phenol yielded the phenol coefficient. A value of 1 indicated equivalent activity, greater than 1 indicated activity less than phenol, and less than 1 indicated activity greater than phenol. These tests are limited because phenol is not sporicidal at room temperature (but is sporicidal at temperatures approaching 100°C) and has poor activity against non–lipid-containing viruses. This is understandable because phenol is believed to act by disrupting lipid-containing membranes, resulting in leakage of cellular contents. Phenolic compounds are active against the normally resilient mycobacteria, because the cell wall of these organisms has a very high concentration of lipids. Exposure of phenolics to alkaline compounds significantly reduces their activity, whereas halogenation of the phenolics enhances their activity. The introduction of aliphatic or aromatic groups into the nucleus of halogen phenols also increases their activity. Bis-phenols are two phenol compounds linked together. The activity of these compounds can also be potentiated by halogenation. One example of a halogenated bis-phenol is **hexachlorophene,** an antiseptic with activity against gram-positive bacteria.

QUATERNARY AMMONIUM COMPOUNDS

Quaternary ammonium compounds consist of four organic groups covalently linked to nitrogen. The germicidal activity of these cationic compounds is determined by the nature of the organic groups, with the greatest activity observed with compounds with 8 to 18 carbon long groups. Examples of quaternary ammonium compounds include **benzalkonium chloride** and **cetylpyridinium chloride**. These compounds act by denaturing cell membranes to release the intracellular components. Quaternary ammonium compounds are bacteriostatic at low concentrations and bactericidal at high concentrations. However, organisms such as *Pseudomonas, Mycobacterium,* and the fungus *Trichophyton,* among others, are resistant to these compounds. Indeed, some *Pseudomonas* strains can grow readily in quaternary ammonium solutions. Many viruses and all bacterial spores are also resistant. Ionic detergents, organic matter, and dilution neutralize quaternary ammonium compounds.

ALCOHOLS

The germicidal activity of alcohols increases with increasing chain length (maximum of five to eight carbons). The two most commonly used alcohols are **ethanol** and **isopropanol**. These alcohols are rapidly bactericidal against vegetative bacteria, mycobacteria, some fungi, and lipid-containing viruses. Unfortunately, alcohols have no activity against bacterial spores and have poor activity against some fungi and non–lipid-containing viruses. Activity is greater in the presence of water. Thus 70% alcohol is more active than is 95% alcohol. Alcohol is a common disinfectant for skin surfaces and, when followed by treatment with an iodophor, is extremely effective for this purpose. Alcohols are also used to disinfect items such as thermometers.

QUESTIONS

1. Define the following terms and give three examples of each: *sterilization, disinfection,* and *antisepsis.*
2. Define the three levels of disinfection and give examples of each. When would each type of disinfectant be used?
3. What factors influence the effectiveness of sterilization with moist heat, dry heat, and ethylene oxide?
4. Give examples of each of the following disinfectants and their mode of action: iodine compounds, chlorine compounds, phenolic compounds, and quaternary ammonium compounds.

Bibliography

Block SS: *Disinfection, sterilization, and preservation,* ed 2, Philadelphia, 1977, Lea and Febiger.

Brody TM, Larner J, Minneman KP: *Human pharmacology: Molecular to clinical,* ed 3, St Louis, 1998, Mosby.

Widmer A, Frei R: Decontamination, disinfection, and sterilization. In Murray P et al, editors: *Manual of clinical microbiology,* ed 8, Washington, 2003, American Society for Microbiology.

SECTION II

Basic Concepts of the Immune Response

CHAPTER 11

Elements of Host Protective Responses

We live in a microbial world, and our bodies are constantly being exposed to bacteria, fungi, parasites, and viruses. Our bodies' defenses to this onslaught are similar to a military defense. The initial defense mechanisms are **barriers,** such as the skin, acid and bile of the gastrointestinal tract, and mucus that inactivate and prevent entry of the foreign agents. If these barriers are compromised or the agent gains entry in another way, the local militia of **innate responses** (e.g., complement, natural killer cells, neutrophils, macrophages) must quickly rally to the challenge and prevent expansion of the invasion. Once activated, these responses send an alarm (complement and chemokines) and open the vasculature to provide access (complement) to the site. Finally, if these steps are not effective, the innate responses activate a major, specifically directed campaign against the invader by **antigen-specific immune responses** (antibody and T cells) at whatever cost (immunopathogenesis). Similarly, knowledge of the characteristics (antigens) of the enemy through immunization enables the body to mount a faster, more effective response (activation of memory B and T cells) on rechallenge.

The different elements of the immune system interact and communicate using soluble molecules and by direct cell-to-cell interaction. These interactions provide the mechanisms for activation and control of the protective responses. Unfortunately, the protective responses to some infectious agents are insufficient; in other cases the response to the challenge is excessive. In either case, disease occurs.

Activators and Stimulators of Immune Function

Immune cells communicate by direct cell-to-cell interactions (touch) and by the sensing of soluble molecules (similar to taste or smell) from microbes, including lipopolysaccharide and other cell wall components, and bacterial and viral nucleic acids. These and other molecules have **pathogen-associated molecular patterns (PAMP)** recognized by receptors on immune cells that trigger the release of cytokines, interferons, and chemokines. **Cytokines** are proteins that stimulate and regulate the immune response (Table 11–1 and Box 11–1). They are produced by lymphoid and other cells. **Interferons** are proteins produced in response to viral infections (interferon-α and interferon-β) or on activation of the immune response (interferon-γ); they promote antiviral and antitumor responses and stimulate immune responses (see Chapter 14). **Chemokines** are small proteins (approximately 8000 Da) that are associated with inflammatory responses. Neutrophils, basophils, monocytes, and T cells express receptors and can be activated by specific chemokines. The chemokines and other proteins (e.g., the C3a and C5a products of the complement cascade) are chemotactic factors that establish a chemical path to attract phagocytic and inflammatory cells to the site of infection.

Cells of the Immune Response

Immune responses are mediated by specific cells with defined functions. The characteristics of the most important cells of the immune system and their appearances are presented in Figure 11–1 and in Tables 11–2 and 11–3.

The white blood cells can be distinguished on the basis of (1) morphology, (2) histologic staining, (3) immunologic functions, and (4) intracellular and cell surface markers. Monoclonal antibodies are used to distinguish subsets of the different types of cells according to their cell surface markers. These markers have been defined within

TABLE 11–1. Cytokines and Chemokines

Factor	Source	Major Target	Function
Interferon-α, interferon-β	Leukocytes, fibroblasts	Virally infected cells, tumor cells, NK cells	Induction of antiviral state; activation of NK cells, enhancement of cell-mediated immunity
Interferon-γ	CD4 TH1 cells, NK cells	Macrophages,* T cells, B cells	Activation of macrophage, promotion of inflammation, promotion of TH1 and inhibition of TH2 responses
IL-1α, IL-1β	Macrophage, fibroblasts, epithelial cells, endothelial cells	T cells, B cells, PMN, tissue, central nervous system	Many actions: promotion of inflammatory and acute phase responses, fever, activation of T cells
TNF-α (cachectin)	Similar to IL-1	—	Similar to IL-1, antitumor and wasting (cachexia, weight loss) functions
TNF-β	T cells	PMN, tumors	Lymphotoxin: tumor killing, activation of PMN
Colony-stimulating factors (e.g., GM-CSF)	T cells, stromal cells	Stem cells	Growth and differentiation of specific cell types
IL-2	CD4 T cells (TH0, TH1)	T cells, B cells, NK cells	T and B cell growth
IL-3	CD4 T cells, keratinocytes	Stem cells	Differentiation
IL-4	CD4 (TH0, TH2), T cells	B and T cells	B cell growth and differentiation; Ig production; TH2 responses
IL-5	CD4 TH2 cells	B cells, eosinophils	B cell growth and differentiation, IgA and IgE production, eosinophil production, allergic responses
IL-6	Macrophages, T and B cells, fibroblast, epithelial cells, endothelial cells	T and B cells, hepatocytes	Stimulation of acute-phase and inflammatory responses, fever, Ig secretion, B cell growth and development
IL-7	Bone marrow, stroma	Precursor cells and stem cells	Growth of pre-B cell, thymocyte, T cell, and cytotoxic lymphocyte
IL-10	CD4 TH2 cells	B cells, CD4 TH1 cells	B cell growth, inhibition of TH1 response
IL-12, IL-18	DC, macrophage	NK cells, CD4 TH1 cells	Activation of TH1 response
TGF-β	CD4 TH3 cells	B cells	Immunosuppression of B, T, and NK cells and macrophages; promotion of oral tolerance, wound healing, IgA production
α-chemokines: C-X-C chemokines—two cysteines separated by one amino acid (IL-8; IP-10; GRO-α, GRO-β, GRO-γ)	Many cells	Neutrophils, T cells, macrophages	Chemotaxis, activation
β-chemokines: C-C chemokines—two adjacent cysteines (MCP-1; MIP-α; MIP-β; RANTES)	Many cells	T cells, macrophages, basophils	Chemotaxis, activation

GM-CSF, Granulocyte-macrophage colony-stimulating factor; GRO, growth-related oncogene; Ig, immunoglobulin; IL, interleukin; IP, interferon-α protein; MCP, monocyte chemoattractant protein; MIP, macrophage inflammatory protein; NK, natural killer; PMN, polymorphonuclear leukocyte; RANTES, regulated on activation, normal T expressed and secreted; TNF, tumor necrosis factor.

*Applies to one or more cells of the monocyte-macrophage lineage.

TABLE 11–2. Cells of the Immune Response

Cells	Characteristics	Markers	Functions
Natural Cytolytic Cells			
Natural killer cells	Large, granular lymphocytes	Fc receptors for antibody; CD16, CD56, CD57	Kill antibody-decorated cells and virus-infected or tumor cell **(no MHC restriction)**
Phagocytic Cells			
Neutrophils (polymorphonuclear leukocytes)	Granulocytes with short life span, multilobed nucleus and granules, segmented band forms (more immature)	—	*Phagocytose* and kill *bacteria*
Eosinophils	Bilobed nucleus, heavily granulated cytoplasm	Staining with eosin	Involved in parasite defense and allergic response
Macrophages	See other entry for macrophages in this table	—	—
Antigen- Presenting Cells (APCS)		***Class II MHC Expressing Cells***	***Present Antigen to CD4 T cells***
Monocytes*	Found in lymphocytes, blood, lungs, and other organs	Horseshoe-shaped nucleus, lysosomes, granules	*Precursors to macrophage-lineage,* cytokine release
Predendritic cells	Blood and tissue	—	Cytokine response to infection, process antigen
Dendritic cells*	Lymph nodes, tissue	—	Efficient antigen presenters
Langerhans cells*	Presence in skin	—	Transport antigen to lymph nodes
Macrophages*	Possible residence in tissue, spleen, lymph nodes, and other organs; activated by IFN-γ and TNF	Large, granular cells; Fc and C3 receptors	Initiate inflammatory and acute phase response; activated cells are antibacterial and have antiviral and antitumor activities
Microglial cells*	CNS and brain	—	Produce cytokines
Kupffer cells*	Presence in liver	—	Filter particles from blood (e.g., viruses)
B cells	See other entry for B cells in this table	—	
Antigen-Responsive Cells			
T cells (all)	Mature in thymus; large nucleus, small cytoplasm	CD2, CD3, T-cell receptor	
$\alpha\beta$TCR CD4 T cells	Helper/DTH cells; **activation** by APCs through **class II MHC antigen presentation**	CD2, CD3, $\alpha\beta$T-cell receptor, CD4	Produce IL-2, other cytokines; stimulate T and B cell growth; promote B-cell differentiation (class switching, antibody production)
	TH1 subtype	IL-2, IFN-γ, LT production	Promote initial defenses (local), DTH, T killer cells
	TH2 subtype	IL-4, IL-5, IL-6, IL-10 production	Promote later humoral responses
$\alpha\beta$TCR CD8 T killer cells	**Recognition** of antigen presented by **class I MHC antigens**	CD2, CD3, $\alpha\beta$T-cell receptor, CD8	Kill viral, tumor, non-self (transplant) cells; secrete TH1 cytokines

TABLE 11–2. Cells of the Immune Response—*cont'd*

Cells	Characteristics	Markers	Functions
CD8 T cells (suppressor cells)	**Recognition** of antigen presented by **class I MHC antigens**	CD2, CD3, T-cell receptor, CD8	Suppress T- and B-cell response
γδ* TCR T cells	CD2, CD3, γδ T cell receptor	Early sensor of some bacterial infections in tissue and blood	
Antibody-Producing Cells			
B cells	Mature in Peyer's patches, bone marrow, bursal equivalent; large nucleus, small cytoplasm; activation by antigens and T cell factors	Surface antibody, **class II MHC antigens**	Produce antibody and present antigen
Plasma cells	Small nucleus, large cytoplasm	—	Terminally differentiated, antibody factories
Other Cells			
Basophils/mast cells	Granulocytic	Fc receptors for IgE	Release histamine, provide allergic response, are antiparasitic

APCs, antigen-presenting cells; CNS, central nervous system; DTH, delayed-type hypersensitivity; IFN, interferon; Ig, immunoglobulin; IL, interleukin; LT, lymphotoxin; MHC, major histocompatibility complex; TNF, tumor necrosis factor.
*Monocyte/macrophage lineage.

BOX 11–1. Major Cytokine-Producing Cells

Innate (acute phase responses)
- Dendritic cells and macrophages: IL-1, TNF-α, TNF-β, IL-6, IL-12, GM-CSF, chemokines, interferons α,β

Immune: T cells (CD4 and CD8)
- TH1 cells: IL-2, IL-3, GM-CSF, interferon-γ, TNF-α, TNF-β
- TH2 cells: IL-4, IL-5, IL-6, IL-10, IL-3, IL-9, IL-13, GM-CSF, TNF-α

GM-CSF, Granulocyte-macrophage colony-stimulating factor; IL, interleukin; TNF, tumor necrosis factor.

TABLE 11–3. Normal Blood Cell Counts

	Mean Number per Microliter	Normal Range
White blood cells (leukocytes)	7,400	4,500-11,000
Neutrophils	4,400	1,800-7,700
Eosinophils	200	0-450
Basophils	40	0-200
Lymphocytes	2,500	1,000-4,800
Monocytes	300	0-800

From Abbas AK, Lichtman AH, Pober JS: *Cellular and molecular immunology*, ed 4, Philadelphia, 2000, WB Saunders.

clusters of differentiation and the markers indicated by **"CD"** (cluster of differentiation) numbers (Table 11–4). In addition, **all nucleated cells express class I MHC (MHC I) antigens** (HLA-A, HLA-B, HLA-C).

A special class of cells that are **antigen-presenting cells (APCs) express class II major histocompatibility complex (MHC) antigens** (HLA-DR, HLA-DP, HLA-DQ). APCs include dendritic cells, macrophage family cells, B lymphocytes, and a limited number of other cell types.

HEMATOPOIETIC CELL DIFFERENTIATION

Differentiation of a common progenitor cell, termed the pluripotent **stem cell,** gives rise to all blood cells. Differentiation of these cells begins during development of the fetus and continues throughout life. The pluripotent stem cell differentiates into stem cells (sometimes referred to as colony-forming units) for different lineages of blood cells, including the lymphoid (T and B cells), myeloid, erythrocytic, and megakaryoblastic (source of platelets) lineages (see Fig. 11–1). The stem cells reside primarily in the bone marrow but can also be isolated from the fetal blood in umbilical cords and as rare cells in adult blood. Differentiation of stem cells into the functional blood cells is triggered by specific cell surface interactions with the stromal

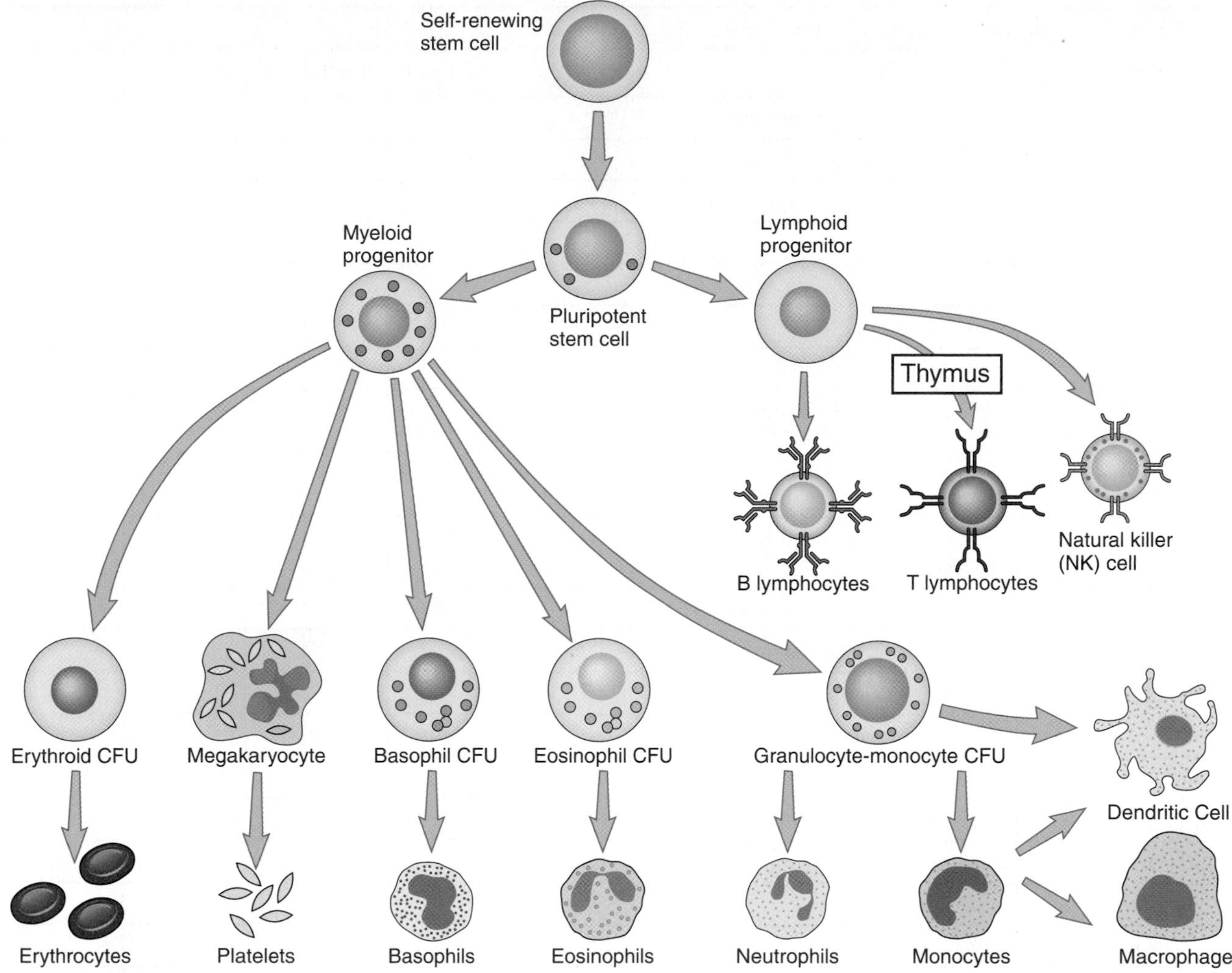

FIGURE 11–1. Morphology and lineage of cells involved in the immune response. Pluripotent stem cells and colony-forming units are long-lived cells capable of replenishing the more differentiated functional and terminally differentiated cells. (From Abbas K et al: *Cellular and molecular immunology,* ed 5, Philadelphia, 2003, WB Saunders.)

cells of the marrow and specific cytokines produced by these and other cells. The **thymus and the "bursal equivalent" in the Peyer's patches promote development of T cells and B cells, respectively.** Helper T cells, macrophages, and other cells release specific cytokines that promote hematopoietic cell growth and terminal differentiation in response to infections and on activation.

The bone marrow and thymus are considered **primary lymphoid organs** (Figure 11–2). These sites of initial lymphocyte differentiation are essential to the development of the immune system. **Secondary lymphoid organs** include the **lymph nodes, spleen,** and **mucosa-associated lymphoid tissue (MALT),** which also include gut-associated lymphoid tissue (GALT) (e.g., Peyer's patches) and bronchus-associated lymphoid tissue (BALT) (e.g., tonsils, appendix). These sites are where B and T cells reside and respond to antigenic challenges. Proliferation of the lymphocytes in response to infectious challenge causes these tissues to swell (i.e., "swollen glands"). The cells of the primary and secondary lymphoid organs express cell surface adhesion molecules **(addressins)** that interact with homing receptors **(cell adhesion molecules)** expressed on B and T cells.

The spleen and lymph nodes are encapsulated organs in which the macrophages and B and T cells reside in defined regions. Their location facilitates interactions that promote immune responses to antigen (Figure 11–3). The **lymph nodes** are kidney-shaped organs 2 to 10 mm in diameter that filter the fluid that passes from intercellular spaces into the lymphatic system, almost like a sewage processing plant. The lymph node is constructed to optimize the meeting of the innate (dendritic cells and macrophages) and the immune response (B and T) cells to initiate and expand specific immune

TABLE 11–4. Selected CD Markers of Importance

CD Markers	Identity and Function	T Cell	B cell	NK	Monocyte	Macrophage
CD1	non-peptide antigen presentation		*			
CD2 (LFA-3R)	Erythrocyte receptor	**				
CD3	TCR subunit (γ, δ, ε, ζ, η); activation	**				
CD4	Class II MHC receptor	**				
CD5						
CD8	Class I MHC receptor	**				
CD11b (CR3)	C3b complement receptor 3 (α chain)					
CD14	LPS-binding protein receptor				**	**
CD16 (Fc-γ RIII)	Phagocytosis and ADCC			**		
CD21 (CR2)	C3d complement receptor, EBV receptor, B cell activation		**			
CD25 (TAC)	IL-2 receptor (α chain), early activation marker, marker for regulatory cells	*	*		*	*
CD28	Receptor for B-7 costimulation: activation	**	*			
CD32 (Fc-γ RII)	Low-affinity receptor for immune complexes					**
CD35 (CR1)	C3b and C4b complement receptor					
CD40	Stimulation of B cell		**			
CD40 L	Ligand for CD40	**				
CD45 (LCA)	Augments activation of B and T cells			*		
CD45RO	Isoform (on memory cells)					
CD56 (NKH1)	Adhesion molecule	*		**		
CD57 (leu-7)	Adhesion molecule		*	**		
CD64 (Fc-γ RI)	High-affinity IgG receptor					
CD70	CD27-ligand: costimulation of B and T cells	*	*			
CD80	B 7-1: costimulation of T cells on APCs		+			+
CD86	B 7-2: costimulation of T cells on APCs		+			+
CD152 (CTLA-4)	Receptor for B-7; tolerance	**				
Adhesion Molecules						
CD11a	LFA-1 (α chain)					
CD29	VLA (β chain)					
VLA-1, VLA-2, VLA-3	α integrins	*				
VLA-4	α_4 integrin homing receptor	+	+		+	
CD50	ICAM-3	+	+	+	+	+
CD54	ICAM-1					
CD58	LFA-3					

ADCC, antibody-dependent cellular cytotoxicity; APCs, antigen-presenting cells; CTLA, cytotoxic T-lymphocyte associated protein; EBV, Epstein Barr virus; ICAM, intercellular adhesion molecule; Ig, immunoglobulin; IL, interleukin; LCA, leukocyte common antigen; LFA, leukocyte function–associated antigen; LPS, lipopolysaccharide; MHC, major histocompatibility complex; TAC, T-cell activation complex; TCR, T-cell antigen receptor; VLA, very late activation (antigen).

Modified from Male D et al: *Advanced immunology*, ed 3, St Louis, 1996, Mosby.

This table shows the recognized CD markers of hemopoietic cells and their distribution. A filled rectangle or + means cell population present; a half-filled triangle is subpopulation; *, activated cells only; **, markers that identity or are critical to the cell type.

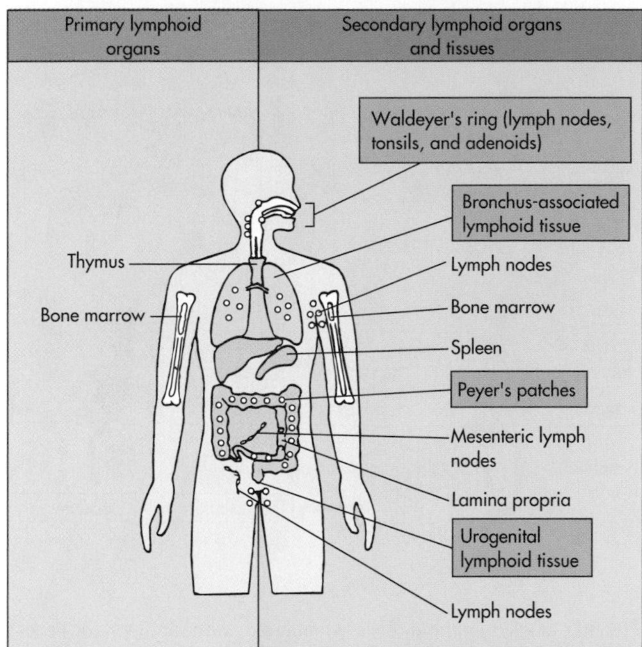

FIGURE 11–2. Organs of the immune system. Thymus and bone marrow are primary lymphoid organs. They are sites of maturation for T and B cells, respectively. Cellular and humoral immune responses develop in the secondary (peripheral) lymphoid organs and tissues; effector and memory cells are generated in these organs. The spleen responds predominantly to blood-borne antigens. Lymph nodes mount immune responses to antigens in intercellular fluid and in the lymph, absorbed either through the skin (superficial nodes) or from internal viscera (deep nodes). Tonsils, Peyer's patches, and other mucosa-associated lymphoid tissues *(blue boxes)* respond to antigens that have penetrated the surface mucosal barriers. (From Roitt I et al: *Immunology,* ed 4, St Louis, 1996, Mosby.)

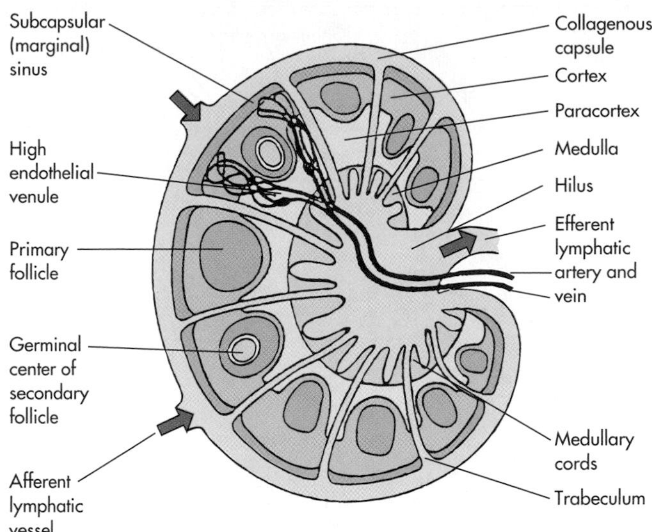

FIGURE 11–3. Organization of the lymph node. Beneath the collagenous capsule is the subcapsular sinus, which is lined with phagocytic cells. Lymphocytes and antigens from surrounding tissue spaces or adjacent nodes pass into the sinus via the afferent lymphatic system. The cortex contains aggregates of B cells (primary follicles), most of which are stimulated (secondary follicles) and have a site of active proliferation or germinal center. The paracortex contains mainly T cells and dendritic cells (antigen-presenting cells). Each lymph node has its own arterial and venous supplies. Lymphocytes enter the node from the circulation through the specialized high endothelial venules in the paracortex. The medulla contains both T and B cells, as well as most of the lymph node plasma cells organized into cords of lymphoid tissue. Lymphocytes can leave the node only through the efferent lymphatic vessel. (From Roitt I et al: *Immunology,* ed 4, St Louis, 1996, Mosby.)

responses. A lymph node consists of the following three layers:

1. The cortex, the outer layer that contains mainly B cells and macrophages arranged in clusters called follicles.
2. The paracortex, which contains dendritic cells that bring antigens from the tissues to be presented to the T cells to initiate immune responses.
3. The medulla, which contains B and T cells and antibody-producing plasma cells.

The **spleen** is a large organ that acts like a lymph node and also filters antigens, encapsulated bacteria, and viruses from blood and removes aged blood cells and platelets (Figure 11–4). The spleen consists of two types of tissue, the white pulp and the red pulp. The white pulp consists of arterioles surrounded by lymphoid cells (periarteriolar lymphoid sheath), in which the T cells surround the central arteriole. B cells are organized into primary unstimulated or secondary stimulated follicles that have a germinal center. The germinal center contains memory cells, macrophages, and follicular dendritic cells (APCs of lymphoid origin). The red pulp is a storage site for blood cells and the site of turnover of aged platelets and erythrocytes. **MALT** contains less structured aggregates of lymphoid cells (Figure 11–5). For example, the **Peyer's patches** along the intestinal wall have special cells in the epithelium (M cells) that deliver antigens to the lymphocytes contained in defined regions (T [interfollicular] and B [germinal]). Once thought to be expendable, the **tonsils** are an important part of the MALT. These lymphoepithelial organs sample the microbes in the oral and nasal area. The tonsils contain a large number of mature and memory B cells (50% to 90% of the lymphocytes) that use their antibodies to sense specific pathogens and, with dendritic cells and T cells, can initiate immune responses. Swelling of the tonsils may be caused by infection or a response to infection.

POLYMORPHONUCLEAR LEUKOCYTES

Polymorphonuclear leukocytes (neutrophils) constitute 50% to 70% of circulating white blood cells (see Figure 11–1) and are a primary **phagocytic defense** against bacterial infection. These short-lived cells circulate in the blood for 7 to 10 hours and then migrate into the tissue, where they live for 3 days. **Neutrophils** are 11 to

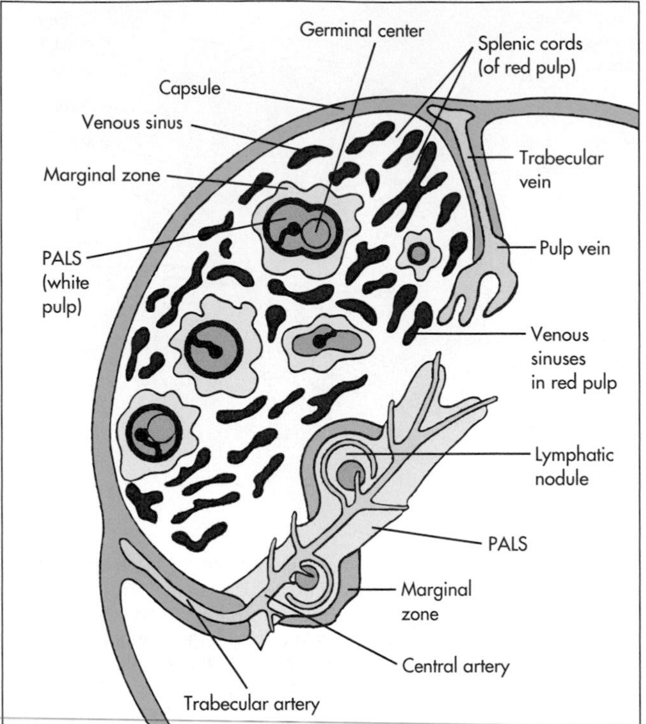

FIGURE 11–4. Organization of lymphoid tissue in the spleen. The white pulp contains germinal centers and is surrounded by the marginal zone, which contains numerous macrophages, antigen-presenting cells, slowly recirculating B cells, and natural killer cells. The red pulp contains venous sinuses separated by splenic cords. Blood enters the tissues via the trabecular arteries, which give rise to the many-branched central arteries. Some end in the white pulp, supplying the germinal centers and mantle zones, but most empty into or near the marginal zones. PALS, Periarteriolar lymphoid sheath. (From Roitt I et al: *Immunology,* ed 4, St Louis, 1996, Mosby.)

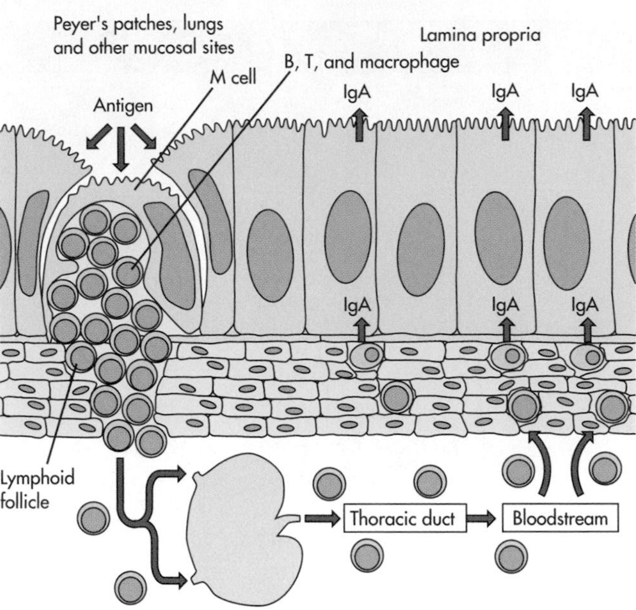

FIGURE 11–5. Lymphoid cells stimulated with antigen in Peyer's patches (or the lungs or another mucosal site) migrate via the regional lymph nodes and thoracic duct into the bloodsteam, then to the lamina propria of the gut and probably other mucosal surfaces. Thus lymphocytes stimulated at one mucosal surface may become distributed throughout the MALT (mucosa-associated lymphoid tissue) system. IgA, Immunoglobulin A. (From Roitt I et al: *Immunology,* ed 4, St Louis, 1996, Mosby.)

14 μm in diameter, lack mitochondria, have a granulated cytoplasm in which granules stain with both acidic and basic stains, and have a multilobed nucleus. Neutrophils leave the blood and concentrate at the site of infection in response to chemotactic factors. During infection, the neutrophils in the blood increase in number and include precursor forms. These precursors are termed **band forms,** in contrast to the terminally differentiated and **segmented neutrophils.** The finding of such an increase and change in neutrophils by a blood count is sometimes termed *a left shift with an increase in bands versus segs.* Neutrophils ingest bacteria by phagocytosis and expose the bacteria to antibacterial substances and enzymes contained in **primary (azurophilic)** and **secondary (specific) granules.** Azurophilic granules are reservoirs for enzymes such as myeloperoxidase, β-glucuronidase, elastase, and cathepsin G. Specific granules serve as reservoirs for lysozyme and lactoferrin.

Eosinophils are heavily granulated cells (11 to 15 μm in diameter) with a bilobed nucleus that stain with the acid dye eosin Y. They are also phagocytic, motile, and granulated. The granules contain acid phosphatase, peroxidase, and eosinophilic basic proteins. Eosinophils play a role in the defense against **parasitic infections.** The eosinophilic basic proteins are toxic to many parasites. **Basophils,** another type of granulocyte, are not phagocytic but release the contents of their granules during allergic responses (type 1 hypersensitivity).

MONONUCLEAR PHAGOCYTE SYSTEM

The **mononuclear phagocyte system** (previously called the reticuloendothelial system) are myeloid cells and consist of monocytes (see Fig. 11–1) in the blood and cells derived from **monocytes,** such as **macrophages, alveolar macrophages in the lungs, Kupffer cells in the liver, intraglomerular mesangial cells in the kidney, histiocytes in connective tissue, osteoclasts, synovial A cells, and microglial cells in the brain. Alveolar and serosal (e.g., peritoneal) macrophages** are examples of "wandering" macrophages. **Brain microglia** are cells that enter the brain around the time of birth and differentiate into fixed cells. Some **dendritic cells** are myeloid cells and may be derived from monocytes.

Monocytes are 10 to 18 μm in diameter, with a single-lobed, kidney bean–shaped nucleus. They represent 3% to 8% of peripheral blood leukocytes. Different cytokines

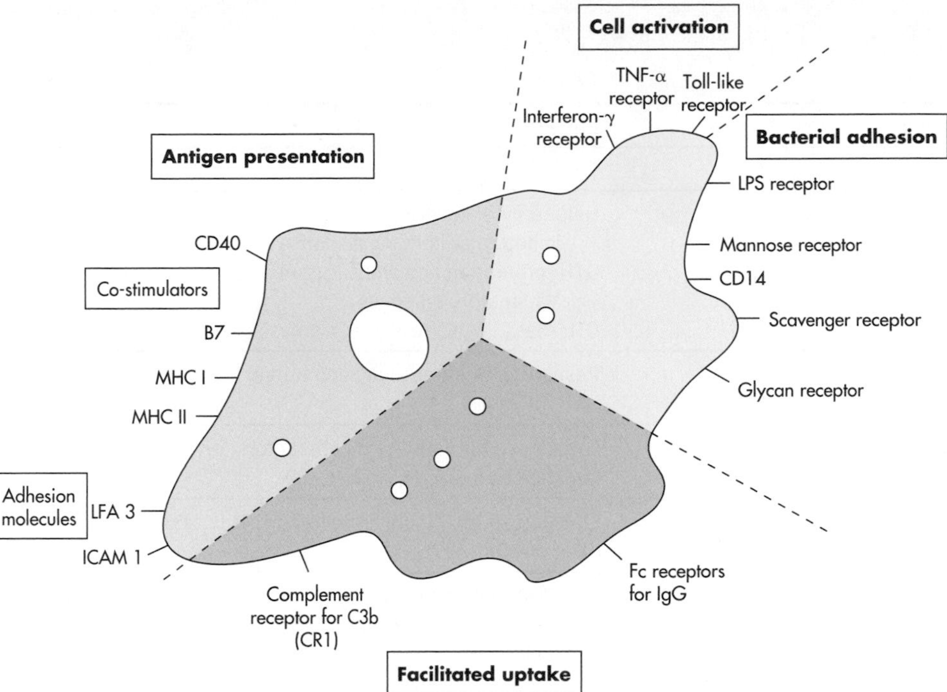

FIGURE 11–6. Macrophage surface structures mediate cell function. Bacteria and antigens either bind directly to receptors or through antibody or complement receptors (opsonization) and can then be phagocytized; the cell is activated and presents antigen to T cells. The dendritic cell shares many of these characteristics.

or tissue environments promote myeloid stem cells and monocytes to differentiate into the various macrophages and dendritic cells. These mature forms have different morphologies corresponding to their ultimate tissue location and function and may express a subset of macrophage activities or cell surface markers.

Macrophages are long-lived cells that are phagocytic, contain lysosomes and, unlike neutrophils, have mitochondria. Macrophages have the following basic functions: (1) phagocytosis, (2) antigen presentation to T cells to initiate specific immune responses, and (3) secretion of cytokines to activate and promote innate and immune responses (Figure 11–6). Macrophages express cell surface receptors for the Fc portion of immunoglobulin (Ig) G **(Fc-γ RI, Fc-γ RII, Fc-γ RIII)** and for the C3b product of the complement cascade **(CR1, CR3).** These receptors facilitate the phagocytosis of antigen, bacteria, or viruses coated with these proteins. **Toll-like and other pattern-recognition receptors** recognize pathogen-associated molecular patterns and activate protective responses. Macrophages also express the **class II MHC antigen,** which allows these cells to present antigen to CD4 helper T cells to initiate the immune response. Macrophages secrete **interleukin-1, interleukin-6, tumor necrosis factor, interleukin-12,** and other molecules in response to bacterial interaction, which stimulates immune and inflammatory responses, including fever. A T cell–derived lymphokine, **interferon-γ,** activates macrophages. **Activated macrophages** have enhanced phagocytic, killing, and antigen-presenting capabilities.

DENDRITIC CELLS

Dendritic cells (DCs) of myeloid and lymphoid origins have octopus-like tendrils and are professional APCs that can also produce cytokines. Different immature dendritic cells are found in tissue and blood; they include **Langerhans cells** in the skin, **dermal interstitial cells, splenic marginal dendritic** cells, and dendritic cells in the **liver, thymus, germinal centers of the lymph nodes,** and **blood.** Immature DCs capture and phagocytose antigen efficiently, release cytokines to activate and steer the subsequent immune response, and then mature into dendritic cells. These cells move to lymph node regions rich in T cells to present antigen on class I and class II MHC antigens.

LYMPHOCYTES

The lymphocytes are 6 to 10 μm in diameter, which is smaller than leukocytes. The two major classes of lymphocytes, **B cells** and **T cells,** have a large nucleus and smaller, agranular cytoplasm. Although B and T cells are indistinguishable by their morphologic features, they can be distinguished on the basis of function and surface markers (Table 11–5). Lymphoid cells that are not B or T cells (non-B/non-T cells, or null cells) are large, granular lymphocytes (LGLs), also known as **natural killer (NK) cells.**

The primary function of **B cells** is to **make antibody,** but they also internalize antigen, process the antigen, and

TABLE 11–5. Comparison of B and T Cells

Property	T Cells	B Cells
Origin	Bone marrow	Bone marrow
Maturation	Thymus	Bursal equivalent: bone marrow, Peyer's patches
Functions	Helper: cytokine production for initiation and promotion of immune response DTH: promotion and amplification of inflammatory response CTL: class I MHC–restricted cytolysis	**Antibody production** Antigen presentation to T cells —
Protective response	Resolution of intracellular and fungal infections	Protect against rechallenge, block spread of agent in blood, opsonize, etc.
Products*	Cytokines, interferon-γ, growth factors, cytolytic substances (perforin, granzymes)	IgM, IgD, IgG, IgA, or IgE
Distinguishing surface markers	CD2 (sheep red blood cell receptor), TCR, CD3, CD4, or CD8	Surface antibody, complement receptors, class II MHC antigens
Subsets	CD4 TH0: helper precursor CD4 TH1: activates growth, macrophage, and CTLs (DTH) CD4 TH2: B cell growth, class switching CD4 TH3: class switching-IgA, suppression CD8: cytotoxic T cells (CTL) CD8: suppressor cells Memory cells: long-lived, anamnestic response	B cells: antibody, antigen presentation Plasma cell: terminally differentiated antibody factories Memory cells: long-lived, anamnestic response

CTL, Cytotoxic lymphocyte; DTH, delayed-type hypersensitivity; Ig, immunoglobulin; MHC, major histocompatibility complex; TCR, T-cell receptor.
*Depending on subset.

present the antigen to T cells to initiate or enhance the immune response. B cells can be identified by the presence of immunoglobulins, class II MHC molecules, and receptors for the C3b and C3d products of the complement cascade (CR1, CR2) on their cell surfaces (Figure 11–7). The B-cell name is derived from its site of differentiation in birds, the *b*ursa of Fabricius and the *b*one marrow of mammals. B-cell differentiation also takes place in the fetal liver and fetal spleen. Activated B cells either develop into **memory cells,** which express the CD45RO cell surface marker and circulate until activated by specific antigen, or terminally differentiate into plasma cells. **Plasma cells** have small nuclei and a large cytoplasm for their job as producers of antibody.

T cells acquired their name because they develop in the *t*hymus. T cells have the following two major functions in response to foreign antigen:

1. Control, suppress (when necessary), and activate immune and inflammatory responses by releasing cytokines.
2. Directly kill virally infected cells, foreign cells (e.g., tissue grafts), and tumors.

T cells make up 60% to 80% of peripheral blood lymphocytes.

T cells were initially distinguished from B cells on the basis of their ability to bind and surround themselves (forming rosettes) with sheep erythrocytes through the CD2 molecule. All T cells express an antigen-binding **T-cell receptor (TCR),** which resembles but differs from antibody, and **CD2-** and **CD3-associated** proteins on their cell surface (see Figure 11–7). T cells are divided into three major groups on the basis of the type of TCR and the cell surface expression of two proteins, CD4 and CD8. Most lymphocytes express the αβ **TCR. CD4-expressing T cells** are primarily cytokine-producing cells, which help initiate and mature immune responses, activate macrophages to induce delayed-type hypersensitivity responses (DTH), and a subset of these cells suppress responses. The CD4 T cells can be further divided into TH0, TH1, TH2, and TH3 subgroups according to the spectrum of cytokines they secrete and the type of immune response that they promote. TH1 cells promote local, cellular inflammatory, and DTH responses, whereas TH2 cells promote antibody production. TH3 cells promote IgA production and T-cell tolerance. The **CD8 T cells** also release cytokines but are better known for their ability to recognize and kill virally infected cells, foreign tissue transplants (non–self-grafts), and tumor cells as cytotoxic killer T cells. CD8 T cells are also responsible for suppressing

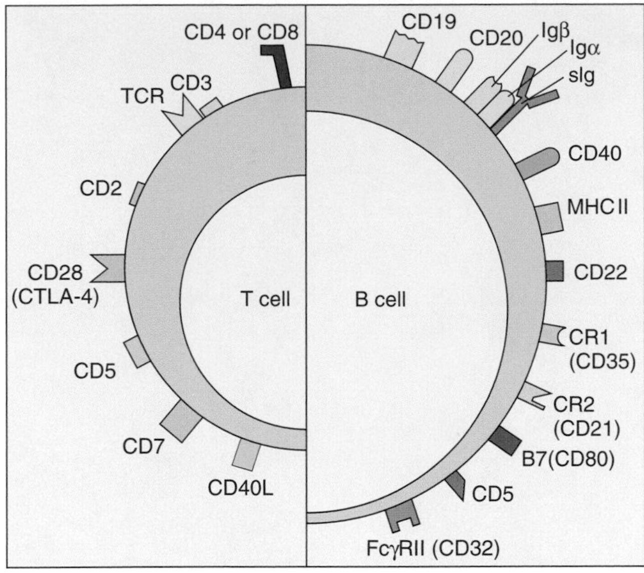

FIGURE 11–7. Surface markers of human B and T cells.

immune responses. T cells also produce **memory cells** that express CD45RO. Terminally differentiated effector CD4 and CD8 T cells express the class II MHC antigen. A variable number of T cells express the γδ **TCR** but do not express CD4 or CD8. These cells generally reside in skin and mucosa and are important for innate immunity.

The **large, granular lymphocyte NK cells** resemble the CD8 T cells in cytolytic function toward virally infected and tumor cells, but they differ in the mechanism for identifying the target cell. NK cells also have Fc receptors, which are used in antibody-dependent killing and hence are also called **antibody-dependent cellular cytotoxicity (ADCC or K) cells.** The cytoplasmic granules contain cytolytic proteins to mediate the killing.

QUESTIONS

A professor was teaching an introductory course and described the different immune cells with the following nicknames. Explain why the nicknames are appropriate or, why they are not.

1. Macrophage: Pac-man (a computer game character who normally eats dots but eats bad guys when activated)
2. Lymph node: Police department
3. CD4 T cell: Desk sergeant/dispatch officer
4. CD8 T cell: "Cop on the beat"/patrol officer
5. B cell: Product design and building company
6. Plasma cell: factory
7. Mast cell: Activatable chemical warfare unit
8. Neutrophil: Trash collector and disinfector
9. Dendritic cell: Billboard display

Bibliography

Abbas AK et al: *Cellular and molecular immunology,* ed 5, Philadelphia, 2003, WB Saunders.

Goldsby RA, Kindt TJ, Osborne BA: *Kuby immunology,* ed 5, New York, 2003, WH Freeman.

Trends in Immunology: Issues contain understandable reviews on current topics in immunology.

Janeway CA et al: *Immunobiology: The immune system in health and disease,* ed 6, New York, 2004, Current Biology Publications and Garland Press.

Male D. *Immunology,* ed 4. London, 2004, Elsevier.

Male D et al: *Advanced immunology,* ed 3, St Louis, 1996, Mosby.

Roitt I, Brostoff J, Male D: *Immunology,* ed 4, St Louis, 1996, Mosby.

Sompayrac L: *How the immune system works,* ed 2, Malden, Mass, 2003, Blackwell Scientific.

CHAPTER 12

The Humoral Immune Response

The primary molecular component of the humoral immune response is antibody. B cells and plasma cells synthesize antibody molecules in response to challenge by antigen. Antibodies provide protection from rechallenge by an infectious agent, block spread of the agent in the blood, and facilitate elimination of the infectious agent. To accomplish these tasks, an incredibly large repertoire of antibody molecules must be available to recognize the tremendous number of infectious agents and molecules that challenge our bodies. In addition to interacting specifically with foreign structures, antibodies must interact with host systems and cells (e.g., complement, macrophages) to promote clearance of antigen and activation of subsequent immune responses (Box 12–1). Antibody molecules also serve as the cell surface receptors that stimulate the appropriate B cell antibody factories to grow and produce more antibody in response to antigenic challenge.

Immunogens, Antigens, and Epitopes

Almost all of the proteins and carbohydrates associated with an infectious agent, whether a bacterium, fungus, virus, or parasite, are considered foreign to the human host and have the potential to induce an immune response. A protein or carbohydrate that challenges the immune system and can initiate an immune response is called an **immunogen** (Box 12–2). Immunogens may contain more than one antigen (e.g., bacteria). An **antigen** is a molecule that is recognized by specific antibody or T cells. An **epitope (antigenic determinant)** is the actual molecular structure that interacts with a single antibody molecule. Within a protein, an epitope may be formed by a specific sequence **(linear epitope)** or a three-dimensional structure **(conformational epitope).** Antigens and immunogens usually contain several epitopes, each capable of binding to a different antibody molecule. As described later in this chapter, a **monoclonal antibody** recognizes a single epitope.

Not all molecules are immunogens. In general, *proteins are the best immunogens, carbohydrates are weaker immunogens, and lipids and nucleic acids are poor immunogens.* In general the immunogen must be of sufficient size, and proteins must be degradable by phagocytes so that they can be presented to lymphocytes, to initiate an immune response. **Haptens (incomplete immunogens)** are often too small to immunize (i.e., initiate a response) an individual but can be recognized by antibody. Haptens can be made immunogenic by attachment to a **carrier molecule,** such as a protein. For example, dinitrophenol conjugated to bovine serum albumin is an immunogen for the dinitrophenol hapten.

During artificial immunization (e.g., vaccines), an adjuvant is used to enhance the response to antigen. **Adjuvants** usually prolong the presence of antigen in the tissue and activate or promote uptake of the immunogen by dendritic cells (DCs), macrophages, and lymphocytes. Ideally, an adjuvant activates responses that mimic a natural antigenic challenge, such as would occur during an infection. Most vaccines are precipitated onto alum to promote the slow release of antigen and the uptake by macrophages. Cells are stimulated and antigen is released slowly when emulsified in complete Freund's adjuvant (consisting of heat-killed mycobacteria in mineral oil). Complete Freund's adjuvant is not for human use, but newer, less toxic adjuvants are being tested for use with human vaccines. These include liposomes (defined lipid complexes), bacterial cell wall components, molecular cages for antigen, and polymeric surfactants. Cholera toxin and *Escherichia coli* lymphotoxin are potent adjuvants for secretory antibody (immunoglobulin [Ig] A).

BOX 12–1. Antimicrobial Action of Antibodies

Are opsonic: promote ingestion and killing by phagocytic cells (IgG)
Neutralize (block attachment) toxins and virus
Agglutinate bacteria: may aid in clearing
Render motile organisms nonmotile
Combine with antigens on the microbial surface and activate the complement cascade, thus inducing an inflammatory response, bringing fresh phagocytes and serum antibodies into the site
Combine with antigens on the microbial surface, activate the complement cascade, and anchor the membrane attack complex involving C5b to C9

BOX 12–2. Definitions

Adjuvant: Substance that promotes immune response to immunogen
Antigen: Substance *recognized* by immune response
Carrier: Protein modified by hapten to elicit response
Epitope: Molecular structure recognized by immune response
Hapten: Incomplete immunogen that cannot initiate response but that can be recognized by antibody
Immunogen: Substance capable of *eliciting* an immune response
T-dependent antigens: Antigens that must be presented to T and B cells for antibody production
T-independent antigens: Antigens with large, repetitive structures (e.g., bacteria, flagellin, lipopolysaccharide, polysaccharide)

Some molecules will not elicit an immune response in an individual. During growth of the fetus, the body develops **immune tolerance** toward self-antigens and any foreign antigens that may be introduced before maturation of the immune system. Later in life, tolerance may develop under special conditions; for example, ingestion of high concentrations of bovine myelin can cause an individual to develop tolerance to myelin. This has been proposed as a potential therapy for the autoimmunopathogenesis that causes multiple sclerosis.

The type of immune response initiated by an immunogen depends on its molecular structure. A primitive but rapid antibody response can be initiated toward *bacterial polysaccharides, peptidoglycan, or flagellin.* Termed **T-independent antigens,** these molecules have a large, repetitive structure, which is sufficient to activate B cells directly to make antibody without the participation of T-cell help. In these cases the response is limited to production of **IgM** antibody and fails to stimulate an anamnestic (booster) response. The transition from an IgM response to an IgG, IgE, or IgA response is a big change in the B cell and is equivalent to differentiation of the cell. This requires help, in the form of cytokines, from T cells. The antigen must therefore be recognized and stimulate both T and B cells. **T-dependent antigens** are usually proteins; they stimulate all five classes of immunoglobulins and can elicit an **anamnestic** (secondary-booster) response.

In addition to the structure of the antigen, the amount, route of administration, and other factors influence the type of immune response, including the types of antibody produced. For example, oral or nasal administration of a vaccine promotes production of a secretory form of **IgA** (sIgA) that would not be produced on intramuscular challenge.

Immunoglobulin Types and Structures

Immunoglobulins are composed of at least two heavy chains and two light chains, a dimer of dimers. They are subdivided into classes and subclasses based on the structure and antigenic distinction of their heavy chains. IgG, IgM, and IgA are the major antibody forms, whereas IgD and IgE make up less than 1% of the total immunoglobulins. The IgA and IgG classes of immunoglobulin are divided further into subclasses based on differences in the Fc portion. There are four subclasses of IgG, designated as IgG1 through IgG4, and two IgA subclasses (IgA1 and IgA2) (Figure 12–1).

Antibody molecules are Y-shaped molecules with two major structural regions that mediate the two major functions of the molecule (Figure 12–1 and Table 12–1). The **variable-region/antigen-combining site** must be able to identify and specifically interact with an epitope on an antigen. A large number of different antibody molecules, each with a different variable region, are produced in every individual to recognize the seemingly infinite number of different antigens in nature. The **Fc portion** (stem of the antibody Y) interacts with host systems and cells to promote clearance of antigen and activation of subsequent immune responses. The Fc portion is responsible for fixation of complement and binding of the molecule to cell surface immunoglobulin receptors **(FcR)** on macrophages, natural killer cells, and T cells. For IgG and IgA, the Fc portion interacts with other proteins to promote transfer across the placenta and the mucosa, respectively (Table 12–2). In addition, each of the different types of antibody can be synthesized with a **membrane-spanning portion** to make it a cell surface antigen receptor.

IgG and IgA have a flexible **hinge region** rich in proline and susceptible to cleavage by proteolytic enzymes. Digestion of IgG molecules with **papain** yields two **Fab** fragments and one **Fc** fragment (see Figure 12–2). Each Fab fragment has one antigen-binding site. **Pepsin** cleaves the molecule, producing an **F(ab′)$_2$** fragment with two antigen-binding sites and a **pFc′** fragment.

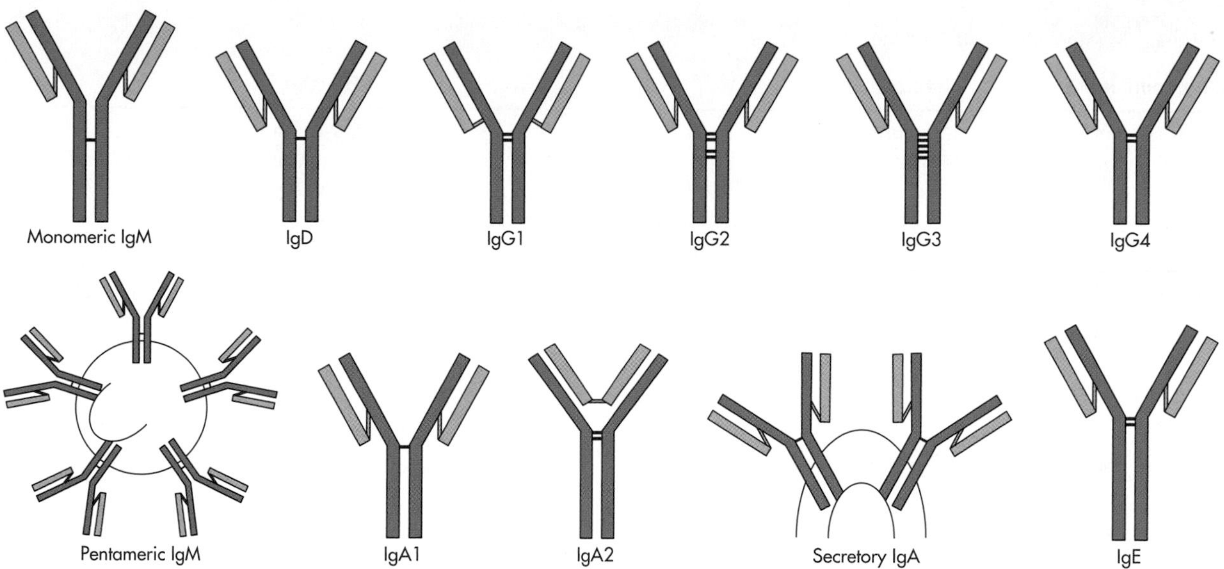

FIGURE 12–1. Comparative structures of the immunoglobulin (Ig) classes and subclasses in humans. IgA and IgM are held together in multimers by the J chain. IgA can acquire the secretory component for the traversal of epithelial cells.

TABLE 12–1. Immunoglobulins

Ig	IgM	IgD	IgG	IgE	IgA
CD4 T-helper subclass association	T independent and TH1	—	TH1, TH2	TH2	TH2, TH3
Total Ig (%)	5–10	<1	85	<1	5–15
Molecular mass (kDa)	900	185	154	190	160 (+dimer)
H-chain class	μ	δ	γ	ε	α
Subclass	—	—	γ-1, γ-2, γ-3, γ-4	—	α-1, α-2
Serum half-life (days)	5	2–3	23	2–3	6
Principal site of action	Serum	Receptor for B cells	Serum and tissue	Mast cells	Secretions
Principal biologic effect	Resistance: precipitin, primary response	B-cell activation	Resistance: opsonin, secondary response	Anaphylaxis	Resistance: protection of mucous membranes
Complement fixation	++++	–	+++	–	+
Opsonin for macrophage, PMN			+		
Mucosal secretion	–	–	–	–	+
Crossing of placenta	–	–	+	–	–

PMN, Polymorphonuclear neutrophil (leukocyte); +/–, relative activity.

The different types and parts of immunoglobulin can also be distinguished using antibodies directed against different portions of the molecule. **Isotypes (IgM, IgD, IgG, IgA, IgE)** are determined by antibodies directed against the Fc portion of the molecule (*iso* meaning the same for all people.) **Allotypic** differences occur for antibody molecules with the same isotype but contain protein sequences that differ from one person to another (in addition to the antigen-binding region). *(Every one ["allo"] of them cannot have the same IgG.)* The **idiotype** refers to the

TABLE 12–2. Fc Interactions with Immune Components

Immune Component	Interaction	Function
Fc receptor	Macrophages	Opsonization
	PMNs	Opsonization
	T cells	Activation
	NK cells (antibody-dependent cellular cytotoxicity)	Killing
	Mast cells for immunoglobulin E	Allergic reactions, antiparasitic
Complement	Complement system	Opsonization, killing (especially bacteria)

NK, Natural killer; PMN, polymorphonuclear neutrophils.

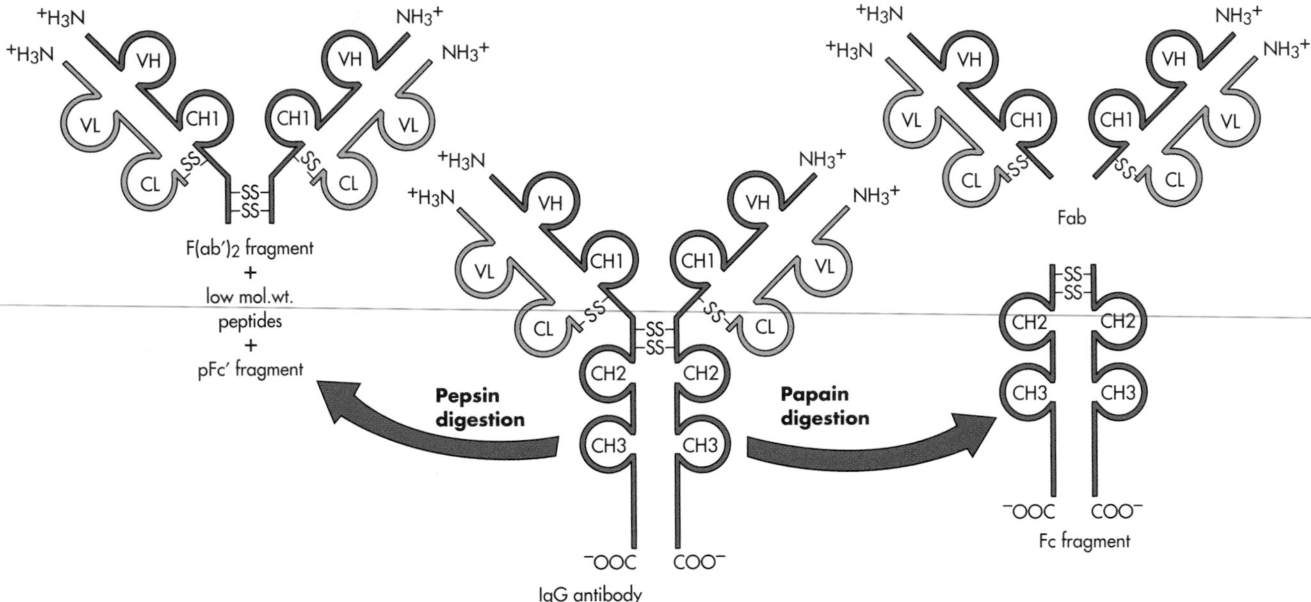

FIGURE 12–2. Proteolytic digestion of immunoglobulin G (IgG). Pepsin treatment produces a dimeric F(ab′)$_2$ fragment. Papain treatment produces monovalent Fab fragments and an Fc fragment. The F(ab′)$_2$ and the Fab fragments bind antigen but lack a functional Fc region. The heavy chain is depicted in blue; the light chain in orange.

protein sequences in the variable region that generate the large number of antigen-binding regions. *(There are many different idiots.)*

On a molecular basis, each antibody molecule is made up of heavy and light chains encoded by separate genes. The basic immunoglobulin unit consists of **two heavy (H)** and **two light (L) chains.** IgM and IgA consist of multimers of this basic structure. The heavy and light chains of immunoglobulin are fastened together by **interchain disulfide bonds.** Two types of light chains—**κ and λ**—are present in all five immunoglobulin classes, although only one type is present in an individual molecule. Approximately 60% of human immunoglobulin molecules have κ light chains, and 40% have λ light chains. There are **five types of heavy chains,** one for each isotype of antibody **(IgM, μ; IgG, γ; IgD, δ; IgA, α; and IgE, ε).** Intrachain disulfide bonds define molecular domains within each chain. Light chains have a variable and a constant domain. The heavy chains have a variable and three (IgG, IgA) or four (IgM, IgE) constant domains. The variable domains on the heavy and light chains interact to form the antigen-binding site. The constant domains from each chain provide the molecular structure to the immunoglobulin and define the interaction of the antibody molecule with host systems, hence its ultimate function. The heavy chain of the different antibody molecules can also be synthesized with a membrane-spanning region to make the antibody an antigen-specific cell surface receptor for the B cell.

IMMUNOGLOBULIN D

IgD, which has a molecular mass of 185 kDa, accounts for less than 1% of serum immunoglobulins. IgD exists primarily as membrane IgD, which serves with IgM as an antigen receptor on early B-cell membranes to help initiate antibody responses by activating B cell growth. IgD and IgM are the only isotypes that can be expressed together by the same cell.

IMMUNOGLOBULIN M

IgM is the first antibody produced in response to antigenic challenge and can be produced in a T-cell–independent manner. IgM makes up 5% to 10% of the total immunoglobulins in adults and has a half-life of 5 days. It is a **pentameric molecule** with five immunoglobulin units joined by disulfide bonds and the **J chain,** with a total molecular mass of 900 kDa. Theoretically, this immunoglobulin has 10 antigen-binding sites. IgM is the most efficient immunoglobulin for fixing (binding) complement. A single IgM pentamer can activate the classical complement pathway. Monomeric IgM is found with IgD on the B-cell surface, where it serves as the receptor for antigen. Because IgM is relatively large, it cannot spread from the blood into tissue. IgM is particularly important for immunity against polysaccharide antigens on the exterior of pathogenic microorganisms. It also promotes phagocytosis and promotes bacteriolysis by activating complement through its Fc portion. IgM is also a major component of rheumatoid factors (autoantibodies).

IMMUNOGLOBULIN G

IgG comprises approximately 85% of the immunoglobulins in adults. It has a molecular mass of 154 kDa, based on two L chains of 22,000 Da each and two H chains of 55,000 Da each. The four subclasses of IgG differ in structure (see Figure 12–1), relative concentration, and function. Production of IgG requires T-cell help. IgG, as a class of antibody molecules, has the longest half-life (23 days) of the five immunoglobulin classes, crosses the placenta, and is the principal antibody in the **anamnestic or booster response.** IgG shows high avidity (binding capacity) for antigens, fixes complement, stimulates chemotaxis, and acts as an opsonin to facilitate phagocytosis.

IMMUNOGLOBULIN A

IgA comprises 5% to 15% of the serum immunoglobulins and has a half-life of 6 days. It has a molecular mass of 160 kDa and a basic four-chain monomeric structure. However, it can occur as monomers, dimers, trimers, and multimers combined by the J chain (similar to IgM). In addition to serum IgA, a **secretory IgA** appears in body secretions and provides localized immunity. IgA production requires specialized T-cell help and mucosal stimulation. Adjuvants, such as cholera toxin and attenuated *Salmonella* bacteria, can promote an IgA response. IgA binds to a **poly-Ig receptor** on epithelial cells for transport across the cell. The poly-Ig receptor remains bound to IgA and is then cleaved to become the **secretory component** when secretory IgA is secreted from the cell. An adult secretes approximately 2 g of IgA per day. Secretory IgA appears in colostrum, intestinal and respiratory secretions, saliva, tears, and other secretions. IgA-deficient individuals have an increased incidence of respiratory tract infections.

IMMUNOGLOBULIN E

IgE accounts for less than 1% of the total immunoglobulins and has a half-life of approximately 2.5 days. Most IgE is bound to Fc receptors on **mast cells,** on which it serves as a receptor for allergens and parasite antigens. When sufficient antigen binds to the IgE on the mast cell, the mast cell releases histamine, prostaglandin, platelet-activating factor, and cytokines. IgE is important for protection against parasitic infection and is responsible for **anaphylactic hypersensitivity** (type 1) (rapid allergic reactions).

Immunogenetics

The antibody response can recognize as many as 10^8 structures but can still specifically amplify and focus a response directed to a specific challenge. The mechanisms for generating this antibody repertoire and the different immunoglobulin subclasses are tied to the genetic events that accompany the development (differentiation) of the B cell (Figures 12–3 and 12–4).

Human chromosomes 2, 22, and 14 contain immunoglobulin genes for κ, λ, and H chains, respectively. The **germline forms** of these genes consist of different and separate sets of genetic building blocks for the light **(V and J gene segments)** and heavy chains **(V, D, and J gene segments),** which are genetically recombined to produce the immunoglobulin variable regions. These variable regions are then associated with the constant-region C gene segments. For the κ light chain, there are 300 V gene segments, 5 J gene segments, and 1 C gene segment. The number of λ gene segments for V and J is more limited. For the heavy chain, there are 300 to 1000 V genes, 12 D genes, and 6 (heavy-chain) J genes, but only 9 C genes (one for each class and subclass of antibody [μ; δ; γ_3, γ_1, γ_2, and γ_4; ε; α_1 and α_2]). In addition, gene segments for membrane-spanning peptides can be attached to the heavy-chain genes to allow the antibody molecule to insert into the B-cell membrane as an antigen-activation receptor.

Production of the final antibody molecule in the pre-B and B cell requires genetic recombination at the deoxyribonucleic acid (DNA) level and post-transcriptional processing at the ribonucleic acid (RNA) level to assemble the immunoglobulin gene and messenger RNA (mRNA)

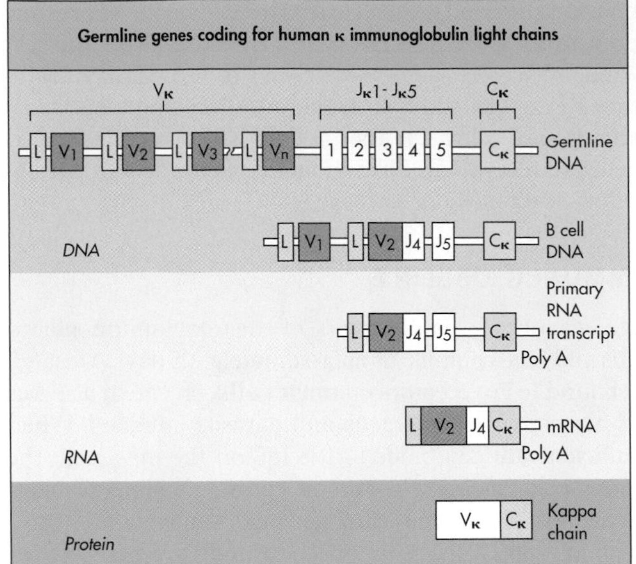

FIGURE 12–3. Rearrangement of the germline genes to produce the human immunoglobulin κ light chains. Genetic recombination juxtaposes one of the 100 V-region genes with a J-region gene and a Cκ gene during differentiation into a pre-B cell. The remaining intervening sequences are removed by splicing the messenger RNA. L, Leader sequence.

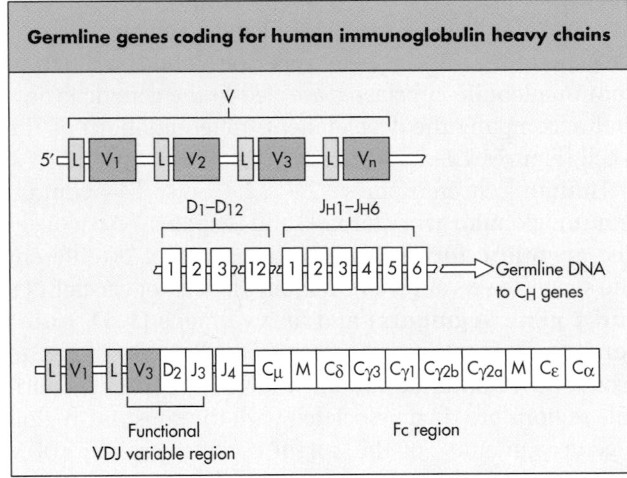

FIGURE 12–4. Rearrangement of the germline genes to produce the human immunoglobulin (Ig) heavy chains. A V-region gene (of 100 possible) combines with a D-region gene (of 12 possible) and a J-region gene (of six possible). Constant-region genes (corresponding to IgM [μ], IgD [δ], IgG [γ], IgE [ε], and IgA [α]) are attached to the VDJ region. M, Membrane-spanning segment.

(Figure 12–5). Each of the V, D, and J segments is surrounded by DNA sequences that promote **directional recombination and loss of the intervening DNA sequences.** Juxtaposition of randomly chosen V and J gene segments of the light chains and the V, D, and J gene segments of the heavy chains produces the variable region of the immunoglobulin chains. These recombination reactions are analogous to matching and sewing together similar patterns from a long swatch of cloth, then cutting out the intervening loops of extra cloth. **Somatic mutation** of the immunoglobulin gene occurs later in activated, growing B cells to add to the enormous number of possible coding sequences for the variable region and to fine-tune a specific immune response. Attachment of the variable-region sequences (VDJ) to the beginning of the C gene segments by recombination produces a heavy-chain gene containing the μ; δ; γ_3, γ_1, γ_2, and γ_4; ε; and α_1 and α_2 sequences in the indicated order. In the pre-B and immature B cells, mRNAs are produced and contain the variable-region gene segments connected to the C gene sequences for μ and δ. Processing of the mRNA removes either the μ or δ, as if it were an intron, to produce the final immunoglobulin. The pre-B cell expresses cytoplasmic IgM, whereas the B cell expresses cytoplasmic and cell surface IgM and cell surface IgD. IgM and IgD are the only pair of isotypes that can be expressed on the same cell.

Class switching (IgM to IgG, IgE, or IgA) occurs in mature B cells in response to different cytokines produced by TH1, TH2, or TH3 CD4 helper T cells. Genetic recombination juxtaposes the appropriate constant-region sequence with the variable-region sequences and in the process deletes the intervening C-region gene segments (see Figure 12–5). Each of the C gene segments, except for δ, is preceded by a DNA sequence, called the **switch site.** After the appropriate cytokine signal, the switch in front of the μ sequence recombines with the switch in front of the γ_3, γ_1, γ_2, or γ_4; ε; or α_1, or α_2 sequences, creating a DNA loop that is subsequently removed. Processing of the RNA transcript yields the final mRNA for the immunoglobulin heavy-chain protein. For example, IgG1 production would result from excision of DNA containing the C gene segments C_μ, C_δ, and $C\gamma_3$ to attach the variable region to the γ_1 C gene segment. **Class switching does not change the variable region.**

The final steps in B-cell differentiation to memory cells or plasma cells do not change the antibody gene. **Memory cells** are long-lived, antigen-responsive B cells expressing the CD45RO surface marker. Memory cells can be activated in response to antigen later in life to divide and then produce its specific antibody. **Plasma cells** are terminally differentiated B cells with a small nucleus but a large cytoplasm filled with endoplasmic reticulum. Plasma cells are antibody factories.

Antibody Response

An initial repertoire of IgM and IgD immunoglobulins is generated in pre-B cells by the genetic events previously described (Figure 12–6). Expression of cell surface IgM and IgD accompany differentiation of the pre-B cell to the B cell. Cell surface antibody is associated with signal

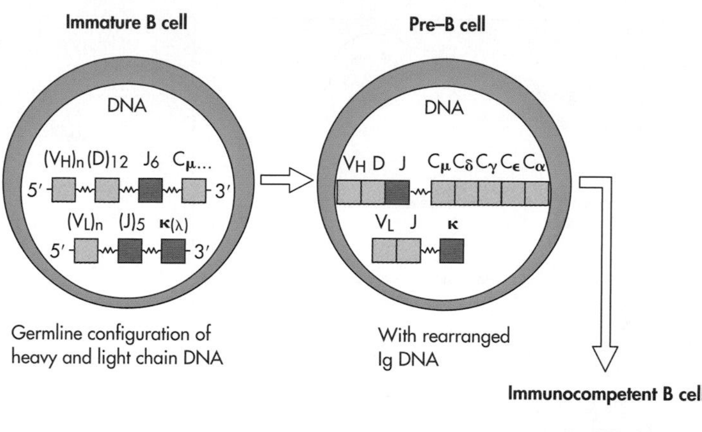

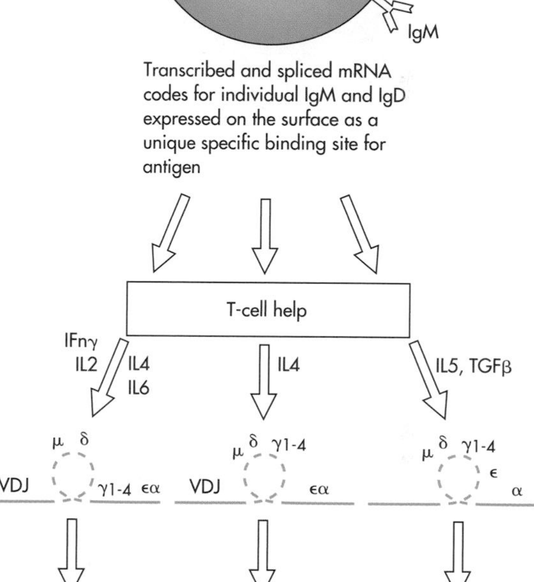

FIGURE 12–5. Differentiation of the B cell promotes genetic recombination and class switching. Switch regions in front of the constant-region genes (including immunoglobulin [Ig] G subclasses) allow attachment of a preformed VDJ region with different heavy-chain constant-region genes, genetically removing the μ, δ, and other intervening genes. This produces an immunoglobulin gene with the same VDJ region (except for somatic mutation) but different heavy-chain genes. Splicing of messenger RNA (mRNA) produces the final IgM and IgD mRNA.

transduction receptors, Ig-α (CD79a) and Ig-β (CD79b), in the membrane through which antigen binding initiates an activation signal. A cascade of protein tyrosine kinases, phospholipase C, and calcium fluxes that activate transcription and cell growth mediate the activation signal. Other surface molecules, including the CR2 (CD21) complement (C3d) receptor, amplify the activation signal. T-independent antigens cross-link sufficient numbers of surface antibody to stimulate growth of the antigen-specific B cells. In this manner, the B cells that best recognize the different epitopes of the antigen are selected to increase in number in a process termed **clonal expansion.** Production of antibody to T-dependent antigens requires interaction of the B cell with the helper T cell through CD40 (on the B cell), CD40L (T cell), and the action of cytokines (interleukin-4 [IL-4], IL-5, IL-2, or interferon-γ) and the C3d component of complement.

Clonal expansion of the antigen-specific B cells increases the number of antibody factories making the relevant antibody, and the strength of the antibody response is thus increased. Activation of the B cells also promotes ***somatic mutation*** *of the variable region, increasing the diversity of antibody molecules* directed at the specific antigen. The B-cell clones that express antibody with the strongest antigen binding are preferentially stimulated, selecting for a better antibody response.

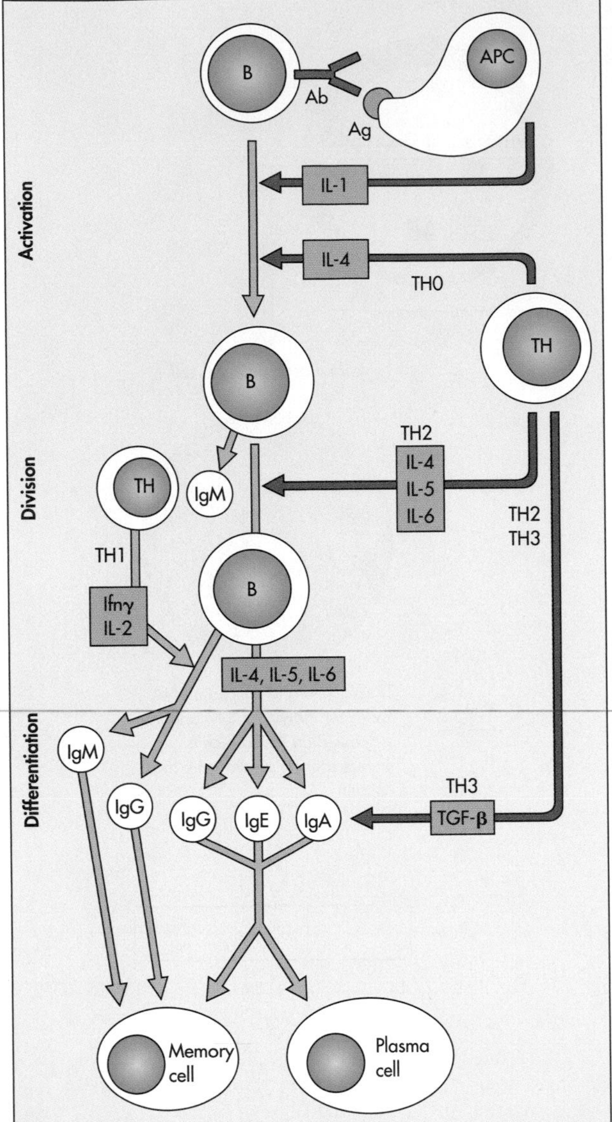

FIGURE 12–6. B-cell activation. Binding of antigen, cross-linking of cell surface receptors, and the C3d product of complement, endotoxin, and cytokines activate the growth and differentiation of B cells. Specific cytokines direct the development of the B cell to produce TH1, TH2, or TH3 associated antibodies. APC, Antigen-presenting cell; Ifnγ, interferon-γ; Ig, immunoglobulin; IL, interleukin; TGF-β, transforming growth factor-β.

Different combinations of cytokines produced by helper T cells induce class switching. **TH1-helper responses (IL-2, interferon-γ) promote production of IgM and IgG. TH2-helper responses (IL-4, IL-5, IL-6, IL-10) promote production of IgM, IgG, IgE, and IgA. IgA production is especially promoted by IL-5 and transforming growth factor-β (TGF-β).** Memory cells are developed with T-cell help. Terminal differentiation produces the ultimate antibody factory, the plasma cell.

The primary antibody response is characterized by the initial production of IgM. As the response matures, IgG antibodies rapidly increase in concentration (Figure 12–7). IgM antibodies appear in the blood within 3 days to 2 weeks after exposure to a novel immunogen. The first antibodies that are produced react with residual antigen and therefore are rapidly cleared. After the initial lag phase, however, the antibody titer increases logarithmically to reach a plateau.

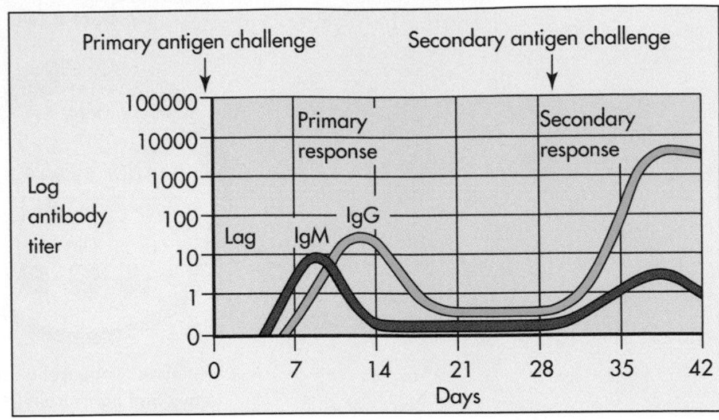

FIGURE 12–7. Time course of immune responses. The primary response occurs after a lag period. The immunoglobulin (Ig) M response is the earliest response. The secondary immune response (anamnestic response) reaches a higher titer, lasts longer, and consists predominantly of IgG.

Reexposure to an immunogen, a **secondary response,** induces a heightened antibody response (also termed **anamnestic response**). The antibodies develop more rapidly, last longer, and reach a higher titer. The antibodies in a secondary response are principally of the IgG class, although IgM antibodies can also be detected in response to some infections.

During an immune response, antibodies are made against different epitopes of the foreign object, protein, or infectious agent. *Specific antibody is a mixture of many different immunoglobulin molecules made by many different B cells* **(polyclonal antibody),** each immunoglobulin molecule differing in the epitope that it recognizes and the strength of the interaction. Different antibody molecules are made against different epitopes on the antigen, and each binds with different strengths (**avidity,** multivalent binding of antibody to antigen; **affinity,** monovalent binding to an epitope) for the same antigen.

Monoclonal antibodies are identical antibodies produced by a single clone of cells or by myelomas (cancers of plasma cells) or hybridomas. Hybridomas are cloned, laboratory-derived cells obtained by the fusion of antibody-producing spleen cells and a myeloma cell. In 1975, Kohler and Millstein developed the technique for producing monoclonal antibodies from B-cell hybridomas. The hybridoma is immortal and produces a single (monoclonal) antibody. This technique has revolutionized the study of immunology because it allows selection (cloning) of individual antibody-producing cells and their

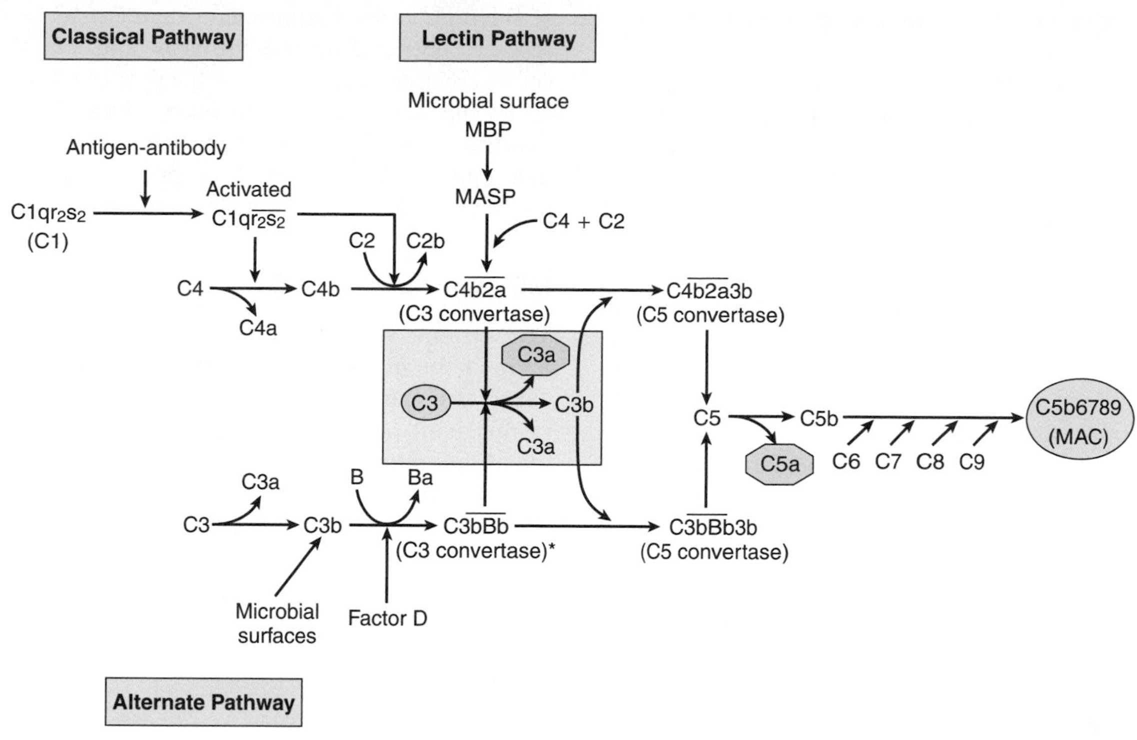

FIGURE 12–8. The classical, lectin, and alternate complement pathways. Despite different activators, the goal of these pathways is cleavage of C3 and C5 to provide chemoattractants and anaphylotoxins (C3a, C5a), an opsonin (C3b) that adheres to membranes, and to initiate the membrane attack complex to kill cells. MASP, MBP-associated serine protease; MBP, mannose-binding protein. (Redrawn from Rosenthal KS, Tan JS: *Rapid review microbiology and immunology,* St. Louis, 2002, Mosby.)

development into cellular factories for production of large quantities of that antibody. Monoclonal antibodies have been commercially produced for both diagnostic reagents and therapeutic purposes.

Complement

The complement system is an alarm and a weapon against infection, especially bacterial infection. The complement system is activated directly by bacteria and bacterial products **(alternate or properdin pathway)**, by lectin binding to sugars on the bacterial cell surface **(mannose-binding protein)**, or by complexes of antibody and antigen **(classical pathway)** (Figure 12–8). Activation by either pathway initiates a cascade of proteolytic events that produce chemotactic factors to attract phagocytic and inflammatory cells to the site, increase vascular permeability to allow access to the site of infection, bind to the agent to promote their phagocytosis **(opsonization)** and elimination, and directly kill the infecting agent. The three activation pathways of complement coalesce at a common junction point, the activation of the **C3 component.**

ALTERNATE PATHWAY

The alternate pathway is activated directly by bacterial cell surfaces and their components (e.g., endotoxin, microbial polysaccharides), as well as other factors. This pathway can be activated before the establishment of an immune response to the infecting bacteria because it does not depend on antibody and does not involve the early complement components (C1, C2, and C4). The initial activation of the alternate pathway is mediated by *properdin factor B* binding to C3b and then with *properdin factor D,* which splits *factor B* in the complex to yield the *Bb active fragment* that remains linked to *C3b (activation unit).* The C3b sticks to the cell surface and anchors the complex. Inactive *Ba* is split from this complex, leading to cleavage and activation of many C3 molecules (amplification). The complement cascade continues in a manner analogous to the classical pathway.

CLASSICAL PATHWAY

The classical complement cascade is initiated by *binding to the Fc portion of antibody that is bound to cell surface antigens, or in an immune complex with soluble antigens.* Aggregation of antibody **(IgG or IgM, not IgA or IgE)** changes the structure of the heavy chain to allow binding to complement (see Figure 12–8).

The first complement component, designated *C1*, consists of a complex of three separate proteins designated *C1q, C1r, and C1s* (see Figure 12–8). One molecule each of C1q and C1s with two molecules of C1r comprises the C1 complex or **recognition unit.** C1q facilitates binding of the recognition unit to cell surface antigen-antibody complexes. Activation of the classical complement cascade requires linkage of C1q to two IgG antibodies through their Fc regions. In contrast, one pentameric IgM molecule attached to a cell surface may interact with C1q to initiate the classical pathway. Binding of C1q activates C1r (referred to now as C1r*) and in turn C1s (C1s*). C1s* then cleaves *C4* to C4a and C4b, and *C2* to C2a and C2b. The ability of a single recognition unit to split numerous C2 and C4 molecules represents an amplification mechanism in the complement cascade. The union of *C4b* and *C2a* produces **C4b2a,** which is known as **C3 convertase.** This complex binds to the cell membrane and cleaves *C3* into *C3a* and *C3b* fragments. The C3b protein has a unique thioester bond that will covalently attach C3b to a cell surface or be hydrolyzed. The C3 convertase amplifies the response by splitting many C3 molecules. The interaction of C3b with C4b2a bound to the cell membrane produces **C4b3b2a,** which is termed **C5 convertase.** This activation unit splits *C5* into *C5a* and *C5b* fragments and represents yet another amplification step.

LECTIN PATHWAY

The lectin pathway is also a bacterial and fungal defense mechanism. **Mannose-binding protein** (previously known as RaRF) is a large serum protein that binds to nonreduced mannose, fucose, and glucosamine on bacterial and other cell surfaces. Mannose-binding protein resembles and replaces the C1q component and on binding to bacterial surfaces, activates the cleavage of mannose-binding protein–associated serine protease. Mannose-binding protein–associated serine protease cleaves the C4 and C2 components to produce the C3 convertase, the junction point of the complement cascade.

BIOLOGIC ACTIVITIES OF COMPLEMENT COMPONENTS

Cleavage of the C3 and C5 components produces important factors that enhance clearance of the infectious agent by promoting access to the infection site and by attracting the cells that mediate protective inflammatory reactions. **C3b** is an **opsonin** that promotes clearance of bacteria by binding directly to the cell membrane to make the cell more attractive to phagocytic cells such as neutrophils and macrophages, which have receptors for C3b. C3b can be cleaved further to generate **C3d,** which is an activator of B lymphocytes. Complement fragments **C3a** and **C5a** serve as powerful **anaphylatoxins** that stimulate mast cells to release histamine, which *enhances vascular permeability and smooth muscle contraction.* **C3a** and **C5a** also act as attractants **(chemotactic factors)** for neutrophils and macrophages. These cells also express receptors for C3b, are phagocytic, and promote inflammatory reactions.

MEMBRANE ATTACK COMPLEX

The terminal stage of the classical pathway involves creation of the **membrane attack complex,** which is also called **the lytic unit** (Figure 12–9). The five terminal complement proteins (C5 through C9) associate into a membrane attack complex on target cell membranes to mediate injury. Initiation of membrane attack complex assembly begins with C5 cleavage into C5a and C5b fragments. A $(C5b,6,7,8)_1(C9)_n$ complex forms and drills a hole in the membrane, leading to the hypotonic lysis of

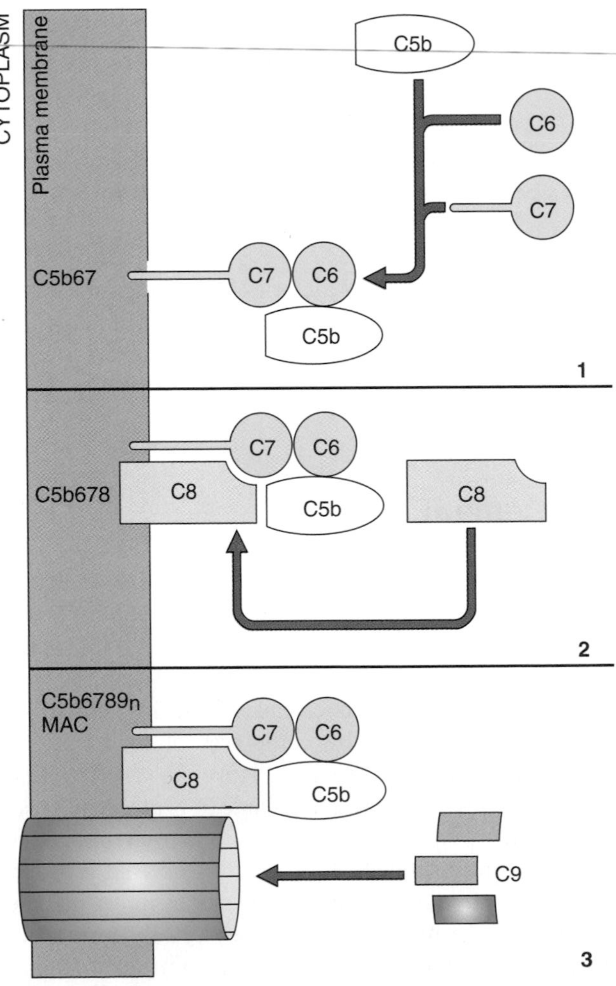

FIGURE 12–9. Cell lysis by complement. Activation of C5 initiates the molecular construction of an oil-well–like membrane attack complex (MAC).

cells. The C9 component is similar to perforin, which is produced by cytolytic T cells and natural killer cells.

REGULATION OF COMPLEMENT ACTIVATION

Humans have several mechanisms for preventing generation of the C3 convertase to protect against inappropriate complement activation. These include C1 inhibitor, C4 binding protein, Factor H, Factor I, and the cell surface proteins, which are decay-accelerating factor (DAF) and membrane cofactor protein. In addition, CD59 (protectin) prevents formation of the membrane attack complex. Most infectious agents lack these protective mechanisms and remain susceptible to complement. A genetic deficiency in these protection systems can result in disease.

QUESTIONS

What is wrong with each of the following statements, and why?

1. The laboratory tested a baby for IgM maternal antibodies.
2. An investigator attempted to use fluorescent-labeled $F(ab')_2$ fragments to locate class II major histocompatibility complex molecules on the cell surface of antigen-presenting cells without cross-linking (binding two molecules together) these cell surface molecules.
3. A patient is diagnosed as having been infected with a specific strain of influenza A (A/Bangkok/1/79/H3N2) on the basis of the presence of anti-influenza IgG in serum taken from the patient at the initial visit (within 2 days of symptoms).
4. A patient with a T-cell deficiency, unable to promote class switching of B cells, was also considered unable to use the complement systems.
5. Analysis of immunoglobulin genes from B cells taken from the patient described in statement 4 did not contain recombined VDJ variable-region gene sequences.
6. A patient was considered to have a B-cell deficiency because serum levels of IgE and IgD were undetectable despite proper concentrations of IgG and IgM.

Bibliography

Abbas AK et al: *Cellular and molecular immunology*, ed 5, Philadelphia, 2003, WB Saunders.

Goldsby RA, Kindt TJ, Osborne BA: *Kuby immunology*, ed 5, New York, 2003, WH Freeman.

Trends in Immunology: Issues contain understandable reviews on current topics in immunology.

Janeway CA et al: *Immunobiology: The immune system in health and disease*, ed 6, New York, 2004, Current Biology Publications and Garland Press.

Male D et al: *Advanced immunology*, ed 3, St Louis, 1996, Mosby.

Male D: *Immunology*, ed 4. London, 2004, Elsevier.

Roitt I, Brostoff J, Male D: *Immunology*, ed 4, St Louis, 1996, Mosby.

Sompayrac L: *How the immune system works, ed 2*, Malden, Mass, 2003, Blackwell Scientific.

CHAPTER 13

Cellular Immune Responses

The drama of the immune response unfolds after an antigenic challenge in several acts. The actors include neutrophils, monocyte-macrophage lineage cells, predendritic and dendritic cells (DCs), large, granular lymphocytes (LGLs) (natural killer [NK] cells), T and B lymphocytes, and other cells. Act 1 occurs at the site of infection and involves innate responses. Neutrophils and activated macrophages act directly on bacteria and infection. The LGLs provide early responses to infection and kill virally infected and tumor cells. In the second act, LGLs kill cells decorated with antibody (antibody-dependent cellular cytotoxicity [ADCC]). Immature dendritic cells (iDCs) bridge the gap between the innate and the antigen-specific protective responses by first producing cytokines to enhance the action, and then taking their phagocytosed and pinocytosed cargo to the lymph node as the only antigen-presenting cell (APC) that can **initiate** an immune response. Act 2 includes the adaptive immune responses and commences in the lymph node, where the mature DCs present antigen to the T lymphocytes. The plot of this story may proceed to reinforce local site inflammatory responses (TH1) or initiate systemic, humoral responses (TH2), depending on the cytokine dialogue of the DC and the T cell. The T cells play a central role in activating and controlling (helping) immune and inflammatory responses through the release of cytokines. In Act 3, the cast of T cells and B lymphocytes responding to the infection expands to deliver antigen-specific immune responses and then terminally differentiates. Macrophages and B cells refine and strengthen the direction of the response, as APCs. Certain members of the B- and T-cell cast maintain a low profile and become memory cells, to be able to replay the drama more quickly and efficiently in the future. This chapter will introduce the cast of cellular actors and the roles that they play in the immune response drama.

Immature-Dendritic and Dendritic Cells

Immature dendritic cells (iDCs) provide an early cytokine-mediated warning system and then mature into **dendritic cells,** which are the ultimate antigen-presenting cell, the only antigen-presenting cell that can initiate an antigen-specific immune response (Box 13–1). DCs may be of myeloid or lymphoid origin (plasmacytoid DCs), both of which have octopus-like arms (dendrites), an antigen-sticky cell surface, produce cytokines, and present antigen on major histocompatibility complex (MHC) I and MHC II molecules.

Precursor DCs and monocytes circulate in the blood and then differentiate into immature DCs in tissue. Some of the various immature DCs found in tissue and blood are specialized and include: (1) **Langerhans cells** in the skin, (2) **dermal interstitial cells,** (3) **follicular DCs** (lymph node and spleen), (4) **interdigitating cells** (lymph node and spleen), and (5) **splenic marginal DCs,** but DCs are also present in the **liver, thymus, germinal centers of the lymph nodes,** and **blood.**

Immature DCs sense the presence of microbes and release cytokines, which determine whether the subsequent immune response will develop into a TH1 or a TH2 type of immune response, depending on the nature of the activation signals. These cells express different combinations of microbial sensors from the **Toll-Like Receptors (TLRs)** family of proteins, as well as other receptors. The TLRs include 10 different cell surface proteins that sense the presence of microbial infection by binding to the characteristic patterns within molecules on the outside of bacteria, fungi, and viruses, and even to forms of the deoxyribonucleic acid (DNA) and ribonucleic acid (RNA) of these microbes, termed **pathogen-associated**

TABLE 13–1. Toll-Like Receptors

Toll-Like Receptor*	Cell Types†	Activators. Microorganism	Ligand
TLR 1	MDTBcG	Bacteria, Mycobacteria Neisseria Meningitidis	Lipopeptides Soluble factors
TLR2	MDG	Bacteria Fungi Cells	LPS, LTA, PGN, etc. Zymosan Necrotic cells
TLR3	MDT	Viruses	Double-stranded RNA
TLR4	MDTGBc	Bacteria Viruses	**LPS**, LTA RSV, HCV glycoproteins
TLR5	MDG	Bacteria	Flagellin
TLR6	MDBc	Bacteria Fungi	LTA, lipopeptides, zymosan
TLR7	MDBc	Viruses	Single-stranded RNA Imidazoquinolines
TLR8	MD	Viruses	Single-stranded RNA Imidazoquinolines
TLR9	MDBc	Bacteria Viruses	Unmethylated DNA (CpG)

Activators: CMV, Cytomegalovirus; dsRNA, double-stranded RNA; gram +/–, gram-positive and gram-negative bactera; HCV, hepatitis C virus; LPS, lipopolysaccharide; LTA, lipoteichoic acid; PGN, peptidoglycan; RSV, respiratory syncytial virus.

*Information about Toll-Like Receptors from Takeda A, Kaisho T, Akira S: *Annu Rev Immunol* 21:335-376, 2003; Akira S, Takeda K: *Nature Rev Immunol* 4:499-511, 2003.

†Cell types: Bc, B cell; D, dendritic cell; G, granulocyte; M, macrophage; T, T cell.

BOX 13–1. Dendritic Cells

Lineage: Myeloid and lymphoid
Morphology: Octopus-like with tendrils
Activities:
- Immature DC:
  - In blood and tissue
  - Phagocytosis and cytokine production directs TH1 or TH2 responses
- Mature DC:
  - In lymphoid tissues (Up-regulated MHC II and B7-1 and B7-2 molecules)
  - Move to T cell areas of lymph node, process and present antigen to initiate T cell response
- MHC I-peptide: CD8 T cells
- CD1-glycolipids: CD8 T cells
- MHC II-peptide: CD4 T cells
- Follicular DC:
  - In B cell areas of lymphoid tissues (Fc and CR1, CR2, and CR3 complement receptors, lack MHC II)
  - Presentation of antigen stuck to membrane to B cells

molecular patterns (PAMPs) (Table 13–1). These patterns are present within the endotoxin component of lipopolysaccharide (LPS), in teichoic acid, fungal glycans, unmethylated cytosine-guanosine units of DNA (CpG ODN) commonly found in bacteria, double-stranded RNA produced during the replication of some viruses, and other molecules. Activation of the TLR triggers a cascade of protein kinases and other responses that result in the activation of the cell and production of cytokines.

The iDCs are constantly acquiring antigenic material by macropinocytosis, pinocytosis, or phagocytosis of apoptotic cells, debris, and proteins in normal tissue and at the site of infection or tumor. However, on activation of the iDC by a TLR cascade in response to infection, the iDC matures into a DC and its role changes. The DC loses its ability to phagocytize, preventing it from acquiring irrelevant antigenic material, and progresses to the lymph node. As an analogy, the immature DC is like a clam, constantly surveying its environment by filter feeding the cellular and microbial debris (if present), but when triggered by a TLR signal that microbes are present, it releases a local cytokine alarm, closes its shell, and moves to the lymph node to trigger a response to the challenge. The mature DC moves to T cell areas of lymph nodes and up-regulates cell surface molecules involved in antigen presentation (class II MHC and B7-1 and B7-2 [costimulatory] molecules). DCs can present antigenic material attached to MHC class I and CD1 molecules to CD8 T cells, on MHC class II molecules to CD4 T cells, and antigen stuck to the outside of the cell to B cells. DCs are so effective at presenting antigen that 10 cells loaded with antigen are sufficient to initiate protective immunity in a mouse to a lethal bacterial challenge.

Cells of the Monocyte-Macrophage Lineage

Monocytes are myeloid cells that develop from the same lineage as polymorphonuclear granulocytes. Monocytes mature into different types of macrophages, dentritic, and other cells of the macrophage lineage that differ in function and tissue location. The surface markers on monocyte-macrophages correspond to the cells' functions. These cells express the following proteins:

1. **Receptors for opsonins** (e.g., immunoglobulin Fc receptors [Fc-γ RI, Fc-γ RII, Fc-γ RIII] and **complement receptors** [CR1, CR3])
2. **Lectins** (specific sugar-binding proteins, such as mannosyl-fucosyl receptors)
3. **Toll-Like Receptors,** which recognize **pathogen-associated molecular patterns** and provide signals for cell activation
4. A **receptor (CD14) for the lipopolysaccharide-binding protein** to facilitate bacterial uptake and promote activation
5. Adhesion molecules to promote cell-to-cell interactions; for example, leukocyte function–associated (antigen)-1 (LFA-1)
6. The B7 and class II MHC proteins to allow **antigen presentation** to T cells

Binding and ingestion of microbes to monocytes and macrophages promote the release of interleukin-1 (IL-1), IL-12, and tumor necrosis factor (TNF), which initiate inflammatory reactions. Interferon-γ (IFN-γ), made by NK or T cells, activates killing mechanisms in the macrophage (activated/angry macrophage) and the production of more IL-12, which reinforces CD4 TH1 immune responses. The CD4 TH1 cells make much more IFN-γ to solidify the activity of the macrophage. The **activated macrophages** reinforce local inflammatory reactions by producing various chemokines to attract neutrophils, immature DCs, NK cells, and activated T cells. Activation of the macrophages makes them more efficient killers of phagocytosed microbes, virally infected cells, and tumor cells. Macrophages activated by IL-4 and IL-13 support TH2 antiparasitic responses. Continuous stimulation of macrophages by T cells, as in the case of an unresolved mycobacterial infection, promotes the fusion of macrophages into **multinucleate giant cells** and large macrophages called epithelioid cells that surround the infection and form a **granuloma.**

Natural Killer Cells

NK cells are an important part of the natural immune (innate) system. NK cells provide an early cellular response to a viral infection, have antitumor activity, and amplify inflammatory reactions after bacterial infection. NK cells are also responsible for **ADCC,** in which they bind and kill antibody-coated cells.

NK cells are LGLs that share many characteristics with T cells, except the mechanism for target cell recognition. NK cells are stimulated by (1) IFN-α and IFN-β (produced early in response to viral and other infections), (2) TNF-α, and (3) IL-12, IL-15, and IL18 (produced by pre-DCs and activated macrophages), and (4) IL-2 (produced by CD4 TH1 cells). The NK cells express many of the same cell surface markers as T cells (e.g., CD2, CD7, IL-2 receptor [IL-2R], and **FasL** [Fas ligand]) but also the **Fc receptor for IgG (CD16),** and complement receptors for ADCC. Activated NK cells produce IFN-γ, IL-1, and granulocyte-macrophage colony-stimulating factor (GM-CSF), which reinforce local initial protective responses (TH1) by encouraging the production of IL12 by pre-DCs and activated macrophages. The granules in an NK cell contain **perforin,** a pore-forming protein, and **granzymes** (esterases), which are similar to the contents of the granules of a CD8 cytotoxic T lymphocyte (CTL). These molecules promote the death of the target cell.

Unlike T cells, NK cells do not express a TCR or CD3. They neither recognize a specific antigen nor require presentation of antigen by MHC molecules. The NK system does not involve memory or require sensitization and cannot be enhanced by specific immunization.

The NK cell sees every cell as a potential victim unless it receives an inhibitory signal from the target cell. NK cells interact closely with the target cell by binding to carbohydrates and surface proteins on the cell surface. Interaction of a Class I MHC molecule on the target cell with a **killer-cell inhibitory receptor on the NK cell** is like a secret password, indicating that all is normal, and sends an inhibitory signal to prevent NK killing of the target cell. Binding of the NK cell to antibody-coated target cells (ADCC) also initiates killing, but this is not controlled by an inhibitory signal. The **killing mechanisms** are similar to those of CTLs. A synapse (pocket) is formed between the NK and target cell, and **perforin and granzymes** are released to disrupt the target cell and induce apoptosis. In addition, the interaction of the **FasL** on the NK cell with **Fas** protein on the target cell can also induce apoptosis (see discussion of CD8 T cells, later in this chapter).

CYTOKINE-ACTIVATED KILLER CELLS

Cytokine-activated killer (**LAK** [L from earlier term *lymphokine*]) cells are IL-2–activated effectors that are able to bind and kill many types of tumor and virally infected cells. Most LAK cell activity is derived from NK cells, but some T cells also become LAK cells.

T Cells

The T cells are directors and play a starring role in the immune response drama. T cells were initially distinguished from B cells on the basis of their ability to bind sheep red blood cells through the CD2 molecule and form rosettes. These cells communicate through direct cell-to-cell interactions and with cytokines. T cells are defined through the use of antibodies that distinguish their cell surface molecules. The T-cell surface proteins include: (1) the **T-cell receptor (TCR)**, (2) the CD4 and CD8 co-receptors, (3) accessory proteins that promote recognition and activation, (4) cytokine receptors, and (5) adhesion proteins. All of these proteins determine the types of cell-to-cell interactions for the T cell and therefore the functions of the cell.

Development of T Cells

T-cell precursors develop into T cells in the thymus (Figure 13–1; Box 13–2). Contact with the thymic epithelium and hormones such as thymosin, thymulin, and thymopoietin II in the thymus promote extensive proliferation and differentiation of the individual's T-cell population during fetal development. While T cell precursors are in the thymus, genetic events generate numerous TCRs, each expressed on a different T-cell clone. T cells that react with the host (self-reactive) are forced into committing suicide (apoptosis), and the remaining T cells differentiate into the subpopulations of T cells. T cells can be distinguished by the type of T-cell antigen receptor, either the **TCR 1**, consisting of **γ and δ chains**, or the **TCR 2**, consisting of **α and β chains.**

T cells expressing TCR1 (**γδ T cells**) are present in blood, mucosal epithelium, and other tissue locations and are important for stimulating innate and mucosal immunity. These cells make up 5% of circulating lymphocytes but expand to between 20% and 60% of T cells during

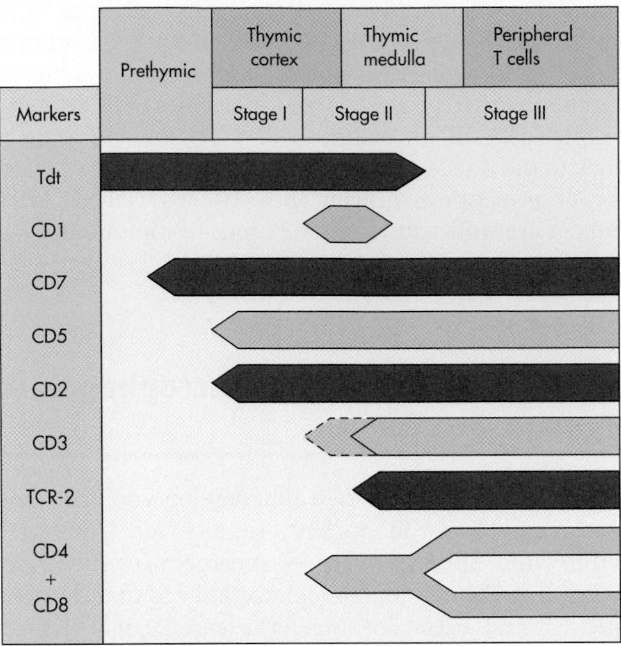

FIGURE 13–1. Human T-cell development. T-cell markers are useful for the identification of the differentiation stages of the T cell and for characterizing T-cell leukemias and lymphomas. Tdt, Cytoplasmic terminal deoxynucleotide transferase.

BOX 13–2. T Cells

γδ T cells:
γδ TCR reactive to microbial metabolites
Local responses: resident in blood and tissue
Quicker responses than αβ T cells
Produce IFN-γ; activate DCs and macrophages
αβ T cells:
CD4: αβ TCR reactive with APC presented peptides on MHC II
- Activated in lymph nodes, then progresses to tissue
- Cytokines activate and direct immune response (TH1, TH2, TH3)
- Cytotoxic through Fas-Fas ligand interactions

CD4 CD25: Suppressor/Regulator cells
- Limit expansion of immune response; promote memory cell development.

CD8: αβ TCR reactive with APC presented peptides on MHC I
- Activated in lymph nodes, then progress to tissue
- Produce similar cytokines as CD4 cells
- Cytotoxic through perforin and granzymes and fas-fas ligand induction of apoptosis

NK-1 T cells: αβ TCR reactive with glycolipids (mycobacteria) on CD1 molecules
- Kill tumor and viral infected cells similar to NK cells
- Provide early support to antibacterial responses

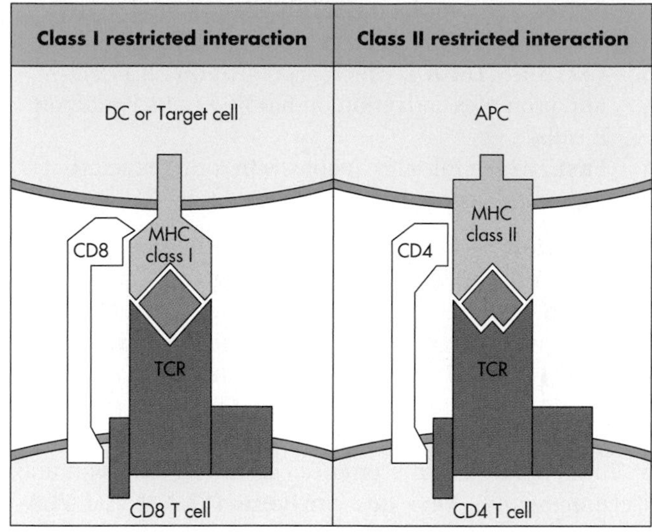

FIGURE 13–2. MHC restriction and antigen presentation to T cells. *Left,* Antigenic peptides bound to class I MHC molecules are presented to the T-cell receptor (TCR) on CD8 T killer/suppressor cells. *Right,* Antigenic peptides bound to class II MHC molecules on the antigen-presenting cell (APC) (B cell, dendritic cell, or macrophage) are presented to CD4 helper cells and delayed-type hypersensitivity T cells.

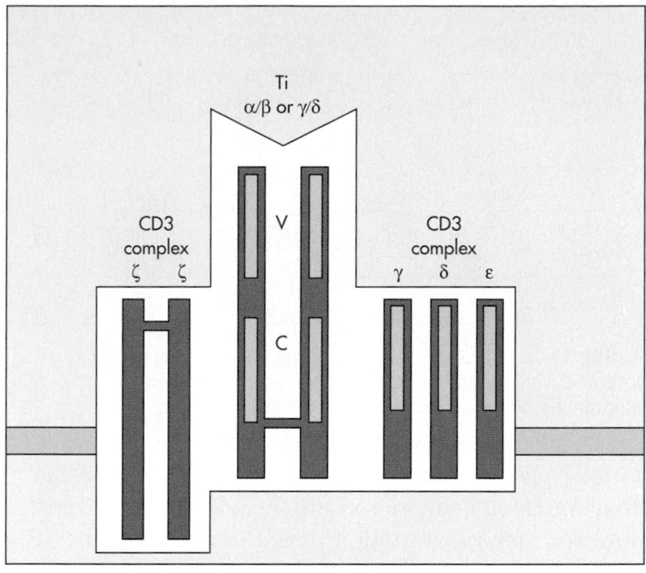

FIGURE 13–3. T-cell receptor (TCR). The TCR consists of different subunits. Antigen recognition occurs through the α/β or γ/δ subunits. The CD3 complex of γ, δ, ε, and ζ subunits promotes T-cell activation. C, Constant region; V, variable region.

certain bacterial and other types of infections. The γδ TCR senses unusual microbial metabolites, produce cytokines, and initiate immune responses.

TCR2 is expressed on most T cells **(αβ T cells),** and these cells are primarily responsible for antigen-activated immune responses. T cells with the αβ TCR are distinguished further by the expression of either a CD4 or a CD8 molecule.

The helper T cells (CD4) activate and control immune and inflammatory responses by releasing cytokines (soluble messengers). Helper T cells interact with peptide antigens presented on class II MHC molecules expressed on APCs (DCs, macrophages, and B cells) (Figure 13–2). The vocabulary of cytokines secreted by a specific CD4 T cell in response to antigenic challenge further distinguishes the CD4 T cell as a TH0, TH1, or TH2 cell. **TH0** cells respond to antigen and can be converted to either TH1 or TH2 cells, depending on the cytokines produced by the antigen presenting cells. **TH1 cells** promote inflammatory responses, which are especially important for controlling intracellular (mycobacterial and viral) and fungal infections and promoting certain types of antibody production. **TH2 cells** promote antibody and memory responses. A TH3 subtype has also been described; it helps promote production of immunoglobulin (Ig) A. The TH1 and TH2 responses are antagonistic, and TH3 responses suppress TH1 and TH2 responses.

CD8 T cells are characterized as cytolytic and suppressor T cells but can also make cytokines similar to CD4 cells. Activated CD8 T cells "patrol" the body for virus-infected or tumor cells, which are identified by antigenic peptides presented by class I MHC molecules. Class I MHC molecules are found on all nucleated cells.

NK-1 T cells are like a hybrid between NK cells and T cells. They express a TCR, but it is the same for all NK-1 T cells. They may express CD4, but most lack CD4 and CD8 molecules ($CD4^-CD8^-$). The TCR of these cells react with CD1 molecules, which present microbial glycolipids and glycopeptides. NK-1 T cells help in the initial responses to infection.

Cell Surface Receptors of T cells

The **TCR complex** is a combination of the antigen recognition structure (TCR) and cell-activation machinery **(CD3)** (Figure 13–3). The specificity of the TCR determines the antigenic response of the T cell. Each TCR molecule is made up of two different polypeptide chains. As with antibody (as described in Chapter 12), each TCR chain has a constant region and a variable region. The repertoire of TCRs is very large and can identify a tremendous number of antigenic specificities (estimated to be able to recognize 10^{15} separate epitopes). The genetic mechanisms for the development of this diversity are also similar to those for antibody (Figure 13–4). The TCR gene is made up of multiple V ($V_1V_2V_3 \ldots V_n$), D, and J segments. In the early stages of T cell development, a particular V segment genetically recombines with a D segment, deleting intervening V and D segments, and then recombines with a J segment to form a unique TCR gene. Unlike

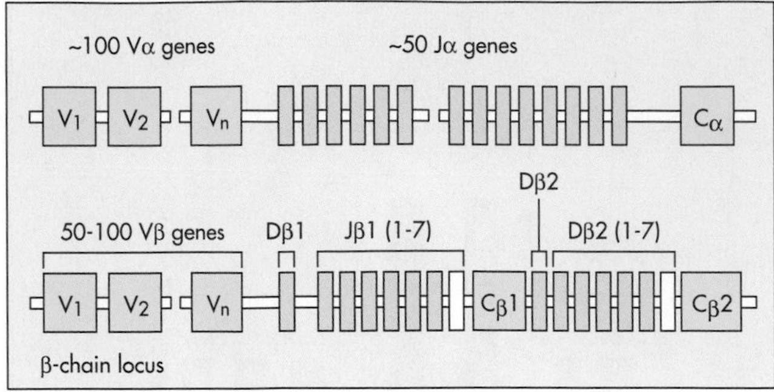

FIGURE 13–4. Structure of the embryonic T-cell receptor (TCR) gene. Note the similar approach to generation of a diverse recognition repetoire as for the immunoglobulin genes.

antibody genes, however, TCR genes can contain more than one D segment, increasing the potential for diversity. However, somatic mutation does not occur for the TCR gene. Each T cell clone expresses a unique TCR.

The **CD3 complex** is found on all T cells and consists of the γ, ε_2, δ, and ζ_2 polypeptide chains. The CD3 complex is the **signal transduction unit** for the TCR. **Tyrosine protein kinases** associate with the CD3 complex when antigen is bound to the TCR complex, promoting a cascade of protein phosphorylations and other events that lead to activation of the T cell and production of IL-2 and its receptor, IL-2R.

The **CD4 and CD8 proteins** are co-receptors for the TCR, because they facilitate the interaction of the TCR with the antigen-presenting MHC molecule and can enhance the activation response. The **CD4** molecule is present on and identifies the helper or delayed-type hypersensitivity (DTH) T cells. CD4 binds to class II MHC molecules on the surface of APCs. **CD8** is present on and identifies the cytotoxic (CTL) and suppressor T cells. CD8 binds to class I MHC molecules on the surface of the target cell. Class I MHC molecules are expressed on all nucleated cells (see more on MHC later in this chapter). The cytoplasmic tails of CD4 and CD8 associate with a protein tyrosine kinase ($p56^{lck}$), which enhances the TCR-induced activation of the cell on binding to the APC or target cell. CD4 or CD8 is found on α/β T cells but not on γ/δ T cells.

Accessory molecules expressed on the T cell include several protein receptors on the cell surface that interact with proteins on APCs and target cells, leading to activation of the T cell, promoting tighter interactions between the cells, or facilitating the killing of the target cell. These accessory molecules are as follows:

1. **CD45RA (native T cells)** or **CD45RO (memory T cells)**, a transmembrane protein tyrosine phosphatase.
2. **CD28** or cytotoxic T lymphocyte associated protein–4 **(CTLA-4)** (on activated T cells), which binds to the B7 protein on APCs to deliver a costimulation or inhibitory signal to the T cell.
3. **CD154 (CD40L)**, which is present on all T cells and promotes activation on binding to its ligand on B cells.
4. **FasL**, which initiates apoptosis in a target cell that expresses **Fas** on its cell surface.

Adhesion molecules tighten the interaction of the T cell with the APC or target cell and may also promote activation. Adhesion molecules include **LFA-1**, which interacts with the **intercellular adhesion molecules (ICAM-1, ICAM-2,** and **ICAM-3)** on the target cell. **CD2** was originally identified by its ability to bind to sheep red blood cells **(erythrocyte receptors)**. CD2 binds to LFA-3 on the target cell and promotes cell-to-cell adhesion and T-cell activation. **Very late antigens (VLA-4** and **VLA-5)** are expressed on activated cells later in the response and bind to fibronectin on target cells to enhance the interaction.

T cells express receptors for many cytokines that activate and regulate T-cell function. The **cytokine receptors** activate protein kinase cascades on binding of cytokine to deliver their signal to the nucleus. *IL-1 and IL-2 receptors are activation receptors.* **The IL-2 receptor (IL-2R)** is composed of three subunits. β/γ subunits are on most T cells (also NK cells) and have intermediate affinity for IL-2. The α subunit (CD25) is induced by cell activation (a marker of activation) to form a high-affinity $\alpha/\beta/\gamma$ IL-2R. Binding of IL-2 to the IL-2R initiates a growth-stimulating signal to the T cell, which also promotes the production of more IL-2 and IL-2R. CD25 is also expressed on a subset of CD4 T cells ($CD4^+CD25^+$), which regulate and suppress the immune response. Other cytokine receptors regulate the growth and cytokine expression of the T cell.

Antigen Presentation to T Cells

Unlike cell surface immunoglobulin on the B cell, which senses ("tastes" or "sniffs") the presence of soluble foreign molecules floating past the cell, the TCR on the T cell must be presented with the relevant epitope, which is cleaved from the protein and cradled in a molecular holder on the surface of an APC, allowing the T cell to "touch" and respond to it. **Class I** and **II MHC** molecules provide the molecular cradle for the peptide. The **CD8** molecule on cytolytic/suppressor T cells binds to and promotes the interaction with class I MHC molecules on target cells. The **CD4** molecule on helper/DTH T cells binds to and promotes interactions with class II MHC molecules on APCs.

Class I MHC molecules are found on all nucleated cells and are the major determinant of "self." The class I

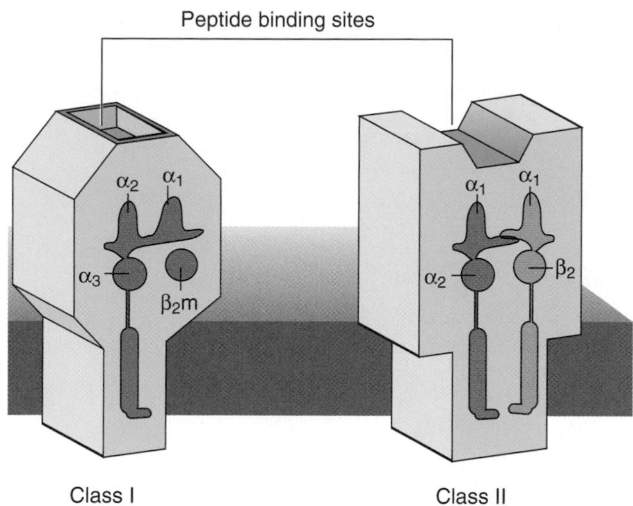

FIGURE 13–5. Structure of class I and class II major histocompatibility (MHC) molecules. The class I MHC molecules consist of two subunits, the heavy chain and β_2-microglobulin. The binding pocket is closed at each end and can only hold peptides of eight to nine amino acids. Class II MHC molecules consist of two subunits, α and β and hold 11 or more amino acid peptides.

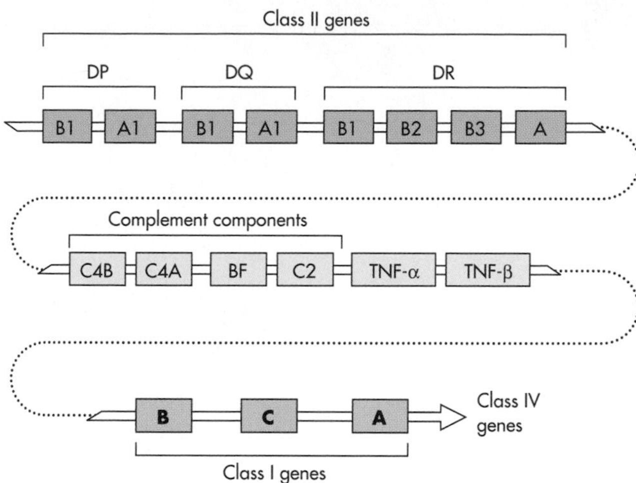

FIGURE 13–6. Genetic map of the major histocompatibility complex (MHC). Genes for class I and class II molecules, as well as complement components and tumor necrosis factor (TNF), are within the MHC gene complex.

MHC molecule, also known as **HLA** for human and H-2 for mouse, consists of two chains, a **variable heavy chain** and a **light chain (β_2-microglobulin)** (Figure 13–5). Differences in the heavy chain of the HLA molecule between individuals (*allotypic differences*) elicit the T-cell response that prevents graft (tissue) transplantation. There are three major HLA genes and proteins: HLA-A, HLA-B, and HLA-C (Figure 13–6). Each cell expresses a pair of different **HLA-A, HLA-B,** and **HLA-C** genes, one from each parent. *The class I MHC molecule binds an antigenic peptide of eight or nine amino acids in a cleft formed by the heavy chain.* The class I MHC molecule presents antigenic peptides from within the cell **(endogenous)** to CD8-expressing T cells. Up-regulation of class I MHC molecules makes the cell a better target for T cell action. Some cells (brain) and some virus infections (cytomegalovirus) down-regulate the expression of MHC I antigens to reduce their potential as targets for T cells.

Class II MHC molecules are normally expressed on APCs, cells that interact with CD4 T cells (e.g., macrophages, dendritic cells, B cells). The class II MHC molecule (once known as **HLA-D**) is encoded by the **DP, DQ,** and **DR** loci. The class II MHC molecule is a dimer of **α and β subunits** (see Figure 13–5). The class II MHC molecule binds an antigenic peptide of 11 or more amino acids in a cleft formed by the α and β subunits. The class II MHC molecule presents ingested **(exogenous)** antigenic peptides to CD4-expressing T cells.

CD1 MHC molecules resemble MHC I molecules, have a heavy chain and a light chain (β_2-microglobulin), but bind glycolipids rather than peptides. These molecules are primarily expressed on DC and present antigen to the αβ TCR on CD8T or NKT cells ($CD4^-CD8^-$) cells. CD1 molecules are especially important for defense against mycobacterial infections.

PEPTIDE PRESENTATION BY CLASS I AND CLASS II MHC MOLECULES

Unlike antibodies that can recognize conformational epitopes, T-cell antigenic peptides must be linear epitopes. A T-cell antigen must be a peptide of 8 to 11 amino acids that is able to bind to the molecular cleft of the class I or class II MHC molecule and still expose a T-cell epitope to the TCR. Because of these constraints, there may be only one T-cell antigenic peptide in a protein. All nucleated cells proteolytically process a set of intracellular proteins and express the peptides to CD8 T cells **(endogenous route of antigen presentation)** to distinguish "self" and "nonself," whereas APCs process and present phagocytized proteins to CD4 T cells **(exogenous route of antigen presentation)** (Figure 13–7). Dendritic cells can cross these routes **(cross-presentation)** to present exogenous antigen to CD8 T cells to initiate antiviral and antitumor responses.

Class I MHC molecules bind and present peptides that are degraded from cellular proteins (trash) by the **proteosome** (a protease machine) and then shuttled into the endoplasmic reticulum (ER) through the **TAP** (transporter associated with antigen processing). Most of these peptides come from misfolded proteins marked by attachment of the **ubiquitin** protein. The antigenic peptide binds to the heavy chain of the class I MHC molecule. Then the MHC heavy chain can assemble properly with β_2-microglobulin, exit the ER, and proceed to the cell membrane.

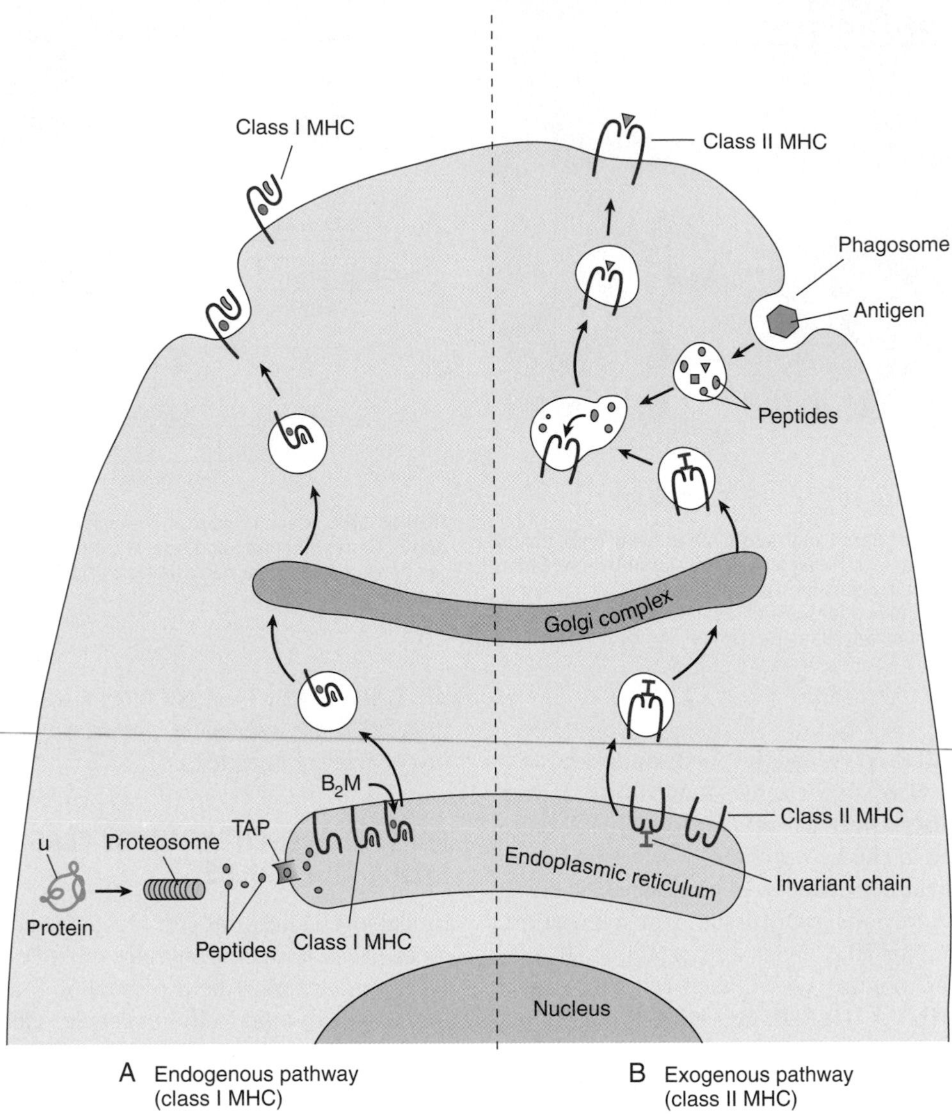

FIGURE 13–7. Antigen presentation. **A, Class I MHC:** Endogenous antigen (produced by the cell and analogous to cell trash) is targeted by attachment of ubiquitin (*u*) for digestion in the proteosome. Peptides of eight to nine amino acids are transported through the TAP (transporter associated with antigen processing) into the endoplasmic reticulum (ER). The peptide binds to a groove in the heavy chain of the class I MHC molecule, allowing association with β_2 microglobulin. The complex is processed through the Golgi apparatus and delivered to the cell surface for presentation to CD8 T cells. **B, Class II MHC:** Class II MHC molecules assemble in the ER with an invariant chain protein and are transported in a vesicle through the Golgi apparatus. Exogenous antigen (phagocytosed) is degraded in lysosomes, which then fuse with a vesicle containing the class II MHC molecules. The invariant chain is degraded, and peptides of 11 to 13 amino acids bind to the class II MHC molecule. The complex is then delivered to the cell surface for presentation to CD4 T cells.

Each MHC I molecule can bind a repertoire of peptides expressing a specific backbone structure **(agretope).** The peptide-binding cleft of the class I MHC molecule is closed-ended, like a pita bread pocket, and holds a peptide of eight to nine amino acids. During a **viral infection,** large quantities of viral proteins are produced and degraded into peptides and become the predominant source of peptides occupying the class I MHC molecules to be presented to CD8 T cells. **Transplanted cells (grafts)** express peptides on their MHC molecules, which differ from those of the host and therefore may be recognized as foreign. **Tumor cells** often express peptides derived from abnormal or embryonic proteins, which may elicit responses in the host because the host was not tolerized to these proteins.

Class II MHC molecules present peptides from exogenous proteins that were phagocytosed and then degraded in lysosomes by APCs, macrophages, or B cells. The class II MHC protein acquires its antigenic peptide as a result of a merging of the vesicular transport pathway (carrying newly synthesized class II MHC molecules) and the lysosomal degradation pathway (carrying phagocytosed and proteolysed proteins). The antigenic peptides displace a peptide (invariant chain) attached in the ER and associate with the cleft formed in the class II MHC protein; the complex is then delivered to the cell surface. With open ends, the class II MHC peptide-binding cleft is more like a hot dog bun and holds a peptide of 11 to 12 amino acids.

Cross-presentation of antigen is used by dendritic cells to present antigen to naïve CD8 T cells, initiating the response to viruses and tumor cells. After picking up antigen (including debris from apoptotic cells) in the periphery by macropinocytosis, pinocytosis, or phagocytosis, the protein, or its peptides, enters the cytoplasm and is then shuttled through the TAP into the ER to bind to MHC I molecules. Alternatively, the MHC I molecule may acquire exogenous peptides as it progresses through the Golgi apparatus to the plasma membrane. The DCs present the antigenic peptide to CD8 T cells in the lymph node to initiate the response from cells.

The following analogy might aid in the understanding of antigen presentation: All cells degrade their protein "trash" and then display it on the cell surface on class I MHC trash cans. CD8 T cells "policing" the neighborhood are not alarmed by the normal, everyday peptide trash. A viral intruder would produce large amounts of viral peptide trash (e.g., beer cans, pizza boxes) displayed on class I MHC molecular garbage cans, which would alert the policing CD8 T cells. APCs (dendritic cells, macrophages, and B cells) are similar to garbage collectors; they gobble up the neighborhood trash or sewage, degrade it, display it on class II MHC molecules, and then move to a lymph node to present the antigenic peptides to the CD4 T cells in the "police station." Foreign antigens would alert the CD4 T cells to release cytokines and activate an immune response.

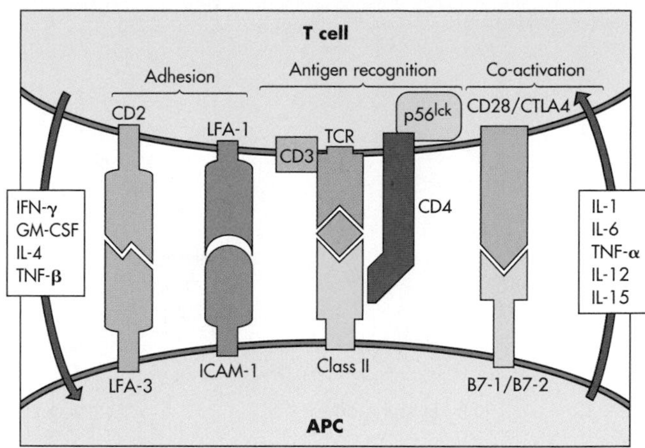

FIGURE 13–8. The molecules involved in the interaction between T cells and antigen-presenting cells (APCs). The various cytokines and their direction of action are also shown. GM-CSF, Granulocyte-macrophage colony-stimulating factor; ICAM-1, intercellular adhesion molecule 1, IFN-γ, interferon-γ; TNF, tumor necrosis factor. (From Roitt I et al: *Immunology,* ed 4, St Louis, 1996, Mosby.)

Activation of CD4 T Cells and Their Response to Antigen

CD4 helper T cells are activated by the interaction of the TCR with antigenic peptide presented by class II MHC molecules on the APC (Figure 13–8). The interaction is strengthened by the binding of CD4 to the class II MHC molecule and the linkage of adhesion proteins on the T cell and the APC. The signal is transmitted to the nucleus through the CD3 complex by activation of phospholipase C and protein kinase C, release of intracellular calcium, and the activation of specific protein kinase cascades. The CD3 complex also activates several tyrosine protein kinase cascades. The result is the activation of specific transcription factors in the nucleus.

A **costimulatory signal** is required to induce growth of the T cell as a fail-safe mechanism to ensure legitimate activation. Costimulatory signals are generated by the interaction of CD28 on the T cell, with the B7-1 and B7-2 molecules on the macrophage, dendritic, or B cell APC, or by cytokines binding to their receptors. Resting T cells require cytokine signals (e.g., IL-1, IL-2) to initiate growth of the cell. Proper activation of the helper T cell promotes production of IL-2 to promote growth of other T cells and increases expression of IL-2Rs on the cell surface, enhancing the cell's own ability to bind and maintain activation by IL-2. Once activated, the IL-2 sustains the growth of the cell, and other cytokines influence whether the helper T cell matures into a TH1 or TH2 helper cell (see following section).

Partial activation (T-cell receptor interaction with MHC peptide) without appropriate cytokine or CD28-B7 costimulation leads to **anergy** (unresponsiveness) or apoptotic death (cell suicide) of the T cell. This is a mechanism for (1) eliminating self-reactive immature and other T cells in the developing thymus and (2) promoting the development of **tolerance** to self proteins. In addition, binding of the CTLA-4 costimulator molecule on T cells with B7 on target or APC cells can result in anergy toward the antigen.

CD4 T cells are known as helper T cells because they trigger the activation and differentiation of B lymphocytes and other cells by their contact and cytokines. In the lymph node or spleen, antigen presentation initiates close interactions between the T cell and APC that allow the CD40L or CD154 molecule on the T cell to bind and activate CD40 on the APC. These interactions stimulate the activation of the T cell. For the B lymphocyte, this interaction and the cytokines produced by the T cell determine which immunoglobulin the B cell will produce.

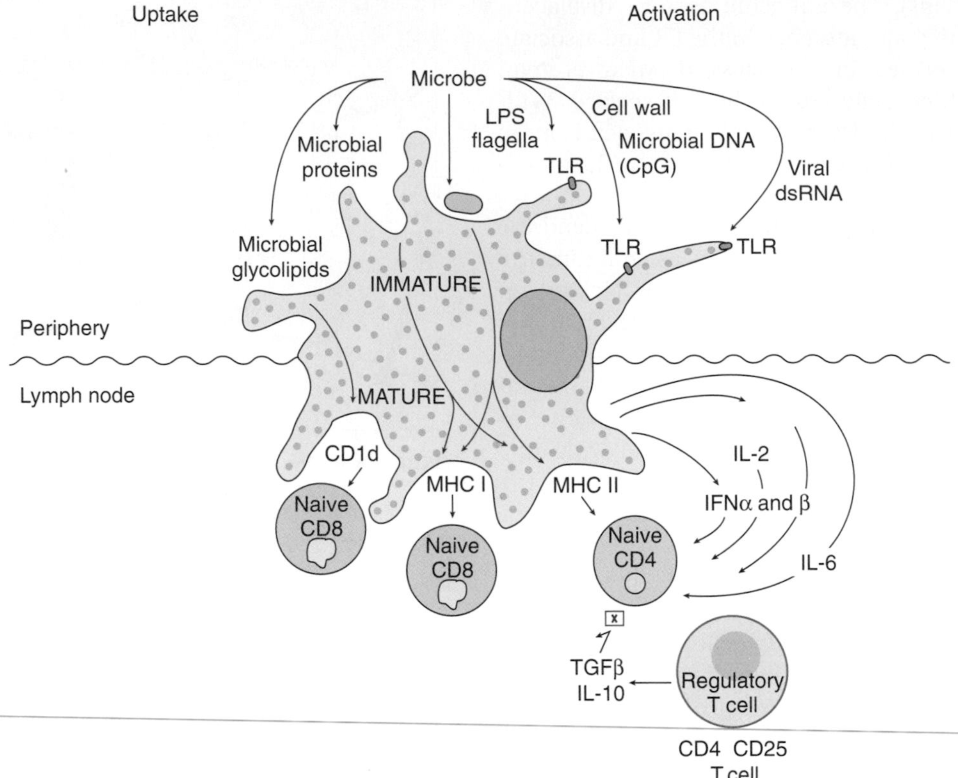

FIGURE 13–9. Dendritic cells initiate immune responses. Immature dendritic cells constantly internalize and process proteins, debris, and microbes, when present. Binding of microbial components to Toll-Like Receptors (TLRs) activates the maturation of the DC so that it ceases to internalize any new material, moves to the lymph node, up-regulates MHC II, B7 and B7.1 molecules for antigen presentation, and produces cytokines to activate T cells. Release of IL-6 inhibits release of TGF β and IL-10 by T regulatory cells. The cytokines produced by DC and its interaction with TH0 cells initiate immune responses. IL-12 and IL-2 promote TH1 responses while IL-4 promotes TH2 responses. Most of the T cells divide to enlarge the response, but some remain as memory cells. Memory cells can be activated by DC, macrophage, or B cell presentation of antigen for a secondary response.

TH1 AND TH2 CELLS

The CD4 T cells start as a TH0 cell that can develop into TH1, TH2, or TH3 cells, as defined by the cytokines that they secrete and thus the responses that they induce (Figures 13–9 and 13–10; Table 13–2). Understanding the TH0, TH1, and TH2 division of cytokine production is the basis for understanding the generation of immune responses. All three types of T cells produce GM-CSF, IL3, TNFα, and some chemokines. TH0 cells have not committed to TH1 or TH2 and produce cytokines of both responses, including IL-2, IFN-γ, and IL-4. The T cell response is initiated by DC presentation of antigenic peptide. TH0 cells mature into either TH1 or TH2 cells, depending on the antigen, how it is presented, the type of APC, the concentration of antigen, and the cytokine environment. Once activated, the TH1 and TH2 cells produce cytokines that stimulate their own growth and development (autocrine) but inhibit the development of the other type of CD4 T cell.

TH1 cells are activated by dendritic cells and macrophages, which secrete IL-12 or IL-15 and present antigen to the CD4 T cell. TH1 cells are characterized by secretion of **IL-2, IFN-γ,** and **TNF-β (lymphotoxin).** These cytokines stimulate inflammatory responses and the production of IgM and specific subclasses of IgG that can fix complement. **IFN-γ,** also known as **macrophage activation factor,** reinforces TH1 responses by promoting more IL-12 production, creating a self-sustaining cycle. TH1 cells are inhibited by IL-10, which is produced by TH2 cells. Activated TH1 cells also express the **FasL,** which can interact with **Fas** on target cells to promote apoptosis (killing) of the target cell.

The **TH1 response (1 meaning first)** *usually occurs first and promotes local responses.* It often occurs early in an infection. The TH1 responses amplify local inflammatory reactions and DTH reactions by activating macrophages, NK cells, and CD8 cytotoxic T cells and also expand the immune response by stimulating growth of B and T cells with IL-2. The inflammatory responses and complement-binding antibody stimulated by TH1 responses are important for eliminating intracellular infections (e.g., viruses, bacteria, and parasites) and fungi but are also associated with autoimmune inflammatory diseases (e.g., multiple sclerosis, Crohn's disease, rheumatoid arthritis).

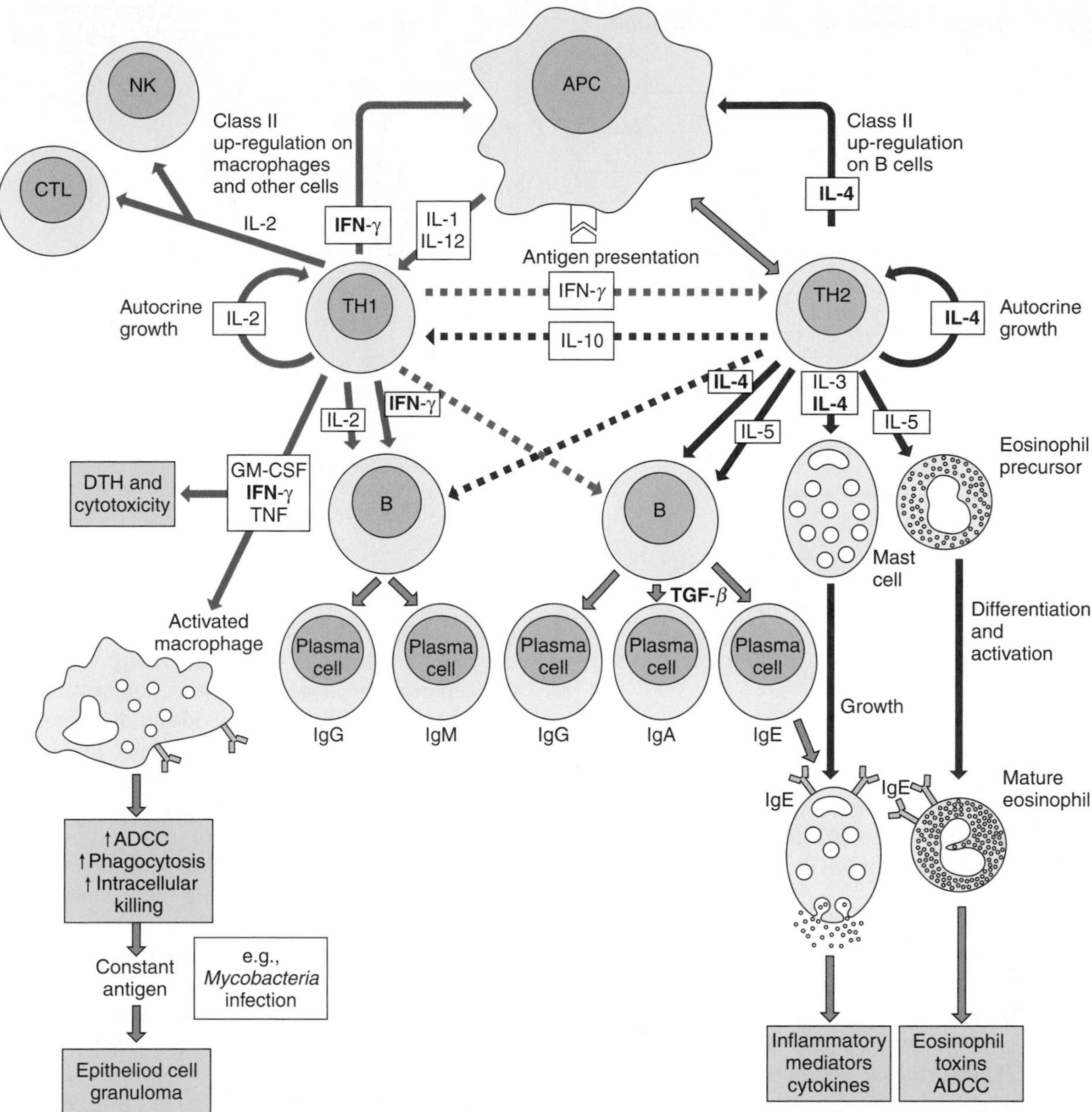

FIGURE 13–10. Cytokines produced by TH1 and TH2 cells and their effects on the immune system. TH1 responses are initiated by IL-12 and interferon-γ, and TH2 responses by IL-4. TH1 cells promote inflammation and production of complement and macrophage-binding antibody *(solid blue lines)* and inhibit TH2 responses *(dotted blue lines)*. TH2 cells promote humoral responses *(solid red lines)* and inhibit TH1 responses *(dotted red lines)*. Colored square denotes end result. ADCC, Antibody-dependent cellular cytotoxicity; APC, antigen-presenting cell; CTL, cytotoxic T cell; DTH, delayed-type hypersensitivity; GM-CSF, granulocyte-macrophage colony-stimulating factor; TNF, tumor necrosis factor.

The **TH2 response (2 meaning second)** *occurs later and acts systemically.* The TH2 response occurs in the absence of an IL-12/ IFN-γ signal from innate responses, and then IL-4 reinforces the continuation of TH2 responses. TH2 cell development is inhibited by IFN-γ. The TH2 response may be stimulated later in an infection, when antigen reaches the lymph nodes and is presented by DCs, macrophages, and B cells. B cells expressing specific cell surface antibody can capture, process, and present antigen to TH2 cells to initiate an antigen-specific circuit, stimulating the growth of and clonally expanding the helper T cells and B cells, which are specific for the same antigen. TH2 cells release IL-4, IL-5, IL-6, and IL-10 cytokines that promote humoral (systemic) responses. These cytokines stimulate B-cell differentiation, resulting in deletions in the immunoglobulin gene to switch from production of IgM and IgD to production of specific subtypes of IgG, IgE, or IgA. TH2 responses can limit the development of inflammatory and autoimmune diseases but can exacerbate an intracellular infection (e.g., *Mycobacterium leprae*) by prematurely shutting off protective TH1 responses.

TABLE 13–2. Cytokines Produced by TH0, TH1, and TH2 Cells*

Cytokine	TH0	TH1	TH2
IFN-γ	+	++	–
IL-2	+	++	–
TNF-β (LT)	+	++	–
Chemokines	+	+	–
GM-CSF	+	++	+
TNF-α	+	++	+
IL-3	+	++	++
IL-4	+	–	++
IL-5	+	–	++
IL-6		–	++
IL-10	+	–	++

GM-CSF, Granulocyte-macrophage colony-stimulating factor; IFN, interferon; IL, interleukin; LT, lymphotoxin; TNF, tumor necrosis factor; +, minor product; ++, major product; –, no product.

*The relative ability of TH0, TH1, and TH2 cells to produce different cytokines after activation. The cytokines that differentiate TH1 and TH2 cells are boxed.

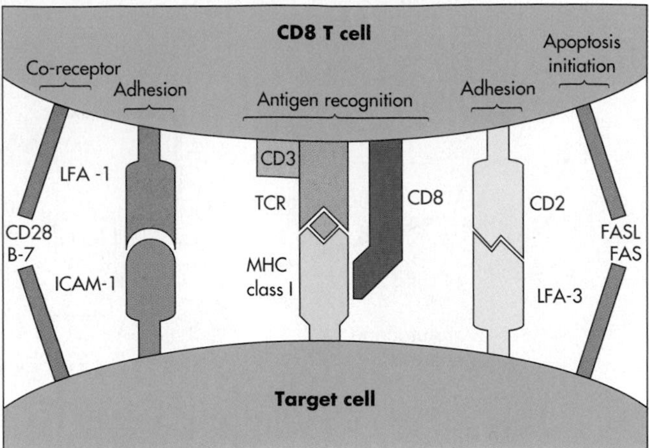

FIGURE 13–11. Interactions between CD8 cytotoxic T lymphocyte (CTL) and target cells. The Fas-FasL interaction promotes apoptosis. ICAM-1, Intercellular adhesion molecule 1. (From Roitt I et al: *Immunology,* ed 4, St Louis, 1996, Mosby.)

TH3 cells are characterized by their production of IL-5 and transforming growth factor β (TGF-β), which are important for promoting B-cell differentiation to produce IgA. TGF-β inhibits TH1 and TH2 cell action to promote tolerance.

CD4$^+$CD25$^+$ T cells express the α component of the IL-2 (βγ) receptor and are antigen-specific suppressor cells. These cells prevent the development of autoimmune responses by producing TGF-β and IL-10, help to keep T cell responses under control, and promote memory cell development. The normal secretion of TGF-β and IL-10 by CD4$^+$ CD25$^+$ T cells is inhibited by IL-6, which is produced by DC and macrophage in response to infection. This allows the T cell response to develop.

CD8 T Cells

CD8 T cells include **CTLs** and **suppressor cells.** CTLs are part of the TH1 response and are important for eliminating virally infected cells and tumor cells. CD8 T cells can also secrete TH1-like cytokines. Less is known about suppressor cells.

The CTL response is initiated when CTL precursors in the lymph node are stimulated by binding of their TCR and CD8 to the antigenic peptide on class I MHC molecules and a costimulatory signal from IL-2 or a CD28-B7 interaction with dendritic cells or macrophages (Figure 13–11). Presentation of the antigen may be the result of a virus infection of the APC or caused by cross-presentation of an antigen acquired at the site of infection or tumor by a DC. The activated CD8 T cells divide and differentiate into mature CTLs. During a viral challenge of mice, the numbers of specific CTLs will increase up to 100,000 times. When the activated CTL finds a target cell, it binds tightly through interactions of the TCR with antigen-bearing class I MHC proteins and adhesion molecules on both cells (similar to the closing of a zipper). **Granules** containing toxic molecules, **granzymes (esterases),** and a pore-forming protein (perforin) move to the site of interaction and release their contents into the pocket **(immune synapse)** formed between the T cell and target cell. **Perforin** generates holes in the target cell membrane to allow the granule contents to enter and induce **apoptosis (programmed cell death)** in the target cell. CD8 T cells can also initiate apoptosis in target cells through the interaction of the **FasL on the T cell with the Fas protein on the target cell surface.** FasL is a member of the TNF family of proteins, and Fas is a member of the TNF receptor family of proteins. Apoptosis is characterized by degradation of the target cell DNA into discrete fragments of approximately 200 base pairs and disruption of internal membranes. The cells shrink into apoptotic bodies, which are readily phagocytosed by macrophages and dendritic cells. Apoptosis is a clean method of cell death, unlike necrosis, which signals neutrophil action and further tissue damage. TH1 CD4 T cells also express FasL and can initiate apoptosis in target cells.

Suppressor T cells provide antigen-specific regulation of helper T cell function through inhibitory cytokines and other means. Like CTLs, suppressor T cells interact with class I MHC (class I MHC restricted).

QUESTIONS

1. The importance of specific molecules can be determined through development of genetically deficient strains of mice (knockout mice) and then testing the immune systems of these mice. Describe the immune functions that should be missing and the cell types that should be affected for the mice deficient in the following molecules:
   a. Class I MHC
   b. Class II MHC
   c. TCR γ/δ
   d. IL-2 receptor
   e. CD4
   f. B7-1 and B7-2
   g. IFN-γ
   h. IL-1
2. The division of helper T cell responses into TH1, TH2, and TH3 subsets provides one of the most useful approaches to understanding immune responses to challenge. What would be the consequence of each of the following?
   a. Initiation of TH2 response to an intracellular infection (e.g., *Mycobacterium leprae*) before a TH1 response
   b. Uncontrolled TH1 response to a vaginal yeast infection (e.g., *Candida albicans*)
   c. Insufficient TH1 response to viral infection of a neonate as a result of low levels of IFN-γ (e.g., herpes simplex virus).
   d. Immunization with a mixture of IL-2, GM-CSF, and IFN-γ and human immunodeficiency virus glycoprotein 120 antigen, rather than the antigen alone.

Bibliography

Abbas AK et al: *Cellular and molecular immunology,* ed 5, Philadelphia, 2003, WB Saunders.

Akira S, Takeda K: Toll-Like Receptor Signalling, *Nature Rev Immunol* 4:499-511, 2004.

Goldsby RA, Kindt TJ, Osborne BA: *Kuby immunology,* ed 5, New York, 2003, WH Freeman.

Immunology Today: Issues contain understandable reviews on current topics in immunology.

Janeway CA et al: *Immunobiology: The immune system in health and disease,* ed 6, New York, 2004, Current Biology Publications and Garland Press.

Male D et al: *Advanced immunology,* ed 3, St Louis, 1996, Mosby.

Male D: *Immunology,* ed 4, London, 2004, Elsevier.

Roitt I, Brostoff J, Male D: *Immunology,* ed 4, St Louis, 1996, Mosby.

Sompayrac L: *How the immune system works,* ed 2, Malden, Mass, 2003, Blackwell Scientific.

Takeda K, Kaisho T, Akira S: Toll-Like Receptors, *Annu. Rev Immunol* 21: 335-376, 2003.

CHAPTER 14

Immune Responses to Infectious Agents

The previous chapters in this section introduced the different immunologic actors and their characteristics. This chapter describes the different roles they play in host protection from infection, their interactions, and the immunopathogenic consequences that may arise as a result of the response. The importance of each of the components of the host response differs for different infectious agents (Table 14–1), and their importance becomes obvious when it is genetically deficient or is blocked by chemotherapy, disease, or infection (e.g., acquired immune deficiency syndrome [AIDS]).

Human beings have three basic lines of protection against invasion by infectious agents, which are as follow:

1. **Natural barriers,** such as skin, mucus, ciliated epithelium, gastric acid, and bile, which restrict entry of the agent
2. **Innate, antigen-nonspecific immune defenses,** such as fever, interferon, complement, neutrophils, macrophages and natural killer (NK) cells, which provide rapid, local responses to challenge by an invader
3. **Adaptive, antigen-specific immune responses,** such as antibody and T cells, which specifically target, attack, and eliminate the invaders that succeed in passing the first two defenses

Barriers to Infection

The **skin** and **mucous membranes** serve as barriers to most infectious agents (Figure 14–1 and Table 14–2), with few exceptions (e.g., papillomavirus, dermatophytes ["skin-loving" fungi]). Free fatty acids produced in sebaceous glands and by organisms on the skin surface, lactic acid in perspiration, and the low pH and relatively dry environment of the skin all form unfavorable conditions for the survival of most organisms.

The mucosal epithelium covering the orifices of the body is protected by mucus secretions and cilia. For example, pulmonary airways are coated with mucus, which is continuously transported toward the mouth by ciliated epithelial cells. Large, airborne particles get caught in the mucus, whereas small particles (0.05 to 3 microns [μm]), the size of viruses or bacteria) that reach the alveoli are phagocytosed by macrophages and transported out of the airspaces. Some bacteria and viruses (e.g., *Bordetella pertussis,* influenza virus), cigarette smoke, or other pollutants can interfere with this clearance mechanism by damaging the ciliated epithelial cells, thus rendering the patient susceptible to secondary bacterial pneumonia. Antimicrobial substances (cationic peptides, lysozyme, lactoferrin, and secretory [IgA]) found in secretions at mucosal surfaces (e.g., tears, mucus, saliva) also provide protection. Lysozyme induces lysis of bacteria by cleaving the polysaccharide backbone of the peptidoglycan of gram-positive bacteria. Lactoferrin, an iron-binding protein, deprives microbes of the free iron they need for growth.

The **acidic environment** of the stomach, bladder, and kidneys and the **bile** of the intestines inactivate many viruses and bacteria. **Urinary flow** also limits the establishment of infection.

Body temperature, and especially **fever,** limits or prevents the growth of many microbes. In addition, the immune response is more efficient at elevated temperatures.

Antibacterial Responses

Figure 14–2 illustrates the progression of protective responses to a bacterial challenge. Protection is initiated by activation of innate responses on a local basis and

TABLE 14–1. Antimicrobial Defenses for Infectious Agents

	Bacteria	Intracellular Bacteria	Viruses	Fungi	Parasites
Complement	+	–	–	–	–
Interferon-α/β	–	–	++++	–	–
Neutrophils	++++	–	–	+	+
Macrophages	++	+++	++	++	+
NK cells	–	–	+++	–	–
CD4 TH1, DTH	–	++	+++	+*	+
CD8 CTL	–	–	++++	–	–
Antibody	++	+	+	+	++ (IgE)†

CTL, Cytotoxic T lymphocytes; NK, natural killer.
*By activation of macrophages.
†Immunoglubulin E and mast cells are especially important for worm infections.

TABLE 14–2. Nonspecific Humoral Defense Mechanisms

Factor	Function	Source
Lysozyme	Catalyzes hydrolysis of bacterial peptidoglycan	Tears, saliva, nasal secretions, body fluids, lysosomal granules
Lactoferrin, transferrin	Bind iron and compete with microorganisms for it	Specific granules of PMNs
Lactoperoxidase	May be inhibitory to many microorganisms	Milk and saliva
β-lysin	Is effective mainly against gram- positive bacteria	Thrombocytes, normal serum
Chemotactic factors	Induce directed migration of PMNs, monocytes, and other cells	Bacterial substances, products of cell injury, denatured proteins, complement, and chemokines
Properdin	Activates complement in the absence of antibody-antigen complex	Normal plasma
Cationic peptides (defensins, etc.)	Disrupt membranes, block cell- transport activities	Polymorphonuclear granules

PMNs, Polymorphonuclear neutrophils (leukocytes).

progresses to acute-phase and antigen-specific responses on a systemic scale. A summary of antibacterial responses is presented in Box 14–1.

Acute inflammation is an early defense mechanism to contain an infection, prevent its spread from the initial focus, and signal subsequent specific immune responses. Inflammatory responses are beneficial but can also cause tissue damage and, as a result, contribute to the symptoms of disease. The three major events in acute inflammation are (1) expansion of capillaries to increase blood flow (seen as blushing or a rash); (2) increase in permeability of the microvasculature structure to allow escape of fluid, plasma proteins, and leukocytes from the circulation (source of edema); and (3) exit of leukocytes from the capillaries, and their accumulation and response to infection at the site of injury (pus).

ACTIVATION OF RESPONSE

Bacterial components are excellent activators of the innate antigen-nonspecific protective responses (Box 14–2). The peptidoglycan layer in bacterial cell walls (teichoic acid and peptidoglycan fragments of gram-positive bacteria) and lipopolysaccharide (LPS) in gram-negative bacterial cell walls can activate the **alternative complement pathway (properdin)** in the absence of antibody and, with **mannose-binding protein,** can activate the classic complement pathway. Macrophages and

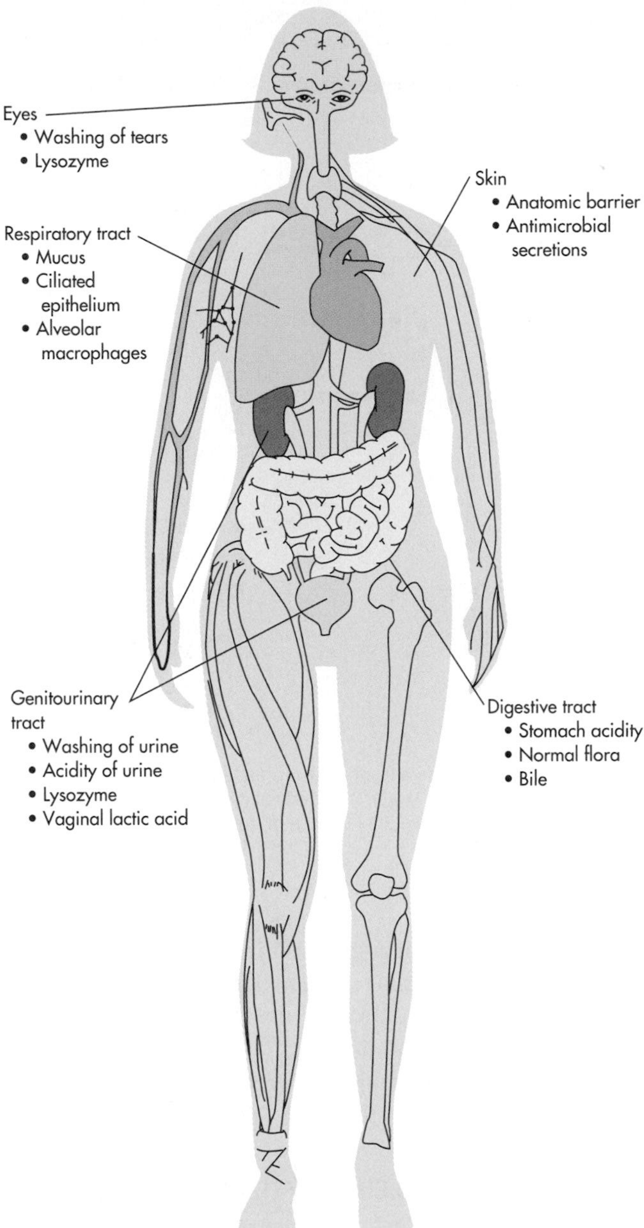

FIGURE 14–1. Barrier defenses of the human body.

BOX 14–1. Summary of Antibacterial Responses

Complement
Alternative and lectin pathways activated by bacterial surfaces
Classic pathway activated later by antibody-antigen complexes
Production of chemotactic and anaphylotoxic proteins (C3a, C5a)
Opsonization of bacteria (C3b)
Promotion of killing of gram-negative bacteria
Activation of B cells (C3d)

Neutrophils
Important antibacterial phagocytic cell
Killing by oxygen-dependent and oxygen-independent mechanisms

Dendritic Cells
Production of cytokines
Initiation of specific immune responses

Macrophages
Important antibacterial phagocytic cell
Killing by oxygen-dependent mechanisms
Production of interleukins IL-1, IL-6, and IL-12; tumor necrosis factor (TNF)-α and TNF-β, and interferon (INF)-α
Activation of acute-phase and inflammatory responses
Presentation of antigen to CD4 T cell

T Cells
$\gamma\lambda$ T-cell response to bacterial metabolites
Natural killer (NK)-1 T-cell response to CD1 presentation of mycobacterial glycolipids
TH1 CD4 response important for intracellular bacterial infections
TH2 CD4 response important for all bacterial infections
CD8 cytolytic T cells not very important

Antibody
Binding to surface structures of bacteria (fimbriae, lipoteichoic acid, capsule)
Blocking of attachment
Opsonization of bacteria for phagocytosis
Promotion of complement action
Promotion of clearance of bacteria
Neutralization of toxins and toxic enzymes

dendritic cells express **pathogen-associated pattern-recognition receptors,** including the **Toll-Like Receptors (TLRs),** which recognize these bacterial structures and activate cytokine production and protective responses. **LPS (endotoxin)** binds to TLR4 and is a very strong activator of dendritic cells, macrophages, B cells, and selected other cells (e.g., endothelial cells).

Activation of the **complement system** by the alternative pathway or via the mannose-binding protein (see Chapter 12) is a very early and important antibacterial defense. Complement activates inflammatory responses and can also directly kill gram-negative bacteria and, to a much lesser extent, gram-positive bacteria (the thick peptidoglycan of gram-positive bacteria shields them from lysis). Activation of the complement cascade by gram-positive or gram-negative bacteria provides the following protective factors:

1. **Chemotactic factors (C5a)** to attract neutrophils and macrophages to the site of infection
2. **Anaphylotoxins (C3a and C5a)** to stimulate mast cell release of histamine and thereby increase

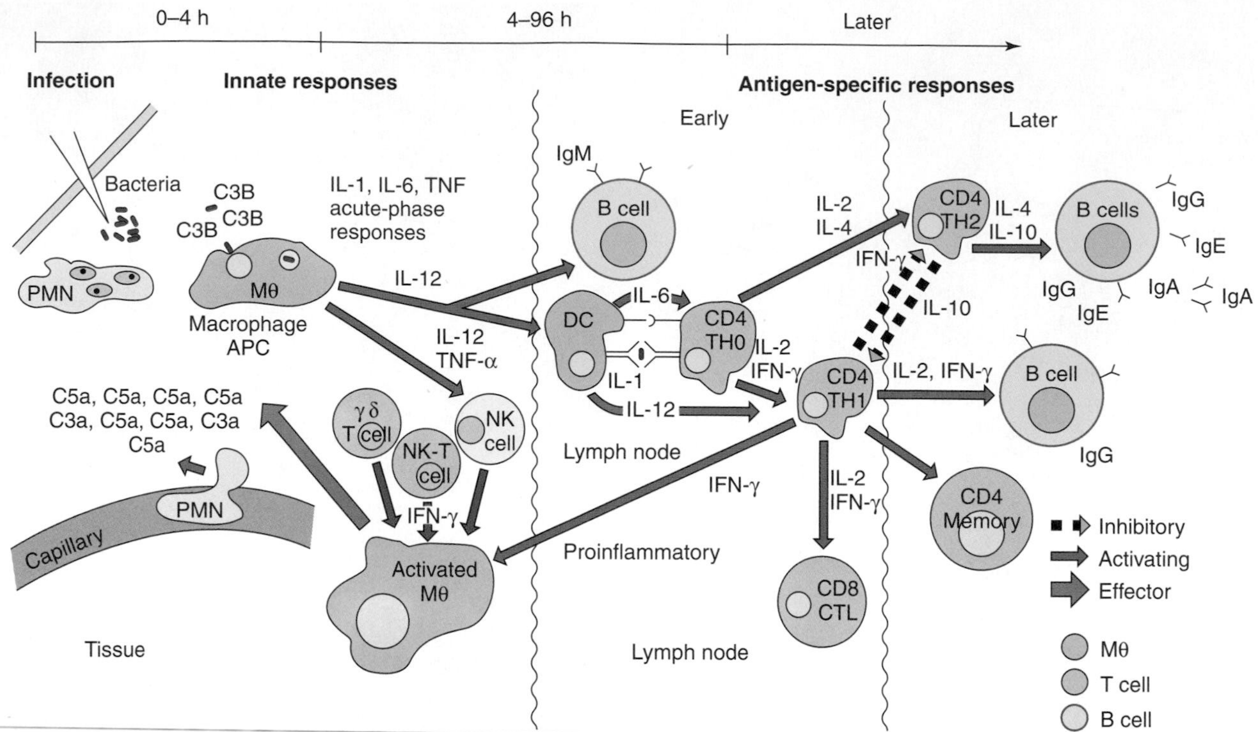

FIGURE 14–2. Antibacterial responses. First, innate antigen-nonspecific responses attract and promote polymorphonuclear neutrophil (PMN) and macrophage (Mθ) responses. Antigen-presenting cells (APCs) and antigen reach the lymph node to activate early immune responses (TH1 and immunoglobulin M[IgM]). Later, TH2 systemic antibody responses and memory cells are developed. The time course of events is indicated at the top of the figure. CTL, Cytotoxic T lymphocyte; IFN, interferon; IL, interleukin, TNF, tumor necrosis factor.

BOX 14–2. Bacterial Components That Activate Protective Responses

Direct Activation through TLRs and Other Receptors:
Lipopolysaccharide (endotoxin)
Lipoteichoic acid
Lipoarabinomannan
Glycolipids and glycopeptides
Polyanions
N-Formyl peptides (formyl-methionyl-leucyl-phenylalanine)
Peptidoglycan fragments

Chemotaxis via C3a, C5a, and Other Mechanisms:
Peptidoglycan fragments
Cell surface activation of alternative pathways of complement

vascular permeability, allowing access to the infection site

3. **Opsonins (C3b),** which bind to bacteria and promote their phagocytosis
4. A **B-cell activator (C3d)**

Antibody **(IgM** or **IgG),** which is present later in an infection, enhances the complement response through activation of the **classical complement cascade.**

Kinins and clotting factors induced by tissue damage (e.g., factor XII [Hageman factor], bradykinin, fibrinopeptides) are also involved in inflammation. These factors increase vascular permeability and are chemotactic for leukocytes. Products of arachidonic acid metabolism also affect inflammation. These products include prostaglandins and leukotrienes, which can mediate essentially every aspect of acute inflammation.

CHEMOTAXIS AND LEUKOCYTE MIGRATION

Chemotactic factors produced in response to infection and inflammatory responses, such as complement components (C3a, C5a), bacterial products (e.g., formyl-methionyl-leucyl-phenylalanine [f-met-leu-phe]), and chemokines, are powerful chemoattractants for neutrophils, macrophages, and, later in the response, lymphocytes. **Chemokines** are sticky proteins that establish a chemically lighted "runway" to guide these cells to the site of an infection and also activate them. The chemokines and tumor necrosis factor-α (TNF-α) cause the endothelial cells lining the capillaries (near the inflammation) and the leukocytes passing by to express complementary adhesion molecules (molecular "Velcro"). The leukocytes slow, roll, attach to the lining, and then extravasate across (i.e., pass through) the capillary wall to the site of inflammation (in a process called **diapedesis**) (Figure 14–3).

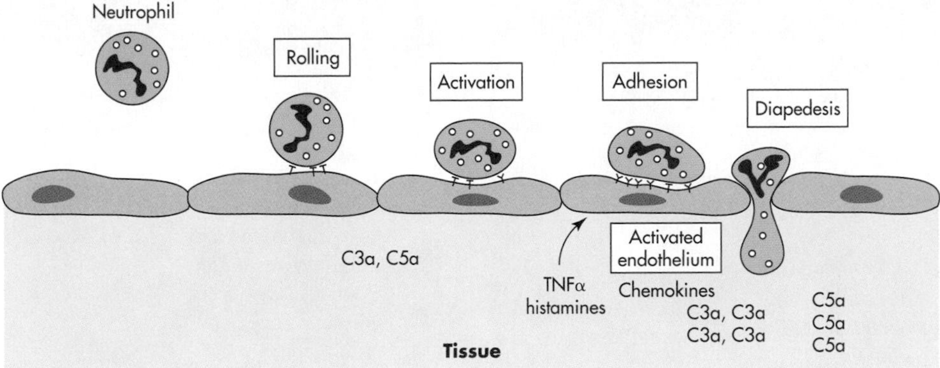

FIGURE 14–3. Neutrophil diapedesis in response to inflammatory signals. Tumor necrosis factor-α (TNF-α) and chemokines activate the expression of selectins and intercellular adhesion molecules (ICAM-1) on the endothelium near the inflammation, and their ligands on the neutrophil: integrins, L-selectin, and LFA-1 (leukocyte function-associated antigen). The neutrophil binds progressively tighter to the endothelium until it finds its way through the endothelium.

INNATE CELLULAR RESPONSES

The earliest cellular responses to infection are mediated by immature dendritic cells, Langerhans cells, NK cells, and γδ T cells that reside in tissue. Polymorphonuclear neutrophils (PMNs), monocytes, and occasionally eosinophils are the first cells to arrive at the site in response to acute inflammation; they are followed later by macrophages.

Neutrophils are polymorphonuclear and provide a major antibacterial response. They are attracted to the site of infection, where they phagocytose and then kill the internalized bacteria. An increased number of neutrophils in the blood, body fluids (e.g., cerebrospinal fluid), or tissue indicates a bacterial infection. The mobilization of neutrophils is accompanied by a "left shift," an increase in the number of immature **band forms** released from the bone marrow (*left* refers to the beginning of a chart of neutrophil development).

Phagocytosis of bacteria by macrophages and neutrophils involves three steps: attachment, internalization, and digestion. **Attachment of the bacteria** to the macrophage is mediated by receptors for bacterial carbohydrates (**lectins** [specific sugar-binding proteins]), fibronectin receptors (especially for *Staphylococcus aureus*), and **receptors for opsonins,** including complement [C3b], mannose-binding protein receptors, and Fc receptors for antibody. After attachment, a portion of plasma membrane surrounds the particle, which forms a **phagocytic vacuole** around the microbe. This vacuole fuses with the **primary lysosomes** (macrophages) or **granules** (PMNs) to allow inactivation and digestion of the vacuole contents. Phagocytic killing may be oxygen dependent or oxygen independent, depending on the antimicrobial chemicals produced by the granules (Figure 14–4). Activation of macrophages is promoted by interferon-γ (IFN-γ) (best), granulocyte-macrophage colony-stimulating factor (GM-CSF), TNF-α, and lymphotoxin (TNF-β), which are produced early in the infection by NK cells or later by CD4 T cells. Activation of macrophages is required for macrophages to kill internalized microbes.

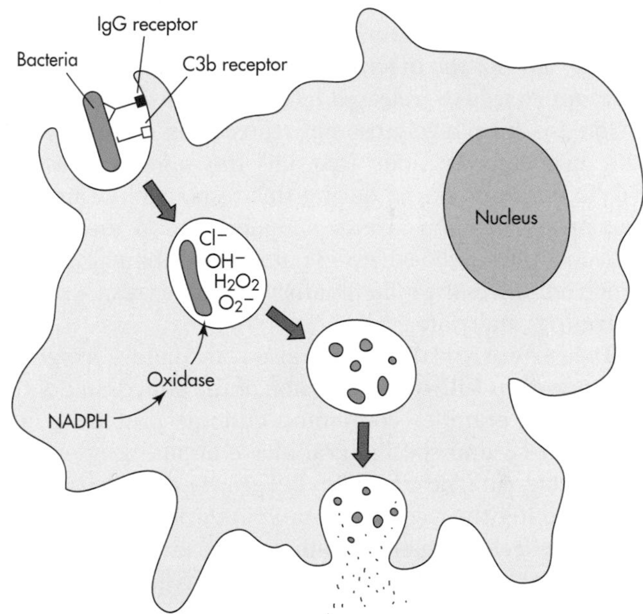

FIGURE 14–4. Phagocytosis and killing of bacteria. Bacteria are bound directly or are opsonized by mannose-binding protein, immunoglobulin G (IgG) and/or C3b receptors promoting their adherence and uptake by phagocytes. Within the phagosome, oxygen-dependent and oxygen-independent mechanisms kill and degrade the bacteria. NADPH, reduced form of nicotinamide-adenine dinucleotide phosphate.

Oxygen-dependent killing is activated by a powerful oxidative burst that culminates in the formation of hydrogen peroxide and other antimicrobial substances (Box 14–3). The fusion of specific lysosomal granules and phagosomes permits the interaction of NADPH (reduced form of nicotinamide-adenine dinucleotide phosphate) oxidase with cytochrome b. With the aid of quinone, this

BOX 14–3. Antibacterial Compounds of the Phagolysosome

Oxygen-Dependent Compounds
Hydrogen peroxide: NADPH oxidase and NADH oxidase
Superoxide
Hydroxyl radicals (OH)
Activated halides (Cl^-, I^-, Br^-): myeloperoxidase (neutrophil)
Nitrous oxide

Oxygen-Independent Compounds
Acids
Lysosome (degrades bacterial peptidoglycan)
Lactoferrin (chelates iron)
Defensins and other cationic proteins (damage membranes)
Proteases, elastase, cathepsin G

combination reduces oxygen to superoxide anion (O_2^-), which in the presence of a catalyst (e.g., superoxide dismutase) is converted to hydrogen peroxide. In the neutrophil, but not the macrophage, hydrogen peroxide with **myeloperoxidase** (released by primary granules during fusion to the phagolysosome) transforms chloride ions into hypochlorous ions that kill the microorganisms. **Nitric oxide** produced during this response has antimicrobial activity and is also a major second messenger molecule (like cyclic adenosine monophosphate [cAMP]), which enhances the inflammatory and other responses by activating guanylate cyclase.

The **neutrophil** can also mediate **oxygen-independent killing** upon fusion of the phagosome with azurophilic granules containing cationic proteins (e.g., cathepsin G) and specific granules containing lysozyme and lactoferrin. These proteins kill gram-negative bacteria by disrupting their cell membrane integrity, but they are far less effective against gram-positive bacteria, which are killed principally through the oxygen-dependent mechanism.

Splenic macrophages are important for clearing bacteria, especially encapsulated bacteria, from blood. Asplenic (congenically or surgically) individuals are highly susceptible to pneumonia, meningitis, and other manifestations of *Streptococcus pneumoniae, Neisseria meningitidis,* and other encapsulated bacteria.

CYTOKINE-INDUCED RESPONSES

LPS and other bacterial cell wall components stimulate immature dendritic cells and macrophages to release interleukins IL-1 and IL-6, TNF-α, and chemokines. These cytokines are **endogenous pyrogens** because they promote **fever** production and enhance the inflammatory response by further activating macrophages and promoting the acute-phase response. The **acute-phase response** (Box 14–4) is triggered by IL-1, IL-6, TNF-α, inflammation, tissue injury (produced by macrophages), prostaglandin E_2, and interferons associated with infection (Box 14–5). The acute-phase response promotes changes that support host defenses and include fever, anorexia, sleepiness, metabolic changes, and production of proteins. Acute-phase proteins that are produced and released into the serum include C-reactive protein, complement components, coagulation proteins, LPS-binding proteins, transport proteins, protease inhibitors, and adherence proteins. **C-reactive protein** complexes with

BOX 14–4. Secreted Products of Macrophages with a Protective Effect on the Body

Acute-phase cytokines: IL6, TNFα, and IL-1 (endogenous pyrogens)
Other cytokines: IL-12, GM-CSF, G-CSF, M-CSF, interferon-α
Cytotoxic factors
- Oxygen metabolites:
  - Hydrogen peroxide
  - Superoxide anion
  - Nitric oxide
- Hydrolytic enzymes:
  - Collagenase
  - Lipase
  - Phosphatase
- Complement components:
  - C1 through C5
  - Properdin
  - Factors B, D, H, and I

Coagulation factors
Plasma proteins
Arachidonic acid metabolites:
Prostaglandin
Thromboxane
Leukotrienes

CSF, Colony-stimulating factor; G, granulocyte; IL, interleukin; M, macrophage.

BOX 14–5. Acute-Phase Reactants

α_1-antitrypsin
α_1-glycoprotein
Amyloids A and P
Antithrombin III
C-reactive protein
C1 esterase inhibitor
C3 complement
Ceruloplasmin
Fibrinogen
Haptoglobin
Orosomucoid
Plasminogen
Transferrin
Lipopolysaccharide-binding proteins

the polysaccharides of numerous bacteria and fungi and activates the complement pathway, facilitating removal of these organisms from the body through greater phagocytosis. The acute-phase proteins reinforce the innate defenses against infection, but their excessive production during sepsis (induced by endotoxin) can cause serious problems, such as shock.

Immature dendritic cells, macrophages, and other cells of the macrophage lineage play many roles in addition to the phagocytosis of bacteria and antigen (Figure 14–5), including a major role in the transition between the antigen-nonspecific and antigen-specific responses. The immature dendritic cells and macrophages produce IL-12, which activates NK cells at the site of infection and initiates the TH1 response.

γδ T cells in tissue and in the blood sense phosphorylated amine metabolites from some bacteria (*Escherichia coli*, mycobacteria) but not others (streptococci, staphylococci), and with NK cells produce IFN-γ to further activate macrophages, enforcing a TH1 cycle of cytokines. Dendritic cells can present bacterial glycolipids to activate **NK1-T** cells, which can also produce IFN-γ.

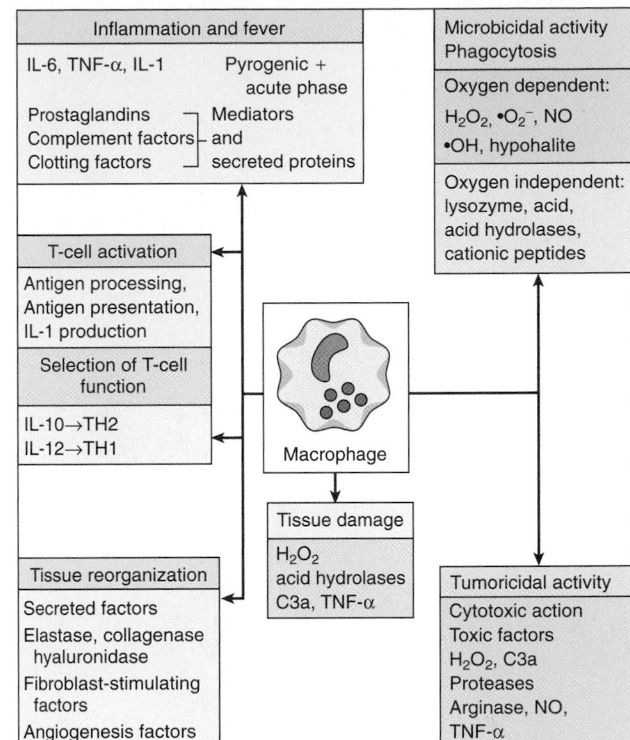

FIGURE 14–5. The many functions of macrophages and members of the macrophage family. IL, Interleukin; TNF, tumor necrosis factor. (From Roitt et al: *Immunology*, ed 4, St Louis, 1996, Mosby.)

ANTIGEN-SPECIFIC RESPONSE TO BACTERIAL CHALLENGE

On ingestion of bacteria and stimulation of TLRs by bacterial components, the immature dendritic cell (iDC) matures to a dendritic cell (DC), ceases to phagocytize, and moves to the lymph nodes to deliver and process their internalized antigen for presentation to T cells (see Fig. 14–2; Figure 14–6). Antigenic peptides (having more than 11 amino acids) produced from phagocytosed proteins (exogenous route) are bound to class II major histocompatibility complex (MHC) molecules and presented by these antigen-presenting cells (APCs) to naïve CD4 TH0 cells. The CD4 T cells are activated by a combination of (1) antigenic peptide in the MHC II complex with the T-cell antigen receptor and CD4, (2) costimulatory signals provided by the interaction of CD28 molecules on the T cells with the B7 molecule on the DC or macrophage, and (3) IL-1, IL-12, and other cytokines produced by the DC. In addition, IL-6 produced by the DC inhibits the production of suppressive cytokines (transforming growth factor-β [TGF-β] and IL-10) by $CD4^+CD25^+$ regulatory T cells to allow the activation of the naïve T cells. The TH0 cells produce IL-2, IFN-γ, and IL-4. Simultaneously, bacterial antigens stuck to the surface of the DC or free antigen interacts with B cells expressing surface IgM and IgD specific for the antigen and activates the cell to grow and produce IgM. Microbial cell wall polysaccharides, especially LPS, activate B cells and promote the specific IgM antibody responses. Swollen lymph nodes are an indication of lymphocyte activation in response to antigenic challenge.

The conversion of TH0 cells to TH1 cells is promoted by IL-12 and reinforced by IFN-γ. **TH1 CD4 T cells** (1) promote and reinforce inflammatory responses (e.g., IFN-γ activation of macrophage) and growth of T and B cells (IL-2) to expand the immune response; and (2) promote B cells to produce complement-binding antibodies (IgM, IgG1, and IgG3 upon class-switching). These responses are important for the early phases of an antibacterial defense. TH1 responses are also essential for combating intracellular bacterial infections and mycobacteria, which are hidden from antibody. IFN-γ activates macrophage and other inflammatory processes (DTH) to kill the infected cell. Alternatively, the continuous stimulation induced by a chronic infection (e.g., tuberculosis) can promote fusion of macrophage to giant cells and epithelioid cells, forming a granuloma around the infection. CD8 T cells are not very important for antibacterial immunity.

CD4 TH2 T-cell responses occur later and are often initiated by the B-cell presentation of antigen. Binding of antigen to the cell surface antibody on B cells activates the B cells and also promotes uptake, processing of the antigen, and presentation of antigenic peptides on class II MHC molecules to the CD4 TH2 cell. The TH2 cell produces IL-4, IL-5, IL-6, IL-10, and IL-13, which enhance IgG production and, depending on other factors, the production of IgE or IgA. The TH2 response also promotes terminal differentiation of B cells to plasma-cell antibody

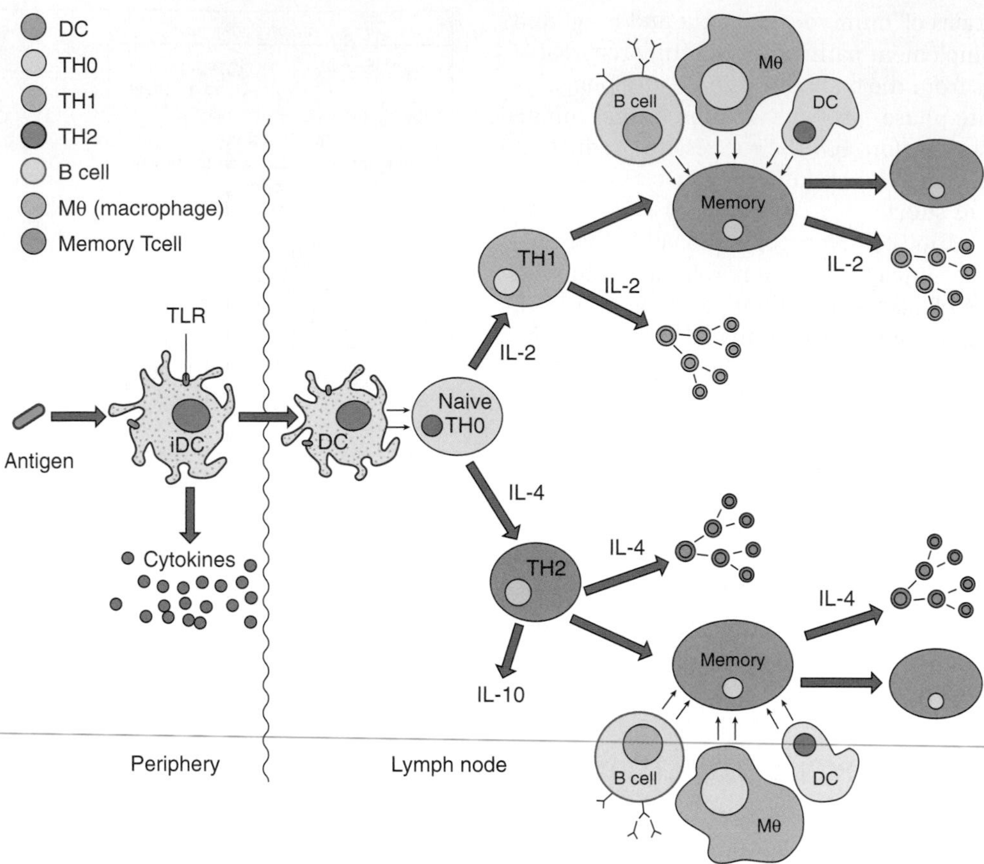

FIGURE 14–6. Initiation and expansion of specific immune responses. Immature dendritic cells at the site of infection acquire bacteria and debris, bacterial components activate the cell through Toll-Like Receptors, and DCs mature, move to the lymph node, and present antigen to naïve T cells to initiate the antigen-specific response. During a secondary or memory response, B cells, macrophages, and DCs can present antigen to initiate the response.

factories. **CD4$^+$CD25$^+$ regulatory T cells** curtail both TH1 and TH2 responses and promote the development of some of the antigen-specific cells into memory T cells.

Antibodies are the primary protection against extracellular bacteria and reinfection. Antibody is important for promoting complement activation, opsonizing the bacteria for phagocytosis, blocking bacterial adhesion, and neutralizing (inactivating) exotoxins (e.g., tetanospasmin, botulinum toxin) and other cytotoxic proteins produced by bacteria (e.g., degradative enzymes). Vaccine immunization with inactivated exotoxins (toxoids) is the primary means of protection against the potentially lethal effects of exotoxins.

IgM antibodies are produced early in the antibacterial response. IgM bound to bacteria activates the classical complement cascade, promoting both the direct killing of gram-negative bacteria and the inflammatory responses. The large size of IgM limits its ability to spread into the tissue. Later in the immune response, T-cell help promotes differentiation of the B cell and immunoglobulin class-switching to produce IgG. **IgG** antibodies are the predominant antibody, especially on rechallenge. IgG antibodies, except IgG4, fix complement and promote phagocytic uptake of the bacteria through Fc receptors on macrophages. The production of **IgA** requires TH2 and TH3 (TGF-β) cytokines. IgA is the primary secretory antibody and is important for protecting mucosal membranes. Secretory IgA acquires the secretory component that promotes interaction and passage of IgA through mucosal epithelial cells. IgA neutralizes the binding of bacteria and their toxins at epithelial cell surfaces.

A primary antigen-specific response to bacterial infection takes at least 5 to 7 days. Movement of the DC to the lymph node may take 1 to 3 days, followed by activation, expansion, and maturation of the response. On rechallenge to infection, memory T cells can respond quickly to antigen presentation by DC, macrophage, or B cells, not just DC; memory B cells can respond to antigen; and the secondary response occurs within 2 to 3 days.

BACTERIAL IMMUNOPATHOGENESIS

Activation of the inflammatory and acute-phase responses can initiate significant tissue and systemic damage. Although IL-1, IL-6, and TNF-α promote protective responses to a local infection, these same responses can be life threatening when activated by systemic infection. Activation of macrophages in the liver and spleen by endotoxin can promote release of TNF-α into the blood, causing many of the symptoms of **sepsis,** including hemodynamic failure, shock, and death (see Chapter 19). Antibodies produced against bacterial antigens that share determinants with human proteins can initiate tissue destruction (e.g., antibodies produced in post-streptococcal glomerulonephritis and rheumatic fever). Nonspecific activation of CD4 T cells by **superantigens** (e.g., toxic shock syndrome toxin of *S. aureus*) promotes the production of large amounts of cytokines and eventually the death of the activated T cell. The sudden, massive release of cytokines can cause shock and severe tissue damage (e.g., toxic shock syndrome) (see Chapter 19).

BACTERIAL EVASION OF PROTECTIVE RESPONSES

The mechanisms used by bacteria to evade host-protective responses are discussed in Chapter 19 as virulence factors. These mechanisms include: (1) the inhibition of phagocytosis and intracellular killing in the phagocyte, (2) inactivation of complement function, (3) cleavage of IgA, (4) intracellular growth (avoidance of antibody), and (5) change in bacterial antigenic appearance. Some microorganisms, including but not limited to mycobacteria (also *Listeria* and *Brucella* species), survive and multiply within macrophages, and use the macrophages as a protective reservoir or transport system to help spread the organisms throughout the body. However, on activation the macrophages can kill the intracellular pathogens.

Antiviral Responses

HOST DEFENSES AGAINST VIRAL INFECTION

The immune response is the best and, in most cases, the only means of controlling a viral infection (Figure 14–7). Unfortunately, it is also the source of pathogenesis for many viral diseases. The humoral and cellular immune responses are important for antiviral immunity. Unlike for a bacterial infection, the ultimate goal of the immune response in a viral infection is to eliminate both the virus and the host cells harboring or replicating the virus. Interferons, NK cells, CD4 TH1 responses, and CD8 cytotoxic T-killer cells are more important for viral infections than for bacterial infections. Failure to resolve the infection may lead to persistent or chronic infection or death.

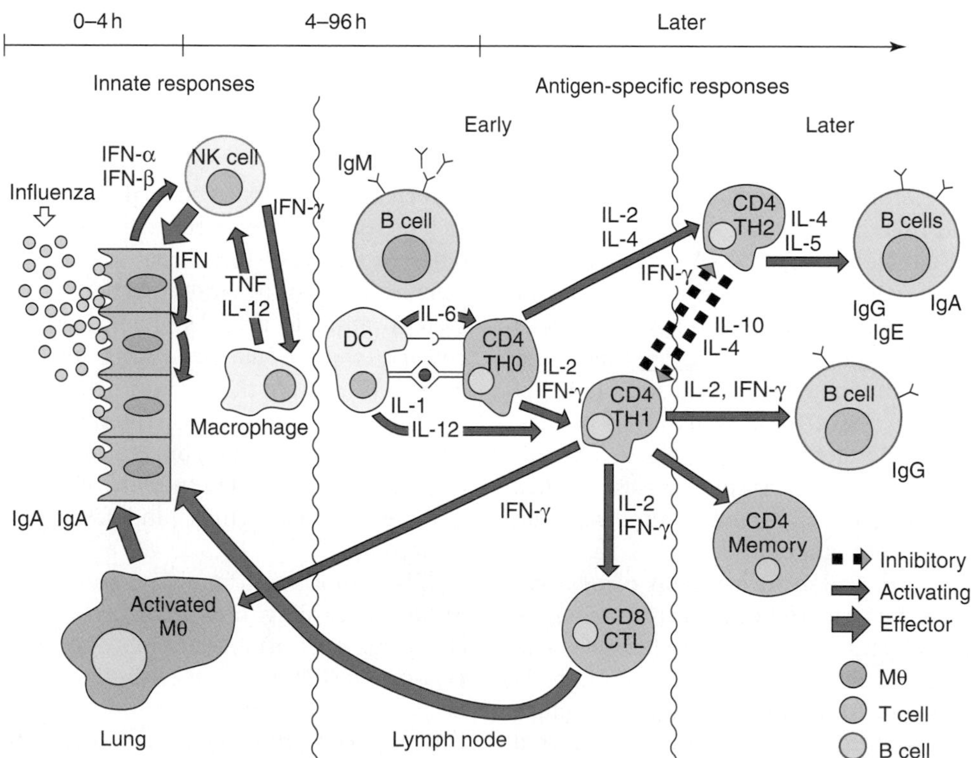

FIGURE 14–7. Antiviral responses. The response to a virus (e.g., influenza virus) initiates with interferon production and action and NK cells. Activation of antigen-specific immunity resembles the antibacterial response, except that CD8 cytotoxic T lymphocytes (CTLs) are important antiviral responses. The time course of events is indicated at the top of the figure. APC, Antigen-presenting cell; HLA, human leukocyte antigen; IFN, interferon, Mθ, macrophage; NK, natural killer, TNF, tumor necrosis factor.

TABLE 14–3. Basic Properties of Human Interferons (IFNs)

Property	IFN-α	IFN-β	IFN-γ
Previous designations	Leukocyte IFN Type I	Fibroblast IFN Type I	Immune IFN Type II
Genes	>20	1	1
Molecular mass (Da)*			
Major subtypes	16,000–23,000	23,000	20,000–25,000
Cloned[†]	19,000	19,000	16,000
Glycosylation	No[‡]	Yes	Yes
pH 2 stability	Stable[‡]	Stable	Labile
Induction	Viruses	Viruses	Immune activation
Principal source	Epithelium, leukocytes	Fibroblast	Lymphocyte
Introns in gene	No	No	Yes
Homology with human IFN-α	100%	30%–50%	<10%

From White DO: *Antiviral chemotherapy, interferons and vaccines,* Basel, Switzerland, 1984, Karge; and Samuel CE: *Virology* 183:1-11, 1991.
*Molecular mass of monomeric form.
[†]Nonglycosylated form, as produced in bacteria by recombinant DNA technology.
[‡]Most subtypes but not all.

INNATE DEFENSES

Body temperature, fever, interferons, other cytokines, the mononuclear phagocyte system, and NK cells provide a local, rapid response to viral infection and also activate the specific immune defenses. Often the nonspecific defenses are sufficient to control a viral infection, thus preventing the occurrence of symptoms.

Viral infection can induce the release of cytokines (e.g., TNF, IL-1) and interferon from infected cells, immature dendritic cells, and macrophages. Viral ribonucleic acid (RNA) (especially double-stranded RNA), deoxyribonucleic acid (DNA), and some viral glycoproteins are potent activators of TLRs to promote the release of these cytokines. These soluble protein factors trigger local and systemic responses. Induction of fever and stimulation of the immune system are two of these systemic effects.

Body temperature and fever can limit the replication of or destabilize some viruses. Many viruses are less stable (e.g., herpes simplex virus) or cannot replicate (rhinoviruses) at 37° C or higher.

Cells of the **dendritic and mononuclear phagocyte system** phagocytose the viral and cell debris from virally infected cells. Macrophages in the liver (Kupffer cells) and spleen rapidly filter many viruses from the blood. Antibody and complement bound to a virus facilitate its uptake by macrophages (opsonization). Dendritic cells and macrophages also present antigen to T cells and release IL-1, IL12, and IFN-α to expand the innate and initiate the antigen-specific immune responses. Activated macrophages can also distinguish and kill infected target cells.

NK cells are activated by interferon and specific cytokines to kill virally infected cells. Viral infection may reduce the expression of MHC antigens or may alter the carbohydrates on cell surface proteins to provide cytolytic signals to the NK cell.

INTERFERON

Interferon was first described by Isaacs and Lindemann as a factor that "interferes with" the replication of many different viruses. Interferon is the body's *first* active defense against a viral infection, an "early warning system" at the local and systemic levels. *In addition to activating a target-cell antiviral defense to block viral replication, interferons activate the immune response and enhance T-cell recognition of the infected cell.* Interferon is a very important defense against infection but is also a cause of the systemic symptoms associated with many viral infections, such as malaise, myalgia, chills, and fever (nonspecific flulike symptoms).

IFN comprises a family of proteins that can be subdivided according to several properties, including size, stability, cell of origin, and mode of action (Table 14–3). **IFN-α** and **IFN-β** are Type 1 interferons that share many properties, including structural homology and mode of action. B cells, monocytes, macrophages, and immature dendritic cells make **IFN-α.** Fibroblasts and other cells make **IFN-β** in response to viral infection and other stimuli. **IFN-γ** is a Type 2 interferon, a cytokine produced by activated T and NK cells later in the infection. Although

BOX 14–6. Interferons

Induction

- Double-stranded ribonucleic acid (dsRNA) (e.g., RNA virus intermediate)
- Viral inhibition of cellular protein synthesis
- Enveloped virus interaction with immature dendritic cell

Mechanism of Action

- Initial infected cell releases interferon
- Interferon binds to a specific cell surface receptor on another cell
- Interferon induces the "antiviral state":
  - Synthesis of protein kinase R (PKR), 2′-5′ oligoadenylate synthetase, and ribonuclease L
  - Viral infection of the cell activates these enzymes
  - Messenger RNA (mRNA) is degraded and protein synthesis inhibited to block viral replication
  - Degradation of mRNA (2′-5′ oligoadenylate synthase and RNAse L)
  - Inhibition of ribosome assembly (PKR)
  - Initiation of innate and immune antiviral responses

IFN-γ inhibits viral replication, its structure and mode of action differ from those of the other interferons. IFN-γ is also known as **macrophage activation factor** and is the defining component of the TH1 response.

The best inducer of IFN-α and IFN-β production is **double-stranded RNA (dsRNA),** *produced as the replicative intermediates of RNA viruses* or from the interaction of sense/antisense messenger RNAs (mRNAs) for some DNA viruses (Box 14–6). One dsRNA molecule per cell is sufficient to induce the production of interferon. Interaction of some enveloped viruses (e.g., herpes simplex virus and human immunodeficiency virus [HIV]) with immature dendritic cells can promote production of *IFN-α*. Inhibition of protein synthesis in a virally infected cell can decrease the production of a repressor protein of the interferon gene, allowing expression of the interferon gene. Nonviral interferon inducers include the following:

1. Intracellular microorganisms (e.g., mycobacteria, fungi, protozoa)
2. Activators of certain TLRs or mitogens (e.g., endotoxins, phytohemagglutinin)
3. Double-stranded polynucleotides (e.g., poly I:C, poly dA:dT)
4. Synthetic polyanion polymers (e.g., polysulfates, polyphosphates, pyran)
5. Antibiotics (e.g., kanamycin, cycloheximide)
6. Low-molecular-weight synthetic compounds (e.g., tilorone, acridine dyes)

IFN-α and IFN-β can be induced and released within hours of infection (Figure 14–8). The interferon binds to specific receptors on the neighboring cells and induces the production of antiviral proteins—**the antiviral state.** However, these antiviral proteins are not activated until they bind dsRNA. The major antiviral effects of interferon are produced by two enzymes, 2′-5′ oligoadenylate synthetase (an unusual polymerase) and protein kinase R (PKR) (Figure 14–9). Viral infection of the cell and production of dsRNA activate these enzymes and trigger a cascade of biochemical events that leads to (1) the inhibition of protein synthesis by PKR phosphorylation of an important ribosomal initiation factor (eukaryotic initiation factor [eIF-2α]), and (2) the degradation of mRNA (preferentially, viral mRNA) by ribonuclease L, activated by 2′,5′ oligoadenosine. This process essentially puts the cellular protein synthesis factory "on strike" and prevents viral replication. It must be stressed that interferon induces an antiviral state but does not directly block viral replication. The antiviral state lasts for 2 to 3 days, which may be sufficient for the cell to degrade and eliminate the virus without being killed.

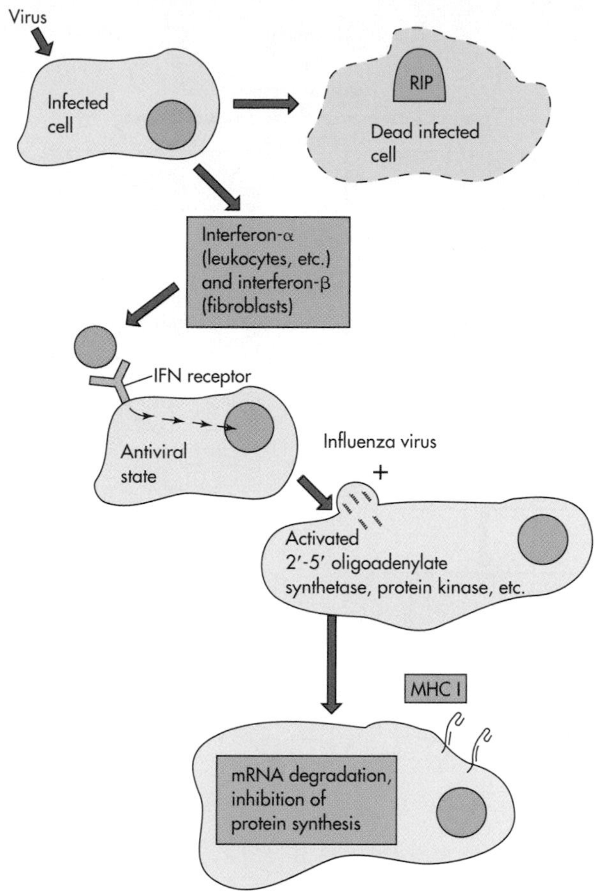

FIGURE 14–8. Induction of the antiviral state by interferon-α or interferon-β. Interferon is produced in response to viral infection but does not affect the initially infected cell. The interferon binds to a cell surface receptor on other cells and induces production of antiviral enzymes (antiviral state). The infection and production of double-stranded RNA activates the antiviral activity. MHC I, Major histocompatibility antigen type 1.

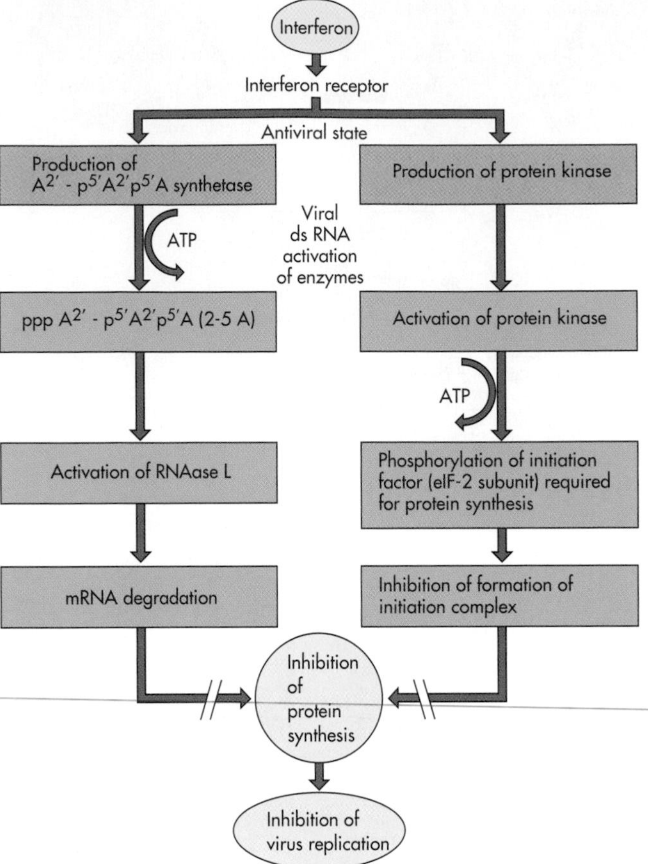

FIGURE 14–9. The two major routes for interferon inhibition of viral protein synthesis. One mechanism involves the induction of an unusual polymerase (2′-5′ oligoadenylate synthetase [2-5A]) that is activated by double-stranded RNA (dsRNA). The activated enzyme synthesizes an unusual adenine chain with a 2′,5′-phosphodiester linkage. The oligomer activates RNAase L that degrades messenger RNA (mRNA). The other mechanism involves the induction of protein kinase R (PKR) that inactivates the eukaryotic initiation factor (eIF-2α) by phosphorylating one of the subunits to prevent initiation of protein synthesis. ATP, Adenosine triphosphate.

Interferons stimulate cell-mediated immunity by activating effector cells and enhancing recognition of the virally infected target cell. Interferons stimulate pre-NK cells to differentiate to NK cells to *activate an early, local, natural defense against infection.* Activation of macrophages by IFN-γ promotes production of more interferon, secretion of other biologic response modifiers, phagocytosis, recruitment, and inflammatory responses. IFN-γ increases the expression of class II MHC antigens on the macrophage to help promote antigen presentation to T cells. IFN-α and IFN-β increase the expression of class I MHC antigens, enhancing the cell's ability to present antigen and making the cell a better target for cytotoxic T cells (CTLs). However, IFN-β suppresses dendritic cell function.

Interferon also has widespread regulatory effects on cell growth, protein synthesis, and the immune response. All three interferon types block cell proliferation at appropriate doses.

Genetically engineered recombinant interferon is being used as an antiviral therapy for some viral infections (e.g., human papilloma and hepatitis C viruses). Effective treatment requires the use of the correct interferon subtype(s) and its prompt delivery at the appropriate concentration. The use of IFN-β for treatment of multiple sclerosis is based on prevention of myelin basic protein presentation by DCs. Interferons have also been used in clinical trials for the treatment of certain cancers. However, interferon treatment has flulike side effects, such as chills, fever, and fatigue.

Antigen-Specific Immunity

Humoral immunity and cell-mediated immunity play different roles in resolving viral infections (i.e., eliminating the virus from the body). Humoral immunity (antibody) acts mainly on extracellular virions, whereas cell-mediated immunity (T cells) is directed at the virus-producing cell (see Figure 14–6).

HUMORAL IMMUNITY

Practically all viral proteins are foreign to the host and are immunogenic (i.e., capable of eliciting an antibody response). However, not all immunogens elicit protective immunity.

Antibody blocks the progression of disease through the **neutralization and opsonization** of cell-free virus. *Protective antibody responses are generated toward the viral capsid proteins of naked viruses and the glycoproteins of enveloped viruses that interact with cell surface receptors (viral attachment proteins).* These antibodies can neutralize the virus by preventing viral interaction with target cells or by destabilizing the virus, thus initiating its degradation. Binding of antibody to these proteins also opsonizes the virus, promoting its uptake and clearance by macrophages. Antibody recognition of infected cells can also promote antibody-dependent cellular cytotoxicity (ADCC) by NK cells. Antibodies to other viral antigens may be useful for serologic analysis of the viral infection (Box 14–7).

The major antiviral role of antibody is to *prevent the spread of extracellular virus to other cells.* Antibody is especially important in limiting the spread of the virus by **viremia,** *preventing the virus from reaching the target tissue for disease production. Antibody is most effective at resolving cytolytic infections.* Resolution occurs because the virus kills the cell factory and the antibody eliminates the extracellular virus. Antibody is the primary defense initiated by vaccination.

BOX 14–7. Summary of Antiviral Responses

Interferon
Interferon is induced by double-stranded RNA, inhibition of cellular protein synthesis, or enveloped virus.
Interferon initiates the antiviral state in surrounding cells.
Interferon blocks local viral replication.
Interferon initiates systemic antiviral responses.

Natural Killer (NK) Cells
NK cells are activated by interferon-α (INF-α) and IL-12 and activate macrophages (INF-γ).
NK cells target and kill virus-infected cells (especially enveloped viruses).

Macrophage and Dendritic Cells
Macrophages filter viral particles from blood.
Macrophages inactivate opsonized virus particles.
Immature dendritic cells (iDCs) produce INF-α and other cytokines.
DC initiate CD4 and CD8 T-cell response.
DC and macrophage present antigen to CD4 T cells.

T Cells
T cells are essential for controlling enveloped and noncytolytic viral infections.
T cells recognize viral peptides presented by major histocompatibility complex (MHC) molecules on cell surfaces.
Antigenic viral peptides (linear epitopes) can come from any viral protein (e.g., glycoproteins, nucleoproteins).
TH1 CD4 responses are more important than TH2 responses.
CD8 cytotoxic T cells respond to viral peptide-class I MHC protein complexes on the cell surface.
TH2 CD4 responses are important for the maturation of the antibody response.
TH2 CD4 responses may be detrimental if they prematurely limit the TH1 inflammatory and cytolytic responses.

Antibody
Antibody neutralizes extracellular virus:
It blocks viral attachment proteins (e.g., glycoproteins, capsid proteins).
It destabilizes viral structure.
Antibody opsonizes virus for phagocytosis.
Antibody promotes killing of target cell by the complement cascade and antibody-dependent cellular cytotoxicity.
Antibody resolves lytic viral infections.
Antibody blocks viremic spread to target tissue.
Immunoglobulin M (IgM) is an indicator of recent or current infection.
IgG is a more effective antiviral than IgM.
Secretory IgA is important for protecting mucosal surfaces.

T-CELL IMMUNITY

T cell–mediated immunity promotes antibody and inflammatory responses (CD4 helper T cells) and kills infected cells (cytotoxic T cells [CD4 and CD8]) (see Box 14–7). The **CD4 TH1** response is generally more important than TH2 responses for controlling a viral infection, especially noncytolytic and enveloped viruses. **CTLs** induce apoptosis on interaction of their Fas ligand protein with the Fas protein on the target cell. **CD8** killer T cells can also kill cells after their T-cell receptor binds to a viral peptide presented by a class I MHC protein. The peptides expressed on class I MHC antigens are obtained from viral proteins synthesized within the infected cell (endogenous route), *which include peptides derived from viral proteins that may not elicit protective antibody* (e.g., intracellular or internal virion proteins, nuclear proteins, improperly folded or processed proteins [cell trash]), in addition to viral glycoproteins. For example, the matrix and nucleoproteins of the influenza virus and the ICP4 (nuclear) protein of herpes simplex virus are targets for CTL lysis but do not elicit protective antibody. Perforin, a complement-like membrane poreformer, is released into the space between the CTL and target cell and induces apoptosis in the target cell.

The CD8 CTL response probably evolved as a defense against virus infection. Cell-mediated immunity is especially important for resolving infections by syncytia-forming viruses (e.g., measles, herpes simplex, and varicella-zoster viruses), which can spread from cell to cell without exposure to antibody, and noncytolytic viruses (e.g., hepatitis A and measles viruses), and for controlling latent viruses (herpes viruses and papillomaviruses). *CTLs kill infected cells and, as a result, eliminate the source of new virus.*

Immune Response to Viral Challenge

PRIMARY VIRAL CHALLENGE

The innate host responses are the earliest responses to viral challenge and are often sufficient to limit viral spread (see Figure 14–6). The **interferon** produced in response to most viral infections initiates the protection of adjacent cells, enhances antigen presentation by increasing the expression of MHC antigens, and initiates the clearance of infected cells by activating NK cells and antigen-specific responses. Virus and viral components released from the infected cells are phagocytosed by **immature dendritic cells** that produce cytokines and then move to the lymph nodes. Macrophages in the liver and spleen are especially important for clearing virus from the bloodstream (filters). These phagocytic cells degrade and process the viral antigens. The appropriate peptide fragments bound to class II MHC antigens are presented to CD4 T cells. Dendritic cells process phagocytosed viral antigens and cross-present these antigens on MHC I molecules to CD8 T cells. The APCs also release IL-1, IL-6, and TNF to induce fever and, with IL-12, promote activation of helper T cells and specific cytokine production (TH1 response).

Antiviral antigen–specific responses are similar to antibacterial antigen–specific responses, except that the CD8 T cell plays a more important role. **IgM** is produced approximately 3 days after infection. Its production indicates a primary infection. **IgG** and **IgA** are produced 2 to 3 days after IgM. Secretory IgA is made in response to a viral challenge through the natural openings of the body (i.e., eyes, mouth, and respiratory and gastrointestinal systems). **CD8 killer** T cells are present at approximately the same time as serum IgG. During infection, the number of CD8 T cells specific for antigen may increase 50,000 to 100,000 times. The antigen specific CD8 T cells move to the site of infection and kill virally infected cells. Recognition and binding to class I MHC viral peptide–expressing target cells promotes apoptotic killing of the target cells either through the release of perforin and granzymes (to disrupt the cell membrane) or through the binding of the Fas ligand with Fas on the target cell. Resolution of the infection occurs later, when sufficient antibody is available to neutralize all virus progeny or when cellular immunity has been able to reach and eliminate the infected cells. For the resolution of most enveloped and noncytolytic viral infections, TH1-mediated responses are required (in addition to antibody) to kill the viral factory.

Viral infections of the brain and the eye can cause serious damage, because these tissues cannot repair tissue damage and are **immunologically privileged sites** of the body. T-cell responses are suppressed to prevent the serious tissue destruction that accompanies inflammation. These sites depend on innate, cytokine, and antibody control of infection. If cell-mediated responses become necessary, permanent tissue damage often results.

Cell-mediated and IgG immune responses do not arise until 6 to 8 days after viral challenge. For many viral infections, this is after innate responses have controlled viral replication. However, for other viral infections, this period allows the virus to expand the infection, spread through the body and infect the target tissue, and cause disease (e.g., brain:encephalitis, liver:hepatitis). The response to the expanded infection may require a larger and more intense immune response, which often includes the immunopathogenesis and tissue damage that cause disease symptoms.

SECONDARY VIRAL CHALLENGE

In any war it is easier to eliminate an enemy if its identity and origin are known and if establishment of its foothold can be prevented. Similarly, in the human body, prior immunity, established by prior infection or vaccination, allows rapid, specific mobilization of defenses to prevent disease symptoms, promote rapid clearance of the virus, and block viremic spread from the primary site of infection to the target tissue to prevent disease. As a result, most secondary viral challenges are asymptomatic. Antibody and memory B and T cells are present in an immune host to generate a more rapid and extensive anamnestic (booster) response to the virus. Secretory IgA is produced quickly to provide an important defense to reinfection through the natural openings of the body, but it is produced only transiently.

Host, viral, and other factors determine the outcome of the immune response to a viral infection. Host factors include genetic background, immune status, age, and the general health of the individual. Viral factors include viral strain, infectious dose, and route of entry. The time required to initiate immune protection, the extent of the response, the level of control of the infection, and the potential for immunopathology (see Chapter 49) resulting from the infection differ after a primary infection and a rechallenge.

VIRAL MECHANISMS FOR ESCAPING THE IMMUNE RESPONSE

A major factor in the virulence of a virus is its ability to escape immune resolution. Viruses may escape immune resolution by evading detection, preventing activation, or blocking the delivery of the immune response. Specific examples are presented in Table 14–4. Some viruses even encode special proteins that suppress the immune response.

Viral Immunopathogenesis

The symptoms of many viral diseases are the consequence of cytokine action or overzealous immune responses. The flulike symptoms of influenza and any virus that establishes a viremia (e.g., arboviruses) are a result of the interferon and other cytokine responses induced by the virus. Antibody interactions with large amounts of viral antigen in blood, such as occurs with hepatitis B virus infection, can lead to immune complex diseases. The measles rash, the extensive tissue damage to the brain associated with herpes simplex virus encephalitis ("-itis" means inflammation), and the tissue damage and symptoms of hepatitis are a result of cell-mediated immune responses. The more aggressive NK-cell and T-cell responses of adults exacerbate some diseases that are benign in children, such as varicella-zoster virus, Epstein-Barr virus infectious mononucleosis, and hepatitis B infec-

TABLE 14–4. Examples of Viral Evasion of Immune Responses

Mechanism	Viral Examples	Action
Humoral Response		
Hidden from antibody	Herpesviruses, retroviruses	Latent infection
	Herpes simplex virus, varicella-zoster virus, paramyxoviruses, human immunodeficiency virus	Cell-to-cell infection (syncytia formation)
Antigenic variation	Lentiviruses (human immunodeficiency virus)	Genetic change after infection
	Influenza virus	Annual genetic changes
Secretion of blocking antigen	Hepatitis B virus	Hepatitis B surface antigen
Decay of complement	Herpes simplex virus	Glycoprotein C, which binds and promotes C3 decay
Interferon		
Block production	Hepatitis B virus	Inhibition of IFN transcription
	Epstein-Barr virus	IL-10 analogue (BCRF-1) blocks IFN-γ production
Block action	Adenovirus	Inhibits up-regulation of MHC expression, VA1 RNA blocks double-stranded RNA activation of interferon- induced protein kinase (PKR)
	Herpes simplex virus	Inactivates PKR and activates phosphatase (PP1) to reverse inactivation of initiation factor for protein synthesis
Immune Cell Function		
Impairment of dendritic cell (DC) function	Measles, hepatitis C	Induction of IFN-β, which inhibits DC function
Impairment of lymphocyte function	Herpes simplex virus	Prevention of CD8 T-cell killing
	Human immunodeficiency virus	Kills CD4 T cells and alteration of macrophages
	Measles virus	Suppression of NK, T, and B cells
Immunosuppressive factors	Epstein-Barr virus	BCRF-1 (similar to IL-10) suppression of TH1 CD4 helper T-cell responses
Decreased Antigen Presentation		
Reduced class I MHC expression	Adenovirus 12	Inhibition of class I MHC transcription
		19-kDa protein (E3 gene) binds class I MHC heavy chain, blocking translocation to surface
	Cytomegalovirus	H301 protein blocks surface expression of β_2-microglobulin and class I MHC molecules
	Herpes simplex virus	ICP47 blocks TAP, preventing peptide binding to class I MHC molecules
Inhibition of Inflammation		
	Poxvirus, adenovirus	Blocking of action of IL-1 or tumor necrosis factor

IFN, interferon; IL, interleukin; MHC I, major histocompatibility complex, antigen type 1; NK, natural killer; PMN, polymorphonuclear neutrophil; TAP, transporter associated with antigen production.

tion. Yet, the lack of such a response in children makes them prone to chronic hepatitis B infection, because the response is insufficient to kill the infected cells and resolve the infection.

Specific Immune Responses to Fungi

The primary protective responses to fungal infection are promoted by **TH1-mediated inflammatory reactions.** Patients deficient in these responses (e.g., patients with AIDS) are most susceptible to fungal (opportunistic) infections. **Macrophages activated by IFN-γ** are important for killing the fungi. Neutrophil production of cationic proteins may be important for some fungal infections (e.g., mucormycosis), and nitric oxide may be important against *Cryptococcus* and other fungi. Antibody, as an opsonin, may facilitate clearance of the fungi.

Specific Immune Responses to Parasites

It is difficult to generalize about the mechanisms of antiparasitic immunity, because there are many different parasites that have different forms and reside in different tissue locations during their life cycles (Table 14–5). Stimulation of *CD4 TH1, CD8 T-cell, and macrophage responses are important for intracellular infections, and TH2 antibody responses are important for extracellular parasites in blood and fluids.* **IgE, eosinophil,** and **mast cell** action are especially important for eliminating worm (cestode and nematode) infections. The efficiency of control of the infection may depend on which response is initiated in the host. Initiation of a TH2 response to *Leishmania* infection results in the inhibition of protective inflammatory responses and a poor outcome. This observation provided the basis for the discovery that TH1 and TH2 responses are separate and antagonistic. Parasites have developed sophisticated mechanisms for avoiding immune clearance and often establish chronic infections.

Extracellular parasites, such as *Trypanosoma cruzi, Toxoplasma gondii,* and *Leishmania* species, are phagocytosed by **macrophage. Antibody** may facilitate the uptake of (opsonize) the parasites. Killing of the parasites follows activation of the macrophage by IFN-γ (produced by NK, γδ T, or CD4 TH1 cells) or TNF-α (produced by other macrophages) and induction of **oxygen-dependent killing mechanisms** (peroxide, superoxide, nitric oxide). The parasites may replicate in the macrophage and hide from subsequent immune detection, unless the macrophage is activated by TH1 responses.

TH1 production of IFN-γ and activation of macrophages are also essential for defense against intracellular protozoa and for the development of **granulomas** around *Schistosoma mansoni* eggs and worms in the liver. The

TABLE 14–5. Examples of Antiparasitic Immune Responses

Parasite	Habitat	Main Host Effector Mechanism*	Method of Avoidance
Trypanosoma brucei	Bloodstream	Antibody + complement	Antigenic variation
Plasmodium species	Hepatocyte, blood cell	Antibody, cytokines (TH1)	Intracellular, antigenic variation
Toxoplasma gondii	Macrophage	O_2 metabolites, NO, lysosomal enzymes (TH1)	Inhibition of fusion with lysosomes
Trypanosoma cruzi	Many cells	O_2 metabolites, NO, lysosomal enzymes (TH1)	Escape into cytoplasm, thus avoiding digestion in lysosome
Leishmania species	Macrophage	O_2 metabolites, NO, lysosomal enzymes (TH1)	Impairment of O_2 burst and scavenging of products; avoidance of digestion
Trichinella spiralis	Gut, blood, muscle	Myeloid cells, antibody + complement (TH2)	Encystment in muscle
Schistosoma mansoni	Skin, blood, lungs, portal vein	Myeloid cells, antibody + complement (TH2)	Acquisition of host antigens, blockade by antibody; soluble antigens and immune complexes; antioxidants
Wuchereria bancrofti	Lymphatic system	Myeloid cells, antibody + complement (TH2)	Thick, extracellular cuticle; antioxidants
Helminths	Gut	IgE	Extracellular cuticle

From Roitt, et al: *Immunology,* ed 4, St Louis, 1996, Mosby.

*Antibody is most important for extracellular pathogens. Cell-mediated immunity (TH1 response) is most important for intracellular pathogens.

granuloma, formed by layers of inflammatory cells, protects the liver from toxins produced by the eggs. However, the granuloma also causes fibrosis, which interrupts the venous blood supply to the liver, leading to hypertension and cirrhosis.

Neutrophils phagocytose and kill extracellular parasites through both oxygen-dependent and oxygen-independent mechanisms. **Eosinophils** localize near parasites, bind to IgG or IgE on the surface of larvae or worms (e.g., helminths, *S. mansoni, Trichinella spiralis*), degranulate by fusing their intracellular granules with the plasma membrane, and release the **major basic protein** into the intercellular space. The major basic protein is toxic to the parasite.

For parasitic worm infections, cytokines produced by TH2 CD4 T-cells are very important for stimulating the production of IgE and the activation of mast cells (Figure 14–10). IgE bound to Fc receptors on mast cells targets the cells to antigens of the infecting parasite. In the lumen of the intestine, antigen binding and cross-linking of the IgE on the mast cell surface stimulate the release of histamine and substances toxic to the parasite and promote mucus secretion to coat and promote expulsion of the worm.

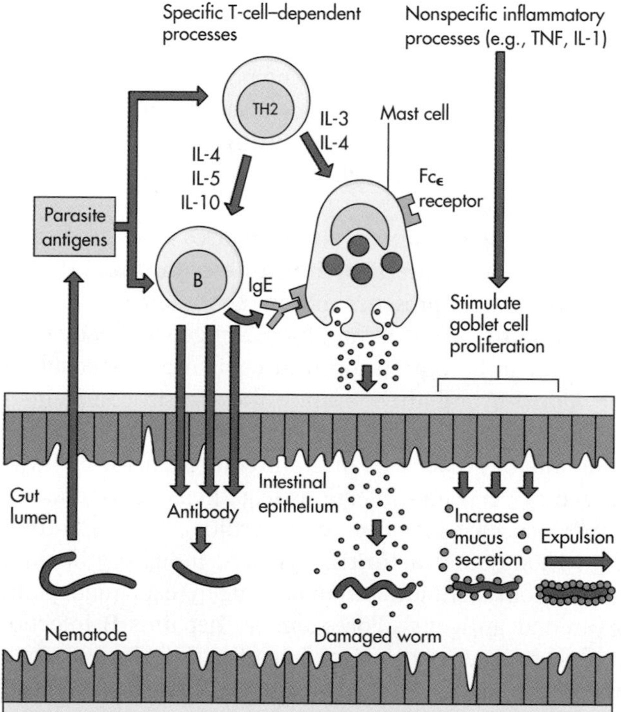

FIGURE 14–10. Elimination of nematodes from the gut. TH2 responses are important for stimulating the production of antibody. Antibody can damage the worm. Immunoglobulin E (IgE) is associated with mast cells, the release of histamine, and toxic substances. Increased mucus secretion also promotes expulsion. IL, Interleukin; TNF, tumor necrosis factor. (From Roitt I et al: *Immunology,* ed 4, St Louis, 1996, Mosby.)

IgG antibody also plays an important role in antiparasitic immunity as an opsonin and by activating complement on the surface of the parasite.

EVASION OF IMMUNE MECHANISMS BY PARASITES

Animal parasites have developed remarkable mechanisms for establishing chronic infections in the vertebrate host (see Table 14–5). These mechanisms include intracellular growth, inactivation of phagocytic killing, release of blocking antigen (e.g., *Trypanosoma brucei, Plasmodium falciparum*), and development of cysts (e.g., protozoa: *Entamoeba histolytica;* helminths: *T. spiralis*) to limit access by the immune response. The African trypanosomes can reengineer the genes for their surface antigen (variable surface glycoprotein) and therefore change their antigenic appearance. Schistosomes can coat themselves with host antigens, including MHC molecules.

Other Immune Responses

Antitumor responses and **rejection of tissue transplants** are primarily mediated by T cells. CD8 cytolytic T cells recognize and kill tumors expressing peptides from embryologic proteins, mutated proteins, or other proteins on class I MHC molecules (endogenous route of peptide presentation). These proteins may be expressed inappropriately by the tumor cell, and the host immune response may not be tolerized to them. In addition, IL-2 treatment in vitro generates lymphokine-activated killer (LAK) cells and NK cells that target tumor cells, and IFN-γ–activated ("angry") macrophages can also distinguish and kill tumor cells.

Rejection of **allografts** used for tissue transplants is triggered by recognition of foreign peptides expressed on foreign class I MHC antigens. In addition to host rejection of the transplanted tissue, cells from the donor of a blood transfusion or a tissue transplant can react against the new host in a **graft versus host (GVH) response.** An in vitro test of T-cell activation and growth in a GVH-like response is the **mixed lymphocyte reaction.** Activation is usually measured as DNA synthesis (radioactive thymidine uptake).

Immunopathogenesis

HYPERSENSITIVITY RESPONSES

Once activated, the immune response is sometimes difficult to control and causes tissue damage.

TABLE 14–6. Hypersensitivity Reactions

Reaction Type	Onset Time	Key Features	Beneficial Effects	Pathologic Effects
Type I	<30 min	Soluble antigen–triggered, immunoglobulin E–dependent release of vasoactive mediators	Antiparasitic responses and toxin neutralization	Localized allergies (e.g., hay fever, asthma) Systemic anaphylaxis
Type II	<8 h	Cell-bound antibody–promoting C′-mediated cytotoxicity	Direct lysis and phagocytosis of extracellular bacteria and other susceptible microbes	Destruction of red blood cells (e.g., transfusion reactions, Rh disease) Organ-specific tissue damage in some autommune diseases (e.g., Goodpasture's syndrome)
Type III	<8 h	Soluble antigen-antibody complexes activate C′	Acute inflammatory reaction at site of extracellular microbes and their clearance	Arthus reaction (localized) Serum sickness and drug reactions (generalized) Systemic autoimmune diseases
Type IV	24-72 h (acute) >1 week (chronic)	Soluble antigen presented to CD4 T cells by MHC II leads to release of TH1 cytokines, activating macrophages and cytotoxic T lymphocytes	Protection against infection by fungi, intracellular bacteria, and viruses	Acute: contact dermatitis, tuberculosis skin test Chronic: granuloma formation, graft rejection

Hypersensitivity reactions are responsible for many of the symptoms associated with microbial infections, especially viral infections. *The mediator and the time course* primarily distinguish the four types of hypersensitivity responses (Table 14–6).

Type I hypersensitivity is caused by **IgE** and is associated with **allergic, atopic,** and **anaphylactic reactions** (Figure 14–11). IgE allergic reactions are rapid-onset reactions. IgE binds to Fc receptors on mast cells and becomes the cell surface receptor for antigens **(allergens).** Cross-linking of several cell surface IgE molecules by an allergen (e.g., pollen) triggers degranulation, releasing **chemoattractants** (cytokines, leukotrienes) to attract eosinophils, neutrophils, and mononuclear cells; **activators** (histamine, platelet-activating factor, tryptase, kininogenase) to promote vasodilation and edema; and **spasmogens** (histamine, prostaglandin D_2, leukotrienes) to directly affect bronchial smooth muscle and promote mucus secretion. Desensitization (allergy shots) produces IgG to bind the allergen and prevent allergen binding to IgE.

Type II hypersensitivity is caused by **antibody binding** to cell surface molecules and the subsequent activation of *cytolytic responses by the* **classic complement cascade** *or by cellular mechanisms* (Figure 14–12). These reactions occur as early as 8 hours following a tissue or blood transplant or as part of a chronic disease. Examples of these reactions are (1) myasthenia gravis (due to antibodies to acetylcholine receptors on neurons), (2) autoimmune hemolytic anemia, and (3) Goodpasture's syndrome (lung and kidney basement membrane damage). Another example is hemolytic disease of newborns (blue babies), which is caused by the reaction of maternal antibody generated during the first pregnancy to Rh factors on fetal erythrocytes of a second baby (Rh incompatibility).

Type III hypersensitivity responses result from activation of **complement** by **immune complexes** (Figure 14–13). In the presence of an abundance of soluble antigen in the bloodstream, large antigen-antibody complexes form, become trapped in capillaries (especially in the kidney), and then initiate the classic complement cascade. Activation of the complement cascade initiates inflammatory reactions. Immune complex disease may be caused by persistent infections (e.g., hepatitis B, malaria, staphylococcal infective endocarditis), autoimmunity (e.g., rheumatoid arthritis, systemic lupus erythematosus), or consistent inhalation of antigen (e.g., mold, plant, or animal antigens). For example, hepatitis B infection produces large amounts of hepatitis B surface antigen, which may form immune complexes that lead to glomerulonephritis. Type III hypersensitivity reactions can be induced in presensitized people by the intradermal injection of antigen to cause an **Arthus reaction,** a skin reaction characterized by redness and swelling. Serum sickness, extrinsic allergic alveolitis (a reaction to inhaled

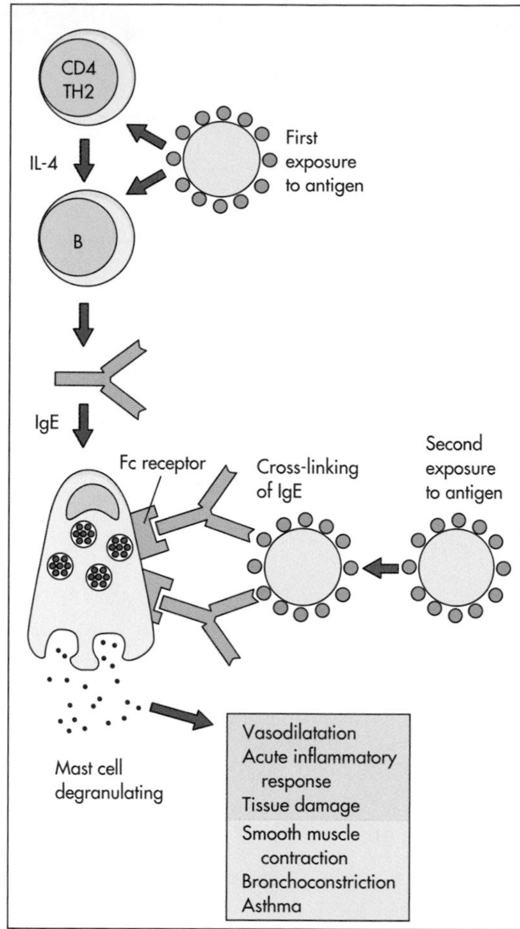

FIGURE 14–11. Type I hypersensitivity: immunoglobulin E (IgE)–mediated atopic and anaphylactic reactions. IgE produced in response to the initial challenge binds to Fc receptors on mast cells and basophils. Allergen binding to the cell surface IgE promotes the release of histamine and prostaglandins from granules to produce symptoms. Examples are hay fever, asthma, penicillin allergy, and reaction to bee stings. IL, Interleukin.

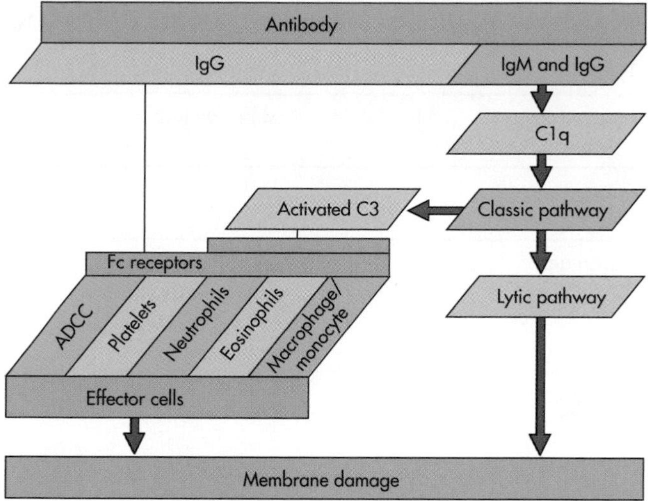

FIGURE 14–12. Type II hypersensitivity: mediated by antibody and complement. Complement activation promotes direct cell damage through the complement cascade and by the activation of effector cells. Examples are Goodpasture's syndrome, the response to Rh factor in newborns, and autoimmune endocrinopathies. ADCC, Antibody-dependent cellular cytotoxicity; Ig, immunoglobulin.

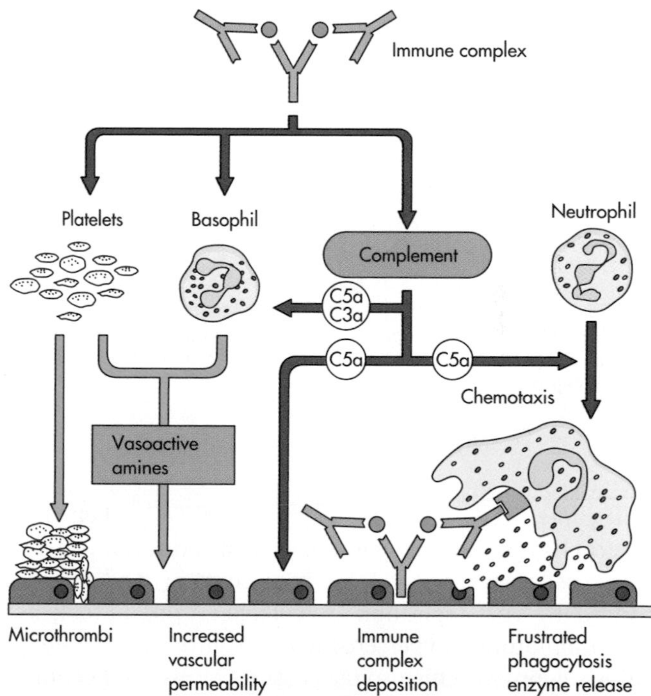

FIGURE 14–13. Type III hypersensitivity: immune complex deposition. Immune complexes can be trapped in the kidney and elsewhere in the body, can activate complement, and can cause other damaging responses. Examples are serum sickness, nephritis associated with chronic hepatitis B infection, and Arthus reaction.

fungal antigen), and glomerulonephritis result from type III hypersensitivity reactions.

Type IV hypersensitivity responses are **delayed-type hypersensitivity (DTH)** inflammatory responses (Figure 14–14 and Table 14–7). It usually takes 24 to 48 hours for antigen to be presented o **CD4 T cells,** and for them to **activate macrophages** to induce the response. Although essential for the control of fungal infections and intracellular bacteria (e.g., mycobacteria), DTH is also responsible for **contact dermatitis** (e.g., cosmetics, nickel) and the response to poison ivy. Intradermal injection of **tuberculin antigen** (purified protein derivative) elicits firm swelling that is maximal 48 to 72 hours after injection and is indicative of prior exposure to *Mycobacterium tuberculosis* (Figure 14–15). **Granulomas** form in response to the intracellular growth and to contain the spread of *M. tuberculosis.* These structures consist of

TABLE 14–7. Important Characteristics of Four Types of Delayed-Type Hypersensitivity Reactions

Type	Reaction Time	Clinical Appearance	Histologic Appearance	Antigen
Jones-Mote	24 h	Skin swelling	Basophils, lymphocytes, mononuclear cells	Intradermal antigen: ovalbumin
Contact	48 h	Eczema	Mononuclear cells, edema, raised epidermis	Epidermal: nickel, rubber, poison ivy
Tuberculin	48 h	Local induration and swelling with or without fever	Mononuclear cells, lymphocytes and monocytes, reduced macrophages	Dermal: tuberculin, mycobacterial, and leishmanial
Granulomatous	4 wk	Skin induration	Epithelioid cell granuloma, giant cells, macrophages, fibrosis with or without necrosis	Persistent antigen or antigen-antibody complexes in macrophages or "nonimmunologic" (e.g., talcum powder)

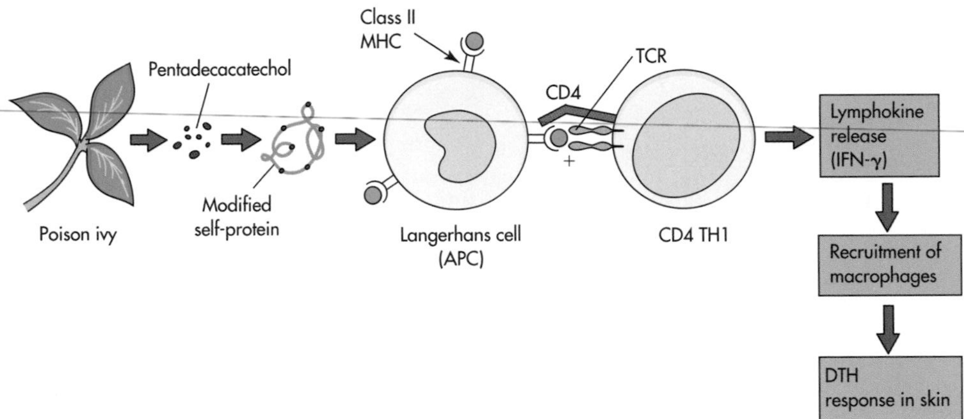

FIGURE 14–14. Type IV hypersensitivity: delayed-type hypersensitivity (DTH) mediated by CD4 T cells (TH1). In this case, chemically modified self-proteins are processed and presented to CD4 T cells, which release cytokines (including interferon-γ [IFN-γ]) that promote inflammation. Other examples of DTH are the tuberculin response (purified protein derivative test) and reaction to metals such as nickel. APC, antigen-presenting cell; TCR, T-cell receptor.

epithelioid cells created from chronically activated macrophages, fused epithelioid cells (multinucleated giant cells) surrounded by lymphocytes, and fibrosis caused by the deposition of collagen from fibroblasts. Granulomatous hypersensitivity occurs with tuberculosis, leprosy, schistosomiasis, sarcoidosis, and Crohn's disease.

Autoimmune Responses

Normally a person is tolerized to self-antigens during the development of the immune system as a fetus and later in life by other mechanisms (e.g., oral tolerization). However, deregulation of the immune response may be initiated by cross-reactivity with microbial antigens (e.g., group A streptococcal infection, rheumatic fever), polyclonal activation of lymphocytes induced by tumors or infection (e.g., malaria, Epstein-Barr virus infection), or a genetic predisposition caused by lack of tolerization to specific antigens.

Autoimmune reactions result from the presence of autoantibodies, activated T cells, and hypersensitivity reactions. People with certain MHC antigens are at higher risk for autoimmune responses (e.g., HLA-B27 [human leukocyte antigen], juvenile rheumatoid arthritis, ankylosing spondylitis). Many of these responses are associated with inflammatory TH1-type responses. Multiple sclerosis, an inflammatory response directed against myelin basic protein, may be triggered by immune responses to one or more viruses, such as human herpesvirus 6 or measles.

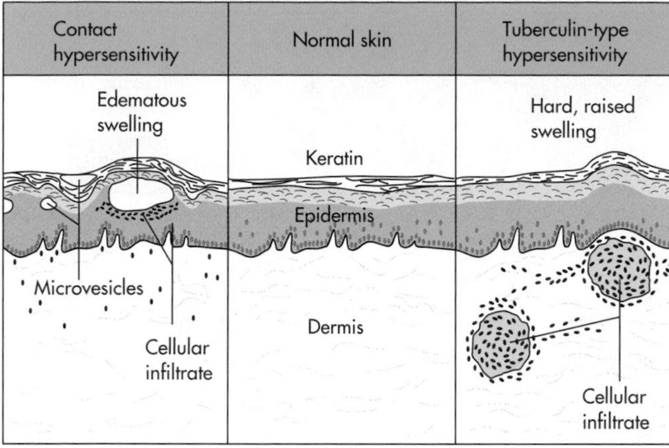

FIGURE 14–15. Contact and tuberculin hypersensitivity responses. These type IV responses are cell mediated but differ in the site of cell infiltration and in the symptoms. Contact hypersensitivity occurs in the epidermis and leads to the formation of blisters; tuberculin-type hypersensitivity occurs in the dermis and is characterized by swelling.

Immunodeficiency

Immunodeficiency may result from genetic deficiencies, starvation, drug-induced immunosuppression (e.g., steroid treatment, cancer chemotherapy, chemotherapeutic suppression of tissue graft rejection), cancer (especially of immune cells), or disease (e.g., AIDS), and naturally occurs in neonates and pregnant women. Deficiencies in specific protective responses put a patient at high risk for serious disease because of the infectious agents that would be controlled by that response (Table 14–8). These "natural experiments" illustrate the importance of specific responses in controlling specific infections.

IMMUNOSUPPRESSION

Immunosuppressive therapy is important for reducing excessive inflammatory or immune responses of macrophages and T cells or for preventing the rejection of tissue transplants by T cells. **Anti-inflammatory treatments** primarily target the production and action of TNF, IL12, and IL-1. Corticosteroids prevent their production by macrophages and may be toxic to T cells. Soluble forms of the TNF receptor and antibody to TNF can be used to block the binding of TNF and prevent its action. **Immunosuppressive therapy for transplantation** generally inhibits the action or causes the lysis of T cells. Cyclosporin, tacrolimus (FK-506), and rapamycin prevent the activation of T cells. Anti-CD3 and anti-CD25 prevent activation of T cells to prevent a response. Administration of antibody to costimulatory molecules such as B7 or CD40 ligand at the time of transplant can block proper T-cell activation and promote anergy rather than responsiveness.

TABLE 14–8. Infections Associated with Defects in Immune Responses

Defect	Pathogen
Induction by physical means (e.g., burns, trauma)	*Pseudomonas aeruginosa* *Staphylococcus aureus* *Staphylococcus epidermidis* *Streptococcus pyogenes* *Aspergillus* species *Candida* species Splenectomy Encapsulated bacteria and fungi
Granulocyte and monocyte defects in movement, phagocytosis, or killing or decreased number of cells (neutropenia)	*S. aureus* *S. pyogenes* *Haemophilus influenzae* Gram-negative bacilli *Escherichia coli* *Klebsiella* species *P. aeruginosa* *Nocardia* species *Aspergillus* species *Candida* species
Individual components of complement system	*S. aureus* *Streptococcus pneumoniae* *Pseudomonas* species *Proteus* species *Neisseria* species *Neisseria meningitidis*
T cells	Cytomegalovirus Herpes simplex virus Herpes zoster virus *Listeria monocytogenes* *Mycobacterium* species *Nocardia* species *Aspergillus* species *Candida* species *Cryptococcus neoformans* *Histoplasma capsulatum* *Pneumocystis carinii* *Strongyloides stercoralis*
B cells	Enteroviruses *S. aureus* *Streptococcus* species *H. influenzae* *N. meningitidis* *E. coli* *Giardia lamblia* *Pneumocystis carinii*
Combined immunodeficiency	See pathogens listed for T cells and B cells

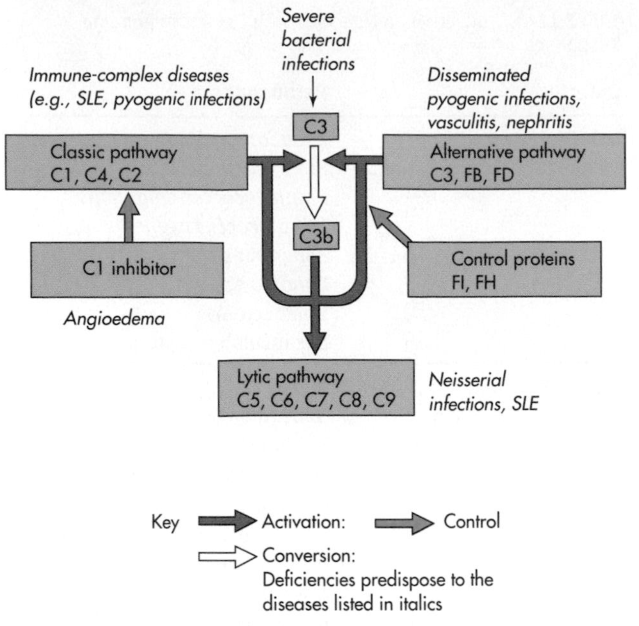

FIGURE 14–16. Consequences of deficiencies in the complement pathways. Factor B binds to C3b on cell surfaces, and the plasma serine protease D cleaves and activates B-C3b as part of the alternative pathway. Factors FI and FH limit the inappropriate activation of complement. FH binds to C3b and prevents activation and is a cofactor for FI. FI is a serine protease that cleaves C3b and C4b. C1 inh, C1 inhibitor; SLE, systemic lupus erythematosus.

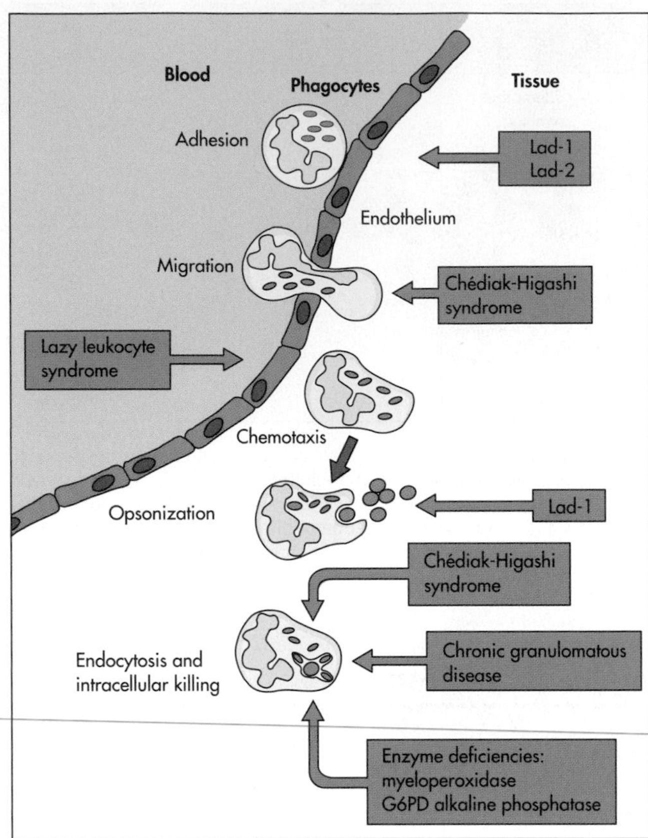

FIGURE 14–17. Consequences of phagocyte dysfunction. G6PD, Glucose-6-phosphate dehydrogenase; Lad, leukocyte adhesion deficiency.

HEREDITARY COMPLEMENT DEFICIENCIES AND MICROBIAL INFECTION

Inherited **deficiencies of C1q, C1r, C1s, C4,** and **C2** components are associated with defects in activation of the classic complement pathway that lead to greater susceptibility to pyogenic (pus-producing) staphylococcal and streptococcal infections (Figure 14–16). These bacteria escape detection by γδ T cells. A **deficiency of C3** leads to a defect in activation of both the classic and the alternative pathways, which also results in a higher incidence of pyogenic infections. **Defects of the properdin factors** impair activation of the alternative pathway, which also results in an increased susceptibility to pyogenic infections. Finally, **deficiencies of C5 through C9** are associated with defective cell killing, which raises the susceptibility to disseminated neisserial infections.

DEFECTS IN PHAGOCYTE ACTION

People with defective phagocytes are more susceptible to bacterial infections but not to viral or protozoal infections (Figure 14–17). The clinical relevance of oxygen-dependent killing is illustrated by **chronic granulomatous disease** in children who have diminished levels of cytochrome b and fail to form superoxide anions. Although phagocytosis is normal, these children have an impaired ability to oxidize NADPH and destroy bacteria through the oxidative pathway. In patients with **Chédiak-Higashi syndrome,** the neutrophil granules fuse when the cells are immature in the bone marrow. Thus neutrophils from these patients can phagocytose bacteria but have greatly diminished ability to kill them. **Asplenic individuals** are at risk for infection with encapsulated organisms because such people lack the filtration mechanism of spleen macrophages. Other deficiencies are shown in Figure 14–17.

DEFICIENCIES IN ANTIGEN-SPECIFIC IMMUNE RESPONSES

People deficient in **T-cell function** are susceptible to **opportunistic infections** by (1) viruses, especially enveloped and noncytolytic viruses and recurrences of viruses that establish latent infections, (2) intracellular bacteria, and (3) fungi. T-cell deficiencies can also prevent the maturation of B-cell antibody responses. T-cell deficiencies can arise from genetic disorders (e.g., X-linked immunodeficiency syndrome, Duncan's disease, DiGeorge syndrome) (Table 14–9), infection (e.g., HIV and AIDS),

TABLE 14–9. Immunodeficiencies of Lymphocytes

Condition	T Cell No.	T-Cell Function	B Cell No.	Serum Antibodies	Incidence*
XLA, Bruton's syndrome	✓	✓	↓↓	IgG, IgA, IgM↓↓	Rare
X-SCID	↓↓	↓	✓	↓	Rare
XLP, Duncan's syndrome	✓	↓	✓	✓ or ↓	Rare
X-hyper IgM	✓	↓	✓	IgG↓↓, IgA↓↓, IgM↑	Rare
Wiskott-Aldrich syndrome	✓	↓	✓	IgA↑, IgE↑, IgM↓	Rare
ADA deficiency (SCID)	↓↓	↓↓	↓	↓	Very rare
PNP deficiency (SCID)	↓	↓	✓	✓	Very rare
HLA deficiency	✓	↓	✓	Poor Ag response	Very rare
Ataxia telangiectasia	↓	↓	✓	IgE↓, IgA↓, IgG2↓	Uncommon
DiGeorge syndrome	↓↓	↓	✓	✓	Very rare
IgA deficiency	✓	✓	✓	IgA↓	Common

From Brostoff J, Male DK: *Clinical immunology: an illustrated outline,* St Louis, 1994, Mosby.

ADA, Adenosine deaminate; Ag, antigen; HLA, human leukocyte antigen; Ig, immunoglobulin; PNP, purine nucleoside phosphorylase; XLA, X-linked agammaglobulinemia; XLP, X-linked lymphoproliferative (syndrome); X-SCID, X-linked severe, combined immunodeficiency disease; ✓ = normal; ↑ = increased; ↓ = decreased or defective.

*Approximate incidence: Very rare = $<10^{-6}$; rare = 10^{-5} to 10^{-6}; common = 10^{-2} to 10^{-3}.

cancer chemotherapy, or immunosuppressive therapy for tissue transplantation.

The immaturity of the immune system of **neonates** increases their susceptibility to infections resolved by TH1-associated responses, including infections by herpesviruses. Neonates are deficient in TH1 responses as a result of insufficient production of IFN-γ. Similarly, the less-pronounced cell-mediated immune and inflammatory responses of **children** decrease the severity (in comparison with adults) of herpes (e.g., infectious mononucleosis, chickenpox) and hepatitis B infections but also increase the potential for the establishment of a chronic hepatitis B virus infection because of incomplete resolution. Pregnancy also induces immunosuppressive measures to prevent rejection of the fetus (a foreign tissue).

B-cell deficiencies may result in a complete lack of antibody production (hypogammaglobulinemia), inability to undergo class-switching, or inability to produce specific subclasses of antibody. People deficient in antibody production are very susceptible to **bacterial infection.** IgA deficiency, which occurs in 1 of 700 Caucasians, results in a greater susceptibility to **respiratory infections.** A deficiency in IgG2 antibodies raises the risk for capsular bacterial infections, because IgG2 antibodies constitute the primary anticapsule response.

QUESTIONS

1. Describe the types of immune responses that would be generated to the following different types of vaccines. Consider the route of processing and presentation of the antigens and the cells and cytokines involved in generating each response.
   a. Tetanus toxoid: intramuscular injection of formalin-fixed, heat-inactivated tetanus toxin protein
   b. Inactivated polio vaccine: intramuscular injection of chemically inactivated poliovirus incapable of replication
   c. Live, attenuated measles vaccine: intramuscular injection of virus that replicates in cells and expresses antigen in cells and on cell surfaces
2. Reproduce (i.e., write out on a separate piece of paper) the following table and fill in the appropriate columns:

Immunodeficiency Disease	Immune Defect	Susceptibility to Specific Infections
Chédiak-Higashi syndrome		
Chronic granulomatous disease		
Complement C5 deficiency		
Complement C3 deficiency		
Complement C1 deficiency		
IgA deficiency		
X-linked agammaglobulinemia		
X-linked T-cell deficiency		
AIDS		
DiGeorge syndrome		
IgE deficiency		

Bibliography

Alcami A, Koszinowski UH: Viral mechanisms of immune evasion, *Trends Microbiol* 8:410-418, 2000.

Abbas AK et al: *Cellular and molecular immunology,* ed 5, Philadelphia, 2003, WB Saunders.

Goldsby RA, Kindt TJ, Osborne BA: *Kuby immunology,* ed 5, New York, 2003, WH Freeman.

Trends in Immunology: Issues contain understandable reviews on current topics in immunology.

Janeway CA et al: *Immunobiology: The immune system in health and disease,* ed 6, New York, 2004, Current Biology Publications and Garland Press.

Male D et al: *Advanced immunology,* ed 3, St Louis, 1996, Mosby.

Male D: *Immunology,* ed 4, London, 2004, Elsevier.

Mims C et al: *Medical microbiology,* ed 3, London, 2004, Elsevier.

Roitt I, Brostoff J, Male D: *Immunology,* ed 4, St Louis, 1996, Mosby.

CHAPTER 15

Antimicrobial Vaccines

Immunity, whether generated in reaction to immunization or administered as therapy, can prevent or lessen the serious symptoms of disease by **blocking the spread** of a bacterium, bacterial toxin, virus, or other microbe to its target organ or by acting rapidly at the site of infection. The immunization of a population, like personal immunity, stops the spread of the infectious agent by reducing the number of susceptible hosts **(herd immunity)**. Immunization programs on national and international levels have achieved the following goals:

1. Protection of population groups from the symptoms of pertussis, diphtheria, tetanus, and rabies
2. Control of the spread of measles, mumps, rubella, varicella-zoster virus, *Haemophilis influenzae B*, and *Streptococcus pneumoniae*
3. Elimination of wild-type poliomyelitis in the Western Hemisphere and smallpox worldwide.

In conjunction with immunization programs, measures can be taken to prevent disease by limiting the exposure of healthy people to infected people **(quarantine)** and by eliminating the source (e.g., water purification) or means of spread (e.g., mosquito eradication) of the infectious agent. Smallpox is an example of an infection that was controlled by such means. As of 1977, natural smallpox was eliminated through a successful World Health Organization (WHO) program that combined vaccination and quarantine.

Vaccine-preventable diseases still occur, however, where immunization programs (1) are unavailable or too expensive (developing countries) or (2) are neglected (e.g., the United States). An example is measles, which causes 2 million deaths annually worldwide for the first reason and outbreaks of which are becoming more common in the United States for the second reason.

Types of Immunization

The injection of purified antibody or antibody-containing serum to provide rapid, temporary protection or treatment of a person is termed **passive immunization.** Newborns receive natural passive immunity from maternal immunoglobulin that crosses the placenta or is present in the mother's milk.

Active immunization occurs when an immune response is stimulated because of challenge with an immunogen, such as exposure to an infectious agent **(natural immunization)** or through exposure to microbes or their antigens in **vaccines.** On subsequent challenge with the virulent agent, a secondary immune response is activated that is faster and more effective at protecting the individual, or antibody is present to block the spread or function of the agent.

PASSIVE IMMUNIZATION

Passive immunization may be used as follows:

1. To prevent disease after a known exposure (e.g., needlestick injury with blood that is contaminated with hepatitis B virus
2. To ameliorate the symptoms of an ongoing disease
3. To protect immunodeficient individuals
4. To block the action of bacterial toxins and prevent the diseases they cause (i.e., as therapy)

Immune serum globulin preparations derived from seropositive humans or animals (e.g., horses) are available as prophylaxis for several bacterial and viral diseases (Table 15–1). Human serum globulin is prepared from pooled plasma and contains the normal repertoire of antibodies for an adult. Special high-titer immune globulin preparations are available for hepatitis B virus (HBIg),

TABLE 15–1. Immune Globulins Available for Postexposure Prophylaxis*

Disease	Source
Hepatitis A	Human
Hepatitis B	Human[d]
Measles	Human
Rabies	Human[†]
Chickenpox, varicella-zoster	Human[†]
Cytomegalovirus	Human
Tetanus	Human,[†] equine
Botulism	Equine
Diphtheria	Equine

*Immune globulins to other agents may also be available.
[†]Specific, high-titer antibody is available and is the preferred therapy.

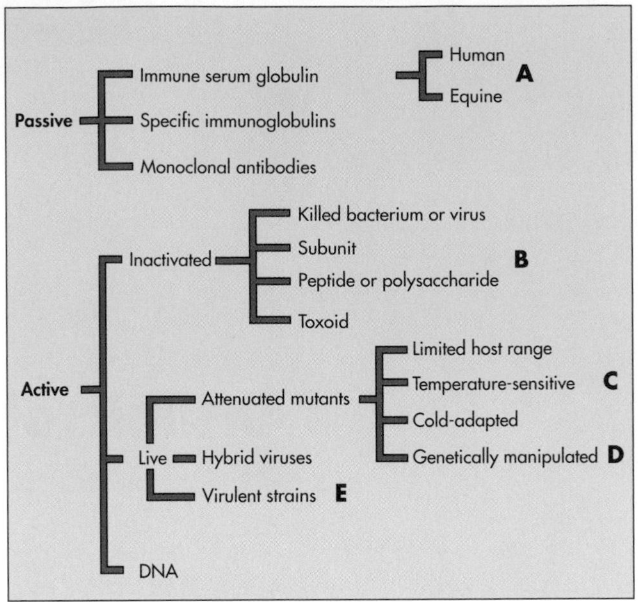

FIGURE 15–1. Types of immunizations. Antibodies (passive immunization) can be provided to block the action of an infectious agent, or an immune response can be elicited (active immunization) by natural infection or vaccination. The different forms of passive and active immunization are indicated. *A,* Equine antibodies can be used if human antibody is not available. *B,* Vaccine can consist of components purified from the infectious agent or can be developed through genetic engineering. *C,* Vaccine selected by passage in animals, embryonated eggs, or tissue culture cells. *D,* Deletion, insertion, reassortment, and other laboratory-derived mutants. *E,* Vaccine composed of a virus from a different species, which has a common antigen with the human virus.

varicella-zoster virus (VZIg), rabies (RIg), and tetanus (TIg). Human immunoglobulin is preferable to animal immunoglobulin, because there is little risk of a hypersensitivity reaction (serum sickness).

Monoclonal antibody preparations are being developed for protection against various agents and diseases. Also in development are monoclonal antibodies that can block the pathogenic mechanisms associated with infection, such as neutrophil adherence and septic shock.

ACTIVE IMMUNIZATION

The term *vaccine* is derived from vaccinia virus, a less virulent member of the poxvirus family that is used to immunize people against smallpox. Classical vaccines can be subdivided into two groups on the basis of whether they elicit an immune response on infection (**live vaccines** such as vaccinia) or not **(inactivated-subunit-killed vaccines)** (Figure 15–1). Deoxyribonucleic acid (DNA) vaccines represent a new potential means of immunization. In this approach, plasmid DNA is injected into muscle or skin, then taken up by dendritic, muscle, or macrophage cells, which express the gene for the immunogen as if for a natural infection.

INACTIVATED VACCINES

Inactivated vaccines utilize a large amount of antigen to produce a protective antibody response but without the risk of infection by the agent. Inactivated vaccines can be produced by chemical (e.g., formalin) or heat inactivation of bacteria, bacterial toxins, or viruses or by purification or synthesis of the components or subunits of the infectious agents.

These vaccines are usually administered with an adjuvant, such as alum, which boosts their immunogenicity. Better adjuvants are being developed that use bacterial cell wall components, synthetic polymers, or liposomes. The adjuvant also influences the type of immune response induced by the vaccine (TH1 or TH2). Attenuated forms of cholera toxin (CT) and *Escherichia coli* lymphotoxin (LT) are being developed as potent adjuvants that promote production of secretory immunoglobulin A (IgA) after intranasal or oral immunization.

Inactivated rather than live vaccines are used to confer protection against most bacteria and viruses that cannot be attenuated, may cause recurrent infection, or have oncogenic potential. Inactivated vaccines are generally safe, except in people who have allergic reactions to vaccine components. For example, many antiviral vaccines are produced in eggs and therefore cannot be administered to people who are allergic to eggs. The immune response evoked by inactivated vaccines is predominantly a TH2 (antibody) immune response, does not elicit effective immune memory, and is more limited than that evoked by live vaccines. The disadvantages of inactivated vaccines are listed below and compared to live vaccines in Table 15–2.

TABLE 15–2. Advantages and Disadvantages of Live versus Inactivated Vaccines

Property	Live	Inactivated
Route of administration	Natural* or injection	Injection
Dose of virus, cost	Low	High
Number of doses	Single†	Multiple
Need for adjuvant	No	Yes‡
Duration of immunity	Long-term	Short-term
Antibody response	IgG, IgA§	IgG
Cell-mediated immune response	Good	Poor
Heat lability in tropics	Yes‖	No
Interference¶	Occasional	None
Side effects	Occasional mild symptoms#	Occasional sore arm
Reversion to virulence	Rarely	None

From White DO, Fenner FJ: *Medical virology*, ed 3, New York, 1986, Academic Press.
Ig, Immunoglobulin.
*Oral or respiratory, in certain cases.
†A single booster may be required (yellow fever, measles, rubella) after 6 to 10 years.
‡However, the commonly used alum is inefficient.
§IgA if delivered via the oral or respiratory route. Oral polio vaccine can prevent wild-type poliovirus from multiplying in the gut.
‖Magnesium chloride and other stabilizers and cold storage assist preservation.
¶Interference from other viruses or diseases.
#Especially rubella and measles.

1. Immunity is not usually life long.
2. Immunity may be only humoral and not cell mediated.
3. The vaccine does not elicit a local IgA response.
4. Booster shots are required.
5. Larger doses must be used.

There are three major types of inactivated bacterial vaccines: **toxoid** (inactivated toxins), **inactivated (killed)** bacteria, and **capsule or protein subunits** of the bacteria. The bacterial vaccines currently available are listed in Table 15–3. Most antibacterial vaccines protect against the pathogenic action of toxins.

Inactivated viral vaccines are available for **polio, hepatitis A, influenza, and rabies,** among other viruses. The Salk polio vaccine (inactivated poliomyelitis vaccine, or **IPV**) and the influenza vaccine are prepared through the formaldehyde inactivation of virions. The influenza vaccine, which is formulated annually, is a mixture of viruses predicted to threaten the population for the coming year. In the past, a rabies vaccine was prepared by means of formalin inactivation of infected rabbit neurons or duck embryos. Now, however, it is prepared through the chemical inactivation of virions grown in human diploid tissue culture cells. Because of the slow course of rabies, the vaccine can be administered immediately after a person is exposed to the virus and still elicit a protective antibody response.

A **subunit vaccine** consists of the bacterial or viral components that elicit a protective immune response. Surface structures of bacteria and the viral attachment proteins (capsid or glycoproteins) elicit protective antibodies. T-cell epitopes may also be included in a subunit vaccine. The immunogenic component can be isolated from the bacterium, virus, or virally infected cells by biochemical means, or the vaccine can be prepared through genetic engineering by the expression of cloned viral genes in bacteria or eukaryotic cells. For example, the hepatitis B virus subunit vaccine was initially prepared from surface antigen obtained from human sera of chronic carriers of the virus. Today the form of vaccine used in the United States is purified from yeast bearing the gene for the antigen. The antigen is purified, chemically treated, and absorbed onto alum to be used as a vaccine.

Vaccines against ***Haemophilus influenzae B, Neisseria meningitidis, Salmonella typhi,*** and ***Streptococcus pneumoniae*** are prepared from **capsular polysaccharides.** Unfortunately, **polysaccharides are generally poor immunogens** (T-independent antigens). The meningococcal vaccine contains the polysaccharides of four major serotypes (A, C, Y, and W-135). The pneumococcal vaccine contains polysaccharides from 23

TABLE 15–3. Bacterial Vaccines*

Bacteria (Disease)	Vaccine Components	Who Should Receive Vaccinations
Corynebacterium diphtheriae (diphtheria)	Toxoid	Children and adults
Clostridium tetani (tetanus)	Toxoid	Children and adults
Bordetella pertussis (pertussis)	Killed cell or acellular	Children
Haemophilus influenzae B (Hib)	Capsule polysaccharide; capsule polysaccharide–protein conjugate	Children
Neisseria meningitidis A and C (meningococcal disease)	Capsule polysaccharide	People at high risk (e.g., those with asplenia), travelers to epidemic areas (e.g., military personnel), children
Streptococcus pneumoniae (pneumococcal disease; meningitis)	Capsule polysaccharides; capsule polysaccharide–protein conjugate	People at high risk (e.g., those with asplenia), children, the elderly
Vibrio cholerae (cholera)	Killed cell	Travelers at risk to exposure
Salmonella typhi (typhoid)	Killed cell; polysaccharide	Travelers at risk to exposure, household contacts, sewage workers
Bacillus anthracis (anthrax)	Killed cell	Handlers of imported fur, military personnel
Yersinia pestis (plague)	Killed cell	Veterinarians, animal handlers
Francisella tularensis (tularemia)	Live attenuated	Animal handlers in endemic areas
Coxiella burnetii (Q fever)	Inactivated	Sheep handlers, laboratory personnel working with *C. burnetii*
Mycobacterium tuberculosis (TB)	Live attenuated bacille Calmette-Guérin *(Mycobacterium bovis)*	Not recommended in United States
Borrelia burgdorferi (Lyme disease)	Subunit	People in endemic regions

*Listed in order of frequency of use.

serotypes. The immunogenicity of polysaccharides can be enhanced by chemical linkage to a protein carrier **(conjugate vaccine)** (e.g., diphtheria toxoid, *N. meningitidis* outer membrane protein, or *Corynebacterium diphtheriae* protein). The *H. influenzae B* (Hib) polysaccharide–diphtheria toxoid carrier complex is approved for administration to infants and children. An *S. pneumoniae* "pneumococcal" conjugate vaccine has been developed in which polysaccharide from the seven most prevalent strains in the United States is attached to a nontoxic form of the diphtheria toxin. This vaccine is available for use in infants and young children. The other polysaccharide vaccines are less immunogenic and should be administered only to children older than 2 years.

Lyme disease (*Borrelia burgdorferi*) vaccine is a subunit vaccine that initiates protection in a unique manner. The immunogen consists of an outer membrane protein (OspA) of the bacteria that is expressed while the bacteria are in the vector (deer tick). When the tick takes it blood meal from a human, it ingests antibodies that are generated in the human, and these antibodies inactivate the bacteria to prevent infection and disease. This vaccine was withdrawn from the market due to limited demand.

LIVE VACCINES

Live vaccines are prepared with organisms limited in their ability to cause disease (e.g., **avirulent** or **attenuated** organisms). Live vaccines are especially useful for protection against infections caused by enveloped viruses, which require T-cell immune responses for resolution of the infection. Immunization with a live vaccine resembles the natural infection in that the immune response progresses through TH1 and then TH2 immune responses, and humoral, cellular, and memory immune responses are developed. Immunity is generally long lived and, depending on the route of administration, can mimic the normal immune response to the infecting agent. However, the following list includes three problems with live vaccines:

1. The vaccine virus may still be dangerous for immunosuppressed people or pregnant women, who

do not have the immunologic resources to resolve even a weakened virus infection.
2. The vaccine may revert to a virulent viral form.
3. The viability of the vaccine must be maintained.

Live bacterial vaccines include the orally administered live, attenuated *S. typhi* strain (Ty2la) vaccine for typhoid; the Calmette-Guérin bacillus vaccine for tuberculosis, which consists of an attenuated strain of *Mycobacterium bovis;* and an attenuated tularemia vaccine. A combination of antibody and cell-mediated immune responses elicited by a live vaccine may be required against intracellularly growing bacteria. The Calmette-Guérin bacillus vaccine is not routinely used in the United States because people vaccinated with it show a false-positive reaction to the purified protein derivative (PPD) test, which is the screening test used to control tuberculosis in the United States.

Live virus vaccines consist of less virulent mutants **(attenuated)** of the wild-type virus, viruses from other species that share antigenic determinants (vaccinia for smallpox), or genetically engineered viruses lacking virulence properties (see Figure 15–1). Wild-type viruses are attenuated by growth in embryonated eggs or tissue culture cells, at nonphysiologic temperatures (32°C to 34°C), and away from the selective pressures of the host immune response. These conditions **select** for, or allow the growth of, viral strains (mutants) that (1) are less virulent because they grow poorly at 37°C (**temperature-sensitive strains** [e.g., measles vaccine] and cold-adapted strains), (2) do not replicate well in any human cell **(host-range mutants)**, (3) cannot escape immune control, or (4) can replicate at a benign site but do not disseminate, bind, or replicate in the target tissue characteristically affected by the disease (e.g., polio vaccine replicates in the gastrointestinal tract but does not reach or infect the brain). Table 15–4 lists examples of attenuated live virus vaccines currently in use.

The first vaccine—that for smallpox—was developed by Edward Jenner. The idea for the vaccine came to him when he noted that cowpox (vaccinia), a virulent virus from another species that shares antigenic determinants with smallpox, caused benign infections in humans but conferred protective immunity against smallpox. Similarly, the vaccine for the first identified tumor virus, Marek's disease virus of chickens, consists of the turkey herpesvirus. In addition, vaccines consisting of bovine, simian, or a reassortment of these rotaviruses have shown success in protecting infants against human rotavirus in clinical trials.

Albert Sabin developed the first live **oral polio vaccine (OPV)** in the 1950s. The attenuated virus vaccine was obtained by multiple passage of the three types of poliovirus through monkey kidney tissue culture cells. At least 57 mutations accumulated in the polio type 1 vaccine strain. When this vaccine is administered orally, IgA is secreted in the gut and IgG in the serum, providing protection along the normal route of infection by the wild-type virus. This vaccine is inexpensive, easy to administer, and relatively stable. The vaccination program has been so successful that wild-type polio has been eliminated in the Western Hemisphere. Unfortunately, because of the risk of vaccine virus–induced polio disease, the IPV rather than the OPV is used for routine well-baby immunizations (Figure 15–2).

Live vaccines for measles, mumps, rubella (administered together as the MMR vaccine), **varicella-zoster,** and now **influenza** have been developed. Protection against these infections requires a potent cellular immune response, so if the vaccine is administered at 2 years of age, which is late enough to elicit a mature T-cell response, there will be no interference by maternal antibodies. A killed measles vaccine proved to be a failure because it conferred an incomplete immunity that induced more serious symptoms (atypical measles) on challenge with wild-type measles virus than the symptoms associated with the natural infection.

The initial live measles vaccine consisted of the Edmonston B strain, which was developed by Enders and colleagues. This virus underwent extensive passage at 35°C through primary human kidney cells, human amnion cells, and chicken embryo cells. The currently used Moraten (United States) and Schwarz (other countries) vaccine strains of measles were obtained by further passage of the Edmonston B strain in chick embryos at 32°C.

The mumps vaccine (Jeryl Lynn strain) and rubella vaccine (Wistar RA 27/3) viruses were also attenuated by extensive passage of the virus in cell culture. The varicella-zoster vaccine uses the Oka strain, an attenuated virus. The varicella-zoster vaccine also requires a mature T-cell response and is administered along with the MMR vaccine.

A new live influenza vaccine is administered nasally within a mist. Unlike the previous inactivated vaccine, T- and B-cell responses and mucosal immunity are elicited by this vaccine.

FUTURE DIRECTIONS FOR VACCINATION

Molecular biology techniques are being used to develop new vaccines. New live vaccines can be created by genetic engineering mutations to inactivate or delete a virulence gene instead of through random attenuation of the virus by passage through tissue culture. Genes from infectious agents that cannot be properly attenuated can be inserted into safe viruses (e.g., vaccinia, canarypox) to form **hybrid virus vaccines** (see Figure 55–3). This approach holds the promise of allowing the development of a polyvalent vaccine to many agents in a single, safe,

TABLE 15–4. Viral Vaccines*

Virus	Vaccine Components	Who Should Receive Vaccinations
Polio	Inactivated (inactivated polio vaccine, Salk vaccine) Attenuated (oral polio vaccine, Sabin vaccine)	Children Children
Measles	Attenuated	Children
Mumps	Attenuated	Children
Rubella	Attenuated	Children
Varicella-zoster	Attenuated	Children
Influenza	Inactivated Attenuated (nasal spray)	Adults, especially medical personnel and the elderly Older children, adults <50 yrs
Hepatitis B	Subunit	Newborns, health care workers, high-risk groups (e.g., promiscuous people, intravenous drug users)
Hepatitis A	Inactivated Live (China)	Children, child-care workers, travelers to endemic areas, Native Americans and Alaskans
Adenovirus	Attenuated	Military personnel
Yellow fever	Attenuated	Travelers at risk to exposure, military personnel
Rabies	Inactivated	Anyone exposed to virus Preexposure: veterinarians, animal handlers
Rotavirus	Rhesus-bovine-human hybrids	In development
Smallpox	Live vaccinia virus	Protection from bioterrorism
Japanese encephalitis	Inactivated	Travelers at risk to exposure
Eastern and Western equine encephalitis, Russian spring-summer encephalitis	Inactivated	Military personnel

*Listed in order of frequency of use.

inexpensive, and relatively stable vector. On infection the hybrid virus vaccine need not complete a replication cycle but simply promote the expression of the inserted gene to initiate an immune response to the antigens. The vaccinia and canarypox virus vector systems have been used in several experimental hybrid vaccines and for the rabies vaccine for forest animals. Other vectors that have been considered are attenuated retroviruses, adenovirus, and herpes simplex virus.

A new **defective infectious single-cycle (DISC) virus** vaccine would immunize an individual but can proceed through only one round of virus replication. A virus with a deletion of an essential gene is grown in a tissue culture cell that expresses the gene to "complement" the defect in the virus. On vaccination, the progeny virus infects the host and produces only one round of virus, which is sufficient for immunization. However, the new virus cannot replicate.

Genetically engineered **subunit vaccines** are being developed through cloning of genes that encode immunogenic proteins into bacterial and eukaryotic vectors. The greatest difficulties in the development of such vaccines are (1) identifying the appropriate subunit or peptide immunogen that can elicit protective antibody and, ideally, T-cell responses and (2) presenting the antigen in the correct conformation. Once identified, the gene can be isolated, cloned, and expressed in bacteria or yeast cells, and then large quantities of these proteins can be produced. Genes for protective immunogens, such as the surface antigen of hepatitis B *(in use)*, the envelope protein gp120 of the human immunodeficiency virus (HIV), the hemagglutinin of influenza, the G antigen of rabies, and the glycoprotein D of herpes simplex virus, have been cloned, and their proteins have been generated in bacteria or eukaryotic cells for use (or potential use) as subunit vaccines. Use of a viruslike particle (VLP), assembled from the

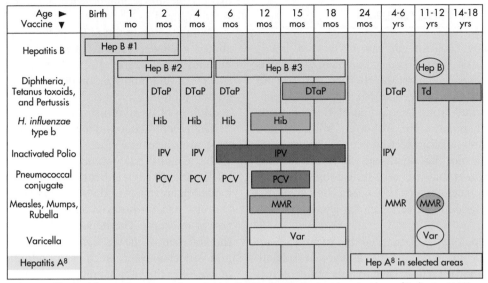

Recommended Childhood Immunization Schedule
United States, January - December 2000

Vaccines are listed under routinely recommended ages. [Bars] indicate range of recommended ages for immunization. Any dose not given at the recommended age should be given as a "catch-up" immunization at any subsequent visit when indicated and feasible. (Ovals) indicate vaccines to be given if previously recommended doses were missed or given earlier than the recommended minimum age.

Age ► / Vaccine ▼	Birth	1 mo	2 mos	4 mos	6 mos	12 mos	15 mos	18 mos	24 mos	4-6 yrs	11-12 yrs	14-18 yrs
Hepatitis B	Hep B #1											
		Hep B #2				Hep B #3					(Hep B)	
Diphtheria, Tetanus toxoids, and Pertussis			DTaP	DTaP	DTaP		DTaP			DTaP	Td	
H. influenzae type b			Hib	Hib	Hib	Hib						
Inactivated Polio			IPV	IPV		IPV				IPV		
Pneumococcal conjugate			PCV	PCV	PCV	PCV						
Measles, Mumps, Rubella						MMR				MMR	(MMR)	
Varicella							Var				(Var)	
Hepatitis A[8]									Hep A[8] in selected areas			

Approved by the Advisory Committee on Immunization Practices (ACIP), the American Academy of Pediatrics (AAP), and the American Academy of Family Physicians (AAFP).

FIGURE 15–2. Recommended immunization schedule from the Centers for Disease Control and Prevention. Vaccines are listed at the ages routinely recommended for their administration. Bars indicate the range of acceptable ages for vaccination. For example, hepatitis B vaccine should be administered to children at 11 to 12 years of age who have not been previously vaccinated; varicella-zoster virus vaccine should be administered to children who were not previously vaccinated and who lack a reliable history of chickenpox. DtaP, Diphtheria and tetanus toxoids and acellular pertussis vaccines; Td, tetanus and diphtheria toxoids, absorbed, for adult use.

genetically engineered capsid proteins of papillomavirus, has shown promise in animal trials.

Peptide subunit vaccines consist of *specific epitopes* of microbial proteins that elicit neutralizing antibody or desired T-cell responses. To generate such a response, the peptide must contain sequences that bind to MHC I or MHC II (class I or class II major histocompatibility complex) proteins for presentation and recognition by T cells to initiate an immune response. The immunogenicity of the peptide can be enhanced by its covalent attachment to a carrier protein (e.g., tetanus toxoid or keyhole limpet hemocyanine) or an immunologic peptide that can specifically present the epitope to the appropriate immune response. Better vaccines are being developed as the mechanisms of antigen presentation and T-cell receptor–specific antigens are better understood.

Anti-idiotype antibodies are also being investigated as potential vaccines. Such antibodies recognize the variable region of a monoclonal antiviral antibody, which is like a cast of the viral epitope. The anti-idiotype antibody resembles the original viral epitope, as if it were molded in the cast. Immunization with an anti-idiotype antibody or the viral peptide would therefore elicit the production of similar antibodies.

Adjuvants in addition to alum are being developed to enhance the immunogenicity and direct the response of vaccines to a TH1 or TH2 type of response. These include activators of Toll-Like Receptors, such as the oligodeoxynucleotide CpG, derivatives of Lipid A from lipopolysaccharide, cytokines, liposomes, etc.

DNA vaccines offer great potential for immunization against infectious agents that require T-cell and antibody responses but that are not appropriate for use in live vaccines. For these vaccines, the gene for a protein that elicits protective responses is cloned into a plasmid that allows the protein to be expressed in eukaryotic cells. The naked DNA is injected into the muscle or skin of the vaccine recipient, where the DNA is taken up by cells, the gene is expressed, and the protein is produced and presented to the immune response to elicit TH1 and TH2 responses. Often it is easier to develop a DNA vaccine than other types of vaccines.

With the advent of new technology, it should be possible to develop vaccines against infectious agents such as *Streptococcus mutans* (to prevent tooth decay), the herpesviruses, HIV, and parasites such as *Plasmodium falciparum* (malaria) and *Leishmania.* In fact, it should be possible to produce a vaccine to almost any infectious agent once the appropriate protective immunogen is identified and its gene isolated.

Immunization Programs

An effective vaccine program can save millions of dollars in health care costs. Such a program not only protects each vaccinated person against infection and disease but also reduces the number of susceptible people in the population, thereby preventing the spread of the infectious agent within the population. Although immunization may be the best means of protecting people against infection, vaccines cannot be developed for all infectious agents. One reason is that it is very time consuming and costly to develop vaccines. Box 15–1 lists the considerations that are weighed in the choice of a candidate for a vaccine program.

Natural smallpox was eliminated by means of an effective vaccine program because it was a good candidate for such a program; the virus existed in only one serotype, symptoms were always present in infected people, and the vaccine was relatively benign and stable. However, its elimination came about only as the result of a concerted, cooperative effort on the part of the WHO and local health agencies worldwide. Rhinovirus is an example of a poor candidate for vaccine development, because the viral disease is not serious and there are too many serotypes for vaccination to be successful. Practical aspects of and problems with vaccine development are listed in Box 15–2.

From the standpoint of the individual, the ideal vaccine should elicit dependable, lifelong immunity to infection without serious side effects. Factors that influence the success of an immunization program include not only the composition of the vaccine but also the timing, site, and conditions of its administration.

The recommended schedules of vaccinations for children are given in Figure 15–2. Infants are immunized with the diphtheria, tetanus toxoid, and acellular pertussis vaccines (DTaP), Hib inactivated vaccine, and the inactivated polio vaccine. The inactivated hepatitis A vaccine can also be administered on this schedule or to adults at risk of infection. The hepatitis B vaccine is suggested for the first year of life, as well as later in life. The live MMR and varicella-zoster vaccines are administered at 2 years of age, after the baby's immune response has matured and maternal antibodies have dissipated. Booster immunizations of inactivated vaccines and the live measles vaccine are required later in life. Adults should be immunized with vaccines for *S. pneumoniae* (pneumococcus), influenza, rabies, hepatitis B virus, and other diseases, depending on their jobs, the type of traveling they do, and other risk factors that may make them particularly susceptible to specific infectious agents.

BOX 15–1. Properties of a Good Candidate for Vaccine Development

Organism causes significant illness.
Organism exists as only one serotype.
Antibody blocks infection or systemic spread.
Organism does not have oncogenic potential.
Vaccine is heat stable, so that it can be transported to endemic areas.

BOX 15–2. Problems with Vaccine Use

Live vaccine can occasionally revert to virulent forms.
Interference by other organisms may prevent the infection produced by a live virus vaccine; for example, rubella prevents replication of poliovirus.
Vaccination of an immunocompromised person with a live vaccine can be life threatening.
Side effects to vaccination can occur; these include hypersensitivity and allergic reactions to the antigen, to nonmicrobial material in the vaccine, and to contaminants (e.g., eggs).
Vaccine development and liability insurance for the manufacturer are very expensive with limited profit.
Organisms with many serotypes are difficult to control with vaccination.

QUESTIONS

1. Why is an inactivated rather than a live vaccine used for the following immunizations: rabies, influenza, tetanus, hepatitis B virus, *H. influenzae* B, diphtheria, polio, and pertussis?
2. Tetanus is treated with passive immunization and prevented by active immunization. Compare the nature and function of each of these therapies.
3. The inactivated polio vaccine is administered intramuscularly, whereas the live polio vaccine is administered as an oral vaccine. How do the course of the immune response and the immunoglobulins produced in response to each vaccine differ? What step in poliovirus infection is blocked in a person vaccinated by each vaccine?
4. Why have large-scale vaccine programs not been developed for rhinovirus, herpes simplex virus, and respiratory syncytial virus?
5. Describe the public or personal health benefits that justify the development of the following major vaccine programs: measles, mumps, rubella, polio, smallpox, tetanus, and pertussis.

Bibliography

Advisory Committee on Immunization Practices (ACIP): Statements available online at www.cdc.gov/nip/acip.

Centers for Disease Control and Prevention (CDC): Immunization information page, available online at www.cdc.gov.

Conrad DA, Jensen HB: New and improved vaccines, *Postgrad Med* 100:113-127, 1996.

Hill DR: Immunizations, *Infect Dis Clin North Am* 6:291, 1992.

National Coalition for Adult Immunization, online at www.nfid.org/ncai/

Plotkin SA, Orenstein WA: *Vaccines*, ed 4, Philadelphia, 2004, WB Saunders.

Vaccination information statements, available online at www.immunize.org/vis.

Vaccines: National Insititue of Allergy and Infectious Diseases (NIAID) fact sheet, available online at www.niaid.nih/gov/publications/vaccine.htm.

World Health Organization: Diseases and vaccines, available online at www.who.int/vaccines-diseases/index.html.

SECTION III

General Principles of Laboratory Diagnosis

CHAPTER 16

Microscopic Principles and Applications

The true complexity of our surroundings was not appreciated until the first microbes were observed through the lens of a microscope. Indeed, the use of microscopy has helped define the relationships among a diversity of organisms, ranging from the smallest viruses consisting of a few proteins and minimal genetic information to multicellular parasites almost 10 meters long.

In general, microscopy is used in microbiology for two basic purposes: the initial detection of microbes and the preliminary or definitive identification of microbes. The microscopic examination of clinical specimens is used to detect bacterial cells, fungal elements, parasites (eggs, larvae, or adult forms), and viral inclusions present in infected cells. Characteristic morphologic properties can be used for the preliminary identification of most bacteria and are used for the definitive identification of many fungi and parasites. The microscopic detection of organisms stained with antibodies labeled with fluorescent dyes or other markers has proved to be very useful for the specific identification of many organisms. Five general microscopic methods have been used (Box 16–1).

Microscopic Methods

BRIGHTFIELD (LIGHT) MICROSCOPY

The basic components of light microscopes consist of a light source used to illuminate the specimen positioned on a stage, a condenser used to focus the light on the specimen, and two lens systems (**objective lens** and **ocular lens**) used to magnify the image of the specimen. In brightfield microscopy the specimen is visualized by transillumination, with light passing up through the condenser to the specimen. The image is then magnified, first by the objective lens, then by the ocular lens. The total magnification of the image is the product of the magnifications of the objective and ocular lenses. Three different objective lenses are commonly used: low power (10-fold magnification), which can be used to scan a specimen; high dry (40-fold), which is used to look for large microbes such as parasites and filamentous fungi; and oil immersion (100-fold), which is used to observe bacteria, yeasts (single-cell stage of fungi), and the morphologic details of larger organisms and cells. Ocular lenses can further magnify the image (generally 10-fold to 15-fold).

The limitation of brightfield microscopy is the resolution of the image (i.e., the ability to distinguish that two objects are separate and not one). The **resolving power** of a microscope is determined by the wavelength of light used to illuminate the subject and the angle of light entering the objective lens (referred to as the **numerical aperture**). The resolving power is greatest when oil is placed between the objective lens (typically the 100× lens) and the specimen because oil reduces the dispersion of light. The best brightfield microscopes have a resolving power of approximately 0.2 μm, which allows most bacteria but not viruses to be visualized. Although most bacteria and larger microorganisms can be seen with brightfield microscopy, the **refractive indices** of the organisms and background are similar. Thus organisms must be stained with a dye so that they can be observed, or an alternative method must be used.

DARKFIELD MICROSCOPY

The same objective and ocular lenses used in brightfield microscopes are used in darkfield microscopes; however, a special **condenser** is used that prevents transmitted light

BOX 16–1. Microscopic Methods

Brightfield (light) microscopy
Darkfield microscopy
Phase-contrast microscopy
Fluorescent microscopy
Electron microscopy

from directly illuminating the specimen. Only oblique, scattered light reaches the specimen and passes into the lens systems, which causes the specimen to be brightly illuminated against a black background. The advantage of this method is that the resolving power of darkfield microscopy is significantly improved compared with that of brightfield microscopy (i.e., 0.02 µm versus 0.2 µm), which makes it possible for extremely thin bacteria, such as *Treponema pallidum* (etiologic agent of syphilis), *Borrelia burgdorferi* (Lyme disease), and *Leptospira* spp. (leptospirosis), to be detected. The disadvantage of this method is that because light passes around rather than through organisms, their internal structure cannot be studied.

PHASE-CONTRAST MICROSCOPY

Phase-contrast microscopy enables the internal details of microbes to be examined. In this form of microscopy, as parallel beams of light are passed through objects of different densities, the wavelength of one beam moves out of "phase" relative to the other beam of light (i.e., the beam moving through the more dense material is retarded more than the other beam). Through the use of **annular rings** in the condenser and the objective lens, the differences in phase are amplified so that in-phase light appears brighter than out-of-phase light. This creates a three-dimensional image of the organism or specimen, which permits more detailed analysis of the internal structures.

FLUORESCENT MICROSCOPY

Some compounds called **fluorochromes** can absorb short-wavelength ultraviolet or ultrablue light and emit energy at a higher visible wavelength. Although some microorganisms show natural fluorescence **(autofluorescence),** fluorescent microscopy typically involves staining organisms with fluorescent dyes and then examining them with a specially designed fluorescent microscope. The microscope uses a high-pressure mercury, halogen, or xenon vapor lamp that emits a shorter wavelength of light than that emitted by traditional brightfield microscopes. A series of filters are used to block the heat generated from the lamp, eliminate infrared light, and select the appropriate wavelength for exciting the fluorochrome. The light emitted from the fluorochrome is then magnified through traditional objective and ocular lenses. Organisms and specimens stained with fluorochromes appear brightly illuminated against a black background, although the colors vary depending on the fluorochrome selected. The contrast between the organism and background is great enough that the specimen can be screened rapidly under low magnification and then the material examined under higher magnification once fluorescence is detected.

ELECTRON MICROSCOPY

Unlike other forms of microscopy, **magnetic coils** (rather than lenses) are used in electron microscopes to direct a beam of electrons from a tungsten filament through a specimen and onto a screen. Because a much shorter wavelength of light is used, magnification and resolution are improved dramatically. Individual viral particles (as opposed to viral inclusion bodies) can be seen with electron microscopy. Samples are usually stained or coated with metal ions to create contrast. There are two types of electron microscopes: **transmission electron microscopes,** in which electrons such as light pass directly through the specimen, and **scanning electron microscopes,** in which electrons bounce off the surface of the specimen at an angle and a three-dimensional picture is produced.

Examination Methods

Clinical specimens or suspensions of microorganisms can be placed on a glass slide and examined under the microscope (i.e., direct examination of a wet mount). Although large organisms and cellular material can be seen using this method, analysis of the internal detail is often difficult. Phase-contrast microscopy can overcome some of these problems; alternatively, the specimen or organism can be stained by a variety of methods (Table 16–1).

DIRECT EXAMINATION

Direct-examination methods are the simplest for preparing samples for microscopic examination. The sample can be suspended in water or saline **(wet mount),** mixed with alkali to dissolve background material **(potassium hydroxide [KOH] method),** or mixed with a combination of alkali and a contrasting dye (e.g., **lactophenol cotton blue, iodine**). The dyes nonspecifically stain the cellular material, increasing the contrast with the background, and permit examination of the detailed structures. A variation is the **India ink method,** in which the ink darkens the background rather than the cell. This method is used to detect capsules surrounding organisms, such as the yeast *Cryptococcus* (the dye is excluded by the

Table 16–1. Microscopic Preparations and Stains Used in the Clinical Microbiology Laboratory

Staining Method	Principle and Applications
Direct Examination	
Wet mount	Unstained preparation examined by brightfield, darkfield, or phase-contrast microscopy.
10% KOH	KOH used to dissolve proteinaceous material and facilitate detection of fungal elements that are not affected by strong alkali solution. Dyes such as lactophenol cotton blue can be added to increase contrast between fungal elements and background.
India ink	Modification of KOH procedure in which ink is added as contrast material. Dye primarily used to detect *Cryptococcus* spp. in cerebrospinal fluid and other body fluids. Polysaccharide capsule of *Cryptococcus* spp. excludes ink, creating halo around yeast cell.
Lugol's iodine	Iodine is added to wet preparations of parasitology specimens to enhance contrast of internal structures. Facilitates differentiation of ameba and host white blood cells.
Differential Stains	
Gram stain	Most commonly used stain in microbiology laboratory, forming basis for separating major groups of bacteria (e.g., gram-positive, gram-negative). After fixation of specimen to glass slide (by heating or alcohol treatment), specimen is exposed to crystal violet, and then iodine is added to form complex with primary dye. During decolorization with alcohol or acetone, complex is retained in gram-positive bacteria but lost in gram-negative organisms; counterstain safranin is retained by gram-negative organisms (hence their red color). Degree to which organism retains stain is function of organism, culture conditions, and staining skills of microscopist.
Iron hematoxylin stain	Used for detection and identification of fecal protozoa. Helminth eggs and larvae retain too much stain and are more easily identified with wet-mount preparation.
Methenamine silver stain	Generally performed in histology laboratories rather than in microbiology laboratories. Used primarily for detection of fungal elements in tissue, although other organisms, such as bacteria, can be detected. Silver staining requires skill because nonspecific staining can render slides unable to be interpreted.
Toluidine blue O stain	Used primarily for detection of *Pneumocystis* organisms in respiratory specimens. Cysts stain reddish-blue to dark purple on light-blue background. Background staining is removed by sulfation reagent. Yeast cells stain and are difficult to distinguish from *Pneumocystis* cells. Trophozoites do not stain. Many laboratories have replaced this stain with specific fluorescent stains.
Trichrome stain	Alternative to iron hematoxylin for staining protozoa. Protozoa have bluish-green to purple cytoplasms with red or purplish-red nuclei and inclusion bodies; specimen background is green.
Wright-Giemsa stain	Used to detect blood parasites; viral and chlamydial inclusion bodies; and *Borrelia, Toxoplasma, Pneumocystis,* and *Rickettsia* spp. Polychromatic stain that contains mixture of methylene blue, azure B, and eosin Y. Giemsa stain combines methylene blue and eosin. Eosin ions are negatively charged and stain basic components of cells orange to pink, whereas other dyes stain acidic cell structures various shades of blue to purple. Protozoan trophozoites have red nucleus and grayish-blue cytoplasm; intracellular yeasts and inclusion bodies typically stain blue; rickettsiae, chlamydiae, and *Pneumocystis* spp. stain purple.
Acid–Fast Stains	
Ziehl-Neelsen stain	Used to stain mycobacteria and other acid-fast organisms. Organisms are stained with basic carbolfuchsin and resist decolorization with acid-alkali solutions. Background is counterstained with methylene blue. Organisms appear red against light-blue background. Uptake of carbolfuchsin requires heating specimen (hot acid-fast stain).
Kinyoun stain	Cold acid-fast stain (does not require heating). Same principle as Ziehl-Neelsen stain.
Auramine-rhodamine stain	Same principle as other acid-fast stains, except that fluorescent dyes (auramine and rhodamine) are used for primary stain and potassium permanganate (strong oxidizing agent) is the counterstain and inactivates unbound fluorochrome dyes. Organisms fluoresce yellowish-green against black background.

Table 16–1. Microscopic Preparations and Stains Used in the Clinical Microbiology Laboratory—*cont'd*

Staining Method	Principle and Applications
Modified acid-fast stain	Weak decolorizing agent is used with any of three acid-fast stains listed. Whereas mycobacteria are strongly acid-fast, other organisms stain weaker (e.g., *Nocardia, Rhodococcus, Tsukamurella, Gordonia, Cryptosporidium, Isospora, Sarcocystis,* and *Cyclospora*). These organisms can be stained more efficiently by using weak decolorizing agent. Organisms that retain this stain are referred to as partially acid-fast.
Fluorescent Stains	
Acridine orange stain	Used for detection of bacteria and fungi in clinical specimens. Dye intercalates into nucleic acid (native and denatured). At neutral pH, bacteria, fungi, and cellular material stain reddish-orange. At acid pH (4.0), bacteria and fungi remain reddish-orange, but background material stains greenish-yellow.
Auramine-rhodamine stain	Same as acid-fast stains.
Calcofluor white stain	Used to detect fungal elements and *Pneumocystis* spp. Stain binds to cellulose and chitin in cell walls; microscopist can mix dye with KOH. (Many laboratories have replaced traditional KOH stain with this stain.)
Direct fluorescent antibody stain	Antibodies (monoclonal or polyclonal) are complexed with fluorescent molecules. Specific binding to an organism is detected by presence of microbial fluorescence. Technique has proved useful for detecting or identifying many organisms (e.g., *Streptococcus pyogenes, Bordetella, Francisella, Legionella, Chlamydia, Pneumocystis, Cryptosporidium, Giardia,* influenza virus, herpes simplex virus). Sensitivity and specificity of the test are determined by the number of organisms present in the test sample and quality of antibodies used in reagents.

KOH, Potassium hydroxide.

capsule, creating a clear halo around the yeast cell), and is a rapid method for the preliminary detection and identification of this important fungus.

DIFFERENTIAL STAINS

A variety of differential stains are used to stain specific organisms or components of cellular material. The **Gram stain** is the best known and most widely used stain and forms the basis for the phenotypic classification of bacteria. Yeasts can also be stained with this method (yeasts are gram-positive). The **iron hematoxylin** and **trichrome** stains are invaluable for the identification of protozoan parasites, and the **Wright-Giemsa** stain is used to identify blood parasites and other selected organisms. Stains such as methenamine silver and toluidine blue O have largely been replaced by more sensitive or technically easier differential or fluorescent stains.

ACID-FAST STAINS

At least three different acid-fast stains are used, each exploiting the fact that some organisms retain a primary stain even when exposed to strong decolorizing agents such as mixtures of acids and alcohols. The **Ziehl-Neelsen** is the oldest method used but requires heating the specimen during the staining procedure. Many laboratories have replaced this method with either the cold acid-fast stain **(Kinyoun method)** or the fluorochrome stain **(auramine-rhodamine method).** The fluorochrome method is the stain of choice because a large area of the specimen can be examined rapidly by simply searching for fluorescing organisms against a black background. Some organisms are "partially acid-fast," retaining the primary stain only when they are decolorized with a weakly acidic solution. This property is characteristic of only a few organisms (see Table 16–1), making it quite valuable for their preliminary identification.

FLUORESCENT STAINS

The auramine-rhodamine acid-fast stain is a specific example of a fluorescent stain. Numerous other fluorescent dyes have also been used to stain specimens. For example, the **acridine orange stain** can be used to stain bacteria and fungi, and **calcofluor white** stains the chitin in fungal cell walls. Although the acridine orange stain is rather limited in its applications, the calcofluor white stain has replaced the potassium hydroxide stains. Another procedure is the examination of specimens with specific antibodies labeled with fluorescent dyes **(fluorescent antibody stains).** The presence of fluorescing organisms is a rapid method for both the detection and identification of the organism.

QUESTIONS

1. Explain the principles underlying brightfield, darkfield, phase-contrast, fluorescent, and electron microscopy. Give one example in which each method would be used.
2. List examples of direct microscopic examinations, differential stains, acid-fast stains, and fluorescent stains.

Bibliography

Chapin K, Murray P: Reagents, stains, and media. In Murray P et al, editors: *Manual of clinical microbiology,* ed 8, Washington, 2003, American Society for Microbiology.

Murray P, Shea Y: *ASM pocket guide to clinical microbiology,* ed. 3, Washington, 2004, American Society for Microbiology.

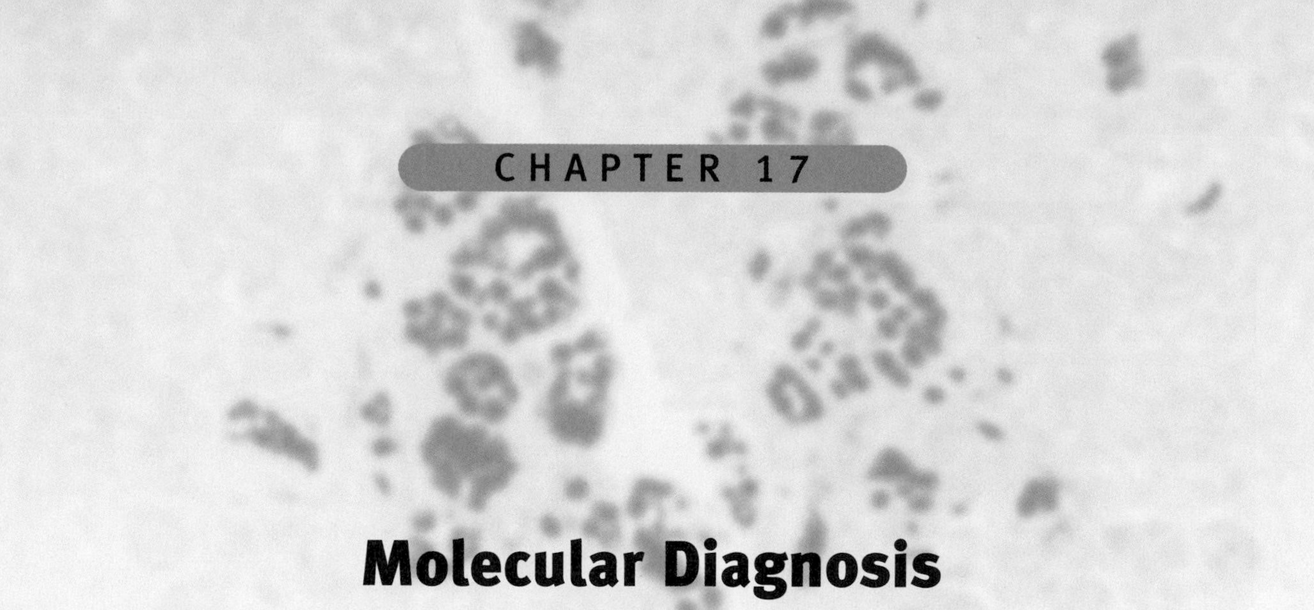

CHAPTER 17

Molecular Diagnosis

Like the evidence left at the scene of a crime, the DNA (deoxyribonucleic acid), RNA (ribonucleic acid), or proteins of an infectious agent in a clinical sample can be used to help identify the agent. In many cases the agent can be detected and identified in this way, even if it cannot be isolated or detected by immunologic means. New techniques and applications of the techniques are being developed for the analysis of infectious agents.

The advantages of molecular techniques are their sensitivity, specificity, and safety. From the standpoint of safety, these techniques do not require isolation of the infectious agent and can be performed on chemically fixed (inactivated) samples or extracts. Because of their sensitivity, very dilute samples of microbial DNA can be detected in a tissue even if the agent is not replicating or producing other evidence of infection. These techniques distinguish stains on the basis of differences in their genotype (i.e., mutants). This is especially useful for distinguishing antiviral drug-resistant strains, which may differ by a single nucleotide.

Detection of Microbial Genetic Material

ELECTROPHORETIC ANALYSIS OF DNA AND RESTRICTION FRAGMENT LENGTH POLYMORPHISM

The genome structure and genetic sequence are major distinguishing characteristics of the family, type, and strain of microorganism. Specific strains of microorganisms can be distinguished on the basis of their DNA or RNA or by the DNA fragments produced when the DNA is cleaved by specific restriction endonucleases **(restriction enzymes).** Restriction enzymes recognize specific DNA sequences that have a palindromic structure; an example follows:

$$\begin{matrix} \overrightarrow{G} & A & A & T & T & C \\ C & T & T & A & A & \underleftarrow{G} \end{matrix}$$

EcoR1 recognition sequence and cleavage

The DNA sites recognized by different restriction endonucleases differ in their sequence, length, and frequency of occurrence. As a result, different restriction endonucleases cleave the DNA of a sample in different places, yielding fragments of different lengths. The cleavage of different DNA samples with one restriction endonuclease can also yield fragments of many different lengths. The differences in the length of the DNA fragments among the different strains of a specific organism produced on cleavage, with one or more restriction endonucleases, is termed **restriction fragment length polymorphism** (RFLP).

DNA or RNA fragments of different sizes or structures can be distinguished by their electrophoretic mobility in an agarose or polyacrylamide gel. Different forms of the same DNA sequence and different lengths of DNA move through the mazelike structure of an agarose gel at different speeds, allowing their separation. The DNA can be visualized by staining with ethidium bromide. Smaller fragments (fewer than 20,000 base pairs), such as those from bacterial plasmids or from viruses, can be separated and distinguished by normal electrophoretic methods. Larger fragments, such as those from whole bacteria, can be separated only by using a special electrophoretic technique called pulsed-field gel electrophoresis.

RFLP is useful, for example, for distinguishing different strains of herpes simplex virus (HSV). Comparison of the restriction endonuclease cleavage patterns of DNA from different isolates can identify a pattern of virus transmission from one person to another or can distinguish HSV-1 from HSV-2. RFLP has also been used to show the spread

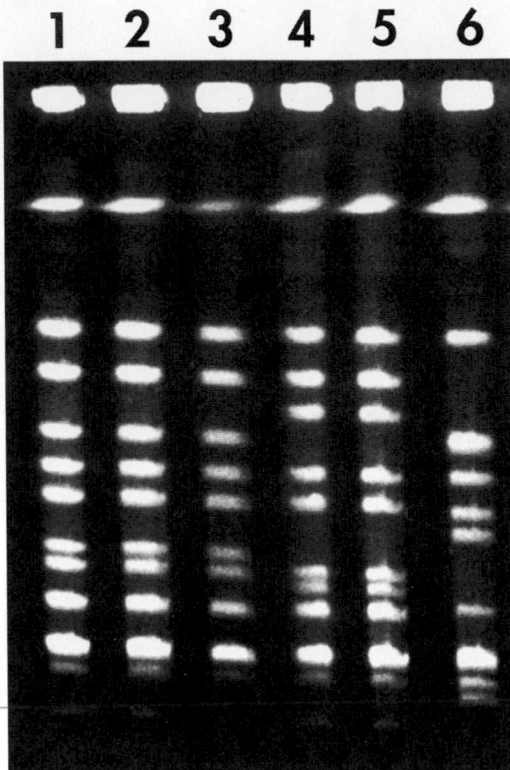

FIGURE 17–1. Restriction fragment length polymorphism distinction of DNA from bacterial strains separated by pulsed-field gel electrophoresis. Lanes *1* to *3* show Sma 1 restriction endonuclease digested DNA isolated from two family members with necrotizing fasciitis and from their physician (pharyngitis). Lanes *4* to *6* are from unrelated *Streptococcus pyogenes* strains. (Courtesy of Dr. Joe DiPersio, Akron, Ohio.)

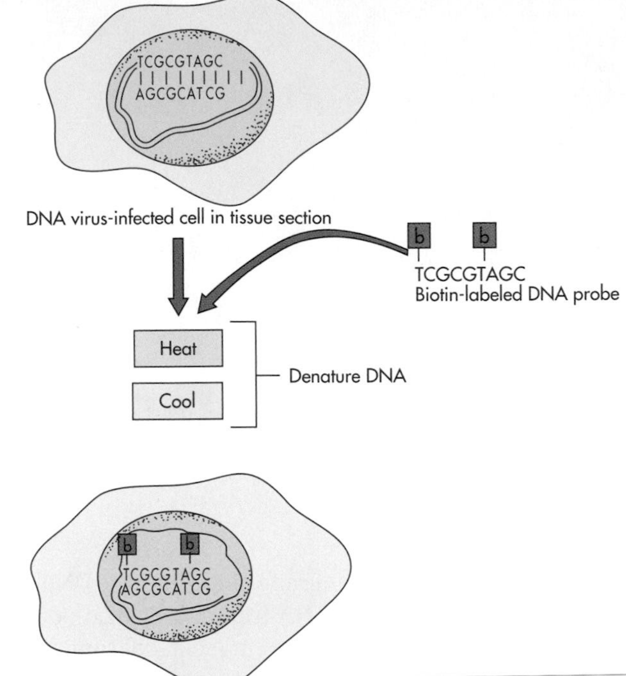

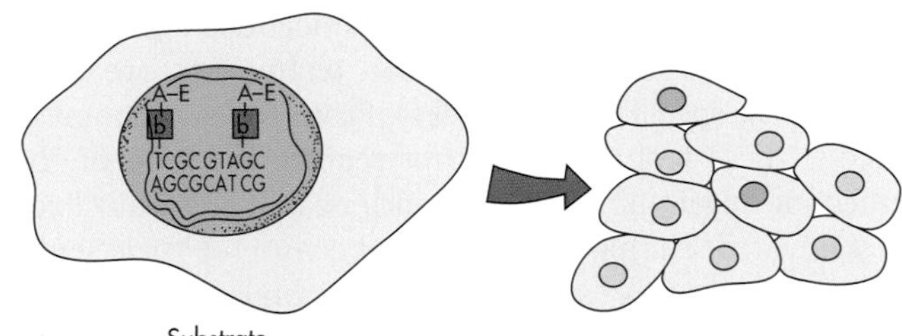

FIGURE 17–2. DNA probe analysis of virus-infected cells. Such cells can be localized in histologically prepared tissue sections using DNA probes consisting of as few as nine nucleotides or bacterial plasmids containing the viral gene. A tagged DNA probe is added to the sample. In this case the DNA probe is labeled with biotin-modified thymidine, but radioactive agents can also be used. The sample is heated to denature the DNA and cooled to allow the probe to hybridize to the complementary sequence. Horseradish peroxidase–labeled avidin is added to bind to the biotin on the probe. The appropriate substrate is added to color the nuclei of virally infected cells. A, Adenine; b, biotin; C, cytosine; G, guanine.

of a strain of *Streptococcus* producing necrotizing fasciitis from one patient to other patients, an emergency medical technician, and the emergency department and attending physicians (Figure 17–1).

GENETIC PROBES

DNA probes can be used like antibodies as sensitive and specific tools to detect, locate, and quantitate specific nucleic acid sequences in clinical specimens (Figure 17–2). Because of the specificity and sensitivity of DNA probe techniques, individual species or strains of an infectious agent can be detected even if they are not growing or replicating.

DNA probes are chemically synthesized or obtained by cloning specific genomic fragments or an entire viral genome into bacterial vectors (plasmids, cosmids). DNA copies of RNA viruses are made with the retrovirus reverse transcriptase and then cloned into these vectors. After chemical or heat treatments to melt (separate) the DNA strands in the sample, the DNA probe is added and allowed to **hybridize** (bind) with the identical or nearly identical sequence in the sample. The **stringency** (the requirement for an exact sequence match) of the interaction can be varied so that related sequences can be detected or different strains (mutants) can be distinguished. The DNA probes are labeled with radioactive or chemically modified nucleotides (e.g., biotinylated uridine), so that they can be detected and quantitated. The use of a biotin-labeled DNA probe allows the use of a fluorescent- or enzyme-labeled avidin or streptavidin (a protein that binds tightly to biotin) molecule to detect viral nucleic acids in a cell in a way similar to which indirect

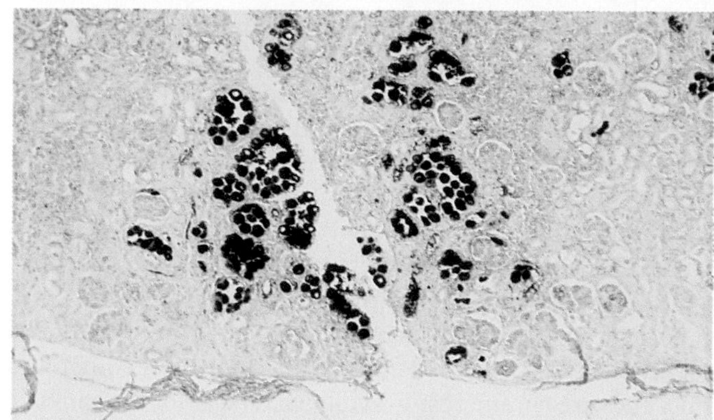

FIGURE 17–3. In situ localization of cytomegalovirus (CMV) infection using a genetic probe. CMV infection of the renal tubules of a kidney is localized with a biotin-labeled, CMV-specific DNA probe and is visualized by means of the horseradish peroxidase–conjugated avidin conversion of substrate, in a manner similar to enzyme immunoassay. (Courtesy of Donna Zabel, Akron, Ohio.)

immunofluorescence or an enzyme immunoassay localizes an antigen.

The DNA probes can detect specific genetic sequences in fixed, permeabilized tissue biopsy specimens by **in situ hybridization.** The localization of cytomegalovirus- (Figure 17–3) or papillomavirus-infected cells by in situ hybridization is preferable to an immunologic means of doing so and is the only commercially available means of localizing papillomavirus. There are now many commercially available viral probes and kits for detecting viruses.

Specific nucleic acid sequences in extracts from a clinical sample can be detected by applying a small volume of the extract to a nitrocellulose filter **(dot blot)** and then probing the filter with labeled, specific viral DNA. Alternatively, the electrophoretically separated restriction endonuclease cleavage pattern can be transferred onto a nitrocellulose filter (**Southern blot**—DNA:DNA probe hybridization), and then the specific sequence can be identified by hybridization with a specific genetic probe and by its characteristic electrophoretic mobility. Electrophoretically separated RNA (**Northern blot**—RNA:DNA probe hybridization) blotted onto a nitrocellulose filter can be detected in a similar manner.

The **polymerase chain reaction (PCR)** amplifies single copies of viral DNA millions of times over and is one of the newest techniques of genetic analysis (Figure 17–4). In this technique a sample is incubated with two short DNA oligomers, termed **primers**, that are complementary to the ends of a known genetic sequence within the total DNA, a heat-stable DNA polymerase (Taq or other polymerase obtained from thermophilic bacteria), nucleotides, and buffers. The oligomers hybridize to the appropriate sequence of DNA and act as primers for the polymerase, which copies that segment of the DNA. The sample is then heated to denature the DNA

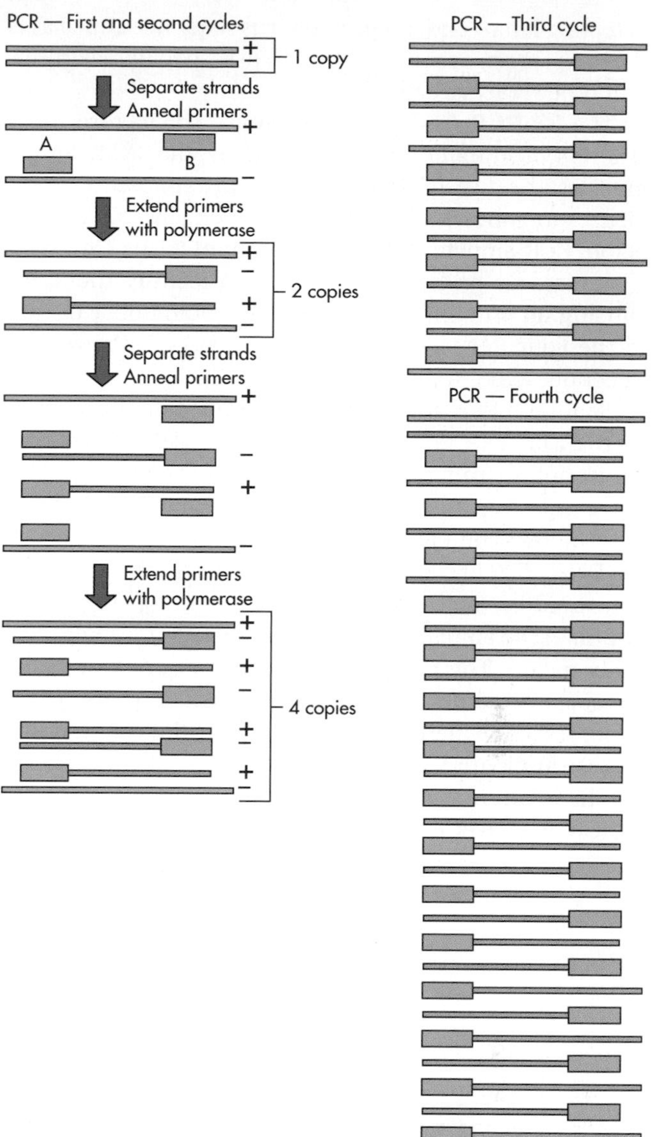

FIGURE 17–4. Polymerase chain reaction (PCR). This technique is a rapid means of amplifying a known sequence of DNA. A sample is mixed with a heat-stable DNA polymerase, excess deoxyribonucleotide triphosphates, and two DNA oligomers **(primers),** which complement the ends of the target sequence to be amplified. The mixture is heated to denature the DNA, then cooled to allow binding of the primers to the target DNA and extension of the primers by the polymerase. The cycle is repeated 20 to 40 times. After the first cycle, only the sequence bracketed by the primers is amplified. In the **RT-PCR** technique, RNA can also be amplified after its conversion to DNA by reverse transcriptase. A and B, DNA oligomers used as primers; + and –, DNA strands. (Modified from Blair GE, Blair Zajdel ME: *Biochem Educ* 20:87-90, 1992.)

(separating the strands of the double helix) and cooled to allow hybridization of the primers to the new DNA. Each copy of DNA becomes a new template. The process is repeated many (20 to 40) times to amplify the original DNA sequence in an exponential manner. A target sequence can be amplified a millionfold in a few hours using this method. This technique is especially useful for detecting latent and integrated virus sequences, such as is the case for retroviruses, herpesviruses, papillomaviruses, and other DNA viruses.

The **RT-PCR** (reverse transcriptase polymerase chain reaction) technique is a variation of the PCR, and it involves the use of the reverse transcriptase of retroviruses to convert viral RNA or messenger RNA to DNA before PCR amplification. In 1993, hantavirus sequences were used as primers for RT-PCR to identify the agent causing an outbreak of hemorrhagic pulmonary disease in the Four Corners area of New Mexico. It showed the infectious agent to be a hantavirus.

Real-time PCR was invented to quantitate the amount of DNA or RNA, after it is converted to DNA by reverse transcriptase, in a sample. Simply put, the more DNA in the sample the faster new DNA is made in a PCR reaction, and the reaction kinetics are proportional to the amount of DNA. The production of double-stranded DNA is measured by the increase in fluorescence of a molecule bound to the amplified double-strand DNA molecule or by other means. This procedure is useful for quantitating the number of human immunodeficiency virus (HIV) genomes in a patient's blood to evaluate the course of the disease and antiviral drug efficacy.

The **branched-chain DNA assay** is a new alternative to PCR and RT-PCR for detecting small amounts of specific RNA or DNA sequences. This technique is especially useful for quantitating plasma levels of HIV RNA. In this case, plasma is incubated in a special tube that is lined with a short complementary DNA (cDNA) sequence to capture the viral RNA. Another cDNA sequence is added to bind to the sample, but this DNA is attached to an artificially branched chain of DNA. On development, each branch is capable of initiating a detectable signal. This amplifies the signal from the original sample.

Assay kits that use variations on the aforementioned techniques to detect, identify, and quantitate different microbes are commercially available. The ability to rapidly determine DNA sequences allows identification of certain bacteria, including the slow-growing Nocardia and Mycobacterium by sequencing the 16S ribosomal RNA gene, or various housekeeping genes, such as the heat shock protein gene.

Detection of Proteins

In some cases, viruses and other infectious agents can be detected on the basis of the finding of certain characteristic enzymes or specific proteins. For example, the detection of reverse transcriptase enzyme activity in

TABLE 17–1. Molecular Techniques

Technique	Purpose	Clinical Examples
RFLP	Comparison of DNA	Molecular epidemiology, HSV-1 strains
DNA electrophoresis	Comparison of DNA	Viral strain differences (up to 20,000 bases)
Pulsed-field gel electrophoresis	Comparison of DNA (large pieces of DNA)	Streptococcal strain comparisons
In situ hybridization	Detection and localization of DNA sequences in tissue	Detection of nonreplicating DNA virus (e.g., cytomegalovirus, human papillomavirus)
Dot blot	Detection of DNA sequences in solution	Detection of viral DNA
Southern blot	Detection and characterization of DNA sequences by size	Identification of specific viral strains
Northern blot	Detection and characterization of RNA sequences by size	Identification of specific viral strains
PCR	Amplification of very dilute DNA samples	Detection of DNA viruses
RT-PCR	Amplification of very dilute RNA samples	Detection of RNA viruses
Real-time PCR	Quantification of very dilute DNA and RNA samples	Quantitation of HIV genome:virus load
Branched-chain DNA	Amplification of very dilute DNA or RNA samples	Quantitation of DNA and RNA viruses
SDS-PAGE	Separation of proteins by molecular weight	Molecular epidemiology of HSV

HSV, Herpes simplex virus; PCR, polymerase chain reaction; RFLP, restriction fragment length polymorphism; RT-PCR, reverse transcriptase polymerase chain reaction; SDS-PAGE, sodium dodecyl sulfate–polyacrylamide gel electrophoresis.

serum or cell culture indicates the presence of a retrovirus. The pattern of proteins from a virus or another agent after sodium dodecyl sulfate–polyacrylamide gel electrophoresis (SDS-PAGE) can also be used to identify and distinguish different strains of viruses or bacteria. In the SDS-PAGE technique, SDS binds to the backbone of the protein to generate a uniform peptide structure and peptide length-to-charge ratio, such that the mobility of the protein in the gel is inversely related to the logarithm of its molecular weight. For example, the patterns of electrophoretically separated HSV proteins can be used to distinguish different types and strains of HSV-1 and HSV-2. Antibody can be used to identify specific proteins separated by SDS-PAGE using a Western blot technique (see Chapter 51). The molecular techniques used to identify infectious agents are summarized in Table 17–1.

Bibliography

DiPersio JR et al: Spread of serious disease-producing M3 clones of group A *Streptococcus* among family members and health care workers, *Clin Infect Dis* 22:490-495, 1996.

Forbes BA, Weissfeld AS, Sahm DF: *Baily and Scott's diagnostic microbiology,* ed 11, St Louis, 2002, Mosby.

Fredericks DN, Relman DA: Application of polymerase chain reaction to the diagnosis of infectious diseases, *Clin Infect Dis* 29:475-486, 1999.

Murray PR: *ASM pocket guide to clinical microbiology,* ed 2, Washington, 1998, American Society for Microbiology.

Specter S, Hodinka RL, Young SA: *Clinical virology manual,* ed 3, Washington, 2000, ASM Press.

Strauss JM, Strauss EG: *Viruses and human disease,* San Diego, Academic Press, 2002.

CHAPTER 18

Serologic Diagnosis

Immunologic techniques are used to detect, identify, and quantitate antigen in clinical samples, as well as to evaluate the antibody response to infection and a person's history of exposure to infectious agents. The specificity of the antibody-antigen interaction and the sensitivity of many of the immunologic techniques make them powerful laboratory tools (Table 18–1). In most cases the same technique can be used to evaluate antigen and antibody. Because many serologic assays are designed to give a positive or negative result, quantitation of the antibody strength is obtained as a **titer.** The titer of an antibody is defined as the lowest dilution of the sample that retains a detectable activity.

Antibodies

Antibodies can be used as sensitive and specific tools to detect, identify, and quantitate the antigens from a virus, bacterium, fungus, or parasite. Specific antibodies may be obtained from convalescent patients (e.g., antiviral antibodies) or prepared in animals. These antibodies are **polyclonal;** that is, they are heterogeneous antibody preparations that can recognize many epitopes on a single antigen. **Monoclonal** antibodies recognize individual epitopes on an antigen. Monoclonal antibodies for some antigens are commercially available, especially for lymphocyte cell surface antigens.

The development of monoclonal antibody technology revolutionized the science of immunology. For example, because of the specificity of these antibodies, lymphocyte subsets (e.g., CD4 and CD8 T cells) and lymphocyte cell surface antigens were identified. Monoclonal antibodies are the products of hybrid cells generated by the fusion and cloning of spleen cells from an immunized mouse and myeloma cells, which produces a hybridoma. The myeloma provides immortalization to the antibody-producing B cells of the spleen. *Each hybridoma clone is a factory for one antibody molecule, yielding a monoclonal antibody that recognizes only one epitope.* Monoclonal antibodies can also be prepared through genetic engineering.

The advantages of monoclonal antibodies are that their specificity can be confined to a single epitope on an antigen and that they can be prepared in "industrial-sized" tissue culture preparations. A major disadvantage of monoclonal antibodies is that they are often too specific, such that a monoclonal antibody specific for one epitope on a viral antigen of one strain may not be able to detect different strains of the same virus.

Methods of Detection

Antibody-antigen complexes can be detected directly, by precipitation techniques or by labeling the antibody with a radioactive, fluorescent, or enzyme probe, or they can be detected indirectly, through measurement of an antibody-directed reaction, such as complement fixation. *Most of the procedures for detecting and identifying antigen can also be used for serologically evaluating antibody levels.*

PRECIPITATION AND IMMUNODIFFUSION TECHNIQUES

Specific antigen-antibody complexes and cross-reactivity can be distinguished by immunoprecipitation techniques. Within a limited concentration range for both antigen and antibody, termed the **equivalence zone,** the antibody cross-links the antigen into a complex that is too large to stay in solution and therefore precipitates. This technique is based on the multivalent nature of antibody molecules (e.g., immunoglobulin [Ig] G has two antigen-binding

TABLE 18–1. Selected Immunologic Techniques

Technique	Purpose	Clinical Examples
Ouchterlony immunodouble diffusion	Detect and compare antigen and antibody	Fungal antigen and antibody
Immunofluorescence	Detection and localization of antigen	Viral antigen in biopsy (e.g., rabies, herpes simplex virus)
Enzyme immunoassay (EIA)	Same as immunofluorescence	Same as for immunofluorescence
Immunofluorescence flow cytometry	Population analysis of antigen-positive cells	Immunophenotyping
Enzyme-linked immunosorbent assay (ELISA)	Quantitation of antigen or antibody	Viral antigen (rotavirus); viral antibody (anti-HIV)
Western blot	Detection of antigen-specific antibody	Confirmation of anti-HIV seropositivity
Radioimmunoassay (RIA)	Same as ELISA	Same as for ELISA
Complement fixation	Quantitate specific antibody titer	Fungal, viral antibody
Hemagglutination inhibition	Antiviral antibody titer; serotype of virus strain	Seroconversion to current influenza strain; identification of influenza
Latex agglutination	Quantitation and detection of antigen and antibody	Rheumatoid factor; fungal antigens; streptococcal antigens

HIV, Human immunodeficiency virus.

domains). The antigen-antibody complexes are soluble at concentration ratios of antigen to antibody that are above and below the equivalence concentration.

Various immunodiffusion techniques make use of the equivalence concept to determine the identity of an antigen or the presence of antibody. **Single radial immunodiffusion** can be used to detect and quantify an antigen. In this technique, antigen is placed into a well and allowed to diffuse into antibody-containing agar. The higher the concentration of antigen, the farther it diffuses before it reaches equivalence with the antibody in the agar and precipitates as a ring around the well.

The **Ouchterlony immunodouble diffusion** technique is used to determine the relatedness of different antigens, as shown in Figure 18–1. In this technique, solutions of antibody and antigen are placed in separate wells cut into agar, and the antigen and antibody are allowed to diffuse toward each other to establish concentration gradients of each substance. A visible precipitin line occurs where the concentrations of antigen and antibody reach equivalence (see Figure 18–1). On the basis of the pattern of the precipitin lines, this technique can also be used to determine whether samples are identical, share some but not all epitopes (partial identity), or are distinct. This technique is used to detect antibody to fungal antigens (e.g., *Histoplasma* species, *Blastomyces* species, coccidioidomycoses).

In other immunodiffusion techniques the antigen may be separated by electrophoresis in agar and then reacted with antibody (immunoelectrophoresis), it may be pushed into agar that contains antibody by means of electrophoresis (rocket electrophoresis), or antigen and antibody may be placed in separate wells and allowed to move electrophoretically toward each other (countercurrent immunoelectrophoresis).

Immunoassays for Cell-Associated Antigen (Immunohistology)

Antigens on the cell surface or within the cell can be detected by **immunofluorescence** and **enzyme immunoassay (EIA).** In **direct immunofluorescence,** a fluorescent molecule is covalently attached to the antibody (e.g., fluorescein isothiocyanate–labeled rabbit antiviral antibody). In **indirect immunofluorescence,** a second fluorescent antibody specific for the primary antibody (e.g., fluorescein isothiocyanate–labeled goat antirabbit antibody) is used to detect the primary antiviral antibody and locate the antigen (Figures 18–2 and 18–3). In EIA, an enzyme such as horseradish peroxidase or alkaline phosphatase is conjugated to the antibody and converts a substrate into a chromophore to mark the antigen. Alternatively, an antibody modified by the attachment of a **biotin** (the vitamin) molecule can be localized by the very high affinity binding of avidin or streptavidin molecules. A fluorescent molecule or an enzyme can modify the

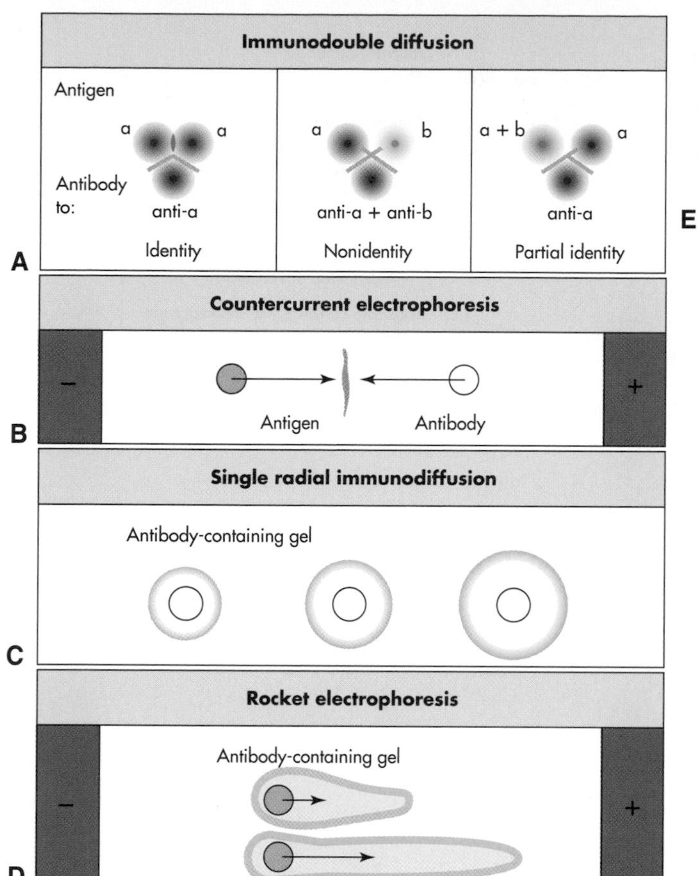

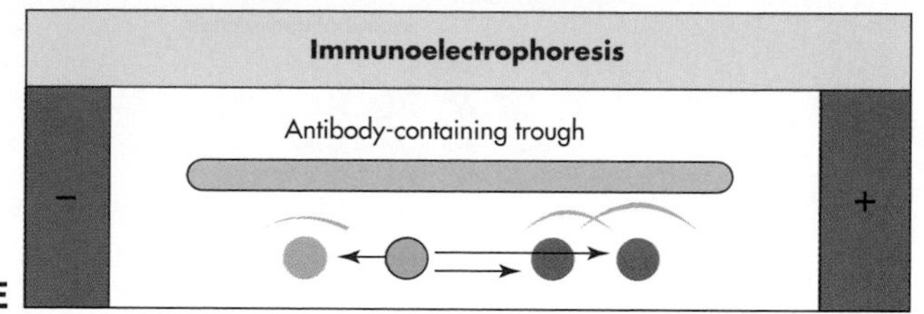

FIGURE 18–1. Analysis of antigens and antibodies by immunoprecipitation. The precipitation of protein occurs at the equivalence point, at which multivalent antibody forms large complexes with antigen. **A,** Ouchterlony immunodouble diffusion. Antigen and antibody diffuse from wells, meet, and form a precipitin line. If identical antigens are placed in adjacent wells, the concentration of antigen between them is doubled, and precipitation does not occur in this region. If different antigens are used, two different precipitin lines are produced. If one sample shares antigen but is not identical, then a single spur results for the complete antigen. **B,** Countercurrent electrophoresis. This technique is similar to the Ouchterlony method, but antigen movement is facilitated by electrophoresis. **C,** Single radial immunodiffusion. This technique involves the diffusion of antigen into an antibody-containing gel. Precipitin rings indicate an immune reaction, and the area of the ring is proportional to the concentration of antigen. **D,** Rocket electrophoresis. Antigens are separated by electrophoresis into an agar gel that contains antibody. The length of the "rocket" indicates concentration of antigen. **E,** Immunoelectrophoresis. Antigen is placed in a well and separated by electrophoresis. Antibody is then placed in the trough, and precipitin lines form as antigen and antibody diffuse toward each other.

avidin and streptavidin to promote detection. These techniques are useful for the analysis of tissue biopsy specimens, blood cells, and tissue culture cells.

The **flow cytometer** can be used to analyze the immunofluorescence of cells in suspension and is especially useful for identifying and quantitating lymphocytes (immunophenotyping). A laser is used in the flow cytometer to excite the fluorescent antibody attached to the cell and to determine the size of the cell by means of light-scattering measurements. The cells flow past the laser at rates of more than 5000 cells per second, and analysis is performed electronically. The **fluorescence-activated cell sorter (FACS)** is a flow cytometer that can also isolate specific subpopulations of cells for tissue culture growth on the basis of their size and immunofluorescence.

The data obtained from a flow cytometer are usually presented in the form of a histogram, with the fluorescence intensity on the x-axis and the number of cells on the y-axis, or in the form of a dot plot, in which more than one parameter is compared for each cell. The flow cytometer can perform a differential analysis of white blood cells and compare CD4 and CD8 T-cell populations simultaneously (Figure 18–4). Flow cytometry is also useful for analyzing cell growth after the fluorescent labeling of deoxyribonucleic acid (DNA) and other fluorescent applications.

Immunoassays for Antibody and Soluble Antigen

The **enzyme-linked immunosorbent assay (ELISA)** uses antigen immobilized on a plastic surface, bead, or

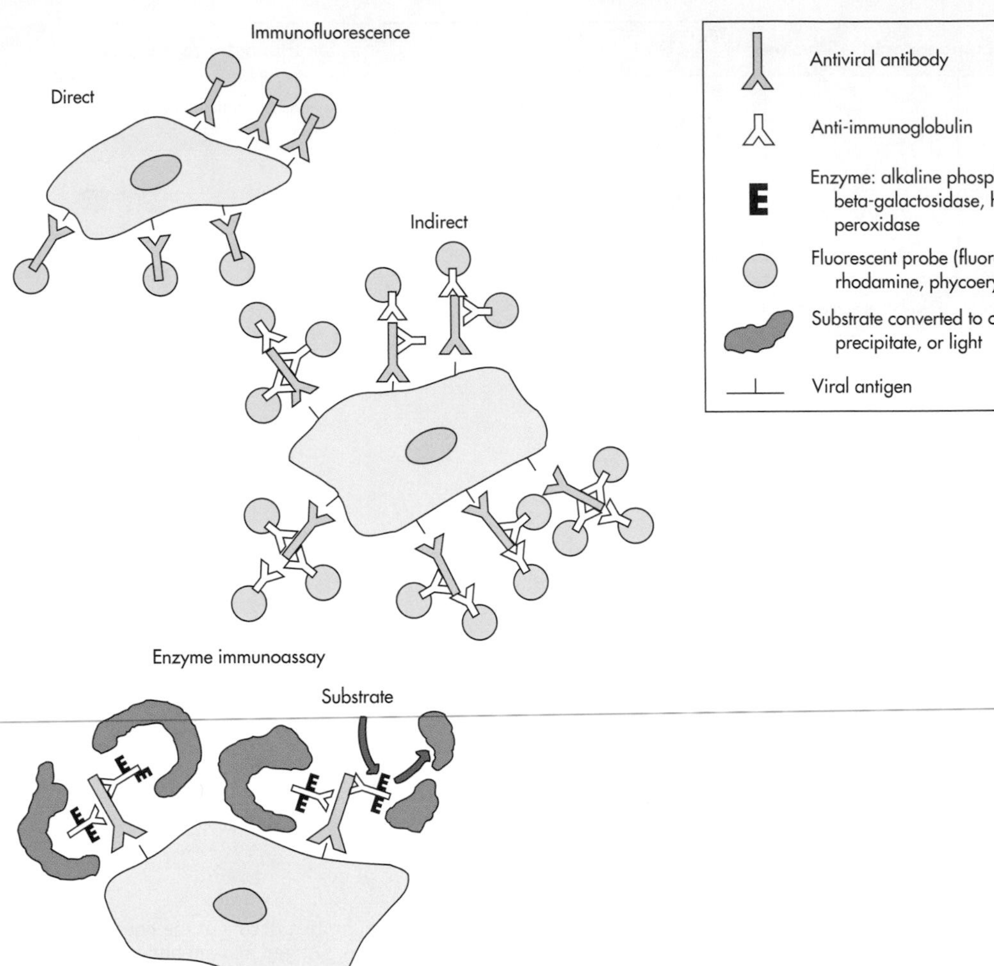

FIGURE 18–2. Immunofluorescence and enzyme immunoassays for antigen localization in cells. Antigen can be detected by *direct* assay with antiviral antibody modified covalently with a fluorescent or enzyme probe, or by *indirect* assay using antiviral antibody and chemically modified anti-immunoglobulin. The enzyme converts substrate to a precipitate, chromophore, or light.

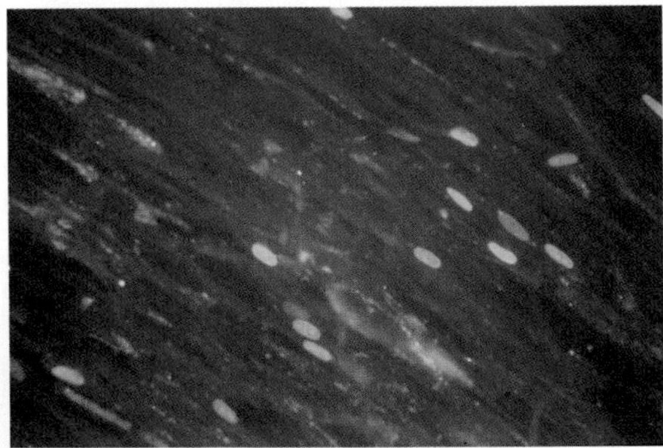

FIGURE 18–3. Immunofluorescence localization of herpes simplex virus (HSV)-infected nerve cells in a brain section from a patient with herpes encephalitis. (From Emond RT, Rowland HAK: *A color atlas of infectious diseases,* ed 2, London, 1987, Wolfe.)

filter to capture and separate the specific antibody from other antibodies in a patient's serum (Figure 18–5). An anti-human antibody with a covalently linked enzyme (e.g., horseradish peroxidase, alkaline phosphatase, β-galactosidase) then detects the affixed patient antibody. It is quantitated spectrophotometrically according to the intensity of the color produced in response to the enzyme conversion of an appropriate substrate. The actual concentration of specific antibody can be determined by comparison with the reactivity of standard human antibody solutions. The many variations of ELISAs differ in the way in which they capture or detect antibody or antigen.

ELISAs can also be used to quantitate the soluble antigen in a patient's sample. In these assays, soluble antigen is captured and concentrated by an immobilized antibody and then detected with a different antibody labeled with the enzyme. An example of a commonly used ELISA is the home pregnancy test for the human chorionic gonadotropin hormone.

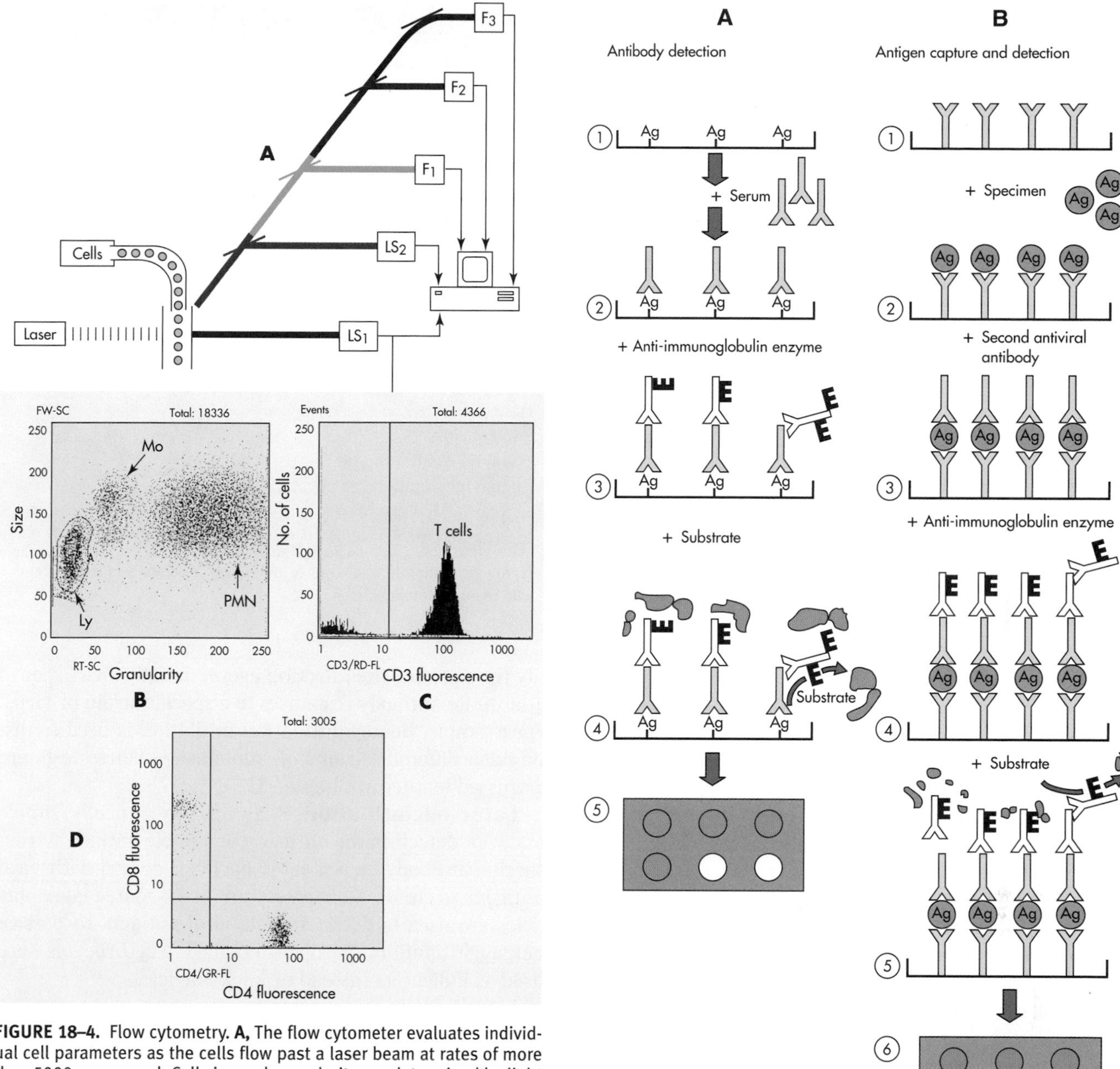

FIGURE 18–4. Flow cytometry. **A,** The flow cytometer evaluates individual cell parameters as the cells flow past a laser beam at rates of more than 5000 per second. Cell size and granularity are determined by light scattering *(LS)*, and antigen expression is evaluated by immunofluorescence *(F)*, using antibodies labeled with different fluorescent probes. Parts **B** to **D** depict T-cell analysis of a normal patient. **B,** Light-scatter analysis was used to define the lymphocytes *(Ly)*, monocytes *(Mo)*, and polymorphonuclear (neutrophil) leukocytes *(PMN)*. **C,** The lymphocytes were analyzed for CD3 expression to identify T cells (presented in a histogram). **D,** CD4 and CD8 T cells were identified. Each dot represents one T cell. (Data provided by Dr. Tom Alexander, Akron, Ohio.)

FIGURE 18–5. Enzyme immunoassays for quantitation of antibody or antigen. **A,** Antibody detection. *1,* Viral antigen, obtained from infected cells, virions, or genetic engineering, is affixed to a surface. *2,* Patient serum is added and allowed to bind to the antigen. Unbound antibody is washed away. *3,* Enzyme-conjugated antihuman antibody is added, and unbound antibody is washed away. *4,* Substrate is added and converted *(5)* into chromophore, precipitate, or light. **B,** Antigen capture and detection. *1,* Antiviral antibody is affixed to a surface. *2,* A specimen that contains antigen is added, and unbound antigen is washed away. *3,* A second antiviral antibody is added to detect the captured antigen. *4,* Enzyme-conjugated anti-antibody is added, washed, and followed by substrate *(5)*, which is converted *(6)* into chromophore, precipitate, or light.

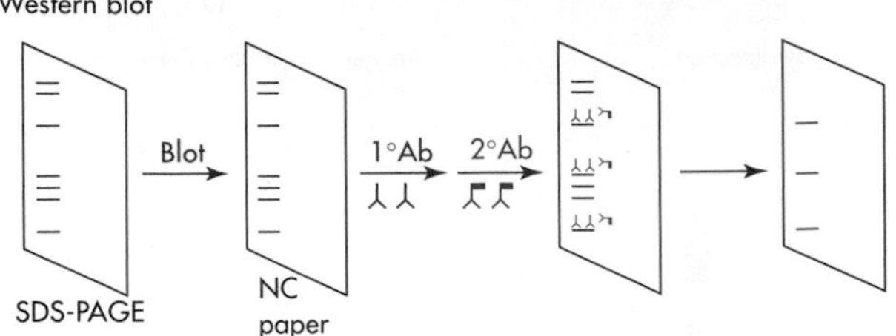

FIGURE 18–6. Western blot analysis. Proteins are separated by sodium dodecyl sulfate–polyacrylamide gel electrophoresis (SDS-PAGE), electroblotted onto nitrocellulose (NC) paper, and incubated with antigen-specific or patient's antisera (1°Ab) and then enzyme-conjugated anti-human serum (2°Ab). Enzyme conversion of substrate identifies the antigen.

BOX 18–1. Serologic Assays

Complement fixation
Hemagglutination inhibition*
Neutralization*
Immunofluorescence (direct and indirect)
Latex agglutination
In situ enzyme immunoassay (EIA)
Enzyme-linked immunosorbent assay (ELISA)
Radioimmunoassay (RIA)

*For detection of antibody or serotyping of virus.

BOX 18–2. Viruses Diagnosed by Serology*

Epstein-Barr virus
Rubella virus
Hepatitis A, B, C, D, and E viruses
Human immunodeficiency virus
Human T-cell leukemia virus
Arboviruses (encephalitis viruses)

*Serologic testing is also used to determine a person's immune status with regard to other viruses.

Western blot analysis is a variation of an ELISA. In this technique, viral proteins separated by electrophoresis, according to their molecular weight or charge, are transferred (blotted) onto a filter paper (e.g., nitrocellulose, nylon). When exposed to a patient's serum, the immobilized proteins capture virus-specific antibody and are visualized with an enzyme-conjugated antihuman antibody. This technique shows the proteins recognized by the patient serum. Western blot analysis is used to confirm ELISA results in patients suspected to be infected with the human immunodeficiency virus (HIV) (Figure 18–6; also see Figure 51–7).

In **radioimmunoassay (RIA),** radiolabeled (e.g., with iodine-125) antibody or antigen is used to quantitate antigen-antibody complexes. RIA can be performed as a capture assay, as described previously for ELISA, or as a competition assay. In a competition assay, antibody in a patient's serum is quantitated according to its ability to compete with and replace a laboratory-prepared, radiolabeled antibody from antigen-antibody complexes. The antigen-antibody complexes are precipitated and separated from free antibody, and the radioactivity is measured for both fractions. The amount of the patient's antibody is then quantitated from standard curves prepared with use of known quantities of competing antibody. The radioallergosorbent assay is a variation of an RIA capture assay, in which radiolabeled anti-IgE is used to detect allergen-specific responses.

Complement fixation is a standard but technically difficult serologic test (Box 18–1). In this test the patient's serum sample is reacted with laboratory-derived antigen and extra complement. Antibody-antigen complexes bind, activate, and fix (use up) the complement. The residual complement is then assayed through the lysis of red blood cells coated with antibody. Antibodies measured by this system generally develop slightly later in an illness than those measured by other techniques.

Antibody inhibition assays make use of the specificity of an antibody to prevent infection **(neutralization)** or other activity **(hemagglutination inhibition)** to identify the strain of the infecting agent, usually a virus, or to quantitate antibody responses to a specific strain of virus. For example, hemagglutination inhibition is used to distinguish different strains of influenza A. These tests are discussed further in Chapter 51.

Latex agglutination is a rapid, technically simple assay for detecting the antibody or soluble antigen. Virus-specific antibody causes latex particles coated with viral antigens to clump. Conversely, antibody-coated latex particles are used to detect soluble viral antigen. In passive hemagglutination, antigen-modified erythrocytes are used as indicators instead of latex particles.

Serology

The humoral immune response provides a history of a patient's infections. Serology can be used to identify the infecting agent, evaluate the course of an infection, or determine the nature of the infection—whether it is a primary infection or a reinfection, and whether it is acute or chronic. The antibody type and titer and the identity of the antigenic targets provide serologic data about an infection. Serologic testing is used to identify viruses and other agents that are difficult to isolate and grow in the laboratory or that cause diseases with slower courses (Box 18–2).

The relative antibody concentration is reported as a titer. A **titer** is the inverse of the greatest dilution, or lowest concentration (e.g., dilution of 1 : 64 = titer of 64), of a patient's serum that retains activity in one of the immunoassays just described. The amount of IgM, IgG, IgA, or IgE reactive with antigen can also be evaluated through the use of a labeled second antihuman antibody specific for the antibody isotype.

Serology is used to determine the time course of an infection by determining whether **seroconversion** has occurred. Seroconversion occurs when antibody is produced in response to a primary infection. *Specific IgM antibody, found during the first 2 to 3 weeks of a primary infection, is a good indicator of a recent primary infection.* Reinfection, or recurrence later in life, causes an **anamnestic** (secondary or booster) response. Antibody titers may remain high, however, in patients whose disease recurs frequently (e.g., herpesviruses). Seroconversion or reinfection is indicated by the finding *of at least a fourfold increase in the antibody titer between serum obtained during the acute phase of disease and that obtained at least 2 to 3 weeks later, during the convalescent phase.* Because of the inherent imprecision of serologic assays based on twofold serial dilutions, confirmation of seroconversion is defined as a fourfold increase in the antibody titer between acute and convalescent sera. For example, samples with 512 and 1023 units of antibody would both give a reaction on a 512-fold dilution but not on a 1024-fold dilution, and both results would be reported as titers of 512. On the other hand, samples with 1020 and 1030 units are not significantly different but would be reported as titers of 512 and 1024, respectively.

Serology can also be used to determine the stage of a slower or chronic infection (e.g., hepatitis B, or infectious mononucleosis caused by Epstein-Barr virus), based on the presence of antibody to specific microbial antigens. The first antibodies to be detected are those directed against antigens most available to the immune system (e.g., on the virion, on surfaces of infected cells, secreted). Later in the infection, when cells have been lysed by the infecting virus or the cellular immune response, antibodies directed against the intracellular proteins and enzymes are detected.

QUESTIONS

Describe the diagnostic procedure or procedures (molecular or immunologic) that would be appropriate for each of the following applications:

1. Determination of the apparent molecular weights of the HIV proteins
2. Detection of human papillomavirus 16 (a nonreplicating virus) in a Papanicolaou (Pap) smear
3. Detection of herpes simplex virus (a replicating virus) in a Pap smear
4. Presence of *Histoplasma* fungal antigens in a patient's serum
5. CD4 and CD8 T-cell concentrations in blood from a patient infected with HIV
6. The presence of antibody and the titer of anti-HIV antibody
7. Genetic differences between two herpes simplex viruses (DNA virus)
8. Genetic differences between two parainfluenza viruses (ribonucleic acid [RNA] virus)
9. Amount of rotavirus antigen in stool
10. Detection of group A streptococci and their distinction from other streptococci

Bibliography

Forbes BA, Weissfeld AS, Sahm DF: *Baily and Scott's diagnostic microbiology*, ed 11, St Louis, 2002, Mosby.

Murray PR: *ASM pocket guide to clinical microbiology*, Washington, 1996, American Society for Microbiology.

Specter S et al: *Clinical virology manual*, ed 3, Washington, 2000, ASM Press.

Strauss JM, Strauss EG: *Viruses and human disease*, San Diego, 2002, Academic Press.

SECTION IV

Bacteriology

CHAPTER 19

Mechanisms of Bacterial Pathogenesis

To a bacterium, the human body is a collection of environmental niches that provide the warmth, moisture, and food necessary for growth. Bacteria have acquired genetic traits that enable them to enter (invade) the environment, remain in a niche (adhere or colonize), gain access to food sources (degradative enzymes), and escape clearance by host immune and nonimmune protective responses (e.g., **capsule**). Unfortunately, many of the mechanisms that bacteria use to maintain their niche and the by-products of bacterial growth (e.g., acids, gas) cause damage and problems for the human host. Many of these genetic traits are **virulence factors,** which enhance the ability of bacteria to cause disease. Although many bacteria cause disease by directly destroying tissue, some release toxins, which are then disseminated by the blood to cause system-wide pathogenesis (Box 19–1). The surface structures of bacteria are powerful stimulators of host responses (acute phase: interleukin-1 [IL-1], interleukin-6 [IL-6], tumor necrosis factor [TNF]), which can be protective but are often the significant causes of the disease symptoms (e.g., sepsis).

Not all bacteria or bacterial infections cause disease; however, some always cause disease. The human body is colonized with numerous microbes **(normal flora),** many of which serve important functions for their hosts. Normal flora bacteria aid in the digestion of food, produce vitamins (e.g., vitamin K), and can protect the host from colonization with pathogenic microbes. Although many of these endogenous bacteria can cause disease, they normally reside in locations such as the gastrointestinal (GI) tract, mouth, skin, and upper respiratory tract, which are technically outside the body (Figure 19–1). Normal flora bacteria cause disease if they enter normally sterile sites of the body. **Virulent bacteria** have mechanisms that promote their growth in the host at the expense of the host's tissue or organ function. Disease results from the damage or loss of tissue or organ function or the development of host inflammatory responses. **Opportunistic bacteria** take advantage of preexisting conditions that enhance the susceptibility of the patient, such as immunosuppression, to grow and cause more serious disease. For example, *Pseudomonas aeruginosa* infects burn victims and the lungs of patients with cystic fibrosis, and patients with the acquired immune deficiency syndrome (AIDS) are very susceptible to infection by intracellularly growing bacteria, such as the mycobacteria.

The **signs and symptoms of a disease** are determined by the function of the affected tissue. **Systemic responses** are produced by toxins and the cytokines produced in response to the infection. The seriousness of the disease depends on the importance of the affected organ and the extent of the damage caused by the infection. Infections of the central nervous system are always serious. The **bacterial strain** and **inoculum size** are also major factors in determining whether disease occurs; however, this can vary from a relatively small inoculum (e.g., less than 200 *Shigella* for shigellosis) to a very large inoculum (e.g., 10^8 *Vibrio cholerae* or *Campylobacter* organisms for GI tract infections). Host factors can also play a role. For example, although a million or more *Salmonella* organisms are necessary for gastroenteritis to become established in a healthy person, only a few thousand organisms are necessary in a person whose gastric pH is neutral. Congenital defects, immunodeficiency states (see Chapter 14), and other disease-related conditions might also increase a person's susceptibility to infection.

Entry into the Human Body

For infection to become established, bacteria must first gain entry into the body (Figure 19–1 and Table 19–1).

Natural defense mechanisms and barriers, such as skin, mucus, ciliated epithelium, and secretions containing antibacterial substances (e.g., lysozyme), make it difficult for bacteria to gain entry into the body. However, these barriers are sometimes broken (e.g., a tear in the skin, a tumor or ulcer in the bowel), providing a portal of entry for the bacteria, or the bacteria may have the means to compromise the barrier and invade the body. On invasion, the bacteria can travel in the bloodstream to other sites in the body.

The **skin** has a thick, horny layer of dead cells that protects the body from infection. However, cuts in the skin, produced accidentally or surgically or kept open with catheters or other surgical appliances, provide a means for the bacteria to gain access to the susceptible tissue underneath. For example, *Staphylococcus aureus* and *Staphylococcus epidermidis,* which are a part of the normal flora on skin, can enter the body through breaks in the skin and pose a major problem for people with indwelling catheters and intravenous lines.

The *mouth, nose, respiratory tract, ears, eyes, urogenital tract, and anus are sites through which bacteria can enter the body.* These natural openings in the skin, and their associated body cavities, are protected by natural defenses such as the mucus and ciliated epithelium that line the upper respiratory tract, the lysozyme and other antibacterial secretions in tears and mucus, and the acid and bile in the GI tract. However, many bacteria are unaffected or have the means to evade these defenses. For example, the outer membrane of the gram-negative bacteria makes these bacteria more resistant to lysozyme, acid, and bile. The enterobacteria are thus enabled to colonize the GI tract, where they serve the beneficial function of producing the vitamin K that the body needs. These endogenous bacteria are normally benign and restricted to the body cavities that they colonize. However, these bacteria can enter normally sterile sites of the body, such as the peritoneum and the bloodstream, through a break in the normal barrier. An example of this is the patient whose colon tumor was diagnosed after detection of a septicemia (blood-borne infection) caused by enteric bacteria.

BOX 19–1. Bacterial Virulence Mechanisms
Adherence
Invasion
By-products of growth (gas, acid)
Toxins
Degradative enzymes
Cytotoxic proteins
Endotoxin
Superantigen
Induction of excess inflammation
Evasion of phagocytic and immune clearance
Capsule
Resistance to antibiotics
Intracellular growth

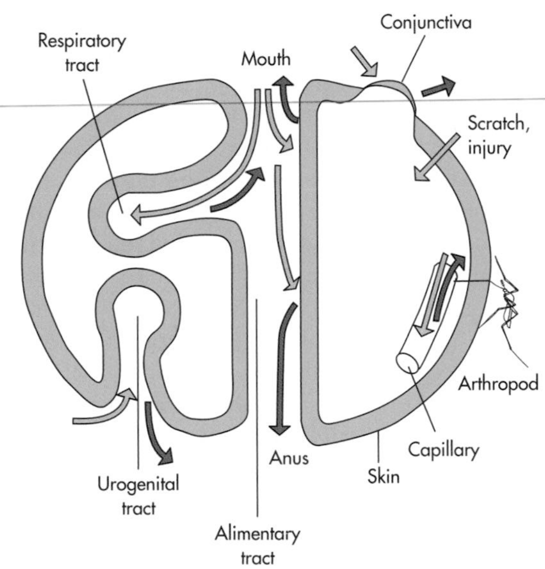

FIGURE 19–1. Body surfaces as sites of microbial infection and shedding. Green arrows indicate infection; purple arrows indicate shedding. (Redrawn from Mims C et al: *Medical microbiology,* London, 1993, Mosby-Wolfe.)

TABLE 19–1. Bacterial Port of Entry

Route	Examples
Ingestion	*Salmonella* sp., *Shigella* sp., *Yersinia enterocolitica,* enterotoxigenic *Escherichia coli, Vibrio* sp., *Campylobacter* sp., *Clostridium botulinum, Bacillus cereus, Listeria* sp., *Brucella* sp.
Inhalation	*Mycobacterium* sp., *Nocardia* sp., *Mycoplasma pneumoniae, Legionella* sp., *Bordetella, Chlamydia psittaci, Chlamydia pneumoniae, Streptococcus* sp.
Trauma	*Clostridium tetani*
Needlestick	*Staphylococcus aureus, Pseudomonas* sp.
Arthropod bite	*Rickettsia, Ehrlichia, Coxiella, Francisella,* and *Borrelia* spp., *Yersinia pestis*
Sexual transmission	*Neisseria gonorrhoeae, Chlamydia trachomatis, Treponema pallidum*

Colonization, Adhesion, and Invasion

As previously mentioned, the GI tract is naturally colonized by benign and potentially beneficial bacteria. In some cases, environmental conditions determine the bacteria that can or will colonize a site. For example, *Legionella* grows in the lungs but does not readily spread because it cannot tolerate high temperatures (e.g., 35°C). Colonization of sites that are normally sterile implies the existence of a defect in a natural defense mechanism or a new portal of entry. Patients with cystic fibrosis have such defects because of the reduction in their ciliary mucoepithelial function and altered mucosal secretions; as a result, their lungs are colonized by *S. aureus* and *P. aeruginosa.*

Bacteria may use specific mechanisms to adhere to and colonize different body surfaces (Table 19–2). If the bacteria can adhere to epithelial or endothelial cell linings of the bladder, intestine, and blood vessels, they cannot be washed away, and this adherence allows them to colonize the tissue. For example, natural bladder function eliminates any bacteria not affixed to the bladder wall. *Escherichia coli* and other bacteria have **adhesins** that bind to specific receptors on the tissue surface, which keep them from being washed away. Many of these adhesin proteins are present at the tips of **fimbriae (pili)** and bind tightly to specific sugars on the target tissue. (This sugar-binding activity defines these proteins as lectins.) For example, most *E. coli* strains that cause pyelonephritis produce a fimbrial adhesin termed *P fimbriae.* This adhesin can bind to receptors for α-d-galactosyl-β-d-galactoside (Gal-Gal), which is part of the P blood group antigen structure on human erythrocytes and uroepithelial cells. *Neisseria gonorrhoeae* pili are also important virulence factors; they bind to oligosaccharide receptors on epithelial cells. *Yersinia* organisms, *Bordetella pertussis,* and *Mycoplasma pneumoniae* express adhesin proteins that are not on fimbriae. *Streptococcus pyogenes* uses **lipoteichoic acid** and the F protein (binds to fibronectin) to bind to epithelial cells.

A special bacterial adaptation that facilitates colonization, especially of surgical appliances such as artificial valves or indwelling catheters, is a **biofilm** produced by the bacteria. Bacteria in biofilms are bound within a sticky web of polysaccharide that binds the cells together and to the surface. Some bacteria, such as *Pseudomonas aeruginosa,* sense that sufficient bacteria are present to make a biofilm (quorum sensing) and create a bacterial community. Dental plaque is an example of a biofilm. The biofilm matrix can also protect the bacteria from host defenses and antibiotics.

Although bacteria do not have mechanisms that enable them to cross skin, several bacteria can cross mucosal membranes and other tissue barriers to enter normally sterile sites and more susceptible tissue. These invasive bacteria either destroy the barrier or penetrate into the cells of the barrier. *Shigella, Salmonella,* and *Yersinia* organisms are enteric bacteria that use fimbriae to bind to M (microfold) cells of the colon and then inject proteins into the M cell that stimulate the cell membrane to surround and take in the bacteria. *Shigella* can then spread to adjacent cells, whereas *Salmonella* can pass through to the other side and initiate systemic infection. *Salmonella* species and enteropathogenic strains of *E. coli* encode the

TABLE 19–2. Examples of Bacterial Adherence Mechanisms

Microbe	Adhesin	Receptor
Staphylococcus aureus	LTA	Unknown
Staphylococcus sp.	Slime	Unknown
Streptococcus, group A	LTA-M protein complex	Fibronectin
Streptococcus pneumoniae	Protein	*N*-acetylhexosamine-gal
Escherichia coli	Type 1 fimbriae Colonization factor antigen fimbriae P fimbriae	D–Mannose GM ganglioside 1 P blood group glycolipid
Other Enterobacteriaceae	Type 1 fimbriae	D–Mannose
Neisseria gonorrhoeae	Fimbriae	GD_1 ganglioside
Treponema pallidum	P_1, P_2, P_3	Fibronectin
Chlamydia sp.	Cell surface lectin	*N*-acetylglucosamine
Mycoplasma pneumoniae	Protein P1	Sialic acid
Vibrio cholerae	Type 4 pili	Fucose and mannose

LTA, Lipoteichoic acid.

protein machinery for virulence within a pathogenicity island of deoxyribonucleic acid (DNA). **Pathogenicity islands** are large, chromosomal regions that contain sets of genes encoding numerous virulence factors. In many cases a virulence process requiring coordinated expression of several genes is encoded in a pathogenicity island. These genes may be turned on by a single stimulus (e.g., the temperature of the gut, pH of a lysosome) and can be transferred as a unit to different sites within a chromosome or to other bacteria. Pathogenicity islands found in other bacteria encode different sets of virulence genes.

Pathogenic Actions of Bacteria

TISSUE DESTRUCTION

By-products of bacterial growth, especially fermentation, result in the production of acids, gas, and other substances that are toxic to tissue. In addition, **many bacteria release degradative enzymes** to break down tissue, thereby providing food for the growth of the organisms and promoting the spread of the bacteria, especially if blood vessels are involved. For example, *Clostridium perfringens* organisms are part of the normal flora of the GI tract but are also opportunistic pathogens that can establish infection in oxygen-depleted tissues and cause gas gangrene. These anaerobic bacteria produce enzymes (e.g., phospholipase C, collagenase, protease, hyaluronidase), several toxins, and acid and gas from bacterial metabolism, which destroy the tissue. Staphylococci produce many different enzymes that modify the tissue environment. These enzymes include hyaluronidase, fibrinolysin, and lipases. Streptococci also produce enzymes, including streptolysins S and O, hyaluronidase, DNAases, and streptokinases; these enzymes facilitate the development of infection and spread into the tissue.

TOXINS

Toxins are bacterial products that directly harm tissue or trigger destructive biologic activities. Toxin and toxinlike activities are caused by degradative enzymes that cause lysis of cells, and specific receptor-binding proteins that initiate toxic reactions in a specific target tissue. In addition, cell wall components initiate a systemic response (e.g., fever) by promoting the inappropriate release of cytokines. In many cases, the toxin is completely responsible for causing the characteristic symptoms of the disease. For example, the **preformed toxin** present in food mediates the food poisoning caused by *S. aureus* and *Bacillus cereus* and the botulism caused by *Clostridium botulinum.* The symptoms caused by preformed toxin occur much sooner than for other forms of gastroenteritis, because the effect is like eating a poison and the bacteria do not need to grow for the symptoms to occur. Because a toxin can be spread systemically through the bloodstream, symptoms may arise at a site distant from the site of infection, such as occurs in tetanus, which is caused by *Clostridium tetani,* or the toxin can be disseminated throughout the body, as occurs in the staphylococcal scalded skin syndrome.

ENDOTOXIN AND OTHER CELL WALL COMPONENTS

The presence of bacterial cell wall components is a powerful multialarm warning to the body as a signal of infection to activate the host's protective systems. The molecular patterns in these structures **(pathogen-associated molecular patterns [PAMPs])** bind to Toll-Like Receptor (TLR) molecules on myeloid cells and stimulate the production of cytokines. In some cases, the host response is excessive and may even be life threatening. On infection with gram-positive bacteria, **peptidoglycan** and its breakdown products, as well as **teichoic** and **lipoteichoic acids,** are released, and these stimulate endotoxin-like **pyrogenic acute-phase responses.** The **lipopolysaccharide** (LPS) produced by gram-negative bacteria is an even more powerful activator of acute-phase and inflammatory reactions and is termed **endotoxin. The lipid A portion of LPS** is responsible for endotoxin activity. It is important to appreciate that endotoxin is not the same as exotoxin and that *only gram-negative bacteria make endotoxin.*

Gram-negative bacteria release endotoxin during infection. Endotoxin binds to specific receptors (CD14 and TLR4) on macrophages, B cells, and other cells and stimulates the production and release of **acute-phase cytokines,** such as IL-1, TNF-α, IL-6, and prostaglandins (Figure 19–2). Endotoxin also stimulates the growth (mitogenic) of B cells.

At low concentrations, endotoxin stimulates the mounting of protective responses, such as fever, vasodilatation, and the activation of immune and inflammatory responses (Box 19–2). However, the endotoxin levels in the blood of patients with **gram-negative bacterial sepsis** (bacteria in the blood) can be very high, and the response to these can be overpowering, resulting in shock and possibly death. High concentrations of endotoxin can also activate the alternative pathway of complement; promote high fever, hypotension, and shock, produced by vasodilatation and capillary leakage; and disseminate intravascular coagulation stemming from the activation of blood coagulation pathways. The high fever, petechiae (skin lesions resulting from capillary leakage), and potential symptoms of shock (resulting from

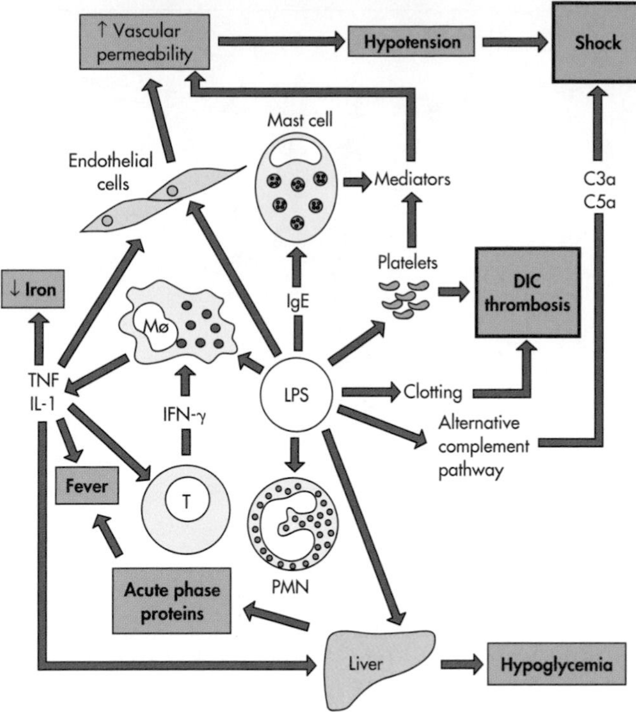

FIGURE 19–2. The many activities of lipopolysaccharide (LPS). This bacterial endotoxin activates almost every immune mechanism, as well as the clotting pathway, which together make LPS one of the most powerful immune stimuli known. DIC, Disseminated intravascular coagulation; IFN-γ interferon-γ; IgE, immunoglobulin E; IL-1, interleukin-1; PMN, polymorphonuclear (neutrophil) leukocytes; TNF, tumor necrosis factor. (Redrawn from Mims C et al: *Medical microbiology,* London, 1993, Mosby-Wolfe.)

BOX 19–2. Endotoxin-Mediated Toxicity

- Fever
- Leukopenia, followed by leukocytosis
- Activation of complement
- Thrombocytopenia
- Disseminated intravascular coagulation
- Decreased peripheral circulation and perfusion to major organs
- Shock
- Death

increased vascular permeability) associated with *Neisseria meningitidis* infection can be related to the large amounts of endotoxin released during infection.

EXOTOXINS

Exotoxins are proteins that can be produced by gram-positive or gram-negative bacteria and include cytolytic enzymes and receptor-binding proteins that alter a function or kill the cell. In many cases, the toxin gene is encoded on a plasmid (tetanus toxin of *C. tetani,* LT and ST toxins of enterotoxigenic *E. coli*) or a lysogenic phage (*Corynebacterium diphtheriae* and *C. botulinum*). An example of a cytolytic enzyme is the α-toxin (phospholipase C) produced by *C. perfringens,* which breaks down sphingomyelin and other membrane phospholipids, resulting in cell lysis.

Many toxins are dimeric with A and B subunits **(A-B toxins).** The B portion of the A-B toxins binds to a specific cell surface receptor, and then the A subunit is transferred into the interior of the cell, where cell injury is induced. The tissues targeted by these toxins are very defined and limited (Figure 19–3 and Table 19–3). The biochemical targets of A-B toxins include ribosomes, transport mechanisms, and intracellular signaling (cyclic adenosine monophosphate [cAMP] production, G protein function), with effects ranging from diarrhea to loss of neuronal function to death. The functional properties of cytolytic and other exotoxins are discussed in greater detail in the chapters dealing with the specific diseases involved.

Superantigens are a special group of toxins (Figure 19–4). These molecules activate T cells by binding simultaneously to a T-cell receptor and a major histocompatibility complex class II (MHC II) molecule on another cell without requiring antigen. *This nonspecific means of activating T cells can trigger life-threatening autoimmune-like responses by stimulating the release of large amounts of interleukins,* such as IL-1 and IL-2. This superantigen stimulation of T cells can also lead to death of the activated T cells, resulting in the loss of specific T-cell clones and the loss of their immune responses. Superantigens include the toxic shock syndrome toxin of *S. aureus,* staphylococcal enterotoxins, and the erythrogenic toxin A or C of *S. pyogenes.*

Immunopathogenesis

In many cases, the symptoms of a bacterial infection are produced by excessive immune and inflammatory responses triggered by the infection. As described earlier, the acute-phase response to cell wall components, especially endotoxin, is a protective antibacterial response when limited and controlled. However, when systemic and out of control, the acute-phase response can cause life-threatening symptoms associated with sepsis and meningitis (see Figure 19–2). Tissue damage induced by neutrophils, macrophage, and complement at the site of the infection and granuloma formation induced by CD4 T cells and macrophages for *Mycobacterium tuberculosis* can lead to tissue destruction. The bacterial M protein of *S. pyogenes* antigenically mimics heart tissue, such that anti-M protein antibodies cross-react with and can initiate damage to the heart to cause rheumatic fever. Immune complexes deposited in the glomeruli of the kidney cause poststreptococcal glomerulonephritis. For *Chlamydia,*

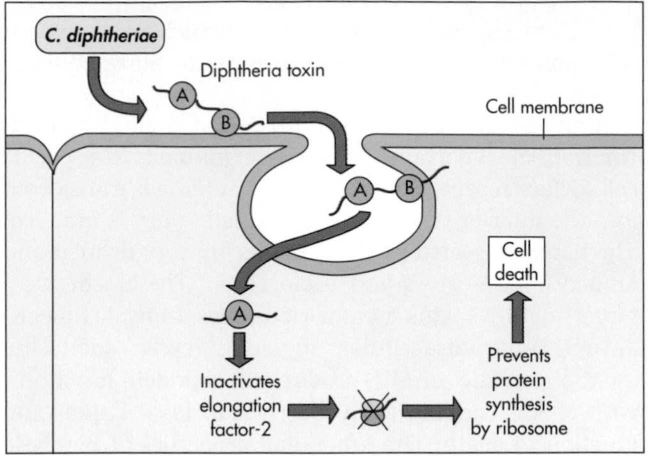

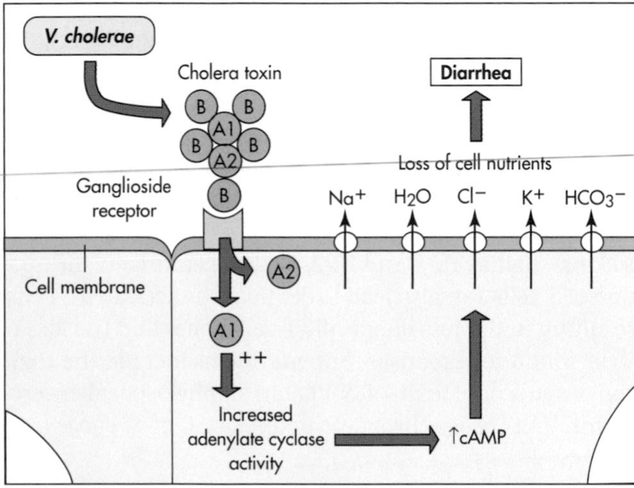

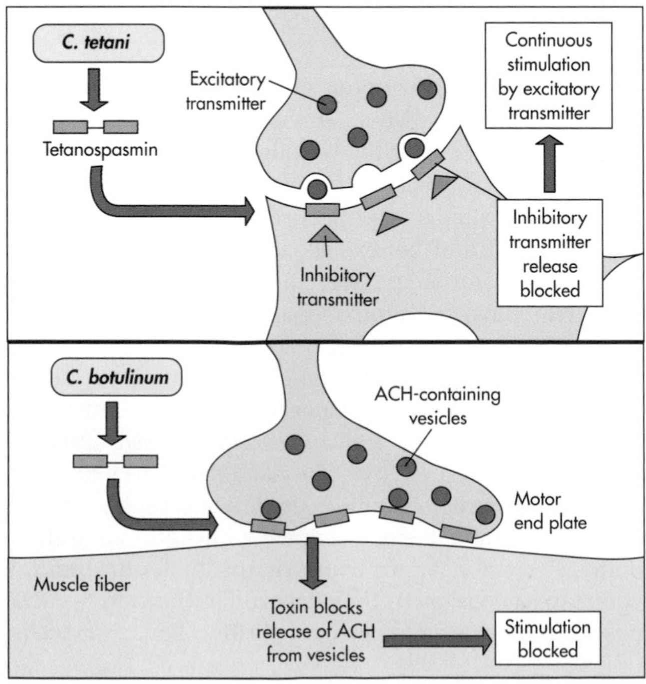

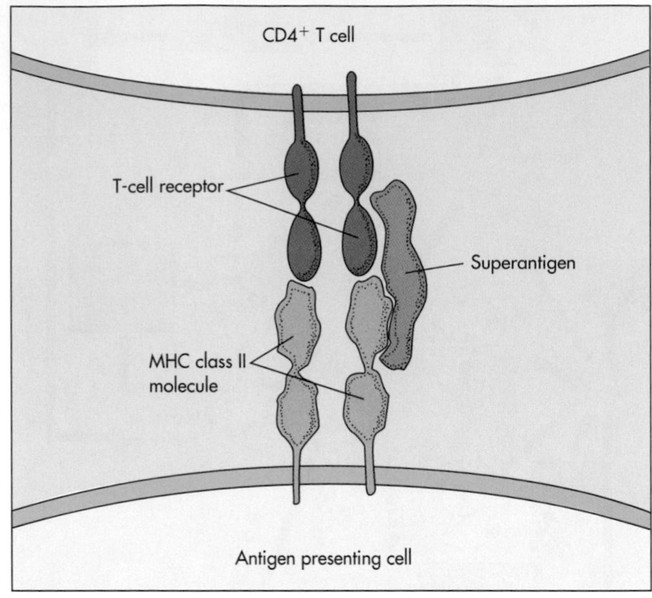

FIGURE 19–4. Superantigen binding to the external regions of the T-cell receptor and the major histocompatibility complex class II (MHC II) molecules.

Treponema (syphilis), *Borrelia* (Lyme disease), and other bacteria the host immune response is an important cause of disease symptoms in patients.

Mechanisms for Escaping Host Defenses

Logically, the longer a bacterial infection remains in a host, the more time the bacteria have to grow and also cause damage. Therefore, bacteria that can evade or incapacitate the host defenses have a greater potential for causing disease. Bacteria have developed ways to avoid the major antibacterial defenses by evading recognition and killing by phagocytic cells, by inactivating or evading the complement system and antibody, and even by growing inside cells to hide from these host responses (Box 19–3).

The capsule is one of the most important virulence factors (Box 19–4). These slime layers function by shielding the bacteria from immune and phagocytic responses. Capsules are usually made of polysaccharides, which are usually poor immunogens. The *S. pyogenes* capsule, for example, is made of hyaluronic acid, which mimics human connective tissue, thereby masking the bacteria

FIGURE 19–3. The mode of action of dimeric A-B exotoxins. The bacterial A-B toxins often consist of a two-chain molecule. The B chain promotes entry of the bacteria into cells, and the A chain has inhibitory activity against some vital function. ACH, Acetylcholine; cAMP, cyclic adenosine monophosphate. (Redrawn From Mims C et al: *Medical microbiology,* London, 1993, Mosby-Wolfe.)

TABLE 19–3. Properties of A-B Type Bacterial Toxins

Toxin	Organism	Gene Location	Subunit Structure	Target Cell Receptor	Biologic Effects
Anthrax toxins	*Bacillus anthracis*	Plasmid	Three separate proteins (EF, LF, PA)	Unknown, probably glycoprotein	EF + PA: increase in target cell cAMP level, localized edema; LF + PA: death of target cells and experimental animals
Bordetella adenylate cyclase toxin	*Bordetella* sp.	Chromosomal	A-B	Unknown, probably glycolipid	Increase in target cell cAMP level, modified cell function or cell death
Botulinum toxin	*Clostridium* botulinum	Phage	A-B	Possibly ganglioside (GD_{1b})	Decrease in peripheral, presynaptic acetylcholine release, flaccid paralysis
Cholera toxin	*Vibrio cholerae*	Chromosomal	A-5B	Ganglioside (GM_1)	Activation of adenylate cyclase, increase in cAMP level, secretory diarrhea
Diphtheria toxin	*Corynebacterium diphtheriae*	Phage	A-B	Growth factor receptor precursor	Inhibition of protein synthesis, cell death
Heat-labile enterotoxins	*Escherichia coli*	Plasmid	Similar or identical to cholera toxin		
Pertussis toxin	*Bordetella pertussis*	Chromosomal	A-5B	Unknown, probably glycoprotein	Block of signal transduction mediated by target G proteins
Pseudomonas exotoxin A	*Pseudomonas aeruginosa*	Chromosomal	A-B	Unknown, but different from diphtheria toxin	Similar or identical to diphtheria toxin
Shiga toxin	*Shigella dysenteriae*	Chromosomal	A-5B	Glycoprotein or glycolipid	Inhibition of protein synthesis, cell death
Shiga toxins	*Enterohemorrhagic E. coli*	Phage	Similar or identical to Shiga toxin		
Tetanus toxin	*Clostridium tetani*	Plasmid	A-B	Ganglioside (GT_1) and/or GD_{1b}	Decrease in neurotransmitter release from inhibitory neurons, spastic paralysis

Modified from Mandell G, Douglas G, Bennett J: *Principles and practice of infectious disease,* ed 3, New York, 1990, Churchill Livingstone.
cAMP, Cyclic adenosine monophosphate.

BOX 19–3. Microbial Defenses Against Host Immunologic Clearance

Encapsulation
Antigenic mimicry
Antigenic masking
Antigenic shift
Production of antiimmunoglobulin proteases
Destruction of phagocyte
Inhibition of chemotaxis
Inhibition of phagocytosis
Inhibition of phagolysosome fusion
Resistance to lysosomal enzymes
Intracellular replication

BOX 19–4. Examples of Encapsulated Microorganisms

Staphylococcus aureus
Streptococcus pneumoniae
Streptococcus pyogenes (group A)
Streptococcus agalactiae (group B)
Bacillus anthracis
Bacillus subtilis
Neisseria gonorrhoeae
Neisseria meningitidis
Haemophilus influenzae
Escherichia coli
Klebsiella pneumoniae
Salmonella sp.
Yersinia pestis
Campylobacter fetus
Pseudomonas aeruginosa
Bacteroides fragilis
Cryptococcus neoformans (yeast)

and keeping them from being recognized by the immune system. The capsule also acts like a slimy football jersey, in that it is hard to grasp and tears away when grabbed by a phagocyte. The capsule also protects a bacterium from destruction within the phagolysosome of a macrophage or leukocyte. All of these properties can extend the time bacteria spend in blood (bacteremia) before being eliminated by host responses. Mutants of normally encapsulated bacteria that lose the ability to make a capsule also lose their virulence; examples of such bacteria are *Streptococcus pneumoniae* and *N. meningitidis.* A biofilm, which is made from capsular material, can prevent antibody and complement from getting to the bacteria.

Bacteria can evade antibody responses by **intracellular growth, antigenic variation,** or by **inactivation of antibody or complement.** Bacteria that grow intracellularly include mycobacteria, francisellae, brucellae, chlamydiae, and rickettsiae. Unlike most bacteria, control of these infections requires TH1 T-helper cell immune responses, which activate macrophages to kill or create a wall around the infected cell (as for *Mycobacterium tuberculosis*). *Neisseria gonorrhoeae* can vary the structure of surface antigens to evade antibody responses and also produces a protease that degrades immunoglobulin A (IgA). By degrading the C5a component of complement, *Streptococcus pyogenes* can limit the chemotaxis of leukocytes to the site of infection.

Phagocytes (neutrophil, macrophage) are an important antibacterial defense, but many bacteria can circumvent phagocytic killing in various ways. They can produce enzymes capable of lysing phagocytic cells (e.g., the streptolysin produced by *S. pyogenes* or the α-toxin produced by *C. perfringens*). They can inhibit phagocytosis (e.g., the effects of the **capsule** and the **M protein** produced by *S. pyogenes*) or block intracellular killing. Bacterial mechanisms for protection from intracellular killing include blocking phagolysosome fusion to prevent contact with its bactericidal contents (*Mycobacterium* species), capsule-mediated or enzymatic resistance to the bactericidal lysosomal enzymes or substances, and the ability to exit the phagosome into the host cytoplasm before being exposed to lysosomal enzymes (Table 19–4 and Figure 19–5). For example, staphylococci produce catalase, an enzyme that makes the myeloperoxidase system less effective. Many of the bacteria that are internalized but survive phagocytosis can use the cell as a place to grow and to hide from immune responses and as a means of being disseminated throughout the body.

Other important host defenses subverted by bacteria include the alternate pathway of complement and antibody. Bacteria evade complement action by masking themselves and by inhibiting activation of the cascade. The long O antigen of LPS prevents the complement from

TABLE 19–4. Methods That Circumvent Phagocytic Killing

Method	Example
Inhibition of phagolysome fusion	*Legionella* sp., *Mycobacterium tuberculosis, Chlamydia* sp.
Resistance to lysosomal enzymes	*Salmonella typhimurium, Coxiella* sp., *Ehrlichia* sp., *Mycobacterium leprae, Leishmania* sp.
Adaptation to cytoplasmic replication	*Listeria, Francisella,* and *Rickettsia* spp.

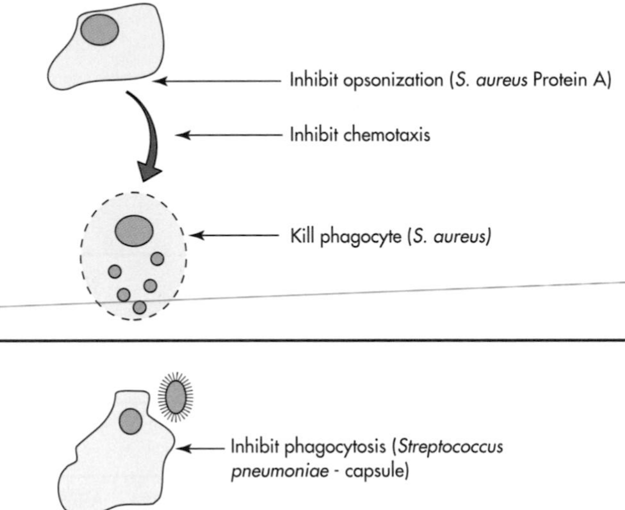

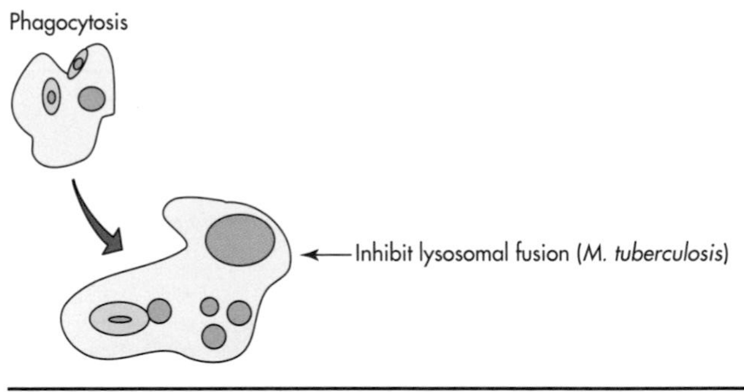

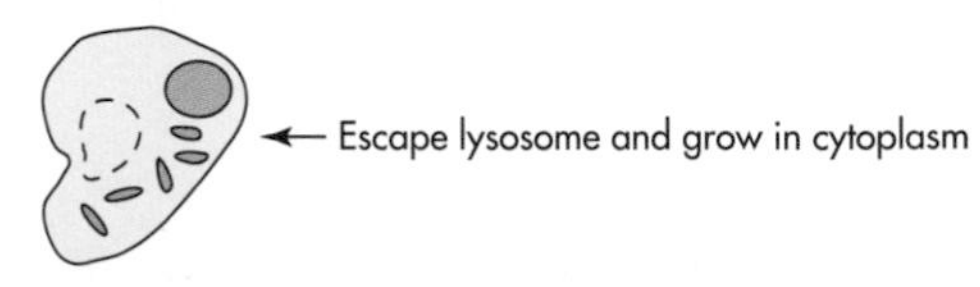

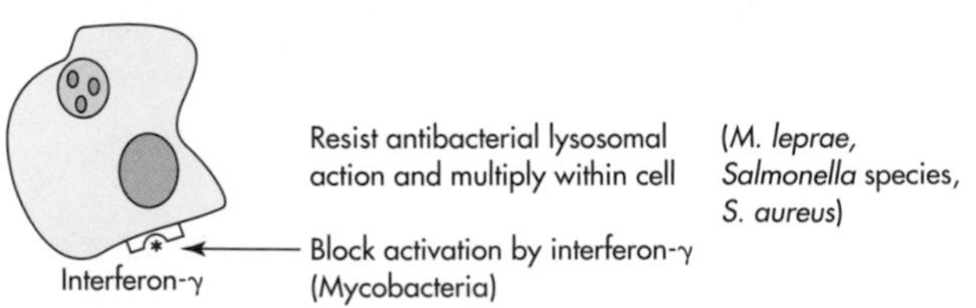

FIGURE 19–5. Bacterial mechanisms for escaping phagocytic clearance. Selected examples of bacteria that use the indicated antiphagocytic mechanisms are given.

BOX 19–5. Examples of Intracellular Pathogens

Mycobacterium sp.	*Listeria monocytogenes*
Brucella sp.	*Salmonella typhi*
Francisella sp.	*Shigella dysenteriae*
Rickettsiae sp.	*Yersinia pestis*
Chlamydia sp.	*Legionella pneumophila*

gaining access to the membrane and protects gram-negative bacteria from damage. Immunoglobulin A antibody is inactivated by an IgA-specific protease made by *N. gonorrhoeae. S. aureus* makes an immunoglobulin G–binding protein, protein A, which masks the bacteria and thereby prevents antibody action.

S. aureus can also escape host defenses by walling off the site of infection. *S. aureus* can produce coagulase, an enzyme that promotes the conversion of fibrin to fibrinogen to produce a clotlike barrier; this feature distinguishes *S. aureus* from *S. epidermidis. M. tuberculosis* is able to survive in a host by promoting the development of a granuloma, within which viable bacteria may reside for the life of the infected person. The bacteria may resume growth if there is a decline in the immune status of the person.

Summary

The primary virulence factors of bacteria are the capsule, adhesins, invasins, degradative enzymes, toxins, and mechanisms for escaping elimination by host defenses. Bacteria may only have one virulence mechanism. For example, *C. diphtheriae* has only one virulence mechanism, which is diphtheria toxin. Other bacteria express many virulence factors. *S. aureus* is an example of such a bacterium; it expresses adhesins, degradative enzymes, toxins, catalase, and coagulase, which are responsible for producing a spectrum of diseases. In addition, different strains within a bacterial species may express different virulence mechanisms. For example, the symptoms and sequelae of gastroenteritis (diarrhea) caused by *E. coli* may include invasion and bloody stools, cholera-like watery stools, and even severe hemorrhagic disease, depending on the specific infecting strain.

QUESTIONS

1. Name three routes by which exogenous pathogens can infect a person. List five examples of organisms that use each route.
2. How are microbes able to resist immunologic clearance? Give at least one specific example of each mechanism.
3. What are the two general types of exotoxins? List examples of each type.

Bibliography

Finlay BB, Falkow S: Common themes in microbial pathogenicity revisited, *Microbiol Mol Biol Rev* 61:136-169, 1997.

Gorbach SL, Bartlett JG, Blacklow NR: *Infectious diseases,* ed 2, Philadelphia, 1997, WB Saunders.

Groisman EA, Ochman H: How *Salmonella* became a pathogen, *Trends Microbiol* 5:343-349, 1997.

Lee CA: Pathogenicity islands and the evolution of bacterial pathogens, *Infect Agents Dis* 5:1-7, 1996.

Mandell GL, Bennet JE, Dolin R, editors: *Principles and practice of infectious diseases,* ed 6, Philadelphia, 2005, Churchill Livingstone.

McClane BA et al: *Microbial pathogenesis: A principles-oriented approach,* Madison, Conn, 1999, part of Blackwell Science Inc. Fence Creek Publishing.

McGee J et al: *Oxford textbook of pathology,* vol 1, Oxford, England, 1992, Oxford University Press.

Papageorgiou AC, Acharya KR: Microbial superantigens: From structure to function, *Trends Microbiol* 8:369-375, 2000.

Strauss JM, Strauss EG: *Viruses and human disease,* San Diego, 2002, Academic Press.

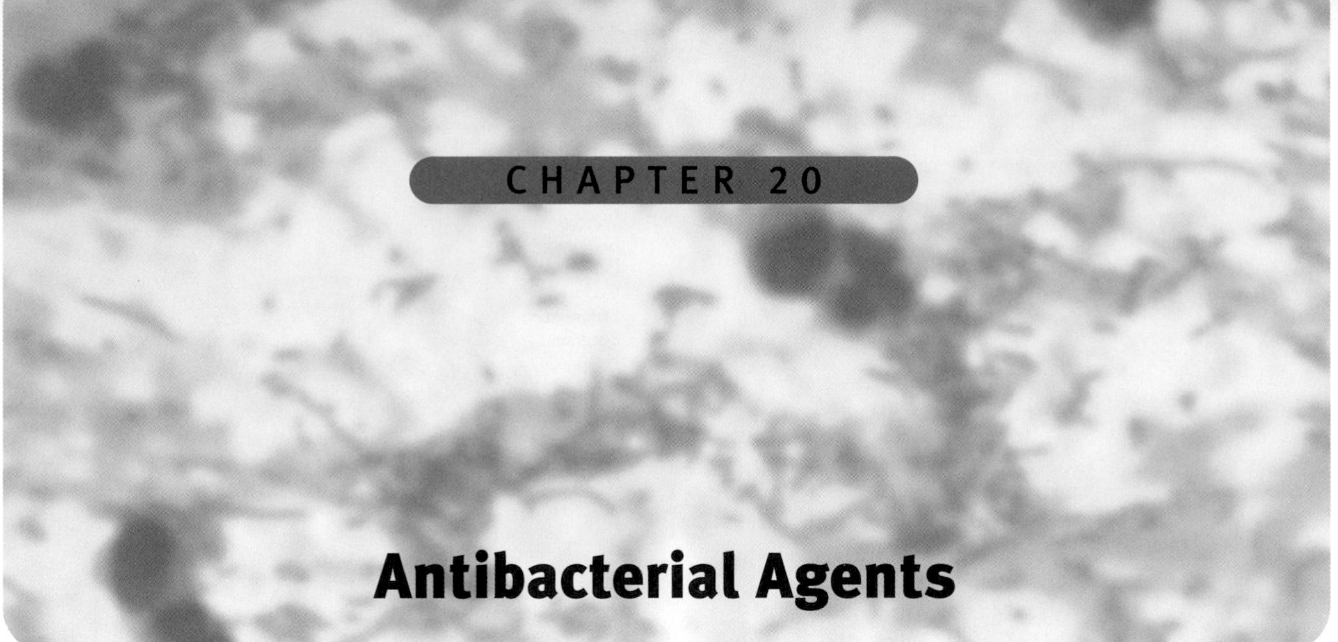

CHAPTER 20

Antibacterial Agents

This chapter provides an overview of the mechanisms of action and antibacterial spectrum of the most commonly used antibiotics, as well as a description of the common mechanisms of bacterial resistance. The terminology appropriate for this discussion is summarized in Box 20–1.

The year 1935 was an important one for the chemotherapy of systemic bacterial infections. Although antiseptics had been applied topically to prevent the growth of microorganisms, systemic bacterial infections had not as yet responded to any existing agents. In 1935, the red azo dye protosil was shown to protect mice against systemic streptococcal infection and to be curative in patients suffering from such infections. It was soon found that protosil was cleaved in the body to release *p*-aminobenzene sulfonamide, or sulfanilamide, which was subsequently shown to have antibacterial activity. These observations regarding the first "sulfa" drug ushered in a new era in medicine. Compounds (antibiotics) produced by microorganisms were eventually discovered to inhibit the growth of other microorganisms. For example, Alexander Fleming was the first to note that the mold *Penicillium* prevented the multiplication of staphylococci. A concentrate from a culture of this mold was prepared, and the remarkable antibacterial activity and lack of toxicity of the first antibiotic, penicillin, were demonstrated. Streptomycin and the tetracyclines were developed in the 1940s and 1950s, followed rapidly by the development of additional aminoglycosides, semisynthetic penicillins, cephalosporins, quinolones, and other antimicrobials. All these antibacterial agents greatly increased the range of infectious diseases that could be prevented or cured.

Despite the rapidity with which new chemotherapeutic agents are introduced, bacteria have shown a remarkable ability to develop resistance to these agents. Thus antibiotic therapy will not be the magical cure for all infections, as predicted; rather, it is only one weapon, albeit an important one, against infectious diseases. It is also important to recognize that because resistance to antibiotics is often not predictable, physicians must rely on their clinical experience for the initial selection of empirical therapy. Guidelines for the management of infections caused by specific organisms are discussed in the relevant chapters of this text.

The results of in vitro antimicrobial susceptibility testing are valuable for selecting chemotherapeutic agents active against the infecting organism. Extensive work has been performed in an effort to standardize the testing methods and improve the clinical predictive value of the results. Despite these efforts, the in vitro tests are simply a measurement of the effect of the antibiotic against the organism under specific conditions. The selection of an antibiotic and the patient's outcome are influenced by a variety of interrelated factors, including the pharmacokinetic properties of the antibiotic, drug toxicity, the clinical disease, and the patient's general medical status. The basic mechanisms and sites of antibiotic activity are summarized in Table 20–1 and Figure 20–1, respectively.

Inhibition of Cell Wall Synthesis

By far, the most common mechanism of antibiotic activity is interference with bacterial cell wall synthesis. Most of the cell wall–active antibiotics are classified as β-lactam antibiotics (e.g., penicillins, cephalosporins, cephamycins, carbapenems, monobactams, β-lactamase inhibitors), so named because they share a common β-lactam ring structure. Other antibiotics that interfere with construction of the bacterial cell wall include vancomycin, bacitracin, and the following antimycobacterial agents: isoniazid, ethambutol, cycloserine, and ethionamide.

BOX 20–1. Terminology

Antibacterial spectrum: Range of activity of an antimicrobial against bacteria. A **broad-spectrum** antibacterial drug can inhibit a variety of gram-positive and gram-negative bacteria, whereas a **narrow-spectrum** drug is active only against a limited variety of bacteria.

Bacteriostatic activity: Level of antimicrobial activity that **inhibits** the growth of an organism. This is determined in vitro by testing a standardized concentration of organisms against a series of antimicrobial dilutions. The lowest concentration that inhibits the growth of the organism is referred to as the **minimum inhibitory concentration (MIC).**

Bactericidal activity: Level of antimicrobial activity that **kills** the test organism. This is determined in vitro by exposing a standardized concentration of organisms to a series of antimicrobial dilutions. The lowest concentration that kills 99.9% of the population is referred to as the **minimum bactericidal concentration (MBC).**

Antibiotic combinations: Combinations of antibiotics that may be used to (1) broaden the antibacterial spectrum for empirical therapy or the treatment of polymicrobial infections, (2) prevent the emergence of resistant organisms during therapy, and (3) achieve a synergistic killing effect.

Antibiotic synergism: Combinations of two antibiotics that have enhanced bactericidal activity when tested together compared with the activity of each antibiotic.

Antibiotic antagonism: Combination of antibiotics in which the activity of one antibiotic interferes with the activity of the other (e.g., the sum of the activity is less than the activity of the most active individual drug).

β-Lactamase: An enzyme that hydrolyzes the β-lactam ring in the β-lactam class of antibiotics, thus inactivating the antibiotic. The enzymes specific for penicillins, cephalosporins, and carbapenems are the **penicillinases, cephalosporinases,** and **carbapenemases** (metallo-β-lactamases), respectively.

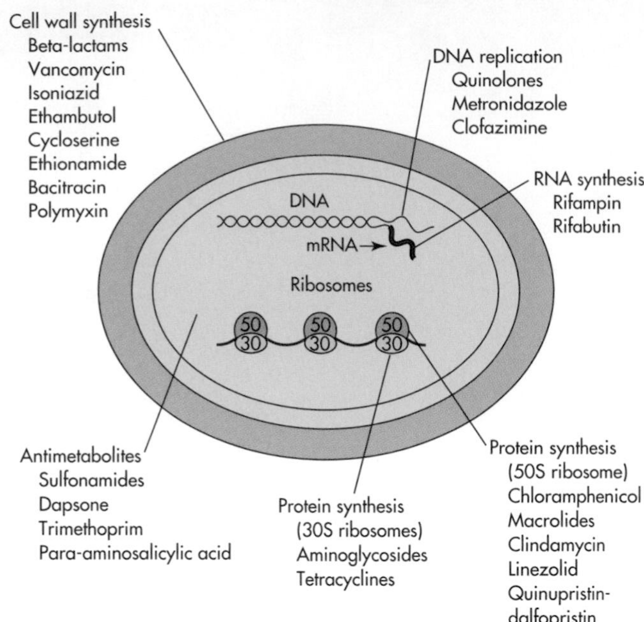

FIGURE 20–1. Basic sites of antibiotic activity.

β-LACTAM ANTIBIOTICS

The major structural component of bacterial cell walls is the peptidoglycan layer. The basic structure is a chain of 10 to 65 disaccharide residues consisting of alternating molecules of *N*-acetylglucosamine and *N*-acetylmuramic acid. These chains are then cross-linked with peptide bridges that create a rigid mesh coating for the bacteria. The building of the chains and cross-links is catalyzed by specific enzymes (e.g., transpeptidases, transglycosylases, carboxypeptidases) that are members of a large family of serine proteases. These regulatory enzymes are also called **penicillin-binding proteins (PBPs)** because they can be bound by β-lactam antibiotics. When growing bacteria are exposed to these antibiotics, the antibiotic binds to specific PBPs in the bacterial cell wall and inhibits formation of cross-links between peptidoglycan chains. This in turn activates autolysins that degrade the cell wall, resulting in bacterial cell death. Thus the β-lactam antibiotics generally act as bactericidal agents.

Bacteria can become resistant to β-lactam antibiotics by three general mechanisms: (1) prevention of the interaction between the antibiotic and the target PBP, (2) modification of the binding of the antibiotic to the PBP, and (3) hydrolysis of the antibiotic by β-lactamases. The first mechanism of resistance is seen only in gram-negative bacteria (particularly *Pseudomonas* species), because they have an outer membrane that overlies the peptidoglycan layer. Penetration of β-lactam antibiotics into gram-negative rods requires transit through pores in the outer membrane. Changes in the proteins **(porins)** that form the walls of the pores can alter the size or charge of these channels and result in the exclusion of the antibiotic.

Resistance can also be acquired by modification of the β-lactam antibiotic binding to the PBP. This can be mediated by (1) an overproduction of PBP (a rare occurrence); (2) acquisition of a new PBP (e.g., methicillin resistance in *Staphylococcus aureus*); or (3) modification of an existing PBP through recombination (e.g., penicillin resistance in *Streptococcus pneumoniae*) or a point mutation (penicillin resistance in *Enterococcus faecium*).

Finally, bacteria can produce **β-lactamases** that inactivate the β-lactam antibiotics. Interestingly, the β-lactamases are in the same family of serine proteases as the PBPs. More than 200 different β-lactamases have been described. Some are specific for penicillins (i.e., penicillinases), cephalosporins (i.e., cephalosporinases), or carbapenems (i.e., carbapenemases), whereas others have a broad range of activity, including some that are capable of inactivating most β-lactam antibiotics. An

TABLE 20–1. Basic Mechanisms of Antibiotic Action

Antibiotic	Action
Disruption of Cell Wall	
Penicillin Cephalosporin Cephamycin Carbapenem Monobactam	Binds PBPs and enzymes responsible for peptidoglycan synthesis
β-lactam/β-lactamase inhibitor	Binds β-lactamases and prevents enzymatic inactivation of β-lactam
Vancomycin	Inhibits cross-linkage of peptidoglycan layers
Isoniazid Ethionamide	Inhibits mycolic acid synthesis
Ethambutol	Inhibits arabinogalactan synthesis
Cycloserine	Inhibits cross-linkage of peptidoglycan layers
Polymyxin	Inhibits bacterial membranes
Bacitracin	Inhibits bacterial cytoplasmic membrane and movement of peptidoglycan precursors
Inhibition of Protein Synthesis	
Aminoglycoside	Produces premature release of aberrant peptide chains from 30S ribosome
Tetracycline	Prevents polypeptide elongation at 30S ribosome
Oxazolidinone	Prevents initiation of protein synthesis at 50S ribosome
Macrolide Clindamycin Streptogramins	Prevents polypeptide elongation at 50S ribosome
Inhibition of Nucleic Acid Synthesis	
Quinolone	Binds α subunit of DNA gyrase
Rifampin Rifabutin	Prevents transcription by binding DNA-dependent RNA polymerase
Metronidazole	Disrupts bacteria DNA (is cytotoxic compound)
Antimetabolite	
Sulfonamide	Inhibits dihydropteroate synthase and disrupts folic acid synthesis
Dapsone	Inhibits dihydropteroate synthase
Trimethoprim	Inhibits dihydrofolate reductase and disrupts folic acid synthesis

DNA, Deoxyribonucleic acid; PBPs, penicillin-binding proteins; RNA, ribonucleic acid.

exhaustive discussion of β-lactamases is beyond the scope of this chapter; however, a brief discussion is germane for understanding the limitations of β-lactam antibiotics. By one classification scheme, β-lactamases have been separated into four classes (A to D). The most common class A β-lactamases are SHV-1 and TEM-1, penicillinases found in common gram-negative rods (e.g., *Escherichia, Klebsiella*), with minimal activity against cephalosporins. Unfortunately, simple point mutations in the genes encoding these enzymes have created β-lactamases with activity against all penicillins and cephalosporins. These β-lactamases are referred to as **extended-spectrum β-lactamases (ESBLs)** and are particularly troublesome because they are encoded on plasmids that can be transferred from organism to organism. The class B β-lactamases are zinc-dependent metalloenzymes that have a broad spectrum of activity against all β-lactam antibiotics, including the cephamycins and carbapenems. The class C β-lactamases are primarily cephalosporinases that are encoded on the bacterial chromosome. Expression of these enzymes is generally repressed, although this can be altered by exposure to certain "inducing" β-lactam antibiotics or by mutations in the genes controlling expression of the enzymes. Expression of this class of β-lactamases is particularly troublesome because they are active against the most potent expanded-spectrum cephalosporins. The class D β-lactamases are penicillinases found primarily in gram-negative rods.

Penicillins

Penicillin antibiotics (Table 20–2) are highly effective antibiotics with an extremely low toxicity. The basic compound is an organic acid with a β-lactam ring obtained from culture of the mold *Penicillium chrysogenum.* If the mold is grown by a fermentation process, large amounts of 6-aminopenicillanic acid (the β-lactam ring is fused with a thiazolidine ring) are produced. The biochemical modification of this intermediate yields derivatives that have decreased acid lability and increased absorption in the gastrointestinal tract, resistance to destruction by penicillinase, or a broader spectrum of activity that includes gram-negative bacteria.

Penicillin G is incompletely absorbed because it is inactivated by gastric acid. Thus it is used mainly as an intravenous drug for the treatment of infections caused by the limited number of susceptible organisms. Penicillin V is more resistant to acid and is the preferred oral form for the treatment of susceptible bacteria. **Penicillinase-resistant penicillins** such as methicillin and oxacillin are used to treat infections caused by susceptible staphylococci. Ampicillin was the first **broad-spectrum penicillin,** although the spectrum of activity against gram-negative rods was limited primarily to *Escherichia, Proteus,* and *Haemophilus* species. Other penicillins (e.g., carbenicillin, ticarcillin, piperacillin) that have been developed are effective against a broader range of gram-negative bacteria, including *Klebsiella, Enterobacter,* and *Pseudomonas* species.

Selected penicillins have been combined with **β-lactamase inhibitors.** The β-lactamase inhibitors (e.g., clavulanic acid, sulbactam, tazobactam) are relatively inactive by themselves but, when combined with some penicillins (i.e., ampicillin, amoxicillin, ticarcillin, piperacillin), are effective in treating some infections caused by β-lactamase–producing bacteria. The inhibitors irreversibly bind and inactivate susceptible bacterial β-lactamases (although not all are bound by these inhibitors), permitting the companion drug to disrupt bacterial cell wall synthesis.

Cephalosporins and Cephamycins

The cephalosporins (Table 20–3) are β-lactam antibiotics derived from 7-aminocephalosporanic acid (the β-lactam ring is fused with a dihydrothiazine ring) that was originally isolated from the mold *Cephalosporium.* The cephamycins are closely related to the cephalosporins, except that they contain oxygen in place of sulfur in the dihydrothiazine ring, rendering them more stable to β-lactamase hydrolysis. The cephalosporins and cephamycins have the same mechanism of action as the penicillins; however, they have a wider antibacterial spectrum, are resistant to many β-lactamases, and have improved pharmacokinetic properties (e.g., longer half-life).

Biochemical modifications in the basic antibiotic molecule resulted in the development of antibiotics with improved activity and pharmacokinetic properties. The cephalosporins have enhanced activity against gram-negative bacteria compared with the penicillins. This activity in turn varies among the different "generations" of cephalosporins. The activity of **narrow-spectrum,** first-generation antibiotics is primarily restricted to *Escherichia coli, Klebsiella* species, *Proteus mirabilis,* and oxacillin-susceptible gram-positive cocci. Many of the

TABLE 20–2. Penicillins

Antibiotics	Spectrum of Activity
Natural penicillins: benzylpenicillin (penicillin G), phenoxymethyl penicillin (penicillin V)	Active against all β-hemolytic streptococci and most other species; limited activity against staphylococci; active against meningococci and most gram-positive anaerobes; poor activity against aerobic and anaerobic gram-negative rods
Penicillinase-resistant penicillins: methicillin, nafcillin, oxacillin, cloxacillin, dicloxacillin	Similar to the natural penicillins, except enhanced activity against staphylococci
Broad-spectrum penicillins: aminopenicillins (ampicillin, amoxicillin, carbenicillin, ticarcillin); ureidopenicillins (piperacillin)	Activity against gram-positive cocci equivalent to the natural penicillins; active against some gram-negative rods with piperacillin the most active
β-Lactam with β-lactamase inhibitor (ampicillin-sulbactam, amoxicillin-clavulanate, ticarcillin-clavulanate, piperacillin-tazobactam)	Activity similar to natural β-lactams, plus improved activity against β-lactamase producing staphylococci and selected gram-negative rods; not all β-lactamases are inhibited; piperacillin/tazobactam is the most active

TABLE 20–3. Selected Examples of Cephalosporins and Cephamycins

Antibiotics	Spectrum of Activity
Narrow spectrum (cephalexin, cephalothin, cefazolin, cephapirin, cephradine)	Activity equivalent to oxacillin against gram-positive bacteria; some gram-negative activity (e.g., *Escherichia coli, Klebsiella, Proteus mirabilis*)
Expanded-spectrum cephalosporins (cefaclor, cefuroxime)	Activity equivalent to oxacillin against gram-positive bacteria; improved gram-negative activity to include *Enterobacter, Citrobacter,* and additional *Proteus* species
Expanded-spectrum cephamycins (cefotetan, cefoxitin)	Activity similar to expanded-spectrum cephalosporins but less susceptible to β-lactamases
Broad spectrum (cefixime, cefotaxime, ceftriaxone, ceftazidime)	Activity equivalent to oxacillin against gram-positive bacteria; improved gram-negative activity to include *Pseudomonas*
Extended spectrum (cefepime, cefpirome)	Activity equivalent to oxacillin against gram-positive bacteria; marginally improved gram-negative activity

TABLE 20–4. Other β-Lactam Antibiotics

Antibiotics	Spectrum of Activity
Carbapenems (imipenem, meropenem, ertapenem)	Broad-spectrum antibiotics active against most aerobic and anaerobic gram-positive and gram-negative bacteria except oxacillin-resistant staphylococci, most *Enterococcus faecium,* and selected gram-negative rods (e.g., some *Burkholderia, Stenotrophomonas,* some *Pseudomonas*)
Monobactam (aztreonam)	Active against selected aerobic gram-negative rods but inactive against anaerobes or gram-positive cocci

expanded-spectrum, second-generation antibiotics have additional activity against *Haemophilus influenzae; Enterobacter, Citrobacter,* and *Serratia* species; and some anaerobes, such as *Bacteroides fragilis.* The **broad-spectrum,** third-generation antibiotics and **extended-spectrum,** fourth-generation antibiotics are active against most Enterobacteriaceae and *Pseudomonas aeruginosa.* Extended-spectrum antibiotics offer the advantage of increased stability to β-lactamases. Unfortunately, gram-negative bacteria have rapidly developed resistance to most cephalosporins and cephamycins (primarily as the result of β-lactamase production), which has significantly compromised the use of all these agents.

Other β-Lactam Antibiotics

Other classes of β-lactam antibiotics (Table 20–4) are the **carbapenems** (e.g., imipenem, meropenem, ertapenem) and **monobactams** (e.g., aztreonam). The carbapenems are important, widely prescribed broad-spectrum antibiotics that are active against virtually all groups of organisms, with only a few exceptions (e.g., resistance has been reported for all oxacillin-resistant staphylococci, selected Enterobacteriaceae and *Pseudomonas,* and other gram-negative rods). In contrast, the monobactams are narrow-spectrum antibiotics that are active only against aerobic, gram-negative bacteria. Anaerobic bacteria and gram-positive bacteria are resistant. The advantage of narrow-spectrum antibiotics is that they can be used to treat susceptible organisms without disruption of the patient's normal, protective bacterial population. Despite this advantage, monobactams are not widely used.

GLYCOPEPTIDES

Vancomycin, originally obtained from *Streptomyces orientalis,* is a complex glycopeptide that disrupts cell wall peptidoglycan synthesis in growing gram-positive bacteria. Vancomycin interacts with the D-alanine–D-alanine termini of the pentapeptide side chains, which interferes sterically with the formation of the bridges between the peptidoglycan chains. Vancomycin is used for the management of infections caused by oxacillin-resistant staphylococci and other gram-positive bacteria resistant to β-lactam antibiotics. Vancomycin is inactive against gram-negative bacteria because the molecule is too large to pass through the outer membrane pores and reach the peptidoglycan target site. In addition, some organisms are intrinsically resistant to vancomycin (e.g., *Leuconostoc, Lactobacillus, Pediococcus,* and *Erysipelothrix*) because the pentapeptide terminates in D-alanine–D-lactate, which does not bind vancomycin. Intrinsic resistance is also found in some species of enterococci that contain a D-alanine–D-serine terminus (i.e., *Enterococcus gallinarum, Enterococcus casseliflavus*). Finally, some species of enterococci (particularly *Enterococcus faecium* and *Enterococcus* *faecalis*) have acquired resistance to vancomycin. The genes for this resistance (primarily *van*A and *van*B), which also mediate changes in the pentapeptide terminus, can be carried on plasmids and have seriously compromised the usefulness of vancomycin for the treatment of enterococcal infections. More importantly, the gene for vancomycin resistance contained within a transposon on a multiresistance conjugative plasmid has been transferred in vivo from *E. faecalis* to a multiresistant *S. aureus*. The transposon then moved from the *E. faecalis* plasmid and recombined and integrated into the *S. aureus* multiresistance plasmid. This resulted in an *S. aureus* plasmid that encoded resistance to β-lactams, vancomycin, aminoglycosides, and other antibiotics—a plasmid that could be transferred to other staphylococci by conjugation. Obviously, if this resistance becomes widespread, the medical implications are profound.

POLYPEPTIDES

Bacitracin, which was isolated from *Bacillus licheniformis*, is a mixture of polypeptides used in topically applied products (e.g., creams, ointments, sprays) for the treatment of skin infections caused by gram-positive bacteria (particularly those caused by *Staphylococcus* and group A *Streptococcus*). Gram-negative bacteria are resistant to this agent. Bacitracin inhibits cell wall synthesis by interfering with dephosphorylation and the recycling of the lipid carrier responsible for moving the peptidoglycan precursors through the cytoplasmic membrane to the cell wall. It may also damage the bacterial cytoplasmic membrane and inhibit ribonucleic acid (RNA) transcription. Resistance to the antibiotic is most likely caused by failure of the antibiotic to penetrate into the bacterial cell.

The **polymyxins** are a group of cyclic polypeptides derived from *Bacillus polymyxa*. These antibiotics insert into bacterial membranes like detergents, by interacting with lipopolysaccharides and the phospholipids in the outer membrane, producing increased cell permeability and eventual cell death. Polymyxins B and E (colistin) are capable of causing serious nephrotoxicity. Thus their use has been limited chiefly to the external treatment of localized infections such as external otitis, eye infections, and skin infections caused by sensitive organisms. Oral administration is used to sterilize the gut. These antibiotics are most active against gram-negative rods, because gram-positive bacteria do not have an outer membrane.

ISONIAZID, ETHIONAMIDE, ETHAMBUTOL, AND CYCLOSERINE

Isoniazid, ethionamide, ethambutol, and cycloserine are cell wall–active antibiotics used for the treatment of mycobacterial infections. **Isoniazid** (isonicotinic acid hydrazide [INH]) is bactericidal against actively replicating mycobacteria. Although the exact mechanism of action is unknown, the synthesis of mycolic acid is affected (the desaturation of the long-chain fatty acids and the elongation of fatty acids and hydroxy lipids are disrupted). **Ethionamide,** a derivative of INH, also blocks mycolic acid synthesis. **Ethambutol** interferes with the synthesis of arabinogalactan in the cell wall, and **cycloserine** inhibits two enzymes, d-alanine–d-alanine synthetase and alanine racemase, which catalyze cell wall synthesis. Resistance to these four antibiotics results primarily from reduced drug uptake into the bacterial cell or alteration of the target sites.

Inhibition of Protein Synthesis

The primary action of the agents in the second largest class of antibiotics is the inhibition of protein synthesis (see Table 20–1).

AMINOGLYCOSIDES

The aminoglycoside antibiotics (Table 20–5) consist of amino sugars linked through glycosidic bonds to an aminocyclitol ring. Streptomycin, neomycin, kanamycin, and tobramycin were originally isolated from *Streptomyces* species, and gentamicin and sisomicin were isolated from *Micromonospora* species. Amikacin and netilmicin are synthetic derivatives of kanamycin and sisomicin, respectively. These antibiotics exert their effort by passing through the bacterial outer membrane (in gram-negative bacteria), cell wall, and cytoplasmic membrane to the cytoplasm, where they inhibit bacterial protein synthesis by irreversibly binding to the 30S ribosomal proteins. This attachment to the ribosomes has two effects: production of aberrant proteins as the result of misreading of the messenger RNA (mRNA), and interruption of protein synthesis by causing the premature release of the ribosome from mRNA.

The aminoglycosides are bactericidal because of their ability to bind irreversibly to ribosomes and are commonly used to treat serious infections caused by many gram-negative rods (e.g., Enterobacteriaceae, *Pseudomonas*, *Acinetobacter*) and some gram-positive organisms. Penetration through the cytoplasmic membrane is an aerobic, energy-dependent process, so anaerobes are resistant to aminoglycosides. Streptococci and enterococci are resistant to aminoglycosides because the aminoglycosides fail to penetrate through the cell wall of these bacteria. Treatment of these organisms requires coadministration of an aminoglycoside with an inhibitor of cell wall synthesis (e.g., penicillin, ampicillin, vancomycin) that facilitates uptake of the aminoglycoside.

TABLE 20–5. Aminoglycosides and Aminocyclitol

Antibiotics	Spectrum of Activity
Aminoglycosides (streptomycin, kanamycin, gentamicin, tobramycin, amikacin)	Primarily used to treat infections with gram-negative rods; kanamycin with limited activity; tobramycin slightly more active than gentamicin vs. *Pseudomonas;* amikacin most active; streptomycin and gentamicin combined with cell wall–active antibiotic to treat enterococcal infections; streptomycin active vs. mycobacteria and selected gram-negative rods
Aminocyclitol (spectinomycin)	Active vs. *Neisseria gonorrhoeae*

TABLE 20–6. Macrolides, Lincosamide, and Tetracyclines

Antibiotics	Spectrum of Activity
Macrolides (erythromycin, azithromycin, clarithromycin)	Broad-spectrum antibiotics active against gram-positive and some gram-negative bacteria, *Neisseria, Legionella, Mycoplasma, Chlamydia, Chlamydophila, Treponema,* and *Rickettsia;* clarithromycin and azithromycin active against some mycobacteria
Lincosamide (clindamycin)	Broad-spectrum activity against aerobic gram-positive cocci and anaerobes
Tetracyclines (tetracycline, doxycycline, minocycline)	Broad-spectrum antibiotics with activity similar to that of macrolides

The most commonly used antibiotics in this class are **amikacin, gentamicin,** and **tobramycin.** All three aminoglycosides are used to treat systemic infections caused by susceptible gram-negative bacteria. **Amikacin** has the best activity and is frequently reserved for treatment of infections caused by gram-negative bacteria that are resistant to gentamicin and tobramycin. **Streptomycin** is not readily available but has been used for the treatment of tuberculosis, tularemia, and gentamicin-resistant streptococcal or enterococcal infections (in combination with a penicillin).

Resistance to the antibacterial action of aminoglycosides can develop in one of four ways: (1) mutation of the ribosomal binding site, (2) decreased uptake of the antibiotic into the bacterial cell, (3) increased expulsion of the antibiotic from the cell, or (4) enzymatic modification of the antibiotic. The most common mechanism of resistance is enzymatic modification of aminoglycosides. This is accomplished by the action of phosphotransferases (APHs; seven described), adenyltransferases (ANTs; four described), and acetyltransferases (AACs; four described) on the amino and hydroxyl groups of the antibiotic. The differences in the antibacterial activity among the aminoglycosides are determined by their relative susceptibility to these enzymes. The other mechanisms by which bacteria develop resistance to aminoglycosides are relatively uncommon. Resistance caused by alteration of the bacterial ribosome requires systematic mutation of the multiple copies of the ribosomal genes that exist in the bacterial cell. Resistance caused by inhibited transport of the antibiotic into the bacterial cell is occasionally observed with *Pseudomonas* but is more commonly seen with anaerobic bacteria. This mechanism produces low-level cross-resistance to all aminoglycosides. Active efflux of aminoglycosides occurs only in gram-negative bacteria and is rarely observed.

TETRACYCLINES

The tetracylines (Table 20–6) are broad-spectrum, bacteriostatic antibiotics that inhibit protein synthesis in bacteria by binding reversibly to the 30S ribosomal subunits, thus blocking the binding of aminoacyl–transfer RNA (tRNA) to the 30S ribosome–mRNA complex. Tetracyclines (i.e., **tetracycline, doxycycline, minocycline**) are effective in the treatment of infections caused by *Chlamydia, Mycoplasma,* and *Rickettsia* species and other selected gram-positive and gram-negative bacteria. All tetracyclines have a similar spectrum of activity, with the primary difference among the antibiotics in their pharmacokinetic properties (doxycycline and minocycline are easily absorbed and have a long half-life). Resistance to the tetracyclines can stem from decreased penetration of the antibiotic into the bacterial cell, active efflux of the antibiotic out of the cell, alteration of the ribosomal target site, or enzymatic modification of the antibiotic. Mutations in the chromosomal gene encoding the outer membrane porin protein, OmpF, can lead to low-level resistance to the tetracyclines, as well as to other antibiotics (e.g., β-lactams, quinolones, chloramphenicol).

Researchers have identified a variety of genes in different bacteria that control the active efflux of the tetracyclines from the cell. This is the most common cause of resistance. Resistance to the tetracyclines can also result from the production of proteins similar to elongation factors that protect the 30S ribosome. When this happens, the antibiotic can still bind to the ribosome, but protein synthesis is not disrupted.

OXAZOLIDINONES

The oxazolidinones are a narrow-spectrum class of antibiotics, with **linezolid** being the agent currently used. Linezolid blocks initiation of protein synthesis by interfering with the formation of the initiation complex consisting of tRNA, mRNA, and the ribosome. The drug binds to the 50S ribosomal subunit, which distorts the binding site for tRNA, thus inhibiting formation of the 70S initiation complex. Because of this unique mechanism, cross-resistance with other protein inhibitors does not occur. Linezolid has activity against all staphylococci, streptococci, and enterococci (including those strains resistant to penicillins, vancomycin, and the aminoglycosides). Because the multidrug-resistant enterococci are difficult to treat, use of linezolid is generally reserved for these infections.

CHLORAMPHENICOL

Chloramphenicol has a broad antibacterial spectrum similar to that of tetracycline but is not commonly used in the United States. The reason for its limited use is that besides interfering with bacterial protein synthesis, it disrupts protein synthesis in human bone marrow cells and can produce blood dyscrasias such as aplastic anemia (one per 24,000 treated patients). Chloramphenicol exerts its bacteriostatic effect by binding reversibly to the peptidyl transferase component of the 50S ribosomal subunit, thus blocking peptide elongation. Resistance to chloramphenicol is observed in bacteria producing plasmid-encoded chloramphenicol acetyltransferase, which catalyzes the acetylation of the 3-hydroxy group of chloramphenicol. The product is incapable of binding to the 50S subunit. Less commonly, chromosomal mutations alter the outer membrane porin proteins, causing the gram-negative rods to be less permeable.

MACROLIDES

Erythromycin, derived from *Streptomyces erythreus,* is the model macrolide antibiotic (see Table 20–6). The basic structure of this class of antibiotics is a macrocyclic lactone ring bound to two sugars, desosamine and cladinose. Modification of the macrolide structure led to the development of newer agents, including **azithromycin** and **clarithromycin.** Macrolides are bacteriostatic antibiotics with a broad spectrum of activity. They have been used to treat pulmonary infections caused by *Mycoplasma, Legionella,* and *Chlamydia* species, as well as to treat infections caused by *Campylobacter* species and gram-positive bacteria in patients allergic to penicillin. Most gram-negative bacteria are resistant to the macrolides. Azithromycin and clarithromycin have also been used to treat infections caused by mycobacteria (e.g., *Mycobacterium avium* complex). Macrolides exert their effect by their reversible binding to the 23S rRNA of the 50S ribosomal subunit, which blocks polypeptide elongation. Resistance to macrolides most commonly stems from the methylation of the 23S ribosomal RNA, preventing binding by the antibiotic. Other mechanisms of resistance include inactivation of the macrolides by enzymes (e.g., esterases, phosphorylases, glycosidase) or mutations in the 23S rRNA and ribosomal proteins.

CLINDAMYCIN

Clindamycin (in the family of lincosamide antibiotics) is a derivative of lincomycin, which was originally isolated from *Streptomyces lincolnensis.* Like chloramphenicol and the macrolides, clindamycin blocks protein elongation by binding to the 50S ribosome. It inhibits peptidyl transferase by interfering with the binding of the amino acid–acyl-tRNA complex. Clindamycin is active against staphylococci and anaerobic gram-negative rods but is generally inactive against aerobic gram-negative bacteria. Methylation of the 23S ribosomal RNA is the source of bacterial resistance. Because both erythromycin and clindamycin can induce this enzymatic resistance (also plasmid mediated), cross-resistance between these two classes of antibiotics is observed.

STREPTOGRAMINS

The streptogramins are a class of cyclic peptides produced by *Streptomyces* species. These antibiotics are administered as a combination of two components, group A and group B streptogramins, which act synergistically to inhibit protein synthesis. The antibiotic currently available in this class is **quinupristin-dalfopristin** (known by the trade name Synercid). Dalfopristin binds to the 50S ribosomal subunit and induces a conformational change that facilitates binding of quinupristin. Dalfopristin prevents peptide chain elongation, and quinupristin initiates premature release of peptide chains from the ribosome. This combination drug is active against staphylococci, streptococci, and *E. faecium* (but not *E. faecalis*). Use of the antibiotic has been restricted primarily to treating vancomycin-resistant *E. faecium* infections.

Inhibition of Nucleic Acid Synthesis

QUINOLONES

The quinolones (Table 20–7) are one of the most widely used classes of antibiotics. These are synthetic

TABLE 20–7. Quinolones

Antibiotics	Spectrum of Activity
Narrow spectrum (nalidixic acid)	Active against selected gram-negative rods; no useful gram-positive activity
Broad spectrum (ciprofloxacin, levofloxacin, ofloxacin)	Broad-spectrum antibiotics with activity against gram-positive and gram-negative bacteria
Extended spectrum (gatifloxacin, grepafloxacin, clinafloxacin, moxifloxacin)	Broad-spectrum antibiotics with enhanced activity against gram-positive bacteria (particularly streptococci and enterococci) compared with early quinolones; activity against gram-negative rods similar to that of ciprofloxacin and related quinolones

chemotherapeutic agents that inhibit bacterial DNA topoisomerase type II (gyrase) or topoisomerase type IV, which are required for DNA replication, recombination, and repair. The DNA gyrase-A subunit is the primary quinolone target in gram-negative bacteria, whereas topoisomerase type IV is the primary target in gram-positive bacteria. The first quinolone used in clinical practice was **nalidixic acid.** This drug was used to treat urinary tract infections caused by a variety of gram-negative bacteria, but resistance to the drug developed rapidly, causing it to fall out of use. This drug has now been replaced by newer, more active quinolones, such as **ciprofloxacin, levofloxacin, gatifloxacin,** and **moxifloxacin.** Modifying the two-ring quinolone nucleus made these newer quinolones (referred to as fluoroquinolones). These antibiotics have excellent activity against gram-positive and gram-negative bacteria, although resistance can develop rapidly in *Pseudomonas,* oxacillin-resistant staphylococci, and enterococci. In particular, the newer extended-spectrum quinolones have significant activity against gram-positive bacteria.

Resistance to the quinolones is mediated by chromosomal mutations in the structural genes for DNA gyrase and topoisomerase type IV. Other mechanisms include decreased drug uptake caused by mutations in the membrane permeability regulatory genes, and overexpression of efflux pumps that actively eliminate the drug. Each of these mechanisms is primarily chromosomally mediated.

RIFAMPIN AND RIFABUTIN

Rifampin, a semisynthetic derivative of rifamycin B produced by *Streptomyces mediterranei,* binds to DNA-dependent RNA polymerase and inhibits the initiation of RNA synthesis. Rifampin is bactericidal for *Mycobacterium tuberculosis* and is very active against aerobic gram-positive cocci, including staphylococci and streptococci.

Because resistance can develop rapidly, rifampin is usually combined with one or more other effective antibiotics. Rifampin resistance in gram-positive bacteria results from a mutation in the chromosomal gene that codes for the b subunit of RNA polymerase. Gram-negative bacteria are resistant intrinsically to rifampin, as the result of decreased uptake of the hydrophobic antibiotic. **Rifabutin,** a derivative of rifamycin, has a similar mode and spectrum of activity. It is particularly active against *M. avium.*

METRONIDAZOLE

Metronidazole was originally introduced as an oral agent for the treatment of *Trichomonas* vaginitis. However, it was also found to be effective in the treatment of amebiasis, giardiasis, and serious anaerobic bacterial infections (including those caused by *B. fragilis*). Metronidazole has no significant activity against aerobic or facultatively anaerobic bacteria. The antimicrobial properties of metronidazole stem from the reduction of its nitro group by bacterial nitroreductase, thereby producing cytotoxic compounds that disrupt the host DNA. Resistance results either from decreased uptake of the antibiotic or from elimination of the cytotoxic compounds before they can interact with host DNA.

Antimetabolites

The **sulfonamides** are antimetabolites that compete with *p*-aminobenzoic acid, thereby preventing the synthesis of the folic acid required by certain microorganisms. Because mammalian organisms do not synthesize folic acid (required as a vitamin), sulfonamides do not interfere with mammalian cell metabolism. **Trimethoprim** is another antimetabolite that interferes with folic acid metabolism by inhibiting dihydrofolate reductase, thereby preventing the conversion of dihydrofolate to tetrahydrofolate. This inhibition blocks the formation of thymidine, some purines, methionine, and glycine. Trimethoprim is commonly combined with sulfamethoxazole to produce a synergistic combination active at two steps in the synthesis of folic acid. **Dapsone** and ***p*-aminosalicylic** acid are also antifolates that have proved to be useful for treating mycobacterial infections.

Sulfonamides are effective against a broad range of gram-positive and gram-negative organisms, such as

Nocardia, Chlamydia, and some protozoa. Short-acting sulfonamides such as sulfisoxazole are among the drugs of choice for the treatment of acute urinary tract infections caused by susceptible bacteria, such as *E. coli.* Trimethoprim-sulfamethoxazole is effective against a large variety of gram-positive and gram-negative microorganisms and is the drug of choice for the treatment of acute and chronic urinary tract infections. The combination is also effective in the treatment of infections caused by *Pneumocystis carinii,* bacterial infections of the lower respiratory tract, otitis media, and uncomplicated gonorrhea.

Resistance to these antibiotics can stem from a variety of mechanisms. Bacteria such as *Pseudomonas* are resistant as the result of permeability barriers. A decreased affinity of dihydrofolate reductase can be the source of trimethoprim resistance. In addition, bacteria that use exogenous thymidine (e.g., enterococci) are also intrinsically resistant.

Other Antibiotics

Clofazimine is a lipophilic antibiotic that binds to mycobacterial deoxyribonucleic acid (DNA). It is highly active against *M. tuberculosis,* is a first-line drug for the treatment of *Mycobacterium leprae* infections, and has been recommended as a secondary antibiotic for the treatment of infections caused by other mycobacterial species.

Pyrazinamide (PZA) is active against *M. tuberculosis* at a low pH, such as that found in phagolysosomes. The active form of this antibiotic is pyrazinoic acid, produced when PZA is hydrolyzed in the liver. The mechanism by which PZA exerts its effect is unknown.

QUESTIONS

1. Describe the mode of action of the following antibiotics: penicillin, vancomycin, isoniazid, gentamicin, tetracycline, erythromycin, polymyxin, ciprofloxacin, and sulfamethoxazole.
2. Name the three mechanisms bacteria use to become resistant to β-lactam antibiotics. What is the mechanism responsible for oxacillin resistance in *Staphylococcus?* Imipenem resistance in *Pseudomonas?* Penicillin resistance in *S. pneumoniae?*
3. By what three mechanisms have organisms developed resistance to aminoglycosides?
4. What mechanism is responsible for resistance to the quinolones?
5. How do trimethoprim and the sulfonamides differ in their mode of action?

Bibliography

Kucers A, Bennett NM: *The use of antibiotics: A comprehensive review with clinical emphasis,* ed 4, Philadelphia, 1989, Lippincott.

Mandell GL, Bennet JE, Dolin R, editors: *Principles and practice of infectious diseases,* ed 6, Philadelphia, 2005, Churchill Livingstone.

Murray P et al: *Manual of clinical microbiology,* ed 8, Washington, 2003, American Society for Microbiology.

CHAPTER 21

Laboratory Diagnosis of Bacterial Diseases

Many of the tests performed in microbiology laboratories require the recovery of viable organisms. This means that the proper specimen must be collected, delivered expeditiously to the laboratory in the appropriate transport system, and inoculated onto media that will support the growth of the most likely pathogens. Care must also be taken to keep the specimen from being contaminated with clinically insignificant organisms that are present in the environment or that normally colonize the patient. Collection of the proper specimen and its rapid delivery to the clinical laboratory are primarily the responsibility of the patient's physician, whereas the clinical microbiologist selects the appropriate transport systems and culture method. These responsibilities are not mutually exclusive, however. The microbiologist should be prepared to instruct the physician about what specimens should be collected if a particular diagnosis is suspected, and the physician must provide the microbiologist with information about the clinical diagnosis, so that the right culture media and growth conditions are selected. The chapters and bibliographic citations that follow provide information about the selection of culture media for specific pathogens. The primary focus of this chapter, however, is to provide guidelines for the proper collection and transport of different specimens (Table 21–1) and general information about the laboratory processing of specimens. Whenever an unusual or fastidious pathogen is suspected (e.g., *Bordetella pertussis*, *Francisella tularensis*), the laboratory should be notified so that the appropriate transport system and culture media can be used.

Blood

The culture of blood is one of the most important procedures performed in the clinical microbiology laboratory. The success of this test is directly related to the methods used to collect the blood sample. The most important factor that determines the success of a blood culture is the volume of blood processed. For example, there is a 40% increase in the rate of cultures positive for organisms if 20 ml rather than 10 ml of blood are cultured, because more than half of all septic patients have less than one organism per milliliter of blood. Therefore, approximately 20 ml of blood should be collected from an adult for each blood culture and proportionally smaller volumes should be collected from children and neonates. Because many hospitalized patients are susceptible to infections with organisms colonizing their skin, careful disinfection of the patient's skin is important.

Bacteremia and fungemia are defined as the presence of bacteria and fungi, respectively, in the blood, and these infections are referred to collectively as septicemia. Clinical studies have shown that septicemia can be continuous or intermittent. **Continuous septicemia** occurs primarily in patients with intravascular infections (e.g., endocarditis, septic thrombophlebitis, infections associated with intravascular catheter) or with overwhelming sepsis (e.g., septic shock). **Intermittent septicemia** occurs in patients with infections localized at a distal site (e.g., lungs, urinary tract, soft tissues). The timing of blood collection is not important for patients with continuous septicemias, but it is important for patients with intermittent septicemia. In addition, because clinical signs of sepsis (e.g., fever, chills, hypotension) are a response to the release of endotoxins or exotoxins from the organisms, these signs occur as long as 1 hour after the organisms entered the blood. Thus few to no organisms may be in the blood when the patient becomes febrile. For this reason, it is recommended that two to three blood samples should be collected at random times during a 24-hour period.

Most blood samples are inoculated into bottles filled with enriched nutrient broths. This should be done when

TABLE 21–1. Bacteriology Specimen Collection for Bacterial Pathogens

Specimen	Transport System	Specimen Volume	Other Considerations
Blood—routine bacterial culture	Blood culture bottle with nutrient media	Adults: 20 ml/culture Children: 5–10 ml/culture Neonates: 1–2 ml/culture	Skin should be disinfected with 70% alcohol followed by 2% iodine; 2-3 cultures collected every 24 hr unless patient is in septic shock or antibiotics will be started immediately; blood collections should be separated by 30-60 min; blood is divided equally into two bottles of nutrient media.
Blood—intracellular bacteria (e.g., *Brucella, Francisella, Neisseria* spp.)	Same as that for routine blood cultures; lysis-centrifugation system	Same as that for routine blood cultures	Considerations are same as those for routine blood cultures; release of intracellular bacteria may improve organism's recovery; *Neisseria* species is inhibited by some anticoagulants (sodium polyanethoesulfonate).
Blood—*Leptospira* sp.	Sterile heparinized tube	1–5 ml	Specimen is useful only during the first week of illness; afterward, urine should be cultured.
Cerebrospinal fluid	Sterile screw-capped tube	Bacteria culture: 1–5 ml Mycobacterial culture: as large a volume as possible	Specimen must be collected aseptically and delivered immediately to laboratory; it should not be exposed to heat or refrigeration.
Other normally sterile fluids (e.g., abdominal, chest, synovial, pericardial)	Small volume: sterile screw-capped tube; large volume: blood culture bottle with nutrient medium	As large a volume as possible	Specimens are collected with needle and syringe; swab is not used because quantity of collected specimen is inadequate; air should not be injected into culture bottle because it will inhibit growth of anaerobes.
Catheter	Sterile screw-capped tube or specimen cup	N/A	The entry site should be disinfected with alcohol; catheter should be aseptically removed on receipt of specimen in laboratory; catheter is rolled across blood agar plate and then discarded.
Respiratory—throat	Swab immersed in transport medium	N/A	Area of inflammation is swabbed; exudate is collected if present; contact with saliva should be avoided because it can inhibit recovery of group A streptococci.
Respiratory—epiglottis	Collection of blood for culture	Same as for blood culture	Swabbing the epiglottis can precipitate complete airway closure; blood cultures should be collected for specific diagnosis.
Respiratory—sinuses	Sterile anaerobic tube or vial	1–5 ml	Specimens must be collected with needle and syringe; culture of nasopharynx or oropharynx has no value; specimen should be cultured for aerobic and anaerobic bacteria.
Respiratory—lower airways	Sterile screw-capped bottle; anaerobic tube or vial only for specimens collected by avoiding upper tract flora	1–2 ml	Expectorated sputum: If possible, patient rinses mouth with water before collection of the specimen; patient should cough deeply and expectorate lower airway secretions directly into sterile cup; collector should avoid contamination with saliva. Bronchoscopy specimen: anesthetics can inhibit growth of bacteria, so specimens should be processed immediately; if "protected" bronchoscope is used, anaerobic cultures can be performed. Direct lung aspirate: specimens can be processed for aerobic and anaerobic bacteria.
Ear	Capped, needleless syringe; sterile screw-capped tube	Whatever volume is collected	Specimen should be aspirated with needle and syringe; culture of external ear has no predictive value for otitis media.

TABLE 21–1. Bacteriology Specimen Collection for Bacterial Pathogens—*cont'd*

Specimen	Transport System	Specimen Volume	Other Considerations
Eye	Inoculate plates at bedside (seal and transport to laboratory immediately)	Whatever volume is collected	For infections on surface of eye, specimens are collected with swab or by corneal scrapings; for deep-seated infections, aspiration of aqueous or vitreous fluid is performed; all specimens should be inoculated onto appropriate media at collection; delays will result in significant loss of organisms.
Exudates (transudates, drainage, ulcers)	Swab immersed in transport medium; aspirate in sterile screw-capped tube	Bacteria: 1–5 ml Mycobacteria: 3–5 ml	Contamination with surface material should be avoided; specimens are generally unsuitable for anaerobic culture.
Wounds (abscess, pus)	Aspirate in sterile screw-capped tube or sterile anaerobic tube or vial	1–5 ml of pus	Specimens should be collected with sterile needle and syringe; curette is used to collect specimen at base of wound; swabbed specimens should be avoided.
Tissues	Sterile screw-capped tube; sterile anaerobic tube or vial	Representative sample from center and border of lesion	Specimen should be aseptically placed into appropriate sterile container; adequate quantity of specimen must be collected to recover small numbers of organisms.
Urine—midstream	Sterile urine container	Bacteria: 1 ml Mycobacteria: ≥10 ml	Contamination of specimen with bacteria from the urethra or vagina should be avoided; first portion of the voided specimen is discarded; organisms can grow rapidly in urine, so specimens must be transported immediately to laboratory, held in bacteriostatic preservative, or refrigerated.
Urine—catheterized	Sterile urine container	Bacteria: 1 ml Mycobacteria: ≥10 ml	Catheterization is not recommended for routine cultures (risk of inducing infection); first portion of collected specimen is contaminated with urethral bacteria, so it should be discarded (similar to midstream voided specimen); specimen must be transported rapidly to laboratory.
Urine—suprapubic aspirate	Sterile anaerobic tube or vial	Bacteria: 1 ml Mycobacteria: ≥10 ml	This is an invasive specimen, so urethral bacteria are avoided; it is only valid method available for collecting specimens for anaerobic culture; also useful for collection of specimens from children or adults unable to void uncontaminated specimens.
Genitals	Specially designed swabs for *Neisseria gonorrboeae* and *Chlamydia* probes	N/A	Area of inflammation or exudate should be sampled; endocervix (not vagina) and urethra should be cultured for optimal detection.
Feces (stool)	Sterile screw-capped container	N/A	Rapid transport to laboratory is necessary to prevent production of acid (bactericidal for some enteric pathogens) by normal fecal bacteria; it is unsuitable for anaerobic culture; because a large number of different media will be inoculated, swab should not be used for specimen collection.

N/A, Not applicable.

the sample is collected. To ensure the maximal recovery of important organisms, two bottles of media should be inoculated for each culture. When these inoculated bottles of broth are received in the laboratory, they are incubated at 37°C and inspected at regular intervals for evidence of microbial growth. In most laboratories this is accomplished using automated blood culture instruments. When growth is detected, the broths are subcultured to isolate the organism for identification and antimicrobial susceptibility testing. Most clinically significant isolates are detected within the first 1 to 2 days of incubation; however, all cultures should be incubated for a minimum of 5 to 7 days. More prolonged incubation is generally unnecessary, except for fastidious organisms. Because few organisms are typically present in the blood of a septic patient, it is not worthwhile to perform a Gram stain of blood for microscopic analysis.

Cerebrospinal Fluid

Bacterial meningitis is a serious disease that is associated with high morbidity and mortality if the etiologic diagnosis is delayed. Because some common pathogens are labile (e.g., *Neisseria meningitidis, Streptococcus pneumoniae*), specimens of cerebrospinal fluid should be processed immediately after they are collected. Under no circumstance should the specimen be refrigerated or heated. The patient's skin is disinfected with alcohol and iodine before lumbar puncture, and the cerebrospinal fluid is collected into sterile screw-capped tubes. On receipt of the specimen in the microbiology laboratory, it is concentrated by centrifugation, and the sediment is used to inoculate bacteriologic media and prepare a Gram stain. The laboratory technician should notify the physician immediately if organisms are observed microscopically or in culture.

Other Normally Sterile Fluids

A variety of other normally sterile fluids may be collected for bacteriologic culture, including abdominal (peritoneal), chest (pleural), synovial, and pericardial fluids. If a large volume of fluid can be collected by aspiration (e.g., abdominal or chest fluids), it should be inoculated into blood culture bottles containing nutrient media. A small portion should also be sent to the laboratory in a sterile tube so that appropriate stains (e.g., Gram, acid-fast) can be prepared. Many organisms are associated with infections at these sites, including polymicrobial mixtures of aerobic and anaerobic organisms. For this reason, biologic staining is useful for identifying the organisms responsible for the infection. Because relatively few organisms may be in the sample (as a result of the dilution of organisms or microbial elimination by the host immune response), it is important to culture as large a volume of fluid as possible. However, if only small quantities of fluid are collected, the specimen can be inoculated directly onto agar media and a tube of enriched broth media. Because anaerobes may also be present in the sample (particularly samples obtained from patients with intraabdominal or pulmonary infections), the specimen should not be exposed to oxygen.

Upper Respiratory Tract Specimens

Most bacterial infections of the pharynx are caused by group A *Streptococcus*. Other bacteria that may cause pharyngitis include *Corynebacterium diphtheriae, B. pertussis, Neisseria gonorrhoeae, Chlamydophila pneumoniae,* and *Mycoplasma pneumoniae*. However, special techniques are generally required to recover these organisms. Other potentially pathogenic bacteria, such as *Staphylococcus aureus, S. pneumoniae, Haemophilus influenzae,* Enterobacteriaceae, and *Pseudomonas aeruginosa*, may be present in the oropharynx, but they rarely cause pharyngitis.

A Dacron or calcium alginate swab should be used to collect pharyngeal specimens. The tonsillar areas, posterior pharynx, and any exudate or ulcerative area should be sampled. Contamination of the specimen with saliva should be avoided because bacteria in saliva can overgrow or inhibit the growth of group A streptococci. If a pseudomembrane is present (e.g., as with *C. diphtheriae* infections), a portion should be dislodged and submitted for culture. Group A streptococci and *C. diphtheriae* are very resistant to drying, so special precautions are not required for transport of the specimen to the laboratory. In contrast, specimens collected for the recovery of *B. pertussis* and *N. gonorrhoeae* should be inoculated onto culture media immediately after they are collected and before they are sent to the laboratory. Specimens obtained for the isolation of *C. pneumoniae* and *M. pneumoniae* should be transported in a special transport medium.

Group A streptococci can be detected directly in the clinical specimen through the use of immunoassays for the group-specific antigen. Although these tests are very specific and readily available, they are insensitive and cannot be used to reliably exclude the diagnosis of group A streptococcal pharyngitis. In other words, a negative assay must be confirmed by culture.

Other upper respiratory tract infections can involve the epiglottis and sinuses. Complete airway obstruction can be precipitated by attempts to culture the epiglottis (particularly in children); thus these cultures should never be performed. The specific diagnosis of a sinus infection requires (1) the direct aspiration of the sinus, (2) appropriate anaerobic transport of the specimen to the laboratory (using a system that avoids exposing anaerobes to oxygen and drying), and (3) prompt processing. Culture of the nasopharynx or oropharynx is not useful and should not be performed. *S. pneumoniae, H. influenzae, Moraxella catarrhalis, S. aureus*, and anaerobes are the most common pathogens that cause sinusitis.

Lower Respiratory Tract Specimens

A variety of techniques can be used to collect lower respiratory tract specimens; these include expectoration, induction with saline, bronchoscopy, and direct aspiration through the chest wall. Because upper airway bacteria may contaminate expectorated and induced sputa, the specimen should be inspected microscopically to assess the magnitude of oral contamination and the value of processing the specimen. Specimens containing many squamous epithelial cells and no predominant bacteria in association with leukocytes should not be processed for culture. The presence of squamous epithelial cells indicates that the specimen has been contaminated with saliva. Such contamination can be avoided by obtaining the specimen using specially designed bronchoscopes or direct lung aspiration. If an anaerobic lung infection is suspected, these invasive procedures must be used because contamination of the specimen with upper airway microbes would render the specimen worthless. Most lower respiratory tract pathogens grow rapidly (within 2 to 3 days); however, some slow-growing bacteria such as mycobacteria or nocardia may require extended incubation.

Ear and Eye

Tympanocentesis (i.e., the aspiration of fluid from the middle ear) is required to make the specific diagnosis of a middle ear infection. This is unnecessary in most patients, however, because the most common pathogens that cause these infections (*S. pneumoniae, H. influenzae*, and *M. catarrhalis*) can be treated empirically.

Outer ear infections are typically caused by *P. aeruginosa* ("swimmer's ear") or *S. aureus*. The proper specimen to be obtained for culture is a scraping of the involved area of the ear.

Collection of specimens for the diagnosis of ocular infections is difficult because the sample obtained is generally very small and relatively few organisms may be present. Samples of the eye surface should be collected by a swab before topical anesthetics are applied, followed by corneal scrapings when necessary. The eye must be directly aspirated to collect intraocular specimens. The culture media should be inoculated when the specimens are collected and before they are sent to the laboratory. Although most common ocular pathogens grow rapidly (e.g., *S. aureus, S. pneumoniae, H. influenzae, P. aeruginosa, Bacillus cereus*), some may require prolonged incubation (e.g., coagulase-negative staphylococci) or the use of specialized culture media (*N. gonorrhoeae, Chlamydia trachomatis*).

Wounds, Abscesses, and Tissues

Open, draining wounds can often be colonized with potentially pathogenic organisms unrelated to the specific infectious process. Therefore it is important to collect samples from deep in the wound after the surface has been cleaned. Whenever possible, a swab should be avoided because it is difficult to obtain a representative sample without contamination with organisms colonizing the surface. Likewise, aspirates from a closed abscess should be collected from both the center and the wall of the abscess. Simply collecting pus from an abscess is generally nonproductive because most organisms actively replicate at the base of the abscess rather than in the center. Drainage from soft-tissue infections can be collected by aspiration. If drainage material is not obtained, a small quantity of saline can be infused into the tissue and then withdrawn for culture. Saline containing a bactericidal preservative should not be used.

Tissues should be obtained from representative portions of the infectious process, with multiple samples collected whenever possible. The tissue specimen should be transported in a sterile screw-capped container, and sterile saline should be added to prevent drying if a small sample (e.g., biopsy specimen) is collected. A sample of tissue should also be submitted for histologic examination. Because collection of tissue specimens requires invasive procedures, every effort should be made to collect the proper specimen and ensure that it is cultured for all clinically significant organisms that may be responsible for the infection. This requires close communication between the physician and microbiologist.

Urine

Urine is one of the most frequently submitted specimens for culture. Because potentially pathogenic bacteria colonize the urethra, the first portion of urine collected by voiding or catheterization should be discarded. Urinary tract pathogens can also grow in urine, so there should be no delay in the transport of specimens to the laboratory. If the specimen cannot be cultured immediately, it should be refrigerated or placed into a bacteriostatic **urine preservative.** Once the specimen is received in the laboratory, 1 to 10 μl is inoculated onto each culture medium (generally one nonselective agar medium and one selective medium). This is done so that the number of organisms in the urine can be quantitated, which is useful for assessing the significance of an isolate, although small numbers of organisms in a patient with pyuria can be clinically significant. Numerous urine-screening procedures (e.g., biochemical tests, microscopy stains) have been developed and are used widely; however, these procedures cannot be recommended because they are invariably insensitive in detecting a clinically significant, low-grade bacteriuria.

Genital Specimens

Despite the variety of bacteria associated with sexually transmitted diseases, most laboratories concentrate on detecting *N. gonorrhoeae* and *C. trachomatis*. Traditionally, this was done by inoculating the specimen into a culture system selective for these organisms. This is a slow process, however, taking 2 or more days for a positive culture to be obtained and even more time for isolates to be identified definitively. Culture was also found to be insensitive because the organisms are extremely labile and die rapidly during transit under less than optimal conditions. For these reasons a variety of nonculture methods are now used. The most popular methods are nucleic acid amplification procedures (e.g., amplification of species-specific deoxyribonucleic acid [DNA] sequences by the polymerase chain reaction, ligase chain reaction, or other methods) for both organisms. Detection of these amplified sequences with probes is both sensitive and specific. However, cross-contamination can occur if the test procedures are not controlled carefully. If urine is used for these tests, the first portion of voided urine and not the midstream portion should be tested.

The other major bacterium that causes sexually transmitted disease is *Treponema pallidum*, the etiologic agent of syphilis. This organism cannot be cultured in the clinical laboratory, so the diagnosis is made using microscopy or serology. Material from lesions must be examined using darkfield microscopy, because the organism is too thin to be detected using brightfield microscopy. In addition, the organism dies rapidly when exposed to air and drying conditions, so the microscopic examination must be performed at the time the specimen is collected.

Fecal Specimens

A large variety of bacteria can cause gastrointestinal infections. For these bacteria to be recovered in culture, an adequate stool sample must be collected (generally not a problem in a patient with diarrhea), transported to the laboratory in a manner that ensures the viability of the infecting organism, and inoculated onto the appropriate selective media. Rectal swabs should not be submitted, because multiple selective media must be inoculated for the various possible pathogens to be recovered. The quantity of feces collected on a swab would be inadequate.

Stool specimens should be collected in a clean pan and then transferred into a tightly sealed waterproof container. The specimens should be transported promptly to the laboratory to prevent acidic changes in the stool (caused by bacterial metabolism), which are toxic for organisms such as *Shigella*. If a delay is anticipated, the feces should be mixed with a preservative such as phosphate buffer mixed with glycerol or Cary-Blair transport medium (if *Campylobacter* infection is suspected). In general, however, rapid transport of the specimen to the laboratory is always superior to the use of any transport medium.

It is important to notify the laboratory if a particular enteric pathogen is suspected, because this will help the laboratory select the appropriate culture medium. For example, although *Vibrio* species can grow on the common media used for the culture of stool specimens, the use of media selective for *Vibrio* facilitates the rapid isolation and identification of this organism. In addition, some organisms are not isolated routinely by the laboratory procedures. For example, enterotoxigenic *Escherichia coli* can grow on routine culture media but would not be readily distinguished from nonpathogenic *E. coli*. Likewise, other organisms would not be expected to be in a stool sample because their disease is caused by toxin produced in the food and not by growth of the organism in the gastrointestinal tract (e.g., *S. aureus*). The microbiologist should be able to select the appropriate test (e.g., culture, toxin assay) if the specific pathogen is indicated. *Clostridium difficile* is a significant cause of antibiotic-associated gastrointestinal disease. Although the organism can be cultured from stool specimens if the specimens are delivered promptly to the laboratory, the most specific way to diagnose the infection is by detecting the *C. difficile* toxins in fecal extracts. The toxins are responsible for the disease.

Because many bacteria, both pathogenic and nonpathogenic, are present in fecal specimens, it often takes at least 3 days for the enteric pathogen to be isolated and identified. For this reason, stool cultures are used to confirm the clinical diagnosis, and therapy, if indicated, should not be delayed pending the culture results. Indeed, antimicrobial susceptibility testing is usually not performed with most enteric pathogens.

QUESTIONS

1. What is the most important factor that influences the recovery of microorganisms in blood collected from patients with sepsis?
2. Which organisms are important causes of bacterial pharyngitis?
3. What criteria should be used to assess the quality of a lower respiratory tract specimen?
4. What methods are used to detect the three most common bacteria that cause sexually transmitted diseases?

Bibliography

Forbes B et al: *Bailey and Scott's diagnostic microbiology*, ed 11, St Louis, 2002, Mosby.

Mandell G, Bennett J, Dolin R: *Principles and practice of infectious diseases*, ed 6, New York, 2005, Churchill Livingstone.

Murray P et al: *Manual of clinical microbiology*, ed 8, Washington, 2003, American Society for Microbiology.

CHAPTER 22

Staphylococcus and Related Organisms

The gram-positive cocci are a heterogeneous collection of bacteria. Features that they have in common are their spherical shape, their Gram-stain reaction, and an absence of endospores. The presence or absence of **catalase activity** is a simple test that is used to subdivide the various genera. Catalases are enzymes that catabolize hydrogen peroxide into water and oxygen gas. If a drop of a peroxide solution is placed on a catalase-producing bacterial colony, bubbles will appear when the oxygen gas is formed. The aerobic catalase-positive genera (e.g., *Staphylococcus, Micrococcus, Kocuria, Kytococcus, Alloiococcus*) are discussed in this chapter, the aerobic catalase-negative genera (*Streptococcus, Enterococcus,* and related organisms) are discussed in the next two chapters, and the anaerobic gram-positive cocci are discussed in Chapter 41.

The genus name *Staphylococcus* is derived from the Greek term *staphylé,* meaning "a bunch of grapes" (Box 22–1). Therefore, *Staphylococcus* refers to the fact that the cells of these gram-positive cocci grow in a pattern resembling a cluster of grapes (Figure 22–1); however, organisms in clinical material may also appear as single cells, pairs, or short chains. Most staphylococci are 0.5 to 1.5 μm in diameter, nonmotile, facultatively anaerobic (i.e., grow both aerobically and anaerobically), and able to grow in media containing a high concentration of salt (e.g., 10% sodium chloride) and at temperatures ranging from 18°C to 40°C. These bacteria are present on the skin and mucous membranes of humans. The genus currently consists of 35 species and 17 subspecies, many of which are found on humans (Table 22–1). Some species have very specific niches where they are commonly found. For example, *Staphylococcus aureus* colonizes the anterior nares, *Staphylococcus capitis* is found where sebaceous glands are present (e.g., forehead), and *Staphylococcus haemolyticus* and *Staphylococcus hominis* are found in areas where apocrine glands are present (e.g., axilla). Staphylococci are important pathogens in humans, causing a wide spectrum of life-threatening systemic diseases, including infections of the skin, soft tissues, bones, and urinary tract; and opportunistic infections (Table 22–2). The species most commonly associated with human diseases are *S. aureus* (the most virulent and best-known member of the genus), *Staphylococcus epidermidis, S. haemolyticus, Staphylococcus lugdunensis,* and *Staphylococcus saprophyticus. S. aureus* colonies are golden as the result of the carotenoid pigments that form during their growth, hence the species name. It is also the only species found in humans that produces the enzyme **coagulase.** When a colony of *S. aureus* is suspended in a tube of plasma, coagulase binds to a serum factor, and this complex converts fibrinogen to fibrin, resulting in the formation of a clot. Because the other staphylococcal species do not produce coagulase, they are referred to collectively as **coagulase-negative staphylococci.**

The genus *Micrococcus* has been subdivided into six genera, with *Micrococcus, Kocuria,* and *Kytococcus* most commonly colonizing the human skin surface. These cocci resemble staphylococci and can be confused with the coagulase-negative staphylococci. Although these bacteria may cause opportunistic infections in some patients, their isolation in clinical specimens usually represents clinically insignificant contamination.

Alloiococcus otitidis is the only species in this genus. It is an aerobic, gram-positive coccus that has been implicated in chronic middle ear infections in children. Because this organism grows slowly, its role in disease may be underappreciated.

The remainder of this chapter concentrates on a description of *Staphylococcus* and its role in human disease.

BOX 22–1. Important Staphylococci

Organism	Historical Derivation
Staphylococcus	*staphylé*, bunch of grapes; *coccus*, grain or berry (grapelike coccus)
S. aureus	*aureus*, golden (golden or yellow)
S. epidermidis	*epidermidis*, outer skin (of the epidermis or outer skin)
S. lugdunensis	*Lugdunum*, Latin name for Lyon, France, where the organism was first isolated
S. saprophyticus	*sapros*, putrid; *phyton*, plant (saprophytic or growing on dead tissues)

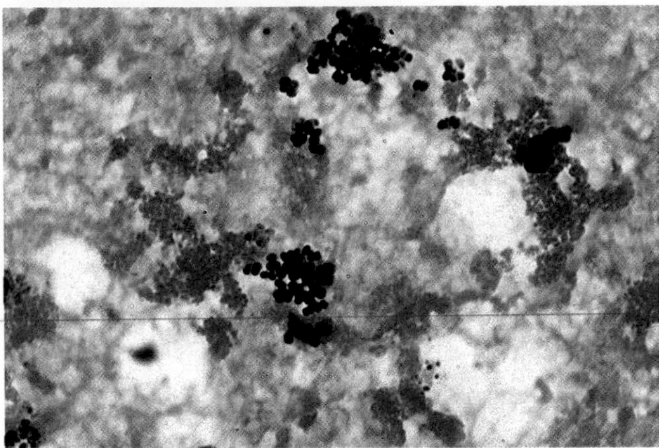

FIGURE 22–1. Gram stain of *Staphylococcus aureus.*

TABLE 22–1. Colonization and Human Diseases Caused by *Staphylococcus*

Species	Human Colonization	Human Disease
S. aureus	Common	Common
S. epidermidis	Common	Common
S. saprophyticus	Common	Common
S. haemolyticus	Common	Common
S. lugdunensis	Common	Common
S. capitis	Common	Uncommon
S. saccharolyticus	Common	Rare
S. warneri	Common	Rare
S. hominis	Common	Rare
S. auricularis	Common	Rare
S. cohnii	Common	Rare
S. xylosus	Uncommon	Rare
S. simulans	Uncommon	Rare
S. caprae	Uncommon	Rare
S. pasteuri	Uncommon	Rare
S. schleiferi	Rare	Rare

TABLE 22–2. *Staphylococcus* Species and Their Diseases

Organism	Diseases
Staphylococcus aureus	Toxin mediated (food poisoning, scalded skin syndrome, toxic shock syndrome); cutaneous (carbuncles, folliculitis, furuncles, impetigo, wound infections); other (bacteremia, empyema, endocarditis, osteomyelitis, pneumonia, septic arthritis)
Staphylococcus epidermidis	Bacteremia; endocarditis; surgical wounds; urinary tract infections; opportunistic infections of catheters, shunts, prosthetic devices, and peritoneal dialysates
Staphylococcus saprophyticus	Urinary tract infections; opportunistic infections
Staphylococcus lugdunensis	Arthritis, bacteremia, endocarditis, opportunistic infections, and urinary tract infections
Staphylococcus haemolyticus	Bacteremia, bone and joint infections, endocarditis, urinary tract infections, wound infections, and opportunistic infections

Physiology and Structure

The structure of the staphylococcal cell wall is illustrated in Figure 22–2.

CAPSULE AND SLIME LAYER

The outermost layer of the staphylococcal cell wall can be covered with a polysaccharide capsule. Eleven capsular serotypes have been identified in *S. aureus,* with serotypes 5 and 7 associated with the majority of infections. Serotypes 1 and 2 are associated with very thick capsules and mucoid-appearing colonies. The capsule protects the bacteria by inhibiting phagocytosis of the organisms by polymorphonuclear leukocytes (PMN). A loose-bound, water-soluble film **(slime layer)** consisting of monosaccharides, proteins, and small peptides is produced by most staphylococci in varying amounts, depending on genetic factors and the growth conditions. This extracellular substance binds the bacteria to tissues and foreign bodies such as catheters, grafts, prosthetic valves and joints, and shunts. This property is particularly important for the survival of relatively avirulent coagulase-negative staphylococci.

PEPTIDOGLYCAN

Half of the cell wall by weight is **peptidoglycan,** a feature common to gram-positive bacteria. The peptidoglycan

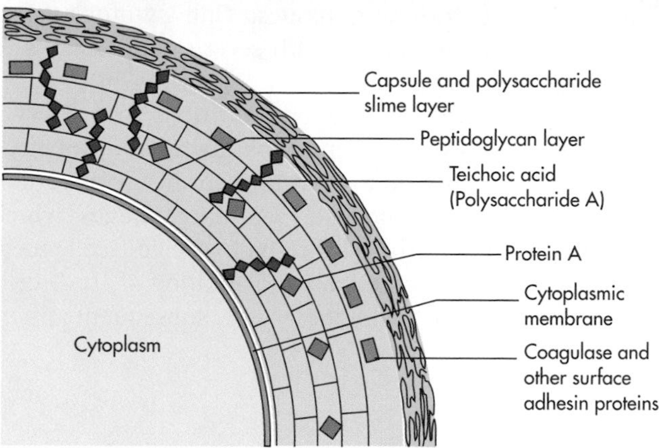

FIGURE 22–2. Structure of staphylococcal cell wall.

consists of layers of glycan chains built with 10 to 12 alternating subunits of *N*-acetylmuramic acid and *N*-acetylglucosamine. Oligopeptide side chains are attached to the *N*-acetylmuramic acid subunits and are then cross-linked with peptide bridges. For example, the glycan chains in *S. aureus* are cross-linked with pentaglycine bridges that are attached to L-lysine in one oligopeptide chain and to D-alanine in an adjacent chain. Unlike gram-negative bacteria, the peptidoglycan layer in gram-positive organisms consists of many cross-linked layers, which makes the cell wall more rigid. The peptidoglycan has endotoxin-like activity, stimulating the production of endogenous pyrogens, activation of complement, production of interleukin-1 from monocytes, and aggregation of PMN (a process responsible for abscess formation).

TEICHOIC ACIDS

Teichoic acids are the other major component of the cell wall, comprising 30% to 50% of the dry weight. Teichoic acids are species-specific, phosphate-containing polymers that are bound covalently to *N*-acetylmuramic acid residues of the peptidoglycan layer or through lipophilic linkage to the cytoplasmic membrane (lipoteichoic acids). Ribitol teichoic acid with *N*-acetylglucosamine residues ("polysaccharide A") is present in *S. aureus*, and glycerol teichoic acid with glucosyl residues ("polysaccharide B") is present in *S. epidermidis*. Teichoic acids mediate the attachment of staphylococci to mucosal surfaces through their specific binding to fibronectin. Although the teichoic acids are poor immunogens, a specific antibody response is stimulated when they are bound to peptidoglycan. The monitoring of this antibody response had been used to detect systemic staphylococcal disease; however, this is less sensitive than other diagnostic tests and is not used today.

PROTEIN A

The surface of most *S. aureus* strains (but not the coagulase-negative staphylococci) is coated with **protein A.** This protein is bound to either the peptidoglycan layer or the cytoplasmic membrane and has a unique affinity for binding to the Fc receptor of immunoglobulin (Ig)G_1, IgG_2, and IgG_4. This effectively prevents antibody-mediated immune clearance of the organism. Extracellular protein A can also bind antibodies, thereby forming immune complexes with the subsequent consumption of the complement. The presence of protein A has been exploited in some serologic tests, in which protein A–coated *S. aureus* is used as a nonspecific carrier of antibodies directed against other antigens. Additionally, detection of protein A can be used as a specific identification test for *S. aureus*.

COAGULASE AND OTHER SURFACE ADHESIN PROTEINS

Numerous surface proteins have been identified in staphylococci. The outer surface of most strains of *S. aureus* contains **clumping factor** (also called **bound coagulase**). This protein is an important virulence factor in *S. aureus*. It binds fibrinogen and converts it to insoluble fibrin, causing the staphylococci to clump or aggregate. Detection of this protein is the primary test for identifying *S. aureus*. Other surface proteins are also important for adherence to host matrix proteins, which in turn bind to host tissues (e.g., fibronectin, fibrinogen, elastin, collagen). These surface adhesion proteins present in staphylococci and other bacteria have been designated MSCRAMM (microbial surface components recognizing adhesive matrix molecules) proteins and have become targets of novel therapeutic interventions.

CYTOPLASMIC MEMBRANE

The **cytoplasmic membrane** is made up of a complex of proteins, lipids, and a small amount of carbohydrates. It serves as an osmotic barrier for the cell and provides an anchorage for the cellular biosynthetic and respiratory enzymes.

Pathogenesis and Immunity

The pathology of staphylococcal infections depends on production of surface proteins that mediate adherence of the bacteria to host tissues (above) and then elaboration of extracellular proteins, such as specific toxins and hydrolytic enzymes. The expression of the exoprotein genes is controlled primarily by a global regulator, *agr*, which in turn is controlled by environmental factors, cell density, and energy availability.

STAPHYLOCOCCAL TOXINS

S. aureus produces many virulence factors (Table 22–3), including five cytolytic or membrane-damaging toxins (alpha, beta, delta, gamma, and Panton-Valentine [P-V] leukocidin), two exfoliative toxins (A and B), eight enterotoxins (A to E, G to I), and toxic shock syndrome toxin-1 (TSST-1). The cytolytic toxins have been described as hemolysins, but this is a misnomer because the activities of the first four toxins are not restricted solely to red blood cells, and P-V leukocidin is unable to lyse erythrocytes. The cytotoxins can lyse neutrophils, resulting in the release of the lysosomal enzymes that subsequently damage the surrounding tissues. One cytotoxin, P-V leukocidin, has been linked with severe pulmonary and cutaneous infections.

Exfoliative toxin A, the enterotoxins, and TSST-1 belong to a class of polypeptides known as **superantigens.** These toxins bind to class II major histocompatibility complex (MHC II) molecules on macrophages, which in turn interact with the β subunit of specific T-cell receptors, leading to the nonspecific proliferation of the T cells and the release of cytokines with subsequent tissue damage.

Alpha Toxin

Alpha (α) toxin, which can be encoded on both the bacterial chromosome and a plasmid, is a 33,000-d

TABLE 22–3. *Staphylococcus aureus* Virulence Factors

Virulence Factors	Biologic Effects
Structural Components	
Capsule	Inhibits chemotaxis and phagocytosis; inhibits proliferation of mononuclear cells; facilitates adherence to foreign bodies
Peptidoglycan	Provides osmotic stability; stimulates production of endogenous pyrogen (endotoxin-like activity); leukocyte chemoattractant (abscess formation); inhibits phagocytosis
Teichoic acid	Regulates cationic concentration at cell membrane; binds to fibronectin
Protein A	Inhibits antibody-mediated clearance by binding IgG_1, IgG_2, and IgG_4 Fc receptors; leukocyte chemoattractant; anticomplementary
Cytoplasmic membrane	Osmotic barrier; regulates transport into and out of cell; site of biosynthetic and respiratory enzymes
Toxins	
Cytotoxins (α, β, δ, γ, leukocidin)	Toxic for many cells, including leukocytes, erythrocytes, fibroblasts, leukocytes, macrophages, and platelets
Exfoliative toxins (ETA, ETB)	Serine proteases that split the intercellular bridges in the stratum granulosum epidermis
Enterotoxins (A-E, G-I)	Superantigens (stimulate proliferation of T cells and release of cytokines); stimulate release of inflammatory mediators in mast cells, increasing intestinal peristalsis and fluid loss, as well as nausea and vomiting
Toxic shock syndrome toxin-1	Superantigen (stimulates proliferation of T cells and release of cytokines); produces leakage or cellular destruction of endothelial cells
Enzymes	
Coagulase	Converts fibrinogen to fibrin
Catalase	Catalyzes removal of hydrogen peroxide
Hyaluronidase	Hydrolyzes hyaluronic acids in connective tissue, promoting the spread of staphylococci in tissue
Fibrinolysin	Dissolves fibrin clots
Lipases	Hydrolyzes lipids
Nucleases	Hydrolyzes DNA
Penicillinase	Hydrolyzes penicillins

polypeptide that is produced by most strains of *S. aureus* that cause human disease. The toxin disrupts the smooth muscle in blood vessels and is toxic to many types of cells, including erythrocytes, leukocytes, hepatocytes, and platelets. It becomes integrated in the hydrophobic regions of host cell membrane, leading to formation of 1- to 2-nm pores. The rapid efflux of K^+ and influx of Na^+, Ca^{2+}, and other small molecules leads to osmotic swelling and cell lysis. The sensitivity to this varies for animal species (rabbit erythrocytes are 1000-fold more sensitive than are human cells) and cell type (e.g., fibroblasts can repair membrane damage more effectively than can erythrocytes). α Toxin is believed to be an important mediator of tissue damage in staphylococcal disease.

Beta Toxin

Beta (β) toxin, also called **sphingomyelinase C,** is a 35,000-d heat-labile protein produced by most strains of *S. aureus* responsible for disease in humans and animals. This enzyme has a specificity for sphingomyelin and lysophosphatidylcholine and is toxic to a variety of cells, including erythrocytes, fibroblasts, leukocytes, and macrophages. It catalyzes the hydrolysis of membrane phospholipids in susceptible cells, with lysis proportional to the concentration of sphingomyelin exposed on the cell surface. This is believed to be responsible for the differences in species susceptibility to the toxin. The role of β toxin in human disease remains to be proved; however, together with α toxin, it is believed to be responsible for the tissue destruction and abscess formation characteristic of staphylococcal diseases.

Delta Toxin

Delta (δ) toxin is a 3000-d polypeptide produced by almost all *S. aureus* strains and other staphylococci (e.g., *S. epidermidis, S. haemolyticus*). The toxin has a wide spectrum of cytolytic activity, affecting erythrocytes, many other mammalian cells, and intracellular membrane structures. This relatively nonspecific membrane toxicity is consistent with the belief that the toxin acts as a surfactant disrupting cellular membranes by means of a detergent-like action.

Gamma Toxin and Panton-Valentine Leukocidin

Gamma (γ) toxin (made by almost all *S. aureus* strains) and **P-V leukocidin** (made by <5% of *S. aureus* strains) are bicomponent toxins, composed of two polypeptide chains: the S (slow-eluting proteins) component and F (fast-eluting proteins) component. Three S proteins (HlgA [hemolysin γ A], HlgC, LukS-PV) and two F proteins (HlgB, LukF-PV) have been identified. Bacteria capable of producing both toxins can encode all these proteins with the potential for producing six distinct toxins. All six toxins can lyse neutrophils and macrophages, whereas the greatest hemolytic activity is associated with HlgA/HlgB, HlgC/HlgB, and HlgA/LukF-PV. The P-V leukocidin toxin (LukS-PV/LukF-PV) is leukotoxic but has no hemolytic activity. Cell lysis by these toxins is mediated by pore formation with subsequent increased permeability to cations and osmotic instability.

Exfoliative Toxins

Staphylococcal scalded skin syndrome (SSSS), a spectrum of diseases characterized by exfoliative dermatitis, is mediated by exfoliative toxins. The prevalence of toxin production in *S. aureus* strains varies geographically but is generally between less than 5% and 10%. Two distinct forms of exfoliative toxin (ETA and ETB) have been identified, and either can produce disease. ETA is heat stable and the gene is chromosomal, whereas ETB is heat labile and plasmid mediated. Ultrastructural studies have shown that exposure to the toxins that are serine proteases is followed by the splitting of the intercellular bridges (desmosomes) in the stratum granulosum epidermis. The precise mechanism for this action is still unknown. The toxins are not associated with cytolysis or inflammation, so neither staphylococci nor leukocytes are typically present in the involved layer of the epidermis (this is an important diagnostic clue). After exposure of the epidermis to the toxin, protective neutralizing antibodies develop, leading to resolution of the toxic process. SSSS is seen mostly in young children and only rarely in older children and adults. One possible explanation for this is that ETA and ETB bind to GM_4-like glycolipids present in the epidermis of susceptible neonates but not in older children or adults.

Enterotoxins

At least 18 serologically distinct **staphylococcal enterotoxins** (A to R) and three subtypes of enterotoxin C have been identified. The enterotoxins are stable to heating at 100°C for 30 minutes and are resistant to hydrolysis by gastric and jejunal enzymes. Thus, once a food product has been contaminated with enterotoxin-producing staphylococci and the toxins have been produced, neither mild reheating of the food nor exposure to gastric acids will be protective. These toxins are produced by 30% to 50% of all *S. aureus* strains. Enterotoxin A is most commonly associated with disease. Enterotoxins C and D are found in contaminated milk products, and enterotoxin B causes staphylococcal pseudomembranous enterocolitis. Less is known about the prevalence of the other enterotoxins. The precise mechanism of toxin activity is not understood because a satisfactory animal model is not available. These toxins are superantigens, capable of inducing nonspecific activation of T cells and cytokine release. Characteristic histologic changes in the stomach and jejunum include infiltration of neutrophils into the epithelium and underlying lamina propria, with loss of the brush border in the jejunum. Stimulation of release of inflammatory mediators from mast cells is believed to be responsible for the emesis that is characteristic of staphylococcal food poisoning.

Toxic Shock Syndrome Toxin-1

TSST-1, formerly called pyrogenic exotoxin C and enterotoxin F, is a 22,000-d heat- and proteolysis-resistant, chromosomally mediated exotoxin. It is estimated that 90% of *S. aureus* strains responsible for menstruation-associated toxic shock syndrome (TSS), and half of the strains responsible for other forms of TSS, produce TSST-1. Only 15% of other strains of *S. aureus* produce TSST-1. Expression of TSST-1 in vitro requires an elevated oxygen concentration and neutral pH. This is likely the reason TSS is relatively uncommon compared with the incidence of *S. aureus* wound infections (a setting where the environment of an abscess is relatively anaerobic and acidic). Enterotoxin B and, rarely, enterotoxin C are responsible for approximately half the cases of nonmenstruation-associated TSS. TSST-1 is a superantigen that stimulates release of cytokines, producing leakage of endothelial cells at low concentrations and a cytotoxic effect to the cells at high concentrations. The ability of TSST-1 to penetrate mucosal barriers, even though the infection remains localized in the vagina or at the site of a wound, is responsible for the systemic effects of TSS. Death in patients with TSS is cause by hypovolemic shock leading to multiorgan failure.

STAPHYLOCOCCAL ENZYMES

Coagulase

S. aureus strains possess two forms of **coagulase:** bound and free. Coagulase bound to the staphylococcal cell wall can directly convert fibrinogen to insoluble fibrin and cause the staphylococci to clump. The cell-free coagulase accomplishes the same result by reacting with a globulin plasma factor (coagulase-reacting factor) to form staphylothrombin, a thrombinlike factor. This factor catalyzes the conversion of fibrinogen to insoluble fibrin. The role of coagulase in the pathogenesis of disease is speculative, but coagulase may cause the formation of a fibrin layer around a staphylococcal abscess, thus localizing the infection and protecting the organisms from phagocytosis. Some other species of staphylococci produce coagulase, but these are primarily animal pathogens and uncommonly recovered in human infections.

Catalase

Hydrogen peroxide can accumulate during bacterial metabolism or after phagocytosis. All staphylococci produce **catalase,** which catalyzes the conversion of hydrogen peroxide to water and oxygen.

Hyaluronidase

Hyaluronidase hydrolyzes hyaluronic acids, the acidic mucopolysaccharides present in the acellular matrix of connective tissue. This enzyme facilitates the spread of *S. aureus* in tissues. More than 90% of *S. aureus* strains produce this enzyme.

Fibrinolysin

Fibrinolysin, also called **staphylokinase,** is produced by virtually all *S. aureus* strains and can dissolve fibrin clots. Staphylokinase is distinct from the fibrinolytic enzymes produced by streptococci.

Lipases

All strains of *S. aureus* and more than 30% of the strains of coagulase-negative *Staphylococcus* produce several different **lipases.** As their name implies, these enzymes hydrolyze lipids, an essential function to ensure the survival of staphylococci in the sebaceous areas of the body. It is believed that these enzymes must be present for staphylococci to invade cutaneous and subcutaneous tissues and for superficial skin infections (e.g., furuncles [boils], carbuncles) to develop.

Nuclease

A thermostable **nuclease** is another marker for *S. aureus*, although some other species produce this enzyme. The role of this enzyme in the pathogenesis of infection is unknown.

Penicillinase

More than 90% of staphylococcal isolates were susceptible to penicillin in 1941, the year the antibiotic was first used clinically. Resistance to penicillin quickly developed, however, primarily because the organisms could produce **penicillinase** (β-lactamase). The widespread distribution of this enzyme was ensured by its presence on transmissible plasmids.

Epidemiology

Staphylococci are ubiquitous. All persons have coagulase-negative staphylococci on their skin, and transient colonization of moist skin folds with *S. aureus* is common (Boxes 22–2 and 22–3). Colonization of the umbilical stump, skin, and perineal area of neonates with *S. aureus* is common. *S. aureus* and coagulase-negative staphylococci are also found in the oropharynx, gastrointestinal tract, and urogenital tract. Short-term or persistent *S. aureus* carriage in older children and adults is more common in the anterior nasopharynx than in the oropharynx. Approximately 15% of normal healthy adults are persistent nasopharyngeal carriers of *S. aureus*, with a higher incidence reported for hospitalized patients, medical personnel, persons with eczematous skin diseases, and those who regularly use needles, either illicitly (e.g., drug abusers) or for medical reasons (e.g., patients with insulin-dependent diabetes, patients receiving allergy injections, or those undergoing hemodialysis). Adherence of the organism to the mucosal epithelium is regulated by the staphylococcal cell surface adhesins.

Because staphylococci are found on the skin and in the nasopharynx, shedding of the bacteria is common and is responsible for many hospital-acquired infections. Staphylococci are susceptible to high temperatures and disinfectants and antiseptic solutions; however, the organisms can survive on dry surfaces for long periods. The organisms can be transferred to a susceptible person either through direct contact or through contact with fomites (e.g., contaminated clothing, bed linens). Therefore, medical personnel must use proper hand-washing techniques to prevent the transfer of staphylococci from themselves to patients or among patients.

BOX 22–2. Summary of *Staphylococcus aureus*

Physiology and Structure

Catalase-positive, gram-positive cocci arranged in clusters
Facultative anaerobe (capable of aerobic and anaerobic growth)
Capsule and slime layer
Coagulase ("clumping factor") and other surface adhesin proteins
Species-specific ribitol teichoic acid with *N*-acetylglucosamine residues ("polysaccharide A")
Species-specific protein A

Virulence

Refer to Table 22–4

Epidemiology

Normal flora on human skin and mucosal surfaces
Organisms can survive on dry surfaces for long periods (owing to thickened peptidoglycan layer and absence of outer membrane—characteristics of all gram-positive bacteria)
Person-to-person spread through direct contact or exposure to contaminated fomites (e.g., bed linens, clothing)
Risk factors include presence of a foreign body (e.g., splinter, suture, prosthesis, catheter), previous surgical procedure, and use of antibiotics that suppress the normal microbial flora
Patients at risk for specific diseases include infants (scalded skin syndrome), young children with poor personal hygiene (impetigo and other cutaneous infections), menstruating women (toxic shock syndrome), patients with intravascular catheters (bacteremia and endocarditis) or shunts (meningitis), and patients with compromised pulmonary function or an antecedent viral respiratory infection (pneumonia)
Infections found worldwide and generally with no seasonal prevalence (except that food poisoning is more common in summer and during late-year holidays)

Diseases

Refer to Table 22–2
Toxin-mediated diseases include food poisoning, toxic shock syndrome, and scalded skin syndrome
Pyogenic diseases include impetigo, folliculitis, furuncles, carbuncles, and wound infections
Other systemic diseases (frequently associated with bacteremia) include pneumonia (typically after viral respiratory infection), empyema (complication of pneumonia or surgical intervention), septic arthritis, osteomyelitis, acute endocarditis, and catheter-related bacteremia

Diagnosis

Microscopy useful for pyogenic infections but not blood infections or toxin-mediated infections
Staphylococci grow rapidly when cultured on nonselective media
Detection of staphylococcal antibodies generally of little value

Treatment, Control, and Prevention

Antibiotics of choice are oxacillin (or other penicillinase-resistant penicillin), or vancomycin for oxacillin-resistant strains
The focus of infection (e.g., abscess) must be identified and drained
Treatment is symptomatic for patients with food poisoning (although the source of infection should be identified so that appropriate preventive procedures can be enacted)
Proper cleansing of wounds and use of disinfectant help prevent infections
Thorough hand washing and covering of exposed skin helps medical personnel prevent infection or spread to other patients

BOX 22–3. Summary of Coagulase-Negative Staphylococci

Physiology and Structure

Catalase-positive, coagulase-negative, gram-positive cocci arranged in clusters

Facultative anaerobe (capable of aerobic and anaerobic growth)

Species-specific teichoic acid

"Slime" layer

Virulence

Refer to Table 22–3

Epidemiology

Normal human flora on skin and mucosal surfaces

Organisms can survive on dry surfaces for long periods

Person-to-person spread through direct contact or exposure to contaminated fomites (although most infections are with the patient's own organisms)

Patients are at risk when a foreign body (e.g., suture, prosthesis, shunt, catheter) is present

The organisms are ubiquitous, so there are no geographic or seasonal limitations

Diseases

Refer to Table 22–2

Catheter-related bacteremia

Subacute endocarditis associated with previously damaged or artificial heart valve

Central nervous system shunt infection

Surgical wound infection when a foreign body (e.g., suture, prosthesis, medical hardware) is present

Diagnosis

As with *S. aureus* infections

Treatment, Control, and Prevention

The antibiotics of choice are oxacillin (or other penicillinase-resistant penicillin), or vancomycin for oxacillin-resistant strains

Removal of the foreign body is often required for successful treatment

Prompt treatment for endocarditis or shunt infections is necessary to prevent further tissue damage or immune complex formation

Maintenance of sterile intravascular catheters helps prevent infections

Clinical Diseases

STAPHYLOCOCCUS AUREUS

S. aureus causes disease through the production of toxin or through the direct invasion and destruction of tissue (Box 22–4). The clinical manifestations of some staphylococcal diseases are almost exclusively the result of toxin activity (e.g., SSSS, staphylococcal food poisoning, and

BOX 22–4. Staphylococcal Diseases: Clinical Summaries

Staphylococcus aureus

Toxin-Mediated Diseases

Scalded skin syndrome: Disseminated desquamation of epithelium in infants; blisters with no organisms or leukocytes

Food poisoning: After consumption of food contaminated with heat-stable enterotoxin, rapid onset of severe vomiting, diarrhea, and abdominal cramping, with resolution within 24 hours

Toxic shock: multisystem intoxication characterized initially by fever, hypotension, and a diffuse, macular erythematous rash; high mortality without prompt antibiotic therapy and elimination of the focus of infection

Suppurative Infections

Impetigo: localized cutaneous infection characterized by pus-filled vesicle on an erythematous base

Folliculitis: impetigo involving hair follicles

Furuncles or boils: large, painful, pus-filled cutaneous nodules

Carbuncles: Coalescence of furuncles with extension into the subcutaneous tissues and evidence of systemic disease (fever, chills, bacteremia)

Bacteremia and endocarditis: Spread of bacteria into the blood from a focus of infection; endocarditis characterized by damage to the endothelial lining of the heart

Pneumonia and empyema: Consolidation and abscess formation in the lungs; seen in the very young and elderly and in patients with underlying or recent pulmonary disease; a severe form of necrotizing pneumonia with septic shock and high mortality is now recognized

Osteomyelitis: Destruction of bones, particularly the metaphyseal area of long bones

Septic arthritis: Painful erythematous joint with collection of purulent material in the joint space

Staphylococcus Species

Wound infections: Characterized by erythema and pus at the site of a traumatic or surgical wound; infections with foreign bodies can be caused by *S. aureus* and coagulase-negative staphylococci

Urinary tract infections: Dysuria and pyuria in young sexually active women (*S. saprophyticus*), in patients with urinary catheters (other coagulase-negative staphylococci), or following seeding of the urinary tract by bacteremia (*S. aureus*)

Catheter and shunt infections: Chronic inflammatory response to bacteria coating a catheter or shunt (most commonly with coagulase-negative staphylococci)

Prosthetic device infections: Chronic infection of device characterized by localized pain and mechanical failure of the device (most commonly with coagulase-negative staphylococci)

TSS), whereas other diseases result from the proliferation of the organisms, leading to abscess formation and tissue destruction (e.g., cutaneous infections, endocarditis, pneumonia, empyema, osteomyelitis, septic arthritis) (Figure 22–3). In the presence of a foreign body (e.g., splinter, catheter, shunt, prosthetic valve or joint), significantly fewer staphylococci are necessary to establish disease. Likewise, patients with congenital diseases associated with an impaired chemotactic or phagocytic response (e.g., Job-Buckley syndrome, Wiskott-Aldrich syndrome, chronic granulomatous disease) are more susceptible to staphylococcal diseases.

Staphylococcal Scalded Skin Syndrome

In 1878, Gottfried Ritter von Rittershain described 297 infants younger than 1-month old, who had bullous exfoliative dermatitis. The disease he described, now called **Ritter's disease** or SSSS, is characterized by the abrupt onset of a localized perioral erythema (redness and inflammation around the mouth) that covers the entire body within 2 days. Slight pressure displaces the skin (a positive Nikolsky's sign), and large bullae or cutaneous blisters form soon thereafter, followed by desquamation of the epithelium (Figure 22–4). The blisters contain clear fluid but no organisms or leukocytes, a finding consistent with the fact that the disease is caused by the bacterial toxin. The epithelium becomes intact again within 7 to 10 days, when protective antibodies appear. Scarring does not occur because only the top layer of epidermis is sloughed. Although this is a disease primarily of neonates and young children, the mortality rate is low. When death does occur, it is a result of secondary bacterial infection of the denuded skin areas.

Bullous impetigo is a localized form of SSSS. In this syndrome, specific strains of toxin-producing *S. aureus* (e.g., phage type 71) are associated with the formation of superficial skin blisters (Figure 22–5). Unlike patients with the disseminated manifestations of SSSS, patients with bullous impetigo have localized blisters that are culture positive. The erythema does not extend beyond the borders of the blister, and Nikolsky's sign is not present. The disease occurs primarily in infants and young children and is highly communicable.

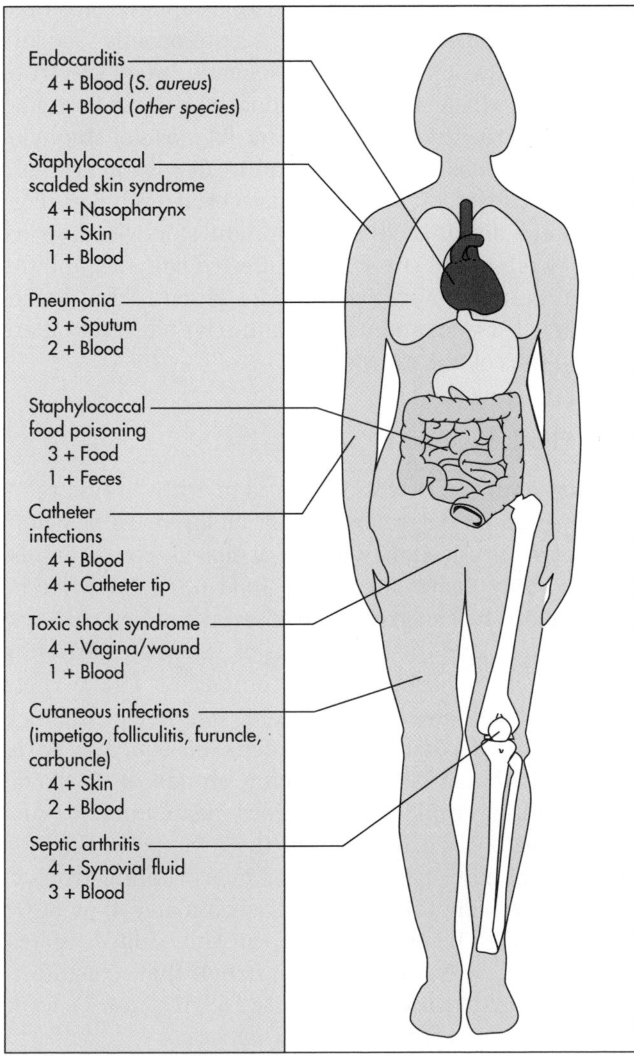

FIGURE 22–3. Staphylococcal diseases. Isolation of staphylococci from sites of infection. *1+*, Less than 10% positive cultures; *2+*, 10% to 50% positive cultures; *3+*, 50% to 90% positive cultures; *4+*, more than 90% positive cultures.

Staphylococcal Food Poisoning

Staphylococcal food poisoning, one of the most common foodborne illnesses, is an intoxication rather than an

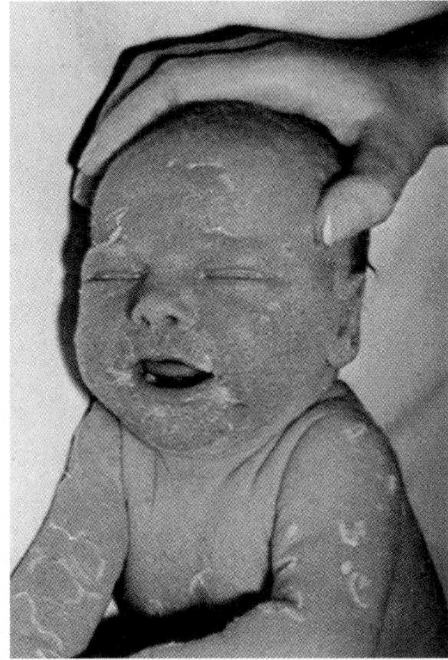

FIGURE 22–4. Staphylococcal scalded skin syndrome. (From Emond RT, Rowland HAK: *A color atlas of infectious diseases,* London, 1987, Wolfe.)

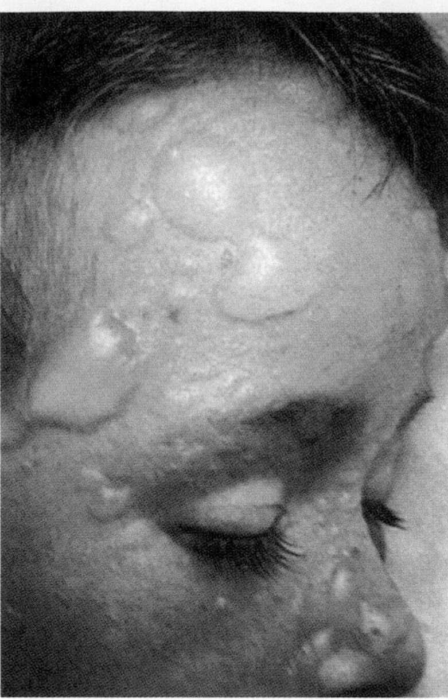

FIGURE 22–5. Bullous impetigo, a localized form of staphylococcal scalded skin syndrome. (From Emond RT, Rowland HAK: *A color atlas of infectious diseases*, London, 1987, Wolfe.)

infection. Disease is caused by bacterial toxin present in food, rather than from a direct effect of the organisms on the patient. The most commonly contaminated foods are processed meats such as ham and salted pork, custard-filled pastries, potato salad, and ice cream. Growth of *S. aureus* in salted meats is consistent with the ability of this organism to grow in the presence of high salt concentrations. Unlike many other forms of food poisoning in which an animal reservoir is important, staphylococcal food poisoning results from contamination of the food by a human carrier. Although contamination can be prevented by not allowing individuals with an obvious staphylococcal skin infection to prepare food, approximately half of the infections originate from carriers with asymptomatic nasopharyngeal colonization. After the staphylococci have been introduced into the food (through a sneeze or contaminated hand), the food must remain at room temperature or warmer for the organisms to grow and release the toxin. The contaminated food will not appear or taste tainted. Subsequent heating of the food will kill the bacteria but not inactivate the heat-stable toxin.

After ingestion of contaminated food, the onset of disease is abrupt and rapid, with a mean incubation period of 4 hours, which is, again, consistent with a disease mediated by preformed toxin. Further toxin is not produced by ingested staphylococci, so the disease has a rapid course, with symptoms generally lasting less than 24 hours. Severe vomiting, diarrhea, and abdominal pain or nausea are characteristic of staphyloccoal food poisoning. Sweating and headache may occur, but fever is not seen. The diarrhea is watery and nonbloody, and dehydration may result from the considerable fluid loss.

The toxin-producing organisms can be cultured from the contaminated food if the organisms are not killed during food preparation. The enterotoxins are heat-stable, so contaminated food can be tested for toxins at a public health facility; however, these tests are rarely performed.

Treatment is for the relief of abdominal cramping and diarrhea and for the replacement of fluids. Antibiotic therapy is not indicated because, as already noted, the disease is mediated by preformed toxin and not by replicating organisms. Neutralizing antibodies to the toxin can be protective, and limited cross-protection occurs among the different enterotoxins. Short-lived immunity means that second episodes of staphylococcal food poisoning can occur, particularly with serologically distinct enterotoxins.

Certain strains of *S. aureus* can also cause enterocolitis, which is manifested clinically by watery diarrhea, abdominal cramps, and fever. The majority of strains producing this disease produce both enterotoxin A and the bicomponent leukotoxin LukE/LukD. Enterocolitis occurs primarily in patients who have received broad-spectrum antibiotics, which suppress the normal colonic flora and permit the growth of *S. aureus*. The diagnosis of staphylococcal enterocolitis can be confirmed only after more common causes of infection have been excluded (e.g., *Clostridium difficile* colitis). Abundant staphylococci are typically present in the stool of affected patients, and the normal gram-negative bacteria are absent. Fecal leukocytes are observed, and white plaques with ulceration are seen on the colonic mucosa.

Toxic Shock Syndrome

The first outbreak of **TSS** occurred in 1928 in Australia, where the disease developed in 21 children, 12 of whom died after an injection with an *S. aureus*–contaminated vaccine. Fifty years later, J. K. Todd observed what he called **toxic shock syndrome** in seven children with systemic disease, and the first reports of TSS in menstruating women were published in the summer of 1980. These reports were followed by a dramatic increase in the incidence of TSS, particularly in women. Subsequently, it was discovered that TSST-1–producing strains of *S. aureus* could multiply rapidly in hyperabsorbent tampons and release toxin. After the recall of these tampons, the incidence of disease, particularly in menstruating women, decreased rapidly. At present, it is estimated that 6000 cases of TSS occur annually in the United States. Although it was originally reported that coagulase-negative staphylococci could cause TSS, it is now believed that this disease is restricted to *S. aureus*.

The disease is initiated with the localized growth of toxin-producing strains of *S. aureus* in the vagina or a wound, followed by release of the toxin into blood. Toxin production requires an aerobic atmosphere and neutral

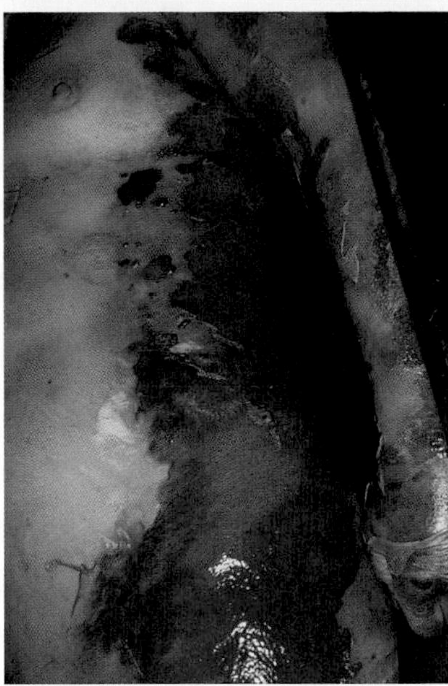

FIGURE 22–6. Toxic shock syndrome. A case of fatal infection with cutaneous and soft-tissue involvement is shown.

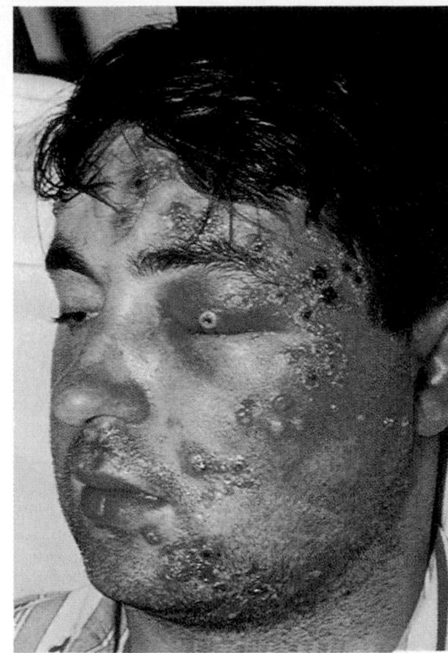

FIGURE 22–7. Pustular impetigo. Note the vesicles at different stages of development, including pus-filled vesicles on an erythematous base and dry, crusted lesions. (From Emond RT, Rowland HAK: *A color atlas of infectious diseases,* London, 1987, Wolfe.)

pH. Clinical manifestations start abruptly and include fever, hypotension, and a diffuse, macular erythematous rash. Multiple organ systems (e.g., central nervous, gastrointestinal, hematologic, hepatic, musculature, renal) are also involved, and the entire skin, including the palms and soles, desquamates (Figure 22–6). As the etiology and epidemiology of this disease have become better understood, the initially high-fatality rate has been decreased to approximately 5%. Unless the patient is specifically treated with an effective antibiotic, however, the risk of recurrent disease is as high as 65%. Serologic studies have demonstrated that more than 90% of adults have antibodies to TSST-1; however, more than 50% of patients with TSS fail to develop protective antibodies after their disease resolves. These unprotected patients are at significant risk for recurrent disease.

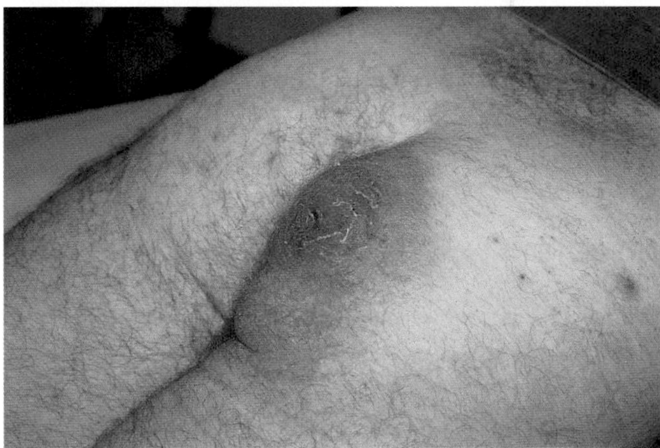

FIGURE 22–8. *Staphylococcus aureus* carbuncle. This carbuncle developed on the buttock over a 7- to 10-day period and required surgical drainage plus antibiotic therapy. (From Cohen J, Powderly WG: *Infectious diseases,* ed 2, St Louis, 2004, Mosby.)

Cutaneous Infections

Localized, **pyogenic staphylococcal infections** include impetigo, folliculitis, furuncles, and carbuncles. **Impetigo,** a superficial infection that mostly affects young children, occurs primarily on the face and limbs. Initially, a small macule (flattened red spot) is seen, and then a pus-filled vesicle (pustule) on an erythematous base develops. Crusting occurs after the pustule ruptures. Multiple vesicles at different stages of development are common, owing to the secondary spread of the infection to adjacent skin sites (Figure 22–7). Impetigo is usually caused by *S. aureus,* although group A streptococci, either alone or with *S. aureus,* are responsible for 20% of cases.

Folliculitis is a pyogenic infection in the hair follicles. The base of the follicle is raised and reddened, and there is a small collection of pus beneath the epidermal surface. If this occurs at the base of the eyelid, it is called a **stye.** **Furuncles** (boils), an extension of folliculitis, are large, painful, raised nodules that have an underlying collection of dead and necrotic tissue. These can drain spontaneously or after surgical incision.

Carbuncles occur when furuncles coalesce and extend to the deeper subcutaneous tissue (Figure 22–8). Multiple sinus tracts are usually present. Unlike patients with folliculitis and furuncles, patients with carbuncles have chills and fevers, indicating the systemic spread of staphylococci via bacteremia to other tissues.

Staphylococcal **wound infections** can also occur in patients after a surgical procedure or after trauma, with organisms colonizing the skin introduced into the wound. The staphylococci are generally not able to establish an infection in an immunocompetent person unless a foreign body (e.g., stitches, a splinter, dirt) is present in the wound. Infections are characterized by edema, erythema, pain, and an accumulation of purulent material. The infection can be easily managed if the wound is reopened, the foreign matter removed, and the purulence drained. If signs such as fever and malaise are observed or if the wound does not clear in response to localized management, antibiotic therapy directed against *S. aureus* is indicated.

Bacteremia and Endocarditis

S. aureus is a common cause of **bacteremia.** Although bacteremias caused by most other organisms originate from an identifiable focus of infection, such as an infection of the lungs, urinary tract, or gastrointestinal tract, the initial foci of infection in approximately a third of patients with *S. aureus* bacteremias are not known. Most likely, the infection spreads to the blood from an innocuous-appearing skin infection. More than 50% of the cases of *S. aureus* bacteremia are acquired in the hospital after a surgical procedure or result from the continued use of a contaminated intravascular catheter. *S. aureus* bacteremias, particularly prolonged episodes, are associated with dissemination to other body sites, including the heart.

Acute **endocarditis** caused by *S. aureus* is a serious disease, with a mortality rate approaching 50%. Although patients with *S. aureus* endocarditis may initially have nonspecific influenza-like symptoms, their condition can deteriorate rapidly and include disruption of cardiac output and peripheral evidence of septic embolization. Unless appropriate medical and surgical intervention is instituted immediately, the patient's prognosis is poor. An exception to this is *S. aureus* endocarditis in parenteral drug abusers, whose disease normally involves the right side of the heart (tricuspid valve) rather than the left. The initial symptoms may be mild, but fever, chills, and pleuritic chest pain caused by pulmonary emboli are generally present. Clinical cure of the endocarditis is the rule, although it is common for complications to occur as the result of secondary spread of the infection to other organs.

Pneumonia and Empyema

S. aureus respiratory disease can develop after the aspiration of oral secretions or from the hematogenous spread of the organism from a distant site. **Aspiration pneumonia** is seen primarily in the very young, the elderly, and patients with cystic fibrosis, influenza, chronic obstructive pulmonary disease, and bronchiectasis. The clinical and radiographic presentations of the pneumonia are not unique. Radiographic examination reveals the presence of patchy infiltrates with consolidation or abscesses, the latter consistent with the organism's ability to secrete cytotoxic toxins and enzymes and to form localized abscesses. **Hematogenous pneumonia** is common for patients with bacteremia or endocarditis. A severe form of community-acquired **necrotizing pneumonia** with massive hemoptysis, septic shock, and a high mortality rate has been observed in recent years. The P-V leukocidin present in strains responsible for this disease appears to be an important virulence factor. Although this disease has been reported most commonly in children and young adults, it is not restricted to these age groups.

Empyema occurs in 10% of patients with pneumonia, and *S. aureus* is responsible for a third of all cases. Because the organism can become consolidated in loculated areas, drainage of the purulent material is sometimes difficult.

Osteomyelitis and Septic Arthritis

S. aureus **osteomyelitis** can result from the hematogenous dissemination to bone, or it can be a secondary infection resulting from trauma or the extension of disease from an adjacent area. Hematogenous spread in children generally results from a cutaneous staphylococcal infection and usually involves the metaphyseal area of long bones, a highly vascularized area of bony growth. This infection is characterized by the sudden onset of localized pain over the involved bone and by high fever. Blood cultures are positive in approximately 50% of cases.

The hematogenous osteomyelitis that is seen in adults commonly occurs in the form of vertebral osteomyelitis and rarely in the form of an infection of the long bones. Intense back pain with fever is the initial symptom. Radiographic evidence of osteomyelitis in children and adults is not seen until 2 to 3 weeks after the initial symptoms appear. **Brodie's abscess** is a sequestered focus of staphylococcal osteomyelitis that arises in the metaphyseal area of a long bone and occurs only in adults. The staphylococcal osteomyelitis that occurs after trauma or a surgical procedure is generally accompanied by inflammation and purulent drainage from the wound or the sinus tract overlying the infected bone. Because the staphylococcal infection may be restricted to the wound, isolation of the organism from this site is not conclusive evidence of bony involvement. With appropriate antibiotic therapy and surgery, the cure rate for staphylococcal osteomyelitis is excellent.

S. aureus is the primary cause of **septic arthritis** in young children and in adults who are receiving intraarticular injections or who have mechanically abnormal joints. Secondary involvement of multiple joints is indicative of hematogenous spread from a localized focus. *S. aureus* is replaced by *Neisseria gonorrhoeae* as the most common cause of septic arthritis in sexually active persons. Staphylococcal arthritis is characterized by a painful, erythematous joint, with purulent material obtained on aspiration. Infection is usually demonstrated in the large joints (e.g., shoulder, knee, hip, elbow). The prognosis in children is excellent, but in adults it depends on the nature of the underlying disease and the occurrence of any secondary infectious complications.

STAPHYLOCOCCUS EPIDERMIDIS AND OTHER COAGULASE-NEGATIVE STAPHYLOCOCCI

Endocarditis

S. epidermidis, S. lugdunensis, and related coagulase-negative staphylococci can infect native and prosthetic heart valves. Infections of native valves are believed to result from the inoculation of organisms onto a damaged heart valve (e.g., a congenital malformation, damage resulting from rheumatic heart disease). This form of staphylococcal endocarditis is relatively rare and is more commonly caused by streptococci.

In contrast, staphylococci are a major cause of endocarditis of artificial valves. The organisms are introduced at the time of valve replacement, and the infection characteristically has an indolent course, with clinical signs and symptoms not developing for as long as 1 year after the procedure. Although the heart valve can be infected, more commonly the infection occurs at the site where the valve is sewn to the heart tissue. Thus infection with abscess formation can lead to separation of the valve at the suture line and to mechanical heart failure. The prognosis is guarded for patients who have this infection, and prompt medical and surgical management is critical.

Catheter and Shunt Infections

More than 50% of all infections of catheters and shunts are caused by coagulase-negative staphylococci. These infections have become a major medical problem because long-dwelling catheters and shunts are used commonly for the medical management of critically ill patients. The coagulase-negative staphylococci are particularly well adapted for causing these infections because they can produce a polysaccharide slime that bonds them to catheters and shunts and protects them from antibiotics and inflammatory cells. A persistent bacteremia is generally observed in patients with infections of shunts and catheters because the organisms have continual access to the blood. Immune complex–mediated glomerulonephritis occurs in patients with long-standing disease.

Prosthetic Joint Infections

Infections of artificial joints, particularly the hip, can be caused by coagulase-negative staphylococci. The patient usually experiences only localized pain and mechanical failure of the joint. Systemic signs such as fever and leukocytosis are not prominent, and blood cultures are usually negative. Treatment consists of joint replacement and antimicrobial therapy. The risk of reinfection of the new joint is considerably increased in such patients.

Urinary Tract Infections

S. saprophyticus has a predilection for causing urinary tract infections in young, sexually active women and is rarely responsible for infections in other patients. It is also infrequently found as an asymptomatic colonizer of the urinary tract. Infected women usually have dysuria (pain on urination), pyuria (pus in urine), and numerous organisms in the urine. Typically, patients respond rapidly to antibiotics and reinfection is uncommon.

Laboratory Diagnosis

MICROSCOPY

Staphylococci are gram-positive cocci that form clusters when grown on agar media but commonly appear as single cells or small groups of organisms in clinical specimens. The successful detection of organisms in a clinical specimen depends on the type of the infection (e.g., abscess, bacteremia, impetigo) and the quality of the material submitted for analysis. If the clinician scrapes the base of the abscess with a swab or curette, then an abundance of organisms should be observed in the Gram-stained specimen. Aspirated pus consists primarily of necrotic material with relatively few organisms, so these specimens are not as useful. Few organisms are generally present in the blood of bacteremic patients (an average of less than 1 organism per milliliter of blood), so blood specimens should be cultured but not stained. Staphylococci are seen in the nasopharynx of patients with SSSS and in the vagina of patients with TSS, but these staphylococci cannot be distinguished from the organisms that normally colonize these sites. Diagnosis of these diseases is made by the clinical presentation of the patient, with isolation of *S. aureus* in culture confirmatory. Staphylococci are implicated in food poisoning by the clinical presentation of the patient (e.g., rapid onset of vomiting and abdominal cramps) and a history of specific food ingestion (e.g., salted ham). Gram stains of the food or patient stool specimens are generally not indicated.

CULTURE

Clinical specimens should be inoculated onto nutritionally enriched agar media supplemented with sheep blood.

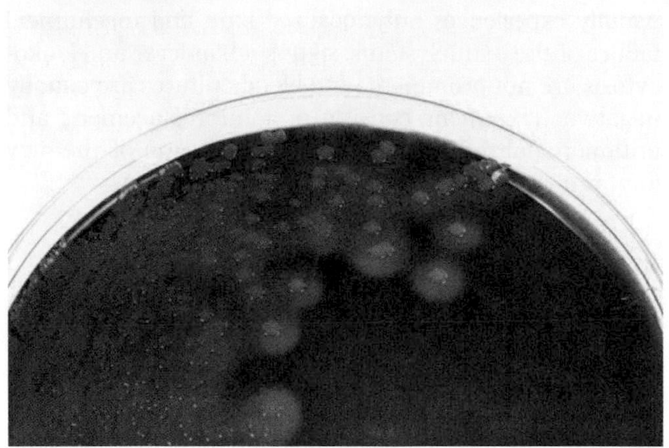

FIGURE 22–9. *Staphylococcus aureus* grown on a sheep blood agar plate. Note the colonies are large and ß hemolytic.

Staphylococci grow rapidly on nonselective media incubated aerobically or anaerobically, with large, smooth colonies seen within 24 hours (Figure 22–9). As noted earlier, *S. aureus* colonies will gradually turn yellow, particularly when the cultures are incubated at room temperature. Almost all isolates of *S. aureus* and some strains of coagulase-negative staphylococci produce hemolysis on sheep blood agar. The hemolysis is caused by cytotoxins, particularly α toxin. If there is a mixture of organisms in the specimen (e.g., wound or respiratory specimen), *S. aureus* can be isolated selectively on agar media supplemented with 7.5% sodium chloride (inhibits the growth of most other organisms) and mannitol (fermented by *S. aureus* but not by most other staphylococci).

SEROLOGY

Antibodies to cell wall teichoic acids are present in many patients with long-standing *S. aureus* infections. Antibodies develop within 2 weeks of the onset of disease and are detected in most patients with staphylococcal endocarditis. This test is less reliable, however, in the detection of antibodies in patients with staphylococcal osteomyelitis or wound infections because the focus of infection is sequestered in these settings and the organisms often do not stimulate a humoral immune response.

IDENTIFICATION

Relatively simple biochemical tests (e.g., positive reactions for coagulase, protein A, heat-stable nuclease, and mannitol fermentation) can be used to identify isolated colonies of *S. aureus* and the other staphylococci. Identification of the coagulase-negative staphylococci is more complex, requiring the use of commercial identification systems. These methods cannot be used to identify staphylococci directly in clinical specimens or when detected in a blood culture broth. Recently, this problem was resolved with the commercial development of a novel method of fluorescent in situ hybridization (FISH). Fluorescent-labeled artificial probes specific for S. aureus are used to discriminate between S. aureus and coagulase-negative staphylococci.

Antibiotic susceptibility patterns (antibiograms), biochemical profiles (biotyping), susceptibility to bacteriophages (phage typing), and nucleic acid analysis can be used for the intraspecies characterization of isolates for epidemiologic purposes. Antibiograms and biotyping are performed in most laboratories as part of the routine identification of an isolate. The tests are not highly discriminatory, however, and are useful only if two isolates have a different antibiotic susceptibility pattern or biochemical profile. Phage typing differentiates among staphylococcal strains by their pattern of susceptibility to lysis by an international collection of specific bacteriophages. This testing is performed only by research laboratories and has been replaced by nucleic acid analysis in epidemiologic studies. The analysis of genomic deoxyribonucleic acid (DNA) by pulsed-field gel electrophoresis or similar techniques has evolved rapidly to be the most sensitive way to characterize isolates at the species and subspecies levels. These methods are currently used in many research and clinical laboratories.

Treatment, Prevention, and Control

Staphylococci quickly developed drug resistance after penicillin was introduced, and today less than 10% of the strains are susceptible to this antibiotic. This resistance is mediated by penicillinase (β-lactamase specific for penicillins), which hydrolyzes the β-lactam ring of penicillin. The genetic information encoding the production of this enzyme is carried on transmissible plasmids, which facilitated the rapid dissemination of resistance among staphylococci.

Because of the problems with penicillin-resistant staphylococci, semisynthetic penicillins resistant to β-lactamase hydrolysis (e.g., methicillin, nafcillin, oxacillin, dicloxacillin) were developed. Unfortunately, the staphylococci developed resistance to these antibiotics as well. Currently, 30% to 50% of the strains of *S. aureus* and more than 50% of the coagulase-negative staphylococci are resistant to these semisynthetic penicillins. Methicillin-resistant *S. aureus* is commonly referred to by the acronym MRSA.

Resistance occurs as the result of acquisition of a gene (*mec*A) that codes for a novel penicillin-binding protein, PBP2′. The penicillins and other β-lactam antibiotics kill bacteria by their ability to bind to penicillin-binding proteins, which are enzymes responsible for construction of the cell wall peptidoglycan. PBP2′ is not bound by penicillins but retains its enzymatic activity. Not all bacteria in a resistant population may express this penicillin-binding protein **(heterogeneous resistance),** so traditional susceptibility methods may not detect resistance. The definitive method for identifying a resistant isolate is detection of the PBP2′ gene, a test that can now be performed in many clinical laboratories (Figure 22–10). Expression of PBP2′ renders the bacteria resistant to all penicillin, cephalosporin, and carbapenem antibiotics.

Until recently, MRSA strains existed almost exclusively in hospitals. However, community outbreaks with MRSA strains have been reported in the last few years. Despite the geographic diversity of the outbreaks, the strains appear to be clonally related and distinct from MRSA strains circulating in hospitals. The majority of these community MRSA strains also carries the P-V leukocidin toxin and has been associated with severe diseases, such as necrotizing pneumonia.

Staphylococci have demonstrated the remarkable ability to develop resistance to most antibiotics. Until recently, the one antibiotic that remained uniformly active against staphylococci was vancomycin, the current antibiotic of choice for treating staphylococci resistant to methicillin. Unfortunately, isolates of *S. aureus* have now been found with two forms of resistance to vancomycin. Low-level resistance is observed in *S. aureus* strains with a thicker, more disorganized cell wall. It is postulated that vancomycin is trapped in the cell wall matrix and is unable to reach the cytoplasmic membrane, where it can disrupt cell wall synthesis. High-level resistance is mediated by the *van*A gene operon that was acquired from vancomycin-resistant enterococci. These bacteria have a modified peptidoglycan layer that does not bind vancomycin. Presently, this resistance is extremely uncommon. However, if these resistant staphylococci become widespread, then antibiotic treatment of these highly virulent bacteria could be difficult.

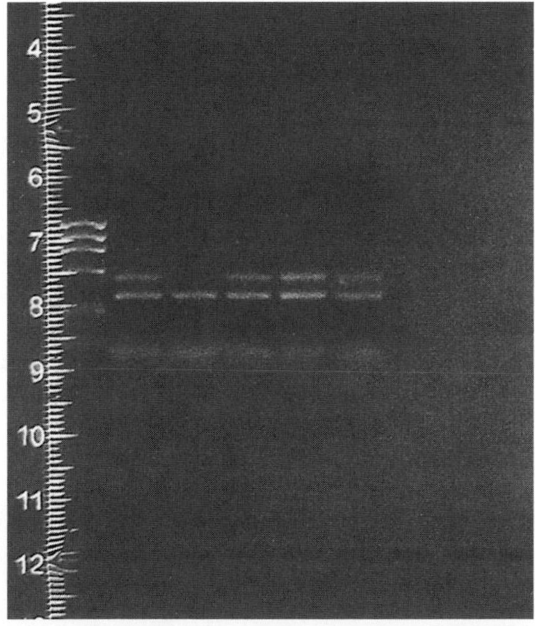

FIGURE 22–10. *mec*A gene analysis by pulsed-field gel electrophoresis (PFGE). After DNA amplification by polymerase chain reaction, the DNA preparation is exposed to a probe for the *mec*A gene. The presence of the gene is detected by PFGE. The first column is a size marker; the second and third columns are positive and negative controls, respectively; and the last three columns are *Staphylococcus aureus* isolates from three patients. All three patients had the *mec*A gene and are therefore resistant to oxacillin, other penicillins, all cephalosporins, carbapenems, and all other β-lactam antibiotics.

A novel approach to the treatment of staphylococcal diseases is the use of human monoclonal antibodies directed against the binding site of MSCRAMM proteins (surface adhesion proteins), such as *S. aureus* clumping factor. Because clumping factor is an important determinant for colonization at the site of infection, prevention of binding has been used successfully to treat experimental staphylococcal infections in animals. The success of this approach in humans remains to be demonstrated.

Staphylococci are ubiquitous organisms present on the skin and mucous membranes, and their introduction through breaks in the skin occurs often. However, the number of organisms required to establish an infection **(infectious dose)** is generally large unless a foreign body (e.g., dirt, a splinter, stitches) is present in the wound. Proper cleansing of the wound and the application of an appropriate disinfectant (e.g., germicidal soap, iodine solution, hexachlorophene) will prevent most infections in healthy individuals.

The spread of staphylococci from person to person is more difficult to prevent. An example of this is surgical wound infections, which can be caused by relatively few organisms, because foreign bodies and devitalized tissue may be present. Although it is unrealistic to sterilize the operating room personnel and environment, the risk of contamination during an operative procedure can be minimized through proper hand washing and the covering of exposed skin surfaces. The spread of methicillin-resistant organisms can also be difficult to control because asymptomatic nasopharyngeal carriage is the most common source of these organisms. However, some success in this regard has been achieved through the use of chemoprophylaxis consisting of vancomycin and rifampin.

CASE STUDY AND QUESTIONS

An 18-year-old man fell on his knee while playing basketball. The knee was painful, but the overlying skin was unbroken. The knee was swollen and remained painful the next day, so he was taken to the local emergency department. Clear fluid was aspirated from the knee, and the physician prescribed symptomatic treatment. Two days later, the swelling returned, the pain increased, and erythema developed over the knee. Because the patient also felt systemically ill and had an oral temperature of 38.8°C, he returned to the emergency department. Aspiration of the knee yielded cloudy fluid, and cultures of the fluid and blood were positive for S. aureus.

1. Name two possible sources of this organism.
2. Staphylococci cause a variety of diseases, including cutaneous infections, endocarditis, food poisoning, SSSS, and TSS. How do the clinical symptoms of these diseases differ from the infection in this patient? Which of these diseases are intoxications?
3. What toxins have been implicated in staphylococcal diseases? Which staphylococcal enzymes have been proposed as virulence factors?
4. Which structures in the staphylococcal cell and which toxins protect the bacterium from phagocytosis?
5. What is the antibiotic of choice for treating staphylococcal infections? (Give two examples.)

Bibliography

Boubaker K et al: Panton-Valentine leukocidin and staphylococcal skin infections in schoolchildren, *Emerg Infect Dis* 10:121-124, 2004.

Boussaud V et al: Life-threatening hemoptysis in adults with community-acquired pneumonia due to Panton-Valentine leukocidin-secreting *Staphylococcus aureus*, Intensive Care Med, 29:1840-1843, 2003.

Dinges MM et al: Exotoxins of *Staphylococcus aureus*, *Clin Microbiol Rev* 13:16-34, 2000.

Gravet A et al: Predominant *Staphylococcus aureus* isolated from antibiotic-associated diarrhea is clinically relevant and produces enterotoxin A and the biocomponent toxin LukE-LukD, *J Clin Microbiol* 37:4012-4019, 1999.

Holmberg SD, Blake PA: Staphylococcal food poisoning in the United States: New facts and old misconceptions, *JAMA* 251:487-489, 1984.

Hovelius B, Mardh PA: *Staphylococcus saprophyticus* as a common cause of urinary tract infections, *Rev Infect Dis* 6:328-337, 1984.

Ladhani S et al: Clinical, microbial, and biochemical aspects of the exfoliative toxins causing staphylococcal scalded skin syndrome, *Clin Microbiol Rev* 12:224-242, 1999.

Lowy FD: *Staphylococcus aureus* infections, *N Engl J Med* 339:520-532, 1998.

Murray PR et al: *Manual of clinical microbiology*, ed 8, Washington, 2003, American Society for Microbiology.

Novick RP. Autoinduction and signal transduction in the regulation of staphylococcal virulence, *Mol Microbiol* 48:1429-1449, 2003.

Patti JM et al: MSCRAMM-mediated adherence of microorganisms to host tissues, *Annu Rev Microbiol* 48:585-617, 1994.

Seenivansan MH, Yu VL: *Staphylococcus lugdunensis* endocarditis—the hidden peril of coagulase-negative Staphylococcus in blood cultures, Eur J Clin Microbiol Infect Dis 22:489-491, 2003.

Shirtliff ME, Mader JT: Acute septic arthritis, *Clin Microbiol Rev* 15:527-544, 2002.

Srinivasan A, Dick JD, Perl TM: Vancomycin resistance in staphylococci, *Clin Microbiol Rev* 15:430-438, 2002.

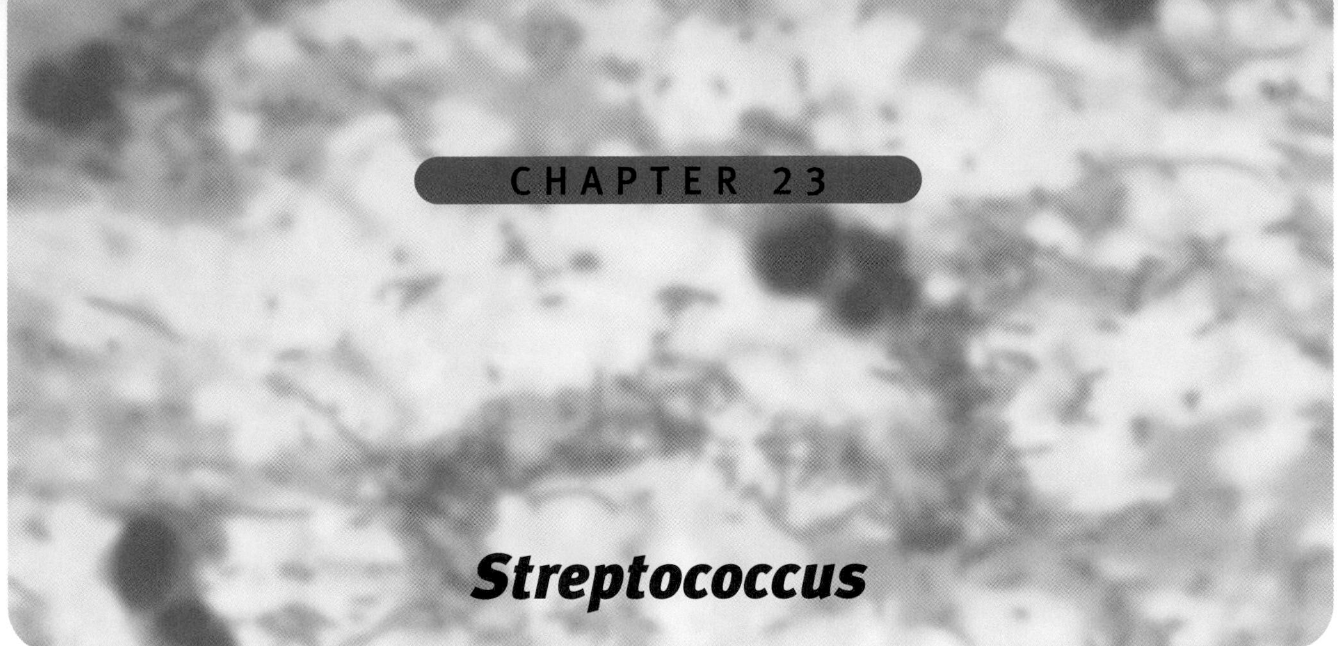

CHAPTER 23

Streptococcus

The genus *Streptococcus* is a diverse collection of gram-positive cocci typically arranged in pairs or chains. Most species are facultative anaerobes, and some grow only in an atmosphere enhanced with carbon dioxide **(capnophilic growth).** Their nutritional requirements are complex, necessitating the use of blood- or serum-enriched media for isolation. Carbohydrates are fermented, resulting in the production of lactic acid, and unlike *Staphylococcus* species, streptococci are catalase-negative.

Numerous streptococci are recognized as important human pathogens, the most common of which are discussed in this chapter (Box 23–1). Unfortunately, the differentiation of species within the genus is complicated, because three different, overlapping schemes are used to classify the organisms (Table 23–1): (1) Serologic properties: Lancefield groupings (originally A to W); (2) hemolytic patterns: complete (beta [β]) hemolysis, incomplete (alpha [α]) hemolysis, and no (gamma) hemolysis; and (3) biochemical (physiologic) properties.

Rebecca Lancefield developed the serologic classification scheme in 1933 for differentiating beta-hemolytic strains. Most β-hemolytic strains and some α-hemolytic and nonhemolytic strains possess group-specific antigens, most of which are cell wall carbohydrates. These antigens can be readily detected by immunologic assays and have been useful for the rapid identification of some important streptococcal pathogens. For example, *Streptococcus pyogenes* (classified as group A *Streptococcus* in the Lancefield typing scheme) is responsible for streptococcal pharyngitis. The group antigen for this organism can be detected by rapid immunoassays directly from throat swab specimens. The Lancefield typing scheme is primarily used today for only a few species of streptococci (e.g., those in groups A, B, C, F, and G).

Most (but not all) α-hemolytic and nonhemolytic streptococci do not possess the group-specific cell wall antigens. These organisms must be identified by biochemical tests. Unfortunately, the classification schemes are not mutually exclusive. For example, members of the *Streptococcus anginosus* group may have any hemolytic pattern and may be nontypable or react with the antisera for groups A, C, F, or G. Likewise, *Streptococcus agalactiae* (Lancefield group B) is usually β-hemolytic but may also be nonhemolytic.

Streptococcus pyogenes (Box 23–2)

The most important species of group A streptococci is *S. pyogenes. S. pyogenes* causes a variety of suppurative and nonsuppurative diseases (Box 23–3). Although this organism is the most common cause of bacterial pharyngitis, the notoriety of *S. pyogenes,* as documented in both the scientific literature and tabloid press, is a product of the dramatic, life-threatening diseases caused by these "flesh-eating" bacteria.

PHYSIOLOGY AND STRUCTURE

Isolates of *S. pyogenes* are spherical cocci, 1 to 2 μm in diameter, arranged in short chains in clinical specimens and longer chains when grown in liquid media (Figure 23–1). Growth is optimal on enriched-blood agar media but is inhibited if the medium contains a high concentration of glucose. After 24 hours of incubation, 1- to 2-mm white colonies with large zones of β-hemolysis are observed (Figure 23–2).

The antigenic structure of *S. pyogenes* has been extensively studied. The basic structural framework of the cell wall is the peptidoglycan layer, which is similar in composition to that found in other gram-positive bacteria. Within the cell wall are the group-specific and type-specific antigens.

BOX 23-1. Important Streptococci

Organism	Historical Derivation
Streptococcus	*streptus,* pliant; *coccus,* grain or berry (a pliant berry or coccus; refers to the appearance of long, flexible chains of cocci)
S. agalactiae	*agalactia,* want of milk (original isolate [called S. mastitidis] was responsible for bovine mastitis)
S. anginosus	*anginosus,* pertaining to angina
S. bovis	*bovis,* bovine (originally associated with disease in cows)
S. constellatus	*constellatus,* studded with stars (original isolate embedded in agar with smaller colonies surrounding the large colony; satellite formation does not occur around colonies on the surface of an agar plate)
S. dysgalactiae	*dys,* ill, hard; *galactia,* pertaining to milk (loss of milk secretion; isolates associated with bovine mastitis)
S. intermedius	*intermedius,* intermediate (initial confusion about whether this was an aerobic or an anaerobic bacterium)
S. mitis	*mitis,* mild (incorrectly thought to cause mild infections)
S. mutans	*mutans,* changing (cocci that may appear rodlike, particularly when initially isolated in culture)
S. pneumoniae	*pneumon,* the lungs (causes pneumonia)
S. pyogenes	*pyus,* pus; *gennaio,* beget or producing (pus producing; typically associated with formation of pus in wounds)
S. salivarius	*salivarius,* salivary (found in the mouth in saliva)

TABLE 23-1. Classification of Common Streptococcal Pathogens

Biochemical Classification	Serologic Classification	Hemolysis Patterns
S. pyogenes	A	β
S. agalactiae	B	β; occasionally nonhemolytic
S. dysgalactiae	C, G	β
S. anginosus group	A, C, F, G, nongroupable	β; occasionally α or nonhemolytic
S. bovis	D	α; nonhemolytic; occasionally β
Viridans group	Nongroupable	α or nonhemolytic
S. pneumoniae	Nongroupable	α

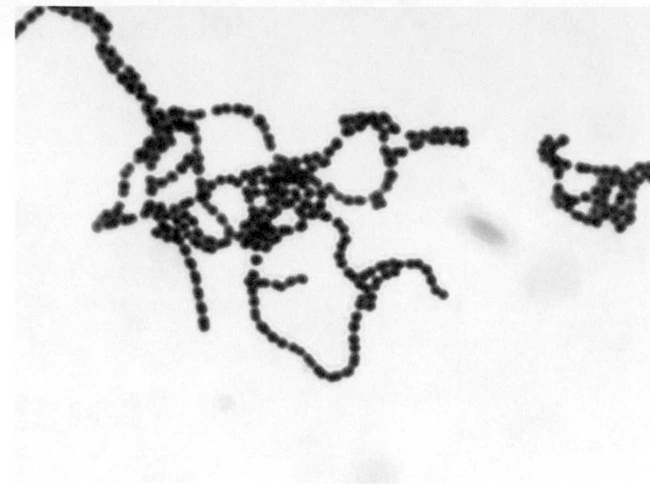

FIGURE 23-1. Gram stain of *Streptococcus pyogenes.*

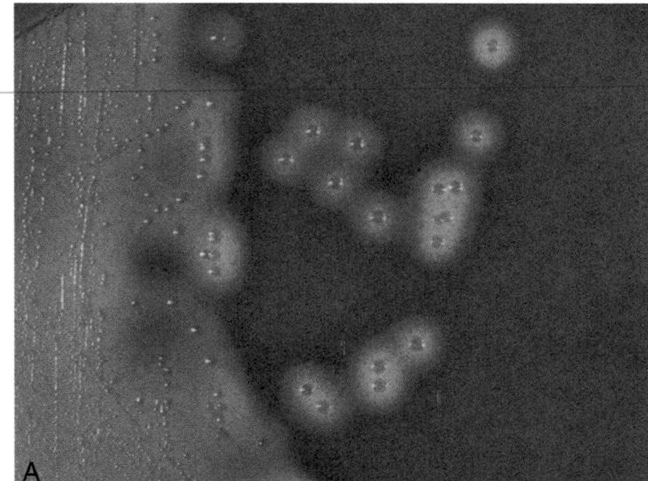

FIGURE 23-2. β-Hemolytic streptococci. **A,** *S. pyogenes* (group A), small colonies with a large zone of hemolysis; **B,** *S. agalactiae* (group B), large colonies with a small zone of hemolysis.

BOX 23–2. Summary of *Streptococcus pyogenes*

Physiology and Structure

Gram-positive cocci arranged in pairs and long chains
β-Hemolytic; more viruluent strains with capsule
Facultative anaerobe
Catalase negative; PYR positive; bacitracin susceptible (important identification tests)
Group-specific carbohydrate (A antigen) and type-specific antigens (M and T proteins) in cell wall
Produce streptolysin O and DNase B (antibodies against these antigens [ASO, anti–DNase B] are clinically important)

Virulence

Refer to Table 23–2

Epidemiology

Asymptomatic colonization in upper respiratory tract and transient colonization of skin
Can survive on dry surfaces for long periods
Person-to-person spread by respiratory droplets (pharyngitis) or through breaks in skin after direct contact with infected person, fomite, or arthropod vector
Individuals at higher risk for disease include children 5 to 15 years old (pharyngitis); patients with extensive soft-tissue infections and bacteremia (streptococcal toxic shock syndrome); children ages 2 to 5 years who have poor personal hygiene (pyoderma); young children and older adults with preexisting respiratory tract or skin infections caused by *S. pyogenes* (erysipelas, cellulitis); children with severe streptococcal disease (rheumatic fever, glomerulonephritis)
Although the organism is ubiquitous, there are seasonal incidences of specific diseases: pharyngitis and associated rheumatic fever or glomerulonephritis (more common in cold months); pyoderma and associated glomerulonephritis (more common in warm months)

Diseases

Refer to Box 23–3

Diagnosis

Microscopy is useful in skin and soft-tissue infections
Direct antigen tests are useful for the diagnosis of streptococcal pharyngitis, but negative results must be confirmed by culture
Culture is highly sensitive
Isolates identified by catalase (negative), positive PYR reaction, susceptibility to bacitracin, and presence of group-specific antigen (group A antigen)
ASO test is useful for confirming rheumatic fever and acute glomerulonephritis; anti–DNase B test should also be performed if acute glomerulonephritis is suspected

Treatment, Control, and Prevention

Penicillin is drug of choice; erythromycin or oral cephalosporin is used for patients allergic to penicillin; antistaphylococcal antibiotics are given for mixed infections
Oropharyngeal carriage occurring after treatment can be re-treated; treatment is not indicated for prolonged asymptomatic carriage, because antibiotics disrupt normal protective flora
Starting antibiotic therapy within 10 days in patients with pharyngitis prevents rheumatic fever
For patients with a history of rheumatic fever, antibiotic prophylaxis is required before procedures (e.g., dental) that can induce bacteremias leading to endocarditis
For glomerulonephritis, no specific antibiotic treatment or prophylaxis is indicated

PYR, *L*-pyrrolidonyl arylamidase.

Group-Specific Carbohydrate

The group-specific carbohydrate that constitutes approximately 10% of the dry weight of the cell (Lancefield group A antigen) is a dimer of *N*-acetylglucosamine and rhamnose. This antigen is used to classify group A streptococci and distinguish them from other streptococcal groups.

Type-Specific Proteins

The **M protein** is a major type-specific protein associated with virulent streptococci. It consists of two polypeptide chains complexed in an alpha helix. The protein is anchored in the cytoplasmic membrane, extends through the cell wall, and protrudes above the cell surface. The carboxyl terminus anchored in the cytoplasmic membrane and the portion of the molecule in the cell wall are highly conserved among all group A streptococci. The amino terminus, which extends above the cell surface, is responsible for the antigenic variability observed among the more than 100 serotypes of M proteins. M proteins are subdivided into class I and class II molecules. The class I M proteins share exposed antigens, whereas the class II M proteins do not have exposed shared antigens. Although strains with both classes of antigens can cause suppurative infections and glomerulonephritis, only bacteria with class I M proteins cause rheumatic fever.

A secondary type-specific protein that is a useful epidemiologic marker for bacterial strains that fail to express the M protein is the **T (trypsin-resistant) protein.** The structural function of this protein is unknown. Although the epidemiologic classification of *S. pyogenes* has been based traditionally on identification of specific M or T types by agglutination with M- or T-specific antibodies, it

BOX 23–3. Streptococcal Diseases—Clinical Summaries

***Streptococcus pyogenes* (group A)**

Suppurative Infections

Pharyngitis: Reddened pharynx with exudates generally present; cervical lymphadenopathy can be prominent

Scarlet fever: Diffuse erythematous rash beginning on the chest and spreading to the extremities; complication of streptococcal pharyngitis

Pyoderma: Localized skin infection with vesicles progressing to pustules; no evidence of systemic disease

Erysipelas: Localized skin infection with pain, inflammation, lymph node enlargement and systemic symptoms

Cellulitis: Infection of the skin that involves the subcutaneous tissues

Necrotizing fasciitis: Deep infection of skin that involves destruction of muscle and fat layers

Streptococcal toxic shock syndrome: Multiorgan systemic infection resembling staphylococcal toxic shock syndrome; however, most patients bacteremic and with evidence of fasciitis

Other suppurative diseases: Variety of other infections recognized including puerperal sepsis, lymphangitis, pneumonia

Nonsuppurative Infections

Rheumatic fever: Characterized by inflammatory changes of the heart (pancarditis), joints (arthralgias to arthritis), blood vessels, and subcutaneous tissues

Acute glomerulonephritis: Acute inflammation of the renal glomeruli with edema, hypertension, hematuria, and proteinuria

***Streptococcus agalactiae* (Group B)**

Early-onset neonatal disease: Within 7 days of birth, infected newborns develop signs and symptoms of pneumonia, meningitis, and sepsis

Late-onset neonatal disease: More than a week after birth, neonates develop signs and symptoms of bacteremia with meningitis

Infections in pregnant women: Most often present as urinary tract infections; bacteremia and disseminated complications may occur

Infections in other adult patients: Most common diseases include bacteremia, pneumonia, bone and joint infections, and skin and soft-tissue infections

Other β-Hemolytic Streptococci

Abscess formation in deep tissues: Associated with *S. anginosus* group

Pharyngitis: Associated with *S. dysgalactiae;* disease resembles that caused by *S. pyogenes;* can be complicated with acute glomerulonephritis

Viridans Streptococci

Abscess formation in deep tissues: Associated with *S. anginosus* group (as above)

Septicemia in neutropenic patients: Associated with *S. mitis* group

Subacute endocarditis: Associated with *S. gordonii, S. mutans, S. mitis, S. oralis,* and *S. sanguis*

Dental caries: Associated with *S. mutans* and *S. sobrinus*

Malignancies of gastrointestinal tract: Associated with *S. bovis*

Streptococcus pneumoniae

Pneumonia: Acute onset with severe chills and sustained fever; productive cough with blood-tinged sputum; lobar consolidation

Meningitis: Severe infection involving the meninges with headache, fever, and sepsis; high mortality and severe neurologic deficits in survivors

Bacteremia: More common in patients with meningitis than with pneumonia, otitis, media, or sinusitis; overwhelming sepsis in asplenic patients

is likely that this procedure will be replaced by sequencing the *emm* gene that encodes the M protein.

Other Cell Surface Components

Other important components in the cell wall of *S. pyogenes* include **M-like surface proteins, lipoteichoic acid,** and **F protein.** A complex of more than 20 genes that comprise the *emm* gene superfamily encode the M-like proteins. These genes code for M proteins, M-like proteins, and other immunoglobulin (Ig)-binding proteins. Lipoteichoic acid and F protein facilitate binding of host cells by complexing with fibronectin, which is present on the host cell surface.

Capsule

Some strains of *S. pyogenes* form an outer hyaluronic acid **capsule** that contains repeating molecules of glucuronic acid and *N*-acetylglucosamine. The capsule is antigenically indistinguishable from hyaluronic acid in mammalian connective tissues. Thus it functions to prevent phagocytosis of the bacteria. Strains of encapsulated *S. pyogenes* are more likely to be responsible for severe systemic infections.

PATHOGENESIS AND IMMUNITY

The virulence of group A streptococci is determined by the ability of the bacteria to adhere to the surface of host cells,

TABLE 23–2. Virulence Factors of *Streptococcus pyogenes*

Virulence Factor	Biologic Effect
Capsule	Antiphagocytic
Lipoteichoic acid	Binds to epithelial cells
M protein	Adhesin; mediates internalization by host cells; antiphagocytic; degrades complement component C3b
M-like proteins	Binds immunoglobulins M and G and α_2-macroglobulin (protease inhibitor); antiphagocytic
F protein	Mediates adherence to epithelial cells and internalization
Pyrogenic exotoxins	Mediate pyrogenicity, enhancement of delayed hypersensitivity and susceptibility to endotoxin, cytotoxicity, nonspecific mitogenicity for T cells, immunosuppression of B-cell function, and production of scarlatiniform rash
Streptolysin S	Lyses leukocytes, platelets, and erythrocytes; stimulates release of lysosomal enzymes; nonimmunogenic
Streptolysin O	Lyses leukocytes, platelets, and erythrocytes; stimulates release of lysosomal enzymes; immunogenic
Streptokinase	Lyses blood clots; facilitates spread of bacteria in tissues
DNase	Depolymerizes cell-free DNA in purulent material
C5a peptidase	Degrades complement component C5a

invade into the epithelial cells, avoid opsonization and phagocytosis, and produce a variety of toxins and enzymes (Table 23–2). More than 10 different bacterial antigens have been demonstrated to mediate adherence to host cells, with lipoteichoic acid, M proteins, and F protein the most important. The initial adherence is a weak interaction between lipoteichoic acid and fatty acid–binding sites on fibronectin and epithelial cells. Subsequent adherence involves M protein, F protein, and other adhesins that interact with specific host cell receptors. *S. pyogenes* can invade into epithelial cells, a process that is mediated by M protein and F protein and other bacterial antigens. This internalization is believed to be important for maintenance of persistent infections (e.g., recurrent streptococcal pharyngitis) and invasion into deep tissues.

S. pyogenes also has multiple mechanisms for avoiding opsonization and phagocytosis. The conserved region of M protein can bind the serum β-globulin factor H, which is a regulatory protein for the alternative complement pathway. The complement component C3b, an important mediator of phagocytosis, is destabilized by factor H. Thus when C3b binds to the cell surface in the region of the M protein, C3b is degraded by factor H and phagocytosis is prevented. The effect is overcome only when the patient produces type-specific opsonic antibodies directed against the specific M protein. The binding of fibrinogen to the surface of M protein also blocks activation of complement by the alternate pathway and reduces the amount of bound C3b. The M-like proteins interfere with phagocytosis. Finally, all strains of *S. pyogenes* can produce C5a peptidase, a serine protease that inactivates C5a. C5a is a chemoattractant of neutrophils and mononuclear phagocytes; thus abscess formation is inhibited until the patient is able to neutralize the peptidase with specific antibodies.

Additionally, a number of enzymes and toxins can mediate the pathology observed with *S. pyogenes* infections.

Pyrogenic Exotoxins

The **streptococcal pyrogenic exotoxins (Spes)**, originally called erythrogenic toxins, are produced by lysogenic strains of streptococci and are similar to the toxin produced in *Corynebacterium diphtheriae.* Four immunologically distinct heat-labile toxins (SpeA, SpeB, SpeC, and SpeF) have been described in *S. pyogenes* and in rare strains of groups C and G streptococci. The toxins act as superantigens, interacting with both macrophages and helper T cells, with the release of (1) interleukin-1 (IL-1), IL-2, and IL-6; (2) tumor necrosis factor-α (TNF-α) and TNF-β; and (3) interferon-γ (Ifn-γ). These cytokines mediate a variety of important effects, including shock and the organ failure seen characteristically in patients with streptococcal toxic shock syndrome. The toxins are also responsible for the rash observed in patients with scarlet fever, although it is unclear whether the rash results from the direct effect of the toxin on the capillary bed or, more likely, is secondary to a hypersensitivity reaction.

Streptolysins S and O

Streptolysin S is an oxygen-stable, nonimmunogenic, cell-bound hemolysin that can lyse erythrocytes, leukocytes, and platelets. It can also stimulate the release of lysosomal contents after engulfment, with subsequent death of the phagocytic cell. Streptolysin S is produced in the presence of serum (the S indicates serum soluble) and is responsible for the characteristic β-hemolysis seen on blood agar media.

Streptolysin O is an oxygen-labile hemolysin capable of lysing erythrocytes, leukocytes, platelets, and cultured cells. Antibodies are readily formed against streptolysin O (anti–streptolysin O [ASO] antibodies), a feature differentiating it from streptolysin S, and are useful for documenting recent group A streptococcal infection **(anti-ASO test).** Because streptolysin O is irreversibly inhibited by cholesterol in skin lipids, however, patients with *S. pyogenes* skin infections do not develop anti-ASO antibodies. This hemolysin is antigenically related to oxygen-labile toxins produced by *Streptococcus pneumoniae, Clostridium tetani, Clostridium perfringens, Bacillus cereus,* and *Listeria monocytogenes.*

Streptokinases

At least two forms of streptokinase (A and B) have been described. These enzymes mediate the cleavage of plasminogen, releasing the protease plasmin that in turn cleaves fibrin and fibrinogen, resulting in the lysis of clots and fibrin deposits. Thus these enzymes can lyse blood clots and fibrin deposits and facilitate the rapid spread of *S. pyogenes* in infected tissues. Antibodies directed against these enzymes (anti-streptokinase antibodies) are a useful marker for infection.

Deoxyribonucleases

Four immunologically distinct deoxyribonucleases **(DNases A to D)** have been identified. These enzymes are not cytolytic but can depolymerize free deoxyribonucleic acid (DNA) present in pus. This process reduces the viscosity of the abscess material and facilitates spread of the organisms. Antibodies developed against DNase B are an important marker of *S. pyogenes* infections, particularly for patients with cutaneous infections, because they fail to make antibodies against streptolysin O (see preceding section).

C5a Peptidase

Complement component C5a mediates inflammation by recruiting and activating phagocytic cells. **C5a peptidase** disrupts this process by degrading C5a.

Other Enzymes

Other enzymes, including hyaluronidase ("spreading factor") and diphosphopyridine nucleotidase (DPNase), have been described for group A streptococci. The role of these enzymes in pathogenesis is unknown.

EPIDEMIOLOGY

The Centers for Disease Control and Prevention estimated that approximately 4500 cases of invasive disease caused by *S. pyogenes* occurred in 2004 in the United States. More than 500 cases of streptococcal toxic shock syndrome (with a 45% fatality rate) were observed. A similar number of cases of necrotizing fasciitis (with a 25% fatality rate) occurred. At least 10 million cases of noninvasive disease occurred, with pharyngitis and pyoderma the most common infections. Group A streptococci commonly colonize the oropharynx of healthy children and young adults (see Box 23–2). Although the incidence of carriage is reported to be 15% to 20%, these figures are misleading. Highly selective culture techniques are necessary to detect small numbers of organisms in oropharyngeal secretions. Additionally, colonization with group A streptococci was assumed to be synonymous with colonization with *S. pyogenes.* However, it is now known that other streptococcal species (e.g., *S. anginosus, S. intermedius, S. constellatus*) can carry the group-specific A antigen and are present in the oropharynx. These species are not believed to cause pharyngitis.

Colonization with *S. pyogenes* is transient, regulated by the person's ability to mount specific immunity to the M protein of the colonizing strain and the presence of competitive organisms in the oropharynx. Untreated patients produce antibodies against the specific bacterial M protein that can result in long-lived immunity; however, this antibody response is diminished in treated patients. Bacteria such as the α-hemolytic and nonhemolytic streptococci are able to produce antibiotic-like substances called **bacteriocins,** which suppress the growth of group A streptococci.

In general, *S. pyogenes* disease is caused by recently acquired strains that can establish an infection of the pharynx or skin before specific antibodies are produced or competitive organisms are able to proliferate. Pharyngitis caused by *S. pyogenes* is primarily a disease of children between the ages of 5 and 15 years, but infants and adults are also susceptible. The pathogen is spread from person to person through respiratory droplets. Crowding, such as in classrooms and daycare facilities, increases the opportunity for the organism to spread, particularly during the winter months. Soft-tissue infections (i.e., pyoderma, erysipelas, cellulitis, fasciitis) are typically preceded by initial skin colonization with group A streptococci, after which the organisms are introduced into the superficial or deep tissues through a break in the skin.

CLINICAL DISEASES

Suppurative Streptococcal Disease

Pharyngitis

Pharyngitis generally develops 2 to 4 days after exposure to the pathogen, with an abrupt onset of sore throat, fever, malaise, and headache. The posterior pharynx can appear erythematous with an exudate, and cervical lymphadenopathy can be prominent. Despite these clinical signs and symptoms, differentiating streptococcal pharyngitis from viral pharyngitis is difficult. For example, approximately only 50% of patients with "strep throat" have pharyngeal or tonsillar exudates. Likewise, many young children with exudative pharyngitis have viral disease. The specific diagnosis can be made only with bacteriologic or serologic tests.

Scarlet fever is a complication of streptococcal pharyngitis that occurs when the infecting strain is lysogenized by a temperate bacteriophage that stimulates production of a pyrogenic exotoxin. Within 1 to 2 days after the initial clinical symptoms of pharyngitis develop, a diffuse erythematous rash initially appears on the upper chest and then spreads to the extremities. The area around the mouth is generally spared **(circumoral pallor),** as are the palms and soles. A yellowish-white coating initially covers the tongue and is later shed, revealing a red, raw surface beneath **("strawberry tongue").** The rash, which blanches when pressed, is best seen on the abdomen and in skin folds **(Pastia's lines).** The rash disappears over the next 5 to 7 days and is followed by desquamation. Suppurative complications of streptococcal pharyngitis (e.g., peritonsillar and retropharyngeal abscesses) have become rare since the advent of antimicrobial therapy.

Pyoderma

Pyoderma (impetigo) is a confined, purulent *("pyo")* infection of the skin *("derma")* that primarily affects exposed areas (i.e., face, arms, legs). Infection begins when the skin is colonized with *S. pyogenes* after direct contact with an infected person or fomites. The organism is introduced into the subcutaneous tissues through a break in the skin (e.g., scratch, insect bite). Vesicles develop, progressing to pustules (pus-filled vesicles), and then rupture and crust over. The regional lymph nodes can become enlarged, but systemic signs of infection (e.g., fever, sepsis, involvement of other organs) are uncommon. Secondary dermal spread of the infection caused by scratching is typical.

Pyoderma is seen primarily during the warm, moist summer months, in young children with poor personal hygiene. Although *S. pyogenes* is responsible for most streptococcal skin infections, groups C and G streptococci have also been implicated. *Staphylococcus aureus* is also commonly present in the lesions. The strains of streptococci that cause skin infections differ from those that cause pharyngitis, although pyoderma serotypes can colonize the pharynx and establish a persistent carriage state.

Erysipelas

Erysipelas (*erythros,* "red"; *pella,* "skin") is an acute infection of the skin. Patients experience localized pain, inflammation (erythema, warmth), lymph node enlargement, and systemic signs (chills, fever, leukocytosis). The involved skin area is typically raised and distinctly differentiated from the uninvolved skin (Figure 23–3). Erysipelas occurs most commonly in young children or older adults, historically on the face but now more commonly on the legs, and usually is preceded by infections of the respiratory tract or skin with *S. pyogenes* (less commonly with group C or G streptococci).

Cellulitis

Unlike erysipelas, **cellulitis** typically involves the skin and deeper subcutaneous tissues, and the distinction between infected and noninfected skin is not as clear. As in erysipelas, local inflammation and systemic signs are observed. Precise identification of the offending organism is necessary, because many different organisms can cause cellulitis.

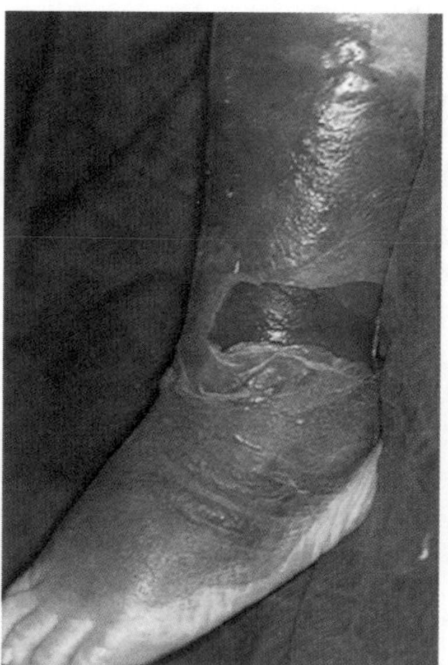

FIGURE 23–3. Acute stage of erysipelas of the leg. Note the erythema in the involved area and bullae formation. (From Emond RTD, Rowland HAK: *A color atlas of infectious diseases,* ed 2, London, 1989, Wolfe.)

Necrotizing Fasciitis

Necrotizing fasciitis (also called streptococcal gangrene) is an infection that occurs deep in the subcutaneous tissue, spreads along the fascial planes, and is characterized by an extensive destruction of muscle and fat (Figure 23–4). The organism (referred to by the news media as "flesh-eating bacteria") is introduced into the tissue through a break in the skin (e.g., minor cut or trauma, vesicular viral infection, burn, surgery). Initially there is evidence of cellulitis, after which bullae form and gangrene and systemic symptoms develop. Systemic toxicity, multiorgan failure, and death are the hallmarks of this disease; thus, prompt medical intervention is necessary to save the patient. Unlike cellulitis, which can be treated with antibiotic therapy, fasciitis must also be treated aggressively with the surgical débridement of infected tissue.

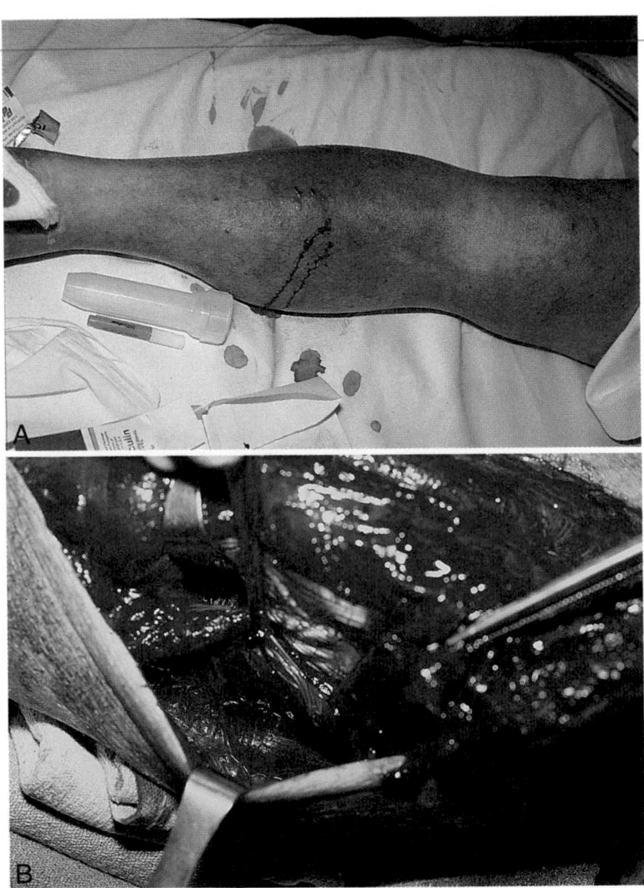

FIGURE 23–4. Necrotizing fasciitis caused by Streptococcus pyogenes. The patient presented with a 3-day history of malaise, diffuse myalgia, and low-grade fever. Over 3 hours, the pain became excruciating and was localized to the calf. **A,** Note the two small, purple bullae over the calf. **B,** Extensive necrotizing fasciitis was present on surgical exploration. The patient died despite aggressive surgical and medical management. (From Cohen J, Powderly W: *Infectious diseases,* ed 2, St Louis, 2004, Mosby).

Streptococcal Toxic Shock Syndrome

Although the incidence of severe *S. pyogenes* disease declined steadily after the advent of antibiotics, this trend changed dramatically in the late 1980s, when infections characterized by multisystem toxicity were reported. Patients with this syndrome initially experience soft-tissue inflammation at the site of the infection, pain, and nonspecific symptoms such as fever, chills, malaise, nausea, vomiting, and diarrhea. The pain intensifies as the disease progresses to shock and organ failure (e.g., kidney, lungs, liver, heart)—features similar to those of staphylococcal toxic shock syndrome. However, patients with streptococcal disease are bacteremic and most have necrotizing fasciitis.

Although people of all age groups are susceptible to **streptococcal toxic shock syndrome,** patients with certain conditions are at increased risk, such as those with human immunodeficiency virus (HIV) infection, cancer, diabetes mellitus, heart or pulmonary disease, and varicella-zoster virus infection, as well as intravenous drug abusers and those who abuse alcohol. The strains of *S. pyogenes* responsible for this syndrome differ from the strains causing pharyngitis, in that most of the former are M serotypes 1 or 3 and many have prominent mucopolysaccharide hyaluronic acid capsules (mucoid strains). The production of pyrogenic exotoxins, particularly SpeA and SpeC, is also a prominent feature of these organisms.

Other Suppurative Diseases

S. pyogenes has been associated with a variety of other suppurative infections, including puerperal sepsis, lymphangitis, and pneumonia. Although these infections are still seen, they became less common after the introduction of antibiotic therapy.

Bacteremia

S. pyogenes is one of the most common β-hemolytic streptococci isolated in blood cultures (Figure 23–5). Patients with localized infections such as pharyngitis, pyoderma, and erysipelas rarely have bacteremia. The blood cultures in most patients with necrotizing fasciitis or toxic shock syndrome, however, are positive for the organism; the mortality in this population of patients approaches 40%.

Nonsuppurative Streptococcal Disease

Rheumatic Fever

Rheumatic fever is a nonsuppurative complication of *S. pyogenes* disease. It is characterized by inflammatory changes involving the heart, joints, blood vessels, and subcutaneous tissues. Involvement of the heart manifests as a pancarditis (endocarditis, pericarditis, myocarditis) and is often associated with subcutaneous nodules. Chronic, progressive damage to the heart valves may occur. Joint manifestations can range from arthralgias to frank arthritis, with multiple joints involved in a migratory pattern (i.e., involvement shifts from one joint to another).

The incidence of rheumatic fever in the United States has decreased from a peak of more than 10,000 cases per year reported in 1961 to 112 cases reported in 1994 (the last year of mandatory reporting). In contrast, disease in developing countries is much more common, with an estimated 100 cases per 100,000 children per year. Specific M types (e.g., types 1, 3, 5, 6, and 18) cause the disease.

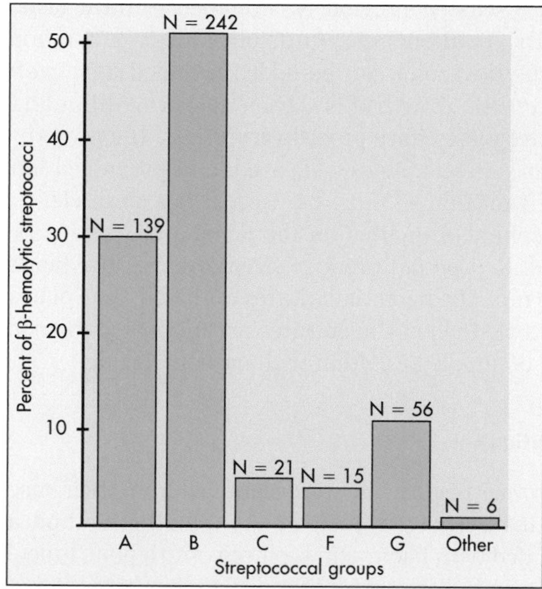

FIGURE 23–5. Distribution of streptococcal groups in bacteremic adults admitted to Barnes Hospital in St. Louis from 1986 to 2000. During this period, 479 patients with β-hemolytic streptococcal bacteremia were seen.

Rheumatic fever is associated with streptococcal pharyngitis but not cutaneous streptococcal infections. As would be expected, the epidemiologic characteristics of the disease mimic those of streptococcal pharyngitis. It is most common in young school-age children, with no male or female predilection, and occurs primarily during the fall or winter. Although disease occurs most commonly in patients with severe streptococcal pharyngitis, as many as a third of patients have asymptomatic or mild infection. Rheumatic fever can recur with subsequent streptococcal infection if antibiotic prophylaxis is not used. The risk for recurrence decreases with time.

Because no specific diagnostic test can identify patients with rheumatic fever, the diagnosis is made on the basis of clinical findings and documented evidence of a recent *S. pyogenes* infection, such as (1) culture results, (2) detection of the group A antigen, or (3) an elevation of anti-ASO, anti–DNase B, or anti-hyaluronidase antibodies. The absence of an elevated or rising antibody titer would be strong evidence against rheumatic fever.

Acute Glomerulonephritis

The second nonsuppurative complication of streptococcal disease is **acute glomerulonephritis,** which is characterized by acute inflammation of the renal glomeruli with edema, hypertension, hematuria, and proteinuria. Specific nephritogenic strains of group A streptococci are associated with this disease. The pharyngeal and pyodermal strains differ. The epidemiologic characteristics of the disease are similar to those of the initial streptococcal infection (Table 23–3). Diagnosis is determined on the basis of the clinical presentation and the finding of evidence of a recent *S. pyogenes* infection. Young patients generally have an uneventful recovery, but the long-term prognosis for adults is unclear. Progressive, irreversible loss of renal function has been observed in adults.

TABLE 23–3. Epidemiologic Features of Acute Streptococcal Glomerulonephritis

Feature	Pharyngitis Associated	Pyoderma Associated
Seasonal occurrence	Winter and spring	Late summer and early autumn
Geographic distribution	Temperate and cold climates	Hot and tropical climates
Age	School-age children	Preschool-age children
Familial occurrence	Common	Common
Attack rate after infection with nephritogenic strain	10%-15%	10%-15%
Carrier state	Pharynx (common)	Skin (rare)
Serologic types	Limited to pharynx	Limited to skin
Anti–streptolysin O response	Common	Uncommon
Anti–DNase B response	Common	Common

LABORATORY DIAGNOSIS

Microscopy

Gram stains of samples of affected tissue can be used to make a rapid, preliminary diagnosis of *S. pyogenes* soft-issue infections or pyoderma. Because streptococci do not normally colonize the skin surface, the finding of gram-positive cocci in pairs and chains in association with leukocytes is important. In contrast, streptococci are part of the normal oropharyngeal flora, so their presence in a respiratory specimen from a patient with pharyngitis has poor predictive value.

Antigen Detection

A variety of immunologic tests using antibodies that react with the group-specific carbohydrate in the bacterial cell wall can be used to detect group A streptococci directly in throat swabs. The antigen is extracted through treatment of the specimen with nitrous acid or pronase for 5 minutes. The extract is then mixed with specific antibodies that are immobilized on a filter membrane (enzyme immunoassay [EIA]) or bound to latex particles. The development of a positive indicator in the EIA or the agglutination of the latex particles represents a positive result.

Although these assays are very specific, the sensitivity of the tests is low (probably no better than 90%); therefore, all negative results must be confirmed by culture. A highly sensitive and specific nucleic acid probe is also available for the direct detection of *S. pyogenes* in clinical specimens.

Culture

Despite the difficulty of collecting throat swab specimens from children, specimens must be obtained from the posterior oropharynx (e.g., tonsils). Fewer bacteria are present in the anterior areas of the mouth, and the mouth (particularly saliva) is colonized with bacteria that inhibit the growth of *S. pyogenes*. Therefore contamination of even a properly collected specimen may obscure or suppress the growth of *S. pyogenes*. The recovery of *S. pyogenes* from patients with impetigo is not a problem. The crusted top of the lesion is raised, and the purulent material and base of the lesion are cultured. Culture specimens should not be obtained from open, draining skin pustules, because they might be superinfected with staphylococci. Organisms are readily recovered in the tissues and blood cultures obtained from patients with necrotizing fasciitis; however, relatively few organisms may be present in the skin of patients with erysipelas or cellulitis.

As discussed previously, streptococci have fastidious growth requirements. Antibiotics (e.g., trimethoprim-sulfamethoxazole) can be added to blood agar plates to suppress the growth of oral bacterial flora. Although these selective plates have proved very useful, the growth of *S. pyogenes* on the plates is delayed, and prolonged incubation (2 to 3 days) must be used. It is also unclear what atmosphere of incubation should be used. Because virtually all *S. pyogenes* produce streptolysin S, the hemolytic pattern of the bacteria cultures on blood agar plates can be detected when the cultures are incubated in room air without supplementation with carbon dioxide.

Identification

S. pyogenes historically were identified from their susceptibility to **bacitracin** (Table 23–4). With this method, a disk saturated with bacitracin is placed onto a plate inoculated with group A streptococci and, after overnight incubation, strains inhibited by bacitracin are considered group A streptococci.

TABLE 23–4. Biochemical Identification of Common Streptococci

Organism	Susceptibility		Hippurate hydrolysis	CAMP reaction	Bile solubility
	Bacitracin	Optochin			
*S. pyogenes**	S	R	–	–	–
S. agalactiae	R	R	+	+	–
S. anginosus†	R	R	–	–	–
S. dysgalactiae‡	R	R	–	–	–
S. pneumoniae	R	S	–	–	+
Viridans group	R	R	–	–	–

CAMP, Christie, Atkins, Munch-Petersen (test); PYR, *L*-pyrrolidonyl arylamidase; R, resistant; S, susceptible.
**S. pyogenes* has a positive PYR reaction.
†*S. anginosus* has negative PYR reaction and a positive Voges-Proskauer (VP) reaction.
‡*S. dysgalactiae* has negative PYR and Voges-Proskauer (VP) reactions.

Group A streptococci are identified definitively through the demonstration of the group-specific carbohydrate, a technique that was not practical until the introduction of direct antigen detection tests.

Differentiation of *S. pyogenes* from *S. anginosus* and all other β-hemolytic streptococci can be accomplished rapidly through demonstration of the presence of the enzyme ***L*-pyrrolidonyl arylamidase (PYR).** This enzyme hydrolyzes *L*-pyrrolindonyl-β-naphthylamide, releasing β-naphthylamine, which is detected in the presence of p-dimethylaminocinnamaldehyde by the formation of a red compound. The advantage of this specific test is that it takes less than 1 minute to determine whether the reaction is positive *(S. pyogenes)* or negative *(S. anginosus).*

Antibody Detection

Patients with *S. pyogenes* disease produce antibodies to many specific enzymes. Although antibodies against the M protein are produced and are important for maintaining immunity, these antibodies appear late in the clinical course of the disease and are type specific. In contrast, the measurement of antibodies against streptolysin O (the **ASO test**) is useful for confirming rheumatic fever or acute glomerulonephritis resulting from a recent streptococcal pharyngeal infection. These antibodies appear 3 to 4 weeks after the initial exposure to the organism and then persist.

An elevated ASO titer is not observed in patients with streptococcal pyoderma. The production of other antibodies against streptococcal enzymes, particularly DNase B, has been documented in patients with streptococcal pyoderma and pharyngitis. The **anti–DNase B test** should be performed if streptococcal glomerulonephritis is suspected.

TREATMENT, PREVENTION, AND CONTROL

S. pyogenes is very sensitive to penicillin. Erythromycin or an oral cephalosporin can be used in patients with a history of penicillin allergy. However, this therapy is ineffective in patients with mixed infections that involve *Staphylococcus aureus.* Treatment in this case should include oxacillin or vancomycin. Newer macrolides (e.g., azithromycin, clarithromcyin) are not more effective than erythromycin, and resistance or poor clinical response has limited the usefulness of the tetracyclines and sulfonamides. Drainage and aggressive surgical débridement must be promptly initiated in patients with serious soft-tissue infections.

Persistent oropharyngeal carriage of *S. pyogenes* can occur after a complete course of therapy. This state may stem from poor compliance with the prescribed course of therapy, reinfection with a new strain, or persistent carriage in a sequestered focus. Because penicillin resistance has not been observed in patients with oropharyngeal carriage, they can be given an additional course of treatment. If carriage persists, re-treatment is not indicated, because prolonged antibiotic therapy can disrupt the normal bacterial flora. Antibiotic therapy in patients with pharyngitis speeds the relief of symptoms and, if initiated within 10 days of the initial clinical disease, prevents rheumatic fever. Antibiotic therapy does not appear to influence the progression to acute glomerulonephritis.

Patients with a history of rheumatic fever require long-term antibiotic prophylaxis to prevent recurrence of the disease. Because damage to the heart valve predisposes these patients to endocarditis, they also require antibiotic prophylaxis before they undergo procedures that can induce transient bacteremias (e.g., dental procedures). Specific antibiotic therapy does not alter the course of acute glomerulonephritis, however, and prophylactic therapy is not indicated because recurrent disease is not observed in these patients.

Streptococcus agalactiae (Box 23–4)

S. agalactiae is the only species that carries the group B antigen. This organism was initially recognized as a cause of puerperal sepsis. Although this disease is now relatively uncommon, *S. agalactiae* has become better known as an important cause of septicemia, pneumonia, and meningitis in newborn children, as well as a cause of serious disease in adults (see Box 23–3).

PHYSIOLOGY AND STRUCTURE

Group B streptococci are gram-positive cocci (0.6 to 1.2 μm) that form short chains in clinical specimens and longer chains in culture, features that make them indistinguishable on Gram stain from *S. pyogenes.* They grow well on nutritionally enriched media, and in contrast with the colonies of *S. pyogenes*, the colonies of *S. agalactiae* are buttery with a narrow zone of β-hemolysis. Some strains (1% to 2%) are nonhemolytic, although their prevalence may be underestimated because nonhemolytic strains are not commonly screened for the group B antigen.

Strains of *S. agalactiae* can be characterized on the basis of three serologic markers: (1) the B antigen or group-specific cell wall polysaccharide antigen (composed of rhamnose, *N*-acetylglucosamine, and galactose), (2) type-specific capsular polysaccharides (Ia, Ia/c, Ib/c, II, IIc, III to VIII), and (3) the surface protein, C protein. The type-specific polysaccharides are important epidemiologic markers, with serotypes Ia, III, and V most commonly associated with colonization and disease. Knowledge of the specific serotypes associated with disease and of shifting patterns of serotype prevalence is important for vaccine development.

BOX 23–4. Summary of Group B Streptococcus

Physiology and Structure
Gram-positive cocci arranged in long chains
Facultative anaerobe
β-Hemolytic or nonhemolytic
Catalase negative; positive CAMP and hippurate hydrolysis reactions (important identification tests)
Classified by group-specific carbohydrate (B antigen) in cell wall, type-specific polysaccharide antigens in capsule, and surface protein (C protein)

Virulence
Thick peptidoglycan layer in cell wall permits survival on dry surfaces
Capsular polysaccharides (types Ia, III, and V) inhibit complement-mediated phagocytosis
Hydrolytic enzymes may facilitate tissue destruction and systemic spread of the bacteria

Epidemiology
Asymptomatic colonization of the upper respiratory tract and genitourinary tract
Most infections in newborns acquired from mother during pregnancy or at time of birth
Neonates are at higher risk for infection if (1) there is premature rupture of membranes, prolonged labor, preterm birth, or disseminated maternal group B streptococcal disease, and (2) mother is without type-specific antibodies and has low complement levels
Women with genital colonization are at risk for postpartum sepsis
Men and nonpregnant women with diabetes mellitus, cancer, or alcoholism are at increased risk for disease
No seasonal incidence

Diseases
Refer to Box 23–3

Diagnosis
Antigen tests are too insensitive
Culture using a selective broth (i.e., LIM) is the current diagnostic test of choice
PCR-based assays are commercially available for screening pregnant women
Isolates identified by catalase (negative), positive CAMP test and hippurate hydrolysis, and present of group-specific carbohydrate (group B antigen)

Treatment, Prevention, and Control
Penicillin G is the drug of choice; a combination of penicillin and aminoglycoside is used in patients with serious infections; vancomycin is used for patients allergic to penicillin
For high-risk babies, penicillin is given at least 4 hours before delivery
The use of polyvalent conjugated vaccines to stimulate maternal antibodies is under evaluation

CAMP, Christie, Atkins, Munch-Petersen; PCR, polymerase chain reaction.

PATHOGENESIS AND IMMUNITY

The following two questions about group B streptococcal disease can be posed: (1) Why are the very young at increased risk, and (2) why are certain serotypes more commonly associated with disease? Antibodies developed against the type-specific capsular antigens of group B streptococci are protective, a factor that partly explains the predilection of this organism for neonates. In the absence of maternal antibodies, the neonate is at risk for disease. Additionally, genital colonization with group B streptococci has been associated with increased risk of premature delivery, and premature infants are at greater risk of disease. Functional classical and alternative complement pathways are required for killing group B streptococci, particularly types Ia, III, and V. As a result, there is a greater likelihood of systemic spread of the organism in colonized premature infants with physiologically low complement levels or for infants in whom the receptors for complement, or for the Fc fragment of IgG antibodies, are not exposed on neutrophils. It has also been found that the type-specific capsular polysaccharides of types Ia, Ib, and II streptococci have a terminal residue of sialic acid. Sialic acid can inhibit activation of the alternative complement pathway, thus interfering with the phagocytosis of these strains of group B streptococci.

Group B streptococci produce several enzymes, including DNases, hyaluronidase, neuraminidase, proteases, hippurase, and hemolysins. Although these enzymes are useful for identifying the organism, their role in the pathogenesis of infection is unknown.

EPIDEMIOLOGY

Group B streptococci colonize the lower gastrointestinal tract and the genitourinary tract. Transient vaginal carriage has been observed in 10% to 30% of pregnant women, although the incidence depends on the time during the gestation period when the sampling is done and the culture techniques used. A similar incidence has been observed in women who are not pregnant.

Approximately 60% of infants born to colonized mothers become colonized with their mothers' organisms. The likelihood of colonization at birth is higher if the mother is heavily colonized. Other risk factors for neonatal colonization are premature delivery, prolonged membrane rupture, and intrapartum fever. The serotypes most commonly associated with neonatal disease are Ia (35% to 40%), III (30%), and V (15%). Serotypes Ia and V are the most common in adult disease, with serotype III less commonly isolated.

Colonization with subsequent development of disease in the neonate can occur in utero, at birth, or during the first few months of life. *S. agalactiae* is the most common cause of septicemia and meningitis in newborns. Disease in infants younger than 7 days of age is called **early-onset disease;** disease appearing between 1 week and 3 months of life is considered **late-onset disease.** The use of intrapartum antibiotic prophylaxis is responsible for a dramatic decline in neonatal disease—from approximately 8000 infections in 1993 to 1800 infections in 2002.

There are more group B streptococcal infections in adults (an estimated 17,000 invasive infections in 2002) than in neonates, but the overall incidence is higher in neonates. The risk of disease is greater in pregnant women than in men and nonpregnant women. Urinary tract infections, amnionitis, endometritis, and wound infections are the most common manifestations in pregnant women. Infections in men and nonpregnant women are primarily skin and soft-tissue infections, bacteremia, urosepsis (urinary tract infection with bacteremia), and pneumonia. Group B streptococci are the most common β-hemolytic streptococci isolated in blood cultures (see Figure 23–5). Conditions that predispose to the development of adult disease include diabetes mellitus, cancer, and alcoholism.

CLINICAL DISEASES

Early-Onset Neonatal Disease

Clinical symptoms of group B streptococcal disease acquired in utero or at birth develop during the first week of life. Early-onset disease, which is characterized by bacteremia, pneumonia, or meningitis, is indistinguishable from sepsis caused by other organisms. Because pulmonary involvement is observed in most infants, and meningeal involvement may be initially inapparent, examination of cerebrospinal fluid is required for all infected children. The mortality rate has decreased to less than 5% as a result of rapid diagnosis and better supportive care; however, 15% to 30% of infants who survive meningitis have neurologic sequelae, including blindness, deafness, and severe mental retardation.

Late-Onset Neonatal Disease

Disease in older infants is acquired from an exogenous source (e.g., mother, another infant). The predominant manifestation is bacteremia with meningitis, which resembles disease caused by other bacteria. Although the survival rate is high, neurologic complications are common in children with meningitis.

Infections in Pregnant Women

Urinary tract infections frequently occur in women during and immediately after pregnancy. Because childbearing women are generally in good health, the prognosis is excellent for those who receive appropriate therapy. Secondary complications of bacteremia, such as endocarditis, meningitis, and osteomyelitis, are rare.

Infections in Men and Nonpregnant Women

Compared with pregnant women who acquire group B streptococcal infection, men and nonpregnant women with group B streptococcal infections are generally older and have debilitating underlying conditions. The most common presentations are bacteremia, pneumonia, bone and joint infections, and skin and soft-tissue infections. Because these patients often have compromised immunity, mortality is higher in this population (i.e., between 15% and 32%).

LABORATORY DIAGNOSIS

Antigen Detection

Commercial tests for the direct detection of the organism in clinical specimens have been developed. A variety of methods are used to detect the group-specific antigen, including staphylococcal coagglutination, latex agglutination, and EIA. Unfortunately, the direct antigen tests are too insensitive to be used to screen mothers and predict which newborns are at increased risk for acquiring neonatal disease.

Culture

Group B streptococci readily grow on a nutritionally enriched medium, producing large colonies after 24 hours of incubation (see Figure 23–2). β-Hemolysis may be difficult to detect or absent, posing a problem in the detection of the organism when other organisms are present in the culture (e.g., vaginal culture). Thus, a selective broth medium, with antibiotics added to suppress the growth of other organisms (e.g., LIM broth with colistin and nalidixic acid), should be used to detect group B streptococcal carriage in pregnant women.

Nucleic Acid–Based Tests

Recently a polymerase chain reaction (PCR)-based assay was approved by the Food and Drug Administration (FDA) for screening pregnant women. Because the test sensitivity and specificity approaches that of culture, this assay may replace standard culture for group B *Streptococcus*. However, additional tests will need to be performed to confirm these preliminary results.

Identification

A preliminary identification of an isolate can be made by demonstration of a positive **CAMP** (Christie, Atkins, Munch-Petersen) **test** (Figure 23–6) or by the **hydrolysis of hippurate.** Group B streptococci are identified definitively by the demonstration of the group-specific carbohydrate or the use of commercially prepared molecular probes.

TREATMENT, PREVENTION, AND CONTROL

Group B streptococci are susceptible to penicillin G, which is the drug of choice. However, the minimum inhibitory concentration (MIC) needed to inhibit the organism is approximately 10 times greater than that needed to inhibit *S. pyogenes.* In addition, tolerance to penicillin (the ability of the antibiotic to inhibit but not kill the organism) has been reported. For these reasons, a combination of penicillin and an aminoglycoside is frequently used in the management of serious infections. Vancomycin is an alternative therapy for patients allergic to penicillin. Antibiotic resistance to erythromycin and tetracycline has been observed.

In an effort to prevent neonatal disease, it is recommended that all pregnant women should be screened for colonization with group B streptococci at 35 to 37 weeks of gestation. Chemoprophylaxis should be used for all women who are either colonized or at high risk. A pregnant woman is considered to be at high risk to give birth to a baby with invasive group B disease if she has previously given birth to an infant with the disease or risk factors for the disease are present at birth. These risk factors are (1) intrapartum temperature of at least 38°C, (2) membrane rupture at least 18 hours before delivery, and (3) vaginal or rectal culture positive for organisms at 35 to 37 weeks of gestation. Intravenous penicillin G administered at least 4 hours before delivery is recommended; clindamycin or cefazolin is used for penicillin-allergic women. This approach ensures high protective antibiotic levels in the infant's circulatory system at the time of birth.

Because newborn disease is associated with decreased circulating antibodies in the mother, efforts have been directed at developing a polyvalent vaccine against serotypes Ia, Ib, II, III, and V. The capsular polysaccharides are poor immunogens; however, complexing them with tetanus toxoid has improved the immunogenicity of the vaccine. Clinical trials with this polyvalent vaccine demonstrated that protective levels of antibodies are induced. However, licensure of the vaccine has been delayed because of concerns associated with testing a vaccine in pregnant women.

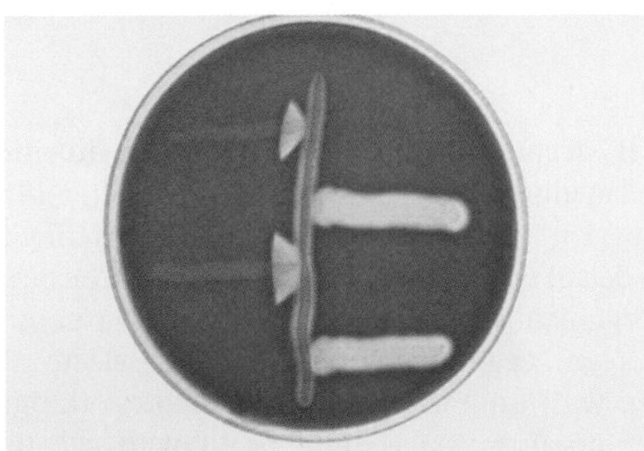

FIGURE 23–6. CAMP (Christie, Atkins, Munch-Petersen) reaction with group B streptococci. Group B streptococci produce a diffusible, heat-stable protein (CAMP factor) that enhances β-hemolysis of *Staphylococcus aureus. S. aureus (streaked from the top to the bottom of the agar plate)* produces sphingomyelinase C, which can bind to erythrocyte membranes. When exposed to the group B CAMP factor, the cells undergo hemolysis (compare the two positive reactions of enhanced hemolysis, to the left of the *S. aureus* streak, with the two negative reactions to the right). (From Howard BJ: *Clinical and pathogenic microbiology,* St Louis, 1987, Mosby.)

Other β-Hemolytic Streptococci

Among the other β-hemolytic streptococci, groups C, F, and G are most commonly associated with human disease. Organisms of particular importance are the *Streptococcus anginosus* group (includes *S. anginosus, S. constellatus,* and *S. intermedius*) and *Streptococcus dysgalactiae.* Members of the *S. anginosus* group can possess the group A, C, F, or G capsular polysaccharide, and *S. dysgalactiae* can have either the group C or G antigen. It should be noted that an individual isolate possesses only one group antigen, a finding consistent with the belief that the species are actually a group of closely related species. Isolates of the *S. anginosus* group grow as small colonies (requiring 2 days of incubation) with a narrow zone of β-hemolysis (Figure 23–7*A*). These species are primarily associated with abscess formation and not pharyngitis, in contrast with the other group A *Streptococcus, S. pyogenes. S. dysgalactiae* produce large colonies with a large zone of β-hemolysis on blood agar media (Figure 23–7*B*), a behavior similar to that of *S. pyogenes.* Like *S. pyogenes, S. dysgalactiae* causes pharyngitis, which is sometimes complicated by acute glomerulonephritis but never rheumatic fever.

Another groupable *Streptococcus* is *Streptococcus bovis.* Although Lancefield classified the original β-hemolytic strain as group D, most strains are α-hemolytic and have been reclassified with the viridans streptococci. *S. bovis* is

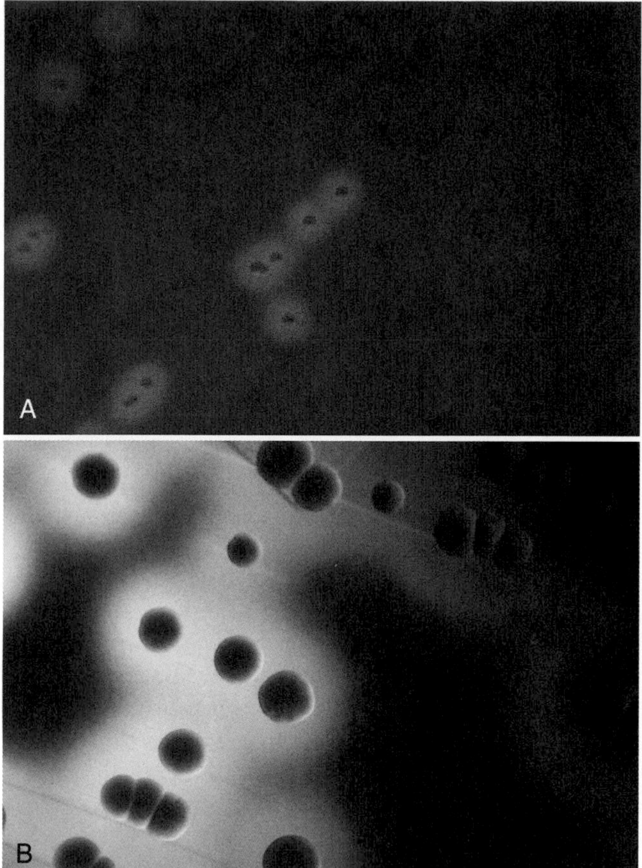

FIGURE 23–7. Group C *Streptococcus*. **A,** *S. anginosus,* small-colony species; **B,** *S. dysgalactiae,* large-colony species.

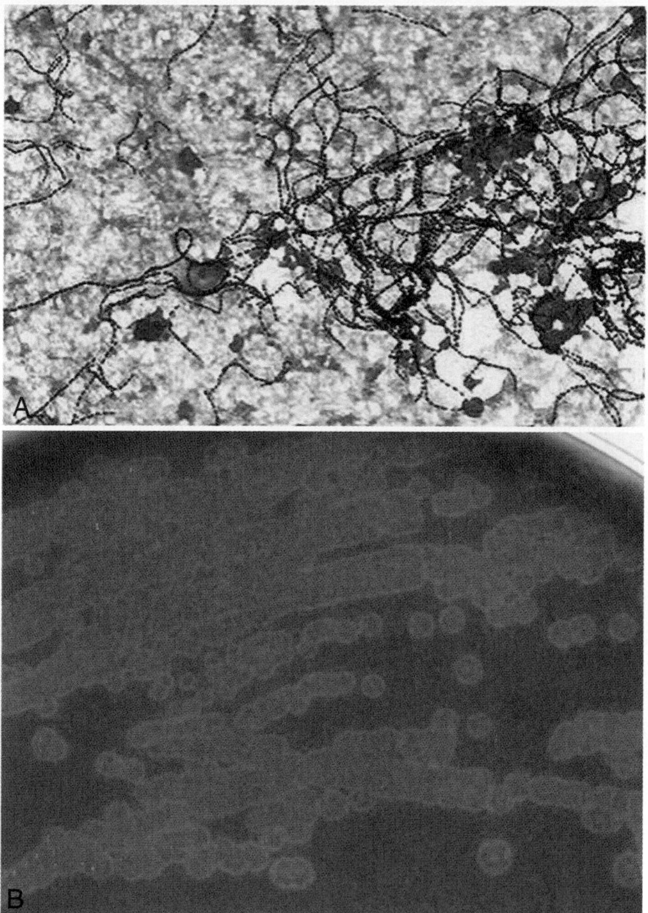

FIGURE 23–8. *Streptococcus mitis*. **A,** Gram stain from blood culture; **B,** α-Hemolytic colonies.

clinically significant, because strains that cause bacteremia have a prominent association with occult malignancy of the colon.

Viridans Streptococci

The viridans group of streptococci is a heterogeneous collection of α-hemolytic and nonhemolytic streptococci. Their group name is derived from *viridis* (Latin for "green"), a reflection of the fact that many of these bacteria produce a green pigment on blood agar media (Figure 23–8). The taxonomic nomenclature for these species is confusing because European and American microbiologists have not reached a consensus on it. Thus different species names are often used interchangeably in the literature. More than 20 species have been identified in the United States, and they are classified into five subgroups (Table 23–5). The precise classification of these bacteria can be problematic and is beyond the scope of this text.

TABLE 23–5. Classification of Viridans Group of *Streptococcus*

Group	Species
Anginosus	*S. anginosus, S. constellatus, S. intermedius*
Mitis	*S. mitis, S. pneumoniae, S. sanguis, S. parasanguis, S. gordonii, S. crista, S. oralis*
Mutans	*S. mutans, S. sobrinus, S. cricetus, S. rattus, S. downei, S. macacae*
Salivarius	*S. salivarius, S. vestibularis, S. thermophilus*
Bovis	*S. bovis, S. alactolyticus, S. equinus*
Ungrouped	*S. acidominimus, S. suis*

Although most isolates of viridans streptococci do not possess a group-specific carbohydrate, their reactivity with some groups of carbohydrates has been reported. This is particularly true for members of the anginosus group and *S. bovis*. It should also be noted that *S. pneumoniae* is a member of the *Streptococcus mitis* group. Although *S. pneumoniae* is discussed separately, it is important to realize that it is very closely related to streptococcal species in the viridans group.

Like most other streptococci, viridans species are nutritionally fastidious, requiring complex media supplemented with blood products and, frequently, an incubation atmosphere augmented with 5% to 10% carbon dioxide. Some strains are "nutritionally deficient," in that they can grow only in the presence of exogenously supplied pyridoxal, the active form of vitamin B_6. These organisms can usually grow initially in blood cultures, but they cannot grow when subcultured unless pyridoxal-supplemented media are used. These strains have been reclassified into two new genera, *Abiotrophia* and *Granulicatella*, although most investigators still refer to them as "nutritionally deficient streptococci."

The viridans streptococci colonize the oropharynx, gastrointestinal tract, and genitourinary tract. They are rarely found on the skin surface, because the surface fatty acids are toxic to them. Although these organisms can cause a variety of infections, they are most commonly associated with dental caries, subacute endocarditis, and suppurative intraabdominal infections. It is important to realize that although the species are collectively classified as viridans streptococci, many of the genera are associated with specific diseases. For example, subacute bacterial endocarditis is associated with *S. gordonii, S. mitis, S. mutans, S. oralis,* and *S. sanguis;* dental caries with *S. mutans* and *S. sobrinus;* abscess formation with *S. anginosus, S. constellatus,* and *S. intermedius;* septicemia in neutropenic patients with mucositis is associated with *S. mitis;* and malignancies of the gastrointestinal tract with *S. bovis.*

In the past, most strains of viridans streptococci were highly susceptible to penicillin, with MICs of less than 0.1 μg/ml. However, moderately resistant (penicillin MIC of 0.2 to 2 μg/ml) and highly resistant (MIC >2 μg/ml) streptococci have become common. Resistance is particularly common in the *S. mitis* group, which includes *S. pneumoniae.* This issue is discussed in greater detail in the next section. Infections with isolates that are moderately resistant can generally be treated with a combination of penicillin and an aminoglycoside. However, alternative antibiotics, such as a broad-spectrum cephalosporin or vancomycin, must be used to treat serious infections caused by penicillin-resistant strains.

Streptococcus pneumoniae (Box 23–5)

S. pneumoniae was isolated independently by Pasteur and Steinberg more than 100 years ago. Since that time, research with this organism has led to a greater understanding of molecular genetics, antibiotic resistance, and vaccine-related immunoprophylaxis. Unfortunately, pneumococcal disease is still a leading cause of morbidity and mortality.

PHYSIOLOGY AND STRUCTURE

The pneumococcus is an encapsulated, gram-positive coccus. The cells are 0.5 to 1.2 μm in diameter, oval or lancet shaped, and arranged in pairs or short chains (Figure 23–9). Older cells decolorize readily and appear gram-negative. Colonial morphology varies. Colonies of encapsulated strains are generally large (1 to 3 mm in diameter on blood agar; smaller on chocolatized or heated blood agar), round, and mucoid; colonies of nonencapsulated strains are smaller and appear flat. All colonies undergo autolysis with aging—that is, the central portion of the colony dissolves, leaving a dimpled appearance. Colonies appear α-hemolytic on blood agar if incubated aerobically and may be β-hemolytic if grown anaerobically. The α-hemolytic appearance results from production of pneumolysin, an enzyme that degrades hemoglobin, producing a green product.

The organism has fastidious nutritional requirements and can grow only on enriched media supplemented with blood products. *S. pneumoniae* can ferment several carbohydrates, with lactic acid the primary metabolic by-product. *S. pneumoniae* grows poorly in media with high glucose concentrations, because lactic acid rapidly reaches toxic levels in such preparations. Like all streptococci, the organism lacks catalase. Unless an exogenous source of catalase is provided (e.g., from blood), the accumulation of hydrogen peroxide inhibits the growth of *S. pneumoniae,* as observed on chocolatized blood agar.

Virulent strains of *S. pneumoniae* are covered with a complex polysaccharide capsule. The capsular polysaccharides have been used for the serologic classification of strains; currently, 90 serotypes are recognized. Purified capsular polysaccharides from the most commonly isolated serotypes are used in a polyvalent vaccine.

The peptidoglycan layer of the cell wall of the pneumococcus is typical of gram-positive cocci. Attached to alternating subunits of *N*-acetylglucosamine and

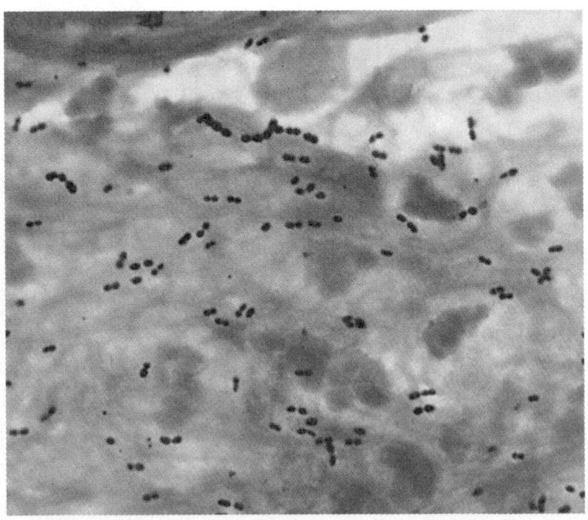

FIGURE 23–9. Gram stain of *Streptococcus pneumoniae.*

BOX 23–5. Summary of *Streptococcus pneumoniae*

Physiology and Structure

Elongated or "lancet-shaped," gram-positive cocci arranged in pairs (diplococci) and short chains

Facultative anaerobe, with fastidious growth requirements

Most strains with an outer capsule

Teichoic acid ("C polysaccharide") in cell wall is rich in choline that can react with a serum protein (referred to as the C-reactive protein)—this is a useful diagnostic test for inflammatory disease

An autolytic enzyme (amidase) is present in the cell wall; older cells undergo spontaneous autolysis, producing colonies with dimpled centers; detection of these dimpled, α-hemolytic colonies and demonstration that the colonies are lysed when exposed to bile constitute an important identification test

Bacteria are inhibited by optochin (useful identification test)

Virulence

Refer to Table 23–6

Epidemiology

Most infections are caused by endogenous spread from the colonized nasopharynx or oropharynx to distal site (e.g., lungs, sinuses, ears, blood, meninges)

Colonization is highest in young children

Person-to-person spread through infectious droplets is rare

Individuals with antecedent viral respiratory tract disease or other conditions that interfere with bacterial clearance from respiratory tract are at increased risk for pulmonary disease

Children and the elderly are at greatest risk for meningitis

People with hematologic disorder (e.g., malignancy, sickle cell disease) or functional asplenia are at risk for fulminant sepsis

Although the organism is ubiquitous, disease is more common in cool months

Diseases

Refer to Box 23–3

Diagnosis

Microscopy is highly sensitive, as is culture, unless the patient has been treated with antibiotics

Culture requires use of enriched-nutrient media (e.g., sheep blood agar); organism highly susceptible to many antibiotics, so culture can be negative in partially treated patients

Isolates identified by catalase (negative), susceptibility to optochin, and solubility in bile

Treatment, Prevention, and Control

Penicillin is the drug of choice for susceptible strains, although resistance is increasingly common

Cephalosporins, erythromycin, chloramphenicol, or vancomycin are used for patients allergic to penicillin or for treatment of penicillin-resistant strains

Immunization with 7-valent conjugated vaccine is recommended for all children younger than 2 years of age; a 23-valent polysaccharide vaccine is recommended for adults at risk for disease

N-acetylmuramic acid are oligopeptide chains, which in turn are cross-linked by pentaglycine bridges. The other major component of the cell wall is teichoic acid, which is rich in galactosamine, phosphate, and choline. The choline is unique to the cell wall of *S. pneumoniae* and plays an important regulatory role in cell wall hydrolysis. Choline must be present for activity of the pneumococcal autolysin, **amidase,** during cell division.

Two forms of **teichoic acid** exist in the pneumococcal cell wall, one exposed on the cell surface and a similar form covalently bound to the plasma membrane lipids. The exposed teichoic acid is linked to the peptidoglycan layer and extends through the overlying capsule. This species-specific structure, called the **C polysaccharide,** is unrelated to the group-specific carbohydrate observed by Lancefield in β-hemolytic streptococci. The C polysaccharide precipitates a serum globulin fraction **(C-reactive protein [CRP])** in the presence of calcium. CRP is present in low concentrations in healthy people but in elevated concentrations in patients with acute inflammatory diseases. The lipid-bound teichoic acid in the bacterial cytoplasmic membrane is called the **F antigen** because it can cross-react with the Forssman surface antigens on mammalian cells.

PATHOGENESIS AND IMMUNITY

Although *S. pneumoniae* has been extensively studied, much remains to be learned about the pathogenesis of pneumococcal disease. The disease manifestations are caused primarily by the host response to infection rather than the production of organism-specific toxic factors. However, an understanding of how *S. pneumoniae* colonizes the oropharynx, spreads into normally sterile tissues, stimulates a localized inflammatory response, and evades being killed by phagocytic cells is crucial (Table 23–6).

Colonization and Migration

S. pneumoniae is a human pathogen that colonizes the oropharynx and then, in specific situations, is able to spread to the lungs, paranasal sinuses, or middle ear. It can also be transported in the blood to distal sites such as

TABLE 23–6. *Streptococcus pneumoniae* Virulence Factors

Virulence Factor	Biologic Effect
Colonization and Migration	
Surface protein adhesions	Bind to epithelial cells
Secretory IgA protease	Disrupts secretory IgA–mediated clearance
Pneumolysin	Possibly destroys ciliated epithelial cells
Tissue Destruction	
Teichoic acid	Activates alternative complement pathway
Peptidoglycan fragments	Activate alternative complement pathway
Pneumolysin	Activates classic complement pathway
Hydrogen peroxide	Allows reactive oxygen intermediates to cause damage
Phosphorylcholine	Binds phosphodiesterase-activating factor, allowing bacteria to enter host cells
Phagocytic Survival	
Capsule	Antiphagocytic
Pneumolysin	Suppresses phagocytic oxidative burst

the brain. The initial colonization of the oropharynx is mediated by the binding of the bacteria to epithelial cells by means of **surface protein adhesins.** Subsequent migration of the organism to the lower respiratory tract can be prevented if the bacteria are enveloped in mucus and removed from the airways by the action of ciliated epithelial cells. The bacteria counteract this envelopment by producing **secretory IgA (sIgA) protease** and **pneumolysin.** Secretory IgA traps bacteria in mucin by attaching itself to the bacteria at the antigen-binding site and to mucin at the Fc region. The bacterial protease prevents this interaction. **Pneumolysin,** a cytotoxin similar to the streptolysin O in *S. pyogenes,* binds cholesterol in the host cell membrane and creates pores. This activity can destroy the ciliated epithelial cells and phagocytic cells.

Tissue Destruction

A characteristic of pneumococcal infections is the mobilization of inflammatory cells to the focus of infection. Pneumococcal teichoic acid, peptidoglycan fragments, and pneumolysin mediate the process. **Teichoic acid** and the **peptidoglycan fragments** activate the alternative complement pathway, producing C5a, which mediates the inflammatory process. This activity is augmented by the bacterial enzyme amidase, which enhances release of the cell wall components. **Pneumolysin** activates the classic complement pathway, resulting in the production of C3a and C5a. In turn, cytokines such as IL-1 and TNF-α are produced by the activated leukocytes, leading to the further migration of inflammatory cells to the site of infection, fever, tissue damage, and other signs characteristic of pneumococcal infection. The production of **hydrogen peroxide** by *S. pneumoniae* can also lead to tissue damage caused by reactive oxygen intermediates.

Finally, **phosphorylcholine** present in the bacterial cell wall can bind to receptors for platelet-activating factor that are expressed on the surface of endothelial cells, leukocytes, platelets, and tissue cells such as those in the lungs and meninges. By binding these receptors, the bacteria can enter the cells, where they are protected from opsonization and phagocytosis, and pass into sequestered areas, such as blood and the central nervous system. This activity facilitates the spread of disease.

Phagocytic Survival

S. pneumoniae survives phagocytosis because of the antiphagocytic protection afforded by its **capsule** and the pneumolysin-mediated suppression of the phagocytic cell oxidative burst, which is required for intracellular killing. The virulence of *S. pneumoniae* is a direct result of this capsule. Encapsulated (smooth) strains can cause disease in humans and experimental animals, whereas non-encapsulated (rough) strains are avirulent. Antibodies directed against the type-specific capsular polysaccharides protect against disease caused by immunologically related strains. The capsular polysaccharides are soluble and have been called **specific soluble substances.** Free polysaccharides can protect viable organisms from phagocytosis by binding with opsonic antibodies.

EPIDEMIOLOGY

S. pneumoniae is a common inhabitant of the throat and nasopharynx in healthy people. A 5% to 75% incidence of such carriage has been reported, but the incidence is significantly affected by the methods used to detect the organism and the population studied. Colonization is more common in children than in adults, and common in adults living in a household with children. Colonization with *S. pneumoniae* initially occurs at approximately 6 months of age. Subsequently, the child is transiently colonized with other serotypes of the organism. The duration of carriage decreases with each successive serotype carried, in part because of the development of serotype-specific immunity. Although new serotypes are acquired throughout the

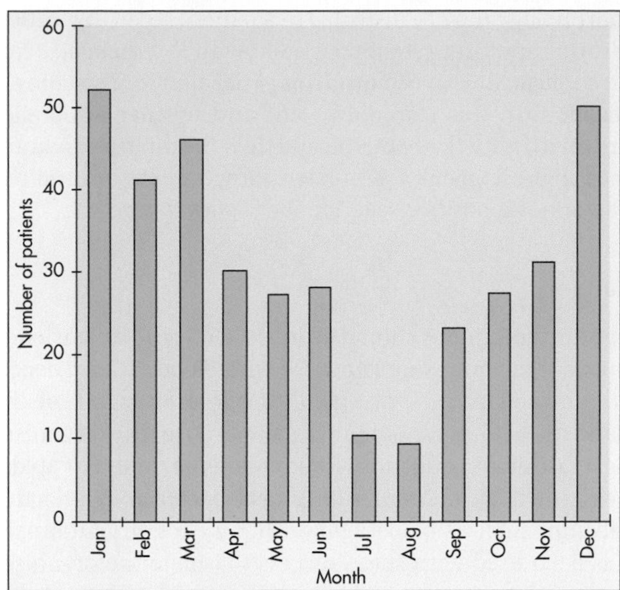

FIGURE 23–10. Seasonal incidence of *Streptococcus pneumoniae* invasive disease. The chart reflects the monthly incidence of bacteremia at Barnes Hospital in St. Louis from 1980 to 1995.

year, the incidence of carriage and associated disease is highest during the cool months (Figure 23–10). The strains of pneumococci that cause disease are the same as those associated with carriage. When infection occurs, the patient acquires a new serotype rather than one associated with prolonged carriage.

Pneumococcal disease occurs when organisms colonizing the nasopharynx and oropharynx spread to distal loci, such as the lungs (pneumonia), paranasal sinuses (sinusitis), ears (otitis media), and meninges (meningitis). Bacteremia, with subsequent spread of the disease to other body sites, can occur with all of these infections.

S. pneumoniae is a common cause of bacterial pneumonia (an estimated 500,000 cases annually in the United States), meningitis (6000 cases annually), otitis media and sinusitis (more than 7 million cases annually), and bacteremia (55,000 cases annually). The incidence of disease is highest in children and the elderly; both populations have low levels of protective antibodies directed against the pneumococcal capsular polysaccharides.

Pneumonia occurs when the endogenous oral organisms are aspirated into the lower airways. Although strains can spread on airborne droplets from one person to another in a closed population, epidemics are rare. Disease occurs when the natural defense mechanisms (e.g., epiglottal reflex, trapping of bacteria by the mucus-producing cells lining the bronchus, removal of organisms by the ciliated respiratory epithelium, and cough reflex) are circumvented, permitting organisms colonizing the oropharynx to gain access to the lungs. Pneumococcal disease is most commonly associated with an antecedent viral respiratory disease, such as influenza or measles, or with other conditions that interfere with bacterial clearance, such as chronic pulmonary disease, alcoholism, congestive heart failure, diabetes mellitus, and chronic renal disease.

CLINICAL DISEASES

Pneumonia

Pneumococcal **pneumonia** develops when the bacteria multiply in the alveolar spaces. After aspiration, the bacteria grow rapidly in the nutrient-rich edema fluid. Erythrocytes, leaking from congested capillaries, accumulate in the alveoli, followed by the neutrophils, then the alveolar macrophages. Resolution occurs when specific anticapsular antibodies develop, facilitating phagocytosis of the organism and microbial killing.

The onset of the clinical manifestations of pneumococcal pneumonia is abrupt, consisting of a severe shaking chill and sustained fever of 39°C to 41°C. The patient often has symptoms of a viral respiratory tract infection 1 to 3 days before the onset. Most patients have a productive cough with blood-tinged sputum, and they commonly have chest pain (pleurisy). Because the disease is associated with aspiration, it is generally localized in the lower lobes of the lungs (hence the name **lobar pneumonia**). However, children and the elderly can have a more generalized bronchopneumonia. Patients usually recover rapidly after the initiation of appropriate antimicrobial therapy, with complete radiologic resolution in 2 to 3 weeks.

The overall mortality rate is 5%, although the likelihood of death is influenced by the serotype of the organism and the age and underlying disease of the patient. The mortality rate is considerably higher in patients with disease caused by *S. pneumoniae* type 3, as well as in elderly patients and patients with documented bacteremia. Patients with splenic dysfunction or splenectomy can also have severe pneumococcal disease, as a result of decreased bacterial clearance from the blood and the defective production of early antibodies. In these patients, disease is associated with a fulminant course and high mortality rate.

Abscesses do not commonly form in patients with pneumococcal pneumonia, except in those infected with specific serotypes (e.g., serotype 3). Pleural effusions are seen in approximately 25% of patients with pneumococcal pneumonia, and empyema (purulent effusion) is a rare complication.

Sinusitis and Otitis Media

S. pneumoniae is a common cause of acute infections of the paranasal sinuses and ear. The disease is usually preceded by a viral infection of the upper respiratory tract, after which polymorphonuclear leukocytes (PMN) infiltrate and obstruct the sinuses and ear canal. Middle ear infection **(otitis media)** is primarily seen in young children, but bacterial **sinusitis** can occur in patients of all ages.

Meningitis

S. pneumoniae can spread into the central nervous system after bacteremia, infections of the ear or sinuses, or head trauma that causes a communication between the subarachnoid space and the nasopharynx. Bacterial **meningitis** can occur in patients of all ages but is primarily a pediatric disease. Although pneumococcal meningitis is relatively uncommon in neonates, *S. pneumoniae* is now a leading cause of disease in children and adults. Mortality and severe neurologic deficits are 4 to 20 times more common in patients with meningitis caused by *S. pneumoniae* than in those with meningitis resulting from other organisms.

Bacteremia

Bacteremia occurs in 25% to 30% of patients with pneumococcal pneumonia and in more than 80% of patients with meningitis. In contrast, bacteria are generally not present in the blood of patients with sinusitis or otitis media. Endocarditis can occur in patients with normal or previously damaged heart valves. Destruction of valve tissue is common.

LABORATORY DIAGNOSIS

Antigen Detection

Pneumococcal C polysaccharide is excreted in urine and can be detected using a commercially prepared immunoassay. Maximum sensitivity requires that the urine be concentrated by ultrafiltation before it is assayed. Sensitivity has been reported to be 70% in patients with pneumococcal pneumonia; however, specificity can be low, particularly in pediatric patients. For this reason, the test is not recommended for patients with pneumonia. The sensitivity and specificity is unknown for patients with disseminated infections such as meningitis.

Microscopy

Gram stain of sputum specimens is a rapid way to diagnose pneumococcal disease. The organisms characteristically appear as lancet-shaped, gram-positive diplococci surrounded by an unstained capsule; however, they may also appear to be gram-negative because they tend not to stain well (particularly older cultures). In addition, their morphology may be distorted in a patient receiving antibiotic therapy. Gram stain consistent with *S. pneumoniae* can be confirmed with the **quellung** (German for "swelling") reaction. In this test, polyvalent anticapsular antibodies are mixed with the bacteria, and then the mixture is examined microscopically. A greater refractiveness around the bacteria is a positive reaction for *S. pneumoniae*.

Culture

Sputum specimens should be inoculated onto an enriched nutrient medium supplemented with blood. *S. pneumoniae* is recovered in the sputum cultures from only half of the patients who have pneumonia, because the organism has fastidious nutritional requirements and is rapidly overgrown by contaminating oral bacteria. A selective medium such as blood agar with 5 μg/ml of gentamicin has been used with some success to isolate the organism from sputum specimens, but it takes some technical skill to distinguish *S. pneumoniae* from the other α-hemolytic streptococci that are often present in the specimen.

For the organism responsible for sinusitis or otitis to be diagnosed definitively, an aspirate must be obtained from the sinus or middle ear. Culture should not be performed for specimens taken from the nasopharynx or outer ear. It is not difficult to isolate *S. pneumoniae* from specimens of cerebrospinal fluid unless antibiotic therapy has been initiated before the specimen is collected. Culture findings are negative in as many as half of infected patients who have received even a single dose of antibiotics.

Identification

Isolates of *S. pneumoniae* are lysed rapidly when the autolysins are activated after exposure to bile **(bile solubility test).** Thus the organism can be identified by placement of a drop of bile on an isolated colony. Most colonies of *S. pneumoniae* are dissolved within a few minutes, whereas other α-hemolytic streptococci remain unchanged. *S. pneumoniae* can also be identified by its susceptibility to **optochin** (ethylhydrocupreine dihydrochloride). The isolate is streaked onto a blood agar plate, and a disk saturated with optochin is placed in the middle of the inoculum. A zone of inhibited bacterial growth is seen around the disk after overnight incubation. Additional biochemical, serologic, or molecular diagnostic tests can be performed for a definitive identification.

TREATMENT, PREVENTION, AND CONTROL

Before the advent of antibiotics, specific treatment of *S. pneumoniae* infection was guided by the passive infusion of type-specific capsular antibodies. These opsonizing antibodies enhanced PMN-mediated phagocytosis and the killing of bacteria. However, this immunotherapy was discontinued once antimicrobial therapy became available.

Penicillin rapidly became the treatment of choice for pneumococcal disease. Alternative effective agents for patients allergic to penicillin have included the cephalosporins, erythromycin, and chloramphenicol (for meningitis). Resistance to tetracycline is well documented. In 1977, researchers in South Africa reported isolates of *S. pneumoniae* resistant to multiple antibiotics, including penicillin. Until 1990, high-level resistance to penicillin (MIC of at least 2 µg/ml) was relatively uncommon, and only 5% of all strains of *S. pneumoniae* isolated in the United States were considered to be moderately resistant (MIC of 0.1 to 1.0 µg/ml). However, this situation has changed dramatically. Resistance to penicillin has now been observed for as many as a third of the strains isolated in the United States and in a higher number of those isolated in other countries. Greater resistance to penicillins is associated with a decreased affinity of the antibiotic for the penicillin-binding proteins present in the bacterial cell wall. Patients infected with resistant bacteria have an increased risk of an adverse outcome.

Efforts to prevent or control the disease have focused on the development of effective anticapsular vaccines. Previously, a 23-valent pneumococcal polysaccharide vaccine (with 23 different capsular polysaccharides) was recommended for children older than 2 years of age and adults. In February 2000, a 7-valent conjugated vaccine was licensed for children younger than 2 years of age. Polysaccharides are T-independent antigens, stimulating mature B lymphocytes but not T lymphocytes. Very young children respond poorly to T-independent antigens, so these polysaccharide vaccines are ineffective for this population. In contrast, conjugation of polysaccharides to proteins stimulates a T-helper cell response, resulting in a strong primary response among infants and effective booster response when reimmunized. This approach of using conjugated vaccines has also been used for other neonatal pathogens, such as *Haemophilus influenzae.* Immunization with the 7-valent pneumococcal vaccine is currently recommended for infants younger than 2 years of age, whereas to 23-valent vaccine is recommend for adults at increased risk for *S. pneumoniae* disease. Approximately 94% of all strains isolated from infected patients either are included in the vaccine or are serologically related to the 23-valent vaccine serotypes. Longitudinal studies have shown that the serotypes of *S. pneumoniae* associated with disease have not been influenced by the use of the vaccine. The 23-valent vaccine is immunogenic in normal adults, and the immunity is long lived. However, the vaccine is less effective in some patients at high risk for pneumococcal disease, including the following: (1) patients with asplenia, sickle cell disease, hematologic malignancy, and HIV infection; (2) patients who have undergone renal transplant; and (3) the elderly.

CASE STUDY AND QUESTIONS

A 62-year-old man with a history of chronic obstructive pulmonary disease (COPD) came to the emergency department because of a fever of 40°C, chills, nausea, vomiting, and hypotension. The patient also produced tenacious, yellowish sputum that had increased in quantity over the preceding 3 days. His respiratory rate was 18 breaths/min, and his blood pressure was 94/52 mmHg. Chest radiographic examination showed extensive infiltrates in the left lower lung that involved both the lower lobe and the lingula. Multiple blood cultures and culture of the sputum yielded S. pneumoniae. The isolate was susceptible to cefazolin, vancomycin, and erythromycin but resistant to penicillin.

1. What predisposing condition made this patient more susceptible to pneumonia and bacteremia caused by *S. pneumoniae?* What other populations of patients are susceptible to these infections? What other infections does this organism cause, and what populations are most susceptible?
2. What is the mechanism most likely responsible for this isolate's resistance to penicillin?
3. What infections are caused by *S. pyogenes, S. agalactiae, S. anginosus, S. dysgalactiae,* and viridans streptococci?
4. What are the major virulence factors of *S. pneumoniae, S. pyogenes,* and *S. agalactiae?*
5. *S. pyogenes* can cause streptococcal toxic shock syndrome. How does this disease differ from the disease produced by staphylococci?
6. What two nonsuppurative diseases can develop after localized *S. pyogenes* disease?

Bibliography

Barry AL: Antimicrobial resistance among clinical isolates of *Streptococcus pneumoniae* in North America, *Am J Med* 107:28S-33S, 1999.

Bisno AL, Stevens DL: Streptococcal infections of skin and soft tissues, *N Engl J Med* 334:240-245, 1996.

Cunningham M: Pathogenesis of group A streptococcal infections, *Clin Microbiol Rev* 13:470-511, 2000.

Fiore AE et al: Clinical outcomes of meningitis caused by *Streptococcus pneumoniae* in the era of antibiotic resistance, *Clin Infect Dis* 30:71-77, 2000.

Hava D, LeMieux J, Camilli A: From nose to lung: The regulation behind *Streptococcus pneumoniae* virulence factors (review), *Mol Microbiol* 50:1103-1110, 2003.

Holm SE: Invasive group A *Streptococcus* infections, *N Engl J Med* 335:590-591, 1996 (editorial).

Jackson LA et al: Risk factors for group B streptococcal disease in adults, *Ann Intern Med* 123:415-420, 1995.

Johnson D et al: A comparison of group A streptococci from invasive and uncomplicated infections: Are virulent clones responsible for serious streptococcal infections? *J Infect Dis* 185:1586-1595, 2002.

Kaul R et al: Population-based surveillance for group A streptococcal necrotizing fasciitis: Clinical features, prognostic indicators, and microbiologic analysis of seventy-seven cases, *Am J Med* 103:18-24, 1997.

Metlay J et al: Impact of penicillin susceptibility on medical outcomes for adult patients with bacteremic pneumococcal pneumonia, *Clin Infect Dis* 30:520-528, 2000.

Schrag S, Schuchat A: Easing the burden: Characterizing the disease burden of neonatal group B streptococcal disease to motivate prevention, *Clin Infect Dis* 38:1209-1211, 2004.

Schuchat A: Epidemiology of group B streptococcal disease in the United States: Shifting paradigms, *Clin Microbiol Rev* 11:497-513, 1998.

Stevens DL: Streptococcal toxic shock syndrome: Spectrum of disease, pathogenesis, and new concepts in treatment, *Emerging Infect Dis* 1:69-78, 1995.

Tuomanen EI, Austriah R, Masure HR: Pathogenesis of pneumococcal infection, *N Engl J Med* 332:1280-1284, 1995.

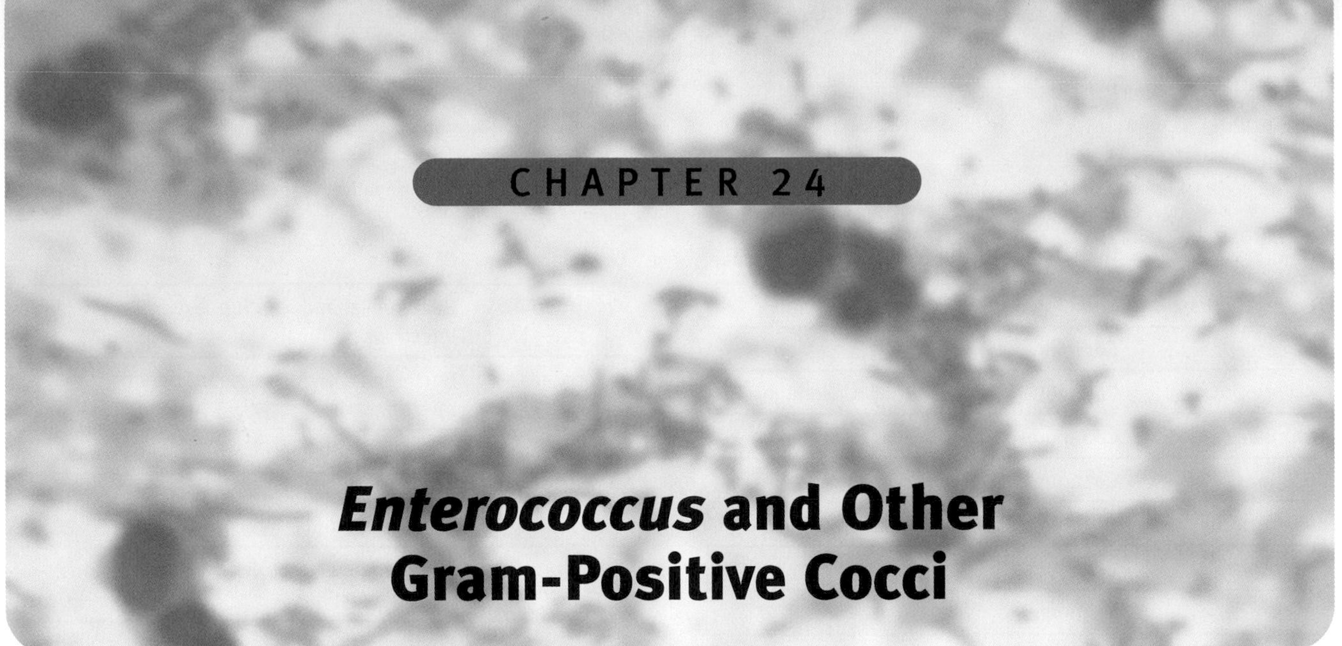

Enterococcus and Other Gram-Positive Cocci

The number of genera of catalase-negative, gram-positive cocci that are recognized as human pathogens continues to increase; however, *Streptococcus* (see Chapter 23) and *Enterococcus* are the genera most frequently isolated and most commonly responsible for human disease (Tables 24–1 and 24–2). The other genera are relatively uncommon and are discussed only briefly here.

Enterococcus

The enterococci ("enteric cocci") were previously classified as group D streptococci because they possess the group D cell wall antigen, a glycerol teichoic acid that is associated with the cytoplasmic membrane (Box 24–1). Despite this observation, it was recognized that these organisms were distinct from other group D streptococci (referred to as *nonenterococcal group D streptococci* [e.g., *Streptococcus bovis*]). The enterococcal and nonenterococcal groups were originally differentiated on the basis of their physiologic properties and with nucleic acid analysis. In 1984, the enterococci were reclassified into the new genus *Enterococcus*, and there are currently 29 species in this genus. The most commonly isolated, clinically important species are *Enterococcus faecalis* and *Enterococcus faecium*. *Enterococcus gallinarum* and *Enterococcus casseliflavus* are also common colonizers of the human intestinal tract and are important because, although they are rarely associated with human disease, these species can be misidentified as vancomycin-resistant *E. faecium*.

PHYSIOLOGY AND STRUCTURE (BOX 24–2)

The enterococci are gram-positive cocci typically arranged in pairs and short chains (Figure 24–1). The microscopic morphology of these isolates frequently cannot be differentiated from that of *Streptococcus pneumoniae*. The cocci are facultatively anaerobic and grow optimally at 35°C, although most isolates can grow in the temperature range 10°C to 45°C. The enterococci have complex nutritional needs, requiring B vitamins, nucleic acid bases, and a carbon source such as glucose. Enriched sheep blood agar supports the growth of enterococci, with large, white colonies appearing after 24 hours of incubation; colonies can appear nonhemolytic, α-hemolytic, or, rarely, β-hemolytic. The enterococci can tolerate exposure to harsh environmental conditions (e.g., grow in the presence of 6.5% NaCl and 40% bile salts). These basic properties can be used to distinguish enterococci from other catalase-negative, gram-positive cocci. Selected phenotypic tests (e.g., fermentation reactions, motility, pigment production) are required to further differentiate the enterococcal species.

PATHOGENESIS AND IMMUNITY

Enterococci are commensal organisms that do not have a potent toxin or other well-defined virulence factors (Table 24–3). For this reason, these bacteria are typically considered to have a limited potential for causing disease, although life-threatening disease, particularly in hospitalized patients, has become a serious problem.

These bacteria have surface adhesin proteins that allow them to bind to the cells lining the human intestine and vagina host tissues, and secrete extracellular proteins with hemolytic activity (cytolysin) and proteolytic activity (e.g., gelatinase, serine protease). The bacteria generally cannot avoid being engulfed and killed by phagocytic cells. Enterococci can also produce protein bacteriocins that inhibit competitive bacteria. Perhaps of greatest significance is that the enterococci either are inherently resistant to many commonly used antibiotics (e.g., oxacillin,

TABLE 24–1. Human Colonization and Disease Caused by Catalase-Negative, Gram-Positive Cocci

Genus	Human Colonization	Human Disease
Enterococcus	Common	Common
Streptococcus	Common	Common
Abiotrophia	Common	Uncommon
Granulicatella	Common	Uncommon
Gemella	Common	Rare
Lactococcus	Uncommon	Uncommon
Leuconostoc	Uncommon	Uncommon
Aerococcus	Uncommon	Rare
Helcococcus	Uncommon	Rare
Pediococcus	Uncommon	Rare
*Alloiococcus**	Rare	Rare
Facklamia	Rare	Rare
Globicatella	Rare	Rare
Ignavigranum	Rare	Rare
Vagococcus	Rare	Rare

*May be catalase positive.

BOX 24–1. Important Enterococci

Organism	Historical Derivation
Enterococcus	*enteron,* intestine; *coccus,* berry (intestinal coccus)
E. faecalis	*faecalis,* relating to feces
E. faecium	*faecium,* of feces
E. gallinarum	*gallinarum,* of hens (original source was intestines of domestic fowl)
E. casseliflavus	*casseli,* Kassel's; *flavus,* yellow (Kassel's yellow)

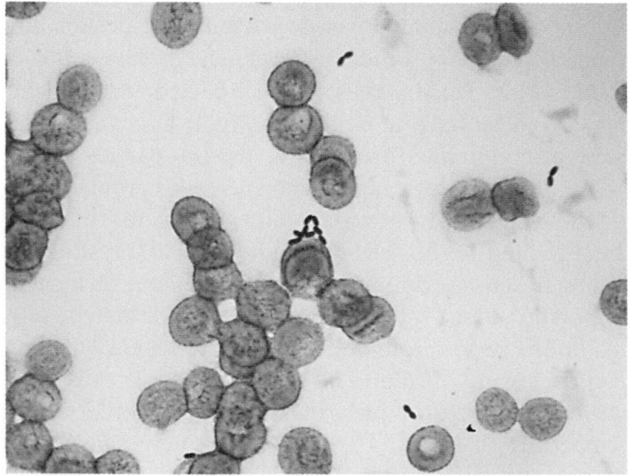

FIGURE 24–1. Gram-stained specimen showing *Enterococcus faecalis.*

TABLE 24–2. Catalase-Negative, Gram-Positive Cocci and Their Diseases

Organism	Diseases
Abiotrophia	Bacteremia, endocarditis, eye infections, oral infections
Aerococcus	Bacteremia, endocarditis, urinary tract infections
Alloiococcus	Chronic middle ear infections
Enterococcus	Bacteremia, endocarditis, urinary tract infections, wound infections
Facklamia	Bacteremia, genitourinary tract infections, wound infections
Gemella	Bacteremia, endocarditis, meningitis, wound infections, osteomyelitis, empyema, lung abscess
Globicatella	Bacteremia, urinary tract infections, meningitis
Granulicatella	Bacteremia, endocarditis, oral infections
Helcococcus	Skin infections, breast abscess
Ignavigranum	Wound infections, ear abscess
Lactococcus	Bacteremia, endocarditis, urinary tract infections, eye infections, osteomyelitis
Leuconostoc	Bacteremia, wound infections, central nervous system infections, peritonitis
Pediococcus	Opportunistic infections
Streptococcus	Refer to Chapter 23
Vagococcus	Bacteremia, peritonitis, wound infections

cephalosporins) or have acquired resistance genes (e.g., to aminoglycosides, vancomycin). Thus in patients who are treated with broad-spectrum antibiotics (and who are typically quite ill), the enterococci that are part of their normal microbial flora are able to proliferate and cause disease.

EPIDEMIOLOGY

As their name implies, enterococci are enteric bacteria, which are commonly recovered in feces collected from humans and from a variety of animals. Many *E. faecalis* organisms are found in the large intestine (e.g., 10^7 organisms per gram of feces) and in the genitourinary tract. The distribution of *E. faecium* is similar to that of *E. faecalis,* but the organisms are found less frequently.

The prevalence of the many other enterococcal species is unknown, although they are believed to colonize the intestines in small numbers. Two species that are commonly recovered in the human intestines are *E. gallinarum* and *E. casseliflavus.* These "nonpathogenic"

BOX 24–2. Summary of Enterococci

Physiology and Structure

Gram-positive cocci arranged in pairs and short chains (similar to *Streptococcus pneumoniae*)

Facultative anaerobe

Cell wall with group-specific antigen (group D glycerol teichoic acid)

Virulence Factors

Refer to Table 24–3

Epidemiology

Colonizes the gastrointestinal tracts of humans and animals

Cell wall structure typical of gram-positive bacteria, which makes it able to survive on environmental surfaces for prolonged periods

Most infections from patient's bacterial flora; some caused by patient-to-patient spread

Patients at increased risk include those hospitalized for prolonged periods and treated with broad-spectrum antibiotics (particularly cephalosporins, to which enterococci are naturally resistant)

Diseases

Urinary tract infections

Wound infections (particularly intraabdominal and usually polymicrobic)

Bacteremia and endocarditis

Diagnosis

Grows readily on common, nonselective media. Differentiated from related organisms by simple tests (catalase negative, PYR positive, resistant to bile and optochin)

Treatment, Prevention, and Control

Therapy for serious infections requires combination of aminoglycosides with a cell wall–active antibiotic (penicillin, ampicillin, or vancomycin); newer agents include linezolid, quinupristin/dalfopristin, and selected fluoroquinolones

Antibiotic resistance is becoming increasingly common, and infections with many isolates (particularly *E. faecium*) are not treatable with any antibiotics

Prevention and control of infections require careful restriction of antibiotic use and implementation of appropriate infection-control practices

TABLE 24–3. Enterococcal Virulence Factors

Virulence Factor	Biologic Effect
Surface Adhesins	
Aggregation substance	Hairlike protein embedded in cytoplasmic membrane that facilitates plasmid exchange and binding to epithelial cells
Enterococcal surface protein	Collagen-binding adhesin present in *E. faecalis*
Carbohydrate adhesins	Present in individual bacterium in multiple types; mediate binding to host cells
Secreted Factors	
Cytolysin	Protein bacteriocin that inhibits growth of gram-positive bacteria (facilitates colonization); induces local tissue damage
Pheromone	Chemoattractant for neutrophils that may regulate inflammatory reaction
Gelatinase	Hydrolyzes gelatin, collagen, hemoglobin, and other small peptides
Antibiotic Resistance	
Multiple plasmid and chromosome genes	Resistant to aminoglycosides, β-lactams, and vancomycin

species are important because they are inherently resistant to vancomycin and can be confused with the more important species, *E. faecalis* and *E. faecium*. Enterococci are not commonly isolated from the respiratory tract or from the skin. Most human infections with enterococci originate from the patient's bowel flora, although the organisms can also be transferred from patient to patient or acquired through the consumption of contaminated food or water.

CLINICAL DISEASES

Despite the paucity of virulence factors, enterococci are well respected for their ability to cause life-threatening infections (Box 24–3). Indeed, enterococci were one of the most feared nosocomial pathogens in the 1990s, because many strains are completely resistant to all conventional antibiotics. Enterococci are one of the leading causes of nosocomial (hospital-acquired) infections, responsible for

BOX 24–3. Enterococcal Diseases: Clinical Summaries

Urinary tract infection: Dyuria and pyuria most commonly in hospitalized patients with an indwelling urinary catheter and receiving broad-spectrum cephalosporin antibiotics
Peritonitis: Abdominal swelling and tenderness after abdominal trauma or surgery; patients are typically acutely ill, febrile, and with positive blood cultures
Endocarditis: Infection of the heart endothelium or valves; associated with persistent bacteremia; can present acutely or chronically

10% of all such infections. The urinary tract, peritoneum, and heart tissue are the sites involved most often. Enterococcal infections are particularly common in patients with urinary or intravascular catheters and in patients who have been hospitalized for prolonged periods and have received broad-spectrum antibiotics. A particularly severe complication of enterococcal bacteremia is endocarditis, a disease with a very high mortality rate. Although enterococci are frequently associated with intraabdominal abscesses (because of their colonization of the intestines) and wound infections, the importance of these isolates is less clear because these infections are generally polymicrobial.

LABORATORY DIAGNOSIS

Enterococci grow readily on nonselective media such as blood agar and chocolate agar. Despite the fact that enterococci may resemble *S. pneumoniae* on Gram-stained specimens, the organisms can be readily differentiated on the basis of simple biochemical reactions; for example, enterococci are resistant to optochin, do not dissolve when exposed to bile, and produces L-pyrrolidonyl arylamidase (the PYR test is a commonly performed "5-minute spot" test). Phenotypic (e.g., pigment production, motility) and biochemical tests and nucleic acid sequencing are necessary to differentiate among *E. faecalis, E. faecium,* and the other *Enterococcus* species, but this topic is beyond the scope of this text.

TREATMENT, PREVENTION, AND CONTROL

Antimicrobial therapy for enterococcal infections is complicated because most antibiotics are not bactericidal at clinically relevant concentrations. Therapy has traditionally consisted of the synergistic combination of an aminoglycoside and a cell wall–active antibiotic (e.g., ampicillin, vancomycin). However, resistance to aminoglycosides, ampicillin, penicillin, and vancomycin has become a major problem. Typically, more than 25% of enterococci are resistant to the aminoglycosides; more than 50% of some species (e.g., *E. faecium*) are resistant to ampicillin, and many medical centers report that more than 20% of enterococci (particularly *E. faecium*) are resistant to vancomycin. The resistance in these strains to aminoglycosides and vancomycin is particularly troublesome because it is mediated by plasmids and can be transferred to other bacteria.

Newer antibiotics have been developed specifically to treat enterococci resistant to ampicillin and vancomycin. They include linezolid, quinupristin/dalfopristin, and selected fluoroquinolones. Although these antibiotics are currently active against many otherwise resistant isolates, the long-term effectiveness of the drugs remains to be determined.

It is difficult to prevent and control enterococcal infections. Careful restriction of antibiotic therapy and the implementation of appropriate infection-control practices (e.g., isolation of infected patients, use of gowns and gloves by anyone in contact with patients) can reduce the risk of colonization with these bacteria, but the complete elimination of infections is unlikely.

Other Catalase-Negative, Gram-Positive Cocci

Other catalase-negative, gram-positive cocci or coccobacilli associated with human disease are *Abiotrophia, Granulicatella, Leuconostoc, Lactococcus, Pediococcus, Aerococcus,* and other less commonly isolated genera. All are relatively avirulent, opportunistic pathogens.

Abiotrophia and *Granulicatella,* formerly called nutritionally deficient streptococci, are problematic because they will initially grow in blood culture broths or in mixed cultures but do not grow when subcultured onto sheep blood agar media, unless the media is supplemented with pyrodoxal (vitamin B_6).

Leuconostoc and *Pediococcus* can resemble streptococci but are resistant to vancomycin, a trait that has not been seen in streptococci.

Lactococcus can be misidentified as *Enterococcus,* and *Aerococcus* ("air coccus") is typically an airborne organism that can contaminate the patient's skin or the specimen while it is being collected or processed in the laboratory. It is difficult to identify most of these organisms precisely, but having knowledge of their presence and clinical features is useful.

CASE STUDY AND QUESTIONS

A 72-year-old man was admitted to the hospital because of a fever that had risen as high as 40°C, myalgias, and respiratory complaints. The clinical diagnosis of influenza was confirmed by the laboratory isolation of influenza virus from respiratory secretions. This patient's hospitalization was complicated by the development of pneumonia caused by oxacillin-resistant Staphylococcus aureus *that was treated with a 2-week course of vancomycin. Declining pulmonary function necessitated the use of a ventilator, which led to the development of a secondary infection with* Klebsiella pneumoniae. *Ceftazidime (a cephalosporin) and gentamicin were added to the patient's treatment. After 4 weeks of hospitalization, the patient became septic.* E. faecium *resistant to vancomycin, gentamicin, and ampicillin was cultured from three blood specimens.*

1. What predisposing conditions made this patient more susceptible to infection with *E. faecium?*
2. What is the most likely source of this organism?
3. What factors contribute to the virulence of enterococci?

Bibliography

Edmond MB et al: Vancomycin-resistant *Enterococcus faecium* bacteremia: Risk factors for infection, *Clin Infect Dis* 20:1126-1133, 1995.

Elsner HA et al: Virulence factors of *Enterococcus faecalis* and *Enterococcus faecium* blood culture isolates, *Eur J Clin Infect Dis* 19:39-42, 2000.

Facklam R, Elliott JA: Identification, classification, and clinical relevance of catalase-negative, gram-positive cocci, excluding the streptococci and enterococci, *Clin Microbiol Rev* 8:479-495, 1995.

Garbutt JM et al: Association between resistance to vancomycin and death in cases of *Enterococcus faecium* bacteremia, *Clin Infec Dis* 30:466-472, 2000.

Gilmore MS et al: *Enterococci: Pathogenesis, molecular biology, and antibiotic resistance,* Washington, 2002, American Society for Microbiology Press.

Handwerger S et al: Infection due to *Leuconostoc* species: Six cases and review, *Rev Infect Dis* 12:602-610, 1990.

Leclercq R, Courvalin P: Resistance to glycopeptides in enterococci, *Clin Infect Dis* 24:545-556, 1997.

Moellering RC: Emergence of *Enterococcus* as a significant pathogen, *Clin Infect Dis* 14:1173-1178, 1992.

Murray BE: Vancomycin-resistant enterococci, *Am J Med* 101:284-293, 1997.

Patterson JE, Zervos MJ: High-level gentamicin resistance in *Enterococcus:* Microbiology, genetic basis, and epidemiology, *Rev Infect Dis* 12:644-652, 1990.

Shay DK et al: Epidemiology and mortality risk of vancomycin-resistant enterococcal bloodstream infections, *J Infect Dis* 172:993-1000, 1995.

Shepard BD, Gilmore, MS: Differential expression of virulence-related genes in Enterococcus faecalis in response to biological cues in serum and urine, *Infect Immun* 70:4344-4352, 2002.

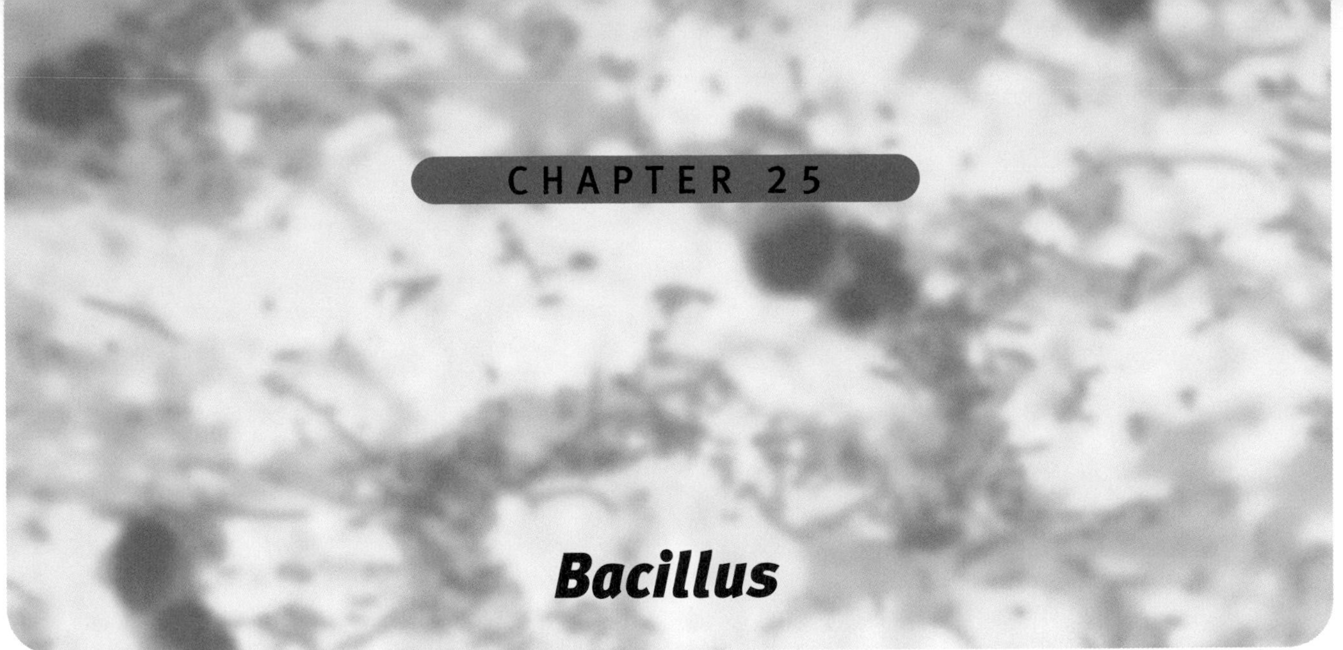

CHAPTER 25

Bacillus

The family Bacillaceae consists of a diverse collection of bacteria comprising obligate aerobes and strict anaerobes, cocci and rods, and gram-positive and gram-negative organisms. The feature they all share is formation of endospores (Figure 25–1). The two clinically important genera are *Bacillus* (the aerobic and facultative anaerobic spore formers; Box 25–1) and *Clostridium* (the strict, anaerobic spore formers; see Chapter 40). In the past few years, the genus *Bacillus* has been subdivided into nine new genera, based on 16S ribosomal ribonucleic acid (rRNA) sequencing studies, and it is expected that a similar taxonomic reorganization awaits *Clostridium.* Most of the medically important aerobic species have been retained in the genus *Bacillus.*

Despite the subdivision of *Bacillus,* more than 70 species remain in the genus. Fortunately, the species that are of medical interest are relatively limited (Table 25–1). *Bacillus anthracis,* the organism responsible for anthrax, is the most important member of this genus. This species is considered one of the most feared agents of biologic warfare and, since the release of weaponized *B. anthracis* spores in the U.S. postal system in 2001, the potential danger associated with this organism has been re-emphasized.

Bacillus anthracis (Box 25–2)

PHYSIOLOGY AND STRUCTURE

B. anthracis is a large (1 × 3 to 8 µm) organism arranged in clinical specimens as single or paired rods or as long, serpentine chains (Figure 25–2). Although spores are readily observed in 2- to 3-day-old cultures, they are not seen in clinical specimens.

Virulent *B. anthracis* carries genes for three toxin protein components on a large plasmid, pXO1. The individual proteins, **protective antigen** (PA), **edema factor** (EF), and **lethal factor** (LF), are nontoxic individually but form important toxins when combined: Protective antigen plus edema factor forms **edema toxin (EdTx),** and protective antigen plus lethal factor forms **lethal toxin (LeTx).** PA is an 83-kDa protein that binds to receptors on host cell surfaces. Two receptors have been identified: tumor endothelial marker 8 (TEM8; also called anthrax toxin receptor, or ATR) and capillary morphogenesis protein 2 (CMG2). Obviously, these protein receptors do not exist to bind anthrax toxin, but their normal functions have not yet been defined. These receptors are present on many cells and tissues (e.g., brain, heart, intestine, lung, skeletal muscle, pancreas, macrophages); therefore, a large range of tissues can be damaged by anthrax toxin. After PA binds to its receptor, host furin proteases cleave PA, releasing a small fragment and retaining the 63-kDa fragment (PA_{63}) on the cell surface. The PA_{63} fragments self-associate on the cell surface, forming a ring-shaped complex of seven fragments (pore precursor or "prepore"). This heptameric complex can then bind up to three molecules of LF and/or EF. Both factors recognize the same binding site of PA_{63}, so the binding is competitive. Formation of the complex stimulates endocytosis and movement to an acidic compartment. In this environment the heptameric complex forms a transmembrane pore and releases LF and EF into the cell cytosol. LF is a 90-kDa zinc metalloprotease that is capable of cleaving mitogen-activated protein (MAP) kinase, leading to cell death by incompletely understood mechanisms. EF is an 89-kDa adenylate cyclase that increases the intracellular cyclic adenosine monophosphate (cAMP) levels, resulting in edema. EF is related to the adenylate cyclases produced by *Bordetella pertussis* and *Pseudomonas aeruginosa.*

A second, important virulence factor carried by *B. anthracis* is a prominent polypeptide **capsule** (consisting of poly-D-glutamic acid). The capsule is observed in

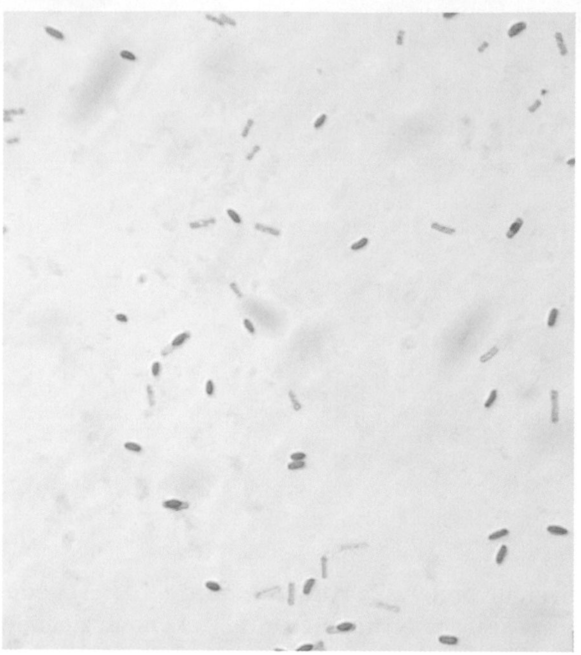

FIGURE 25–1. *Bacillus cereus.* Spores retain the malachite green dye in this special spore stain.

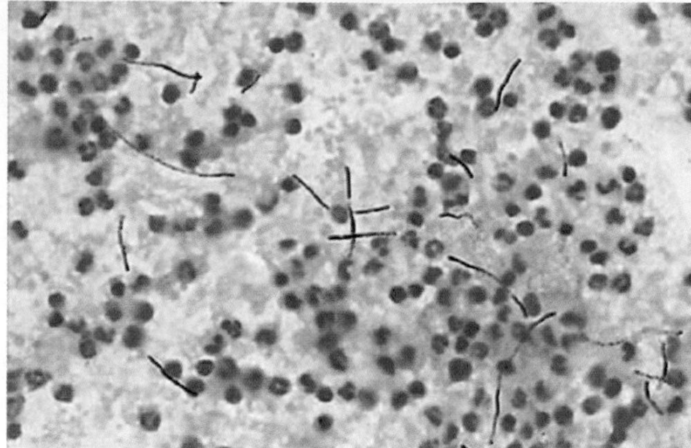

FIGURE 25–2. *Bacillus anthracis* in the blood of a patient with inhalation anthrax.

BOX 25–1. Important *Bacillus* Species

Organism	Historical Derivation
Bacillus	*bacillum,* a small rod
B. anthracis	*anthrax,* charcoal, a carbuncle (refers to the black, necrotic wound associated with cutaneous anthrax)
B. cereus	*cereus,* waxen, wax-colored (refers to colonies with a typical dull or frosted-glass surface)
B. mycoides	*myces,* fungus; *eidus,* shape (rhizoid or funguslike colonies; in *B. cereus* group)
B. sterothermophilus	*stear,* fat; *thermos,* heat; *philus,* loving (fat- and heat-loving; organism used to test effectiveness of autoclaves)
B. subtilis	*subtilis,* slender (a slender rod; common environmental isolate)
B. thuringiensis	*thuringiensis,* of Thuringia (originally isolated in the German province of Thuringia; in *B. cereus* group)

TABLE 25–1. *Bacillus* Species and Their Diseases

Organism	Diseases
*B. anthracis**	Anthrax (cutaneous, gastrointestinal, inhalation)
*B. cereus**	Gastroenteritis (emetic, diarrheal), ocular infections, catheter-related sepsis, opportunistic infections
*B. mycoides**	Gastroenteritis, opportunistic infections
*B. thuringiensis**	Gastroenteritis, opportunistic infections
Other *Bacillus* species	Opportunistic infections

*Members of the *B. cereus* group.

clinical specimens but is not produced in vitro unless special growth conditions are used. Three genes (*cap*A, *cap*B, and *cap*C) are responsible for synthesis of this capsule and are carried on a second plasmid (pXO2). Only one type of capsule has been identified, presumably because it is composed of only glutamic acid.

PATHOGENESIS AND IMMUNITY

The major factors responsible for the virulence of *B. anthracis* are the capsule, edema toxin, and lethal toxin. The capsule inhibits phagocytosis of replicating cells. The adenylate cyclase activity of edema toxin is responsible for the fluid accumulation observed in anthrax. The zinc metalloprotease activity of lethal toxin stimulates macrophages to release tumor necrosis factor-α, interleukin-1β, and other proinflammatory cytokines. This toxin also mediated lysis of macrophages in selected cell cultures. Of the major proteins of *B. anthracis,* PA is the most immunogenic (hence the name). Both LF and EF inhibit the host's innate immune system.

EPIDEMIOLOGY

Anthrax is primarily a disease of herbivores; humans are infected through exposure to contaminated animals or animal products. The disease is a serious problem in countries where animal vaccination is not practiced or is impractical (e.g., disease established in African wildlife). In contrast, natural infections with *B. anthracis* are rarely

BOX 25–2. Summary of *Bacillus anthracis*

Physiology and Structure

Spore-forming, gram-positive rods
Nonmotile, facultative anaerobe
Nonfastidious growth of nonhemolytic colonies that are firmly adherent to the agar surface
Polypeptide capsule consisting of poly-D-glutamic acid observed in clinical specimens

Virulence

Capsule is present in virulent stains
Virulent strains also produce three exotoxins that combine to form edema toxin (combination of protective antigen and edema factor) and lethal toxin (protective antigen with lethal factor)
Spores can survive in soil for years

Epidemiology

B. anthracis primarily infects herbivores with humans as accidental hosts
Rarely isolated in developed countries but is prevalent in impoverished areas where vaccination of animals is not practiced
Individuals at risk include people in endemic areas in contact with infected animals or contaminated soil, people who work with animal materials imported from endemic areas, and military and nonmilitary people exposed to infectious aerosols
The greatest danger of anthrax in industrial countries is the use of *B. anthracis* as an agent of bioterrorism

Diseases

See Box 25–3

Diagnosis

Organism is present in high concentrations in clinical specimens (microscopy typically positive) and grows readily in culture
Preliminary identification is based on microscopic (gram-positive, nonmotile rods) and colonial (nonhemolytic, adherent colonies) morphology. Confirmed by demonstrating capsule and either lysis with gamma phage or a positive DFA test for the specific cell wall polysaccharide

Treatment, Prevention, and Control

Ciprofloxacin is the drug of choice; penicillin, doxycycline, erythromycin, or chloramphenicol may be used (if susceptible), but the bacteria are resistant to sulfonamides and extended-spectrum cephalosporins
Vaccination of animal herds and people in endemic areas can control disease, but spores are difficult to eliminate from contaminated soils
Animal vaccination is effective, but human vaccines have limited usefulness

BOX 25–3. *Bacillus* Diseases: Clinical Summaries

Bacillus Anthracis

Cutaneous anthrax: A painless papule progresses to ulceration with surrounding vesicles and then to eschar formation; painful lymphadenopathy, edema, and systemic signs may develop
Gastrointestinal anthrax: Ulcers form at the site of invasion (e.g., mouth, esophagus, intestine) leading to regional lymphadenopathy, edema, and sepsis
Inhalation anthrax: Initial nonspecific signs are followed by the rapid onset of sepsis with fever, edema, and lymphadenopathy (mediastinal lymph nodes); meningeal symptoms in half the patients and most patients with inhalation anthrax will die unless treatment is initiated immediately

Bacillus Cereus

Gastroenteritis: The emetic form is characterized by a rapid onset of vomiting and abdominal pain and a short duration; the diarrheal form is characterized by a longer onset and duration of diarrhea and abdominal cramps
Ocular infections: Rapid, progressive destruction of the eye after traumatic introduction of the bacteria into the eye

seen in the United States, with only five cases reported between 1981 and 1999. This statistic may now be meaningless, with the deliberate contamination of employees of the U.S. Postal Service with *B. anthracis* spores in 2001. The risk of exposing a large population to the dangerous pathogen has increased dramatically in this era of bioterrorism. A number of nations and independent terrorist groups have biologic warfare programs. Iran, the former Soviet Union, and the Aum Shinrikyo terrorist group in Japan have experimented with using *B. anthracis* as a weapon. Indeed, much of what we know about anthrax acquired via the inhalation route was learned from the accidental release in 1979 of spores in Sverdlovsk in the former Soviet Union (at least 79 cases of anthrax with 68 deaths) and the terrorist contamination of employees of the U.S. Postal Service with letters containing *B. anthracis* (11 patients with inhalation anthrax and 11 patients with cutaneous anthrax).

Human *B. anthracis* disease (Box 25–3) is acquired by one of the following three routes: inoculation, ingestion, and inhalation. Approximately 95% of anthrax infections in humans result from the inoculation of *Bacillus* spores through exposed skin, from either contaminated soil or infected animal products, such as hides, goat hair, and wool.

Ingestion anthrax is very rare in humans, but ingestion is a common route of infection in herbivores. Because the organism can form resilient spores, contaminated soil or animal products can remain infectious for many years.

Inhalation anthrax was historically called **woolsorters' disease** because most human infections resulted from the inhalation of *B. anthracis* spores during the processing of goat hair. This is currently an uncommon source for human infections; however, inhalation is the most likely route of infection with biologic weapons. The infectious dose of the organism is believed to be low, although this depends on the state of the spore preparation. Weaponized spores are treated in a way to minimize clumping so spores can reach the lower airways, where alveolar macrophages can phagocytize the spores and initiate bacterial replication. Person-to-person transmission does not occur because bacterial replication occurs in the mediastinal lymph nodes rather than the bronchopulmonary tree.

CLINICAL DISEASES

Typically, **cutaneous anthrax** starts with the development of a painless papule at the site of inoculation that rapidly progresses to an ulcer surrounded by vesicles, then to a necrotic eschar (Figure 25–3). Systemic signs, painful lymphadenopathy, and massive edema may develop. The mortality rate in patients with untreated cutaneous anthrax is 20%.

Clinical symptoms of **gastrointestinal anthrax** are determined by the site of the infection. If organisms invade the upper intestinal tract, ulcers form in the mouth or esophagus, leading to regional lymphadenopathy, edema, and sepsis. If the organism invades the cecum or terminal ileum, the patient presents with nausea, vomiting, and malaise, which rapidly progress to systemic disease. The mortality associated with gastrointestinal anthrax is believed to approach 100%.

Unlike the other two forms of anthrax, **inhalation anthrax** can be associated with a prolonged latent period (2 months or more), during which the infected patient remains asymptomatic. Spores can remain latent in the nasal passages or reach the lower airways, where alveolar macrophages ingest the inhaled spores and transport them to the mediastinal lymph nodes. The initial clinical symptoms of disease are nonspecific—fever, shortness of breath, cough, headache, vomiting, chills, and chest and abdominal pain. The second stage of disease is more dramatic, with a rapidly worsening course of fever, edema, and massive enlargement of the mediastinal lymph nodes (this is responsible for the widened mediastinum observed on chest radiography; Figure 25–4). Although the route of infection is by inhalation, pulmonary disease rarely develops. Meningeal symptoms are seen in half of patients with inhalation anthrax. Almost all cases progress to shock and death within 3 days of initial symptoms unless anthrax is suspected and treatment is initiated immediately.

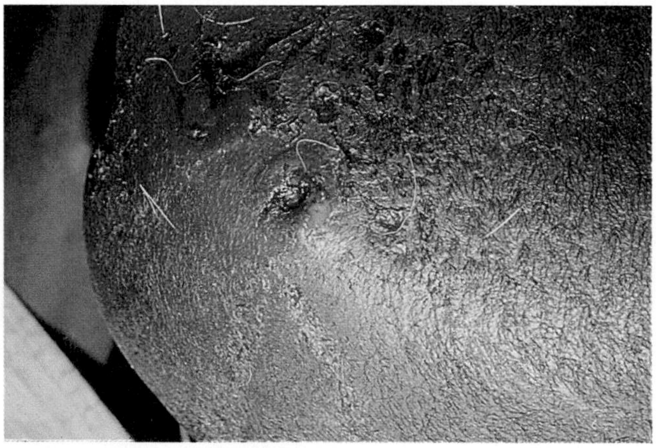

FIGURE 25–3. Cutaneous anthrax demonstrating marked erythema, edema, and vesicle rupture. (From Cohen J, Powderly WG. *Infectious diseases,* ed 2, St Louis, 2004, Mosby.)

LABORATORY DIAGNOSIS

Infections with *B. anthracis* are characterized by overwhelming numbers of organisms present in wounds, involved lymph nodes, and blood. Therefore the detection of organisms by microscopy and culture is not a problem. The diagnostic difficulty is distinguishing *B. anthracis* from other members of the taxonomically related *Bacillus cereus* group. A preliminary identification of *B. anthracis* is based on microscopic and colonial morphology. The organisms appear as long, thin, gram-positive rods arranged singly or in long chains. Spores are not observed in clinical specimens but only in cultures incubated in a low CO_2 atmosphere, and can be best seen with the use of a special spore stain (e.g., malachite green stain; see Figure 25–1). The capsule of *B. anthracis* is produced in vivo but is not typically observed in culture. The capsule can be observed

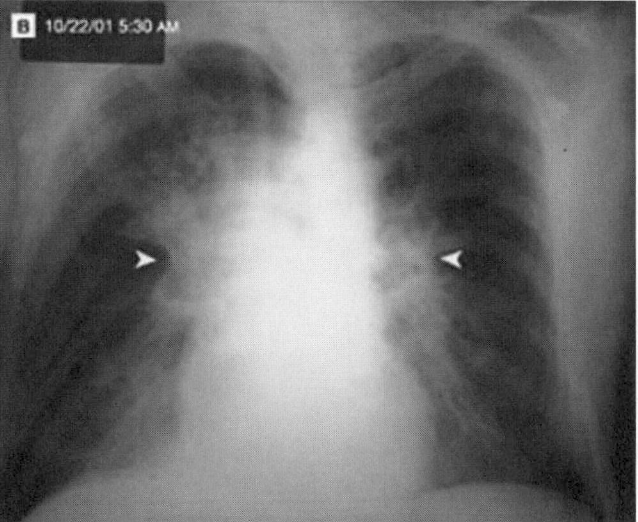

FIGURE 25–4. Inhalation anthrax demonstrating enlarged mediastinal lymph nodes.

with a contrasting stain such as India ink (the ink particles are excluded by the capsule so that the background but not the area around bacteria appears black), M'Fadyean methylene blue stain, or a direct fluorescent antibody (DFA) test developed against the capsular polypeptide. Colonies cultured on sheep blood agar are large, nonpigmented, and have a dry "ground glass" surface and irregular edges with projections along the lines, where the specimen was inoculated onto the agar plate (referred to as "Medusa head" morphology). The colonies are quite sticky and adherent to the agar and, if the edge is lifted with a bacteriologic loop, it will remain standing like a beaten egg white. Colonies are not hemolytic in contrast with *B. cereus*. *B. anthracis* will appear nonmotile in motility tests, such as the microscopic observation of individual rods in a suspended drop of culture medium. The definitive identification of nonmotile, nonhemolytic organisms resembling *B. anthracis* is made in a public health reference laboratory. This is accomplished by demonstrating capsule production (by microscopy or DFA) and either lysis of the bacteria with gamma phage or a positive DFA test for a specific *B. anthracis* cell wall polysaccharide. Additionally, nucleic acid amplification tests (e.g., polymerase chain reaction [PCR]) have been developed and are performed in reference laboratories. The PCR tests are also commercially available.

TREATMENT, PREVENTION, AND CONTROL

In contrast to many other *Bacillus* species, *B. anthracis* is susceptible to penicillin, which has historically been considered the treatment of choice for a suspected infection. Isolates are also susceptible to doxycycline and ciprofloxacin. Because genes encoding resistance to penicillin and doxycycline have been transferred to *B. anthracis*, however, ciprofloxacin is recommended for empirical therapy. *B. anthracis* strains are resistant to sulfonamides and extended-spectrum cephalosporins.

The control of naturally acquired human disease requires the control of animal disease, which involves the vaccination of animal herds in endemic regions and the burning or burial of animals that die of anthrax. Complete eradication of anthrax is unlikely, because the spores of the organism can exist for many years in soil. Furthermore, complete eradication of anthrax infections is unlikely with the threat of bioterrorist-related infections a current reality.

Vaccination of animals is an effective control measure. Vaccination has also been used to protect (1) people who live in areas where the disease is endemic, (2) people who work with animal products imported from countries with endemic anthrax, and (3) military personnel. Although the current vaccine appears to be effective, work to develop less toxic vaccines is a major medical need.

Bacillus cereus and Other *Bacillus* Species

Bacillus species other than *B. anthracis* are primarily opportunistic pathogens that have relatively low capacities for virulence. Although most of these species have been found to cause disease, *B. cereus* is clearly the most important pathogen, with gastroenteritis, ocular infections, and intravenous catheter–related sepsis the diseases most commonly observed (Box 25–4).

PATHOGENESIS

Gastroenteritis caused by *B. cereus* is mediated by one of two enterotoxins (Table 25–2). The heat-stable, proteolysis-resistant enterotoxin causes the **emetic form** of the disease, and the heat-labile enterotoxin causes the **diarrheal form** of the disease. The heat-labile enterotoxin is similar to the enterotoxins produced by *Escherichia*

BOX 25–4. Summary of *Bacillus cereus*

Physiology and Structure

Spore-forming, motile gram-positive rods
Facultative anaerobe
Nonfastidious growth requirements; β-hemolytic on sheep blood agar

Virulence

Heat-stable and heat-labile enterotoxin
Spores can survive in soil
Tissue destruction is mediated by cytotoxic enzymes, including cereolysin and phospholipase C

Epidemiology

Ubiquitous in soils throughout the world
People at risk include those who consume food contaminated with the bacterium (e.g., rice, meat, vegetables, sauces), those with penetrating injuries (e.g., to eye), and those who receive intravenous injections

Diseases

See Box 25–3

Diagnosis

Isolation of the organism in implicated food product or nonfecal specimens (e.g., eye, wound)

Treatment, Prevention, and Control

Gastrointestinal infections are treated symptomatically
Ocular infectious or other invasive diseases require removal of foreign bodies and treatment with vancomycin, clindamycin, ciprofloxacin, or gentamicin
Gastrointestinal disease is prevented by proper preparation of food (e.g., foods should be consumed immediately after preparation or refrigerated)

TABLE 25–2. *Bacillus cereus* Food Poisoning

	Emetic Form	Diarrheal Form
Implicated food	Rice	Meat, vegetables
Incubation period (hours)	<6 (mean, 2)	>6 (mean, 9)
Symptoms	Vomiting, nausea, abdominal cramps	Diarrhea, nausea, abdominal cramps
Duration (hours)	8–10 (mean, 9)	20–36 (mean, 24)
Enterotoxin	Heat stable	Heat labile

coli and *Vibrio cholerae;* each stimulates the adenylate cyclase–cyclic adenosine monophosphate system in intestinal epithelial cells, leading to profuse watery diarrhea. The mechanism of action of the heat-stable enterotoxin is unknown.

The pathogenesis of *B. cereus* ocular infections is also incompletely defined. At least three toxins have been implicated; they are **necrotic toxin** (a heat-labile enterotoxin), **cereolysin** (a potent hemolysin named after the species), and **phospholipase C** (a potent lecithinase). It is likely that the rapid destruction of the eye that is characteristic of *B. cereus* infections results from the interaction of these toxins and other unidentified factors.

Bacillus species can colonize skin transiently and can be recovered as insignificant contaminants in blood cultures. In the presence of an intravascular foreign body, however, these organisms can be responsible for persistent bacteremia and signs of sepsis (i.e., fever, chills, hypotension, shock).

EPIDEMIOLOGY

B. cereus and other *Bacillus* species are ubiquitous organisms, present in virtually all environments. Isolation of bacteria from clinical specimens in the absence of characteristic disease usually represents insignificant contamination.

CLINICAL DISEASES

As mentioned previously, *B. cereus* is responsible for two forms of food poisoning: vomiting disease (emetic form) and diarrheal disease (diarrheal form). The emetic form results from the consumption of contaminated rice. Most bacteria are killed during the initial cooking of the rice, but the heat-resistant spores survive. If the cooked rice is not refrigerated, the spores germinate, and the bacteria can multiply rapidly. The heat-stable enterotoxin that is released is not destroyed when the rice is reheated. After ingestion of the enterotoxin and a 1- to 6-hour incubation period, a disease of short duration (less than 24 hours) develops. Symptoms consist of vomiting, nausea, and abdominal cramps. Fever and diarrhea are generally absent. Fulminant liver failure has also been associated with consumption of food contaminated with large amounts of emetic toxin, which impairs mitochondrial fatty acid metabolism. Fortunately, this is a rare complication.

The diarrheal form of *B. cereus* food poisoning results from the consumption of contaminated meat, vegetables, or sauces. There is a longer incubation period, during which the organism multiplies in the patient's intestinal tract and produces the heat-labile enterotoxin. This enterotoxin is responsible for the diarrhea, nausea, and abdominal cramps that develop. This form of disease generally lasts 1 day or longer.

B. cereus ocular infections usually occur after traumatic, penetrating injuries of the eye with a soil-contaminated object. *Bacillus* panophthalmitis is a rapidly progressive disease that almost universally results in the complete loss of light perception within 48 hours of the injury. Disseminated infections with ocular manifestations can also develop in intravenous drug abusers.

Other infections with *B. cereus* and other *Bacillus* species are intravenous catheter and central nervous system shunt infections and endocarditis (most common in drug abusers), as well as pneumonitis, bacteremia, and meningitis in severely immunosuppressed patients.

LABORATORY DIAGNOSIS

Like *B. anthracis,* other *Bacillus* species can be readily grown in the laboratory. For confirmation of the existence of foodborne disease, the implicated food (e.g., rice, meat, vegetables) should be cultured. Isolation of the organism from the patient should not be attempted, because fecal colonization is common. However, isolation of the organism from the stools of a cluster of epidemiologically related patients is strong evidence implicating *B. cereus* as the causal agent. Tests to detect the heat-stable or heat-labile enterotoxins are not commonly performed. *Bacillus* organisms grow rapidly and are readily detected with Gram stain and culture of specimens collected from infected eyes, intravenous culture sites, and other locations.

TREATMENT, PREVENTION, AND CONTROL

Because the course of *B. cereus* gastroenteritis is short and uncomplicated, symptomatic treatment is adequate. The treatment of other *Bacillus* infections is complicated by the fact that they have a rapid and progressive course and a high incidence of multiple-drug resistance (e.g., *B. cereus* carries genes for resistance to penicillins and cephalosporins). Vancomycin, clindamycin, ciprofloxacin, and gentamicin can be used to treat infections. Penicillins and cephalosporins are ineffective. Rapid consumption of foods after cooking and proper refrigeration of uneaten foods can prevent food poisoning.

CASE STUDY AND QUESTIONS

A 56-year-old female postal worker sought medical care for fever, diarrhea, and vomiting. She was offered symptomatic treatment and discharged from the community hospital emergency department. Five days later she returned to the hospital with complaints of chills, dry cough, and pleuritic chest pain. A chest radiograph showed a small right infiltrate and bilateral effusions but no evidence of a widened mediastinum. She was admitted to the hospital, and the next day her respiratory status and pleural effusions worsened. A computerized tomographic (CT) scan of her chest revealed enlarged mediastinal and cervical lymph nodes. Pleural fluid and blood was collected for culture and was positive within 10 hours for gram-positive rods in long chains.

1. The clinical impression is that this woman has inhalation anthrax. What tests should be performed to confirm the identification of the isolate?
2. What are the three primary virulence factors found in *B. anthracis?*
3. Describe the mechanisms of action of the toxins produced by *B. anthracis.*
4. Describe the two forms of *B. cereus* food poisoning. What toxin is responsible for each form? Why is the clinical presentation of these two diseases different?
5. *B. cereus* can cause eye infections. What are two risk factors for this disease?

Bibliography

Bell CA et al: Detection of *Bacillus anthracis* DNA by LightCycler PCR, *J Clin Microbiol* 40:2897-2902, 2002.

Collier RJ, Young JAT: Anthrax toxin, *Annu Rev Cell Dev Biol* 19:45-70, 2003.

Davey RT Jr, Tauber WB: Posttraumatic endophthalmitis: The emerging role of *Bacillus cereus* infection, *Rev Infect Dis* 9:110-123, 1987.

Drobniewski FA: *Bacillus cereus* and related species, *Clin Microbiol Rev* 6:324-338, 1993.

Ihde DC, Armstrong D: Clinical spectrum of infection due to *Bacillus* species, *Am J Med* 55:839-845, 1973.

Mahler H et al: Fulminant liver failure in association with the emetic toxin of *Bacillus cereus*, *N Engl J Med* 336:1142-1148, 1997.

Mahtab M, Leppla SH: The roles of anthrax toxin in pathogenesis, *Curr Opin. Microbiol* 7:19-24, 2004.

Pickering AK, Merkel TJ: Macrophages release tumor necrosis factor alpha and interleukin-12 in response to intracellular *Bacillus anthracis* spores, *Infect Immun* 72:3096-3072, 2004.

Turnbull, PC: Introduction: Anthrax history, disease and ecology, *Curr Top Microbiol Immunol* 271:1-19, 2002.

Van Ness GB: Ecology of anthrax, *Science* 172:103-109, 1971.

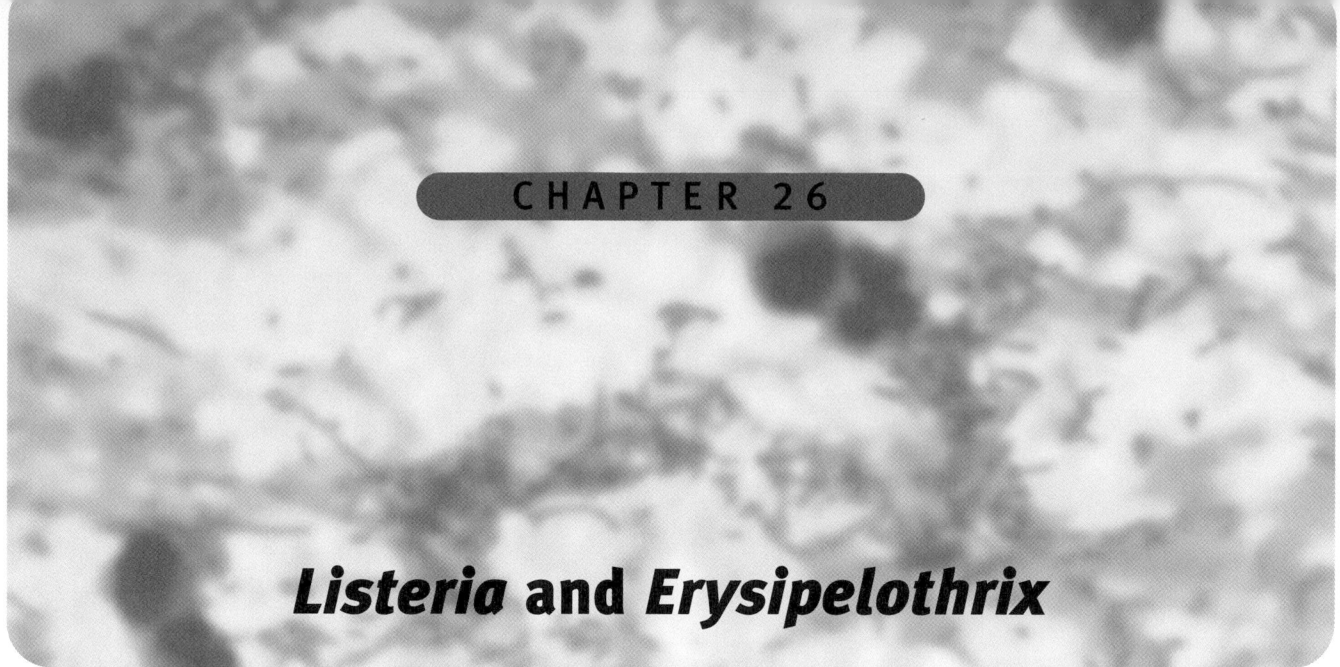

Listeria and *Erysipelothrix*

The aerobic, non–spore-forming, gram-positive rods are a heterogeneous group of bacteria. Some are well-recognized human pathogens (e.g., *Corynebacterium diphtheriae, Mycobacterium tuberculosis*), others are primarily animal pathogens that can cause human disease (e.g., *Erysipelothrix rhusiopathiae, Rhodococcus equi*), and others are opportunistic pathogens typically infecting hospitalized or immunocompromised patients (e.g., *Corynebacterium jeikeium*). Although the clinical presentation of the diseases can be characteristic, detection and identification of the organisms in the laboratory can be problematic. One technique that is useful for the preliminary identification of these bacteria involves their microscopic morphology. Gram-positive rods that are uniform in shape include *Listeria* and *Erysipelothrix* (Box 26–1), the subjects of this chapter. The coryneform rods (which include the genus *Corynebacterium*) comprise a large group of irregularly shaped rods (discussed in Chapter 27). The final group of rod-shaped bacteria is characterized by the presence of long-chain mycolic acids in their cell walls. This cell wall component makes it difficult to stain the bacteria with the Gram stain; thus the acid-fast stain was developed. Bacteria that are partially or completely acid-fast include *Nocardia, Rhodococcus,* and *Mycobacterium* (discussed in Chapters 28 and 29).

Listeria monocytogenes (Box 26–2)

The genus *Listeria* consists of six species, with *Listeria monocytogenes* and *Listeria ivanovii* the only recognized pathogens. *L. monocytogenes* is a significant human pathogen, and *L. ivanovii* is primarily an animal pathogen. *L. monocytogenes* is a short (0.4 to 0.5 × 0.5 to 2.0 μm), nonbranching, gram-positive, facultatively anaerobic rod capable of growth at a broad temperature range (1°C to 45°C) and in a high concentration of salt. The short rods appear singly, in pairs, or in short chains (Figure 26–1) and can be mistaken for *Streptococcus pneumoniae* or *Enterococcus*. This is important because both *S. pneumoniae* and *L. monocytogenes* can cause meningitis. The organisms are motile at room temperature but less so at 37°C, and they exhibit a characteristic end-over-end tumbling motion when a drop of broth is examined microscopically. *L. monocytogenes* exhibits weak β-hemolysis when grown on sheep blood agar plates. These differential characteristics (i.e., Gram-stain morphology, motility, β-hemolysis) are useful for the preliminary identification of *Listeria*. Although the bacteria are widely distributed in nature, human disease is uncommon and is restricted to several well-defined populations: neonates, the elderly, pregnant women, and patients with defective cellular immunity.

PATHOGENESIS AND IMMUNITY

L. monocytogenes is a facultative intracellular pathogen that can grow in macrophages, epithelial cells, and cultured fibroblasts. Studies with animal models have shown that infection is initiated in the enterocytes or M cells in Peyer's patches. Entry into nonphagocytic cells is mediated by a family of six or more leucine-rich proteins, **internalins** (e.g., InlA, InlB, InlC), which interact with glycoprotein receptors on the surface of host cells. After penetration into the cells, the acid pH of the phagolysosome that surrounds the bacteria activates a bacterial exotoxin **(listeriolysin O)** and two different **phospholipase C** enzymes, leading to release of the bacteria into the cell cytosol. The bacteria proceed to replicate and then move to the cell membrane. This movement is mediated by a bacterial protein, **ActA,** localized on the cell surface at one end of a bacterium, that coordinates assembly of actin. The distal ends of the actin tail remain fixed while assembly occurs adjacent to the end of the bacterium. Thus the

BOX 26–1. *Listeria* and *Erysipelothrix*

Organism	Historical Derivation
Listeria	*Listeria*, named after the English surgeon Lord Lister
L. monocytogenes	*monocytum*, a blood cell or monocyte; *gennaio*, produce (monocyte producing; membrane extracts stimulate monocyte production in rabbits, but this is not seen in human disease)
Erysipelothrix	*Erythros*, red; *pella*, skin; *thrix*, hair (thin, hairlike organism that produces a red or inflammatory skin lesion)
E. rhusiopathiae	*rhusios*, red; *pathos*, disease (red disease)

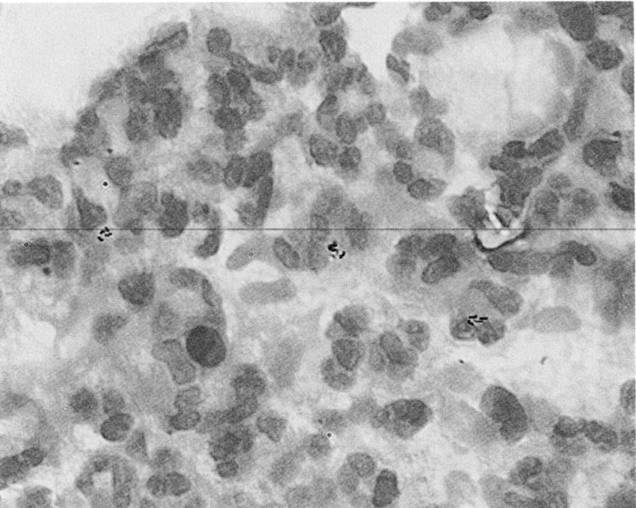

FIGURE 26–1. Gram-stain preparation showing *Listeria monocytogenes* in cerebrospinal fluid.

BOX 26–2. Summary of *Listeria*

Physiology and Structure

Gram-positive coccobacilli often arranged in pairs resembling enterococci

Facultative anaerobe

Motile at room temperature, weakly β-hemolytic, and capable of growth at 4°C and in high-salt concentrations (useful identification features)

Virulence

Facultative intracellular pathogen that can avoid antibody-mediated clearance

Virulent strains produce cell attachment factors (internalins), hemolysins (listeriolysin O, two phospholipase Cs), and a protein that mediates actin-directed motility (ActA)

Growth in contaminated foods in the refrigerator can lead to high concentrations of bacteria

Epidemiology

Isolated in soil, water, and vegetation and from a variety of animals, including humans (low-level gastrointestinal carriage)

Disease associated with consumption of contaminated food products (e.g., soft cheese, milk, turkey, raw vegetables [esp. cabbage]) or transplancental spread from mother to neonate; sporadic cases and epidemics occur throughout the year but peak in warmer months

The young, elderly, and pregnant women, as well as patients with defects in cellular immunity, are at increased risk for disease

Diseases

Refer to Box 26–3

Diagnosis

Microscopy is insensitive; culture may require incubation for 2 to 3 days or enrichment at 4°C

Treatment, Prevention, and Control

The treatment of choice for severe disease is penicillin or ampicillin, alone or in combination with gentamicin

People at high risk should avoid eating raw or partially cooked foods of animal origin, soft cheese, and unwashed raw vegetables

bacterium is pushed to the cell membrane, where a protrusion (filopod) is formed, pushing the bacterium into the adjacent cell. After the adjacent cell ingests the bacterium, the process of phagolysosome lysis, bacterial replication, and directional movement repeats. Entry into macrophages after passage through the intestinal lining carries the bacteria to the liver and spleen, leading to disseminated disease.

Humoral immunity is relatively unimportant for management of infections with *L. monocytogenes*. These bacteria can replicate in macrophages and move within cells, thus avoiding antibody-mediated clearance. For this reason, patients with defects in cellular immunity but not in humoral immunity are particularly susceptible to severe infections.

EPIDEMIOLOGY

L. monocytogenes is isolated from a variety of environmental sources and from the feces of mammals, birds, fish, insects, and other animals. The primary sources of this organism are believed to be soil and decaying vegetable matter. Fecal carriage is estimated to occur in 1% to 5% of healthy people. Because the organism is ubiquitous, exposure and transient colonization are likely to occur in most individuals. An estimated 2500 infections occur annually. However, many mild infections are not reported. Large outbreaks associated with contaminated food products have been documented. For example, 30 million pounds of contaminated meat were recalled in one outbreak in 1999. Many people were exposed to the bacteria before the recall could be accomplished. The incidence of disease is also disproportionate in high-risk populations, such as neonates, the elderly, pregnant women, and patients with severe defects in cell-mediated immunity (e.g., transplants, lymphomas, acquired immune deficiency syndrome [AIDS]).

Human listeriosis is a sporadic disease seen throughout the year, but the incidence peaks in the warmer months. Focal epidemics and sporadic cases of listeriosis have been associated with consumption of contaminated milk, soft cheese, undercooked meat (e.g., turkey franks, cold cuts), unwashed raw vegetables, and cabbage. Because listeria can grow in a wide pH range and in cold temperatures, foods with small numbers of organisms can become grossly contaminated during prolonged refrigeration. Disease can occur if the food is uncooked or inadequately cooked (e.g., microwaved beef and turkey franks) before consumption. The mortality rate of symptomatic listeria infections (20% to 30%) is higher than that of almost all other foodborne diseases.

CLINICAL DISEASES (BOX 26–3)

Neonatal Disease

Two forms of neonatal disease have been described: (1) **early-onset disease,** acquired transplacentally in utero, and (2) **late-onset disease,** acquired at or soon after birth. Early-onset disease, also called **granulomatosis infantiseptica,** is a devastating disease that has a high mortality rate unless treated promptly. It is characterized by the formation of disseminated abscesses and granulomas in multiple organs.

Late-onset disease occurs 2 to 3 weeks after birth, in the form of meningitis or meningoencephalitis with septicemia. The clinical signs and symptoms are not unique; thus other causes of neonatal central nervous system disease, such as group B streptococcal disease, must be excluded.

BOX 26–3. *Listeria* and *Erysipelothrix*: Clinical Summaries

Listeria monocytogenes

Neonatal disease

Early-onset disease ("granulomatosis infantiseptica"): acquired transplacentally in utero and is characterized by disseminated abscesses and granulomas in multiple organs

Late-onset disease: acquired at or shortly after birth and presents as meningitis or meningoencephalitis with septicemia

Disease in healthy adults: typically an influenza-like illness with or without gastroenteritis

Disease in pregnant women or patients with cell-mediated immune defects: can present as a primary bacteremia or as disseminated disease with hypotension and meningitis

Erysipelothrix rhusiopathiae

Erysipeloid: a painful, pruritic inflammatory skin lesion with a raised violaceous edge and central clearing; a diffuse cutaneous infection can develop rarely with systemic manifestations

Septicemic disease: recovery of the bacteria in blood is typically associated with endocarditis (either the acute or the more commonly chronic form); rarely, abscess formation, meningitis, or osteomyelitis may develop

Disease in Healthy Adults

Most listeria infections in healthy adults are asymptomatic or occur in the form of a mild influenza-like illness. Gastrointestinal symptoms develop in some patients. In contrast, illness in patients with compromised cellular immunity is more severe.

Meningitis in Adults

Meningitis is the most common form of listeria infection in adults. Although the clinical signs and symptoms of meningitis caused by this organism are not specific, listeria should always be suspected in patients with organ transplants or cancer and in pregnant women in whom meningitis develops.

Primary Bacteremia

Patients with bacteremia may have an unremarkable history of chills and fever (commonly observed in pregnant women) or a more acute presentation with high-grade fever and hypotension. Only severely immunocompromised patients and the infants of pregnant women with sepsis appear to be at risk of death.

LABORATORY DIAGNOSIS

Microscopy

Gram-stain preparations of cerebrospinal fluid (CSF) typically show no organisms, because the bacteria are generally present in concentrations below the limit of detection (e.g., 10^4 bacteria per ml CSF or less). This is in contrast with most other bacterial pathogens of the central nervous system, which are present in concentrations of 100-fold to 1000-fold higher. If the Gram stain shows organisms, they are intracellular and extracellular gram-positive coccobacilli. Care must be used to distinguish them from other bacteria such as *S. pneumoniae, Enterococcus,* and *Corynebacterium.*

Culture

Listeria grows on most conventional laboratory media, with small, round colonies observed on agar media after incubation for 1 to 2 days. It may be necessary to use selective media and **cold enrichment** (storage of the specimen in the refrigerator for a prolonged period) to detect listeriae in specimens contaminated with rapidly growing bacteria. β-Hemolysis on sheep blood agar media can serve to distinguish *Listeria* from morphologically similar bacteria; however, hemolysis is generally weak and may not be observed initially. Hemolysis is enhanced when the organisms are grown next to β-hemolytic *Staphylococcus aureus* (this enhanced hemolysis is referred to as a positive CAMP [Christie, Atkins, Munch-Petersen] test). The characteristic motility of the organism in a liquid medium or semisolid agar is also helpful for the preliminary identification of listeriae. All gram-positive rods isolated from blood and CSF should be identified to distinguish between *Corynebacterium* (presumably a contaminant) and *Listeria*.

Identification

Selected biochemical and serologic tests are used to identify the pathogen definitively. A total of 13 serotypes have been described, with 1/2a, 1/2b, and 4b responsible for most infections in neonates and adults. Serotyping is generally not useful in epidemiologic investigations, because relatively few serotypes are isolated from humans with disease. Enzyme profiles (i.e., multilocus enzyme electrophoresis [MLEE]) and genomic analysis (e.g., ribotyping, pulsed-field gel electrophoresis [PFGE], random amplified polymorphic DNA [RAPD] typing) are used for epidemiologic investigations. Strains of serotype 1/2a are highly heterogeneous and can be typed by any of the methods mentioned. In contrast, serotype 4b is homogeneous and multiple methods are needed for optimal differentiation.

TREATMENT, PREVENTION, AND CONTROL

Currently, penicillin or ampicillin, either alone or with gentamicin, is the treatment of choice for infections with *L. monocytogenes*. Listeriae are naturally resistant to cephalosporins. Erythromycin can be used in patients allergic to penicillin, but resistance to trimethoprim and the tetracyclines has been observed. Tetracycline resistance was first observed in 1988 and appears to be increasing, in part because of the use of these antibiotics in animal herds. Resistance to aminoglycosides has also been reported. Genes for resistance to tetracyclines and aminoglycosides have been found on conjugative plasmids and transposons that originated in enterococci. The rise in antibiotic resistance is of obvious concern and must be monitored closely.

Because listeriae are ubiquitous and most infections are sporadic, prevention and control are difficult. People at high risk of infection should avoid eating raw or partially cooked foods of animal origin, soft cheeses, and unwashed raw vegetables. A vaccine is not available, and prophylactic antibiotic therapy for high-risk patients has not been evaluated.

Erysipelothrix rhusiopathiae (Box 26–4)

PHYSIOLOGY AND STRUCTURE

The genus *Erysipelothrix* contains three species, of which *E. rhusiopathiae* is responsible for human disease.

BOX 26–4. Summary of *Erysipelothrix*

Physiology and Structure

Slender, pleomorphic gram-positive rods that form long (i.e., 60 μm) filaments

Microaerophilic, facultative anaerobe

Growth is slow, requiring 2 to 3 days of incubation

Virulence

Relatively little is known; production of hyaluronidase and neuraminidase is probably important; capsule-like structure may prevent phagocytosis

Epidemiology

Colonizes a variety of organisms, particularly swine and turkey

Found in soil rich in organic matter or groundwater contaminated with wastes from colonized animals

Uncommon pathogen in the United States

Occupational disease of butchers, meat processors, farmers, poultry workers, fish handlers, and veterinarians

Diseases

Refer to Box 26–3

Diagnosis

Long, filamentous gram-positive rods seen on Gram stain of a biopsy collected at the advancing edge of the lesion

Grows well on blood and chocolate agars incubated in 5% to 10% CO_2

Catalase negative and nonmotile; weakly fermentative; produces H_2S on triple sugar iron (TSI) agar slant (useful identification features)

Treatment, Prevention, and Control

Penicillin is drug of choice; organism is susceptible to cephalosporins, fluoroquinolones, erythromycin, and clindamycin; variable susceptibility to aminoglycosides and sulfonamides; resistant to vancomycin

Workers should cover exposed skin when handling animals and animal products

Swineherds should be vaccinated

E. rhusiopathiae is a gram-positive, non–spore-forming, facultatively anaerobic rod that is distributed worldwide in wild and domestic animals. The rods are slender (0.2 to 0.4×0.8 to 2.5 µm) and sometimes pleomorphic, with a tendency to form filaments as long as 60 µm ("hairlike"). They may decolorize readily and appear gram-negative. The organisms are microaerophilic, preferring a reduced oxygen atmosphere and supplemented carbon dioxide (5% to 10%). Small, grayish, α-hemolytic colonies are observed after 2 to 3 days of incubation. Animal disease—particularly in swine—is widely recognized, but human disease is uncommon.

PATHOGENESIS

Little is known about specific virulence factors in *Erysipelothrix*. Disease in swine has been associated with production of hyaluronidase and neuraminidase. Because this organism is an uncommon human pathogen, similar studies in humans have not been performed. A capsule-like structure has been identified in electron micrographs and could inhibit phagocytosis.

EPIDEMIOLOGY

Erysipelothrix is a ubiquitous organism that is distributed worldwide. It can be recovered on the tonsils or in the digestive tracts of many wild and domestic animals, including mammals, birds, and fish. Colonization is particularly high in swine and turkeys. Soil rich in organic matter or groundwater contaminated with animal wastes can facilitate animal to animal spread. *Erysipelothrix* disease in humans is zoonotic (spread from animals to humans) and primarily occupational. Butchers, meat processors, farmers, poultry workers, fish handlers, and veterinarians are at greatest risk. Cutaneous infections typically develop after the organism is inoculated subcutaneously through an abrasion or puncture wound during the handling of contaminated animal products or soil. The incidence of human disease is unknown because *Erysipelothrix* infection is not a reportable disease.

CLINICAL DISEASES

The following two primary forms of human infection with *E. rhusiopathiae* have been described: (1) a localized skin infection **(erysipeloid)** and (2) a septicemic form. Erysipeloid is an inflammatory skin lesion that develops at the site of trauma after 2 to 7 days of incubation. The lesion most commonly presents on the fingers or hands and appears violaceous with a raised edge. It slowly spreads peripherally as the discoloration in the central area fades. The painful lesion is pruritic, and the patient experiences a burning or throbbing sensation. Suppuration is uncommon, a feature distinguishing erysipeloid from streptococcal erysipelas. The resolution can be spontaneous but can be hastened with appropriate antibiotic therapy. A diffuse cutaneous infection can also develop. It is often associated with systemic manifestations, but blood culture results are typically negative for the organism.

The septicemic form of *Erysipelothrix* infections is uncommon but when present, it is frequently associated with endocarditis. *Erysipelothrix* endocarditis may have an acute onset but is usually subacute. Involvement of previously undamaged heart valves (particularly the aortic valve) is common. Other systemic complications (e.g., abscess formation, meningitis, osteomyelitis) are relatively uncommon.

LABORATORY DIAGNOSIS

The rods are located only in the deep tissue of the lesion. Thus full-thickness biopsy specimens or deep aspirates must be collected from the margin of the lesion. Microscopic studies and the culture of specimens collected from the surface invariably demonstrate the organism. Blood cultures are typically negative. *E. rhusiopathiae* is not fastidious and grows on most conventional laboratory media incubated in the presence of 5% to 10% CO_2. The absence of both motility and catalase production distinguishes this organism from *Listeria*. The organism is weakly fermentative and produces hydrogen sulfide on triple sugar iron agar.

TREATMENT, PREVENTION, AND CONTROL

Erysipelothrix is susceptible to penicillin, which is the antibiotic of choice for both localized and systemic diseases. Cephalosporins, erythromycin, and clindamycin are also active in vitro, but the organism has variable susceptibility to sulfonamides and aminoglycosides and is resistant to vancomycin. Infections in people at a higher occupational risk are prevented by the use of gloves and other appropriate coverings on exposed skin. Vaccination is used to control disease in swine.

CASE STUDY AND QUESTIONS

A 35-year-old man was hospitalized because of headache, fever, and confusion. He had received a kidney transplant 7 months before, after which he had been given immunosuppressive drugs to prevent organ rejection. CSF was collected, which revealed a white blood cell count of 36 cells/mm^3 with 96% polymorphonuclear leukocytes, a glucose concentration of 40 mg/dl, and a protein concentration of 172 mg/dl. A Gram stain preparation of CSF was negative for organisms, but gram-positive coccobacilli grew in cultures of the blood and CSF.

1. What is the most likely cause of this patient's meningitis?
2. What are the potential sources of this organism?
3. What virulence factors are associated with this organism?
4. How would this disease be treated? Which antibiotics are effective in vitro? Which antibiotics are ineffective?

Bibliography

Gorby GL, Peacock JE Jr: *Erysipelothrix rhusiopathiae* endocarditis: Microbiologic, epidemiologic, and clinical features of an occupational disease, *Rev Infect Dis* 10:317-325, 1988.

Hof H, Nichterlein T, Kretschmar M: Management of listeriosis, *Clin Microbiol Rev* 10:345-357, 1997.

Ireton K, Cossart P: Host-pathogen interactions during entry and actin-based movement of *Listeria monocytogenes*, *Annu Rev Genet* 31:113-138, 1997.

Lorber B: Listeriosis, *Clin Infect Dis* 24:1-11, 1997.

Safdar A, Armstrong D: Listeriosis in patients at a comprehensive cancer center, 1955-1997, *Clin Infect Dis* 37:359-364, 2003.

Schlech W: Foodborne listeriosis, *Clin Infect Dis* 31:770-775, 2000.

Verbarg S et al: *Erysipelothrix inopinata* sp. nov., isolated in the course of sterile filtration of vegetable peptone broth, and description of *Erysipelotrichaceae* fam. nov., Int J Syst Evol Microbiol 54:221-225, 2004.

Wing E, Gregory S: *Listeria monocytogenes*: Clinical and experimental update, *J Infect Dis* 185 (suppl 1): S18-S24, 2002.

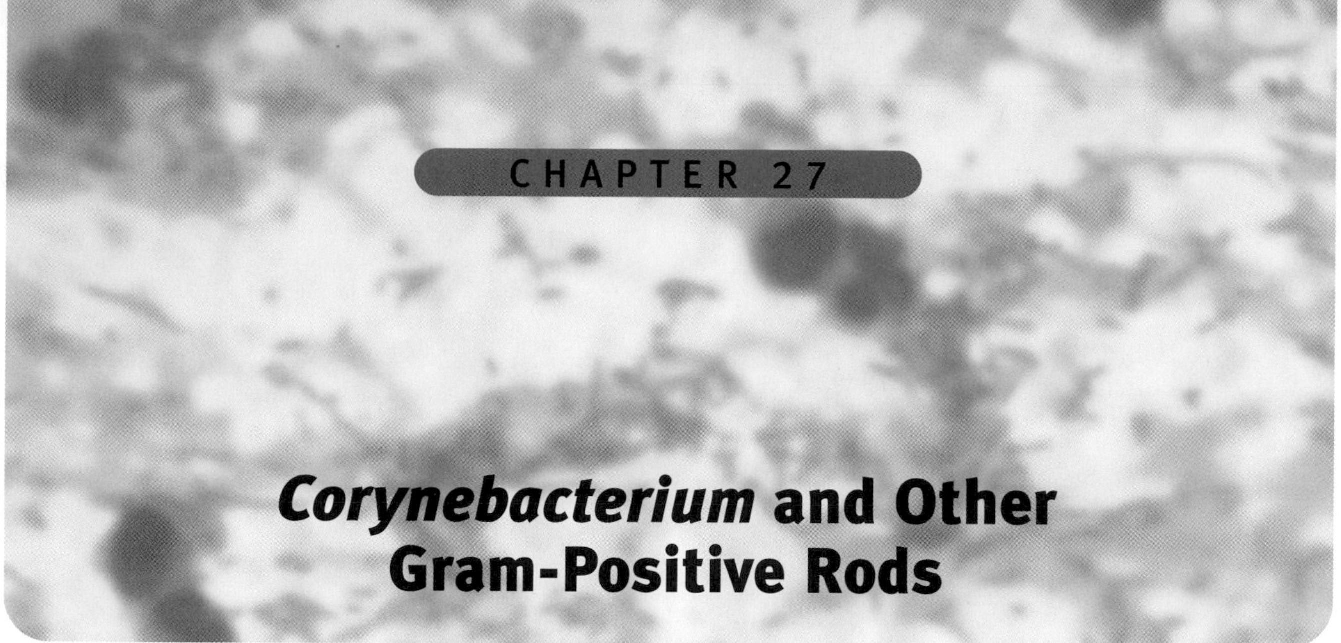

CHAPTER 27

Corynebacterium and Other Gram-Positive Rods

The aerobic gram-positive rods are a heterogeneous group of bacteria that have been loosely grouped on the basis of their cell morphology, staining properties, and guanine plus cytosine (G + C) content. The **coryneform** group (Box 27–1) consists of *Corynebacterium* and related genera that are non–spore-forming, non–acid-fast, gram-positive rods with a high guanine plus cytosine content. These bacteria are the focus of this chapter.

The genus *Corynebacterium* is a large, heterogeneous collection of species that have a cell wall with arabinose, galactose, *meso*-diaminopimelic acid (*meso*-DAP), and (in most species) short-chain mycolic acids (22 to 36 carbon atoms). *Corynebacterium* species are the only coryneform organisms with cell wall mycolic acids (Table 27–1). Gram stains of these bacteria reveal clumps and short chains (V or Y configurations) of irregularly shaped (club-shaped) rods (Figure 27–1). Metachromatic granules (i.e., granules that stain a color different from the primary dye color) within the cells may be seen with special stains. Corynebacteria are aerobic or facultatively anaerobic, nonmotile, and catalase positive. Most (but not all) species ferment carbohydrates, producing lactic acid as a by-product. Many species grow well on common laboratory media; however, some species require supplementation of media with lipids for good growth (lipophilic strains). Currently, more than 60 species of *Corynebacterium* have been defined.

Corynebacteria are ubiquitous in plants and animals, and they normally colonize the skin, upper respiratory tract, gastrointestinal tract, and urogenital tract in humans. Although all species of corynebacteria can function as opportunistic pathogens, a few are more commonly associated with human disease (Table 27–2). The most famous of these is *Corynebacterium diphtheriae*, the etiologic agent of **diphtheria.**

A number of other genera of coryneform bacteria have been characterized. The four genera most commonly associated with human disease are discussed briefly at the end of this chapter.

Corynebacterium diphtheriae (Box 27–2)

PHYSIOLOGY AND STRUCTURE

C. diphtheriae is an irregularly staining, pleomorphic rod (0.3 to 0.8 × 1.0 to 8.0 μm). Metachromatic granules have been observed in rods stained with methylene blue. After overnight incubation, 1- to 3-mm colonies are observed on blood agar medium. More selective, differential media can be used to recover this pathogen from specimens in which other organisms are present. This species is subdivided into four biotypes based on their colonial morphology and biochemical properties: *belfanti, gravis, intermedius,* and *mitis*. Biotypes *intermedius* and *belfanti* are rarely associated with diphtheria.

PATHOGENESIS AND IMMUNITY

C. diphtheriae is a classic model of bacterial virulence. The toxicity observed in diphtheria is directly attributed to an exotoxin secreted by the bacteria at the focus of infection. The organism does not need to enter the blood to produce the systemic signs of disease.

The *tox* gene that codes for the exotoxin is introduced into strains of *C. diphtheriae* by a lysogenic bacteriophage **(β-phage)**. Two processing steps are necessary for the active gene product to be secreted: (1) proteolytic cleavage of the leader sequence from the tox protein during secretion from the bacterial cell; and (2) cleavage of the toxin molecule into two polypeptides (A and B) that remain attached by a disulfide bond. This 58,300-Da protein is an example of the classic **A-B exotoxin.**

BOX 27–1. Important Coryneform Bacteria

Organism	Historical Derivation
Corynebacterium	*coryne*, a club; *bakterion*, a small rod (a small, club-shaped rod)
C. diphtheriae	*diphthera*, leather or skin (reference to the leathery membrane that forms initially on the pharynx)
C. jeikeium	*jeikeium* (species originally classified as group JK)
C. urealyticum	*urea*, urea; *lyticum*, lyse (capable of lysing urea; species rapidly hydrolyzes urea)
C. amycolatum	*a*, without; *mycolatum*, pertaining to mycolic acids (species does not have mycolic acids in the cell wall)
C. minutissimum	*minutissimus*, very small (refers to the relatively short rods and small colonies)
C. pseudotuberculosis	*pseudo*, like; *tuberculosis* (produces chronic purulent infections [e.g., tuberculosis] in sheep and other warm-blooded animals)
C. ulcerans	*ulcerans* (can produce pharyngeal ulcers like *C. diphtheriae*)
Arcanobacterium	*arcanus*, secretive; *bacterium*, rod (secretive bacterium; a slow-growing organism that can prove difficult to isolate)
Brevibacterium	*brevis*, short; *bacterium*, rod (a short rod; this species appears as very small coccobacilli)
Oerskovia	Named after Jeppe Orskov, a Danish microbiologist
Turicella	*Turicella*, pertaining to Turicum (Turicum is the Latin name for Zurich, the city where the first isolates were collected and described)

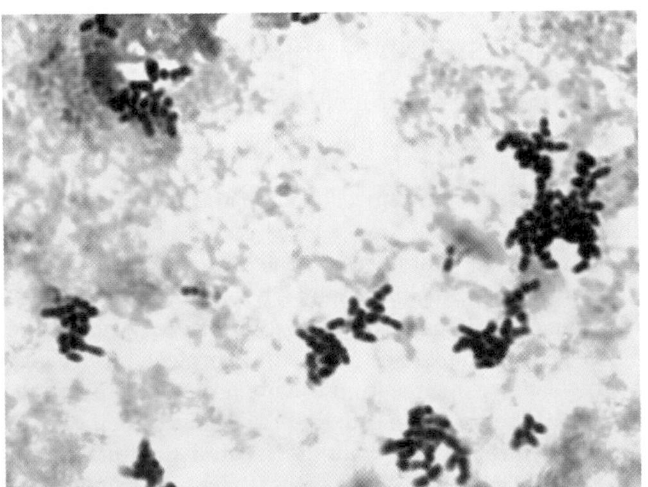

FIGURE 27–1. Gram stain of *Corynebacterium* species in blood culture.

BOX 27–2. Summary of *Corynebacterium diphtheriae*

Physiology and Structure

Gram-positive pleomorphic rod (0.3 to 0.8 × 1.0 to 8.0 um)
Most strains grow well on lipid-free media
Facultative anaerobe (grows aerobically and anaerobically)
Ferments carbohydrates

Virulence

Diphtheria toxin, an A-B exotoxin, inhibits protein synthesis by inactivating elongation factor 2
Additional virulence factors are likely (but unknown) because nontoxigenic strains can cause systemic disease

Epidemiology

Worldwide distribution maintained in asymptomatic carriers and unvaccinated hosts
Humans are the only known reservoir, with carriage in oropharynx or on skin surface
Spread person to person by exposure to respiratory droplets or skin contact
Disease observed in unvaccinated people living in crowded urban areas and in children or adults with waning immunity
Diphtheria is uncommon in the United States

Disease

Refer to Box 27–3

Diagnosis

Microscopy is nonspecific; metachromatic granules observed in *C. diphtheriae* and other corynebacteria
Culture should be performed on nonselective (blood agar) and selective (cysteine-tellurite agar, serum tellurite agar) media
Demonstration of exotoxin is performed by polymerase chain reaction assay or Elek test

Treatment, Prevention, and Control

Infections treated with diphtheria antitoxin to neutralize exotoxin, penicillin or erythromycin to eliminate *C. diphtheriae* and terminate toxin production, and immunization of convalesence patients with diphtheria toxoid to stimulate protective antibodies
Administration of diphtheria vaccine and booster shots to susceptible population

Three functional regions exist on the toxin molecule, a **receptor-binding region** and a **translocation region** on the B subunit and a **catalytic region** on the A subunit. The receptor for the toxin is heparin-binding epidermal growth factor, which is present on the surface of many eukaryotic cells, particularly heart and nerve cells; its presence explains the cardiac and neurologic symptoms observed in patients with severe diphtheria. After the toxin becomes attached to the host cell, the translocation region is inserted into the endosomal membrane, facilitating the movement of the catalytic region into the cytosol. The A

TABLE 27–1. Characteristic Properties of Selected Coryneform Genera

Genus	Catalase	Fermentation/Oxidation	Motility	Cell Wall		Gram Stain
				Mycolic Acids	Diamino Acid	
Corynebacterium	+	Ferm/Oxid	–	+	*meso*-DAP	Club-shaped rods
Arcanobacterium	–	Ferm	–	–	Lysine	Irregularly shaped rods
Brevibacterium	–	Oxid	–	–	*meso*-DAP	Short coccobacilli
Oerskovia	–	Ferm	Variable	–	Lysine	Long branching rods
Turicella	–	Oxid	–	–	*meso*-DAP	Long rods

TABLE 27–2. *Corynebacterium* Species Associated with Human Disease

Organism	Diseases
C. diphtheriae	Diphtheria (respiratory, cutaneous); pharyngitis and endocarditis (nontoxigenic strains)
C. jeikeium (group JK)	Septicemia, endocarditis, wound infections, foreign body (catheter, shunt, prosthesis) infections
C. urealyticum (group D2)	Urinary tract infections (including pyelonephritis and alkaline-encrusted cystitis), septicemia, endocarditis, wound infections
C. amycolatum	Wound infections, foreign body infections, septicemia, urinary tract infections, respiratory tract infections
C. macginleyi	Eye infections
C. minutissimum	Wound infections, respiratory tract infections
C. pseudodiphtheriticum	Respiratory tract infections, endocarditis
C. pseudotuberculosis	Lymphadenitis, ulcerative lymphangitis, abscess formation
C. riegelii	Genitourinary tract infections (females)
C. striatum	Wound infections, respiratory tract infections, foreign body infections
C. ulcerans	Respiratory diphtheria

subunit then terminates host cell protein synthesis by inactivating **elongation factor 2 (EF-2)**, a factor required for the movement of nascent peptide chains on ribosomes. Because the turnover of EF-2 is very slow and approximately only one molecule per ribosome is present in a cell, it has been estimated that one exotoxin molecule can inactivate the entire EF-2 content in a cell, completely terminating host cell protein synthesis. Toxin synthesis is regulated by a chromosomally encoded element, **diphtheria toxin repressor (DTxR)**. This protein, activated in the presence of high-iron concentrations, can bind to the toxin gene operator and prevent toxin production.

EPIDEMIOLOGY

Diphtheria is a disease found worldwide, particularly in poor urban areas where there is crowding and the protective level of vaccine-induced immunity is low. The largest outbreak in the latter part of the 20th century occurred in the former Soviet Union, where in 1994 almost 48,000 cases were documented, with 1746 deaths. *C. diphtheriae* is maintained in the population by asymptomatic carriage in the oropharynx or on the skin of immune people (after either exposure to *C. diphtheriae* or immunization). Respiratory droplets or skin contact transmit it from person to person. Humans are the only known reservoir for this organism.

Diphtheria has become uncommon in the United States as the result of an active immunization program, as shown by the fact that more than 200,000 cases were reported in 1921 but fewer than 5 cases per year have been reported since 1980. Diphtheria is primarily a pediatric disease, but the highest incidence has shifted toward older age groups in areas where there are active immunization programs for children. Skin infection with toxigenic *C. diphtheriae* (cutaneous diphtheria) also occurs, but it is not a reportable disease in the United States, so its incidence is unknown.

BOX 27–3. *Corynebacterium diphtheriae*: Clinical Diseases

Respiratory diphtheria: Sudden onset with exudative pharyngitis, sore throat, low-grade fever, and malaise; a thick pseudomembrane develops over the pharynx; in critically ill patients, breathing obstruction, cardiac arrhythmia, coma, and death can develop

Cutaneous diphtheria: A papule can develop on the skin that progresses to a nonhealing ulcer; systemic signs can develop

CLINICAL DISEASES

The clinical presentation of diphtheria is determined by (1) the site of infection, (2) the immune status of the patient, and (3) the virulence of the organism. Exposure to *C. diphtheriae* may result in asymptomatic colonization in fully immune people, mild respiratory disease in partially immune patients, or a fulminant, sometimes fatal disease in nonimmune patients (Box 27–3).

Respiratory Diphtheria

The symptoms of diphtheria involving the respiratory tract develop after a 2- to 6-day incubation period. Organisms multiply locally on epithelial cells in the pharynx or adjacent surfaces and initially cause localized damage as a result of exotoxin activity. The onset is sudden, with malaise, sore throat, exudative pharyngitis, and a low-grade fever. The exudate evolves into a thick pseudomembrane composed of bacteria, lymphocytes, plasma cells, fibrin, and dead cells that can cover the tonsils, uvula, and palate and can extend up into the nasopharynx or down into the larynx. The pseudomembrane firmly adheres to the respiratory tissue and is difficult to dislodge without making the underlying tissue bleed (unique to diphtheria). As the patient recovers after the approximately 1-week course of the disease, the membrane dislodges and is expectorated. Complications in patients with severe disease include breathing obstruction, cardiac arrhythmia, coma, and, ultimately, death.

Cutaneous Diphtheria

Cutaneous diphtheria is acquired through skin contact with other infected persons. The organism colonizes the skin and gains entry into the subcutaneous tissue through breaks in the skin. A papule develops first and then evolves into a chronic, nonhealing ulcer, sometimes covered with a grayish membrane. Systemic signs of disease can occur as a result of the exotoxin effects.

LABORATORY DIAGNOSIS

The initial treatment of a patient with diphtheria is instituted on the basis of the clinical diagnosis, not laboratory results, because definitive results are not available for at least a week.

Microscopy

The results of microscopic examination of clinical material are unreliable. Metachromatic granules in bacteria stained with methylene blue have been described, but this appearance is not specific to *C. diphtheriae,* and interpretation of the smear requires technical expertise.

Culture

Specimens for the recovery of *C. diphtheriae* should be collected from both the nasopharynx and the throat and should be inoculated onto a nonselective, enriched blood agar plate and a medium developed specifically for this organism (e.g., cysteine-tellurite agar, serum tellurite agar). Tellurite inhibits the growth of most upper respiratory tract bacteria and gram-negative rods and is reduced by *C. diphtheriae* producing characteristic gray to black color on agar containing tellurite. Degradation of cysteine by *C. diphtheriae* cysteinase activity produces a brown halo around the colonies. One of the original media used to recover *C. diphtheriae* was Löffler's medium. The medium is currently not recommended for primary isolation but does enhance production of metachromatic granules in the bacteria.

Toxigenicity Testing

All isolates of *C. diphtheriae* should be tested for the production of exotoxin. This has been done historically by an in vitro immunodiffusion assay **(Elek test),** a tissue culture neutralization assay using specific antitoxin, or an in vivo neutralization assay using guinea pigs injected subcutaneously with the isolate from the patient. Currently, a modification of the Elek test is what is done in most laboratories. An alternative method for detecting toxin is a nucleic acid amplification test developed by the Centers for Disease Control and Prevention (CDC). This test can detect the *tox* gene in clinical isolates and directly in clinical specimens (e.g., swabs from the diphtheritic membrane or biopsy material). Although this test is rapid and specific, strains with the *tox* gene not expressed can give a positive signal. Nontoxigenic strains of *C. diphtheriae* should not be ignored, because these strains have been associated with significant disease, including septicemia, endocarditis, septic arthritis, osteomyelitis, and abscess formation.

TREATMENT, PREVENTION, AND CONTROL

The most important aspect of the treatment for diphtheria is the early administration of diphtheria antitoxin to specifically neutralize the exotoxin before it is bound by the host cell. Once the cell internalizes the toxin, cell death is inevitable. Antibiotic therapy with penicillin or erythromycin is also used to eliminate *C. diphtheriae* and terminate toxin production. Bed rest, isolation to prevent secondary spread, and maintenance of an open airway in patients with respiratory diphtheria are all important. After the patient has recovered, immunization with toxoid is required because most patients fail to develop protective antibodies after a natural infection.

Symptomatic diphtheria can be prevented by actively immunizing people with diphtheria toxoid. The nontoxic, immunogenic toxoid is prepared by formalin treatment of the toxin. Initially, children are given five injections of this preparation with pertussis and tetanus antigens **(DPT vaccine)** at ages 2, 4, 6, 15 to 18 months, and at 4 to 6 years. After that time, it is recommended that booster vaccinations with diphtheria toxoid combined with tetanus toxoid be given every 10 years. Serum antitoxin antibodies can be measured by a rabbit skin or Vero cell neutralization test.

People coming in close contact with patients who have documented diphtheria are at risk for acquiring the disease. Nasopharyngeal specimens for culture should be collected from all close contacts, and antimicrobial prophylaxis with penicillin or erythromycin started immediately. Any contact who has not completed the series of diphtheria immunizations or who has not received a booster dose within the previous 5 years should receive a booster dose of toxoid. People exposed to cutaneous diphtheria should be managed in the same manner as those exposed to respiratory diphtheria. If the respiratory or cutaneous infection is caused by a nontoxigenic strain, it is unnecessary to institute prophylaxis in contacts.

BOX 27–4. Summary of Other *Corynebacterium* Species

Physiology and Structure

Gram-positive rods with an irregular shape

Some species require lipids for good growth (e.g., *C. jeikeium, C. urealyticum, C. macginleyi*)

Most strains are facultative anaerobes

Virulence

Diphtheria A-B exotoxin may be carried by *C. ulcerans* and *C. pseudotuberculosis*

Urinary tract pathogens produce urease (e.g., *C. amycolatum, C. glucuronolyticum, C. riegelii, C. urealyticum*)

Many species able to adhere to foreign bodies (e.g., catheters, shunts, prosthetic devices)

Some species resistant to most antibiotics (e.g., *C. amycolatum, C. jeikeium, C. urealyticum*)

Epidemiology

Most infections are endogenous (produced by species that are part of the host's normal bacterial population on the skin surface and mucosal membranes)

Diseases

Septicemia, endocarditis, foreign body infections, wound infections, urinary tract infections, respiratory infections, including diphtheria

Diagnosis

Culture on nonselective media is reliable, although growth may be slow and media may require supplementation with lipids

Treatment, Prevention, and Control

Treatment with effective antibiotics to eliminate the organism

Removal of foreign body

Other *Corynebacterium* Species

A large number of other *Corynebacterium* species have been found as part of the indigenous human flora and are capable of causing disease. The most common species are listed in Table 27–2 and summarized in Box 27–4.

Corynebacterium jeikeium is a well-recognized opportunistic pathogen in immunocompromised patients, particularly those with hematologic disorders or intravascular catheters. Carriage of this organism is uncommon in healthy people, but the skin of as many as 40% of hospitalized patients can be colonized regardless of their immunologic state. Predisposing conditions for disease include prolonged hospitalization, granulocytopenia, previous or concurrent antimicrobial therapy or chemotherapy, and a mucocutaneous portal of entry. This organism is typically very resistant to antibiotics, so antibiotic therapy during hospitalization may foster colonization of the skin. The organism can then gain access through an intravenous catheter and establish disease in the immunologically compromised patient.

Corynebacterium urealyticum is not a common isolate in healthy people; however, the species is an important pathogen of the urinary tract. As the name implies, *C. urealyticum*, which is a strong urease producer, can produce enough urease to make the urine alkaline, possibly leading to the formation of **struvite calculi** or **renal stones.** Risk factors associated with *C. urealyticum* infections include immunosuppression, underlying genitourinary disorders, an antecedent urologic procedure, and previous antibiotic therapy. Other urease-producing corynebacteria that are associated with urinary tract infections are *Corynebacterium amycolatum, Corynebacterium glucuronolyticum*, and *Corynebacterium riegelii.*

C. amycolatum resides on the skin surface but not in the oropharynx. This species is the most commonly isolated species in clinical specimens, although its importance has been underappreciated because it is frequently misidentified as other corynebacteria species. This species, like *C. jeikeium* and *C. urealyticum*, is resistant to many antibiotics and is an important opportunistic pathogen.

Corynebacterium minutissimum colonizes the skin of healthy people and has been associated with **erythrasma**, a superficial infection of the skin involving the formation of reddish-brown, pruritic macular patches found primarily in the groin. The etiologic role of *C. minutissimum*, however, has been questioned because the methods most commonly used to identify this organism are inadequate. More likely, erythrasma is caused by *C. minutissimum*, as well as other species of *Corynebacterium*.

Corynebacterium pseudotuberculosis and *Corynebacterium ulcerans* are closely related to *C. diphtheriae* and can carry the diphtheria gene. Although *C. ulcerans* can cause a disease indistinguishable from diphtheria, human infections caused by *C. pseudotuberculosis* are rarely observed.

Numerous other *Corynebacterium* species have been associated with opportunistic infections. These bacteria are commonly present on the skin and mucosal surfaces, so their isolation in a clinical specimen may represent an important finding or may simply represent contamination of the specimen.

Treatment of *Corynebacterium* infections can be problematic. *C. jeikeium*, *C. urealyticum*, and *C. amycolatum* are typically resistant to most antibiotics, so infected patients usually must be given vancomycin. The other species tend to be more susceptible to antibiotics, but in vitro testing may be required before a treatment regimen is selected.

Other Coryneform Genera

Other genera of irregularly shaped, gram-positive rods have been found to colonize humans and cause disease (Tables 27–3; also see Table 27–1). *Arcanobacterium* can cause pharyngitis with a "scarlet fever–like: rash, polymicrobic wound infections, and, less commonly, systemic infections such as septicemia and endocarditis. Infections can be treated with penicillin or erythromycin.

Brevibacterium colonize the skin surface and, when grown in culture, produce a cheeselike odor. These bacteria have been blamed for malodorous feet in some colonized people. More important diseases attributed to *Brevibacterium* are septicemia, osteomyelitis, and foreign body infections. Treatment is complicated because many strains are resistant to β-lactam antibiotics, erythromycin, clindamycin, and ciprofloxacin. Use of vancomycin, tetracyclines, or gentamicin has proved effective.

Oerskovia is an environmental organism found in the soil and decaying organic matter. This organism has been associated with septicemia, endocarditis, meningitis, soft-tissue infections, and infections in the presence of foreign bodies. Effective treatment must be guided by in vitro susceptibility tests, because vancomycin-resistant strains have been reported.

Turicella (*Turicella otitidis* is the only species) has been isolated in the ears of healthy and infected individuals. The isolates are susceptible to β-lactam antibiotics but may be resistant to clindamycin and erythromycin.

TABLE 27–3. Less Common Coryneform Gram-Positive Rods Associated with Human Disease

Organism	Diseases
Arcanobacterium	Pharyngitis, cellulitis, wound infections, abscess formation, septicemia, endocarditis
Brevibacterium	Septicemia, osteomyelitis, foreign body (catheter, shunt, prosthesis) infections
Oerskovia	Septicemia, endocarditis, meningitis, soft-tissue infections, foreign body infections
Turicella	Ear infections

CASE STUDY AND QUESTIONS

A 78-year-old man with a history of hypertension was admitted to the hospital because of a severe headache of 4 hours' duration. Evidence of subarachnoid hemorrhage and hydrocephalus was found, and the patient required the placement of a left ventricular-atrial shunt. Fever developed 1 week after the operation. C. jeikeium was isolated from blood cultures and a subsequent culture of fluid collected from the shunt.

1. What risk factors are associated with infections with *C. jeikeium?*
2. What antibiotic therapy could be given for infections with this organism?
3. Name two other *Corynebacterium* species that are commonly resistant to multiple antibiotics. What diseases are associated with these organisms?
4. Explain the synthesis and mode of action of the diphtheria exotoxin.

Bibliography

Coyle MA, Lipsky BA: Coryneform bacteria in infectious diseases: Clinical and laboratory aspects, *Clin Microbiol Rev* 3:227-246, 1990.

Esteban J et al: Microbiological characterization and clinical significance of *Corynebacterium amycolatum* strains, *Eur J Clin Microbiol Infect Dis* 18:518-521, 1999.

Funke G et al: Antimicrobial susceptibility patterns of some recently established coryneform bacteria, *Antimicrob Agents Chemother* 40:2874-2878, 1996.

Funke G et al: *Corynebacterium coyleae* sp. nov., isolated from human clinical specimens, *Int Sys Bacteriol* 47:92-96, 1997.

Funke G et al: Clinical microbiology of coryneform bacteria, *Clin Microbiol Rev* 10:125-159, 1997.

Funke G et al: *Corynebacterium macginleyi* has to date been isolated exclusively from conjunctival swabs, *J Clin Microbiol* 36:3670-3673, 1998.

George MJ: Clinical significance and characterization of *Corynebacterium* species, *Clin Microbiol Newsletter* 17:177-180, 1995.

Gutierrez-Rodero F et al: *Corynebacterium pseudodiphtheriticum:* An easily missed respiratory pathogen in HIV-infected patients, *Diagn Microbiol Infect Dis* 33:209-216, 1999.

Lipsky BA et al: Infections caused by nondiphtheria corynebacteria, *Rev Infect Dis* 4:1220-1235, 1982.

Pascual C et al: Phylogenetic analysis of the genus *Corynebacterium* based on 16S rRNA gene sequences, *Int J Syst Bacteriol* 45:724-728, 1995.

Popovic T et al: Molecular epidemiology of diphtheria in Russia, 1985-1994, *J Infect Dis* 174:1064-1072, 1996.

Soriano F et al: Urinary tract infection caused by *Corynebacterium* group D2: Report of 82 cases and review, *Rev Infect Dis* 12:1019-1034, 1990.

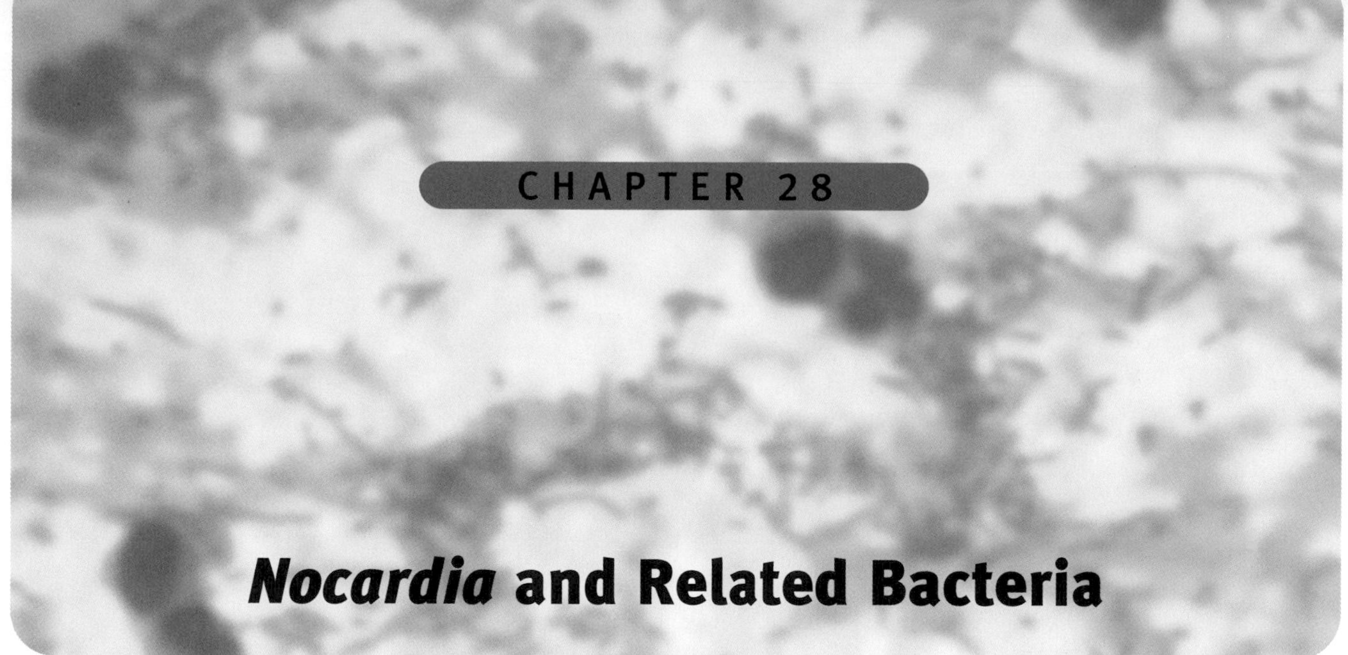

Nocardia and Related Bacteria

The aerobic actinomycetes are gram-positive, catalase-positive rods that can colonize animals and humans and are found commonly in soil and decaying vegetation. Some actinomycetes have delicate filamentous forms (called **hyphae** because they are similar to fungal hyphal forms) in clinical specimens and in culture (thus the fungal reference in the name; Box 28–1). However, the cell structure and antimicrobial susceptibility patterns are typical of bacteria.

Actinomycetales consist of taxonomically diverse genera that were originally classified together because of their morphologic similarities. However, with the increased use of nucleic acid sequencing and DNA-DNA hybridization for resolving taxonomic relationships among microbes, the number of genera and species in the order Actinomycetes has increased at a mind-numbing rate. For our purposes, we can separate the medically important Actinomycetales into two groups based on the presence of cell wall **mycolic acids** (Box 28–2). *Corynebacterium* and *Mycobacterium* are discussed in Chapters 27 and 29, respectively; the other Actinomycetales are discussed in this chapter.

The spectrum of the infections associated with the aerobic actinomycetes is extensive and includes insignificant colonization (many genera), pulmonary disease *(Nocardia, Rhodococcus)*, systemic infections *(Nocardia, Rhodococcus)*, mycetoma *(Actinomadura, Nocardiopsis, Streptomyces,* and *Nocardia)*, other cutaneous infections *(Nocardia, Dermatophilus)*, other opportunistic infections (most genera), Whipple's disease *(Tropheryma)*, and allergic pneumonitis (thermophilic actinomycetes) (Table 28–1).

Nocardia

PHYSIOLOGY AND STRUCTURE

Norcardiae are strict aerobic rods that form branched hyphae in tissues and culture (Box 28–3). The organisms are gram-positive, although many stain poorly and appear to be gram-negative with intracellular gram-positive beads (Figure 28–1). Nocardiae have a cell wall structure similar to that of mycobacteria (see chapter 29), with 10-methyl stearic acid **(tuberculostearic acid)**, *meso*-diaminopimelic acid (*meso*-DAP), arabinose, galactose, and mycolic acids present. The length of the mycolic acids in norcardiae (50 to 62 carbon atoms) is shorter than in mycobacteria (70 to 90 carbon atoms). This difference may explain why even though both genera stain acid-fast, Nocardia is described as **"weakly acid-fast"**; that is, a weak decolorizing solution of hydrochloric acid must be used to demonstrate the acid-fast property of nocardiae (Figure 28–2). This acid-fastness is also a helpful characteristic for distinguishing *Nocardia* organisms from morphologically similar organisms, such as *Actinomyces* (see Chapter 41). Most strains of *Nocardia* have trehalose linked to two molecules of mycolic acid (trehalose-6,6′-dimycolate; **cord factor**). Cord factor is an important virulence factor that facilitates intracellular survival (see Pathogenesis and Immunity Section).

Nocardia species are catalase-positive, use carbohydrates oxidatively, and can grow on most nonselective laboratory media for bacteria, mycobacteria, and fungi; however, their isolation can require 3 to 5 days of incubation. The appearance of colonies varies from dry to waxy and from white to orange. **Aerial hyphae** (hyphae that protrude upward from the surface of a colony) can be observed when the colonies are viewed with a dissecting microscope (Figure 28–3). The presence of aerial hyphae

BOX 28–1. Important Actinomycetes

Organism	Historical Derivation
Actinomycetes	*aktinos,* a ray; *mykes,* fungus (ray fungus referring to the radial arrangement of filaments in colonies)
Actinomadura	*aktinos,* a ray; *Madura,* a province in India (organism first described as the causative agent of "Madura foot")
Dermatophilus	*derma,* skin; *philos,* loving (skin loving)
Gordonia	Named after the American microbiologist Ruth Gordon
Nocardia abscessus	Named after the French veterinarian Edmond Nocard; *abscessus,* associated with abscess formation
N. asteroides	*asteroides,* starlike (arrangement of hyphae)
N. brasiliensis	*brasiliensis,* pertaining to Brazil (first isolate in a Brazilian man)
N. cyriacigeorgica	*cyriaci,* church; *georgicus,* St. George (St. George's church refers to the origin of the name of the town Gelsenkirchen, where the type strain was isolated)
N. farcinica	*farcinica,* farcy or glanders, a disease of horses (the original isolate was thought to be the etiologic agent of bovine farcy)
N. nova	*nova,* new (a new species)
N. otitidiscaviarium	*otitis,* inflammation of the ear; *cavia,* of guinea pigs (ear disease of guinea pigs)
N. paucivorans	*paucus,* little; *vorans,* eating ("eating little"; refers to observation that this species can only use a few compounds as a sole source of carbon and energy)
N. pseudobrasiliensis	*pseudobrasiliensis,* like brasiliensis (phenotypically similar to *N. brasiliensis*)
N. transvalensis	*transvalensis,* pertaining to Transvaal, South Africa
N. veterana	*veteranus,* veteran as in soldier (refers to the veteran's hospital where the organism was isolated)
Nocardiopsis	*Nocardia,* genus of actinomycetes; *opsis,* appearance (organism resembling *Nocardia*)
Rhodococcus equi	*rhodo,* rose or red colored; *coccus,* berry; *equi,* pertaining to horses (red-colored coccus with species originally associated with horses)
Saccharomonospora	*sacchar,* sugar; *mono,* single; *spora,* a seed (single-spore organism from sugar cane)
Saccharopolyspora	*sacchar,* sugar; *polus,* many; *spora,* a seed (many-spored organism from sugar cane)
Streptomyces	*streptos,* pliant or bent; *myces,* fungus (pliant or bent fungus)
Thermoactinomyces	*thermos,* hot; *actinos,* a ray; *myces,* fungus (heat loving or thermophilic ray fungus)
Tropheryma whipplii	*trophe,* nourishment; *eryma,* barrier (barrier to nourishment; malabsorption is characteristic of the clinical syndrome Whipple's disease, first describe by George Whipple)
Tsukamurella	Honoring the Japanese microbiologist, Michio Tsukamura, who first described the original isolate of this genus

BOX 28–2. Pathogenic Aerobic Actinomycetes

Actinomycetes with Mycolic Acids

Corynebacterium
Nocardia
Rhodococcus
Gordonia
Tsukamurella
Mycobacterium

Actinomycetes with No Mycolic Acids

Actinomadura
Nocardiopsis
Streptomyces
Dermatophilus
Tropheryma
Thermophilic actinomycetes
- *Saccharomonospora*
- *Saccharopolyspora*
- *Thermoactinomyces*

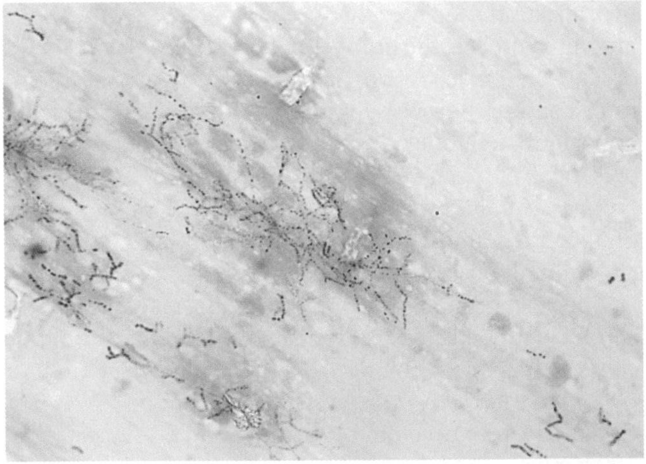

FIGURE 28–1. Gram stain of *Nocardia asteroides* in expectorated sputum. Note that the delicate beaded filaments cannot be distinguished from those of *Actinomyces* organisms (see Chapter 41).

TABLE 28–1. Diseases of Selected Pathogenic Actinomycetes

Organism	Diseases	Frequency
Nocardia	Pulmonary diseases (bronchitis, pneumonia, lung abscesses); primary or secondary cutaneous infections (e.g., mycetoma, lymphocutaneous infections, cellulitis, subcutaneous abscesses); secondary CNS infections (e.g., meningitis, brain abscesses)	Common
Rhodococcus	Pulmonary diseases (pneumonia, lung abscesses); disseminated diseases (e.g., meningitis, pericarditis); opportunistic infections (e.g., wound infections, peritonitis, traumatic endophthalmitis)	Uncommon
Gordonia	Opportunistic infections	Rare
Tsukamurella	Opportunistic infections	Rare
Actinomadura	Mycetoma	Rare (in United States)
Nocardiopsis	Mycetoma	Rare (in United States)
Streptomyces	Mycetoma; opportunistic infections	Rare (in United States)
Dermatophilus	Exudative dermatitis (dermatophilosis)	Rare (in United States)
Tropheryma	Whipple's disease	Common
Saccharomonospora	Allergic pneumonitis	Common
Saccharopolyspora	Allergic pneumonitis	Common
Thermoactinomyces	Allergic pneumonitis	Common

CNS, Central nervous system.

BOX 28–3. Summary of Nocardia

Physiology and Structure

Gram-positive, partially acid-fast, filamentous rods; cell wall with mycolic acid

Strict aerobe capable of growth on most nonselective bacterial media; however, prolonged incubation (7 days or more) may be required

Virulence

Opportunistic pathogen

Cord factor: prevents intracellular killing in phagocytes by interfering with fusion of phagosomes with lysosomes

Catalase and superoxide dismutase: inactivate toxic oxygen metabolites (e.g., hydrogen peroxide, superoxide)

Epidemiology

Worldwide distribution in soil rich with organic matter

Exogenous infections acquired by inhalation (pulmonary) or traumatic introduction (cutaneous)

Disease most common in immunocompetent patients with chronic pulmonary disease (bronchitis, emphysema, bronchiectasis, alveolar proteinosis), immunocompromised patients with T-cell deficiencies (transplant recipients, patients with malignancies, patients infected with the human immunodeficiency virus, patients receiving corticosteroids), and people who have suffered skin wounds through which the organisms could be introduced into subcutaneous tissues

Diseases

Bronchopulmonary disease

Primary or secondary cutaneous infections (e.g., mycetoma, lymphocutaneous infection, cellulitis, subcutaneous abscesses)

Secondary central nervous system infections (e.g., brain abscesses)

Diagnosis

Microscopy is sensitive and relatively specific when branching, partially acid-fast organisms are seen

Culture is slow, requiring incubation for up to 1 week; selective media (e.g., BCYE agar) may be required for isolating *Nocardia* in mixed cultures

Identification at the genus level can be made by the microscopic and macroscopic appearances

Identification at the species level requires genomic analysis for most isolates

Treatment, Prevention, and Control

Infections are treated with antibiotic therapy (e.g., sulfonamides or antibiotics with proven in vivo activity) and proper wound care

Exposure cannot be avoided because nocardiae are ubiquitous

BCYE, Buffered charcoal yeast extract.

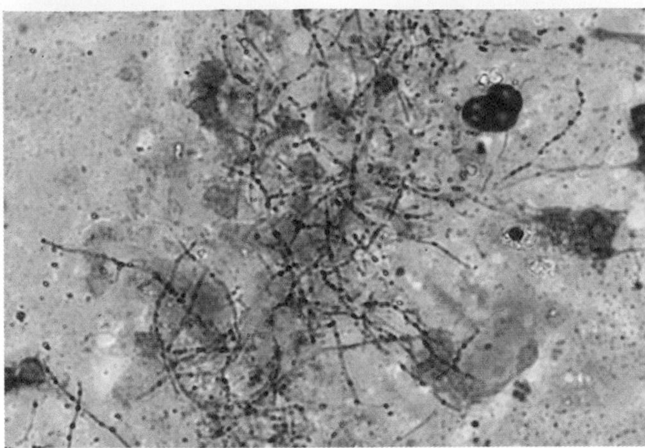

FIGURE 28–2. Acid-fast stain of *Nocardia* species in expectorated sputum. In contrast with the mycobacteria, members of the genus *Nocardia* do not uniformly retain the stain ("partially acid-fast").

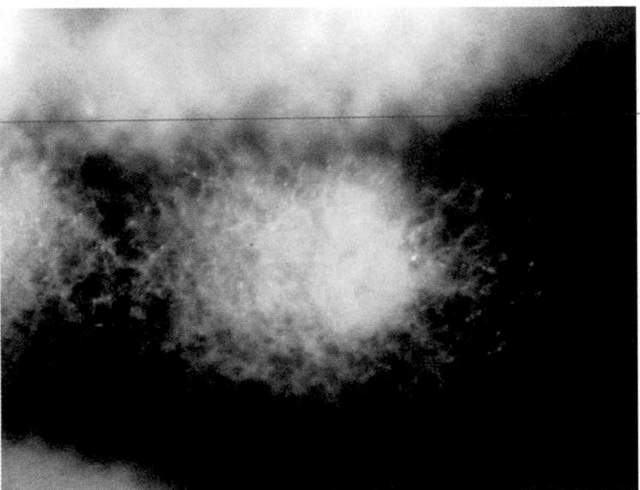

FIGURE 28–3. Aerial hyphae of *Nocardia.*

and acid-fastness is unique to *Nocardia* and can be used as a rapid test for the presumptive identification of the genus.

The taxonomic classification of this genus is—simply stated—a mess, with most of the organisms described in the literature now recognized as incorrectly identified. Historically, these organisms were classified by their ability to use carbohydrates and decompose a variety of substrates (e.g., adenine, casein, hypoxanthine, xanthine, gelatin, urea), as well as their antimicrobial susceptibility patterns. The true taxonomic relationships among the members of the genus were appreciated only recently through the use of gene sequencing and DNA-DNA hybridization. This problem is illustrated with the following example. Historically, *Nocardia asteroides* was reported as the most common human pathogen. It is now recognized that virtually all of the isolates were misnamed and *N. asteroides* is rarely if at all associated with human disease. Approximately 31 species of *Nocardia* have been recognized, with approximately a third of the species associated with human disease (Box 28–4). Although problems exist with the accurate identification of these species, it is generally only necessary to recognize an isolate is in the genus *Nocardia.*

BOX 28–4. *Nocardia* Species Associated with Human Disease

N. abscessus	***N. otitidiscavarium***
N. brasiliensis	***N. paucovorans***
N. brevicatena	***N. pseudobrasiliensis***
N. cyriacigeorgica	***N. transvalensis***
N. facinica	***N. veterna***
N. nova	

PATHOGENESIS AND IMMUNITY

Nocardia cause **bronchopulmonary disease** in immunocompromised patients, with a high predilection for hematogenous spread to the central nervous system (CNS) or skin. Patients at greatest risk for disease are those with T-cell deficiencies produced by disease (e.g., leukemia, acquired immune deficiency syndrome [AIDS]) or immunosuppressive therapy (e.g., corticosteroids for renal, cardiac, or bone marrow transplantation). Chronic localized pulmonary disease can occur in immunocompetent patients with bronchitis, emphysema, asthma, bronchiectasis, and alveolar proteinosis. **Cutaneous nocardiosis** can have four presentations: mycetoma, lymphocutaneous disease, superficial skin infection with abscess formation or cellulitis, and secondary cutaneous involvement following dissemination from a pulmonary site. *Nocardia brasiliensis* most commonly causes primary cutaneous infections in immunocompetent patients.

Bronchopulmonary disease develops after the initial colonization of the upper respiratory tract by inhalation and then aspiration of oral secretions into the lower airways. **Primary cutaneous nocardiosis** develops after traumatic introduction of organisms into subcutaneous tissues. Pulmonary and cutaneous diseases are characterized by necrosis and abscess formation similar to those caused by other pyogenic bacteria. Chronic infections with sinus tract formation can occur, particularly with primary cutaneous infections. Although "sulfur granules" (pigmented microcolonies of bacteria present in wound exudates) are observed with *Actinomyces* species, they are uncommon with nocardiae, being seen in cutaneous disease only.

Although toxins and hemolysins have been described for nocardiae, the role of these factors play in disease has not been defined. It would appear that the primary factor associated with virulence is the ability of pathogenic strains to **avoid phagocytic killing.** When phagocytes contact microbes, an oxidative burst occurs with release of toxic oxygen metabolites (i.e., hydrogen peroxide, superoxide). Pathogenic strains of nocardiae are protected by their secretion of catalase and superoxide dismutase. Surface-associated superoxide dismutase also protects the bacteria. Nocardiae are also able to survive and replicate in macrophages. This is accomplished by (1) preventing fusion of the phagosome-lysosome (mediated by **cord factor**), (2) preventing acidification of the phagosome (by an undefined mechanism), and (3) avoiding acid phosphatase–mediated killing by metabolic utilization of the enzyme as a carbon source.

EPIDEMIOLOGY

Nocardia infections are **exogenous** (i.e., caused by organisms not normally part of the normal human flora but, rather, transient inhabitants). The ubiquitous presence of the organism in soil rich with organic matter and the abundance of immunocompromised patients in hospitals have led to dramatic increases in disease caused by this organism. The increase is particularly noticeable in high-risk populations, such as patients who are infected with human immunodeficiency virus (HIV) or who have received bone marrow or solid organ transplants.

CLINICAL DISEASES (BOX 28–5)

Bronchopulmonary disease caused by *Nocardia* species cannot be distinguished from infections caused by other pyogenic organisms, although *Nocardia* infections tend to develop more slowly. Signs such as cough, dyspnea, and fever are usually present but are not diagnostic. Cavitation and spread into the pleura are common. Although the clinical picture is not specific for *Nocardia*, these organisms should be considered when immunocompromised patients experience pneumonia with cavitation, particularly if there is evidence of dissemination to the CNS or subcutaneous tissues.

Cutaneous infections may be primary infections (e.g., mycetoma, lymphocutaneous infections, cellulitis, subcutaneous abscesses) or may result from the spread of organisms from a primary pulmonary infection. **Actinomycotic mycetoma** is a painless, chronic infection characterized by localized subcutaneous swelling, suppuration, and the formation of multiple sinus tracts. The underlying connective tissues, muscle, and bone can be involved, and draining sinus tracts usually open on the skin surface. A variety of organisms can cause mycetoma, although *N. brasiliensis* is the most common cause of cases in North America, Central America, and South America. **Lymphocutaneous infections** can manifest as cutaneous nodules and ulcerations along the lymphatics and regional lymph node involvement. These infections resemble cutaneous infections caused by species of mycobacteria and by the fungus *Sporothrix schenckii. Nocardia* can also cause chronic ulcerative lesions, subcutaneous abscesses, and cellulitis; Figure 28–4).

As many as a third of all patients with *Nocardia* infections have CNS involvement, most commonly involving the formation of single or multiple brain abscesses. The disease can present initially as chronic meningitis.

BOX 28–5. Nocardiosis: Clinical Summaries

Bronchopulmonary disease: Indolent pulmonary disease with necrosis and abscess formation; dissemination to central nervous system or skin is common

Mycetoma: Chronic destructive, progressive disease, generally of extremities, characterized by suppurative granulomas, progressive fibrosis and necrosis, and sinus tract formation

Lymphocutaneous disease: Primary infection or secondary spread to cutaneous site characterized by chronic granuloma formation and erythematous subcutaneous nodules, with eventual ulcer formation

Cellulitis and subcutaneous abscesses: Granulomatous ulcer formation with surrounding erythema but minimal or no involvement of the draining lymph nodes

Brain abscess: Chronic infection with fever, headache, and focal deficits related to the location of the slowly developing abscess(es)

LABORATORY DIAGNOSIS

Multiple sputum specimens should be collected from patients with pulmonary disease. Because nordicae are usually distributed throughout the tissue and abscess material, it is relatively easy to detect them by microscopy and to recover them in culture of specimens from patients with cutaneous or CNS disease. The delicate hyphae of *Nocardia* in tissues cause them to resemble *Actinomyces* organisms; however, nocardiae stain poorly with Gram stain and are typically partially acid-fast (see Figures 28-1 and 28-2).

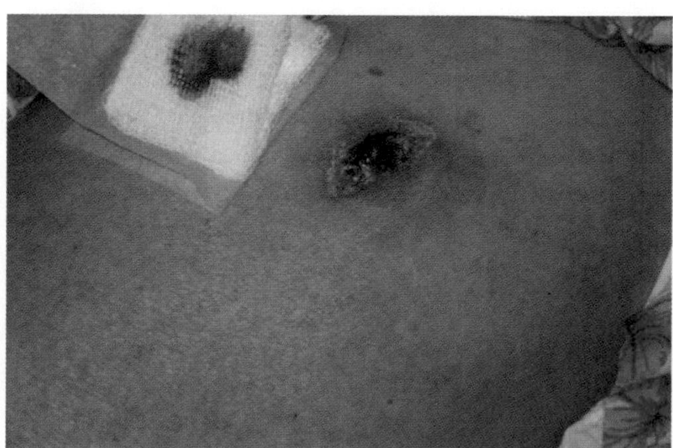

FIGURE 28–4. Cutaneous lesion caused by *Nocardia*.

The organisms grow on most laboratory media incubated in an atmosphere of 5% to 10% carbon dioxide, but the presence of these slow-growing organisms may be obscured by that of more rapidly growing commensal bacteria. If a specimen sent for analysis for *Nocardia* is potentially contaminated with other bacteria (e.g., oral bacteria in sputum), selective media should be inoculated. Success has been achieved with the medium used for the isolation of *Legionella* species (buffered charcoal yeast extract [BCYE] agar; see Figure 28–3). Indeed, this medium can be used to recover both organisms from pulmonary specimens. *Nocardia* occasionally grows on media used for the isolation of mycobacteria and fungi; however, this method is less reliable than the use of special bacterial media. It is important to notify the laboratory that nocardiosis is suspected, because most laboratories do not routinely use special culture media or incubate clinical specimens for more than 1 to 3 days. It takes more time (i.e., as long as a week) for *Nocardia* species to be detected in culture.

The preliminary identification of *Nocardia* is uncomplicated. Members of the genus can be classified initially on the basis of the presence of filamentous, partially acid-fast bacilli and aerial hyphae on the colony surface. Definitive identification at the species level is more difficult. It is recognized that most species cannot be identified accurately by phenotypic (e.g., biochemical) tests, although many laboratories continue to use these tests. The accurate identification of most species requires molecular analysis of ribosomal ribonucleic acid (RNA) genes and "housekeeping" genes (e.g., heat-shock protein gene). Currently, these tests are performed primarily in reference or research laboratories.

TREATMENT, PREVENTION, AND CONTROL

Nocardia infections are treated with the combination of antibiotics and appropriate surgical intervention. Sulfonamides are the antibiotics of choice for treating nocardiosis. Amikacin, imipenem, and broad-spectrum cephalosporins also have good in vitro activity, but their in vivo effectiveness is unproved. Because nocardiae can disseminate and produce significant disease, therapy should be extended for 6 weeks or more. Whereas the clinical response is favorable in patients with localized infections, the prognosis is poor for immunocompromised patients with disseminated disease.

Because nocardiae are ubiquitous, it is impossible to avoid exposure to them. However, bronchopulmonary disease caused by nocardiae is uncommon in immunocompetent persons, and primary cutaneous infections can be prevented with proper wound care. The complications associated with disseminated disease can be minimized if nocardiosis is considered in the differential diagnosis for immunocompromised patients with cavitary pulmonary disease and promptly treated.

Rhodococcus

The genus *Rhodococcus* consists of gram-positive, weakly acid-fast bacteria that initially appear rod-like and then revert to coccoid forms (Figure 28–5). Rudimentary branching may be present, but the delicate, branching filamentous forms commonly seen with nocardiae are not observed with rhodococci. Of the species currently recognized, *Rhodococcus equi* is the most important human pathogen. Originally, *R. equi* (formerly *Corynebacterium equi*) was considered a veterinary pathogen, particularly in herbivores, that occasionally caused occupational disease in farmers and veterinarians. However, this organism has become an increasingly more common pathogen of immunocompromised patients (e.g., patients infected with HIV, transplant recipients). Interestingly, most infected patients do not have a history of contact with grazing animals or of exposure to soil contaminated with herbivore manure. The rise in the incidence of human infection is most likely related to the increase in the number of patients with immunosuppressive diseases, particularly AIDS, and to the enhanced awareness of the organism. It is likely that many isolates were ignored previously or were misidentified as insignificant coryneform bacteria.

Like *Nocardia*, *R. equi* is a facultative, intracellular organism that survives in macrophages and causes granulomatous inflammation, which leads to abscess formation. Although numerous putative virulence factors have been identified, the precise pathophysiology of the infection is incompletely understood. A virulence-associated protein, *vap*A, has been implicated in disease in horses, but its role in human disease is less established. Individuals with depressed production of interferon-γ appear to be unable to clear bacteria from lung infections.

Immunocompromised patients most typically present with invasive pulmonary disease (e.g., pulmonary nodules, consolidation, lung abscesses), and evidence of dissemination in the blood to distal sites (lymph nodes, meninges, pericardium, and skin) is commonly observed. Rhodococci usually cause opportunistic infections in immunocompetent patients (e.g., post-traumatic cutaneous infections, peritonitis in patients undergoing long-term dialysis, traumatic endophthalmitis).

Rhodococci grow readily on nonselective media incubated aerobically, although the characteristic salmon-pink pigment may not be obvious for at least 4 days. Colonies are typically mucoid, although dry forms may also be seen. The organisms can be identified initially by their slow growth, macroscopic and microscopic morphology, and ability to weakly retain the acid-fast stain (particularly when grown on media for mycobacteria). Definitive identification at the species level is problematic because the organisms are relatively inert.

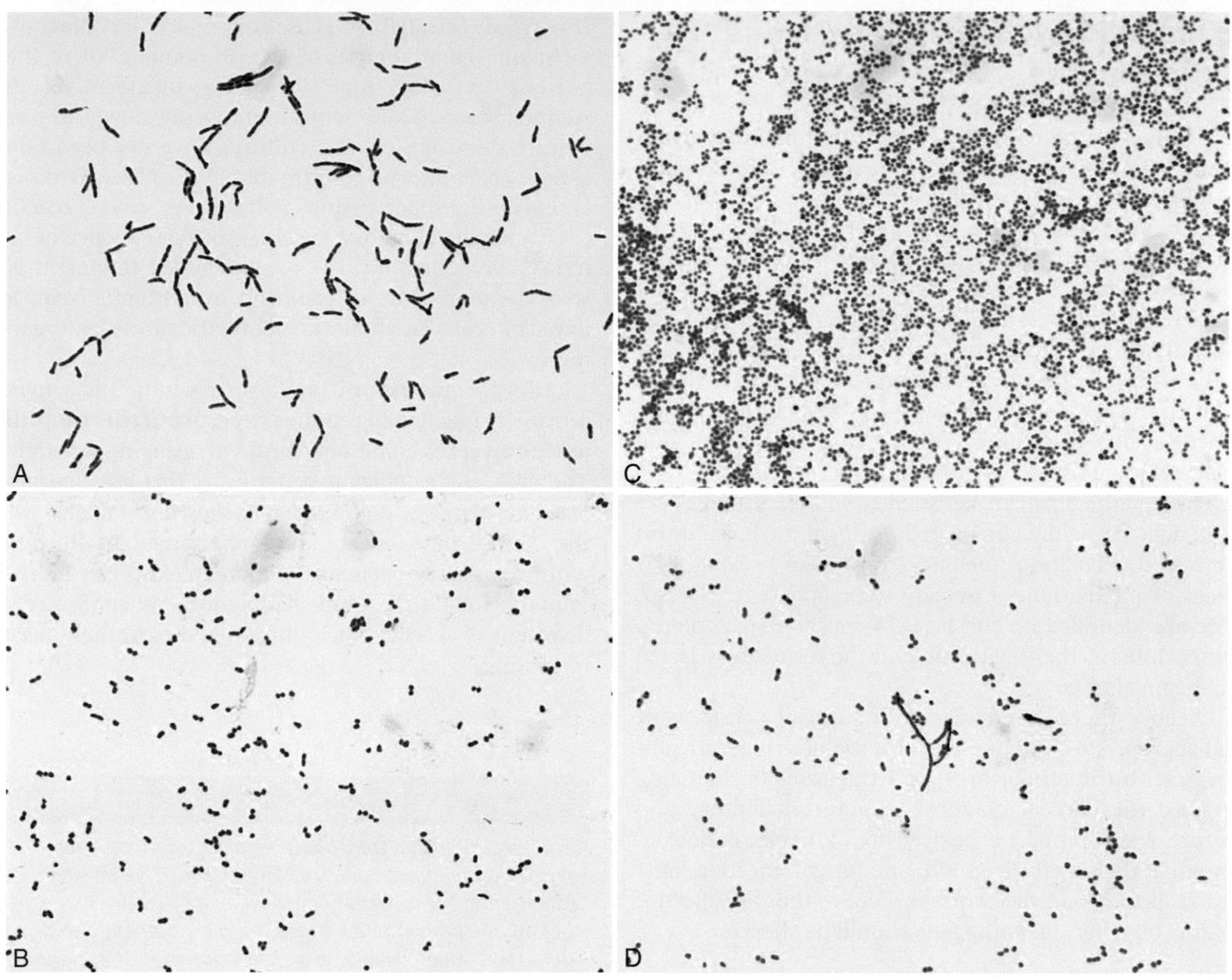

FIGURE 28–5. *Rhodococcus.* **A,** Gram stain after growth in nutrient broth for 4 hours; **B,** Gram stain after growth in nutrient broth for 18 hours; **C,** acid-fast stain of organisms grown on mycobacterial Middlebrook agar for 2 days (note the paucity of red "acid-fast" cells); **D,** Gram stain of branching, filamentous forms.

Rhodococcus infections have proved difficult to treat. Although in vitro tests and tests in animal models have identified specific combinations of drugs as effective, only limited success has been realized in the treatment of human infections, particularly in immunocompromised patients with low CD4 cell counts (50% mortality) compared with immunocompetent patients (20% mortality). The current recommendation for treating localized infections in immunocompetent patients is to use oral antibiotics (e.g., erythromycin, rifampin, and/or ciprofloxacin). Disseminated infections and infections in immunocompromised patients should be managed with combinations of intravenous antibiotics (e.g., vancomycin, imipenem, aminoglycosides, ciprofloxacin, rifampin, and/or erythromycin). Penicillins and cephalosporins should not be used because resistance to these agents is common in rhodococci, and the effectiveness of any antibiotic must be confirmed by in vitro testing.

Gordonia and *Tsukamurella*

Gordonia (formerly *Gordona*) and *Tsukamurella* were previously classified with *Rhodococcus* because they are morphologically similar, contain mycolic acids, and are partially acid-fast. The organisms are present in soil and are rare opportunistic pathogens in humans. *Gordonia* has been associated with pulmonary and cutaneous infections, as well as nosocomial infections such as those resulting from contaminated intravascular catheters. *Tsukamurella* has been associated with catheter infections. The significance of isolating either organism in clinical specimens must be evaluated carefully.

Actinomadura, Nocardiopsis, and *Streptomyces*

Mycetoma can be caused by fungi **("eumycotic mycetoma")** and by bacteria **("actinomycotic mycetoma")** in the genera *Actinomadura, Nocardiopsis, Streptomyces,* and *Nocardia.* The precise etiology of this disease can be determined only by isolation of the pathogen in culture, because (1) many of these bacteria resemble fungi when seen in tissue, and (2) the diseases they cause are clinically indistinguishable. Infection usually results from the traumatic introduction of the bacteria or fungi into tissue, most commonly in an extremity. Chronic cutaneous and subcutaneous infections develop with swelling, tissue destruction, and abscess and sinus tract formation.

These pathogens can be isolated on Sabouraud's dextrose agar (typically considered a fungal medium) or on nonselective bacterial media. It may take as long as 3 weeks of incubation for growth to be apparent. The isolates are identified on the basis of morphologic criteria, composition of their cell wall, and the results of selected biochemical tests.

Effective therapy includes both surgical débridement and appropriate combinations of antibiotics (e.g., streptomycin with trimethoprim-sulfamethoxazole or dapsone). Because the clinical diagnosis is noncontributory and culture results may be delayed for 3 weeks or longer, empirical therapy for bacterial and fungal infection must be initiated. Broad-spectrum antibiotics that are effective against all potential pathogens should be chosen.

Other Actinomycetes

Dermatophilus, an actinomycete found in the soil, causes infections in humans who are exposed to infected animals or contaminated animal products (e.g., slaughterhouse workers, butchers, hunters, dairy farmers, veterinarians). The disease is an **exudative dermatitis** with encrustations that typically involve the hands or feet. This organism is susceptible to many antibiotics, and most infections are treated with the combination of penicillin and an aminoglycoside.

Tropheryma whipplii is the bacterium responsible for **Whipple's disease,** a disorder characterized by arthralgia, diarrhea, abdominal pain, weight loss, lymphadenopathy, fever, and increased skin pigmentation. Historically, the disease was diagnosed on the basis of the clinical presentation and the finding of periodic acid–Schiff positive inclusions in foamy macrophages that infiltrated the lamina propria of the small intestine. Although in vitro cultures of these specimens were uniformly negative, the bacterial etiology of this infection was confirmed through the use of molecular diagnostic techniques, and analysis of the ribosomal DNA of these bacteria revealed that they are members of the Actinomycetes. The organism can grow slowly in tissue culture cells, but cell free cultures have not been established. Laboratory confirmation of clinical disease is currently made using polymerase chain reaction (PCR)-amplification of a species-specific sequence of bacterial DNA. Currently, the recommended treatment is 2 weeks with parenteral penicillin and streptomycin, followed by oral trimethoprim-sulfamethoxazole for a year or more.

Allergic pneumonitis ("farmer's lung") is a hypersensitivity reaction to repeated exposure to **thermophilic actinomycetes** commonly found in decaying vegetation. The clinically significant genera are *Thermoactinomyces, Saccharopolyspora,* and *Saccharomonospora.* Patients with the disease have granulomatous changes in the lung, with pulmonary edema, eosinophilia, and elevations of immunoglobulin E. Clinical diagnosis is confirmed by detection of specific precipitin antibodies to these agents in serum.

CASE STUDY AND QUESTIONS

A 47-year-old renal transplant recipient who had been receiving prednisone and azathioprine for 2 years was admitted to the university medical center. Two weeks before, the patient had noticed the development of a dry, persistent cough. Five days before admission the cough became productive, and pleuritic chest pain developed. On the day of admission the patient was in mild respiratory arrest, and chest radiographs revealed a patchy right upper lobe infiltrate. Sputum specimens were initially sent for bacterial culture; results were reported as negative for organisms after 2 days of incubation. Antibiotic therapy with cephalothin was ineffective, so additional specimens were collected for the culture of bacteria, mycobacteria, Legionella *species, and fungi. After 4 days of incubation,* Nocardia *was isolated on the media inoculated for mycobacteria,* Legionella *species, and fungi.*

1. Why did the organism fail to grow initially? What can be done to correct this problem?
2. If this organism disseminates, what two target tissues are most likely to be involved?
3. What is the most common presentation of disease caused by *N. brasiliensis?*
4. What disease is caused by *Rhodococcus* in immunocompromised patients?
5. What microscopic property does *Rhodococcus* share with *Nocardia?* Which two other genera discussed in this chapter have the same property?
6. Which bacteria cause mycetoma? Which one is the most common cause in the United States?

Bibliography

Baba T, Nishiuchi Y, Yano I: Composition of mycolic acid molecular species as a criterion in nocardial classification, *Int J Syst Bacteriol* 47:795-801, 1997.

Beaman B, Beaman L: *Nocardia* species: Host-parasite relationships, *Clin Microbiol Rev* 7:213-264, 1994.

Chun J, Goodfellow M: A phylogenetic analysis of the genus *Nocardia* with 16S rRNA gene sequences, *Int J Syst Bacteriol* 45:240-245, 1995.

Conville PS et al: Identification of *Nocardia* species by restriction endonuclease analysis of an amplified portion of the 16S rRNA gene, *J Clin Microbiol* 38:158-164, 2000.

Conville P, Witebsky F: *Nocardia* and other aerobic Actinomycetes. In *Topley and Wilson's microbiology and microbial infections,* ed 10, London, 2005.

Giguere S et al: Role of the 85-kilobase plasmid and plasmid-encoded virulence-associated protein A in intracellular survival and virulence of *Rhodococcus equi, Infect Immun* 67:3548-3557, 1999.

Johnson D, Burke C: *Rhodococcus equi* pneumonia, *Semin Respir Infect* 12:57-60, 1997.

La Scola B et al: Description of *Tropheryma whipplei* gen. nov., sp. nov., the Whipple's disease bacillus, *Int J System Evol Microbiol* 51:1471-1479, 2001.

Lerner P: Nocardiosis, *Clin Infect Dis* 22:891-905, 1996.

Marth T, Raoult D: Whipple's disease, *Lancet* 361:239-246, 2003.

McNeil M, Brown J: The medically important aerobic actinomycetes: Epidemiology and microbiology, *Clin Microbiol Rev* 7:357-417, 1994.

Midwald M, Relman D: Whipple's disease and *Tropheryma whippelii:* Secrets slowly revealed, *Clin Infect Dis* 32:457-463, 2001.

Raoult D et al: Cultivation of the bacillus of Whipple's disease, *N Engl J Med* 342:620-625, 2000.

Smego RA, Gallis HA: The clinical spectrum of *Nocardia brasiliensis* infection in the United States, *Rev Infect Dis* 6:164-180, 1984.

Steingrube V et al: Rapid identification of clinically significant species and taxa of aerobic actinomycetes, including *Actinomadura, Gordona, Nocardia, Rhodococcus, Streptomyces,* and *Tsukamurella* isolates, by DNA amplification and restriction endonuclease analysis, *J Clin Microbiol* 35:817-822, 1997.

Torres O et al: Infection caused by *Nocardia farcinica:* Case report and review, *Eur J Clin Microbiol Infect Dis* 19:205-212, 2000.

Weinstock D, Brown A: *Rhodococcus equi:* An emerging pathogen, *Clin Infect Dis* 34:1379-1385, 2002.

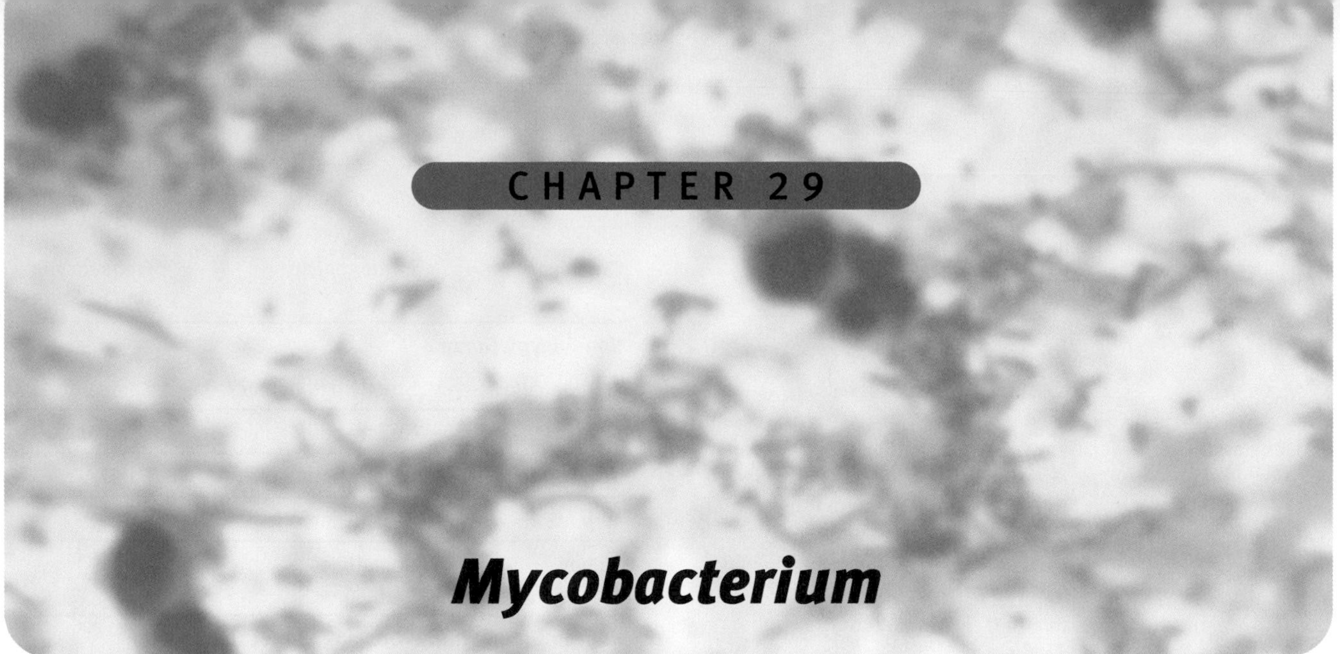

CHAPTER 29

Mycobacterium

The genus *Mycobacterium* (Box 29–1) consists of nonmotile, non–spore-forming, aerobic rods that are 0.2 to 0.6 × 1 to 10 μm in size. The rods occasionally form branched filaments, but these can be readily disrupted. The cell wall is rich in lipids, making the surface hydrophobic and the mycobacteria resistant to many disinfectants and common laboratory stains. Once stained, the rods also cannot be decolorized with acid solutions; hence the name **acid-fast** bacteria. Because the mycobacterial cell wall is complex, and this group of organisms is fastidious, most mycobacteria grow slowly, dividing every 12 to 24 hours. Isolation of the slow-growing organisms (e.g., *Mycobacterium tuberculosis, Mycobacterium avium-intracellulare* [*Mycobacterium avium* complex], *Mycobacterium kansasii*) can require 3 to 8 weeks of incubation, whereas the more "rapidly growing" mycobacteria (e.g., *Mycobacterium fortuitum, Mycobacterium chelonae, Mycobacterium abscessus*) require incubation for 3 days or more. *Mycobacterium leprae,* the etiologic agent of leprosy, cannot be grown in cell-free cultures.

Mycobacteria are still a significant cause of morbidity and mortality, particularly in countries with limited medical resources. Currently, almost 100 species of mycobacteria have been identified, many of which are associated with human disease (Table 29–1). Despite the abundance of mycobacterial species, the following few species or groups cause most human infections: *M. tuberculosis, M. leprae, M. avium* complex, *M. kansasii, M. fortuitum, M. chelonae,* and *M. abscessus.*

Physiology and Structure of Mycobacteria

Bacteria are classified in the genus *Mycobacterium* on the basis of (1) their acid-fastness, (2) the presence of mycolic acids containing 60 to 90 carbons that are cleaved by pyrolysis to C22 to C26 fatty acid methyl esters, and (3) a high (61% to 71%) guanine plus cytosine (G + C) content in their deoxyribonucleic acid (DNA). Although other species of bacteria can be acid-fast (i.e., *Nocardia, Rhodococcus, Tsukamurella, Gordonia*), they stain less intensely (are partially acid-fast) and their mycolic acids chains are shorter.

Mycobacteria possess a complex, lipid-rich cell wall (Figure 29–1). This cell wall is responsible for many of the characteristic properties of the bacteria (e.g., acid-fastness, slow growth, resistance to detergents, resistance to common antibacterial antibiotics, antigenicity, clumping). The basic structure of the cell wall is typical of gram-positive bacteria: an inner plasma membrane overlaid with a thick peptidoglycan layer and no outer membrane. However, the mycobacterial cell wall structure is far more complex than that in other gram-positive bacteria. Anchored in the plasma membrane are proteins, phosphatidylinositol mannosides, and lipoarabinomannan (LAM). LAM is functionally related to the O-antigenic lipopolysaccharides present in other bacteria. The peptidoglycan layer forms the foundation upon which are attached arabinogalactans, a branched polysaccharide consisting of D-arabinose and D-galactose. The terminal D-arabinose residue is esterified to high molecular weight, hydrophobic mycolic acids with attached glycolipid surface molecules. Additional lipids, glycolipids, and peptidoglycolipids are also present. The lipid components comprise 60% of the cell wall weight. Transport proteins and porins are interspersed throughout the cell wall layers, and these constitute 15% of the cell wall weight. The proteins are biologically important antigens, stimulating the patient's cellular immune response to infection. Extracted and partially purified preparations of these protein derivatives **(purified protein derivatives, or PPDs)** are used as skin test reagents to measure exposure to *M. tuberculosis.*

BOX 29–1. Important Mycobacteria

Organism	Historical Derivation
Mycobacterium	*myces,* a fungus; *bakterion,* a small rod (funguslike rod)
M. abscessus	*abscessus,* of abscesses (causes abscess formation)
M. avium	*avis,* of birds (causes tuberculosis-like illness in birds)
M. chelonae	*chelone,* a tortoise
M. fortuitum	*fortuitum,* casual, accidental (refers to fact this is an opportunistic pathogen)
M. haemophilum	*haema,* blood; *philos,* loving (blood loving; refers to requirement for blood or hemin for in vitro growth)
M. intracellulare	*intra,* within, *cella,* small room (within cells; refers to the intracellular location of mycobacteria)
M. kansasii	*kansasii,* of Kansas (where the organism was originally isolated)
M. leprae	*lepra,* of leprosy (the cause of leprosy)
M. marinum	*marinum,* of the sea (bacterium associated with contaminated freshwater and saltwaters)
M. tuberculosis	*tuberculum,* a small swelling or tubercle; *osis,* characterized by (characterized by tubercles; refers to the formation of tubercles in the lungs of infected patients)

Similar preparations from other mycobacteria have been used as species-specific skin test reagents.

Growth properties and colonial morphology are used for the preliminary classification of mycobacteria. As noted earlier, *M. tuberculosis* and closely related species (referred to as *M. tuberculosis* complex) are slow-growing bacteria. The colonies of these mycobacteria are either nonpigmented or buff colored (Figure 29–2). Runyon classified the other mycobacteria ("nontuberculous mycobacteria," or NTM) into four groups on the basis of their rate of growth and their ability to produce pigments in the presence or absence of light. The pigmented mycobacteria produce intensely **yellow carotenoids.** Photochromogenic organisms (Runyon group I) produce these pigments only after exposure to light (Figure 29–3), whereas scotochromogenic organisms (Runyon group II) produce the pigments in the dark and the light. The slow-growing, nonpigmented NTM species are classified as Runyon group III, whereas the relatively rapidly growing mycobacteria are classified as Runyon group IV. Historically, the **Runyon classification** has been a useful differentiation scheme for organizing this diverse collection of clinically important species (see Table 29–1), particularly when detection and identification of mycobacteria in the clinical laboratory would take weeks to months. However, currently used methods for the rapid detection and identification of mycobacteria have made this scheme less important.

TABLE 29–1. Classification of Selected Mycobacteria Pathogenic for Humans

Organism	Pathogenicity	Frequency in United States
Non-Runyon Group		
M. tuberculosis	Strictly pathogenic	Common
M. leprae	Strictly pathogenic	Uncommon
M. africanum	Strictly pathogenic	Rare
M. bovis	Strictly pathogenic	Rare
M. bovis (*BCG strain*)	Sometimes pathogenic	Rare
Runyon Group I (Slow-Growing Photochromogens)		
M. kansasii	Usually pathogenic	Common
M. marinum	Usually pathogenic	Uncommon
M. simiae	Usually pathogenic	Uncommon
Runyon Group II (Slow-Growing Scotochromogens)		
M. szulgai	Usually pathogenic	Uncommon
M. scrofulaceum	Sometimes pathogenic	Uncommon
M. xenopi	Sometimes pathogenic	Uncommon
Runyon Group III (Slow-Growing Nonchromogens)		
M. avium complex	Usually pathogenic	Common
M. genavense	Usually pathogenic	Uncommon
M. haemophilum	Usually pathogenic	Uncommon
M. malmoense	Usually pathogenic	Uncommon
M. ulcerans	Usually pathogenic	Uncommon
Runyon Group IV (Rapid Growers)		
M. abscessus	Sometimes pathogenic	Common
M. chelonae	Sometimes pathogenic	Common
M. fortuitum	Sometimes pathogenic	Common
M. mucogenicum	Sometimes pathogenic	Uncommon

Nonetheless, a pigmented or a rapidly growing mycobacterium should never be mistaken for *M. tuberculosis.*

Mycobacterium Tuberculosis (Box 29–2)

PATHOGENESIS AND IMMUNITY

M. tuberculosis is an intracellular pathogen that is able to establish lifelong infection. The complexity of the

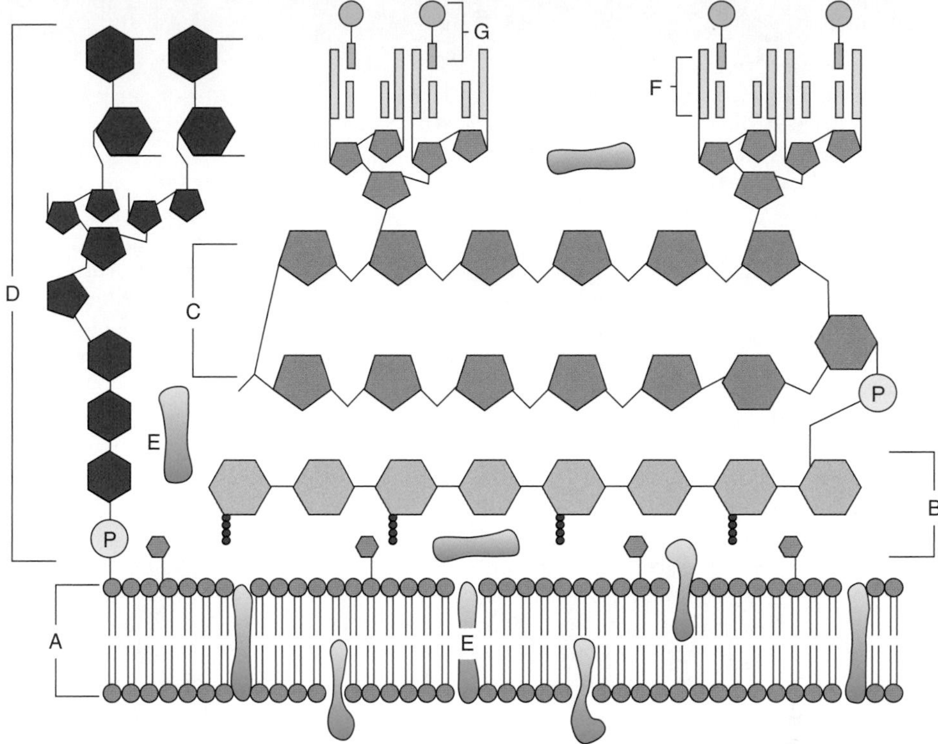

FIGURE 29–1. Mycobacterial cell wall structure. The components include the *(A)* plasma membrane, *(B)* peptidoglycans, *(C)* arabinogalactan, *(D)* mannose-capped lipoarabinomannan, *(E)* plasma-associated and cell wall–associated proteins, *(F)* mycolic acids, and *(G)* glycolipid surface molecules associated with the mycolic acids. (Redrawn from Karakousis et al: *Cell Microbiol* 6:105-116, 2004.)

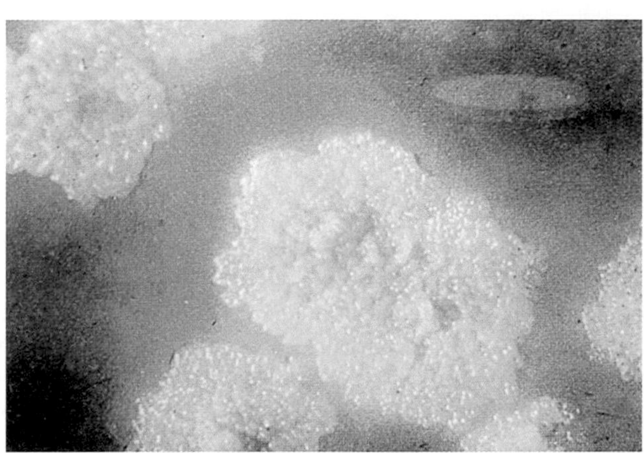

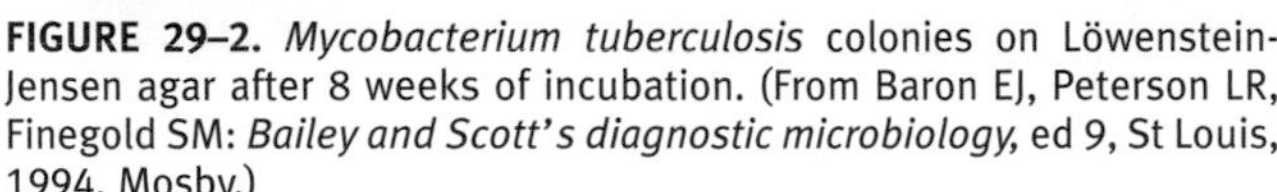

FIGURE 29–2. *Mycobacterium tuberculosis* colonies on Löwenstein-Jensen agar after 8 weeks of incubation. (From Baron EJ, Peterson LR, Finegold SM: *Bailey and Scott's diagnostic microbiology,* ed 9, St Louis, 1994, Mosby.)

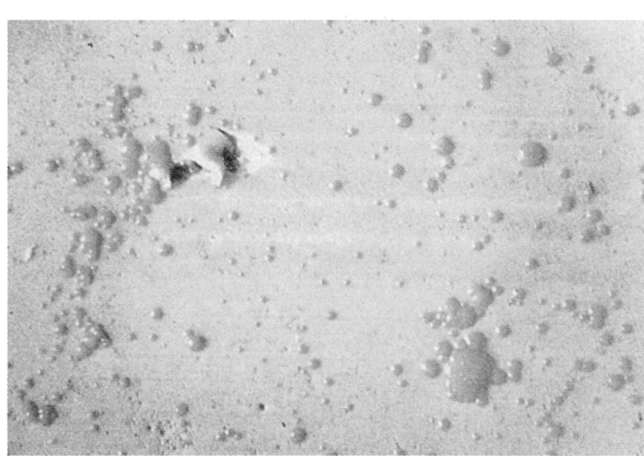

FIGURE 29–3. *Mycobacterium kansasii* colonies on Middlebrook agar 1 day after exposure to light.

intracellular existence of this bacterium is still not completely understood but is slowly being unraveled. At the time of exposure, *M. tuberculosis* enters the respiratory airways and minute infectious particles penetrate to the alveoli, where they are phagocytized by alveolar macrophages. In contrast with most phagocytized bacteria, *M. tuberculosis* prevents fusion of the phagosome with lysosomes (by blocking the specific bridging molecule, early endosomal autoantigen 1 [EEA1]). At the same time the phagosome is able to fuse with other intracellular vesicles, permitting access to nutrients and facilitating intravacuole replication. Phagocytized bacteria are also able to evade macrophage killing mediated by reactive nitrogen intermediates formed between nitric oxide and superoxide anions, by catalytically catabolizing the oxidants that are formed.

Although phagocytosis is initiated by alveolar macrophages, circulating macrophages and lymphocytes are attracted to the infectious focus by the bacteria, cellular debris, and host chemotactic factors (e.g., complement component C5a). The histologic characteristic of this focus is formation of **multinucleated giant cells** of fused macrophages, also called **Langhans cells.** Infected macrophages can also spread during the initial phase of

BOX 29–2. Summary of *Mycobacterium tuberculosis*

Physiology and Structure
Weakly gram-positive, strongly acid-fast, aerobic rods
Lipid-rich cell wall, making the organism resistant to disinfectants, detergents, common antibacterial antibiotics, and traditional stains

Virulence
Capable of intracellular growth in unactivated alveolar macrophages
Disease primarily from host response to infection

Epidemiology
Worldwide; a third of the world's population is infected with this organism
A total of 8.8 million new cases each year and 2 million deaths
Disease most common in Southeast Asia, sub-Saharan Africa, and Eastern Europe
Fewer than 15,000 new cases in United States in 2003
Populations at greatest risk for disease are immunocompromised patients (particularly those with HIV infection), drug or alcohol abusers, homeless persons, and individuals exposed to diseased patients
Humans are the only natural reservoir
Person-to-person spread by infectious aerosols

Diseases
Primary infection is pulmonary
Dissemination to any body site occurs most commonly in immunocompromised patients and untreated patients

Diagnosis
Tuberculin skin test and QuantiFERON-TB test sensitive marker for exposure to organism
Microscopy and culture are sensitive and specific
Direct detection by molecular probes is relatively insensitive
Identification most commonly made using species-specific molecular probes

Treatment, Prevention, and Control
Multiple-drug regimens and prolonged treatment are required to prevent development of drug-resistant strains
Isoniazid (INH), ethambutol, pyrazinamide, and rifampin for 2 months followed by 4 to 6 months of INH and rifampin or alternative combination drugs
Prophylaxis for exposure to tuberculosis can include INH for 9 months, rifampin for 4 months, or rifampin and pyrazinamide for 2 months; pyrazinamide and ethambutol or levofloxacin are used for 6 to 12 months after exposure to drug-resistant *M. tuberculosis*
Immunoprophylaxis with BCG in endemic countries
Control of disease through active surveillance, prophylactic and therapeutic intervention, and careful case monitoring

disease to the local lymph nodes, as well as into the bloodstream and other tissues (e.g., bone marrow, spleen, kidneys, central nervous system).

The histologic signs of mycobacterial infection are primarily the components of the host response to the infection rather than specific virulence factors elaborated by the mycobacteria. The intracellular replication of mycobacteria stimulates both helper (CD4+) T cells and cytotoxic (CD8+) T cells. Activation of CD4+ cells leads to antibody production, but this response is ineffective in controlling mycobacterial disease because the bacteria are protected in their intracellular location. T cells also release interferon-γ and other cytokines that activate macrophages. Activated macrophages can engulf and kill mycobacteria. The cytotoxic T cells can also lyse phagocytic cells with replicating mycobacteria, thus permitting phagocytosis and bacterial killing by activated phagocytic cells.

If a small antigenic burden is present at the time that the macrophages are stimulated, the bacteria are destroyed with minimal tissue damage. If many bacteria are present, however, the cellular immune response results in tissue necrosis. Multiple host factors are involved in this process, including cytokine toxicity, local activation of the complement cascade, ischemia, and exposure to macrophage-derived hydrolytic enzymes and reactive oxygen intermediates. No known mycobacterial toxin or enzyme has been associated with tissue destruction.

The effectiveness of bacterial elimination is in part related to the size of the focus of infection. Localized collections of activated macrophages **(granulomas)** prevent further spread of the bacteria. These macrophages can penetrate into small granulomas (less than 3 mm) and kill all the organisms contained in them. However, larger necrotic or caseous granulomas become encapsulated with fibrin that effectively protects the bacteria from macrophage killing. The bacteria can remain dormant in this stage or can be reactivated years later, when the patient's immunologic responsiveness wanes as the result of old age or immunosuppressive disease or therapy. This process is the reason that disease may not develop until late in life in patients exposed to *M. tuberculosis.*

EPIDEMIOLOGY

Although tuberculosis can be established in primates and laboratory animals, such as guinea pigs, humans are the only natural reservoir. The disease is spread by close person-to-person contact through the inhalation of infectious aerosols. Large particles are trapped on mucosal surfaces and removed by the ciliary action of the respiratory tree. However, small particles containing one to three tubercle bacilli can reach the alveolar spaces and establish infection.

In 2002, the World Health Organization (WHO) estimated that 2 billion people, a third of the world's population, were infected with *M. tuberculosis.* There were 8.8 million new cases and 2 million deaths caused by *M. tuberculosis* that year. Regions with the highest incidence of disease were Southeast Asia, sub-Saharan Africa, and Eastern Europe. In the United States the incidence of tuberculosis has decreased steadily since 1992. In 2003, fewer than 15,000 cases were reported, with more than half the infections in foreign-born persons. Other populations at greater risk for *M. tuberculosis* disease are homeless persons, drug and alcohol abusers, prisoners, and people infected with the human immunodeficiency virus (HIV). Because it is difficult to eradicate disease in these patients, spread of the infection to other populations, including health care workers, poses a significant public health problem. This is particularly true for drug-resistant *M. tuberculosis,* because patients who receive inadequate treatment may remain infectious for a long time.

CLINICAL DISEASES

Although tuberculosis can involve any organ, most infections in immunocompetent patients are restricted to the lungs. The initial pulmonary focus is the middle or lower lung fields, where the tubercle bacilli can multiply freely. The patient's cellular immunity is activated, and mycobacterial replication ceases in most patients within 3 to 6 weeks after exposure to the organism. Approximately 5% of patients exposed to *M. tuberculosis* progress to having active disease within 2 years, and another 5% to 10% experience disease sometime later in life.

The likelihood that infection will progress to active disease is a function of both the infectious dose and the patient's immune competence. For example, active disease develops within 1 year of exposure in approximately 10% of patients who are infected with HIV and have a low CD4 T-cell count, compared with a 10% risk of disease during the lifetime of patients without HIV infection. In patients with HIV infection, disease usually appears before the onset of other opportunistic infections, is twice as likely to spread to extrapulmonary sites, and can progress rapidly to death.

The clinical signs and symptoms of tuberculosis reflect the site of infection, with primary disease usually restricted to the lower respiratory tract. The disease is insidious at onset. Patients typically have nonspecific complaints of malaise, weight loss, cough, and night sweats. Sputum may be scant or bloody and purulent. Sputum production with hemoptysis is associated with tissue destruction (e.g., cavitary disease). The clinical diagnosis is supported by (1) radiographic evidence of pulmonary disease (Figure 29–4), (2) positive skin test reactivity, and (3) the laboratory detection of mycobacteria, either with microscopy or in cultures. One or both upper lobes of the lungs are usually involved in patients with active disease that includes pneumonitis or abscess formation and cavitation.

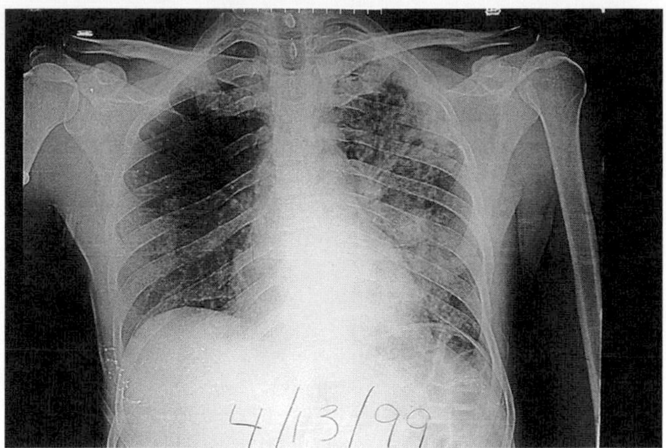

FIGURE 29–4. Pulmonary tuberculosis.

As noted earlier, extrapulmonary tuberculosis can occur as the result of the hematogenous spread of the bacilli during the initial phase of multiplication. There may be no evidence of pulmonary disease in patients with disseminated (military) tuberculosis.

Mycobacterium Leprae (Box 29–3)

PATHOGENESIS AND IMMUNITY

Leprosy (also called **Hansen's disease**) is caused by *M. leprae.* Like the manifestations of infection with *M. tuberculosis,* the clinical manifestations of leprosy depend on the patient's immune reaction to the bacteria. The clinical presentation of leprosy ranges from the tuberculoid form to the lepromatous form. Patients with **tuberculoid leprosy** (also called paucibacillary Hansen's disease) have a strong cellular immune reaction but a weak humoral antibody response. Infected tissues typically have many lymphocytes and granulomas but relatively few bacteria (Figure 29–5; Table 29–2). As in *M. tuberculosis* infections in immunocompetent patients, the bacteria produce cytokines (e.g., interferon-γ, interleukin-2) that mediate macrophage activation, phagocytosis, and bacillary clearance.

Patients with **lepromatous leprosy** (multibacillary Hansen's disease), however, have a strong antibody response but a specific defect in the cellular response to *M. leprae* antigens. Thus an abundance of bacteria are typically observed in dermal macrophages and the Schwann

BOX 29–3. Summary of *Mycobacterium leprae*

Physiology and Structure

Weakly gram-positive, strongly acid-fast rods
Lipid-rich cell wall
Unable to be cultured on artificial media
Diagnosis made with specific skin test (tuberculoid form of disease) or acid-fast stain (lepromatous form)

Virulence

Capable of intracellular growth
Disease primarily from host response to infection

Epidemiology

More than 620,000 new cases were reported in 2002, with most cases in India, Nepal, and Brazil
At the same time, 96 cases were reported in United States
Lepromatous form of disease, but not the tuberculoid form, is highly infectious
Person-to-person spread by direct contact or inhalation of infectious aerosols
People in close contact with patients who have lepromatous disease are at greatest risk

Diseases

Tuberculoid form of leprosy
Lepromatous form of leprosy

Diagnosis

Microscopy is sensitive for the lepromatous form but not the tuberculoid form
Skin testing is required to confirm tuberculoid leprosy
Culture is not useful

Treatment, Prevention, and Control

Tuberculoid form is treated with rifampicin and dapsone for 6 months; clofazimine is added to this regimen for treatment of the lepromatous form, and therapy is extended to a minimum of 12 months
Disease is controlled through the prompt recognition and treatment of infected people

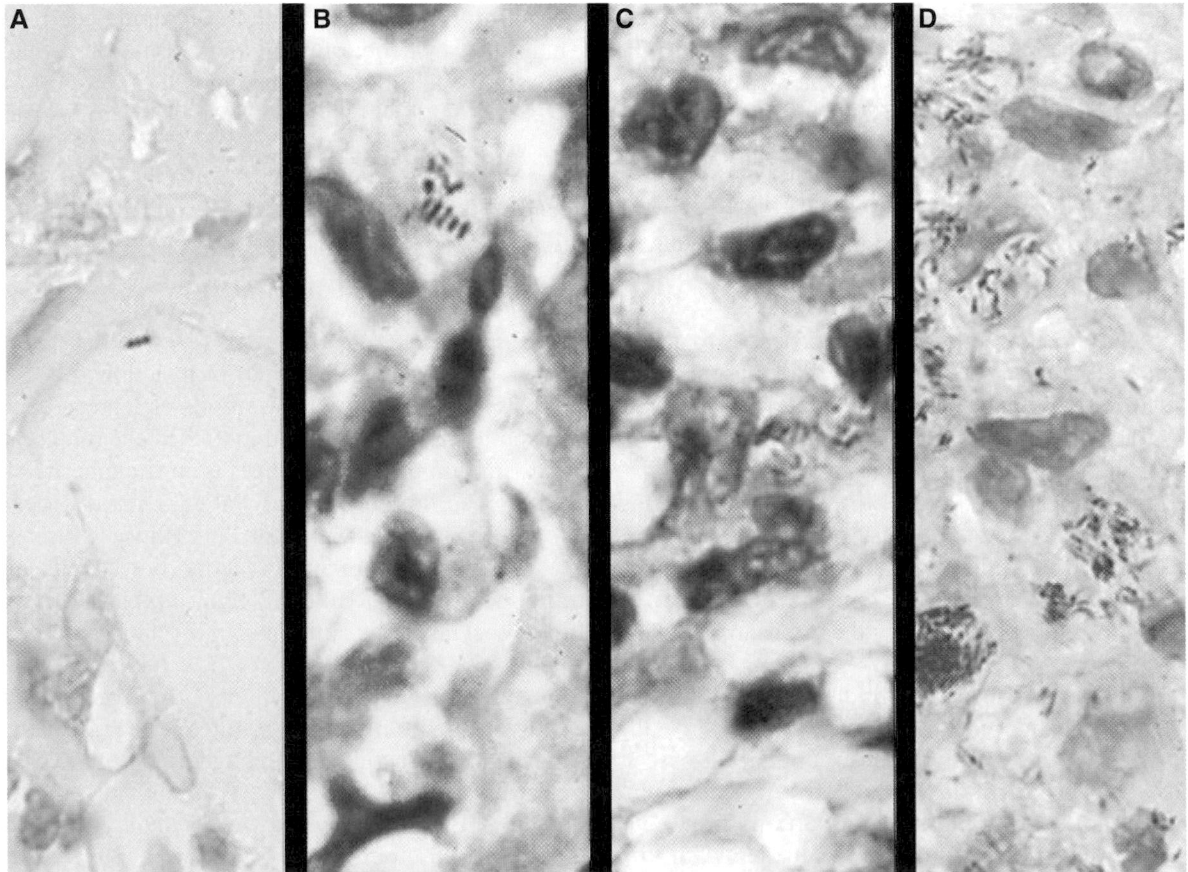

FIGURE 29–5. Acid-fast stains of skin biopsies from patients with **(A)** tuberculoid leprosy, **(B)** borderline tuberculoid leprosy, **(C)** borderline lepromatous leprosy, and **(D)** lepromatous leprosy. Note that there is a progressive increase in bacteria going from the tuberculoid form to the lepromatous form of the disease.

TABLE 29–2. Clinical and Immunologic Manifestations of Leprosy

Features	Tuberculoid Leprosy	Lepromatous Leprosy
Skin lesions	Few erythematous or hypopigmented plaques with flat centers and raised, demarcated borders; peripheral nerve damage with complete sensory loss; visible enlargement of nerves	Many erythematous macules, papules, or nodules; extensive tissue destruction (e.g., nasal cartilage, bones, ears); diffuse nerve involvement with patchy sensory loss; lack of nerve enlargement
Histopathology	Infiltration of lymphocytes around center of of epithelial cells; presence of Langhans cells; few or no acid-fast rods observed	Predominantly "foamy" macrophages with few lymphocytes; lack of Langhans cells; numerous acid-fast rods in skin lesions and internal organs
Infectivity	Low	High
Immune response		
Delayed hypersensitivity	Reactivity to lepromin	Nonreactivity to lepromin
Immunoglobulin levels	Normal	Hypergammaglobulinemia
Erythema nodosum	Absent	Usually present

cells of the peripheral nerves. As would be expected, this is the most infectious form of leprosy.

EPIDEMIOLOGY

Since 1985, the global prevalence of leprosy has fallen by almost 90%. In 1985 the disease was endemic in 122 countries; in 2003 it was endemic in 10 countries in Africa, Asia, and Latin America. The WHO reported that 620,672 new cases of leprosy were documented in 2002. Countries with the highest prevalence of disease were India, Nepal, and Brazil. In the United States, leprosy is uncommon, with 96 cases reported in 2002. Most cases occur in California, Texas, and Hawaii and primarily in immigrants from Mexico, Asia, Africa, and the Pacific Islands. Interestingly, leprosy is endemic in armadillos found in Texas and Louisiana, producing a disease similar to the highly infectious lepromatous form of leprosy in humans. Thus these armadillos represent a potential endemic focus in this country.

Leprosy is spread by person-to-person contact. Although the most important route of infection is unknown, it is believed that *M. leprae* is spread either through the inhalation of infectious aerosols or through skin contact with respiratory secretions and wound exudates. Numerous *M. leprae* are found in the nasal secretions of patients with lepromatous leprosy.

M. leprae cannot grow in cell-free cultures. Thus laboratory confirmation of leprosy requires histopathologic findings consistent with the clinical disease and either skin test reactivity to lepromin or the presence of acid-fast bacteria in the lesions.

CLINICAL DISEASES

Leprosy is a chronic infection that affects the skin and peripheral nerves. The spectrum of tissue involvement is influenced by the patient's immune status, as noted earlier (see Table 29–2). The tuberculoid form (Figure 29–6) is milder and is characterized by hypopigmented skin macules. The lepromatous form (Figure 29–7) is associated with disfiguring skin lesions, nodules, plaques, thickened dermis, and involvement of the nasal mucosa.

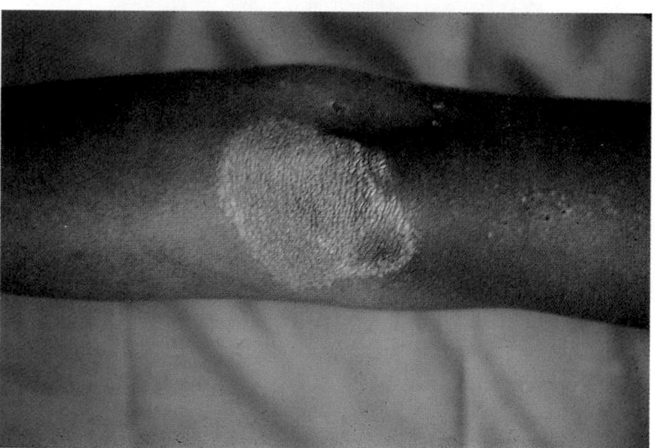

FIGURE 29–6. Tuberculoid leprosy. Early tuberculoid lesions are characterized by anesthetic macules with hypopigmentation. (From Cohen J, Powderly WB: *Infectious diseases,* ed 2, St Louis, 2004, Mosby.)

Mycobacterium Avium Complex (Box 29–4)

M. avium complex consists of two mycobacterial species: *M. avium* and *M. intracellulare.* When these organisms were originally described, they were difficult to differentiate by biochemical tests; thus they were consolidated into the *M. avium* complex (MAC, a term commonly used

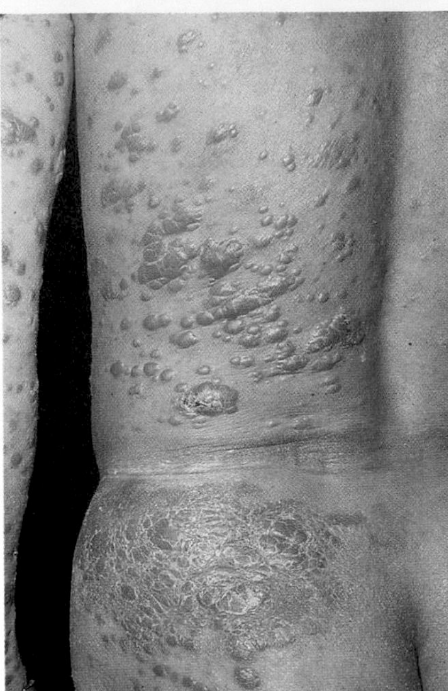

FIGURE 29–7. Lepromatous leprosy. Diffuse infiltration of the skin by multiple nodules of varying size, each with many bacteria. (From Cohen J, Powderly WB: *Infectious diseases*, ed 2, St Louis, 2004, Mosby.)

today). Both species produce disease in immunocompetent patients, whereas disease in HIV-infected patients is primarily caused by *M. avium*. These species are ubiquitous, present in water (fresh, brackish, ocean, drinking water), plants, and soil. Before the acquired immune deficiency syndrome (AIDS) epidemic, recovery of the organisms in clinical specimens typically represented transient colonization or, less commonly, chronic pulmonary disease. Pulmonary disease in immunocompetent patients presents in one of three forms. Most commonly, disease is seen in middle-age or older men with a history of smoking and underlying pulmonary disease. These patients typically have a slowly evolving cavitary disease that resembles tuberculosis on chest radiography. The second form of MAC infection is observed in elderly, female nonsmokers. These patients have lingular or middle lobe infiltrates with a patchy, nodular appearance on radiography and associated bronchiectasis (chronically dilated bronchi). This form of disease is indolent and has been associated with significant morbidity and mortality. It has been postulated that this disease is seen primarily in fastidious elderly women who chronically suppress their cough reflex, leading to nonspecific inflammatory changes in the lungs and predisposing them to superinfection with MAC. This specific disease has been called **Lady Windermere's syndrome** after the principle character in an Oscar Wilde play. The third form of MAC disease is formation of a solitary pulmonary nodule. *M. avium* complex is the most common mycobacterial species that causes solitary the pulmonary nodules.

BOX 29–4. Summary of *Mycobacterium avium* Complex

Physiology and Structure

Weakly gram-positive, strongly acid-fast aerobic rods
Lipid-rich cell wall

Virulence

Capable of intracellular growth
Disease primarily from host response to infection

Epidemiology

Worldwide distribution, but disease is seen most commonly in countries where tuberculosis is less common
Acquired primarily through ingestion of contaminated water or food; inhalation of infectious aerosols is believed to play a minor role in transmission
Patients at greatest risk for disease are those who are immunocompromised (particularly patients with AIDS) and those with long-standing pulmonary disease

Diseases

Asymptomatic colonization
Chronic localized pulmonary disease
Lingular or middle lobe infiltrates with a nodular appearance and bronchiectasis in elderly women
Solitary pulmonary nodule
Disseminated disease, particularly in patients with AIDS

Diagnosis

Microscopy and culture are sensitive and specific

Treatment, Prevention, and Control

Infections treated for prolonged period with clarithromycin or azithromycin combined with ethambutol and rifabutin
Prophylaxis in patients with AIDS who have low CD4+ cell count consists of clarithromycin or azithromycin or rifabutin
Antibiotic prophylaxis has dramatically reduced the incidence of disease in patients with AIDS

A new spectrum of disease has arisen in patients with AIDS, making infection with *M. avium* complex the most common mycobacterial disease in these patients in the United States. (*M. tuberculosis* infections are more common than *M. avium* complex in continents such as Africa and Asia, where tuberculosis is highly endemic.) In contrast to disease in other groups of patients, MAC infection in patients with AIDS is typically disseminated, with virtually no organ spared. The magnitude of these infections is remarkable; the tissues of some patients are literally filled with the mycobacteria (Figure 29–8), and there are hundreds to thousands of bacteria per milliliter of blood. Overwhelming disseminated infections with *M. avium* complex are particularly common in patients who are in the terminal stages of their immune disorder, when their CD4+ T lymphocyte counts fall below 10 cells/mm^3. Fortunately, with more effective antiretroviral therapy and the routine use of prophylactic antibiotics, MAC disease

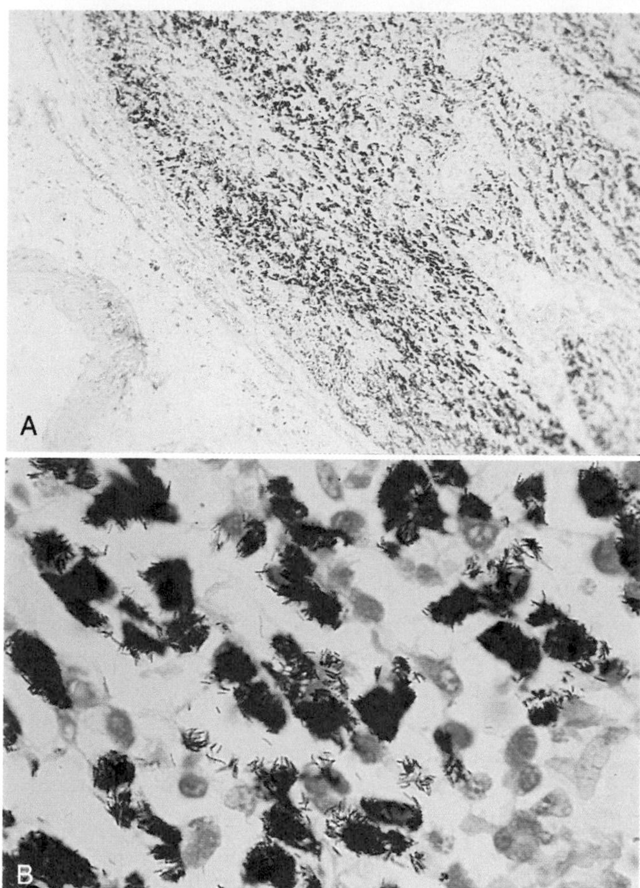

FIGURE 29–8. Tissue from a patient with AIDS who is infected with *Mycobacterium avium* complex photographed under low **(A)** and high **(B)** magnification.

infections are much less common in HIV-infected patients. Although some patients with AIDS develop *M. avium* complex disease after pulmonary exposure (e.g., infectious aerosols of contaminated water), most infections are believed to develop after ingestion of the bacteria. Person-to-person transmission has not been demonstrated. After exposure to the mycobacteria, replication is initiated in localized lymph nodes followed by systemic spread. The clinical manifestations of disease are not observed until the mass of replicating bacteria impairs normal organ function.

Other Slow-Growing Mycobacteria

Many other slow-growing mycobacteria can cause human disease, and new species continue to be reported as better diagnostic test methods are developed. The spectrum of diseases produced by these mycobacteria also continues to expand, in large part because diseases such as AIDS, malignancies, and organ transplantation with concomitant use of immunosuppressive drugs have created a population of patients who are highly susceptible to organisms with relatively low virulence potentials. Some mycobacteria produce disease identical to pulmonary tuberculosis (e.g., *Mycobacterium bovis, M. kansasii*), other species commonly cause infections localized to lymphatic tissue *(Mycobacterium scrofulaceum)*, and others that grow optimally at cool temperatures primarily produce cutaneous infections *(Mycobacterium ulcerans, Mycobacterium marinum, Mycobacterium haemophilum)*. However, disseminated disease can be observed in patients with AIDS who are infected with these same species, as well as with relatively uncommon mycobacteria (e.g., *Mycobacterium genavense, Mycobacterium simiae*).

Most of these mycobacteria have been isolated in water and soil and occasionally from infected animals (e.g., *M. bovis* causes bovine tuberculosis). Often the isolation of these mycobacteria in clinical specimens simply represents transient colonization with organisms that the patient ingested. With the exception of *M. bovis* and other mycobacteria closely related to *M. tuberculosis*, person-to-person spread of these mycobacteria does not occur.

Rapidly Growing Mycobacteria

As discussed previously, nontuberculous mycobacteria can be subdivided into slow-growing species and rapidly growing species (growth in less than 7 days). This distinction is important because the rapidly growing species have a relatively low virulence potential, stain irregularly with traditional mycobacterial stains, and are more susceptible to "conventional" antibacterial antibiotics than to drugs used to treat other mycobacterial infections. The most common species associated with disease are *M. fortuitum, M. chelonae*, and *M. abscessus*.

The rapidly growing mycobacteria rarely cause disseminated infections. Rather, they are most commonly associated with disease occurring after bacteria are introduced into the deep subcutaneous tissues by trauma or iatrogenic infections (e.g., infections associated with an intravenous catheter, contaminated wound dressing, prosthetic device such as a heart valve, peritoneal dialysis, or bronchoscopy). Unfortunately, the incidence of infections with these organisms is increasing as more invasive procedures are performed in hospitalized patients and advanced medical care lengthens the life expectancy of immunocompromised patients.

LABORATORY DIAGNOSIS OF MYCOBACTERIA

The various laboratory tests used in the diagnosis of infections caused by mycobacteria are listed in Box 29–5.

TABLE 29–3. Criteria Defining Positive Purified Protein Derivative Reactivity in Patients Exposed to *Mycobacterium tuberculosis*

Reactivity to PPD	Populations
≥5 mm of induration	HIV-positive patients; patients receiving immunosuppressive therapy; recent contacts of patients with tuberculosis; patients with abnormal chest radiographs consistent with prior tuberculosis
≥10 mm of induration	Recent immigrants from high-prevalence countries; injection drug users; residents and employees of high-risk settings (e.g., prisons; residential facilities for the elderly, patients with AIDS, and homeless persons; health care facilities; mycobacteriology laboratories); persons with conditions of high risk (e.g., silicosis, diabetes, chronic renal failure, hematologic disorders, significant weight loss, gastrectomy, jejunoileal bypass); children younger than 4 years or exposed to adults at high risk
≥15 mm of induration	Persons at low risk for tuberculosis

BOX 29–5. Laboratory Diagnosis of Mycobacterial Disease

Detection
Assessment of cell mediated immunity (e.g., skin test)

Microscopy
Carbolfuchsin acid-fast stain
Fluorochrome acid-fast stain
Direct nucleic acid probes

Culture
Solid agar-based or egg-based media
Broth-based media

Identification
Morphologic properties
Biochemical reactions
Analysis of cell wall lipids
Nucleic acid probes
Nucleic acid sequencing

ASSESSMENT OF CELL MEDIATED IMMUNITY

The traditional test to assess the patient's response to exposure to *M. tuberculosis* is the **tuberculin skin test.** Reactivity to an intradermal injection of mycobacterial antigens can differentiate between infected and noninfected people. The only evidence of infection with mycobacteria in most patients is a lifelong positive skin test reaction and radiographic evidence of calcification of the initial active foci in the lungs or other organs. Tests with protein antigens extracted from *M. tuberculosis* have been used most commonly and are the best-standardized ones, although skin tests with other species-specific mycobacterial antigens have also been developed.

The methods of antigen preparation and skin inoculation have been changed many times since the tests were first developed. The currently recommended tuberculin antigen is the purified protein derivative of the cell wall. In this test, a specific amount of the antigen (0.1 μg [5 tuberculin units] of PPD) is inoculated into the intradermal layer of the patient's skin. Skin test reactivity is measured 48 hours later. Patient population defines the positive reactivity (Table 29–3). A positive PPD reaction usually develops 3 to 4 weeks after exposure to *M. tuberculosis.* Exposure to other mycobacteria may cause a patient to show cross-reactivity with tuberculin, but the reaction is generally less than 10-mm of induration. Patients infected with *M. tuberculosis* may not show a response to the tuberculin skin test if they are anergic (nonreactive to antigens; particularly true of HIV-infected patients); thus control antigens should always be used with tuberculin tests.

Reactivity to lepromin, which is prepared from inactivated *M. leprae,* is valuable for confirming the clinical diagnosis of tuberculoid leprosy. Papular induration develops 3 to 4 weeks after the intradermal injection of the antigen. This test is not useful for identifying patients with lepromatous leprosy, because such patients are anergic to the antigen.

A recently developed and Food and Drug Administration (FDA)-approved alternative to the tuberculin skin test is a test based on the quantification of interferon-γ (IFN-γ) released from sensitized lymphocytes in the patient's blood after incubated overnight with PPD. Although this test (QuantiFERON-TB test) is considered less influenced by reader bias and error, the sensitivity and specificity is no better than the skin test.

MICROSCOPY

The microscopic detection of acid-fast bacteria in clinical specimens is the most rapid way to confirm mycobacterial disease. The clinical specimen is stained with carbolfuchsin (**Ziehl-Neelsen** or **Kinyoun** methods) or fluorescent auramine-rhodamine dyes (Truant **fluorochrome** method), decolorized with an acid-alcohol solution, and then counterstained. The specimens are examined with a light microscope or, if fluorescent dyes are used, a fluorescent microscope (Figure 29–9). The Truant fluorochrome method is the most sensitive method

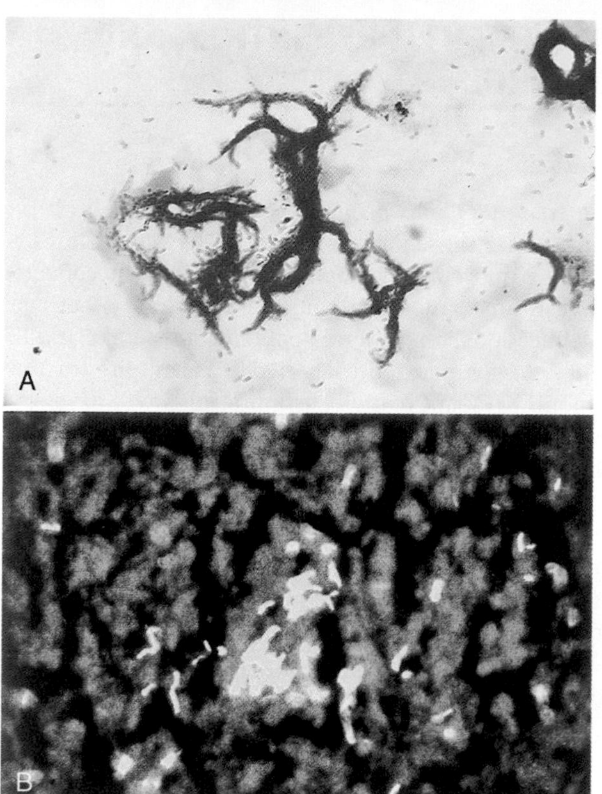

FIGURE 29–9. Acid-fast stains of *Mycobacterium tuberculosis.* **A,** Stained with carbolfuchsin using the Kinyoun method; **B,** Stained with the fluorescent dyes auramine and rhodamine using the Truant fluorochrome method.

because the specimen can be scanned rapidly under low magnification for fluorescent areas, and then the presence of acid-fast bacteria can be confirmed with higher magnification.

In approximately a third to half of all culture-positive specimens, acid-fast bacteria are detected by microscopy. The sensitivity of this test is high for (1) respiratory specimens (particularly from patients with radiographic evidence of cavitation) and (2) specimens for which many mycobacteria are isolated in culture. Thus a positive acid-fast stain reaction corresponds to higher infectivity. The specificity of the test is greater than 95% when it is performed carefully.

NUCLEIC ACID PROBES

Although microscopy provides useful information regarding the presence of mycobacterial disease, it cannot identify the particular mycobacterial species involved. For this reason, techniques have been developed to detect specific mycobacterial nucleic acid sequences present in clinical specimens. Because only a few bacteria may be present, commercial companies have developed a variety of amplification techniques (e.g., polymerase chain reaction, ligase chain reaction, transcription-mediated amplification, strand displacement amplification). The procedures currently used are specific for *M. tuberculosis* but are relatively insensitive. With further refinements, however, these procedures will most likely prove to be useful diagnostic tools. Additionally, alternative gene targets have been identified that can be used to detect and identify a wide range of mycobacterial species. It is likely that over the next decade, the sensitivity and discriminatory power of these methods will be improved sufficiently to allow them to replace microscopy.

CULTURE

Mycobacteria that cause pulmonary disease, particularly in patients with evidence of cavitation, are abundant in the respiratory secretions (e.g., 10^8 bacilli per ml or more). Recovery of the organisms is virtually assured in patients from whom early morning respiratory specimens are collected for 3 consecutive days. However, it is more difficult to isolate *M. tuberculosis* and NTM species from other sites in patients with disseminated disease (e.g., genitourinary tract, tissues, cerebrospinal fluid). In such cases, additional specimens must be collected for cultures and a large volume of fluid or tissue must be processed.

The in vitro growth of mycobacteria is complicated by the fact that most isolates grow slowly and can be obscured by the rapidly growing bacteria that normally colonize people. Thus specimens such as sputum are initially treated with a decontaminating reagent (e.g., 2% sodium hydroxide) to remove organisms that could confound results. Mycobacteria can tolerate brief alkali treatment, which kills the rapidly growing bacteria and permits the selective isolation of mycobacteria. Extended decontamination of the specimen kills mycobacteria, so the procedure is not performed when normally sterile specimens are being tested or when few mycobacteria are expected.

Formerly, when specimens were inoculated onto egg-based (e.g., Löwenstein-Jensen) and agar-based (e.g., Middlebrook) media, it generally took a long time for *M. tuberculosis, M. avium* complex, and other important slow-growing mycobacteria to be detected. However, this time has been shortened through the use of specially formulated broth cultures that support the rapid growth of most mycobacteria. Thus the average time to grow mycobacteria has been decreased from 3 to 4 weeks to 10 to 14 days.

Some mycobacterial species (e.g., *M. marinum, M. haemophilum, M. malmoense*) require a lower incubation temperature than what is used for most cultures (30°C versus 37°C). Additionally, *M. haemophilum* requires supplementation of media with hemin or ferric ammonium citrate for growth.

PRELIMINARY IDENTIFICATION

Growth properties and colonial morphology can be used for the preliminary identification of the most common species of mycobacteria. This step is important, because only mycobacteria in the *M. tuberculosis* complex are transmitted from person to person. Thus only patients infected with these organisms must be isolated and their close contacts given prophylactic antibiotics. The preliminary identification of an isolate can also be used to guide empirical antimicrobial therapy.

DEFINITIVE IDENTIFICATION

The mycobacteria can be identified definitively through the use of a variety of techniques. Biochemical tests were the standard method for identifying mycobacteria but, because results are not available for at least 3 weeks or more, most laboratories do not rely on these tests. Two tests that are useful for the preliminary classification of the most common mycobacteria are production of niacin and reduction of nitrate (Table 29–4). Mycobacterial species can also be identified through chromatographic analysis of their characteristic cell wall lipids. However, species-specific molecular probes are the most useful means of identifying commonly isolated mycobacteria (e.g., *M. tuberculosis, M. avium* complex, *M. kansasii*). Because many organisms are present after in vitro cultivation, it is not necessary to amplify the target genomic sequence. The commercially prepared probe identification systems currently used are rapid (test time, 2 hours), sensitive, and specific.

An additional way to identify mycobacterial species for which probes are not available involves the amplification of the species-specific, hypervariable regions of the 16S ribosomal ribonucleic acid (RNA) genes, followed by sequence analysis to identify the species. This method is rapid (1 to 2 days) and is not limited by the availability of specific probes. It is likely that this method will eventually replace biochemical methods of identifying many mycobacterial species.

TREATMENT, PREVENTION, AND CONTROL

Treatment

The treatment and prophylaxis of mycobacterial infections, unlike those for most other bacterial infections, are complex and controversial. Slow-growing mycobacteria are resistant to most antibiotics used to treat other bacterial infections. In general, patients must take multiple antibiotics for an extended period (e.g., a minimum of 6 to 9 months) or antibiotic-resistant strains will develop. In 1990 the first outbreaks of multiple-drug–resistant *M. tuberculosis* were observed in patients with AIDS and in homeless persons in New York City and Miami. Although there has been a dramatic reduction in infections with these resistant strains, all therapy must be directed against these organisms until antimicrobial susceptibility results are available for the individual patient.

The number of treatment regimens that have been developed for drug-susceptible and drug-resistant tuberculosis is too complex to review here comprehensively (refer to the CDC readings listed in the bibliography at the end of this chapter). Most treatment regimens begin with 2 months of isoniazid (INH), ethambutol, pyrazinamide, and rifampin, followed by 4 to 6 months of INH and rifampin or alternative combination drugs. Modifications to this treatment scheme are dictated by the drug susceptibility of the isolate and the patient population.

In the last decade, treatment of leprosy has successfully reduced the overall incidence of disease. The treatment regimens advanced by the WHO (http://WHO.int/lep) have distinguished between patients with the tuberculoid (paucibacillary) form and the lepromatous (multibacillary) form. The paucibacillary form should be treated with rifampicin and dapsone for a minimum of 6 months, whereas the multibacillary form should have clofazimine added to the regimen and treatment should be extended to 12 months. It should be noted that many investigators

TABLE 29–4. Selected Biochemical Tests for the Preliminary Classification of Common Mycobacterial Species

Organism	Niacin	Nitrate Reductase	Heat-Stable Catalase	Tween-80 Hydrolysis	Iron Uptake	Arylsulfatase	Urease
M. tuberculosis	+	+	–	V		–	V
M. kansasii	–	+	+	+		–	+
M. avium complex	–	–	V	–		–	–
M. fortuitum	–	+	+	V	+	+	+
M. chelonae	V	–	V	V	–	+	+

V, variable.

believe much longer therapy is required for optimum management of patients. Single-drug treatment should not be used for either form.

M. avium complex and many other slow-growing mycobacteria are resistant to common antimycobacterial agents. One regimen recommended currently for MAC infections is clarithromycin or azithromycin, combined with ethambutol and rifabutin. The American Thoracic Society has recommended that *M. kansasii* infections be treated with INH, rifampin, and ethambutol with or without streptomycin. The duration of treatment and final selection of drugs for these species and other slow-growing mycobacteria are determined by (1) the response to therapy and (2) interactions among these drugs and other drugs the patient is receiving (e.g., toxic and pharmacokinetic interactions of these drugs with protease inhibitors used to treat HIV infection).

Unlike the slow-growing mycobacteria, the rapidly growing species are resistant to most commonly used antimycobacterial agents but are susceptible to antibiotics such as clarithromycin, imipenem, amikacin, cefoxitin, and the sulfonamides. The specific activity of these agents must be determined with in vitro tests. Because infections with these mycobacteria are generally confined to the skin or are associated with prosthetic devices, surgical débridement or removal of the prosthesis is also necessary.

CHEMOPROPHYLAXIS

The American Thoracic Society and the Centers for Disease Control and Prevention have examined a number of prophylactic regimens for use in patients (HIV positive and HIV negative) exposed to *M. tuberculosis.* The three regimens that have been recommended are as follows: (1) daily or twice weekly INH for 9 months, (2) daily rifampin for 4 months, and (3) daily rifampin and pyrazinamide for 2 months. Patients who have been exposed to drug-resistant *M. tuberculosis* should receive prophylaxis with pyrazinamide and either ethambutol or levofloxacin for 6 to 12 months. Because *M. avium* complex intracellulare infections are common in patients with AIDS, chemoprophylaxis is recommended for patients whose CD4+ T cell counts fall to less than 50 cells/µl. Prophylaxis with clarithromycin or azithromycin is recommended. Combinations of these drugs with rifabutin have been used, but they are generally more toxic and no more effective than the single agent. Chemoprophylaxis is unnecessary for patients with other mycobacterial infections.

IMMUNOPROPHYLAXIS

Vaccination with attenuated *M. bovis* (bacille Calmette-Guérin **[BCG]**) is commonly used in countries where tuberculosis is endemic and is responsible for significant morbidity and mortality. This practice can lead to a significant reduction in the incidence of tuberculosis if BCG is administered to people when they are young (it is less effective in adults). Unfortunately, BCG immunization cannot be used in immunocompromised patients (e.g., those with HIV infection). Thus it is unlikely to be useful in countries with a high prevalence of HIV infections (e.g., Africa) or to control the spread of drug-resistant tuberculosis. An additional problem with BCG immunization is that positive skin test reactivity develops in all patients and may persist for a prolonged time. However, skin test reactivity is generally low, so a strongly reactive skin test result (e.g., >20 mm of induration) is generally significant. BCG immunization is not widely used in the United States or in other countries where the incidence of tuberculosis is low.

CONTROL

Because a third of the world's population is infected with *M. tuberculosis,* the elimination of this disease is highly unlikely. Disease can be controlled, however, with a combination of active surveillance, prophylactic and therapeutic intervention, and careful case monitoring. The success of this approach was demonstrated in the 44% reduction of drug-resistant tuberculosis in the New York City area from 1991 to 1996.

CASE STUDY AND QUESTIONS

A 35-year-old man with a history of intravenous drug use entered the local health clinic with complaints of a dry, persistent cough; fever; malaise; and anorexia. Over the preceding 4 weeks, he had lost 15 pounds and experienced chills and sweats. A chest radiograph revealed patchy infiltrates throughout the lung fields. Because the patient had a nonproductive cough, sputum was induced and submitted for bacterial, fungal, and mycobacterial cultures, as well as examination for Pneumocystis *organisms. Blood cultures and serologic tests for HIV infection were performed. The patient was found to be HIV positive. The results of all cultures were negative after 2 days of incubation; however, cultures were positive for* M. tuberculosis *after an additional week of incubation.*

1. What is unique about the cell wall of mycobacteria, and what biologic effects can be attributed to the cell wall structure?
2. Why is *M. tuberculosis* more virulent in patients with HIV infection than in non–HIV-infected patients?
3. What is the definition of a positive skin test (PPD) result for *M. tuberculosis?*
4. What are the two clinical presentations of *M. leprae* infections? How do the diagnostic tests differ for these two presentations?
5. Why do mycobacterial infections have to be treated with multiple drugs for 6 months or more?

Bibliography

Centers for Disease Control and Prevention: Targeted tuberculin testing and treatment of latent tuberculosis infection. *MMWR* 49:1 51, 2000.

Centers for Disease Control and Prevention: Guidelines for preventing opportunistic infections among HIV-infected persons—2002 recommendations of the U.S. Public Health Service and the Infectious Diseases Society of America. *MMWR* 51 (No. RR-8):1-53, 2002.

Centers for Disease Control and Prevention: Treatment of tuberculosis, American Thoracic Society, CDC, and Infectious Diseases Society of America. *MMWR* 52 (No. RR-11):1-77, 2003.

Centers for Disease Control and Prevention: Guidelines for using the QuantiFERON-TB test for diagnosing latent *Mycobacterium tuberculosis* infection. *MMWR* 52 (RR-2):15-18, 2003.

Chua J et al. A tale of two lipids: *Mycobacterium tuberculosis* phagosome maturation arrest, *Curr Opin Microbiol* 7:71-77, 2004.

Falkinham J: Epidemiology of infection by nontuberculous mycobacteria, *Clin Microbiol Rev* 9:177-215, 1996.

Flynn JL, Chan J: Immune evasion by *Mycobacterium tuberculosis:* Living with the enemy, *Curr Opin Immunol* 15:450-455, 2003.

Horsburgh C: Epidemiology of *Mycobacterium avium* complex disease, *Am J Med* 102:11-15, 1997.

Jacobson K et al: Clinical and radiological features of pulmonary disease caused by rapidly growing mycobacteria in cancer patients, *Eur J Clin Microbiol Infect Dis* 17:615-621, 1998.

Jacobson K et al: *Mycobacterium kansasii* infections in patients with cancer, *Clin Infect Dis* 30:965-969, 2000.

Karakousis PC, Bishai WR, Dorman SE. Microreview: *Mycobacterium tuberculosis* cell envelope lipids and the host immune response, *Cell Microbiol* 6:105-116, 2004.

Kubica GP, Wayne LG: *The mycobacteria: A sourcebook,* New York, 1984, Marcel Dekker.

Reich JM, Johnson RE: *Mycobacterium avium* complex pulmonary disease presenting as an isolated lingular or middle lobe pattern: The Lady Windermere syndrome, *Chest* 101:1605-1609, 1992.

Russell DG, Mwandumba HC, Rhoades EE: *Mycobacterium* and the coat of many lipids, *J Cell Biol* 158:421-426, 2002.

Sepkowitz KA et al: Tuberculosis in the AIDS era, *Clin Microbiol Rev* 8:180-199, 1995.

Shah MK et al: *Mycobacterium haemophilum* in immunocompromised patients, *Clin Infect Dis* 33:330-337, 2001.

Verdon R et al: Tuberculous meningitis in adults: Review of 48 cases, *Clin Infect Dis* 22:982-988, 1996.

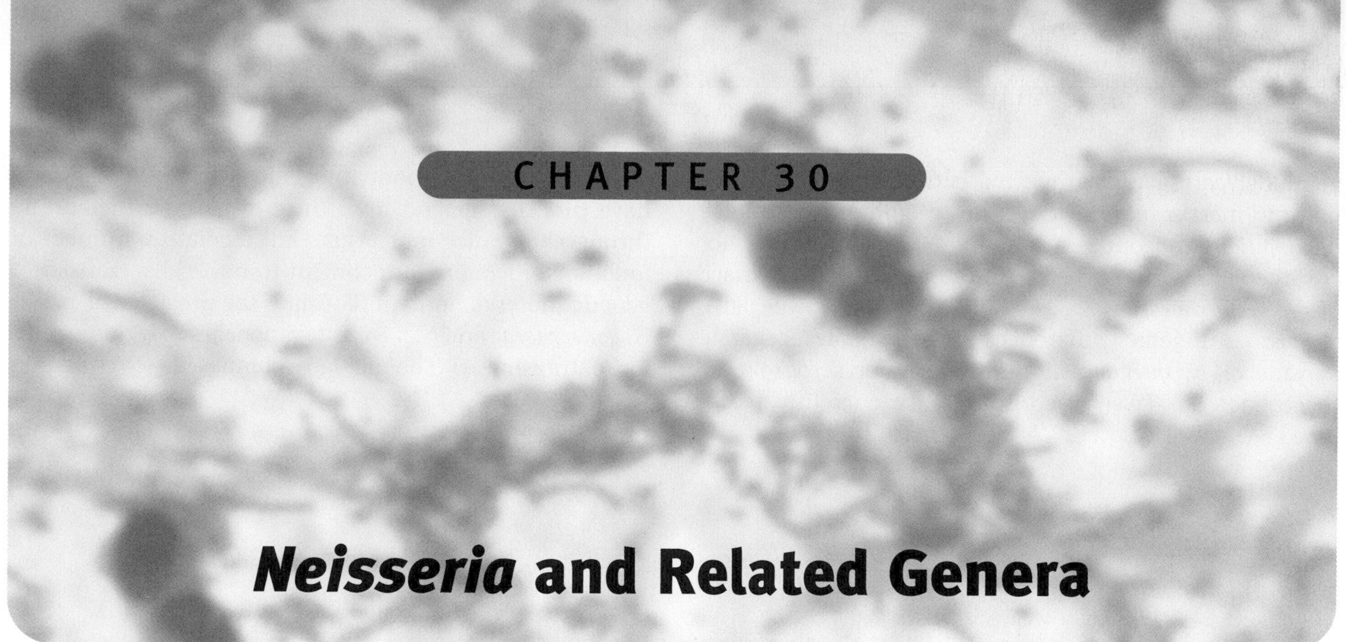

Neisseria and Related Genera

In recent years, the family Neisseriaceae has undergone reorganization, with some genera removed from the family and others added. The three genera of medical interest are *Neisseria, Eikenella,* and *Kingella* (Box 30–1). Other genera in the family are rarely associated with human disease and will not be discussed in this chapter. The genus *Neisseria* consists of 10 species found in humans with two species, *Neisseria gonorrhoeae* and *Neisseria meningitidis,* strictly human pathogens. The remaining species are commonly present on mucosal surfaces of the oropharynx and nasopharynx and occasionally colonize the anogenital mucosal membranes. Although diseases caused by *N. gonorrhoeae* and *N. meningitidis* are well known, the other *Neisseria* species have limited virulence and generally produce disease only in compromised patients. *Eikenella corrodens* and *Kingella kingae* colonize the human oropharynx and are opportunistic pathogens.

Neisseria gonorrhoeae and *Neisseria meningitidis* (Boxes 30–2 and 30–3)

Infection with *N. gonorrhoeae* has been recognized for centuries. Despite effective antibiotic therapy, gonorrhea is still one of the most common sexually transmitted diseases in the United States. *N. meningitidis* is a paradox. This encapsulated, gram-negative diplococcus commonly colonizes the nasopharynx of healthy people. It is also the second most common cause of community-acquired meningitis in adults, and the swift progression from good health to life-threatening disease can cause fear and panic in a community unlike the reaction to almost any other pathogen.

PHYSIOLOGY AND STRUCTURE

Neisseria species are aerobic, gram-negative cocci (0.6 to 1.0 μm in diameter) typically arranged in pairs (diplococci) with adjacent sides flattened together (resembling coffee beans; Figure 30–1). The bacteria are not motile and do not form endospores. All species are oxidase positive, and most produce catalase—properties that combined with the Gram-stain morphology allow for a rapid, presumptive identification of a clinical isolate. Acid is produced by oxidation of carbohydrates (not by fermentation). *N. gonorrhoeae* strains produce acid by oxidizing glucose; *N. meningitidis* strains oxidize both glucose and maltose. Carbohydrate utilization tests are useful for differentiating the pathogenic strains from other *Neisseria* species.

Nonpathogenic species of *Neisseria* can grow on nutrient agar incubated at 35° to 37°C. In contrast, *N. meningitidis* has variable growth on nutrient agar and *N. gonorrhoeae* is a fastidious organism, requiring complex media for growth, and is adversely affected by exposure to dry conditions or fatty acids. All strains of *N. gonorrhoeae* require cystine for growth, and many strains require supplementation of media with amino acids, purines, pyrimidines, and vitamins. Soluble starch is added to the media to neutralize the toxic effect of the fatty acids. The optimum growth temperature is 35° to 37°C, with poor survival of the organism at cooler temperatures. A humid atmosphere supplemented with carbon dioxide (CO_2) is either required or enhances growth of *N. gonorrhoeae.* Although the fastidious nature of this organism makes recovery from clinical specimens difficult, it is nevertheless easy for the organism to be sexually transmitted from person to person.

The structure of *N. gonorrhoeae* and *N. meningitidis* is typical of gram-negative bacteria, with the thin peptidoglycan layer sandwiched between the inner cytoplasmic membrane and the outer membrane. Unlike *N. meningitidis*, the outer surface of *N. gonorrhoeae* is not covered with a true carbohydrate capsule. The cell surface of *N. gonorrhoeae*, however, has a capsule-like negative charge. Antigenic differences in the polysaccharide capsule of *N. meningitidis* is the basis for serogrouping these bacteria. Twelve serogroups are currently recognized (A, B, C, H, I, K, L, W-135, X, Y, Z, 29E).

Pathogenic and nonpathogenic strains of *Neisseria* have **pili** that extend from the cytoplasmic membrane through the outer membrane. Pili mediate a number of functions, including attachment to host cells, transfer of genetic material, and motility, and the presence of pili in *N. gonorrhoeae* and *N. meningitidis* appears to be important for pathogenesis. The pili are composed of repeating

BOX 30–1. Important Neisseriaceae

Organism	Historical Derivation
Neisseria	Named after the German physician Albert Neisser, who originally described the organism responsible for gonorrhea
N. gonorrhoeae	*gone*, seed; *rhoia*, a flow (a flow of seeds; reference to the disease gonorrhea)
N. meningitidis	*meningis*, the covering of the brain; *itis*, inflammation (inflammation of the meninges as in meningitis)
Eikenella	Named after M. Eiken, who first named the type species in this genus
E. corrodens	*corrodens*, gnawing or eating (reference to the observation that colonies of this species eat into the agar)
Kingella	Named after the American bacteriologist Elizabeth King

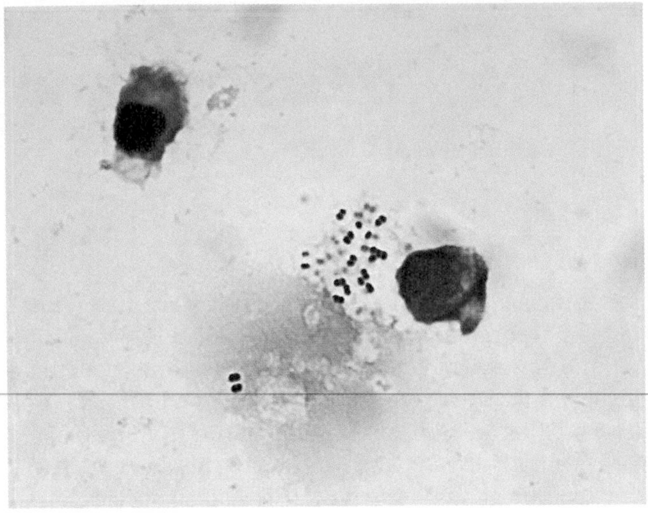

FIGURE 30–1. *Neisseria gonorrhoeae* in urethral exudate. Note the spatial arrangement of the pairs of cocci, with sides pressed together, which is characteristic of this genus.

BOX 30–2. Summary of *Neisseria gonorrhoeae*

Physiology and Structure

Gram-negative diplococci with fastidious growth requirements

Growth best at 35° to 37°C in a humid atmosphere supplemented with CO_2

Oxidase and catalase positive; acid produced from glucose oxidatively

Outer surface with multiple antigens: pili protein; Por proteins; Opa proteins; Rmp protein; protein receptors for transferrin, lactoferrin, and hemoglobin; lipooligosaccharide; immunoglobulin protease; β-lactamase

Virulence

Refer to Table 30–1

Epidemiology

Humans are the only natural hosts

Carriage can be asymptomatic, particularly in women

Transmission is primarily by sexual contact

Almost 310,000 cases reported in United States in 2004 (true incidence of disease believed to be at least twice that)

Disease most common in blacks, people ages 15 to 24 years, residents of southeastern United States, people who have multiple sexual encounters

Higher risk of disseminated disease in patients with deficiencies in late components of complement

Diseases

Refer to Box 30–4

Diagnosis

Gram stain of urethral specimens is accurate for symptomatic males only

Culture is sensitive and specific but has been replaced with nucleic acid amplification assays in most laboratories

Treatment, Prevention, and Control

Ceftriaxone can be administered in uncomplicated cases; fluoroquinolone can be used in susceptible population; penicillin should be avoided because resistance is common

Doxycycline or azithromycin should be added for infections complicated by *Chlamydia*

For neonates, prophylaxis with 1% silver nitrate; ophthalmia neonatorum is treated with ceftriaxone

Prevention consists of patient education, use of condoms or spermicides with nonoxynol-9 (only partially effective), and aggressive follow-up of sexual partners of infected patients

Effective vaccines are not available

BOX 30–3. Summary of *Neisseria meningitidis*

Physiology and Structure

Gram-negative diplococci with fastidious growth requirements
Grows best at 35° to 37°C in a humid atmosphere
Oxidase and catalase positive; acid produced from glucose and maltose oxidatively
Outer surface antigens include polysaccharide capsule, pili, and lipooligosaccharides (LOS)

Virulence

Capsule protects bacteria from antibody-mediated phagocytosis
Specific receptors for meningococcal pili allow colonization of nasopharynx
Bacteria can survive intracellular killing in the absence of humoral immunity
Endotoxin mediates most clinical manifestations

Epidemiology

Humans are the only natural hosts
Person-to-person spread occurs via aerosolization of respiratory tract secretions
Highest incidence of disease is in children younger than 5 years, institutionalized people, and patients with late complement deficiencies
Meningitis and meningococcemia most commonly caused by serogroups B and C; pneumonia most commonly caused by serogroups Y and W135; serogroups A and W135 associated with disease in underdeveloped countries
Disease occurs worldwide, most commonly in the dry, cold months of the year

Diseases

Refer to Box 30–4

Diagnosis

Gram stain of cerebrospinal fluid is sensitive and specific but is of limited value for blood specimens (too few organisms are generally present, except in overwhelming sepsis)
Culture is definitive, but organism is fastidious and dies rapidly when exposed to cold or dry conditions
Tests to detect meningococcal antigens are insensitive and nonspecific

Treatment, Prevention, and Control

Breast-feeding infants have passive immunity (first 6 months)
Treatment is with penicillin (drug of choice), chloramphenicol, ceftriaxone, and cefotaxime
Chemoprophylaxis for contact with persons with the disease is with rifampin, ciprofloxacin, or ceftriaxone
For immunoprophylaxis, vaccination is an adjunct to chemoprophylaxis; it is used only for serogroups A, C, Y, and W135; no effective vaccine is available for serogroup B.
Polysaccharide vaccines conjugated with protein carriers offer protection for infants younger than 2 years

protein subunits **(pilins)**, whose expression is controlled by the *pil* gene complex. Pili expression is associated with virulence, in part because the pili mediate attachment to nonciliated epithelial cells and provide resistance to killing by neutrophils. Pilin proteins have a conserved region at the amino terminal end and a highly variable region at the exposed carboxyl terminus. The lack of immunity to reinfection with *N. gonorrhoeae* results partially from the antigenic variation among the pilin proteins and partially from the phase variation in pilin expression; these factors complicate attempts to develop effective vaccines for gonorrhea.

Other prominent families of proteins are present in the outer membrane. The **Por proteins** are integral outer membrane proteins that form pores or channels for nutrients to pass into the cell and waste products to exit. *N. gonorrhoeae* and *N. meningitidis* have two porin genes, *por*A and *por*B. The gene products, PorA and PorB proteins, are both expressed in *N. meningitidis*, but the *por*A gene is silent in *N. gonorrhoeae*. Thus, not only is PorB the major outer membrane protein in *N. gonorrhoeae*, but it must also be functionally active for *N. gonorrhoeae* to survive. PorB is expressed as two distinct classes of antigens, PIA and PIB, with many distinct serovars. The antigenic differences in the PorB protein are determined by differences in the exposed surface of the protein. PorB is important for the virulence of *N. gonorrhoeae*. Purified PorB proteins can interfere with degranulation of neutrophils (i.e., phagolysosome fusion that would lead to killing of intracellular bacteria) and presumably protect the bacteria from the host's inflammatory response. Additionally, PorB with other adhesins facilitates the bacterial invasion into epithelial cells. Finally, expression of PIA PorB antigens makes the bacteria resistant to complement-mediated serum killing.

Opa proteins (opacity proteins) are a family of membrane proteins that mediate intimate binding to epithelial and phagocytic cells and are important for cell-to-cell signaling. Multiple alleles of these proteins can be expressed by an individual isolate. *N. gonorrhoeae* expressing the Opa proteins appear opaque (versus transparent) when grown in culture. This correlation is not seen in *N. meningitidis*.

The third group of proteins in the outer membrane is the highly conserved **Rmp proteins** (reduction-modifiable proteins). These proteins stimulate antibodies that block serum bactericidal activity against pathogenic neisseriae.

Iron is essential for the growth and metabolism of *N. gonorrhoeae* and *N. meningitidis*. These pathogenic neisseriae are able to complete with their human hosts for iron by binding host cell transferrin to specific bacterial surface receptors. The specificity of this binding for human transferrin is likely the reason these bacteria are strict human pathogens. The presence of this receptor is fundamentally different from most bacteria that synthesize siderophores to scavenge iron. The gonococci also have a variety of additional surface receptors for other host iron complexes, such as lactoferrin and hemoglobin.

Another major antigen in the cell wall is lipooligosaccharide (LOS). This antigen is composed of lipid A and a core oligosaccharide but lack the O-antigen polysaccharide found in lipopolysaccharide (LPS) in most gram-negative rods. The lipid A moiety possesses endotoxin activity. Both *N. gonorrhoeae* and *N. meningitidis* spontaneously release outer membrane blebs during rapid cell growth. These blebs contain LOS and surface proteins and may act to both enhance endotoxin-mediated toxicity and protect replicating bacteria by binding protein-directed antibodies.

N. gonorrhoeae and *N. meningitidis* produce immunoglobulin (Ig) A1 protease, which cleaves the hinge region in IgA1. This action creates immunologically inactive Fc and Fab fragments. Some strains of *N. gonorrhoeae* also produce β-lactamases that can degrade penicillin.

PATHOGENESIS AND IMMUNITY (TABLE 30–1)

Gonococci attach to mucosal cells, penetrate into the cells and multiply, and then pass through the cells into the subepithelial space, where infection is established. Pili, PorB, and Opa proteins mediate attachment and penetration into host cells. The gonococcal LOS stimulates the inflammatory response and release of tumor necrosis factor-α (TNF-α), which causes most of the symptoms associated with gonococcal disease.

IgG_3 is the predominant IgG antibody formed in response to gonococcal infection. Although the antibody response to PorB is minimal, serum antibodies to pilin, Opa protein, and LOS are readily detected. Antibodies to LOS can activate complement, releasing complement component C5a, which has a chemotactic effect on neutrophils. IgG and secretory IgA1 antibodies directed against Rmp protein can block this bactericidal antibody response, however. People with inherited complement deficiencies are at considerably greater risk for systemic disease.

Experiments with nasopharyngeal tissue organ cultures have shown that meningococci attach selectively to specific receptors for meningococcal pili on nonciliated columnar cells of the nasopharynx. Meningococci without pili are less able to bind to these cells.

Meningococcal disease occurs in the absence of specific antibodies directed against the polysaccharide capsule and other expressed bacterial antigens. Infants are initially afforded protection by the passive transfer of maternal antibodies. When the infant has reached age 6 months, however, this protective immunity has waned, a finding that is consistent with the observation that the incidence of disease is greatest in children younger than 2 years. Immunity can be stimulated by colonization with *N. meningitidis* or other bacteria with cross-reactive antigens (e.g., colonization with nonencapsulated *Neisseria* species; exposure to *Escherichia coli* K1 antigen, which cross-reacts with the group B capsular polysaccharide). Bactericidal activity also requires the existence of complement. Patients with deficiencies in C5, C6, C7, or C8 of the complement system are estimated to be at a 6000-fold greater risk for meningococcal disease. Although immunity is mediated primarily by the humoral immune

TABLE 30–1. Virulence Factors in *Neisseria gonorrhoeae*

Virulence Factor	Biologic Effect
Pilin	Protein that mediates initial attachment to nonciliated human cells (e.g., epithelium of vagina, fallopian tube, and buccal cavity); interferes with neutrophil killing
Por protein (protein I)	Porin protein: promotes intracellular survival by preventing phagolysosome fusion in neutrophils
Opa protein (protein II)	Opacity protein: mediates firm attachment to eukaryotic cells
Rmp protein (protein III)	Reduction-modifiable protein: protects other surface antigens (Por protein, LOS) from bactericidal antibodies
Transferrin-binding proteins	Mediate acquisition of iron for bacterial metabolism
Lactoferrin-binding proteins	Mediate acquisition of iron for bacterial metabolism
Hemoglobin-binding proteins	Mediate acquisition of iron for bacterial metabolism
LOS	Lipooligosaccharide: has endotoxin activity
IgA1 protease	Destroys immunoglobulin A1 (role in virulence is unknown)
β-Lactamase	Hydrolyzes the β-lactam ring in penicillin

response, lymphocyte responsiveness to meningococcal antigens is markedly depressed in patients with acute disease.

Like *N. gonorrhoeae*, meningococci are internalized into phagocytic vacuoles and are able to avoid intracellular death, replicate, and then migrate to the subepithelial spaces. The antiphagocytic properties of the polysaccharide capsule protect *N. meningitidis* from phagocytic destruction.

The diffuse vascular damage associated with meningococcal infections (e.g., endothelial damage, inflammation of vessel walls, thrombosis, disseminated intravascular coagulation) is largely attributed to the action of the LOS endotoxin present in the outer membrane.

EPIDEMIOLOGY

Gonorrhea occurs only in humans; it has no other known reservoir. It is second only to chlamydia as the most commonly reported sexually transmitted disease in the United States. Infection rates are the same in males and females, are disproportionately higher in blacks than in Hispanic Americans and whites, and are highest in the southeastern United States. The peak incidence of the disease is in the age group 15 to 24 years. The incidence of disease has decreased from 1975 to 1998; however, between 1998 and 2004 the rate of decrease has slowed. In 2004, almost 310,000 new infections were reported in the United States. However, even this large number is an underestimation of the true incidence of disease because the diagnosis and reporting of gonococcal infections are incomplete. Public health officials believe that at least half of the new infections are not reported.

N. gonorrhoeae is transmitted primarily by sexual contact. Women have a 50% risk of acquiring the infection as the result of a single exposure to an infected man, whereas men have a risk of approximately 20% as the result of a single exposure to an infected woman. The risk of infection rises as the person has more sexual encounters with infected partners.

The major reservoir for gonococci is the asymptomatically infected person. Asymptomatic carriage is more common in women than in men. As many as half of all infected women have mild or asymptomatic infections, whereas most men are initially symptomatic. The symptoms generally clear within a few weeks in people with untreated disease, and asymptomatic carriage may then become established. The site of infection also determines whether carriage occurs, with rectal and pharyngeal infections more commonly asymptomatic than genital infections.

Endemic meningococcal disease occurs worldwide, and epidemics are common in developing countries. Epidemic spread of disease results from the introduction of a new, virulent strain into an immunologically naïve population. Pandemics of disease have been uncommon in developed countries since World War II. Of the 12 serogroups, almost all infections are caused by serogroups A, B, C, Y, and W135. In Europe and the Americas, serogroups B, C, and Y predominate in meningitis or meningococcemia; serogroups A and W135 predominate in developing countries. Serogroups Y and W135 are most commonly associated with meningococcal pneumonia. *N. meningitidis* is transmitted by respiratory droplets among people in prolonged close contact, such as family members living in the same household and soldiers living together in military barracks. Classmates in schools and hospital employees are not considered close contacts and are not at significantly higher risk of acquiring the disease unless they are in direct contact with the respiratory secretions of an infected person.

Humans are the only natural carriers for *N. meningitidis*. Studies of the asymptomatic carriage of *N. meningitidis* have shown that there is a tremendous variation in its prevalence, from less than 1% to almost 40%. The oral and nasopharyngeal carriage rates are highest for school-age children and young adults, are higher in lower socioeconomic populations (caused by person-to-person spread in crowded areas), and do not vary with the seasons, even though disease is most common during the dry, cold months of the year. Carriage is typically transient, with clearance occurring after specific antibodies develop. Endemic disease is most common in children younger than 5 years, particularly infants. People who are older and live in closed populations (e.g., military barracks, prisons) are prone to infection during epidemics.

Neisseria gonorrhoeae

CLINICAL DISEASES (BOX 30–4)

Gonorrhea

Genital infection in men is primarily restricted to the urethra. A purulent urethral discharge (Figure 30–2) and dysuria develop after a 2- to 5-day incubation period. Approximately 95% of all infected men have acute symptoms. Although complications are rare, epididymitis, prostatitis, and periurethral abscesses may occur. The primary site of infection in women is the cervix, because the bacteria infect the endocervical columnar epithelial cells. The organism cannot infect the squamous epithelial cells that line the vagina of postpubescent women. Symptomatic patients commonly experience vaginal discharge, dysuria, and abdominal pain. Ascending genital infections, including salpingitis, tuboovarian abscesses, and pelvic inflammatory disease, are observed in 10% to 20% of women.

BOX 30–4. Neisseriaceae: Clinical Summaries

Neisseria gonorrhoeae

Gonorrhea: Characterized by purulent discharge for involved site (e.g., urethra, cervix, epididymis, prostate, anus) after 2- to 5-day incubation period

Disseminated infections: Spread of infection from genitourinary tract through blood to skin or joints; characterized by pustular rash with erythematous base and suppurative arthritis in involved joints

Ophthalmia neonatorum: Purulent ocular infection acquired by neonate at birth

Neisseria meningitidis

Meningitis: Purulent inflammation of meninges associated with headache, meningeal signs, and fever; high mortality rate unless promptly treated with effective antibiotics

Meningococcemia: Disseminated infection characterized by thrombosis of small blood vessels and multiorgan involvement; small, petechial skin lesions coalesce into larger hemorrhagic lesions

Pneumonia: Milder form of meningococcal disease characterized by bronchopneumonia in patients with underlying pulmonary disease

Eikenella corrodens

Human bite wounds: Infection associated with traumatic (e.g., bite, fistfight injury) introduction of oral organisms into deep tissue

Subacute endocarditis: Infection of endocardium characterized by gradual onset of low grade fevers, night sweats, and chills

Kingella kingae

Subacute endocarditis: As with *E. corrodens*

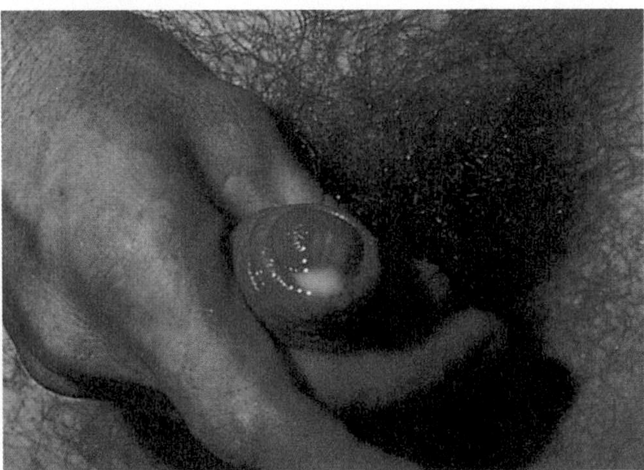

FIGURE 30–2. Purulent urethral discharge in man with urethritis. (From Morse S et al: *Atlas of sexually transmitted diseases and AIDS*, ed 3, St Louis, 2003, Mosby.)

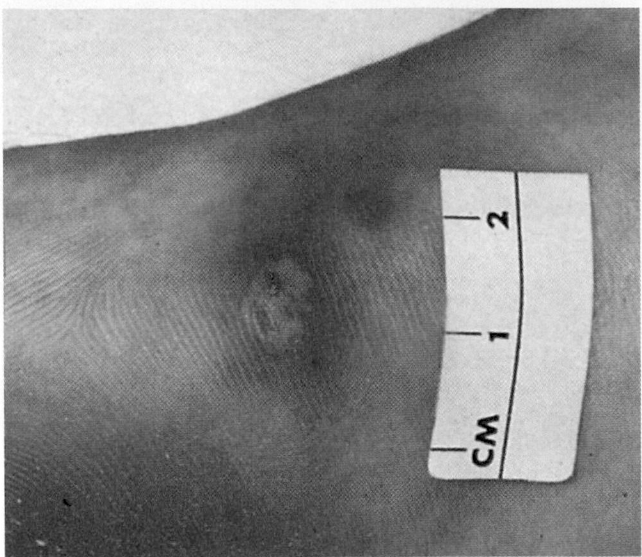

FIGURE 30–3. Skin lesions of disseminated gonococcal infection. Classic large lesions with a necrotic, grayish central lesion on an erythematous base. (From Morse S et al: *Atlas of sexually transmitted diseases and AIDS*, ed 3, St Louis, 2003, Mosby.)

Gonococcemia

Disseminated infections with septicemia and infection of skin and joints occur in 1% to 3% of infected women and in a much lower percentage of infected men. The greater proportion of disseminated infections in women is caused by the numerous untreated asymptomatic infections in this population. The clinical manifestations of disseminated disease include fever; migratory arthralgias; suppurative arthritis in the wrists, knees, and ankles; and a pustular rash on an erythematous base (Figure 30–3) over the extremities but not on the head and trunk. *N. gonorrhoeae* is a leading cause of purulent arthritis in adults.

Other *N. gonorrhoeae* Syndromes

Other diseases associated with N. gonorrhoeae are perihepatitis (Fitz-Hugh–Curtis syndrome); purulent conjunctivitis (Figure 30–4), particularly in newborns infected during vaginal delivery (ophthalmia neonatorum); anorectal gonorrhea in homosexual men; and pharyngitis.

Neisseria meningitidis

CLINICAL DISEASES (see BOX 30–4)

Meningitis

A total of 1254 cases of meningococcal disease (approximately 0.6 cases per 100,000 population) were reported

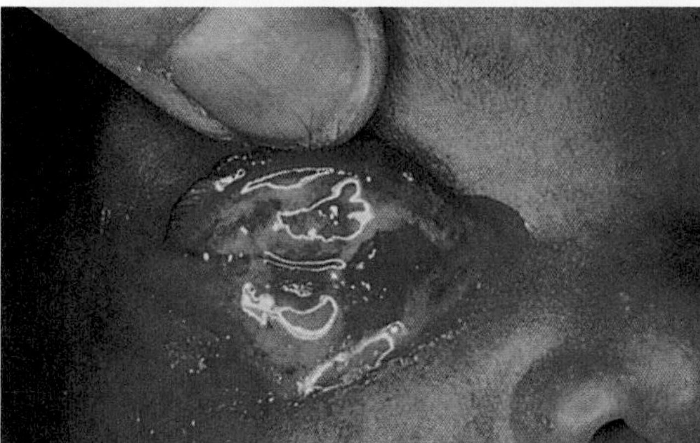

FIGURE 30–4. Gonococcal ophthalmia neonatorum. Lid edema, erythema, and marked purulent discharge are seen. A Gram-stained smear would reveal abundant organisms and inflammatory cells. (From Morse S et al: *Atlas of sexually transmitted diseases and AIDS,* ed 3, St Louis, 2003, Mosby.)

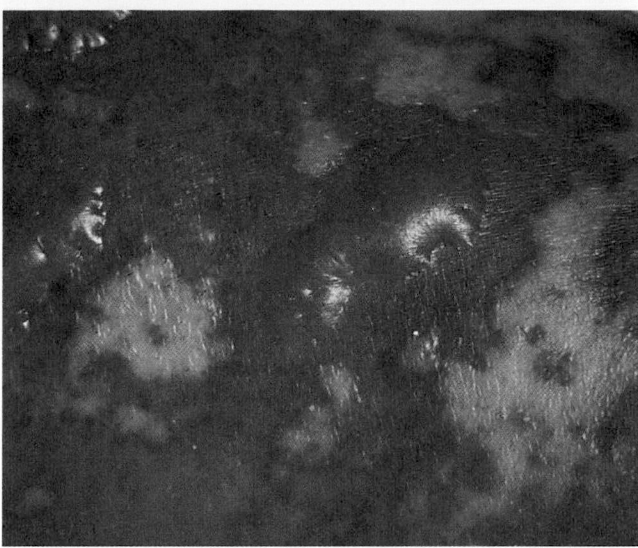

FIGURE 30–5. Skin lesions in a patient with meningococcemia. Note that the petechial lesions have coalesced and formed hemorrhagic bullae.

in the United States in 2004. Most of these infections were meningitis. The disease usually begins abruptly with headache, meningeal signs, and fever. However, very young children may have only nonspecific signs such as fever and vomiting. Mortality approaches 100% in untreated patients but is less than 10% in patients in whom appropriate antibiotic therapy is instituted promptly. The incidence of neurologic sequelae is low, with hearing deficits and arthritis most commonly reported.

Meningococcemia

Septicemia (meningococcemia) with or without meningitis is a life-threatening disease. Thrombosis of small blood vessels and multiorgan involvement are the characteristic clinical features. Small, petechial skin lesions on the trunk and lower extremities are common and may coalesce to form larger hemorrhagic lesions (Figure 30–5). Overwhelming disseminated intravascular coagulation with shock, together with the bilateral destruction of the adrenal glands **(Waterhouse-Friderichsen syndrome),** may ensue.

A milder, chronic septicemia has also been observed. Bacteremia can persist for days or weeks, and the only signs of infection are a low-grade fever, arthritis, and petechial skin lesions. The response to antibiotic therapy in patients with this form of the disease is generally excellent.

Other *N. meningitidis* Syndromes

Additional infections caused by *N. meningitidis* are pneumonia, arthritis, and urethritis. Meningococcal pneumonia is usually preceded by a respiratory tract infection. Symptoms include cough, chest pain, rales, fever, and chills. Evidence of pharyngitis is observed in most affected patients. The prognosis in patients with meningococcal pneumonia is good.

LABORATORY DIAGNOSIS

Microscopy

Gram stain is very sensitive (greater than 90%) and specific (98%) in detecting gonococcal infection in men with purulent urethritis (see Figure 30–1). However, its sensitivity in detecting infection in asymptomatic men is 60% or less. The test is also relatively insensitive in detecting gonococcal cervicitis in both symptomatic and asymptomatic women, although a positive result is considered reliable when an experienced microscopist sees gram-negative diplococci within polymorphonuclear leukocytes. Thus the Gram stain can be reliably used to diagnose infections in men with purulent urethritis, but all negative results in women and asymptomatic men must be confirmed by culture.

Gram stain is also useful for the early diagnosis of purulent arthritis but is insensitive for the detection of *N. gonorrhoeae* in patients with skin lesions, anorectal infections, or pharyngitis. Commensal *Neisseria* species in the oropharynx and morphologically similar bacteria in the gastrointestinal tract can be confused with *N. gonorrhoeae.*

N. meningitidis can be readily seen in the cerebrospinal fluid (CSF) of patients with meningitis (Figure 30–6), unless the patient has received prior antimicrobial therapy. Most patients with bacteremia caused by other organisms have so few organisms present in their blood

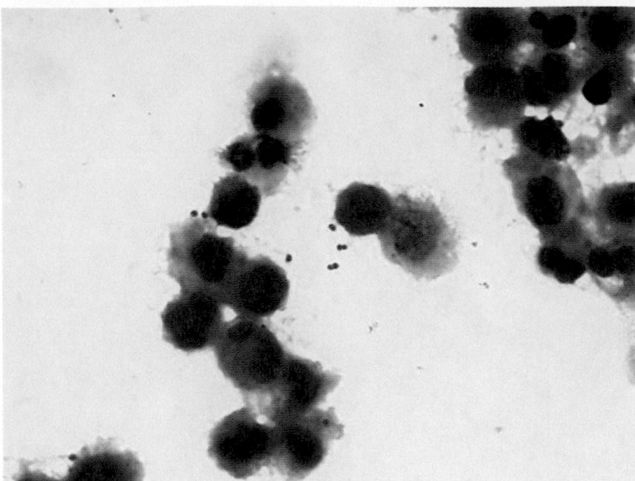

FIGURE 30–6. Gram stain of cerebrospinal fluid showing *Neisseria meningitidis.*

that the Gram stain has no value. In contrast, patients with overwhelming meningococcal disease commonly have large numbers of organisms in their blood, which can be seen when the peripheral blood leukocytes are Gram stained.

Culture

N. gonorrhoeae can be readily isolated from genital specimens if care is taken in collecting and processing the specimens (Figure 30–7). Because other commensal organisms normally colonize mucosal surfaces, all genital, rectal, and pharyngeal specimens must be inoculated onto both selective media (e.g., modified Thayer-Martin medium) and nonselective media (e.g., chocolate blood agar). Selective media suppress the growth of contaminating organisms. A nonselective medium should also be used, however, because some gonococcal strains are inhibited by the vancomycin present in most selective media. The organisms are also inhibited by the fatty acids and trace metals present in the peptone hydrolysates and agar in other common laboratory media (e.g., blood agar, nutrient agar). The gonococci die rapidly if specimens are allowed to dry. Therefore drying and cold temperatures should be avoided through direct inoculation of the specimen onto prewarmed media at the time of collection.

The endocervix must be properly exposed to ensure that an adequate specimen is collected. Although the endocervix is the most common site of infection in women, the rectal specimen may be the only one positive for gonococci in women who have asymptomatic infections, as well as in homosexual and bisexual men. Blood culture results are generally positive for gonococci only during the first week of the infection in patients with disseminated disease. In addition, special handling of blood specimens is required to ensure the adequate recovery of gonococci, because supplements present in the blood culture media can be toxic to *Neisseria.* Culture results of specimens from infected joints are positive for the organism if the specimens are collected at the time the arthritis develops, but skin specimen cultures are generally unrewarding.

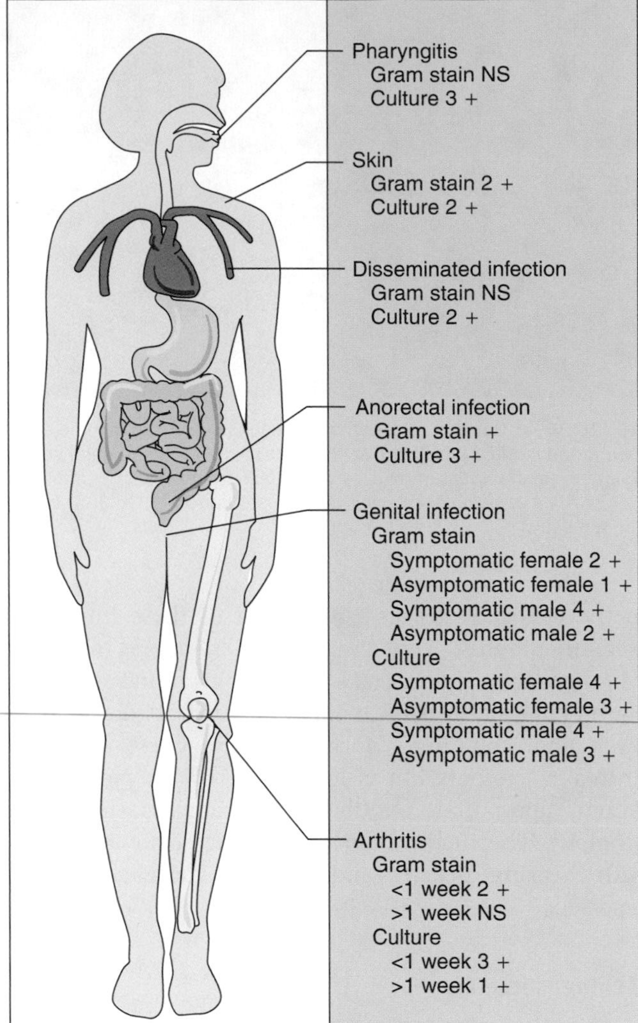

NS, Not specific or sensitive.

FIGURE 30–7. Laboratory detection of *Neisseria gonorrhoeae.*

N. meningitidis is generally present in large numbers in CSF, blood, and sputum. Although the organism is inhibited by toxic factors in media and by the anticoagulant in blood cultures, this appears to be less of a problem than with *N. gonorrhoeae.* Care should be used in processing CSF and blood specimens because bacterial strains responsible for disseminated disease are more virulent and pose a safety risk for the laboratory technologists.

Identification

Pathogenic *Neisseria* species are identified preliminarily on the basis of the isolation of oxidase-positive,

TABLE 30–2. Differential Characteristics of Commonly Isolated *Neisseria* Species

Characteristic	*N. gonorrhoeae*	*N. meningitidis*	*N. lactamica*	*N. sicca*	*N. mucosa*	*N. flavescens*
Growth on:						
CHOC, BA (22°C)	0	0	V	+	+	+
MTM, ML (35°C)	+	+	+	0	0	0
Nutrient agar (35°C)	0	V	+	+	+	+
Acid from:						
Glucose	+	+	+	+	+	0
Maltose	0	+	+	+	+	0
Lactose	0	0	+	0	0	0
Sucrose	0	0	0	+	+	0
Fructose	0	0	0	+	+	0
Nitrate reduction	0	0	0	0	+	0

BA, Blood agar; CHOC, chocolate agar; ML, Martin-Lewis agar; MTM, modified Thayer-Martin agar; V, variable growth; O, unable to grow or utilize substrate.

gram-negative diplococci that grow on chocolate blood agar or on media that are selective for pathogenic *Neisseria* species. Definitive identification is guided by the pattern of oxidation of carbohydrates and other select tests (Table 30–2).

Nucleic Acid Amplification and Antigen Tests

Nucleic acid amplification assays specific for *N. gonorrhoeae* have been developed for the direct detection of bacteria in clinical specimens. Tests using these assays are sensitive, specific, and rapid (results are available in 4 hours). Combination assays for both *N. gonorrhoeae* and *Chlamydia* organisms are also available. In many laboratories, culture for these two pathogens has been replaced with these assays. The primary problem with this approach is that it cannot be used to monitor antibiotic resistance of the identified pathogens.

Commercial tests to detect *N. meningitidis* capsular antigens in CSF, blood, and urine (where the antigens are excreted) were widely used in the past but have fallen into disfavor in recent years because the tests are less sensitive than Gram stains and false-positive reactions particularly with urine specimens can occur.

TREATMENT, PREVENTION, AND CONTROL

Penicillin was historically the antibiotic of choice for treatment of gonorrhea; however, penicillin is not used today because the concentration of drug required to kill "susceptible" strains has steadily increased and frank resistance, because of β-lactamase production (plasmid-mediated) or chromosomally mediated changes in penicillin-binding proteins and in cell wall permeability, has become common. The chromosomally mediated penicillin resistance is also associated with resistance to tetracyclines, erythromycin, and aminoglycosides. Resistance to fluoroquinolones such as ciprofloxacin has also become prevalent in Asia, the Pacific Islands (including Hawaii), California, and in the male homosexual population in some U.S. cities.

Currently, the Centers for Disease Control and Prevention (CDC) recommends that a fluoroquinolone not be used to treat gonorrhea infections acquired in an areas where resistance is common. For these patients, ceftriaxone should be used as initial empiric therapy. If *Chlamydia trachomatis* infection has not been excluded, treatment should be combined with either a single dose of azithromycin or a 1-week course of doxycycline.

N. meningitidis remains susceptible to penicillin, although occasional reports of strains with low-level resistance have been reported. For patients unable to receive penicillin a broad-spectrum cephalosporin (e.g., ceftriaxone) or chloramphenicol can be used.

Although there is tremendous interest in developing a vaccine against *N. gonorrhoeae*, an effective vaccine is not yet available. Immunity to infection with *N. gonorrhoeae* is poorly understood. Antibodies can be detected to pili antigens, Por proteins, and LOS. However, multiple infections are common in sexually promiscuous people. This lack of protective immunity is explained in part by the antigenic diversity of gonococcal strains. The variable region at the carboxyl terminus of the pilin proteins is the immunodominant portion of the molecule. Antibodies developed against this region protect against reinfection with a homologous strain, but cross-protection against heterologous strains is incomplete. This antigenic diversity also explains the ineffectiveness of vaccines developed against pilin proteins.

Chemoprophylaxis is also ineffective, except in the protection of newborns against gonococcal eye infections (ophthalmia neonatorum), in which 1% silver nitrate, 1% tetracycline, or 0.5% erythromycin eye ointments are routinely used. Prophylactic use of penicillin to prevent genital disease is ineffective and may select for infection with a penicillin-resistant strain.

Major efforts to stem the epidemic of gonorrhea encompass education, aggressive detection, and follow-up screening of sexual contacts. It is important to realize that gonorrhea is not an insignificant disease. Chronic infections can lead to sterility, and asymptomatic infections perpetuate the reservoir of disease and lead to a higher incidence of disseminated infections.

Eradication of the pool of healthy carriers of *N. meningitidis* is unlikely. For this reason, efforts have been concentrated on the prophylactic treatment of people exposed to diseased patients and on the enhancement of immunity to the serogroups most commonly associated with disease. Sulfonamides and penicillin are ineffective in eliminating the carrier state. Currently, rifampin, ciprofloxacin, or ceftriaxone are recommended for prophylaxis.

Vaccines directed against the group-specific capsular polysaccharides have been developed for antibody-mediated immunoprophylaxis. A polyvalent vaccine effective against serogroups A, C, Y, and W135, which can be administered to children older than 2 years, has been developed. The vaccine cannot be administered to children in younger age groups, however, because they do not respond to polysaccharide antigens. Conjugation of polysaccharide antigens to protein carriers has been used successfully with the *Haemophilus influenzae* vaccine, and a similar conjugated *N. meningitidis* vaccine is under evaluation. Unfortunately, the group B polysaccharide is a weak immunogen and cannot induce a protective antibody response. Thus immunity to group B *N. meningitidis* must develop naturally after exposure to cross-reacting antigens. Vaccination with a suspension containing serogroup A can be used for control of an outbreak of disease, for travelers to hyperendemic areas, and for people at increased risk for disease (e.g., patients with complement deficiency).

Other *Neisseria* Species

Neisseria species such as *Neisseria sicca* and *Neisseria mucosa* are commensal organisms in the oropharynx. These organisms have been implicated in isolated cases of meningitis, osteomyelitis, endocarditis, bronchopulmonary infections, acute otitis media, and acute sinusitis. The true incidence of respiratory tract infections caused by these organisms is not known because most specimens are contaminated with oral secretions. However, the observation of many gram-negative diplococci associated with inflammatory cells in a well-collected respiratory specimen would support the etiologic role of these organisms. Most isolates of *N. sicca* and *N. mucosa* are susceptible to penicillin, although low-level resistance caused by altered penicillin-binding protein (i.e., PBP2) has been observed.

Eikenella corrodens

In the early 1960s, a collection of small, fastidious, gram-negative rods were classified by workers at the CDC as members of the HB group (named after the patient infected with the original isolate). The organisms were subsequently subdivided into subgroup HB-1 (now known as *E. corrodens*), subgroup HB-2 (*Haemophilus aphrophilus;* see Chapter 35), and subgroups HB-3 and HB-4 (*Actinobacillus actinomycetemcomitans;* see Chapter 35). In addition to being morphologically similar, these organisms colonize the human oropharynx and, in the setting of preexisting heart disease, can cause subacute bacterial endocarditis. In fact, the group of fastidious, gram-negative rods associated with subacute endocarditis is known by the acronym HACEK (*H. aphrophilus, A. actinomycetemcomitans, Cardiobacterium hominis, E. corrodens,* and *K. kingae*).

E. corrodens is a moderate-sized (0.2 by 2.0 µm), nonmotile, non–spore-forming, facultatively anaerobic, gram-negative rod. The organism is named after Eiken, who characterized the bacterium and observed the ability of the organism to pit or "corrode" agar (from its ability to split polygalacturonic acid). *E. corrodens* is a normal inhabitant of the human upper respiratory tract, but because of its fastidious growth requirements, it is difficult to detect unless specific selective culture media are used. It is an opportunistic pathogen that causes infections in patients who are immunocompromised or have diseases or trauma of the oral cavity. *E. corrodens* is most commonly isolated in the settings of a human bite wound or fistfight injury. Other infections are endocarditis, sinusitis, meningitis, brain abscesses, pneumonia, and lung abscesses. Because most infections originate from the oropharynx, polymicrobial mixtures of aerobic and anaerobic bacteria are often present in cultures.

A slow-growing, fastidious organism, *E. corrodens* requires 5% to 10% carbon dioxide to grow. Small (0.5- to 1.0-mm) colonies are observed after 48 hours of incubation on blood or chocolate agar, but the organism grows poorly or not at all on selective media for gram-negative rods. Pitting in agar is a useful differential characteristic, but fewer than half of all isolates exhibit pitting. The organism also produces a characteristic bleach-like odor. Thus, if a slow-growing, gram-negative rod is found to pit blood agar and produce a bleach-like order, a preliminary identification of the organism can be made. *E. corrodens* is susceptible to penicillin, ampicillin, extended-spectrum cephalosporins, tetracyclines, and fluoroquinolone but is resistant to oxacillin, first-generation cephalosporins, clindamycin, erythromycin, and the aminoglycosides. Thus *E. corrodens* is resistant to many antibiotics that are selected empirically to treat bite wound infections.

Kingella kingae

Kingella species are small, gram-negative coccobacilli that morphologically resemble *Neisseria* species and reside in the human oropharynx. The bacteria are facultatively anaerobic, ferment carbohydrates, and have fastidious growth requirements. *K. kingae,* the most commonly isolated species, has been primarily responsible for septic arthritis in children and endocarditis in patients of all ages. Because the organism grows slowly, it may take 3 or more days of incubation for the organism to be detected in clinical specimens. Most strains are susceptible to β-lactam antibiotics, including penicillin, tetracyclines, erythromycin, fluoroquinolones, and aminoglycosides.

CASE STUDY AND QUESTIONS

A 22-year-old female schoolteacher was brought to the emergency room after a 2-day history of headache and fever. On the day of admission the patient had failed to come to school and could not be reached by telephone. When notified of this fact, the patient's mother went to her daughters apartment, where she found her daughter in bed, confused and highly agitated. The patient was rushed to the local hospital, where she was comatose on arrival. Purpuric skin lesions were present on her trunk and arms. Analysis of her CSF revealed the presence of 380 cells/mm^3 (93% polymorphonuclear leukocytes), a protein concentration of 220 mg/dl, and a glucose concentration of 32 mg/dl. Gram stain of CSF showed many gram-negative diplococci, and the same organisms were isolated from blood and CSF. The patient died despite prompt initiation of therapy with penicillin.

1. What is the most likely organism responsible for this fulminant disease? What is the most likely source of this organism?
2. Chemoprophylaxis should be administered to which people? What are the criteria for administering chemoprophylaxis?
3. What other diseases does this organism cause?
4. What virulence factors have been associated with other bacterial species in this genus?

Bibliography

Campos J et al: Genetic diversity of penicillin-resistant *Neisseria meningitidis, J Infect Dis* 166:173-177, 1992.

Jackson LA et al: Prevalence of *Neisseria meningitidis* relatively resistant to penicillin in the United States: 1991, *J Infect Dis* 169:438-441, 1994.

Knapp JS: Antimicrobial resistance in *Neisseria gonorrhoeae* in the United States, *Clin Microbiol Newsletter* 21:1-7, 1999.

MacLennan JM et al: Safety, immunogenicity, and induction of immunologic memory by a serogroup C meningococcal conjugate vaccine in infants: A randomized controlled trial, *JAMA* 283:2795-2801, 2000.

Rosenstein NE et al: The changing epidemiology of meningococcal disease in the United States, 1992-1996, *J Infect Dis* 180:1894-1901, 1999.

Stephens DS et al: Interaction of *Neisseria meningitidis* with human nasopharyngeal mucosa: Attachment and entry into columnar epithelial cells, *J Infect Dis* 148:369-376, 1983.

Van Deuren M et al: Update on meningococcal disease with emphasis on pathogenesis and clinical management, *Clin Microbiol Rev* 13:144-166, 2000.

Winstead JM et al: Meningococcal pneumonia: Characterization and review of cases seen over the past 25 years, *Clin Infect Dis* 30:87-94, 2000.

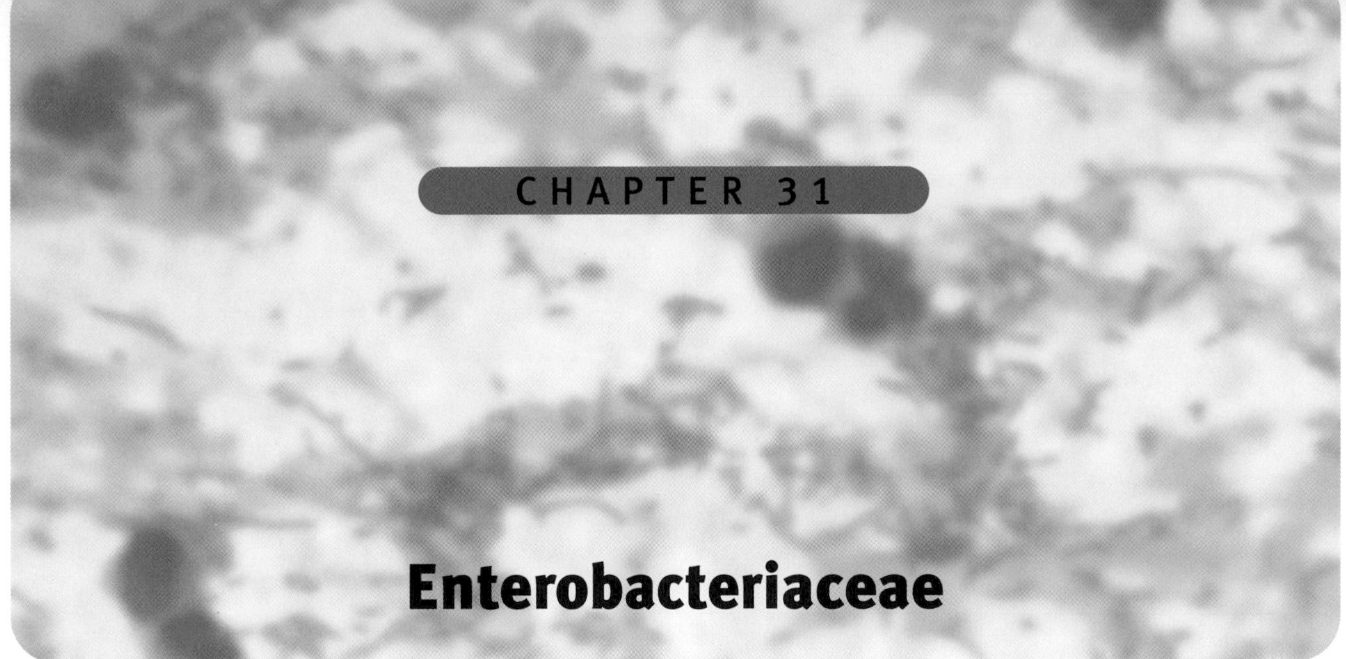

CHAPTER 31

Enterobacteriaceae

The family Enterobacteriaceae is the largest, most heterogeneous collection of medically important gram-negative rods. A total of more than 40 genera and 150 species and subspecies have been described. These genera have been classified based on biochemical properties, antigenic structure, and nucleic acid hybridization and sequencing. Despite the complexity of this family, fewer than 20 species are responsible for more than 95% of the infections (Box 31–1).

Enterobacteriaceae are ubiquitous organisms, found worldwide in soil, water, and vegetation, and are part of the normal intestinal flora of most animals, including humans. These bacteria cause a variety of human diseases, including 30% to 35% of all septicemias, more than 70% of urinary tract infections (UTIs), and many intestinal infections. Some organisms (e.g., *Salmonella typhi*, *Shigella* species, *Yersinia pestis*) are always associated with disease, whereas others (e.g., *Escherichia coli*, *Klebsiella pneumoniae*, *Proteus mirabilis*) are members of the normal commensal flora that can cause opportunistic infections. A third group of Enterobacteriaceae exists—those normally commensal organisms that become pathogenic when they acquire virulence factor genes on plasmids, bacteriophages, or pathogenicity islands (e.g., *E. coli* associated with gastroenteritis). Infections with the Enterobacteriaceae can originate from an animal reservoir (e.g., most *Salmonella* species, *Yersinia* species), from a human carrier (e.g., *Shigella* species, *S. typhi*), or through the endogenous spread of organisms in a susceptible patient (e.g., *E. coli*) and can involve virtually all body sites (Figure 31–1).

Physiology and Structure

Members of the Enterobacteriaceae family are moderately sized (0.3 to 1.0 × 1.0 to 6.0 μm) gram-negative rods (Figure 31–2). They share a common antigen **(enterobacterial common antigen),** are either nonmotile or motile with peritrichous flagella (Figure 31–3), and do not form spores. All members can grow rapidly, aerobically and anaerobically (facultative anaerobes), on a variety of nonselective (e.g., blood agar) and selective (e.g., MacConkey agar) media. The Enterobacteriaceae have simple nutritional requirements, ferment glucose, reduce nitrate, and are catalase positive and **oxidase negative.** The absence of cytochrome oxidase activity is an important characteristic, because it can be measured rapidly with a simple test and is used to distinguish the Enterobacteriaceae from many other fermentative and nonfermentative gram-negative rods. A few exceptions to these rules exist (e.g., *Plesiomonas shigelloides* is oxidase positive; *Klebsiella granulomatis* cannot be cultured on traditional media).

Characteristics of the organisms' colonies on different media have been used to identify common members of the family Enterobacteriaceae. For example, the ability to **ferment lactose** has been used to differentiate lactose-fermenting strains (e.g., *Escherichia, Klebsiella, Enterobacter, Citrobacter,* and *Serratia* spp.) from strains that do not ferment lactose or do so slowly (e.g., *Proteus, Salmonella, Shigella,* and *Yersinia* spp.). Resistance to bile salts in some selective media has been used to separate enteric pathogens (e.g., *Shigella, Salmonella*) from commensal organisms that are inhibited by bile salts (e.g., gram-positive and some gram-negative bacteria present in the gastrointestinal tract). Some Enterobacteriaceae have prominent capsules (e.g., most *Klebsiella*, some *Enterobacter* and *Escherichia* strains), whereas a loose-fitting, diffusible slime layer surrounds other strains.

The heat-stable **lipopolysaccharide (LPS)** is the major cell wall antigen and consists of three components: the outermost somatic O polysaccharide, a core polysaccharide common to all Enterobacteriaceae (enterobacterial common antigen), and lipid A (Figure 31–4). The

BOX 31–1. Common Medically Important Enterobacteriaceae

Citrobacter freundii, Citrobacter koseri
Enterobacter aerogenes, Enterobacter cloacae
Escherichia coli
Klebsiella pneumoniae, Klebsiella oxytoca
Morganella morganii
Proteus mirabilis, Proteus vulgaris
Salmonella enterica
Serratia marcescens
Shigella sonnei, Shigella flexneri
Yersinia pestis, Yersinia enterocolitica, Yersinia pseudotuberculosis

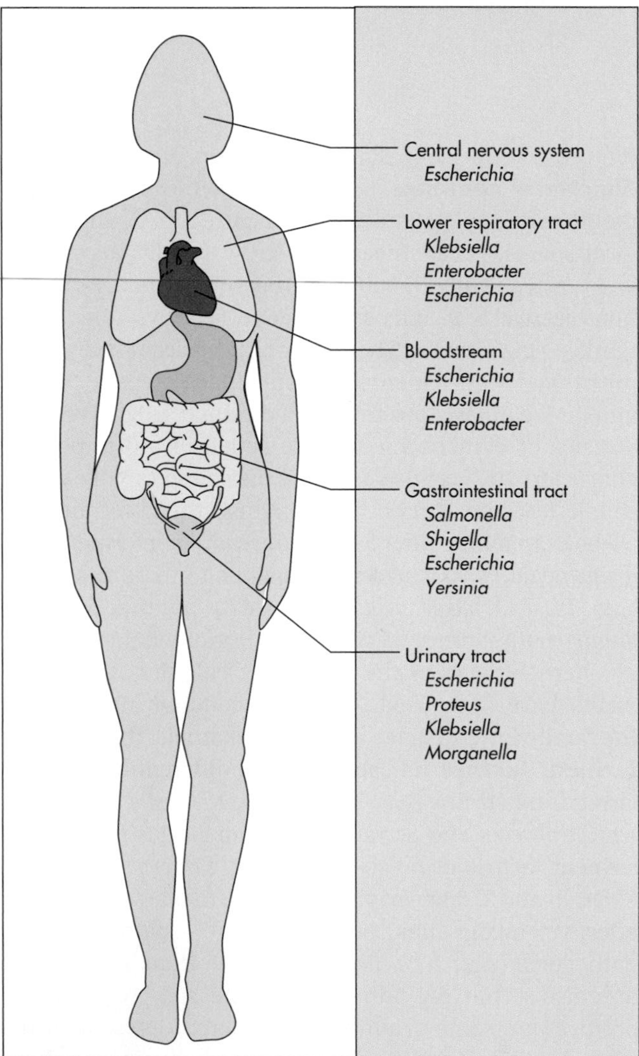

FIGURE 31–1. Sites of infections with common members of the Enterobacteriaceae listed in order of prevalence.

common antigen also occurs as a free glycolipid in the outer membrane. The serologic classification of the Enterobacteriaceae is based on three major groups of antigens: somatic O polysaccharides, capsular K antigens (type-specific polysaccharides), and the flagellar H proteins.

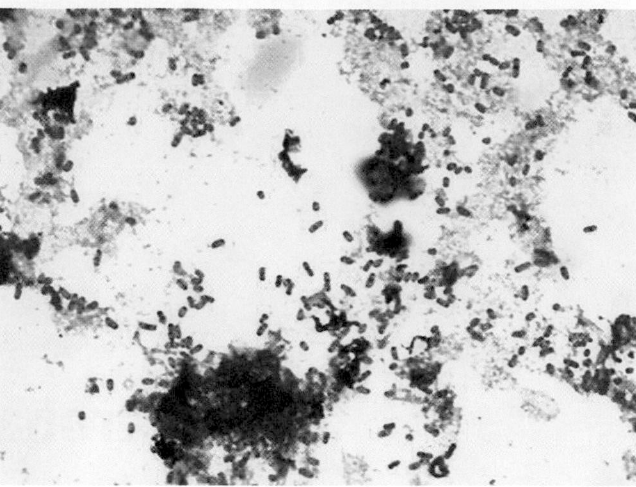

FIGURE 31–2. Gram stain of *Salmonella typhi* from a positive blood culture. Note the intense staining at the ends of the bacteria. This "bipolar staining" is characteristic of the Enterobacteriaceae.

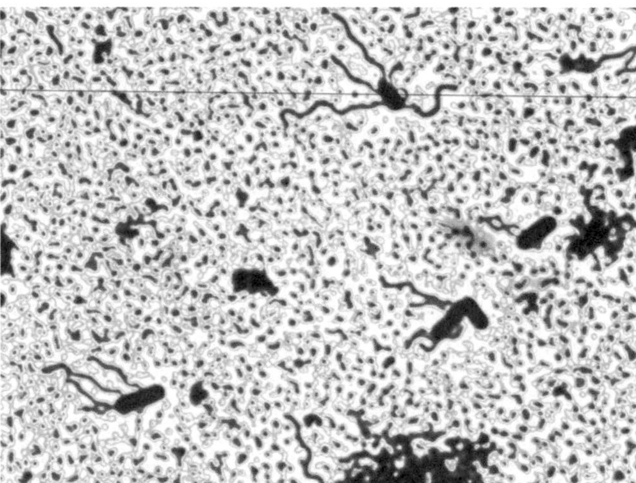

FIGURE 31–3. *Escherichia coli* stained to demonstrate peritrichous flagella.

Specific O antigens are present in each genus, although cross-reactions between closely related genera are common (e.g., *Salmonella* with *Citrobacter, Escherichia* with *Shigella*). The antigens are detected by agglutination with specific antibodies. The heat-labile K antigens may interfere with detection of the O antigens. Boiling of the organism to remove the heat-labile K antigen and expose the heat-stable O antigen circumvents this problem.

Different genera both within and outside the family Enterobacteriaceae possess K antigens; for example, *E. coli* K1 antigen is present in *Neisseria meningitidis* and *Haemophilus influenzae,* and *K. pneumoniae* cross-reacts with *Streptococcus pneumoniae.* The H antigens are heat-labile flagellar proteins. They may be absent from a cell, or they may undergo antigenic variation and be present in two phases.

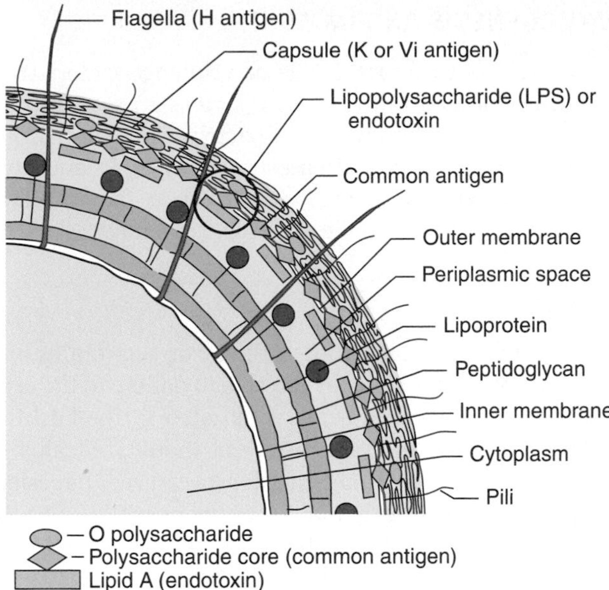

FIGURE 31–4. Antigenic structure of Enterobacteriaceae.

BOX 31–2. Common Virulence Factors Associated with Enterobacteriaceae

- Endotoxin
- Capsule
- Antigenic phase variation
- Sequestration of growth factors
- Resistance to serum killing
- Antimicrobial resistance

Most Enterobacteriaceae are motile with the exception of the common isolates *Klebsiella, Shigella,* and *Yersinia.* The motile strains possess peritrichous **flagella** (distributed over the surface of the bacteria as opposed to polar flagella that are at one or both ends). Many Enterobacteriaceae also possess fimbriae (also referred to as pili), which have been subdivided into two general classes: chromosomally mediated common fimbriae and sex pili that are encoded on conjugative plasmids. The **common fimbriae** are important for the ability of bacteria to adhere to specific host cell receptors, whereas the **sex or conjugative pili** facilitate genetic transfer between bacteria.

Pathogenesis and Immunity

Numerous virulence factors have been identified in the members of the family Enterobacteriaceae. Some are common to all genera (Box 31–2), and others are unique to specific virulent strains.

ENDOTOXIN

Endotoxin is a virulence factor shared among aerobic and some anaerobic gram-negative bacteria. The activity of this toxin depends on the lipid A component of LPS, which is released at cell lysis. Many of the systemic manifestations of gram-negative bacterial infections are initiated by endotoxin, including the following: activation of complement, release of cytokines, leukocytosis, thrombocytopenia, disseminated intravascular coagulation, fever, decreased peripheral circulation, shock, and death.

CAPSULE

Encapsulated Enterobacteriaceae are protected from phagocytosis by the hydrophilic capsular antigens, which repel the hydrophobic phagocytic cell surface. These antigens interfere with the binding of antibodies to the bacteria and are poor immunogens or activators of complement. The protective role of the capsule is diminished, however, if the patient develops specific anticapsular antibodies.

ANTIGENIC PHASE VARIATION

The expression of capsular K and flagellar H antigens is under the genetic control of the organism. Each of these antigens can be alternately expressed or not expressed (phase variation), a feature that protects the bacteria from antibody-mediated cell death.

TYPE III SECRETION SYSTEMS

A variety of distinct bacteria (e.g., *Yersinia, Salmonella, Shigella,* enteropathogenic *Escherichia, Pseudomonas, Chlamydia*) have a common effector system for delivering their virulence factors into targeted eukaryotic cells. Think of the **type III secretion system** as a molecular syringe consisting of approximately 20 proteins that facilitate secretion of bacterial virulence factors when the bacteria come into contact with the host cells. Although the virulence factors and their effects differ among the various gram-negative rods, the general mechanism by which the virulence factors are introduced is the same. In the absence of the type III secretion system, the bacteria lose their virulence.

SEQUESTRATION OF GROWTH FACTORS

Nutrients are provided to the organisms in enriched culture media, but the bacteria must become nutritional scavengers when growing in vivo. Iron is an important growth factor required by bacteria, but it is bound in heme proteins (e.g., hemoglobin, myoglobin) or in iron-chelating proteins (e.g., transferrin, lactoferrin). The bacteria counteract the binding by producing their own competitive siderophores or iron-chelating compounds (e.g., **enterobactin, aerobactin**). Iron can also be released from host cells by hemolysins produced by the bacteria.

RESISTANCE TO SERUM KILLING

Whereas many bacteria can be rapidly cleared from blood, virulent organisms capable of producing systemic infections are often resistant to serum killing. Although the bacterial capsule can protect the organism from serum killing, other factors prevent the binding of complement components to the bacteria and subsequent complement-mediated clearance.

ANTIMICROBIAL RESISTANCE

As rapidly as new antibiotics are introduced, organisms can develop resistance to them. This resistance can be encoded on transferable plasmids and exchanged among species, genera, and even families of bacteria.

Escherichia coli (Box 31–3)

The genus *Escherichia* consists of five species, of which *E. coli* is the most common and clinically most important. This organism is associated with a variety of diseases, including sepsis, UTIs, meningitis, and gastroenteritis. As expected, the multitude of strains capable of causing disease is reflected in the antigenic diversity of the bacteria. Many O, H, and K antigens have been described, and they are used to classify the isolates for epidemiologic purposes. Specific antigenic serogroups are also associated with greater virulence.

BOX 31–3. Specialized Virulence Factors Associated with Escherichia coli

Adhesins
Colonization factor antigens CFA/I, CFA/II, and CFA/III
Aggregative adherence fimbriae AAF/I and AAF/II
Bundle-forming pili (Bfp)
Intimin
P pili
Ipa protein
Dr fimbriae

Exotoxins
Heat-stable toxins STa and STb
Shiga toxins Stx-1 and Stx-2
Hemolysin HlyA
Heat-labile toxins LT-I and LT-II

PATHOGENESIS AND IMMUNITY

E. coli possesses a broad range of virulence factors (Box 31–4). In addition to the general factors possessed by all members of the family Enterobacteriaceae, *Escherichia* strains responsible for diseases such as UTIs and gastroenteritis possess specialized virulence factors. Two general categories are adhesins and exotoxins.

Adhesins

E. coli is able to remain in the urinary or gastrointestinal tract because the organisms are able to adhere to the cells at these sites and avoid being eliminated by the flushing action of voided urine or intestinal motility. Strains of *E. coli* possess numerous highly specialized adhesins. They include colonization factor antigens (CFA/I, CFA/II, CFA/III), aggregative adherence fimbriae (AAF/I, AAF/III), bundle-forming pili (Bfp), intimin, P pili (which also binds to P blood group antigens), Ipa (invasion plasmid antigen) protein, and Dr fimbriae (which bind to Dr blood group antigens).

Exotoxins

E. coli also produces a diverse spectrum of exotoxins. These include Shiga toxins (Stx-1, Stx-2), heat-stable toxins (STa and STb), and heat-labile toxins (LT-I and LT-II). Additionally, hemolysins (HlyA) are considered important in the pathogenesis of disease caused by uropathogenic *E. coli*. The following sections describe the precise mechanisms by which these toxins function.

EPIDEMIOLOGY

Large numbers of *E. coli* are present in the gastrointestinal tract, and the bacteria are common causes of sepsis, neonatal meningitis, infections of the urinary tract, and gastroenteritis. For example, *E. coli* are (1) the most common gram-negative rods isolated from patients with sepsis (Figure 31–5), (2) responsible for causing more than 80% of all community-acquired UTIs, as well as many hospital-acquired infections, and (3) a prominent cause of gastroenteritis in developing countries. Most infections (with the exception of neonatal meningitis and gastroenteritis) are endogenous; that is, the *E. coli* that are part of the patient's normal microbial flora are able to establish infection when the patient's defenses are compromised.

CLINICAL DISEASES

Septicemia

Typically, septicemia caused by gram-negative rods such as *E. coli* originates from infections in the urinary or

BOX 31–4. Summary of Escherichia coli

Physiology and Structure

Gram-negative, facultative anaerobic rods

Fermenter; oxidase negative

Outer membrane makes the organisms susceptible to drying

Lipopolysaccharide consists of outer somatic O polysaccharide, core polysaccharide (common antigen), and lipid A (endotoxin)

Virulence

Refer to Boxes 31–2 and 31–3

Endotoxin

Permeability barrier of outer membrane

Adhesins (e.g., colonization factor antigen, Dr adhesins)

Exotoxins (e.g., heat-stable and heat-labile enterotoxins, Shiga toxins)

Invasive capacity

Epidemiology

Most common aerobic, gram-negative rods in the gastrointestinal tract

Most infections are endogenous (patient's normal microbial flora)

Strains causing gastroenteritis are generally acquired exogenously

Diseases

Bacteremia (most commonly isolated gram-negative rod in the United States)

Urinary tract infection (most common cause of bacterial UTIs); limited to bladder (cystitis) or can spread to kidneys (pyelonephritis) or prostate (prostatitis)

At least five different pathogenic groups cause gastroenteritis (EPEC, ETEC, EHEC, EIEC, EAEC); most cause diseases in developing countries, although EHEC is an important cause of hemorrhagic colitis (HC) and hemolytic uremic syndrome (HUS) in the United States

Neonatal meningitis (usually with strains carrying the K1 capsular antigen)

Intraabdominal infections (associated with intestinal perforation)

Diagnosis

Organisms grow rapidly on most culture media

Enteric pathogens with the exception of EHEC are detected only in reference or research laboratories

Treatment, Prevention, and Control

Enteric pathogens are treated symptomatically unless disseminated disease occurs

Antibiotic therapy is guided by in vitro susceptibility tests

Appropriate infection-control practices are used to reduce the risk of nosocomial infections (e.g., restricting use of antibiotics, avoiding unnecessary use of urinary tract catheters)

Maintenance of high hygienic standards to reduce the risk of exposure to gastroenteritis strains

Proper cooking of beef products to reduce risk of EHEC infections

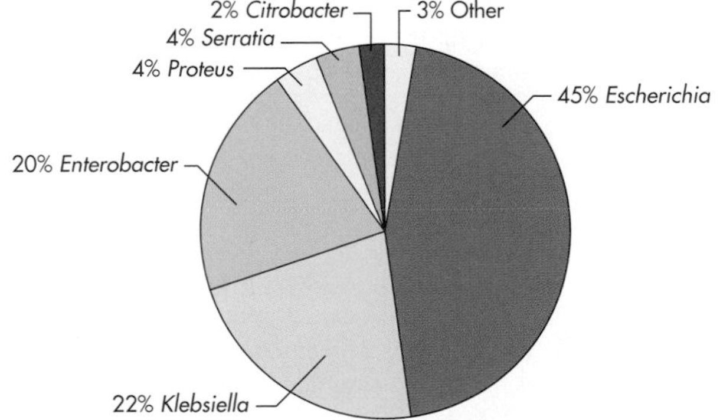

FIGURE 31–5. Incidence of Enterobacteriaceae associated with bacteremia. (Data courtesy Barnes-Jewish Hospital, St. Louis.)

gastrointestinal tract (e.g., intestinal perforation leading to an intraabdominal infection). The mortality associated with *E. coli* septicemia is high for patients in whom immunity is compromised or the primary infection is in the abdomen or central nervous system (CNS).

Urinary Tract Infection

Most gram-negative rods that produce UTIs originate in the colon, contaminate the urethra, ascend into the bladder, and may migrate to the kidney or prostate. Although most strains of *E. coli* can produce UTIs, disease is more common with certain specific serogroups. These bacteria are particularly virulent because of their ability to produce adhesins (primarily P pili, Type I fimbriae, and Dr), which bind to cells lining the bladder and upper urinary tract (preventing the elimination of the bacteria in voided urine), and hemolysin HlyA, which lyses erythrocytes and other cell types (leading to cytokine release and stimulation of an inflammatory response).

Neonatal Meningitis

E. coli and group B streptococci cause the majority of CNS infections in infants younger than 1 month. Approximately 75% of the *E. coli* strains possess the K1 capsular antigen. This serogroup is also commonly present in the gastrointestinal tracts of pregnant women and newborn infants. However, the reason this serogroup has a predilection for causing disease in newborns is not understood.

Gastroenteritis

The strains of *E. coli* that cause gastroenteritis are subdivided into the following five major groups: enteropathogenic (EPEC), enterotoxigenic (ETEC), enterohemorrhagic (EHEC), enteroinvasive (EIEC), and enteroaggregative (EAEC) *E. coli* (Table 31–1).

EPEC

Enteropathogenic *E. coli* was the first *E. coli* associated with diarrheal disease and remains a major cause of infant diarrhea in impoverished countries. Disease is rare in older children and adults, presumably because they have developed protective immunity. Although specific O serogroups have been associated with outbreaks of EPEC diarrhea in nurseries, the serotyping of the *E. coli* isolated in random or endemic disease is discouraged except in epidemiologic investigations.

Disease is characterized by bacterial attachment to epithelial cells of the small intestine, with subsequent effacement (destruction) of the microvillus **(attachment/effacement [A/E] histopathology).** The genes compromising the "locus of enterocyte effacement (LEE)" reside on a pathogenicity island. This island of more than 40 genes mediates attachment and destruction of the host mucosal surface. EPEC strains form microcolonies on the epithelial cell surface with the bacteria attached to the host cells by means of cuplike pedestals. Initially a loose attachment mediated by bundle-forming pili occurs, followed by active secretion of proteins by the bacterial type III secretion system into the host epithelial cell. One protein, **translocated intimin receptor (Tir),** is inserted into the epithelial cell membrane (this process is mediated by two other secreted proteins) and functions as a receptor for an outer membrane bacterial adhesin, **intimin.** The watery diarrhea characteristic of this disease results in part from malabsorption caused by microvilli destruction.

ETEC

Disease caused by **enterotoxigenic *E. coli*** is seen most commonly in developing countries (an estimated 650 million cases per year), although almost 80,000 cases are estimated to occur annually in travelers from the United States. Infections are observed in either young children in developing countries or travelers to these areas. The inoculum for disease is high, so infections are primarily acquired through consumption of fecally contaminated food or water. Person-to-person spread does not occur.

ETEC produce two classes of enterotoxins: heat-labile toxins (LT-I, LT-II) and heat-stable toxins (STa and STb).

TABLE 31–1. Gastroenteritis Caused by *Escherichia coli*

Organism	Site of Action	Disease	Pathogenesis
Enteropathogenic *E. coli* (EPEC)	Small intestine	Infant diarrhea in underdeveloped countries; watery diarrhea and vomiting, nonbloody stools	Chromosomal A/E histopathology with disruption of normal microvillus structure resulting in malabsorption and diarrhea
Enterotoxigenic *E. coli* (ETEC)	Small intestine	Traveler's diarrhea; infant diarrhea in developing countries; watery diarrhea, vomiting, cramps, nausea, low-grade fever	Plasmid-mediated, heat-stable and/or heat-labile enterotoxins that stimulate hypersecretion of fluids and electrolytes
Enterohemorrhagic *E. coli* (EHEC)	Large intestine	Initial watery diarrhea, followed by grossly bloody diarrhea (hemorrhagic colitis) with abdominal cramps; little or no fever; may progress to hemolytic uremic syndrome (HUS)	Mediated by cytotoxic Shiga toxins (Stx-1, Stx-2), which disrupt protein synthesis; A/E lesions with destruction of intestinal microvillus resulting in decreased absorption
Enteroinvasive *E. coli* (EIEC)	Large intestine	Disease in underdeveloped countries; fever, cramping, watery diarrhea; may progress to dysentery with scant, bloody stools	Plasmid-mediated invasion and destruction of epithelial cells lining colon
Enteroaggregative *E. coli* (EAEC)	Small intestine	Infant diarrhea in underdeveloped countries; traveler's diarrhea; persistent watery diarrhea with vomiting, dehydration, and low-grade fever	Plasmid-mediated aggregative adherence of rods ("stacked bricks") with shortening of microvilli, mononuclear infiltration, and hemorrhage; decreased fluid absorption

A/E, Attachment/effacement.

Whereas LT-II is not associated with human disease, LT-I is functionally and structurally similar to cholera toxin (see Chapter 32) and is associated with human disease. This toxin consists of one A subunit and five identical B subunits. The B subunits bind to the same receptor as cholera toxin (GM_1 gangliosides), as well as other surface glycoproteins on epithelial cells in the small intestine.

After endocytosis, the A subunit of LT-I translocates across the membrane of the vacuole. The A subunit has adenosine diphosphate (ADP)-ribosyltransferase activity and interacts with a membrane protein (Gs) that regulates adenylate cyclase. The net effect of this interaction is an increase in cyclic adenosine monophosphate (cAMP) levels, with enhanced secretion of chloride and a decreased absorption of sodium and chloride. These changes are manifested in a watery diarrhea. Exposure to the toxin also stimulates prostaglandin secretion and production of inflammatory cytokines, resulting in further fluid loss.

STa, but not STb, is associated with human disease. STa is a small, monomeric peptide that binds to the transmembrane guanylate cyclase receptor, leading to an increase in the level of cyclic guanosine monophosphate and subsequent hypersecretion of fluids. Genes for LT-I and STa are present on a transferable plasmid, which can also carry the genes for adhesins (CFA/I, CFA/II, CFA/III). The colonization factors are fimbriae that recognize specific host glycoprotein receptors (define the host specificity). Both the toxin and colonization factors are required for disease to develop.

Secretory diarrhea caused by ETEC develops after a 1- to 2-day incubation period and persists for an average of 3 to 4 days. The symptoms (watery diarrhea and abdominal cramps; nausea and vomiting are less commonly observed) are similar to those of cholera but are milder. Neither histologic changes of the intestinal mucosa nor inflammation is observed. Disease mediated by heat-labile toxin is indistinguishable from that mediated by heat-stable toxin. Toxin production is not associated with specific serogroups, so culture combined with immunoassays for the detection of the heat-labile and heat-stable toxins must be performed. Commercial assays have been developed that detect toxin in cell cultures, but these tests are primarily used in reference labs.

EHEC

Enterohemorrhagic *E. coli* strains are the most common strains producing disease in developed countries. It is estimated that these bacteria cause 73,000 infections and 60 deaths each year in the United States. The ingestion of fewer than 100 bacteria can produce disease. The severity of the disease caused by EHEC ranges from mild, uncomplicated diarrhea to **hemorrhagic colitis** with severe abdominal pain, bloody diarrhea, and little or no fever. More than 50 serogroups of EHEC have been isolated; however, the majority that cause human disease in the United States are believed to be serotype O157 : H7.

Hemolytic uremic syndrome (HUS), a disorder characterized by acute renal failure, thrombocytopenia, and microangiopathic hemolytic anemia, is a complication in 5% to 10% of infected children younger than 10 years. EHEC disease is most common in the warm months, and the highest incidence is in children younger than 5 years. Most cases of disease have been attributed to the consumption of undercooked ground beef or other meat products, water, unpasteurized milk or fruit juices (e.g., cider made from apples contaminated with feces from cattle), uncooked vegetables, and fruits.

Initially, a nonbloody diarrhea with abdominal pain develops in patients after 3 to 4 days of incubation. Vomiting is observed in approximately half the patients. Within 2 days of onset, disease in 30% to 65% of patients progresses to a bloody diarrhea with severe abdominal pain. Complete resolution of symptoms typically occurs after 4 to 10 days in most untreated patients; however, HUS is a serious complication, particularly in young children. Death can occur in 3% to 5% of patients with HUS, and severe sequelae (e.g., renal impairment, hypertension, CNS manifestations) can occur in as many as 30% of patients.

EHEC strains express a Shiga toxin (i.e., Stx-1, Stx-2, or both), induce A/E lesions on epithelial cells, and possess a 60-MDa plasmid that carries genes for other virulence factors. Stx-1 is essentially identical to the Shiga toxin produced by *Shigella dysenteriae;* Stx-2 has 60% homology. Both toxins are acquired by lysogenic bacteriophages. Both have one A subunit and five B subunits, with the B subunits binding to a specific glycolipid on the host cell (globotriaosylceramide, GB_3). A high concentration of GB_3 receptors is found in the intestinal villus and renal endothelial cells. After the A subunit is internalized, it is cleaved into two molecules, and the A_1 fragment binds to 28S ribosomal ribonucleic acid (rRNA) and disrupts protein synthesis. Destruction of the intestinal villus results in decreased absorption with a relative increase in fluid secretion.

HUS has been preferentially associated with the production of Stx-2, which has been shown to destroy glomerular endothelial cells. Damage to the endothelial cells leads to platelet activation and thrombin deposition, which in turn results in decreased glomerular filtration and acute renal failure. The Shiga toxins also stimulate expression of inflammatory cytokines (e.g., tumor necrosis factor [TNF]-α, interleukin [IL]-6), which among other effects enhance expression of GB_3.

Two approaches have been used to detect EHEC: culture and toxin detection. In contrast with most *E. coli,* many O157 strains do not ferment sorbitol. Sorbitol-containing MacConkey agar (S-MAC) has been used to screen stool specimens for sorbitol-negative (colorless), gram-negative bacteria that are then confirmed by serogrouping and biochemical tests to be 0157 *E. coli.* The limitations to this approach are some strains of 0157 and many other EHEC serotypes ferment sorbitol and toxin production is not assessed. The preferred method to detect EHEC is to culture stool specimens on nonselective MacConkey agar and then to assay isolated colonies for toxin production by commercially available immunoassays. Unfortunately, the direct detection of toxin in stool samples is currently too insensitive to recommend.

EIEC

Enteroinvasive *E. coli* strains are rare in the United States and uncommon in developing countries. Pathogenic strains are primarily associated with a few restricted O serotypes: O124, O143, and O164. The strains are closely related by phenotypic and pathogenic properties to *Shigella.* The bacteria are able to invade and destroy the colonic epithelium, producing a disease characterized initially by watery diarrhea. A minority of patients progress to the dysenteric form of disease, consisting of fever, abdominal cramps, and blood and leukocytes in stool specimens. A series of bacterial genes carried on a plasmid mediate invasion **(Shingella virulence plasmid)** into the colonic epithelium. The bacteria then lyse the phagocytic vacuole and replicate in the cell cytoplasm. Movement within the cytoplasm and into adjacent epithelial cells is regulated by formation of actin tails (similar to that observed with *Listeria*). This process of epithelial cell destruction with inflammatory infiltration can progress to colonic ulceration. Detection of EIEC strains is restricted to research laboratories. Although immunoassays and nucleic acid based assays have been developed for detecting invasion-related factors, the usefulness of these assays is limited by the fact the genes for these virulence factors reside on a large plasmid that is rapidly lost in vitro.

EAEC

Enteroaggregative *E. coli* strains have been implicated as a cause of often persistent diarrhea in children and adults in both developing and developed countries. The persistence of these bacteria is associated with chronic diarrhea and growth retardation in children in developing countries. The bacteria are characterized by their autoagglutination in a "stacked-brick" arrangement. This process is mediated by bundle-forming fimbriae (aggregative adherence fimbriae I and II), which are carried on a plasmid. EAEC stimulate secretion of mucus, which traps the bacteria in a biofilm overlying the epithelium of the small intestine. Shortening of the microvilli, mononuclear infiltration, and hemorrhage are then observed. A cytotoxin has not been demonstrated but is likely to be present. Diagnosis of these infections is primarily restricted to research laboratories.

Salmonella (Box 31–5)

The taxonomic classification of the genus *Salmonella* is problematic. On one hand deoxyribonucleic acid (DNA) homology studies have revealed that the genus consists of two species: *Salmonella enterica* and *Shigella bongori. S. enterica* is further subdivided into six subspecies, with most human pathogens in the first subspecies, *S. enterica* subsp. *enterica.* Unfortunately, the two species have been subdivided into more than 2500 unique serotypes; historically, the numerous serotypes have been referred to as species (e.g., *S. typhi, Salmonella typhimurium, Salmonella enteritidis*). In an effort to prevent confusion, this approach is used in this section. As a practical matter, it is important to differentiate *S. typhi* from the other *Salmonella* serotypes.

PATHOGENESIS AND IMMUNITY

After ingestion and passage through the stomach, salmonellae are able to invade and replicate in the **M (microfold) cells** that are located in Peyer's patches of the terminal portion of the small intestine. These cells typically transport foreign antigens to the underlying macrophages for clearance. Two separate type III secretion systems mediate the initial invasion into the intestinal mucosa (*Salmonella* pathogenicity island 1 **[SPI-1]**) and subsequent systemic disease **(SPI-2).** Binding to M cells is mediated by species-specific fimbriae. The SPI-1 secretion system then introduces salmonella-secreted invasion proteins (**Sips** or **Ssps**) into the M cells, resulting in rearrangement of the host cell actin with subsequent membrane ruffling. The ruffled membranes surround and engulf salmonellae, leading to intracellular replication in the phagosome with subsequent host cell death and spread to adjacent epithelial cells and lymphoid tissue. The inflammatory response confines the infection to the gastrointestinal tract, mediates the release of prostaglandins, and stimulates cAMP and active fluid secretion.

Salmonella species are also protected from stomach acids and the acid pH of the phagosome by an **acid tolerance response (ATR) gene.** Catalase and superoxide dismutase are other factors that protect the bacteria from intracellular killing.

EPIDEMIOLOGY

Salmonella can colonize virtually all animals, including poultry, reptiles, livestock, rodents, domestic animals, birds, and humans. Animal-to-animal spread and the use

BOX 31–5. Summary of *Salmonella*

Physiology and Structure
Gram-negative, facultative anaerobic rods
Fermenter; oxidase negative
Outer membrane makes the organisms susceptible to drying
Lipopolysaccharide consists of outer somatic O polysaccharide, core polysaccharide (common antigen), and lipid A (endotoxin)
More than 2500 O serotypes (commonly referred to as individual *Salmonella* species)

Virulence
Refer to Box 31–2
Tolerant to acids in phagocytic vesicles
Can survive in macrophages and spread from the intestine to other body sites (particularly true of *S. typhi*)
Endotoxin

Epidemiology
Most infections are acquired by eating contaminated food products (poultry, eggs, and dairy products are the most common sources of infection)
Direct fecal-oral spread in children
S. typhi and *S. paratyphi* are strict human pathogens (no other reservoirs); asymptomatic long-term colonization occurs commonly
Individuals at risk for infection include those who eat improperly cooked poultry or eggs, patients with reduced gastric acid levels, and immunocompromised patients (especially patients infected with AIDS)
Infections occur worldwide, particularly in the warm months of the year

Diseases
Asymptomatic colonization (primarily with *S. typhi* and *S. paratyphi*)
Enteric fever (also called typhoid fever [*S. typhi*] or paratyphoid fever [*S. paratyphi*])
Enteritis characterized by fever, nausea, vomiting, bloody or nonbloody diarrhea, and abdominal cramps
Bacteremia (most commonly seen with *S. typhi, S. paratyphi, S. choleraesuis,* and *S. enteritidis*)

Diagnosis
Isolation from stool specimens requires use of selective media

Treatment, Prevention, and Control
Antibiotic treatment not recommended for enteritis because may prolong duration of disease
Infections with *S. typhi* and *S. paratyphi* or disseminated infections with other organisms should be treated with an effective antibiotic (selected by in vitro susceptibility tests); fluoroquinolones (e.g., ciprofloxacin), chloramphenicol, trimethoprim-sulfamethoxazole, or a broad-spectrum cephalosporin may be used
Most infections can be controlled by proper preparation of poultry and eggs (completely cooked) and avoidance of contamination of other foods with uncooked poultry products
Carriers of *S. typhi* and *S. paratyphi* should be identified and treated
Vaccination against *S. typhi* can reduce the risk of disease for travelers into endemic areas

of *Salmonella*-contaminated animal feeds maintain an animal reservoir. Serotypes such as *S. typhi* and *Salmonella paratyphi* are highly adapted to humans and do not cause disease in nonhuman hosts. Other *Salmonella* strains (e.g., *Salmonella choleraesuis*) are adapted to animals and, when they infect humans, can cause severe disease. Finally, many strains have no host specificity and cause disease in both human and nonhuman hosts.

Most infections result from the ingestion of contaminated food products and, in children, from direct fecal-oral spread. The incidence of disease is greatest in children younger than 5 years and adults older than 60 years, who are infected during the summer and autumn months, when contaminated foods are consumed at outdoor social gatherings. The most common sources of human infections are poultry, eggs, dairy products, and foods prepared on contaminated work surfaces (e.g., cutting boards where uncooked poultry was prepared). Approximately 40,000 cases of nontyphoidal *Salmonella* infections were reported in the United States in 2004, although it has been estimated that more than 1.4 million infections and 600 deaths occur each year. *S. typhi* infections occur when food or water contaminated by infected food handlers is ingested. There is no animal reservoir. A total of 283 *S. typhi* infections was reported in the United States in 2004, most of which were acquired during foreign travel. In contrast, it is estimated that 21 million *S. typhi* infections and 200,000 deaths occur each year worldwide. The risk of disease is highest in children living in poverty in a developing country. For example, in Bamako, Mali, the two most common enteric gram-negative rods causing bacteremia in pediatric patients are *S. typhi* and *S. paratyphi.*

The infectious dose for Salmonella typhi, Salmonella paratyphi, and other Salmonella species that results in symptomatic disease is generally large (e.g., 10^5 to 10^8 bacteria), so person to person spread in the absence of contaminated food or water is uncommon. The organisms can multiply to this high density if contaminated food products are improperly stored (e.g., left at room temperature). The infectious dose is lower for people at high risk for disease because of age, immunosuppression or underlying disease (leukemia, lymphoma, sickle cell disease), or reduced gastric acidity.

CLINICAL DISEASES

The following four forms of *Salmonella* infection exist: gastroenteritis, septicemia, enteric fever, and asymptomatic colonization.

Gastroenteritis

Gastroenteritis is the most common form of salmonellosis, with more than one million annual infections in the U.S. Symptoms generally appear 6 to 48 hours after the consumption of contaminated food or water, with the initial presentation consisting of nausea, vomiting, and nonbloody diarrhea. Fever, abdominal cramps, myalgias, and headache are also common. Colonic involvement can be demonstrated in the acute form of the disease. Symptoms can persist from 2 days to 1 week before spontaneous resolution.

Septicemia

All *Salmonella* species can cause bacteremia, although infections with *S. choleraesuis, S. paratyphi,* and *S. typhi* more commonly lead to a bacteremic phase. The risk for *Salmonella* bacteremia is higher in pediatric and geriatric patients and in patients with the acquired immune deficiency syndrome (AIDS). The clinical presentation of *Salmonella* bacteremia is like that of other gram-negative bacteremias; however, localized suppurative infections (e.g., osteomyelitis, endocarditis, arthritis) can occur in as many as 10% of patients.

Enteric Fever

S. typhi produce a febrile illness called **typhoid fever.** A milder form of this disease, referred to as **paratyphoid fever,** is produced by *S. paratyphi A, Salmonella schottmuelleri* (formerly *S. paratyphi B*), and *Salmonella hirschfeldii* (formerly *S. paratyphi C*). In contrast to other *Salmonella* infections, the bacteria responsible for enteric fever pass through the cells lining the intestines and are engulfed by macrophages. They replicate after being transported to the liver, spleen, and bone marrow. Ten to 14 days after ingestion of the rods, patients experience gradually increasing fever with nonspecific complaints of headache, myalgias, malaise, and anorexia. These symptoms persist for a week or longer and are followed by gastrointestinal symptoms. This cycle corresponds to an initial bacteremic phase that is followed by colonization of the gallbladder and then reinfection of the intestines.

Asymptomatic Colonization

The species of *Salmonella* responsible for causing typhoid and paratyphoid fevers are maintained by human colonization. Chronic colonization for more than 1 year after symptomatic disease develops in 1% to 5% of patients, the gallbladder being the reservoir in most patients. Chronic colonization with other species of *Salmonella* occurs in less than 1% of patients and does not represent an important source of human infection.

Shigella (Box 31–6)

The commonly used taxonomic classification of *Shigella* is simple, although technically incorrect. Four species consisting of more than 45 O antigen–based serogroups have been described: *S. dysenteriae, Shigella flexneri, Shigella boydii,* and *Shigella sonnei. S. sonnei* is the most common cause of shigellosis in the industrial world, and *S. flexneri* is the most common cause in developing countries. However, analysis of DNA has determined that these four species are actually serologically distinct biogroups within *E. coli.* Because it would be confusing to refer to these bacteria as *E. coli,* their historical names have been retained.

PATHOGENESIS AND IMMUNITY

Shigella cause disease by invading and replicating in cells lining the colonic mucosa. Structural gene proteins mediate the adherence of the organisms to the cells, as well as their invasion, intracellular replication, and cell-to-cell spread. These genes are carried on a large virulence plasmid but are regulated by chromosomal genes. Thus the presence of the plasmid does not ensure functional gene activity.

Shigella species appear unable to attach to differentiated mucosal cells; rather, they first attach to and invade the M cells located in Peyer's patches. The type III secretion system mediates secretion of four proteins **(IpaA, IpaB, IpaC, IpaD)** into epithelial cells and macrophages. These proteins induce membrane ruffling on the target cell, leading to engulfment of the bacteria. Shigella lyse the phagocytic vacuole and replicate in the host cell cytoplasm (unlike *Salmonella,* which replicate in the vacuole). With the rearrangement of actin filaments in the host cells, the bacteria are propelled through the cytoplasm to adjacent cells, where cell-to-cell passage occurs. In this way, *Shigella* organisms are protected from immune-mediated clearance. Shigellae survive phagocytosis by inducing programmed cell death **(apoptosis).** This process also leads to the release of IL-1β, resulting in the attraction of polymorphonuclear leukocytes into the infected tissues. This in turn destabilizes the integrity of the intestinal wall and allows the bacteria to reach the deeper epithelial cells.

S. dysenteriae produce an exotoxin, **Shiga toxin.** Like the toxin produced by EHEC, the Shiga toxin has one A subunit and five B subunits. The B subunits bind to a host cell glycolipid (GB_3) and facilitate transfer of the A subunit

BOX 31–6. Summary of *Shigella*

Physiology and Structure

Gram-negative, facultatively anaerobic rods
Fermenter; oxidase negative
Outer membrane makes the organisms susceptible to drying
Lipopolysaccharide consists of somatic O polysaccharide, core polysaccharide (common antigen), and lipid A (endotoxin)
Four species recognized: *S. sonnei* responsible for most infections in developed countries; *S. flexneri* for infections in developing countries; *S. dysenteriae* for the most severe infections; and *S. boydii* is not commonly isolated

Virulence

Refer to Box 31–2
Endotoxin and genes for adherence, invasion, and intracellular replication
Permeability barrier of outer membrane
Exotoxin (Shiga toxin) is produced by *S. dysenteriae;* disrupts protein synthesis and produces endothelial damage
Hemolytic colitis (HC) and hemolytic uremic syndrome (HUS) associated with *S. dysenteriae*

Epidemiology

Humans are only reservoir for these bacteria
Disease spread person to person by fecal-oral route
Patients at highest risk for disease are young children in daycare centers, nurseries, and custodial institutions; siblings and parents of these children; male homosexuals
Relatively few organisms can produce disease (highly infectious)
Disease occurs worldwide with no seasonal incidence (consistent with person-to-person spread involving a low inoculum)

Diseases

Gastroenteritis (shigellosis)
Most common form is an initial watery diarrhea progressing within 1 to 2 days to abdominal cramps and tenesmus (with or without bloody stools)
Asymptomatic carriage develops in a small number of patients (reservoir for future infections)
A severe form of disease is caused by *S. dysenteriae* (bacterial dysentery)

Diagnosis

Isolation from stool specimens requires use of selective media

Treatment, Prevention, and Control

Antibiotic therapy shortens the course of symptomatic disease and fecal shedding
Treatment should be guided by in vitro susceptibility tests
Empiric therapy can be initiated with a fluoroquinolone or trimethoprim-sulfamethoxazole
Appropriate infection control measures should be instituted to prevent spread of the organism, including hand washing and proper disposal of soiled linens

into the cell. The A subunit cleaves the 28S rRNA in the 60S ribosomal subunit, thereby preventing the binding of aminoacyl-transfer RNA and disrupting protein synthesis. The primary manifestation of toxin activity is damage to the intestinal epithelium; however, in a small subset of patients, the Shiga toxin can mediate damage to the glomerular endothelial cells, resulting in renal failure (HUS).

EPIDEMIOLOGY

More than 22,500 *Shigella* infections were reported in the United States in 2003; however, it is estimated that almost 450,000 cases occur each year. This figure pales in comparison with the estimated 150 million cases that occur annually worldwide.

Shigellosis is primarily a pediatric disease; 70% of all infections occur in children younger than 15 years. Endemic disease in adults is common in male homosexuals and in household contacts of infected children. Epidemic outbreaks of disease occur in daycare centers, nurseries, and custodial institutions. Shigellosis is transmitted by the fecal-oral route, primarily by people with contaminated hands and less commonly in water or food. Because as few as 200 bacteria can establish disease, shigellosis spreads rapidly in communities where sanitary standards and the level of personal hygiene are low.

CLINICAL DISEASES

Shigellosis is characterized by abdominal cramps, diarrhea, fever, and bloody stools. The clinical signs and symptoms of the disease appear 1 to 3 days after the bacteria are ingested. Shigella initially colonize the small intestine and begin to multiply within the first 12 hours. The first sign of infection (profuse, watery diarrhea without histologic evidence of mucosal invasion) is mediated by an enterotoxin. However, the cardinal feature of shigellosis is lower abdominal cramps and tenesmus, with abundant pus and blood in the stool. It results from invasion of the colonic mucosa by the bacteria. Abundant neutrophils, erythrocytes, and mucus are found in the stool. Infection is generally self-limited, although antibiotic treatment is recommended to reduce the risk of secondary spread to family members and other contacts. Asymptomatic colonization of the organism in the colon develops in a small number of patients and represents a persistent reservoir for infection.

Yersinia (Box 31–7)

The genus *Yersinia* consists of 11 species, with *Y. pestis, Yersinia enterocolitica,* and *Yersinia pseudotuberculosis* the well-known human pathogens. *Y. enterocolitica* can be subdivided into six biogroups (1A, 1B, 2, 3, 4, and 5). 1A strains are not associated with human disease, but the other biogroups are all capable of causing human disease.

PATHOGENESIS AND IMMUNITY

Y. pestis is a highly virulent pathogen that causes systemic disease with a high mortality rate; *Y. enterocolitica* and *Y. pseudotuberculosis* are primarily enteric pathogens that are rarely isolated from blood. All three species of *Yersinia* carry plasmids with virulence genes.

A common characteristic of the pathogenic *Yersinia* species is their ability to resist phagocytic killing. The type III secretion system mediates this property. On contact with phagocytic cells, the bacteria secrete proteins into the phagocyte that dephosphorylate several proteins required for phagocytosis (YopH gene product), induce cytotoxicity by disrupting actin filaments (YopE gene product), and initiate apoptosis in macrophages (YopJ/P gene product). The type III secretion system also suppresses cytokine production, in turn diminishing the inflammatory immune response to infection.

Y. pestis has two additional plasmids that encode virulence genes: (1) fraction 1 (F1) gene, which codes for an antiphagocytic protein capsule, and (2) plasminogen activator (Pla) protease gene, whose product degrades complement components C3b and C5a, preventing opsonization and phagocytic migration, respectively. The protease also degrades fibrin clots, permitting *Y. pestis* to spread rapidly. Other virulence factors specifically associated with *Y. pestis* are serum resistance and the ability of the organism to absorb organic iron as a result of a siderophore-independent mechanism.

EPIDEMIOLOGY

All *Yersinia* infections are zoonotic, with humans the accidental hosts. There are two forms of *Y. pestis* infection,

BOX 31–7. Summary of *Yersinia*

Physiology and Structure

Gram-negative, facultatively anaerobic rods
Fermenter; oxidase negative
Outer membrane makes the organisms susceptible to drying
Lipopolysaccharide consists of somatic O polysaccharide, core polysaccharide (common antigen), and lipid A (endotoxin)
Y. pestis is covered with a protein capsule
Some species (e.g., *Y. enterocolitica*) can grow at cold temperatures (e.g., can grow to high numbers in contaminated, refrigerated food or blood products)

Virulence

Refer to Box 31–2
Capsule on *Y. pestis* is antiphagocytic
Y. pestis is also resistant to serum killing
Yersinia with genes for adherence, cytotoxic activity, inhibition of phagocytic migration and engulfment, and inhibition of platelet aggregation

Epidemiology

Y. pestis is a zoonotic infection with humans the accidental host; natural reservoirs include rats, squirrels, rabbits, and domestic animals
Disease is spread by flea bites or direct contact with infected tissues or person to person by inhalation of infectious aerosols from a patient with pulmonary disease
Other *Yersinia* infections are spread through exposure to contaminated food products or blood products *(Y. enterocolitica)*
Colonization with other *Yersinia* species can occur

Diseases

Y. pestis causes bubonic plague (most common) and pulmonary plague, both having a high mortality rate
Other *Yersinia* species cause gastroenteritis (acute watery diarrhea or chronic diarrhea) and transfusion-related sepsis
Enteric disease in children may manifest as enlarge mesenteric lymph nodes and mimic acute appendicitis

Diagnosis

Organisms grow on most culture media; prolonged storage at 4°C can selectively enhance isolation

Treatment, Prevention, and Control

Y. pestis infections are treated with streptomycin; tetracyclines, chloramphenicol, or trimethoprim-sulfamethoxazole can be administered as alternative therapy
Enteric infections with other *Yersinia* species are usually self-limited. If antibiotic therapy is indicated, most organisms are susceptible to broad-spectrum cephalosporins, aminoglycosides, chloramphenicol, tetracyclines, and trimethoprim-sulfamethoxazole
Plague is controlled by reduction of the rodent population and vaccination of individuals at risk
Other *Yersinia* infections are controlled by the proper preparation of food products

urban plague, for which rats are the natural reservoirs, and **sylvatic plague,** which causes infections in squirrels, rabbits, field rats, and domestic cats. Pigs, rodents, livestock, and rabbits are the natural reservoirs for *Y. enterocolitica,* whereas rodents, wild animals, and game birds are the natural reservoirs for *Y. pseudotuberculosis.*

Plague, caused by *Y. pestis,* was one of the most devastating diseases in history. Epidemics of the plague were recorded in the Old Testament. The first of three major pandemics (urban plague) started in Egypt in 541 AD and spread throughout North Africa, Europe, central and southern Asia, and Arabia. By the time this pandemic ended in the mid-700s, a major proportion of the population in these countries had died from the plague. The second pandemic, which started in the 1320s, resulted (over a 5-year period) in more than 25 million deaths in Europe alone (30% to 40% of the population). The third pandemic began in China in the 1860s and spread to Africa, Europe, and the Americas. Epidemic and sporadic cases of the disease continue to this day. In the last decade an average of 10 cases annually were reported in the United States, with disease (sylvatic plague) primarily in the western United States.

Urban plague is maintained in rat populations and is spread among rats, or between rats and humans by infected fleas. Fleas become infected during a blood meal from a bacteremic rat. After the bacteria replicate in the flea gut, the organisms can be transferred to another rodent or to humans. Urban plague has been eliminated from most communities by the effective control of rats and better hygiene. In contrast, sylvatic plague is difficult or impossible to eliminate because the mammalian reservoirs and flea vectors are widespread. *Y. pestis* produces a fatal infection in the animal reservoir. Thus cyclic patterns of human disease occur as the opportunity for contact with the reservoir population increases or decreases. Infections can also be acquired through the ingestion of contaminated animals or the handling of contaminated animal tissues. Although the organism is highly infectious, human-to-human spread is uncommon unless the patient has pulmonary involvement.

Y. enterocolitica is a common cause of enterocolitis in Scandinavian and other European countries and in the colder areas of North America. In the United States, approximately one culture-confirmed infection occurs per 100,000 persons each year, with 90% of the infections being associated with consumption of contaminated meat, milk, or water. Most studies show that infections are more common during the cold months. Virulence with this organism is associated with specific serogroups. The most common serogroups found in Europe, Africa, Japan, and Canada are O3 and O9. Serogroup O8 has been identified in the United States. *Y. pseudotuberculosis* is a relatively uncommon cause of human disease.

CLINICAL DISEASES

The two clinical manifestations of *Y. pestis* infection are bubonic plague and pneumonic plague. **Bubonic plague** is characterized by an incubation period of no more than 7 days after a person has been bitten by an infected flea. Patients have a high fever and a painful bubo (inflammatory swelling of the lymph nodes) in the groin or axilla. Bacteremia develops rapidly if patients are not treated, and as many as 75% die. The incubation period (2 to 3 days) is shorter in patients with **pneumonic plague.** Initially, these patients experience fever and malaise, and pulmonary signs develop within 1 day. The patients are highly infectious; person-to-person spread occurs by aerosols. The mortality rate in untreated patients with pneumonic plague exceeds 90%.

Approximately two-thirds of all *Y. enterocolitica* infections are enterocolitis, as the name implies. The gastroenteritis is typically associated with ingestion of contaminated food products or water. After an incubation period of 1 to 10 days (average, 4 to 6 days), the patient experiences disease characterized by diarrhea, fever, and abdominal pain that last for as long as 1 to 2 weeks. A chronic form of the disease can also develop and persist for months. Disease involves the terminal ileum and, if the mesenteric lymph nodes become enlarged, can mimic acute appendicitis. *Y. enterocolitica* infection is most common in children, with pseudoappendicitis posing a particular problem in this age group. *Y. pseudotuberculosis* can also produce an enteric disease with the same clinical features. Other manifestations seen in adults are septicemia, arthritis, intraabdominal abscess, hepatitis, and osteomyelitis.

In 1987, *Y. enterocolitica* was first reported to cause blood transfusion–related bacteremia and endotoxic shock. Because *Yersinia* organisms can grow at 4°C, this organism can multiply to high concentrations in nutritionally rich blood products that are stored in a refrigerator. Currently, there is no reliable method for detecting contaminated blood products.

Other Enterobacteriaceae

KLEBSIELLA

Members of the genus *Klebsiella* have a prominent capsule that is responsible for the mucoid appearance of isolated colonies and the enhanced virulence of the organisms in vivo. The most commonly isolated members of this genus are *K. pneumoniae* and *Klebsiella oxytoca,* which can cause community-acquired primary lobar pneumonia. Alcoholics and people with compromised pulmonary function

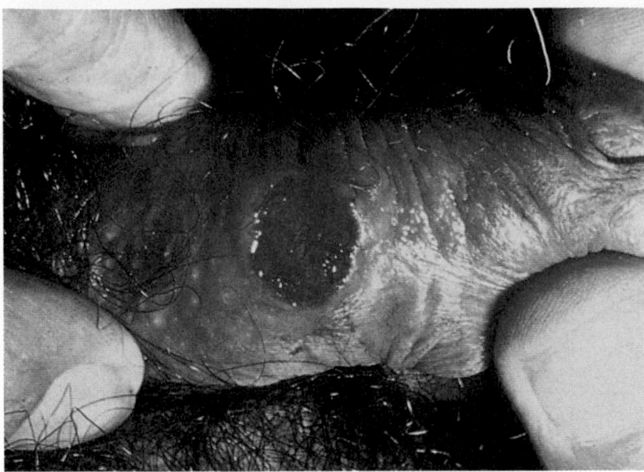

FIGURE 31–6. Penile ulcer caused by *K. granulomatis*. This can mimic the chancre of syphilis. (From Morse SA et al: *Atlas of sexually transmitted diseases*, ed 3, St Louis, 2003, Mosby.)

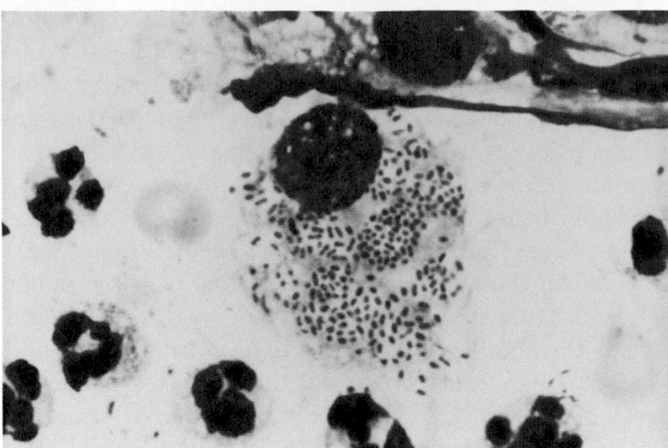

FIGURE 31–7. Light microscopy of impression smear of granulation tissue from genital lesion of patient infected with *K. granulomatis*. Note the numerous bacteria in the cytoplasmic vacuole of the mononuclear cell; modified Giemsa stain. (From Morse SA et al: *Atlas of sexually transmitted diseases*, ed 3, St Louis, 2003, Mosby.)

are at increased risk for pneumonia because of their inability to clear aspirated oral secretions from their lower respiratory tract. Pneumonia caused by *Klebsiella* species frequently involves the necrotic destruction of alveolar spaces, formation of cavities, and the production of blood-tinged sputum. These bacteria also cause wound, soft tissue, and urinary tract infections.

The organism formerly called *Donovania granulomatis* and then *Calymmatobacterium granulomatis* has been reclassified as *Klebsiella granulomatis* based on genomic criteria and the fact this organism produces clinical and pathologic changes similar to two other species of *Klebsiella*—*Klebsiella rhinoscleromatis* (causes a granulomatous disease of the nose) and *Klebsiella ozaenae* (causes chronic atrophic rhinitis). *K. granulomatis* is the etiologic agent of **granuloma inguinale,** a granulomatous disease affecting the genitalia and inguinal area (Figure 31–6). Unfortunately, this disease is commonly called **donovanosis** in reference to the historical origin of the genus name.

K. granulomatis has been isolated in a monocyte culture system but does not appear to grow in cell-free systems. The laboratory diagnosis is made through staining of infected tissues with Giemsa or Wright's stain. The organisms appear as small (0.5 to 1.0 × 1.5 μm) rods in the cytoplasm of histiocytes, polymorphonuclear leukocytes, and plasma cells (Figure 31–7). From 1 to 25 bacteria per phagocytic cell can be seen; a prominent capsule surrounds the organisms.

Granuloma inguinale is a rare disease in the United States but is endemic in parts of Papua New Guinea, the Caribbean, South America, India, southern Africa, Vietnam, and Australia. It can be transmitted after repeated exposure through sexual intercourse or nonsexual trauma to the genitalia. After a prolonged incubation of weeks to months, subcutaneous nodules appear on the genitalia or in the inguinal area. The nodules subsequently break down, revealing one or more painless granulomatous lesions that can extend and coalesce.

Laboratory confirmation of granuloma inguinale is made by scraping the border of the lesion, by spreading the collected tissue on a slide, and by staining it with Giemsa or Wright's stain. Pathognomonic **Donovan bodies** (named after the person who originally discovered this organism) are observed within mononuclear phagocytes. Tetracyclines, erythromycin, and trimethoprim-sulfamethoxazole have been used successfully for treatment, although relapses have occurred with use of these agents. Antibiotic prophylaxis has not proved effective in preventing and controlling infection.

PROTEUS

Infection of the urinary tract with *P. mirabilis* is the most common disease produced by this genus. *P. mirabilis* produces large quantities of urease, which splits urea into carbon dioxide and ammonia. This process raises the urine pH and facilitates the formation of renal stones. The increased alkalinity of the urine is also toxic to the uroepithelium. Despite the serologic diversity of these organisms, infection has not been associated with any specific serogroup. Furthermore, in contrast to *E. coli*, the pili on *P. mirabilis* may decrease its virulence by enhancing phagocytosis of the bacteria.

ENTEROBACTER, CITROBACTER, MORGANELLA, SERRATIA

Primary infections caused by *Enterobacter, Citrobacter, Morganella,* or *Serratia* are rare in immunocompetent patients. They are more common causes of hospital-acquired infections in neonates and immunocompromised patients. For example, *Citrobacter koseri* has been recognized to have a predilection for causing meningitis and brain abscesses in neonates. Antibiotic therapy for these genera can be ineffective, because the organisms are frequently resistant to multiple antibiotics. Resistance is a particularly serious problem with *Enterobacter* species.

Laboratory Diagnosis

CULTURE

Members of the family Enterobacteriaceae grow readily on culture media. Specimens of normally sterile material, such as spinal fluid and tissue collected at surgery, can be inoculated onto nonselective blood agar media. Selective media (e.g., MacConkey agar, eosin–methylene blue [EMB] agar) are used for the culture of specimens normally contaminated with other organisms (e.g., sputum, feces). Use of these selective differential agars enables the separation of lactose-fermenting Enterobacteriaceae from nonfermenting strains, thereby providing information that can be used to guide empirical antimicrobial therapy. Highly selective or organism-specific media are useful for the recovery of organisms such as *Salmonella* and *Shigella* in stool specimens, where an abundance of normal flora can obscure the presence of these important pathogens.

It is difficult to recover *Y. enterocolitica*, because this organism grows slowly at traditional incubation temperatures and prefers cooler temperatures, at which it is more active metabolically. Clinical laboratories have exploited this property, however, by mixing the fecal specimen with saline and then storing the specimen at 4°C for 2 weeks or more before subculturing it to agar media. This **cold** enrichment permits the growth of *Yersinia* but inhibits or kills other organisms in the specimen. Although use of the cold enrichment method does not aid in the initial management of a patient with *Yersinia* gastroenteritis, it has helped elucidate the role of this organism in chronic intestinal disease.

BIOCHEMICAL IDENTIFICATION

There are many diverse species in the family Enterobacteriaceae. The citations listed in the bibliography at the end of this chapter provide additional information about their biochemical identification. Biochemical test systems have become increasingly sophisticated, and now virtually all members of the family can be identified accurately in less than 24 hours with one of the many commercially available identification systems.

SEROLOGIC CLASSIFICATION

Serologic testing is very useful for determining the clinical significance of an isolate (e.g., serotyping specific pathogenic strains, such as *E. coli* O157 : H7 or *Y. enterocolitica* O8) and for classifying isolates for epidemiologic purposes. The usefulness of this procedure is limited, however, by cross-reactions with antigenically related Enterobacteriaceae and with organisms from other bacterial families.

Treatment, Prevention, and Control

Antibiotic therapy for infections with Enterobacteriaceae must be guided by in vitro susceptibility test results and clinical experience. Whereas some organisms such as *E. coli* and *P. mirabilis* are susceptible to many antibiotics, others can be highly resistant. Furthermore, susceptible organisms exposed to subtherapeutic concentrations of antibiotics in a hospital setting can rapidly develop resistance. In general, antibiotic resistance is more common in hospital-acquired infections than in community-acquired infections. Antibiotic therapy is not recommended for some infections. For example, symptomatic relief, but not antibiotic treatment, is usually recommended for patients with enterohemorrhagic *E. coli* and *Salmonella* gastroenteritis because antibiotics can prolong the fecal carriage of these organisms or increase the risk of secondary complications (e.g., HUS with EHEC infections in children). Treatment of *S. typhi* infections or other systemic Salmonella infections is indicated; however, increasing resistance to antibiotics such as the fluoroquinolones has complicated therapy.

It is difficult to prevent infections with Enterobacteriaceae, because these organisms are a major part of the endogenous microbial population. However, some risk factors for the infections should be avoided. These include the unrestricted use of antibiotics that can select for resistant bacteria; the performance of procedures that traumatize mucosal barriers without prophylactic antibiotic coverage; and the use of urinary catheters. Unfortunately, many of these factors are present in patients at greatest risk for infection (e.g., immunocompromised patients confined to the hospital for extended periods).

Exogenous infection with Enterobacteriaceae is theoretically easier to control. For example, the source of infections with organisms such as *Salmonella* is well defined. However, these bacteria are ubiquitous in poultry and eggs. Unless care is taken in the preparation and refrigeration of such foods, little can be done to control these infections. *Shigella* organisms are predominantly transmitted in young children, but it is difficult to interrupt the fecal-hand-mouth transmission responsible for spreading the infection in this population. Outbreaks of these infections can be effectively prevented and controlled only through education and the introduction of appropriate infection-control procedures (e.g., hand washing, proper disposal of soiled diapers and linens) in the settings where these infections typically occur.

A vaccine for *Y. pestis* is no longer available, although this is likely to change in light of the concern that this organism can be used by bioterrorists. Two vaccines for *S. typhi* are available—an oral, live, attenuated vaccine and a Vi capsular polysaccharide vaccine. Both vaccines protect 50% to 80% of the recipients, are administered in multiple doses, and require booster immunization because immunity is short-lived. Refer to the CDC website (www.cdc.gov) for current recommendations.

CASE STUDY AND QUESTIONS

A 25-year-old, previously healthy woman came to the emergency room for the evaluation of bloody diarrhea and diffuse abdominal pain of 24 hours' duration. She complained of nausea and had vomited twice. She reported no history of inflammatory bowel disease, previous diarrhea, or contact with other people with diarrhea. The symptoms began 24 hours after she had eaten an undercooked hamburger at a local fast food restaurant. Rectal examination revealed watery stool with gross blood. Sigmoidoscopy showed diffuse mucosal erythema and petechiae with a modest exudation but no ulceration or pseudomembranes.

1. Name four genera of Enterobacteriaceae that can cause gastrointestinal disease. Name two genera that can cause hemorrhagic colitis.
2. What virulence factor mediates this disease?
3. Name the five groups of *E. coli* that can cause gastroenteritis. What is characteristic of each group of organisms?
4. What are the four forms of *Salmonella* infection?
5. Differentiate between disease caused by *S. typhi* and that caused by *S. sonnei.*
6. Describe the epidemiology of the two forms of disease caused by *Y. pestis.*

Bibliography

Abbott S: *Klebsiella, Enterobacter, Citrobacter,* and *Serratia.* In Murray PR et al, editors: *Manual of clinical microbiology,* ed 8, Washington, 2003, American Society of Microbiology.

Ackers ML et al: Laboratory-based surveillance of *Salmonella* serotype *typhi* infections in the United States: Antimicrobial resistance on the rise, *JAMA* 283:2668-2673, 2000.

Bopp CA et al: *Escherichia, Salmonella,* and *Shigella.* In Murray PR et al, editors: *Manual of clinical microbiology,* ed 8, Washington, 2003, American Society of Microbiology.

Brenner F et al: *Salmonella* nomenclature, *J Clin Microbiol* 38:2465-2467, 2000.

Butler T: *Yersinia* infections: Centennial of the discovery of the plague bacillus, *Clin Infect Dis* 19:655-663, 1994.

Darwin KH, Miller VL: Molecular basis of the interaction of *Salmonella* with the intestinal mucosa, *Clin Microbiol Rev* 12:405-428, 1999.

Farmer JJ: Enterobacteriaceae: Introduction and identification. In Murray PR et al, editors: *Manual of clinical microbiology,* ed 8, Washington, 2003, American Society of Microbiology.

Kehl S. Role of the laboratory in the diagnosis of enterohemorrhagic *Escherichia coli* infections, *J Clin Microbiol* 40:2711-2715, 2002.

Koornhof HJ et al: Yersiniosis II: The pathogenesis of *Yersinia* infections, *Eur J Clin Microbiol Infect Dis* 18:87-112, 1999.

Mead P et al: Food-related illness and death in the United States, *Emerging Infect Dis* 5:607-625, 1999.

Nataro JP, Kaper JB: Diarrheagenic *Escherichia coli, Clin Microbiol Rev* 11:142-201, 1998.

Paton JC, Paton AW: Pathogenesis and diagnosis of Shiga toxin-producing *Escherichia coli* infections, *Clin Microbiol Rev* 11:450-479, 1998.

Perry RD, Fetherston JD: *Yersinia pestis*—etiologic agent of plague, *Clin Microbiol Rev* 10:35-66, 1997.

Podschun R, Ullmann U: *Klebsiella* spp. as nosocomial pathogens: Epidemiology, taxonomy, typing methods, and pathogenicity factors, *Clin Microbiol Rev* 11:589-603, 1998.

Reisner BS: Plague—past and present, *Clin Microbiol Newsletter* 18:153-160, 1996.

Salyers AA, Whitt DD: *Bacterial pathogenesis: A molecular approach,* Washington, 1994, American Society of Microbiology.

Sanders WE, Sanders CC: *Enterobacter* spp.: Pathogens poised to flourish at the turn of the century, *Clin Microbiol Rev* 10:220-241, 1997.

Slutsker L et al: *Escherichia coli* O157:H7 diarrhea in the United States: Clinical and epidemiologic features, *Ann Intern Med* 126:505-513, 1997.

Smego RA et al: Yersiniosis I: Microbiological and clinicoepidemiological aspects of plague and non-plague *Yersinia* infections, *Eur J Clin Microbiol Infect Dis* 18:1-15, 1999.

Su C, Brandt LJ: *Escherichia coli* O157 : H7 infection in humans, *Ann Intern Med* 123:698-714, 1995.

Wong CS et al: The risk of the hemolytic-uremic syndrome after antibiotic treatment of *Escherichia coli* O157 : H7 infections, *N Engl J Med* 342:1930-1936, 2000.

Zaharik ML et al: Delivery of dangerous goods: Type III secretion in enteric pathogens, *Int J Med Microbiol* 291:593-603, 2002.

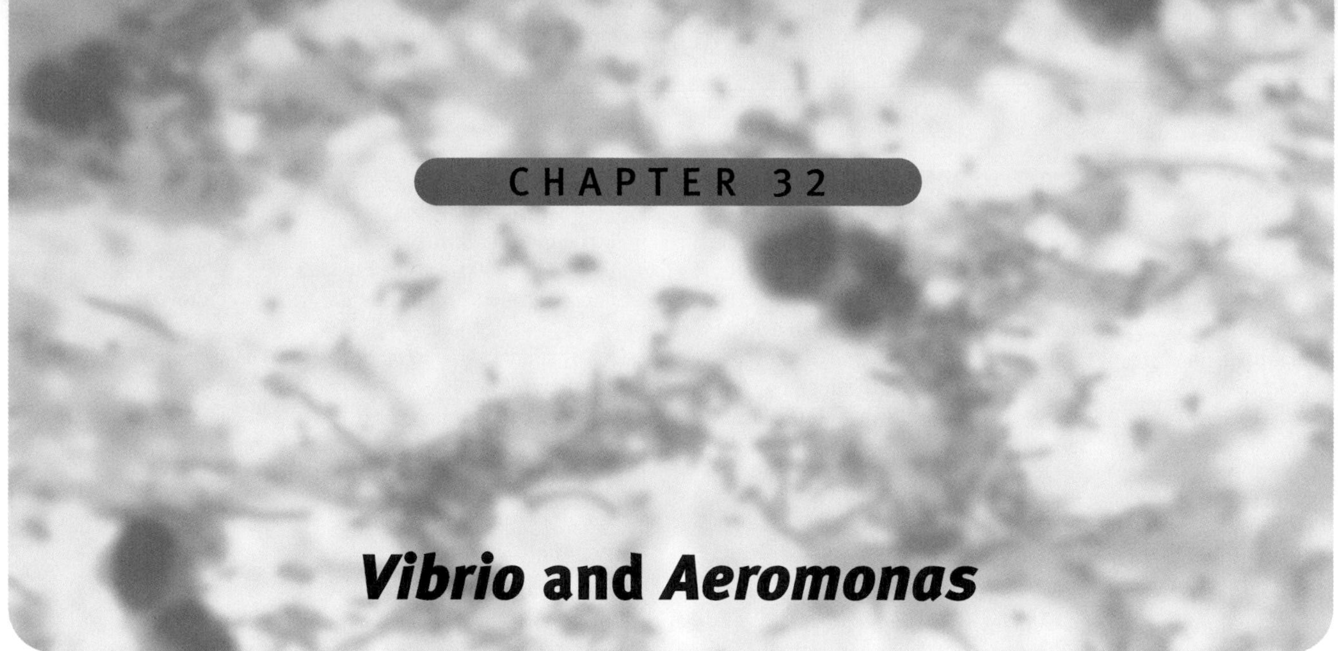

Vibrio and *Aeromonas*

The second major group of gram-negative, facultatively anaerobic, fermentative rods are the genera *Vibrio* and *Aeromonas.* These organisms were at one time classified together in the family Vibrionaceae and were separated from the Enterobacteriaceae on the basis of a positive oxidase reaction and the presence of polar flagella. These organisms were also classified together because they are primarily found in water and are able to cause gastrointestinal disease. However, molecular biology techniques have established that these genera are only distantly related and belong in separate families: *Vibrio* and *Aeromonas* are now classified in the families Vibrionaceae and Aeromonadaceae, respectively (Box 32–1). Despite this taxonomic reorganization, it is appropriate to consider these bacteria together because their epidemiology and range of diseases are similar.

Vibrio

The genus *Vibrio* has undergone numerous changes in recent years, with a number of less common species described or reclassified. Currently, the genus is composed of more than 60 species of curved rods with 10 species implicated in human infections (Table 32–1). *Vibrio cholerae, Vibrio parahaemolyticus,* and *Vibrio vulnificus* are the most important members.

PHYSIOLOGY AND STRUCTURE

Vibrio species can grow on a variety of simple media within a broad temperature range (from 14° to 40°C). *V. cholerae* (Box 32–2) can grow in the absence of salt; most other species that are pathogenic in humans require salt (**halophilic** species). Vibrios tolerate a wide range of pH (e.g., pH of 6.5 to 9.0) but are susceptible to stomach acids. If gastric acid production is reduced or neutralized, patients are more susceptible to *Vibrio* infections.

Most vibrios have a single polar flagellum (in contrast with peritrichous flagella in the family Enterobacteriaceae). These bacteria also have various pili that are important for virulence. For example, epidemic strains of *V. cholerae,* the etiologic agent of cholera, have the **toxin co-regulated pilus** (see the next section). The cell wall structure of vibrios is also important. All strains possess **lipopolysaccharides** consisting of lipid A (endotoxin), core polysaccharide, and an O polysaccharide side chain. The O polysaccharide is used to subdivide *Vibrio* species into serogroups: there are more than 140 serogroups of *V. cholerae* (O1-O140), 7 O serogroups of *V. vulnificus,* and 13 O serogroups of *V. parahaemolyticus.* The interest in this classification scheme is more than academic—***V. cholerae* O1 and O139** produce cholera toxin and are associated with epidemics of cholera. Other strains of *V. cholerae* generally do not produce cholera toxin and do not cause epidemic disease. *V. cholerae* serogroup O1 is further subdivided into serotypes and biotypes. Three serotypes are recognized: **Inaba, Ogawa,** and **Hikojima.** Strains can shift between serotype Inaba and serotype Ogawa, with Hikojima a transitional state in which both Inaba and Ogawa antigens are expressed. Two biotypes of *V. cholerae* O1 are recognized: **classical** and **el tor.** These biotypes are subdivided by differences in phenotypic and morphologic properties. Seven worldwide pandemics of *V. cholerae* infections have been documented. *V. cholerae* strains responsible for the sixth worldwide pandemic of cholera were the classical biotype, whereas most strains responsible for the current seventh pandemic are the el tor biotype.

V. vulnificus and non-O1 *V. cholerae* produce acidic polysaccharide capsules that are important for disseminated infections. *V. cholerae* O1 does not produce a capsule, so

BOX 32–1. Important *Vibrio* and *Aeromonas* Isolates

Organism	Historical Derivation
Vibrio	*vibrio,* move rapidly or vibrate (rapid movement caused by polar flagellae)
V. cholerae	*cholera,* cholera or an intestinal disease
V. parahaemolyticus	*para,* by the side of; *haema,* blood; *lyticus,* dissolving (dissolving blood; Kanagawa toxin positive strains are hemolytic)
V. vulnificus	*vulnificus,* inflicting wounds (associated with prominent wound infections)
Aeromonas	*aero,* gas or air; *monas,* unit or monad (gas-producing bacteria)
A. caviae	*cavia,* guinea pig (first isolated in guinea pigs)
A. hydrophila	*hydro,* water; *phila,* loving (water loving)
A. veronii	*veron,* named after the bacteriologist Veron

TABLE 32–1. *Vibrio* Species Associated with Human Disease

Species	Source of Infection	Clinical Disease
V. alginolyticus	Seawater	Wound infection, external otitis
V. cholerae	Water, food	Gastroenteritis
*V. cincinnatiensis**	Unknown	Bacteremia, meningitis
*V. fluvialis**	Seafood	Gastroenteritis, wound infection, bacteremia
*V. furnissii**	Seawater	Gastroenteritis
*V. harveyi**	Seawater	Wound infection (shark bite)
*V. metschnikovii**	Unknown	Bacteremia
*V. mimicus**	Fresh water	Gastroenteritis, wound infection, bacteremia
V. parahaemolyticus	Shellfish, seawater	Gastroenteritis, wound infection, bacteremia
V. vulnificus	Shellfish, seawater	Bacteremia, wound infection, cellulitis

*Isolates rarely associated with human infection.

BOX 32–2. Summary of *Vibrio cholerae* Infections

Physiology and Structure

Curved gram-negative rods; facultative anaerobe; fermenter

Simple nutritional requirements; do not require salt for growth but can tolerate it

Strains subdivided into more than 140 serogroups (O cell wall antigens)

V. cholerae serogroup O1 is further subdivided into serotypes (Inaba, Ogawa, Hikojima) and biotypes (classical, el tor)

Virulence

Refer to Table 32–2

Epidemiology

Serogroup O1 is responsible for major pandemics (worldwide epidemics) with significant mortality in developing countries; organisms can multiply in brackish water with a high nutrient load

Organism found in estuarine and marine environments worldwide (including along the coast of the United States); associated with chitinous shellfish

Organism can multiply freely in water

Bacterial levels increase in contaminated waters during the warm months

Spread by consumption of contaminated food or water

Direct person-to-person spread is rare because the infectious dose is high; the infectious dose is high because most organisms are killed by stomach acids

Disease

Refer to Box 32–3

Diagnosis

Microscopic examination of stool generally nonproductive

Culture should be performed early in course of disease with fresh stool specimens

Treatment, Prevention, and Control

Fluid and electrolyte replacement are crucial

Antibiotics reduce the bacterial burden and exotoxin production, as well as duration of diarrhea

Doxycycline (adults), trimethoprim-sulfamethoxazole (children), or furazolidone (pregnant women) is administered

Improved hygiene is critical for control

Combination inactivated whole cell and cholera toxin B subunit vaccines provide limited protection; other vaccines are in development

infections with this organism do not spread beyond the confines of the intestine.

V. cholerae and *V. parahaemolyticus* possess two circular chromosomes, each of which contain essential genes for these bacteria. It is not known if other *Vibrio* species have a similar genomic structure. Plasmids, including those encoding antimicrobial resistance, are also commonly found in *Vibrio* species.

PATHOGENESIS AND IMMUNITY

The **bacteriophage CTXϕ** encodes the genes for the two subunits of **cholera toxin** (*ctx*A and *ctx*B). This

TABLE 32–2. Virulence Factors of *Vibrio cholerae* O1 and O139

Virulence Factor	Biologic Effect
Cholera toxin	Hypersecretion of electrolytes and water
Toxin co-regulated pilus	Adherence to intestinal mucosal cells; binding site for CTXϕ
Accessory cholera enterotoxin	Increases intestinal fluid secretion
Zonnula occludens toxin	Increases intestinal permeability
Neuraminidase	Modifies cell surface to increase GM_1 binding sites for cholera toxin

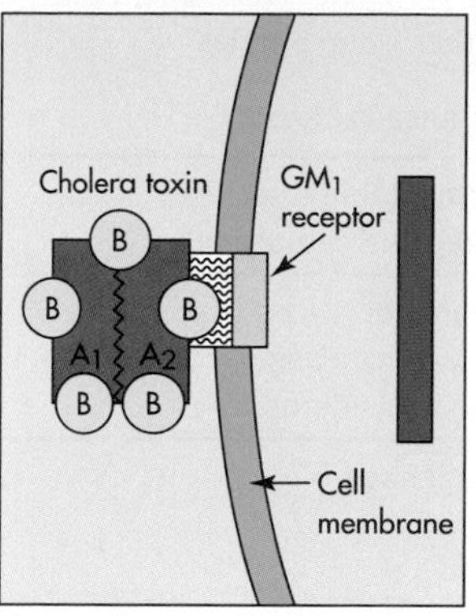

The complete toxin binding to the GM_1-ganglioside receptor on the cell membrane via the binding subunits (B).

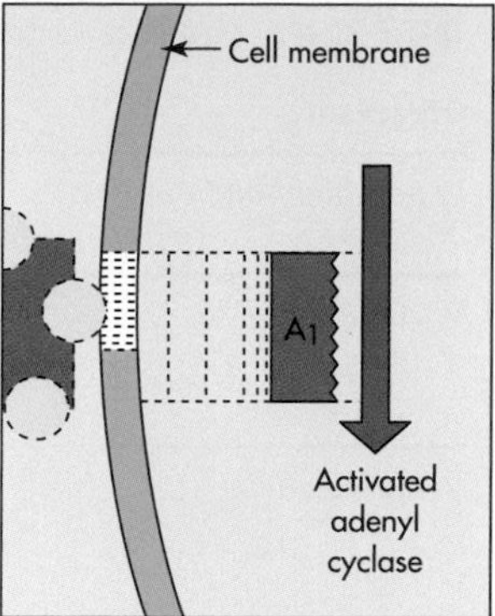

The active portion (A_1) of the A subunit enters the cell and activates adenyl cyclase.

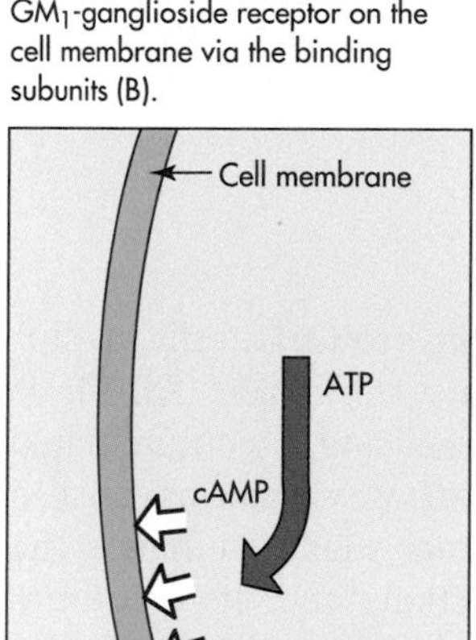

This activity results in accumulation of cyclic adenosine 3′, 5′–monophosphate (cAMP) along the cell membrane.

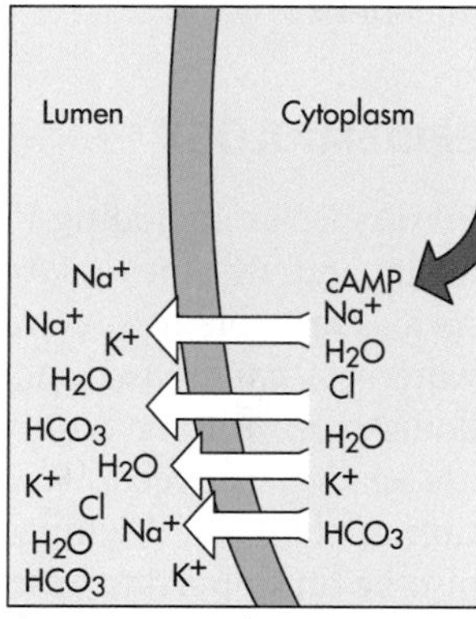

The cAMP causes the active secretion of sodium (Na^+), chloride (Cl), potassium (K^+), bicarbonate (HCO_3), and water (H_2O) out of the cell into the intestinal lumen.

FIGURE 32–1. Mechanism of action of cholera toxin.

bacteriophage binds to the toxin co-regulated pilus (*tcp*) and moves into the bacterial cell, where it becomes integrated into the *V. cholerae* genome. The lysogenic bacteriophage chromosomal locus also contains other potential virulence factors: the *ace* gene for **accessory cholera enterotoxin** and *zot* gene for the **zonnula occludens toxin** (Table 32–2). Multiple copies of these genes are found in *V. cholerae* O1 and O139, and their expression is coordinated by regulatory genes (e.g., *ToxR* regulator).

The cholera toxin is a complex A-B toxin that is structurally and functionally similar to the heat-labile enterotoxin of *Escherichia coli*. A ring of five identical B subunits of cholera toxin binds to the ganglioside GM_1 receptors on the intestinal epithelial cells. The active portion of the A subunit is internalized, interacts with G proteins that control adenylate cyclase, leading to the catabolic conversion of adenosine triphosphate (ATP) to cyclic adenosine monophosphate (cAMP). This results in a hypersecretion of electrolytes (Figure 32–1). Severely infected patients can lose as much as 1 liter of fluid per hour during the height of the disease. Such a tremendous loss of fluid would normally flush the organisms out of the gastrointestinal tract; however, *V. cholerae* are able to adhere to the mucosal cell layer by means of (1) the toxin co-regulated pili encoded by the *tcp* gene complex and (2) chemotaxis proteins. Thus the toxin co-regulated pilus is important both as a receptor for the cholera toxin carrying phage and for adherence to the mucosa lining the intestines. Nonadherent strains are unable to establish infection.

In the absence of cholera toxin, *V. cholerae* O1 may still produce diarrhea through the action of the zonnula occludens toxin and accessory cholera enterotoxin. As the name implies, the zonnula occludens toxin loosens the tight junctions (zonnula occludens) of the small intestine mucosa, leading to increased intestinal permeability, and the enterotoxin produces increased fluid secretion.

Unlike other non-O1 serotypes, *V. cholerae* O139 possesses the same virulence complex as that of the O1 strains. Thus the ability of the O139 strains to adhere to the intestinal mucosa and produce cholera toxin is the reason these strains can produce a watery diarrhea similar to cholera.

The means by which other *Vibrio* species cause disease is less clearly understood, although a variety of potential virulence factors have been identified (Table 32–3). Most virulent strains of *V. parahaemolyticus* produce a thermostable direct hemolysin (TDH; also called Kanagawa hemolysin). TDH is an enterotoxin that induces chloride ion secretion in epithelial cells by increasing intracellular calcium. An important method for classifying virulent strains of *V. parahaemolyticus* is detection of this hemolysin, which produces β-hemolytic colonies on agar media with human blood but not sheep blood. These virulent strains are referred to as **Kanagawa positive.**

TABLE 32–3. Virulence Factors of Other *Vibrio* Species

Organism	Virulence Factors
V. parahaemolyticus	Thermostable direct hemolysin (Kanagawa hemolysin)
V. vulnificus	Antiphagocytic polysaccharide capsule, cytolysins, collagenase, protease, siderophores
V. alginolyticus	Collagenase

Capsule production in *V. vulnificus* is important for the ability of this organism to produce severe, disseminated infections.

EPIDEMIOLOGY

Vibrio species, including *V. cholerae,* grow naturally in estuarine and marine environments worldwide. All *Vibrio* species are able to survive and replicate in contaminated waters with increased salinity. Pathogenic vibrios can also flourish in waters with chitinous shellfish—hence the association between *Vibrio* infections and the consumption of shellfish. Asymptomatically infected humans can also be an important reservoir for this organism in areas where *V. cholerae* disease is endemic.

Seven major pandemics of cholera have occurred since 1817, resulting in thousands of deaths and major socioeconomic changes. Sporadic disease and epidemics occurred before this time, but worldwide spread of the disease became possible only with intercontinental travel resulting from increased commerce and wars.

The seventh pandemic, which is caused by *V. cholerae* O1 biotype el tor, began in Asia in 1961 and spread to Africa, Europe, and Oceania in the 1970s and 1980s. In 1991, the pandemic strain spread to Peru and, subsequently, has caused disease in most countries in South and Central America, as well as in the United States and Canada. A second epidemic strain emerged in 1992 in India. This strain, *V. cholerae* O139 Bengal, produces the cholera toxin and shares other traits with *V. cholerae* O1. This is the first non-O1 strain capable of causing epidemic disease and is capable of producing disease in adults who were previously infected with the O1 strain (showing that no protective immunity is conferred).

Cholera is spread by contaminated water and food. Direct person-to-person spread is unusual because a high inoculum (e.g., more than 10^8 organisms) is required to establish infection in a person with normal gastric acidity. In a person with achlorhydria or hypochlorhydria, the infectious dose can be as low as 10^3 to 10^5 organisms. Cholera is usually seen in communities with poor sanitation. Indeed, one outcome from the cholera pandemics was recognition of the role of contaminated water in the spread of disease and the need to improve community sanitation systems so that the disease could be controlled.

Infections caused by *V. parahaemolyticus, V. vulnificus,* and other pathogenic vibrios result from the consumption of improperly cooked seafood, particularly oysters, or exposure to contaminated seawater. *V. parahaemolyticus* is the most common cause of bacterial gastroenteritis in Japan and Southeast Asia and is the most common *Vibro* species responsible for gastroenteritis in the United States. *V. vulnificus* is not frequently isolated but is responsible for severe wound infections and a high incidence of fatal outcomes. Gastroenteritis caused by vibrios occurs throughout the year, because oysters are typically contaminated with abundant organisms year-round. In contrast, septicemia and wound infections with *Vibrio* occur during the warm months, when the organisms in seawater can multiply to high numbers.

BOX 32–3. Clinical Summaries

Vibrio cholerae

Cholera: Begins with an abrupt onset of watery diarrhea and vomiting and can progress to severe dehydration, metabolic acidosis and hypokalemia, and hypovolemic shock

Gastroenteritis: Milder forms of diarrheal disease can occur in toxin-negative strains of *V. cholerae* O1 and in non-O1 serotypes

Vibrio parahaemolyticus

Gastroenteritis: Generally self-limited with an explosive onset of watery diarrhea and nausea, vomiting, abdominal cramps, headache, and low-grade fever

Wound infection: Associated with exposure to contaminated water

Vibrio vulnificus

Wound infection: Severe, potentially fatal infections characterized by erythema, pain, bullae formation, tissue necrosis, and septicemia

CLINICAL DISEASES (BOX 32–3)

Vibrio Cholerae

Infection with *V. cholerae* O1 can range from asymptomatic colonization or a mild diarrheal disease to severe, rapidly fatal diarrhea. The clinical manifestations of cholera begin an average of 2 to 3 days after ingestion of the bacteria, with the abrupt onset of watery diarrhea and vomiting. As more fluid is lost, the feces-streaked stool specimens become colorless and odorless, free of protein, and speckled with mucus **("rice-water" stools).** The resulting severe fluid and electrolyte loss can lead to

BOX 32–4. Summary of *Vibrio parahaemolyticus* Infections

Physiology and Structure
Curved gram-negative rods, facultative anaerobe; fermenter
Simple nutritional requirements but requires salt for growth

Virulence
Refer to Table 32–3

Epidemiology
Organism found in estuarine and marine environments worldwide
Associated with consumption of contaminated shellfish
Not commonly isolated in the United States but is a major pathogen in countries where raw fish is eaten

Diseases
Refer to Box 32–3

Diagnosis
Culture should be performed as with *V. cholerae*

Treatment, Prevention, and Control
Self-limited disease, although antibiotics can shorten length of symptoms and fluid loss
Disease prevented by proper cooking of shellfish
No vaccines are available

BOX 32–5. Summary of *Vibrio vulnificus* Infections

Physiology and Structure
Curved gram-negative rods; facultative anaerobe; fermenter
Simple nutritional requirements but requires salt for growth

Virulence
Refer to Table 32–3

Epidemiology
Infection associated with exposure of a wound to contaminated salt water or ingestion of improperly prepared shellfish

Diseases
Refer to Box 32–3

Diagnosis
Culture wounds and blood

Treatment, Prevention, and Control
Life-threatening illnesses that must be promptly treated with antibiotics
Minocycline combined with a fluoroquinolone or cefotaxime is the treatment of choice
No vaccine is available

dehydration, metabolic acidosis (bicarbonate loss), and hypokalemia and hypovolemic shock (potassium loss), with cardiac arrhythmia and renal failure. The mortality rate is 60% in untreated patients but less than 1% in patients who are promptly treated with replacement of lost fluids and electrolytes. Cholera can resolve spontaneously after a few days of symptoms. Disease caused by *V. cholerae* O139 can be as severe as disease caused by *V. cholerae* O1. Gastroenteritis caused by other serotypes of *V. cholerae* is milder and is not associated with epidemics.

Vibrio Parahaemolyticus (Box 32–4)

The severity of gastroenteritis caused by *V. parahaemolyticus* can range from a self-limited diarrhea to a mild, cholera-like illness. In general, the disease develops after a 5- to 72-hour incubation period (mean, 24 hours), with explosive, watery diarrhea. No grossly evident blood or mucus is found in stool specimens except in severe cases. Headache, abdominal cramps, nausea, vomiting, and low-grade fever may persist for 72 hours or more. The patient usually experiences an uneventful recovery. Wound infections with this organism can occur in people exposed to contaminated seawater.

Vibrio Vulnificus (Box 32–5)

V. vulnificus is a particularly virulent species of *Vibrio* responsible for rapidly progressive wound infections after exposure to contaminated seawater and for septicemia after consumption of contaminated raw oysters. The wound infections are characterized by initial swelling, erythema, and pain, followed by the development of vesicles or bullae and eventual tissue necrosis. Patients usually experience systemic signs of fever and chills. The mortality in patients with *V. vulnificus* septicemia can be as high as 50% unless antimicrobial therapy is started promptly. Infections are most severe in patients with hepatic disease, hematopoietic disease, or chronic renal failure and in those receiving immunosuppressive drugs.

Other *Vibrio* Species

V. alginolyticus can cause infection in superficial wounds exposed to contaminated seawater. Infections of the ear, eye, and gastrointestinal tract have been reported rarely. *V. mimicus, V. fluvialis,* and *V. furnissii* are responsible for causing gastroenteritis, wound infections, and bacteremia. Single cases of infections with *V. metschnikovii* (bacteremia) and *V. cincinnatiensis* (meningitis) have been documented.

LABORATORY DIAGNOSIS

Microscopy

Vibrio species are small (0.5 to 1.5 to 3 μm), curved, gram-negative rods. The organisms are rarely seen in

Gram-stained stool or wound specimens; however, an experienced observer using darkfield microscopy may be able to detect the characteristic motile bacteria in stool specimens.

Culture

Vibrio organisms survive poorly in an acidic or dry environment. Specimens must be collected early in the disease and inoculated promptly onto culture media. If culture will be delayed, the specimen should be mixed in a Cary-Blair transport medium and refrigerated. Vibrios have low survival rates in buffered glycerol-saline, the transport medium used for most enteric pathogens.

Vibrios grow on most media used in clinical laboratories for stool cultures, including blood agar and MacConkey agar. Special selective agar for vibrios (e.g., thiosulfate citrate bile salts sucrose **[TCBS]** agar), as well as an enrichment broth (e.g., alkaline peptone broth; pH 8.6), can also be used. Isolates are identified with selective biochemical tests and serotyped using polyvalent antisera. In tests performed to identify halophilic vibrios, the media must be supplemented with 1% sodium chloride.

TREATMENT, PREVENTION, AND CONTROL

Patients with cholera must be promptly treated with fluid and electrolyte replacement before the resultant massive fluid loss leads to hypovolemic shock. Antibiotic therapy, although of secondary value, can reduce toxin production and more rapidly eliminate the organism. Doxycycline or tetracycline is the drug of choice for adults, furazolidone is used for pregnant women, and trimethoprim-sulfamethoxazole is used for children. *V. cholerae* O139 strains are often resistant to furazolidone and trimethoprim-sulfamethoxazole.

V. parahaemolyticus gastroenteritis is usually a self-limited disease, although antibiotic therapy can be used in addition to fluid and electrolyte therapy in patients with severe infections. *V. vulnificus* wound infections and septicemia must be promptly treated with antibiotic therapy. The combination of minocycline and a fluoroquinolone or cefotaxime appears to be the most effective treatment.

People infected with *V. cholerae* can shed bacteria for the first few days of acute illness and represent important sources of new infections. Although long-term carriage of *V. cholerae* does not occur, vibrios are free living in estuarine and marine reservoirs. Only improvements in sanitation can lead to effective control of the disease. This involves adequate sewage management, the use of purification systems to eliminate contamination of the water supply, and the implementation of appropriate steps to prevent contamination of food.

A variety of cholera vaccines have been developed, none providing long-term protection. Field trials are underway with an oral vaccine consisting of inactivated whole cell *V. cholerae* combined with B subunits. Multiple doses are required for partial immunity, and protection fades 2 to 3 years after immunization. Other vaccines, including a live, attenuated vaccine, are in development. There is no vaccine for the O139 strains. Tetracycline prophylaxis has also been used to reduce the risk of infection in people traveling to areas where the disease is endemic but has not prevented the spread of cholera. Because the infectious dose of *V. cholerae* is high, antibiotic prophylaxis is generally unnecessary in people who use appropriate hygiene.

Aeromonas

Aeromonas is a gram-negative, facultative anaerobic rod that morphologically resembles members of the family Enterobacteriaceae. As with *Vibrio*, extensive reorganization of the taxonomy of these bacteria has occurred. Fourteen species of *Aeromonas* have been described, most of which are associated with human disease. The most important pathogens are *Aeromonas hydrophila*, *Aeromonas caviae*, and *Aeromonas veronii* biovar *sobria*. The organisms are ubiquitous in fresh and brackish water.

The two major diseases associated with *Aeromonas* are **gastroenteritis** and **wound infections** (with or without bacteremia). Gastrointestinal carriage has been observed in approximately 3% of individuals, with the highest carriage in the warm months. Therefore, the isolation of this organism in enteric specimens does not indicate disease, which is determined by the clinical presentation of the patient. Gastroenteritis typically occurs after the ingestion of contaminated water or food, whereas wound infections result from exposure to contaminated water.

Although numerous potential virulence factors (e.g., endotoxin, hemolysins, enterotoxin, proteases, siderophores, adherence factors) have been identified for *Aeromonas*, their precise role is unknown. *Aeromonas* species cause (1) opportunistic systemic disease in immunocompromised patients (particularly those with hepatobiliary disease or an underlying malignancy), (2) diarrheal disease in otherwise healthy people, and (3) wound infections.

Gastrointestinal disease in children is usually an acute, severe illness, whereas that in adults tends to be chronic diarrhea. Severe *Aeromonas* gastroenteritis resembles shigellosis, in that blood and leukocytes are present in the stool of affected patients. Acute diarrheal disease is self-limited, and only supportive care is indicated in affected patients.

Antimicrobial therapy is necessary in patients with chronic diarrheal disease or systemic infection. *Aeromonas* species are resistant to penicillins, most cephalosporins, and erythromycin. Ciprofloxacin is consistently active against *Aeromonas* strains isolated in the United States and Europe; however, resistance has been reported in strains recovered in Asia. Thus the long-term effectiveness of fluoroquinolones remains to be seen. Gentamicin, amikacin, and trimethoprim-sulfamethoxazole are also active against most aeromonads.

CASE STUDY AND QUESTIONS

A 57-year-old man was hospitalized in New York with a 2-day history of severe, watery diarrhea. The illness had begun 1 day after his return from Ecuador. The patient was dehydrated and suffering from an electrolyte imbalance (acidosis, hypokalemia). The patient made an uneventful recovery after fluid and electrolyte replacement was instituted to compensate for the losses resulting from the watery diarrhea. Stool cultures were positive for V. cholerae.

1. What are the characteristic clinical symptoms of cholera?
2. What is the most important virulence factor in this disease? What other virulence factors have been described? What are the modes of their action?
3. How did this patient acquire this infection? How does this situation differ from the acquisition of infections caused by *V. parahaemolyticus* or *V. vulnificus?*
4. How can cholera be controlled in areas where infection is endemic?

Bibliography

Bhattacharya SK: An evaluation of current cholera treatment, Expert Opin Pharmacother 4:141-146, 2003.

Calia KE: *Vibrio cholerae* O139: An emerging pathogen, *Clin Microbiol Newsletter* 18:17-22, 1996.

Clark RB, Janda JM: *Plesiomonas* and human disease, *Clin Microbiol Newsletter* 13:49-52, 1991.

Holmberg SD, Farmer JJ III: *Aeromonas hydrophila* and *Plesiomonas shigelloides* as causes of intestinal infections, *Rev Infect Dis* 6:633-639, 1984.

Janda JM et al: *Aeromonas* species in septicemia: Laboratory characteristics and clinical observations, *Clin Infect Dis* 19:77-83, 1994.

Kampfer PC et al: In vitro susceptibilities of *Aeromonas* genomic species to 69 antimicrobial agents, *Syst Appl Microbiol* 22:662-669, 1999.

Klose KE: Regulation of virulence in *Vibrio cholerae, Int J Med Microbiol* 291:81-88, 2001.

Ko W-C, Chuang Y-C: *Aeromonas* bacteremia: Review of 59 episodes, *Clin Infect Dis* 20:1298-1304, 1995.

Lacey SW: Cholera: Calamitous past, ominous future, *Clin Infect Dis* 20:1409-1419, 1995.

Lang DR, Guerrant RL: Summary of the 29th United States–Japan Joint Conference on Cholera and Related Diarrheal Diseases, *J Infect Dis* 171:8-12, 1995.

Mahon BE et al: Reported cholera in the United States, 1992-1994: A reflection of global changes in cholera epidemiology, *JAMA* 276:307-312, 1996.

Tauxe RV et al: Epidemic cholera in the new world: Translating field epidemiology into new prevention strategies, *Emerging Infect Dis* 1:141-146, 1995.

Waldor MK, Mekalanos JJ: Emergence of a new cholera pandemic: Molecular analysis of virulence determinants in *Vibrio cholerae* O139 and development of a live vaccine prototype, *J Infect Dis* 170:278-283, 1994.

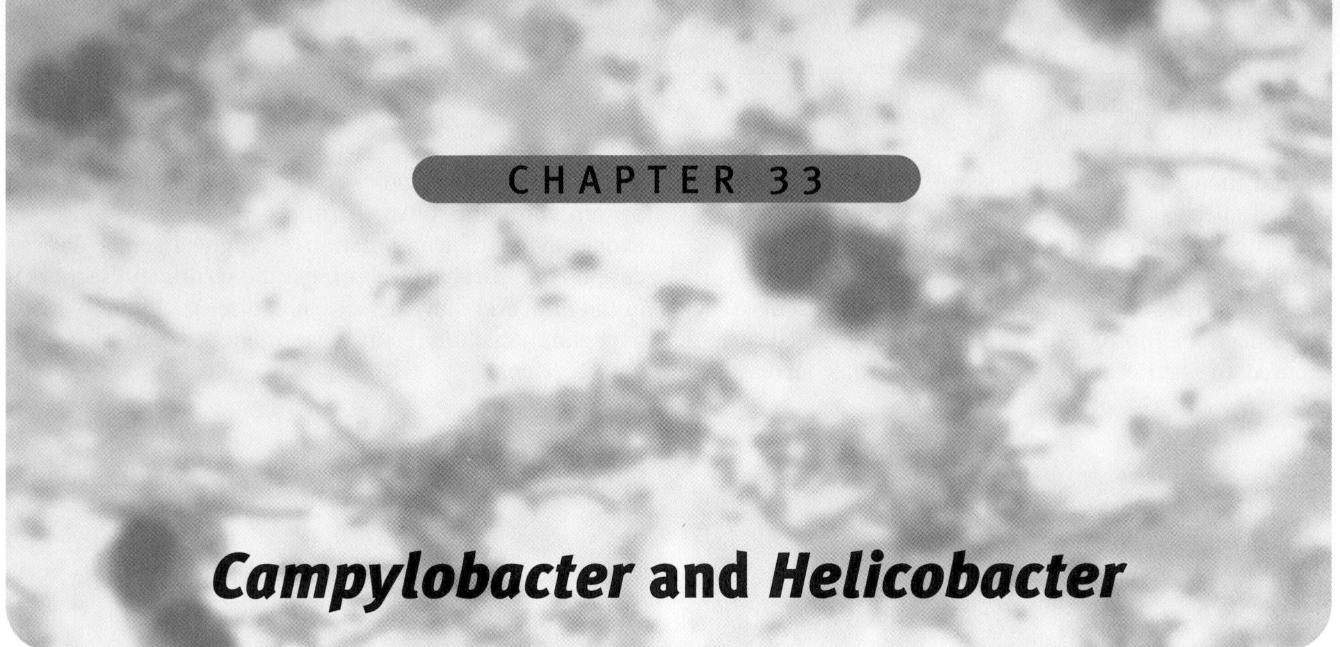

Campylobacter and *Helicobacter*

The classification of *Campylobacter* and *Helicobacter* (Box 33–1) has undergone many changes since the bacteria were first isolated at the beginning of this century. However, molecular biology techniques (e.g., sequence analysis of 16S ribosomal ribonucleic acid [rRNA] genes), characterization of cell wall proteins and lipids, serologic characterization, and analysis of biochemical properties have been used to resolve much of the taxonomic confusion. These genera belong to the same rRNA superfamily, which consists of spiral, gram-negative rods with (1) a low deoxyribonucleic acid (DNA) guanosine plus cytosine base ratio, (2) an inability to ferment or oxidize carbohydrates, and (3) microaerophilic growth requirements (i.e., growth only in the presence of a reduced oxygen level).

Campylobacter (Box 33–2)

The genus *Campylobacter* consists of small (0.2 to 0.5 × 0.5 to 5.0 µm), comma-shaped, gram-negative rods (Figure 33–1) that are motile by means of a polar flagellum. Most species are microaerobic, requiring an atmosphere with decreased oxygen and increased hydrogen and carbon dioxide levels for aerobic growth. A total of 16 species are now recognized, most of which are associated with human disease (Table 33–1).

The primary diseases caused by campylobacters are gastroenteritis and septicemia. *Campylobacter jejuni* is the most common cause of bacterial gastroenteritis in the United States, and *Campylobacter coli* is responsible for 2% to 5% of the cases of *Campylobacter* gastroenteritis. The latter is a more common cause of gastroenteritis in developing countries.

Campylobacter upsaliensis is most likely an important cause of gastroenteritis in humans; however, the true incidence of disease caused by this organism is underestimated by conventional culture methods (*C. upsaliensis* is inhibited by the antibiotics used in isolation media for other campylobacters). A variety of other species are rare causes of gastroenteritis or systemic infections. Unlike other species, *Campylobacter fetus* is most commonly responsible for causing systemic infections such as bacteremia, septic thrombophlebitis, arthritis, septic abortion, and meningitis.

PHYSIOLOGY AND STRUCTURE

Campylobacters have a typical gram-negative cell wall structure. The major antigen of the genus is the lipopolysaccharide of the outer membrane. In addition, the different somatic O polysaccharide antigens and the heat-labile capsular and flagellar antigens have been used for the epidemiologic classification of clinical isolates.

Recognition of the role of campylobacters in gastrointestinal disease was delayed because the organisms grow best in an atmosphere of reduced oxygen (5% to 7%, microaerophilic) and increased carbon dioxide (5% to 10%). In addition, *C. jejuni* grow better at 42°C than at 37°C. These properties have been exploited for the selective isolation of pathogenic campylobacters in stool specimens. The small size of the organisms (0.2 to 0.5 µm in diameter) has also been used to recover the bacteria by filtration of stool specimens. Campylobacters pass through 0.45-µm filters, whereas other bacteria are retained. This method was also used to demonstrate that *C. upsaliensis* causes human gastroenteritis, as well as disease in domestic dogs and cats. Unfortunately, filtration of stool specimens is a cumbersome procedure and is not used in most clinical laboratories.

PATHOGENESIS AND IMMUNITY

Efforts to define the role of specific virulence factors in *Campylobacter* disease have been thwarted by a lack of an animal model to study the disease. *C. jejuni* is the best-studied species. Although adhesins, cytotoxic enzymes, and enterotoxins have been detected in this species, their specific role in disease remains poorly defined. It is clear that the probability of disease is influenced by the infectious dose. The organisms are killed when exposed to gastric acids, so conditions that decrease or neutralize gastric-acid secretion favor disease. The patient's immune status also affects the severity of disease. People living in a population of high endemic disease develop measurable levels of specific serum and secretory antibodies and have less severe disease. Patients with hypogammaglobulinemia have prolonged, severe disease with *C. jejuni*.

BOX 33–1. Common Campylobacters and Helicobacters

Organism	Historical Derivation
Campylobacter	*kampylos*, curved; *bacter*, rod (a curved rod)
C. jejuni	*jejuni*, of the jejunum
C. coli	*coli*, of the colon
C. fetus	*fetus*, refers to the initial observation that these bacteria caused fetal infections
C. upsaliensis	*upsaliensis*, original isolates recovered from the feces of dogs at an animal clinic in Uppsala, Sweden
Helicobacter	*helix*, spiral; *bacter*, rod (a spiral rod)
H. pylori	*pylorus*, lower part of the stomach
H. cinaedi	*cinaedi*, of a homosexual (the organism was first isolated from homosexuals with gastroenteritis)
H. fennelliae	*fennelliae*, named after C. Fennell, who first isolated the organism

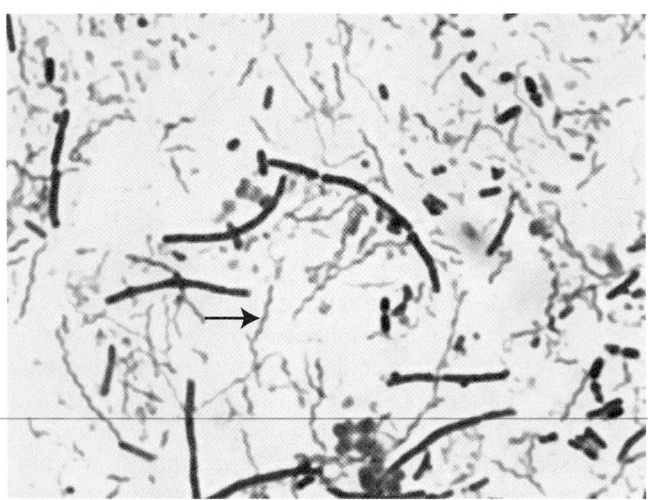

FIGURE 33–1. Mixed culture of bacteria from a fecal specimen. *Campylobacter jejuni* is the thin, curved, gram-negative bacteria (arrow).

BOX 33–2. Summary of *Campylobacter*

Physiology and Structure

Thin, curved, gram-negative rods

Unable to oxidize or ferment carbohydrates

Microaerophilic growth

Virulence

Factors that regulate adhesion, motility, and invasion into intestinal mucosa are poorly defined

S protein in *C. fetus* inhibits C3b binding and subsequent complement-mediated phagocytosis and killing (i.e., resistant to serum killing)

Guillain-Barré syndrome believed to be an autoimmune disease caused by antigenic cross-reactivity between oligosaccharides in bacterial capsule and glycosphingolipids on surface of neural tissues

Epidemiology

Zoonotic infection; improperly prepared poultry is a common source of human infections

Infections acquired by ingestion of contaminated food, unpasteurized milk, or contaminated water

Person-to-person spread is unusual

Dose required to establish infection is high unless the gastric acids are neutralized or absent

Worldwide distribution, with enteric infections most commonly seen in warm months

Diseases

Refer to Table 33–1

Acute enteritis with diarrhea, malaise, fever, and abdominal pain

Most infections are self-limited but can persist for a week or more

C. fetus is associated with septicemia and is disseminated to multiple organs

Diagnosis

Microscopy is insensitive

Culture requires use of specialized media incubated with reduced oxygen, increased carbon dioxide, and (for thermophilic species) elevated temperatures; requires incubation for 2 or more days

Treatment, Prevention, and Control

For gastroenteritis, infection is self-limited and is managed by fluid and electrolyte replacement

Severe gastroenteritis and septicemia are treated with erythromycin (drug of choice), tetracyclines, or fluoroquinolones

Gastroenteritis is prevented by proper preparation of food and consumption of pasteurized milk; preventing contamination of water supplies also controls infection

TABLE 33–1. *Campylobacter* Species Associated with Human Disease

Species	Reservoir Host	Human Disease	Frequency
C. jejuni subsp. *jejuni*	Poultry, pigs, bulls, dogs, cats, rabbits, birds, minks	Gastroenteritis, septicemia, meningitis, spontaneous abortion, proctitis, Guillain-Barré syndrome	Common
C. jejuni subsp. *doylei*	Humans	Gastroenteritis, gastritis, septicemia	Uncommon
C. coli subsp. *fetus*	Pigs, poultry, bulls, sheep, birds	Gastroenteritis, septicemia, gastroenteritis, insects, abortion, spontaneous, meningitis	Uncommon
C. upsaliensis	Dogs, cats	Gastroenteritis, septicemia, abscesses	Uncommon
C. fetus subsp. *fetus*	Cattle, sheep	Septicemia, gastroenteritis, spontaneous abortion, meningitis	Uncommon
C. fetus subsp. *venerealis*	Cattle	Septicemia	Uncommon
C. hyointestinalis	Pigs, cattle, hamsters, deer	Gastroenteritis	Rare
C. concisus	Humans	Periodontal disease, gastroenteritis	Rare
C. sputorum subsp. *sputorum*	Humans, cattle, pigs	Abscesses, gastroenteritis	Rare
C. curvus	Humans	Periodontal disease, gastroenteritis	Rare
C. rectus	Humans	Periodontal disease	Rare
C. showae	Humans	Periodontal disease	Rare
C. lari	Poultry, birds, dogs, cats, monkeys, horses, seals	Gastroenteritis, septicemia	Rare

C. jejuni gastrointestinal disease characteristically produces histologic damage to the mucosal surfaces of the jejunum (as implied by the name of the species), ileum, and colon. The mucosal surface appears ulcerated, edematous, and bloody, with crypt abscesses in the epithelial glands and infiltration of the lamina propria with neutrophils, mononuclear cells, and eosinophils. This inflammatory process is consistent with invasion of the organisms into the intestinal tissue. However, the precise roles of cytopathic toxins, enterotoxins, and endotoxic activity that have been detected in *C. jejuni* isolates have not been defined. For example, strains lacking enterotoxin activity are still fully virulent. An adhesin that mediates the attachment of the organisms to the mucosal layer has been described; however, strains without the adhesin and nonmotile strains are avirulent.

C. jejuni and *C. upsaliensis* have been associated with Guillain-Barré syndrome, an autoimmune disorder of the peripheral nervous system characterized by development of symmetrical weakness over several days and recovery requiring weeks to months. Although this is an uncommon complication of *Campylobacter* disease (approximately one in 1000 diagnosed infections), the syndrome has been associated with specific serotypes (primarily *C. jejuni* serotype O:19). It is believed that the pathogenesis of this disease is related to antigenic cross-reactivity between oligosaccharides of *Campylobacter* and glycosphingolipids present on the surface of neural tissues. Thus antibodies directed against specific strains of *Campylobacter* can damage neural tissue in the peripheral nervous system. Another immune-related late complication of campylobacter infections is **reactive arthritis,** a condition characterized by painful joint swellings that may last for weeks to a year.

Whereas *C. jejuni* and *C. coli* rarely cause bacteremia (1.5 cases per 1000 intestinal infections), *C. fetus* has a propensity to spread from the gastrointestinal tract to the bloodstream and distal foci. This spread is particularly common in debilitated and immunocompromised patients, such as those with liver disease, diabetes mellitus, chronic alcoholism, or malignancies. In vitro studies have shown that *C. fetus* is resistant to complement- and antibody-mediated serum killing, whereas *C. jejuni* and most other *Campylobacter* species are killed rapidly. *C. fetus* is covered with a heat-stable, capsule-like protein **(S protein)** that prevents complement-mediated killing in serum (inhibition of C3b binding to the bacteria). *C. fetus* loses its virulence if this protein layer is removed.

EPIDEMIOLOGY

Campylobacter infections are zoonotic, with a variety of animals serving as reservoirs (see Table 33–1). Humans acquire the infections with *C. jejuni* and *C. coli* after consumption of contaminated food, milk, or water; contaminated poultry are responsible for more than half of the *Campylobacter* infections in developed countries. In contrast, *C. upsaliensis* infections are acquired primarily after contact with domestic dogs (either healthy carriers or pets with diarrheal disease). Food products that neutralize gastric acids (e.g., milk) effectively reduce the infectious dose. Fecal-oral transmission from person-to-person may also occur, but it is uncommon for the disease to be transmitted by food handlers.

The actual incidence of *Campylobacter* infections is unknown, because disease is not reported to public health officials. It has been estimated, however, that more than 2 million infections occur annually in the United States, and these infections are more common than *Salmonella* and *Shigella* infections combined. The number of *Campylobacter* infections may be even higher, because *C. upsaliensis* is believed to be responsible for approximately 10% of the *Campylobacter* infections, and this species would not be isolated by commonly used techniques. Disease is most common in the warm months but occurs throughout the year. The peak incidence of disease is in young adults. In developing countries, symptomatic disease occurs in young children, and persistent, asymptomatic carriage is observed in adults.

C. fetus infections are relatively uncommon, with fewer than 250 cases reported annually. Unlike *C. jejuni*, *C. fetus* primarily infects immunocompromised elderly people.

CLINICAL DISEASES

Gastrointestinal infections with *C. jejuni*, *C. coli*, *C. upsaliensis*, and other enteric pathogens are seen most commonly as acute enteritis with diarrhea, malaise, fever, and abdominal pain. Affected patients can have 10 or more bowel movements per day during the peak of disease, and stools may be bloody on gross examination. The disease is generally self-limited, although symptoms may last for a week or longer. The range of clinical manifestations includes colitis, acute abdominal pain, and bacteremia, and chronic infections can develop. In the most common presentation of *C. fetus* infection the patient experiences initial gastroenteritis, followed by septicemia with dissemination to multiple organs.

LABORATORY DIAGNOSIS

Microscopy

Campylobacters are thin and are not easily seen when specimens are stained. The organism, with its characteristic darting motility, can be detected on dark-field or phase-contrast microscopy in freshly collected stool specimens; however, these examinations are rarely performed. The organisms in cultured specimens appear as small, curved rods, arranged either singly or in end-to-end pairs (either resembling the curved wings of a gull or an S shape; Figure 33–1).

Culture

C. jejuni, *C. coli*, and *C. upsaliensis* went unrecognized for many years because their isolation requires growth in a microaerophilic atmosphere (i.e., 5% to 7% oxygen, 5% to 10% carbon dioxide, and the balance nitrogen), at an elevated incubation temperature (i.e., 42°C), and on selective media. The selective media must contain blood or charcoal to remove toxic oxygen radicals, and antibiotics are added to inhibit the growth of contaminating organisms. Campylobacters are slow-growing organisms, usually requiring incubation for 48 to 72 hours or longer. *C. fetus* is not thermophilic and cannot grow at 42°C; however, its isolation still requires a microaerophilic atmosphere.

Identification

Preliminary identification of isolates is based on growth under selective conditions and typical microscopic morphology. Definitive identification of all isolates is determined from the reactions summarized in Table 33–2.

TREATMENT, PREVENTION, AND CONTROL

Campylobacter gastroenteritis is typically a self-limited infection managed by the replacement of lost fluids and electrolytes. Antibiotic therapy may be used in patients with severe infections or septicemia. Campylobacters are susceptible to a variety of antibiotics, including macrolides (i.e., erythromycin, azithromycin, clarithromycin), tetracyclines, aminoglycosides, chloramphenicol, fluoroquinolones, clindamycin, amoxicillin/clavulanic acid, and imipenem. Most isolates are resistant to penicillins, cephalosporins, and sulfonamide antibiotics. Erythromycin is the antibiotic of choice for the treatment of enteritis, with tetracycline or fluoroquinolones used as secondary antibiotics. Resistance to fluoroquinolones has increased, so these drugs may be less effective. Amoxicillin/clavulanic acid can be used in place of tetracycline, which is contraindicated in young children. Systemic infections are treated with an aminoglycoside, chloramphenicol, or imipenem.

Exposure to enteric campylobacters is prevented by the proper preparation of food (particularly poultry), avoidance of unpasteurized dairy products, and the implementation of safeguards to prevent the contamination of water supplies. It is unlikely that *Campylobacter* carriage in

TABLE 33–2. Phenotypic Properties of Selected *Campylobacter* and *Helicobacter* Species

Characteristics	*C. jejuni*	*C. coli*	*C. upsaliensis*	*C. fetus*	*H. pylori*	*H. cinaedi*	*H. fennelliae*
Oxidase	+	+	+	+	+	+	+
Catalase	+	+	–/W	+	+	+	+
Nitrate reduction	+	+	+	+	–	+	–
Urease	–	–	–	–	+	–	–
Hydrolysis of:							
Hippurate	+	–	–	–	–	–	–
Indoxyl acetate	+	+	+	–	–	–	+
Growth at:							
25°C	–	–	–	+	–	–	–
37°C	+	+	+	+	+	+	+
42°C	+	+	+	–	–	–	–
Growth in 1% glycine	+	+	V	+	–	+	+
Susceptibility to:							
Nalidixic acid	S	S	S	V	R	S	S
Cephalothin	R	R	S	S	S	I	S

Modified from Murray PR et al, editors: *Manual of clinical microbiology,* ed 8, Washington, 2003, American Society for Microbiology.
+, Positive reaction; –, negative reaction; I, intermediate; R, resistant; S, susceptible; V, variable reaction; W, weak reaction.

TABLE 33–3. *Helicobacter* Species Associated with Human Disease*

Species	Reservoir Host	Human Disease	Frequency
H. pylori	Humans, primates, pigs	Gastritis, peptic ulcers, gastric adenocarcinoma	Common
H. cinaedi	Humans, hamsters	Gastroenteritis, septicemia, proctocolitis, cellulitis	Uncommon
H. fennelliae	Humans	Gastroenteritis, septicemia, proctocolitis	Uncommon
H. canadensis	Humans	Gastroenteritis	Rare
H. canis	Dogs	Gastroenteritis	Rare
H. pullorum	Poultry	Gastroenteritis	Rare

*Species associated with only one or two reported infections are not included in this table.

animal reservoirs such as chickens and turkeys will be eliminated, so the risk of infections from these sources remains.

Helicobacter (Box 33–3)

In 1983, spiral, gram-negative rods resembling campylobacters were found in patients with type B gastritis (chronic inflammation of the stomach antrum [pyloric end]). The organisms were originally classified as *Campylobacter* but were subsequently reclassified as a new genus, *Helicobacter.* The bacteria *Helicobacter pylori* have now been associated with gastritis, peptic ulcers, gastric adenocarcinoma, and gastric mucosa–associated lymphoid tissue (MALT) B-cell lymphomas (Table 33–3). Helicobacters have been isolated from the stomachs of many other mammals (e.g., monkeys, dogs, cats, cheetahs, ferrets, mice, rats). The intestinal tract is also colonized by helicobacters, including *Helicobacter cinaedi* and *Helicobacter fennelliae,* which have been isolated from homosexual men with proctitis, proctocolitis, or enteritis.

PHYSIOLOGY AND STRUCTURE

Helicobacter species are characterized according to sequence analysis of their 16S rRNA genes, their cellular fatty acids, and the presence of polar flagella. Currently, 22 species have been characterized, but this taxonomy is

BOX 33–3. Summary of *Helicobacter pylori*

Physiology and Structure
Curved, gram-negative rods
Urease production at very high levels is typical of gastric helicobacters (e.g., *H. pylori*) and uncommon in intestinal helicobacters (important diagnostic test for *H. pylori*)

Virulence
Refer to Table 33–4

Epidemiology
Infections are common, particularly in people in a low socioeconomic class or in developing nations
Humans are the primary reservoir
Person-to-person spread is important (typically fecal-oral)
Ubiquitous and worldwide with no seasonal incidence of disease

Diseases
Refer to Table 33–3

Diagnosis
Microscopy: Histologic examination of biopsy specimens is sensitive and specific
Urease test relatively sensitive and highly specific; urea breath test is a noninvasive test
H. pylori antigen test is sensitive and specific; performed with stool specimens
Culture requires incubation in microaerophilic conditions; growth is slow; relatively insensitive unless multiple biopsies are cultured
Serology useful for demonstrating exposure to *H. pylori*

Treatment, Prevention, and Control
Multiple regimens have been evaluated for treatment of *H. pylori* infections. Combined therapy with tetracycline, metronidazole, bismuth, and omeprazole for 2 weeks has had a high success rate
Prophylactic treatment of colonized individuals has not been useful and potentially has adverse effects, such as predisposing patients to adenocarcinomas of the lower esophagus
Human vaccines are not currently available

changing rapidly. Helicobacters have a bacillary or spiral shape in young cultures but can assume coccoid forms in older cultures (Figure 33–2).

H. pylori is highly motile (corkscrew motility) and produces an abundance of urease. Urease production is a consistent finding in *Helicobacter* species of humans that colonize the stomach but is uncommon in species found in the intestines. Helicobacters do not ferment or oxidize carbohydrates, although they can metabolize amino acids by fermentative pathways. Growth of *H. pylori* and other helicobacters requires a complex medium supplemented with blood, serum, charcoal, starch, or egg yolk, in

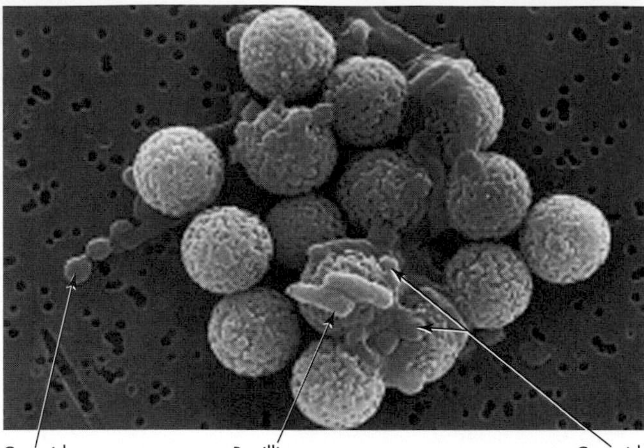

FIGURE 33–2. Scanning electron micrograph of *Helicobacter pylori* in a 7-day culture. Bacillary and coccoid forms (*arrows*) are bound to paramagnetic beads used in immunomagnetic separation. (Courtesy Dr. L. Engstrand, Uppsala, Sweden).

microaerophilic conditions (decreased oxygen and increased carbon dioxide), and in a temperature range between 30°C and 37°C.

PATHOGENESIS AND IMMUNITY

Most research into the virulence factors in helicobacters has focused on *H. pylori*. Multiple factors contribute to the gastric inflammation, alteration of gastric acid production, and tissue destruction that are characteristic of *H. pylori* disease (Table 33–4). Initial colonization is facilitated by (1) blockage of acid production by a bacterial acid–inhibitory protein and (2) neutralization of gastric acids by the ammonia produced by bacterial urease activity. The activity of bacterial urease is enhanced by a **heat shock protein (HspB)** that is coexpressed with **urease** on the bacterial surface. The actively motile helicobacters can then pass through the gastric mucus and adhere to the epithelial cells. Localized tissue damage is mediated by urease by-products, **mucinase, phospholipases,** and the activity of the **vacuolating cytotoxin** that induces epithelial cell damage and, together with urease and bacterial lipopolysaccharide, stimulates the inflammatory response. *H. pylori* is protected from phagocytosis and intracellular killing by production of **superoxide dismutase** and **catalase.** *H. pylori* also produces factors that stimulate (1) secretion of interleukin-8 (IL-8), (2) production of platelet-activating factor that causes hypersecretion of gastric acid, and (3) programmed death of gastric epithelial cells.

EPIDEMIOLOGY

An enormous amount of information about the prevalence of *H. pylori* has been collected since 1984, when the

TABLE 33-4. Virulence Factors of *Helicobacter pylori*

Virulence Factors	Function
Urease	Neutralizes gastric acids; stimulates monocytes and neutrophil chemotaxis; stimulates production of inflammatory cytokines
Heat shock protein (HspB)	Enhances expression of urease
Acid-inhibitory protein	Induces hypochlorhydria during acute infection by blocking acid secretion from parietal cells
Flagella	Allow penetration into gastric mucous layer and protection from acid environment
Adhesins	Mediate binding to host cells; examples of adhesins are hemagglutinins, sialic acid–binding adhesin, Lewis blood group adhesin
Mucinase	Disrupts gastric mucus
Phospholipases	Disrupt gastric mucus
Superoxide dismutase	Prevents phagocytic killing by neutralizing oxygen metabolites
Catalase	Prevents phagocytic killing by neutralizing peroxides
Vacuolating cytotoxin	Induces vacuolation in epithelial cells; stimulates neutrophil migration into mucosa
Poorly defined factors	*H. pylori:* Stimulates interleukin-8 secretion by gastric epithelial cells, which recruits and activates neutrophils Stimulates gastric mucosal cells to produce platelet-activating factor, which stimulates gastric acid secretion Induces nitric oxide synthase in gastric epithelial cells, which mediates tissue injury Induces death of gastric epithelial cells

organism was first isolated in culture. The highest incidence of carriage is found in developing countries, where 70% to 90% of the population is colonized, most before the age of 10 years. In contrast, developed countries such as the United States have documented that the incidence of *H. pylori* colonization in healthy people is relatively low during childhood but increases to approximately 45% in older adults. These studies have also demonstrated that 70% to 100% of patients with gastritis, gastric ulcers, or duodenal ulcers are infected with *H. pylori.* The difference in colonization rates between developing and developed countries is believed to be a result of improved hygienic standards in the latter. Humans are the primary reservoir for *H. pylori,* and transmission is most likely via the fecal-oral route. Thus it is expected that the risk of colonization will decrease with improved hygienic standards.

An interesting observation about *H. pylori* colonization has been made. This organism is clearly associated with diseases such as gastritis, gastric ulcers, gastric adenocarcinoma, and gastric MALT lymphomas. It is anticipated that treatment of colonized or infected individuals will lead to a reduction of these diseases. However, colonization with *H. pylori* appears to offer protection from gastroesophageal reflux disease and adenocarcinomas of the lower esophagus and gastric cardia. Thus it may be unwise to eliminate *H. pylori* in patients without symptomatic disease. Certainly the complex relationship between *H. pylori* and its host remains to be defined.

CLINICAL DISEASES

Helicobacter species can be subdivided into gastric helicobacters (e.g., *H. pylori*) and enteric helicobacters (e.g., *H. cinaedi, H. fennelliae, H. canis, H. canadensis, H. pullorum*). Disease caused by helicobacters is directly related to their site of colonization. For example, H. pylori is associated with gastritis, whereas the enteric species cause gastroenteritis.

Overwhelming clinical evidence shows that *H. pylori* is the etiologic agent in virtually all cases of type B gastritis. This evidence includes (1) virtually a 100% association between gastritis and infection with the bacterium, (2) production of experimental infection in both animals and humans, and (3) histologic resolution of the pathologic changes when specific therapy is used to eradicate the organism. *H. pylori* is also responsible for up to 80% of gastric ulcers and more than 90% of duodenal ulcers, with elimination of the organism leading to healing of the ulcers and a significant reduction in the rate of recurrence.

Chronic gastritis is a risk factor for gastric carcinoma, so it is not surprising that there is a relationship between infection with *H. pylori* and adenocarcinoma of the body and antrum of the stomach but not the cardia (an area of the stomach that is not infected by *H. pylori*). *H. pylori* colonization is also associated with gastric MALT B-cell lymphomas. Supporting the role of *H. pylori* in these malignancies is the observation that therapy directed against the bacteria is associated with regression of the lymphoma.

H. cinaedi and *H. fennelliae* can cause gastroenteritis and proctocolitis with septicemia in homosexual men. *H. cinaedi* also causes recurrent cellulitis with fever and bacteremia in immunocompromised patients.

LABORATORY DIAGNOSIS

Microscopy

H. pylori is detected by histologic examination of gastric biopsy specimens. Although the organism can be seen in specimens stained with hematoxylin-eosin or Gram stain, the Warthin-Starry silver stain is the most sensitive. The sensitivity and specificity of histologic analysis approaches 100% and is considered the diagnostic gold standard; however, this is an invasive test and is not commonly performed for routine diagnosis.

Urease Test

Biopsy specimens can also be tested for the presence of bacterial urease activity. The abundance of urease produced by *H. pylori* permits detection of the alkaline by-product in less than 2 hours. The sensitivity of the direct test with biopsy specimens varies from 75% to 95%; however, the specificity approaches 100%, so a positive reaction is compelling evidence of an active infection. As with microscopy, the limitation of this method is the requirement for a biopsy specimen. Noninvasive urease testing of human breath following consumption of an isotopically labeled urea solution has excellent sensitivity and specificity. Unfortunately, this assay is relatively expensive because of the cost of the detection instruments.

Antigen Detection

H. pylori antigens excreted in stool can be detected in a commercial polyclonal enzyme immunoassay. The assay has a sensitivity and specificity of approximately 90% and 95%, respectively. This test is easy to perform, inexpensive, and relatively accurate for patients with a moderate to high probability of disease.

Culture

H. pylori can grow only in a microaerophilic atmosphere on enriched medium supplemented with blood, hemin, or charcoal. The supplementation of the medium protects the bacteria from oxygen-free radicals, hydrogen peroxide, and fatty acids. Specimens should not be inoculated onto media used for the recovery of *Campylobacter*, because these media are too inhibitory. Culture requires the invasive collection of specimens and is insensitive unless multiple gastric mucosal biopsies are processed. Additionally, the success of culture is influenced by the experience of the microbiologist. Preliminary identification of isolates is based on their growth characteristics under selective conditions, typical microscopic morphologic findings, and detection of oxidase, catalase, and urease activity. Definitive identification of *H. pylori* and related bacteria is guided by the reactions summarized in Table 33–2.

Serology

Serology is considered the diagnostic test of choice, either used alone or in combination with the antigen test. Infection with *H. pylori* stimulates a humoral immune reaction that persists as the result of continuous exposure to the bacteria. Immunoglobulin M (IgM) antibodies appear early in disease and then wane. IgG and IgA antibodies appear soon after IgM and can persist for months or years. Because the antibody titers persist for many years, the test cannot be used to discriminate between past and current infection. Furthermore, the titer of antibodies measured does not correlate with the severity of the disease or the response to therapy. However, the tests are useful for documenting exposure to the bacteria, either for epidemiologic studies or for the initial evaluation of a symptomatic patient.

TREATMENT, PREVENTION, AND CONTROL

Numerous antibiotic regimens have been evaluated for treating *H. pylori* infections. Use of a single antibiotic or an antibiotic combined with bismuth is ineffective. The greatest success in curing gastritis or peptic ulcer disease has been accomplished with the combination of a proton pump inhibitor (e.g., omeprazole) and one or more antibiotics (e.g., tetracycline, clarithromycin, amoxicillin, metronidazole). Bismuth can also be added. At this time, multiple treatment regimens are in use; however, therapy with the combination of tetracycline, metronidazole, bismuth, and omeprazole for 2 weeks has an eradication rate greater than 90%. Growing resistance to metronidazole may necessitate use of an alternative antibiotic mixture. Infections caused by *H. cinaedi* and *H. fennelliae* can generally be treated with ampicillin or gentamicin.

Efforts are under way to develop a vaccine against *H. pylori*. Urease and HspB are expressed uniquely on the surface of the bacteria. The success of using these antigens in a vaccine remains to be demonstrated.

CASE STUDY AND QUESTIONS

A mother and her 4-year-old son came to the local emergency room with a 1-day history of diarrhea and abdominal cramping. Both patients had low-grade fevers, and blood was grossly evident in the child's stool specimen. The symptoms had developed 18 hours after the patients had consumed a dinner consisting of mixed green salad, chicken, corn, bread, and apple pie. Culture of blood samples was negative for organisms, but C. jejuni was isolated from stool specimens of both the mother and the child.

1. Which food that they consumed is most likely responsible for these infections? What measures should be used to prevent these infections?
2. Name three Campylobacter species that have been associated with gastroenteritis. Name the species of Campylobacter that is most commonly associated with septicemia.
3. What diseases have been associated with H. pylori? H. cinaedi? H. fennelliae?
4. H. pylori has multiple virulence factors. Which factors are responsible for interfering with gastric acid secretion? For adhering to the gastric epithelium? For disrupting the gastric mucus? For interfering with phagocytic killing?

Bibliography

Blaser MJ: In a world of black and white, *Helicobacter pylori* is gray, *Ann Intern Med* 130:695-697, 1999.

Bourke B et al: *Campylobacter upsaliensis:* Waiting in the wings, *Clin Microbiol Rev* 1:440-449, 1998.

Dunn B et al: *Helicobacter pylori, Clin Microbiol Rev* 10:720-741, 1997.

Friedman L: *Helicobacter pylori* and nonulcer dyspepsia, *N Engl J Med* 339:1928-1930, 1998 (editorial).

Hunt R, editor: Proceedings of a symposium: *Helicobacter pylori:* From theory to practice, *Am J Med* 100:1-64, 1996.

Nachamkin I et al: *Campylobacter* species and Guillain-Barré syndrome, *Clin Microbiol Rev* 11:555-567, 1998.

NIH Consensus Development Panel: *Helicobacter pylori* in peptic ulcer disease, *JAMA* 272:65-69, 1994.

On SLW: Identification methods for campylobacters, helicobacters, and related organisms, *Clin Microbiol Rev* 9:405-422, 1996.

Parsonnet J et al: Fecal and oral shedding of *Helicobacter pylori* from healthy infected adults, *JAMA* 282:2240-2245, 1999.

Passaro D, Chosy EJ, Parsonnet J: *Helicobacter pylori:* Consensus and controversy, *Clin Infect Dis* 35:298-304, 2002.

Samuel MC et al: Epidemiology of sporadic *Campylobacter* infection in the United States and declining trend in incidence, FoodNet 1996-1999, *Clin Infect Dis* 38:S165-174, 2004.

Solnick J: Clinical significance of *Helicobacter* species other than *Helicobacter pylori, Clin Infect Dis* 36:348-354, 2003.

Staat MA et al: A population-based serologic survey of *Helicobacter pylori* infection in children and adolescents in the United States, *J Infect Dis* 174:1120-1123, 1996.

Wassenaar T: Toxin production by *Campylobacter* spp., *Clin Microbiol Rev* 10:466-476, 1997.

Weingart V et al: Sensitivity of a novel stool antigen test for detection of *Helicobacter pylori* in adult outpatients before and after eradication therapy, *J Clin Microbiol* 42:1319-1321, 2004.

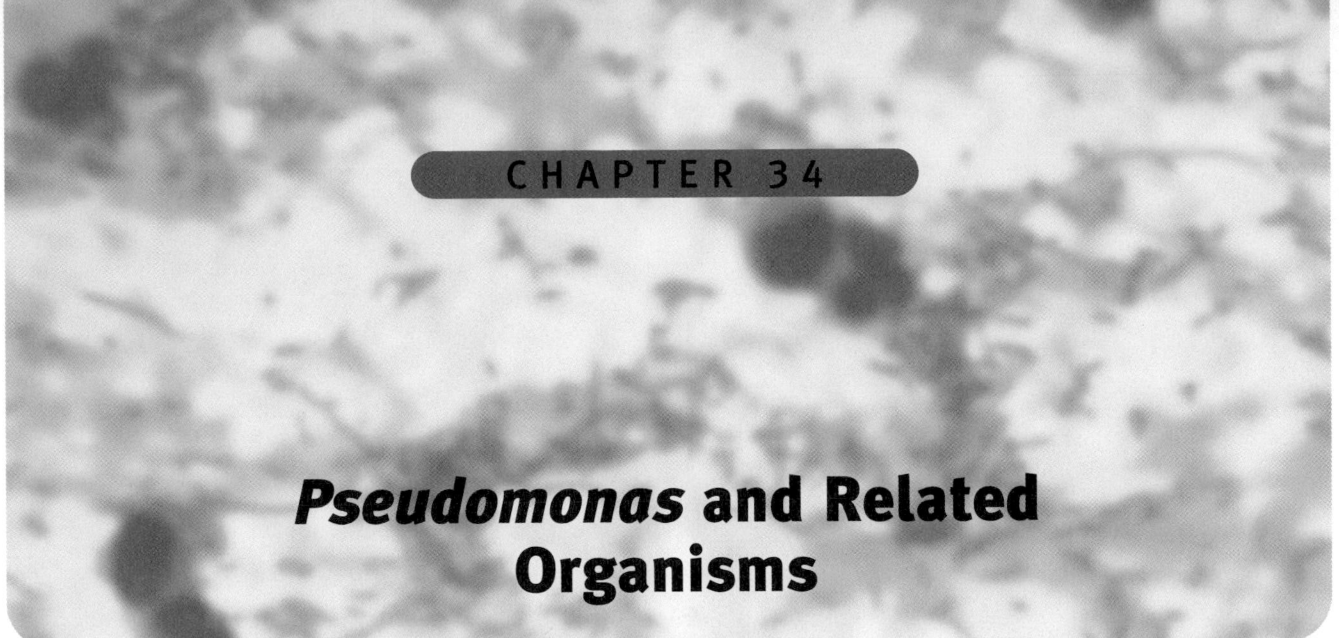

Pseudomonas and Related Organisms

Pseudomonas and related nonfermentative rods are a complex mixture of opportunistic pathogens of plants, animals, and humans. To complicate our understanding of these organisms, their taxonomic classification has undergone numerous changes in recent years. Despite the many genera, only a few are isolated commonly. Specifically, more than 75% of the nonfermenters isolated from clinical specimens are *Pseudomonas aeruginosa, Burkholderia cepacia, Stenotrophomonas maltophilia, Acinetobacter baumannii* and *Acenetobacter lwoffii*, and *Moraxella catarrhalis* (Box 34–1). These organisms will be the focus of this chapter.

Pseudomonas (Box 34–2)

Members of the genus *Pseudomonas* (also called pseudomonads) are ubiquitous organisms found in soil, decaying organic matter, vegetation, and water. Unfortunately, they are also found throughout the hospital environment in moist reservoirs, such as food, cut flowers, sinks, toilets, floor mops, and respiratory therapy and dialysis equipment, and even in disinfectant solutions. It is uncommon for carriage to persist in humans as part of the normal microbial flora, except in hospitalized patients and ambulatory, immunocompromised hosts.

The broad environmental distribution of pseudomonads is made possible by their simple growth requirements and nutritional versatility. They are capable of using many organic compounds as sources of carbon and nitrogen, and some strains can even grow in distilled water by using trace nutrients. Pseudomonads also possess many structural factors, enzymes, and toxins that enhance their virulence and render them resistant to most commonly used antibiotics. Indeed it is surprising that these organisms are not more common pathogens, considering their ubiquitous presence, ability to grow in virtually any environment, virulence properties, and resistance to many antibiotics. Instead, *Pseudomonas* infections are primarily opportunistic (i.e., restricted to patients with compromised host defenses). This fact illustrates the importance of the host's ability to prevent colonization and subsequent invasion with pseudomonads.

PHYSIOLOGY AND STRUCTURE

Pseudomonads are motile, straight or slightly curved, gram-negative rods (0.5 to 1.0 × 1.5 to 5.0 μm) typically arranged in pairs (Figure 34–1). The organisms are nonfermentative, using carbohydrates through respiratory metabolism, with oxygen the terminal electron acceptor. Although pseudomonads are defined as obligate aerobes, they can grow anaerobically using nitrate or arginine as an alternate electron acceptor. The presence of cytochrome oxidase (detected in a rapid, 5-minute test) in *Pseudomonas* species is used to differentiate them from the Enterobacteriaceae. Some strains appear mucoid because of the abundance of a polysaccharide capsule (Figure 34–2); these strains are particularly common in patients with cystic fibrosis. Some pseudomonads produce diffusible pigments (e.g., pyocyanin [blue], fluorescein [yellow], pyorubin [reddish-brown]).

In the past, the genus consisted of a large number of species, but many species have been reclassified in other genera. The genus now consists of approximately 10 species that have been isolated in clinical specimens and numerous other environmental species. *P. aeruginosa* is the most common pseudomonad and the species that is emphasized in this chapter.

PATHOGENESIS AND IMMUNITY

P. aeruginosa has many virulence factors, including structural components, toxins, and enzymes (Table 34–1);

BOX 34–1. Important Nonfermentative Gram-Negative Rods

Organism	Historical Derivation
Acinetobacter baumannii	*akinetos,* unable to move; *bactrum,* rod (nonmotile rods); *baumannii,* named after the microbiologist Baumann
A. lwoffii	*lwoffii,* named after the microbiologist Lwoff
Burkholderia cepacia	*Burkholderia,* named after the microbiologist Burkholder; *cepacia,* like an onion (original strains isolated from rotten onions)
B. mallei	*mallei,* the disease glanders
B. pseudomallei	*pseudes,* false; *mallei* (refers to the fact this species closely resembles *B. mallei*)
Moraxella catarrhalis	*Moraxella,* named after the Swiss ophthalmologist Morax, who first recognized the species; *catarrhus,* downflowing or catarrh (refers to inflammation of the respiratory tract mucus membranes)
Pseudomonas aeruginosa	*pseudes,* false; *monas,* a unit or monas; *aeruginosa,* full of copper rust or green (refers to green pigment produced by this species)
Stenotrophomonas	*maltophilia Stenos,* narrow; *trophos,* one who feeds *monas,* unit (refers to observation that these are narrow bacteria that require few substrates for growth); *malt,* malt; *philia,* friend (friend of malt)

however, defining the role that each factor plays in disease is difficult, and most experts in this field believe that its virulence is multifactorial.

Adhesins

Adherence of *P. aeruginosa* to host cells is mediated by **pili and nonpilus adhesins.** Pili are important for binding to epithelial cells and are similar in structure to the pili found in *Neisseria gonorrhoeae. P. aeruginosa* also produces neuraminidase, which removes sialic acid residues from the pili receptor, thereby enhancing adherence of the bacteria to the epithelial cells.

Polysaccharide Capsule

P. aeruginosa produces a polysaccharide **capsule** (also known as mucoid exopolysaccharide, alginate coat, or glycocalyx) that has multiple functions. The polysaccharide layer anchors the bacteria to epithelial cells and tracheobronchial mucin. The capsule also protects the organism from phagocytosis and activity of antibiotics such as aminoglycosides. The production of this mucoid polysaccharide is under complex regulation. The genes

BOX 34–2. Summary of *Pseudomonas aeruginosa*

Physiology and Structure

Small, gram-negative rods typically arranged in pairs
Obligate aerobe; glucose oxidizer; simple nutritional needs
Mucoid polysaccharide capsule

Virulence

Refer to Table 34–1

Epidemiology

Ubiquitous in nature and moist environmental hospital sites (e.g., flowers, sinks, toilets, respiratory and dialysis equipment)
No seasonal incidence of disease
Can transiently colonize the respiratory and gastrointestinal tracts of hospitalized patients, particularly those treated with broad-spectrum antibiotics, exposed to respiratory therapy equipment, or hospitalized for extended periods

Diseases

Refer to Box 34–3

Diagnosis

Grows rapidly on common laboratory media
Identified by colonial characteristics (e.g., hemolytic, green pigment, grape-like odor) and simple biochemical tests (e.g., positive oxidase reaction; oxidative utilization of carbohydrates).

Treatment, Prevention, and Control

Combined use of effective antibiotics (e.g., aminoglycoside and β-lactam antibiotics) frequently required; monotherapy is generally ineffective and can select for resistant strains
Hospital infection control efforts should concentrate on preventing contamination of sterile medical equipment and nosocomial transmission; unnecessary use of broad-spectrum antibiotics can select for resistant organisms

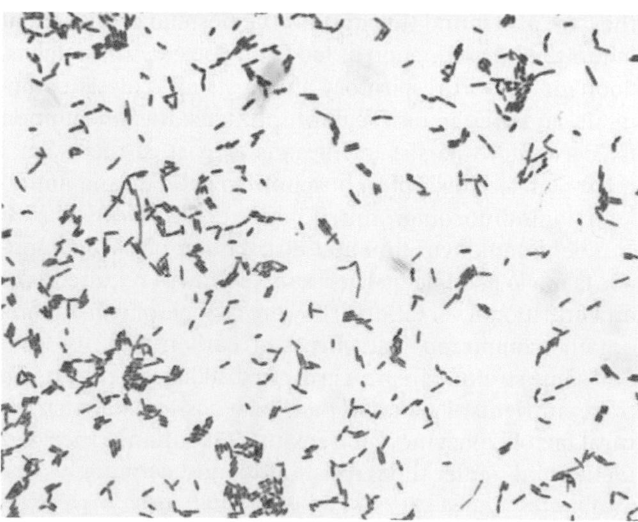

FIGURE 34–1. Gram stain of *Pseudomonas aeruginosa* with cells arranged singly and in pairs.

TABLE 34–1. Virulence Factors Associated with *Pseudomonas aeruginosa*

Virulence Factors	Biologic Effects
Structural Components	
Capsule	Mucoid polysaccharide; adhesin; inhibits antibiotic (e.g., aminoglycoside) killing; suppresses neutrophil and lymphocyte activity
Pili	Adhesin
Lipopolysaccharide	Endotoxin activity
Pyocyanin	Impairs ciliary function; increases release of IL-8, leading to stimulation of inflammatory response; mediates tissue damage through production of toxic oxygen radicals (i.e., hydrogen peroxide, superoxide, hydroxyl radicals)
Toxins and Enzymes	
Exotoxin A	Inhibits protein synthesis; produces tissue damage (e.g., skin, cornea); immunosuppressive
Exotoxin S	Inhibits protein synthesis; immunosuppressive
Cytotoxin (leukocidin)	Cytotoxic for eukaryotic membranes (e.g., disrupts leukocyte function, produces pulmonary microvascular injury)
Elastase	Destruction of elastin-containing tissues (e.g., blood vessels, lung tissue, skin), collagen, immunoglobulins, and complement factors
Alkaline protease	Destruction of tissue; inactivation of INF and TNF-α
Phospholipase C	Heat-labile hemolysin; mediates tissue damage; stimulates inflammatory response
Rhamnolipid	Heat-stable hemolysin; disrupts lecithin-containing tissues; inhibits pulmonary ciliary activity
Antibiotic resistance	Complicates antimicrobial therapy

IL-8, Interleukin-8; INF, interferon, TNF-α, tumor necrosis factor alpha.

controlling production of the alginate polysaccharide can be activated in patients, such as those with cystic fibrosis or other chronic respiratory diseases, who are predisposed to long-term colonization with these mucoid strains of *P. aeruginosa.* The mucoid strains can revert to a nonmucoid phenotype when cultured in vitro.

Endotoxin

Lipopolysaccharide **endotoxin** is a major cell wall antigen in *P. aeruginosa,* as it is in other gram-negative rods. The lipid A component of endotoxin mediates the various biologic effects of the sepsis syndrome.

Pyocyanin

A blue pigment, **pyocyanin,** produced by *P. aeruginosa* catalyzes the production of superoxide and hydrogen peroxide, toxic forms of oxygen. In the presence of pyochelin (an iron-binding siderophore), the more toxic hydroxyl radical is produced, which can mediate tissue damage. This pigment also stimulates interleukin-8 (IL-8) release, leading to enhanced attraction of neutrophils.

Exotoxin A

Exotoxin A (ETA) is believed to be one of the most important virulence factors produced by pathogenic strains of *P. aeruginosa.* This toxin disrupts protein synthesis by blocking peptide chain elongation in eukaryotic cells, much like the diphtheria toxin produced by *Corynebacterium diphtheriae.* However, the toxins produced by these two organisms are structurally and immunologically different, and exotoxin A is less potent than diphtheria toxin. Exotoxin A most likely contributes to the dermatonecrosis that occurs in burn wounds, corneal damage in ocular infections, and tissue damage in chronic pulmonary infections. The toxin is also immunosuppressive.

Exoenzymes S and T

Exoenzymes S and **T** are extracellular toxins produced by *P. aeruginosa.* They possess adenosine diphosphate (ADP)-ribosyltransferase activity, the function of which is unclear. However, when the type III secretion system introduces the proteins into their target eukaryotic cells, epithelial cell damage occurs, facilitating bacterial spread, tissue invasion, and necrosis. This cytotoxicity is mediated by actin rearrangement.

Elastases

Two enzymes, LasA **(serine protease)** and LasB **(zinc metalloprotease),** act synergistically to degrade elastin, resulting in damage to elastin-containing tissues and producing the lung parenchymal damage and hemorrhagic lesions **(ecthyma gangrenosum)** associated with disseminated *P. aeruginosa* infections. These enzymes can also degrade complement components and inhibit neutrophil chemotaxis and function, leading to further spread and tissue damage in acute infections. Chronic *Pseudomonas* infections are characterized by the formation of antibodies to LasA and LasB, with the deposition of immune complexes in the infected tissues.

Alkaline Protease

Like the elastases, **alkaline protease** contributes to tissue destruction and spread of *P. aeruginosa.* It also interferes with the host immune response.

Phospholipase C

Phospholipase C is a heat-labile hemolysin that breaks down lipids and lecithin, facilitating tissue destruction. The exact role of this enzyme in respiratory and urinary tract infections (UTIs) is unclear, although an important association between hemolysin production and disease has been recognized.

Rhamnolipid

Rhamnolipid is a heat-stable hemolysin that disrupts lecithin-containing tissues. This hemolysin is also associated with inhibition of ciliary activity of the respiratory tract.

Antibiotic Resistance

P. aeruginosa is inherently **resistant to many antibiotics** and can mutate to even more resistant strains during therapy. Although numerous resistance mechanisms have been identified, the mutation of porin proteins constitutes the major mechanism of resistance. Penetration of antibiotics into the pseudomonad cell is primarily through pores in the outer membrane. If the proteins forming the walls of these pores are altered to restrict flow into the cell, resistance to many classes of antibiotics can develop simultaneously. *P. aeruginosa* also produces a number of different β-lactamases that can inactivate many β-lactam antibiotics (e.g., penicillins, cephalosporins, carbapenems).

EPIDEMIOLOGY

Pseudomonads are opportunistic pathogens present in a variety of environments. The ability to isolate these organisms from moist surfaces may be limited only by the efforts to look for the organism. Pseudomonads have minimal nutritional requirements, can tolerate a wide range of temperatures (4° to 42°C), and are resistant to many antibiotics and disinfectants. Indeed the recovery of *Pseudomonas* from an environmental source (e.g., hospital sink or floor) means very little unless there is epidemiologic evidence that the contaminated site is a reservoir for infection.

Furthermore, isolation of pseudomonads from a hospitalized patient is worrisome but does not normally justify therapeutic intervention unless there is evidence of disease. The recovery of *Pseudomonas,* particularly species other than *P. aeruginosa,* from a clinical specimen may represent simple transient colonization of the patient or environmental contamination of the specimen during collection or laboratory processing.

CLINICAL DISEASES (Box 34–3)

Pulmonary Infections

P. aeruginosa infections of the lower respiratory tract can range in severity from asymptomatic colonization or benign **tracheobronchitis** to severe **necrotizing bronchopneumonia.** Colonization is seen in patients with cystic fibrosis, other chronic lung diseases, or neutropenia. Infections in patients with cystic fibrosis have been associated with exacerbation of the underlying disease and invasive pulmonary disease. Mucoid strains are commonly isolated from specimens from such patients and are difficult to eradicate with antibiotic therapy.

Conditions that predispose immunocompromised patients to infections with *Pseudomonas* include: (1) previous therapy with broad-spectrum antibiotics that disrupt the normal, protective bacterial population, and (2) use of respiratory therapy equipment, which may introduce the organism to the lower airways. Invasive disease in this population is characterized by a diffuse, typically bilateral bronchopneumonia with microabscess formation and tissue necrosis. The mortality rate is as high as 70%.

Primary Skin Infections

P. aeruginosa can cause a variety of primary skin infections. The most recognized are infections of **burn wounds** (Figure 34–3). Colonization of a burn wound, followed by localized vascular damage, tissue necrosis, and ultimately bacteremia, is common in patients with severe burns. The moist surface of the burn and the lack of a neutrophilic response to tissue invasion predispose

BOX 34–3. Selected Pathogenic, Nonfermentative Gram-Negative Rods: Clinical Summaries

Pseudomonas aeruginosa

Pulmonary infections: Range from mild irritation of the bronchi (tracheobronchitis) to necrosis of the lung parenchyma (necrotizing bronchopneumonia)

Primary skin infections: Opportunistic infections of existing wounds (e.g., burns) to localized infections of hair follicles (e.g., associated with immersion in contaminated waters such as hot tubs)

Urinary tract infections: Opportunistic infections in patients with indwelling urinary catheters and exposure to broad-spectrum antibiotics (selects for these antibiotic-resistant bacteria)

Ear infections: Can range from mild irritation of external ear ("swimmer's ear") to invasive destruction of cranial bones adjacent to the infected ear

Eye infections: Opportunistic infections of exposed, mildly damaged corneas

Bacteremia: Dissemination of bacteria from primary infection (e.g., pulmonary) to other organs and tissues; can be characterized by necrotic skin lesions (ecthyma gangrenosum) *Burkholderia cepacia* complex

Pulmonary infections: The most worrisome infections are in patients with chronic granulomatous disease or cystic fibrosis in whom infections can progress to significant destruction of pulmonary tissue

***Burkholderia cepacia* Complex**

Pulmonary infections: Range from colonization to bronchopneumonia primary in patients with cystic fibrosis or chronic granulomatous disease

Opportunistic infections: Urinary tract infections in catheterized patients; bacteria in immunocompromised patients with contaminated intravascular catheters

Burkholderia pseudomallei

Pulmonary infections: Can range from asymptomatic colonization to abscess formation

Stenotrophomonas maltophilia

Opportunistic infections: A variety of infections (most commonly pulmonary and urinary tract) in immunocompromised patients previously exposed to broad-spectrum antimicrobial therapy

***Acinetobacter* species**

Pulmonary infections: Opportunistic pathogen in patients receiving respiratory therapy

***Moraxella* species**

Pulmonary infections: Tracheobronchitis or bronchopneumonia in patients with chronic pulmonary diseases (most commonly caused by *M. catarrhalis*)

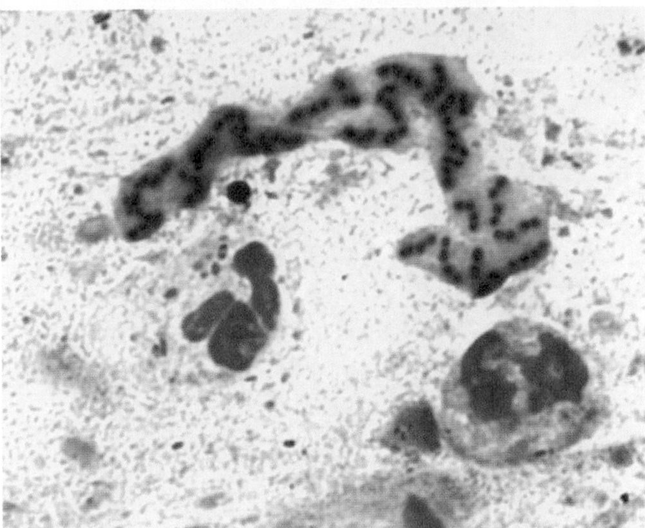

FIGURE 34–2. Gram stain of *Pseudomonas* aeruginosa surrounded by mucoid capsular material in cystic fibrosis patient.

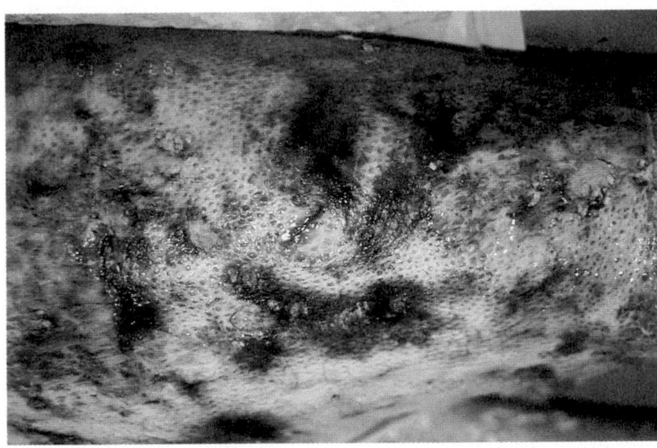

FIGURE 34–3. *Pseudomonas* infection of burn wound (From Cohen J, Powderly WB: *Infectious diseases,* ed 2, St Louis, 2004, Mosby.)

patients to such infections. Wound management with topical antibiotic creams has had only limited success in controlling these infections.

Folliculitis (Figure 34–4) is another common infection caused by *Pseudomonas,* resulting from immersion in contaminated water (e.g., hot tubs, whirlpools, swimming pools). Secondary infections with *Pseudomonas* also occur in people who have acne or who depilate their legs. Finally, *P. aeruginosa* can cause fingernail infections in people whose hands are frequently exposed to water.

Urinary Tract Infections

Infection of the urinary tract is seen primarily in patients with long-term indwelling urinary catheters. Typically, such patients are treated with multiple courses of antibi-

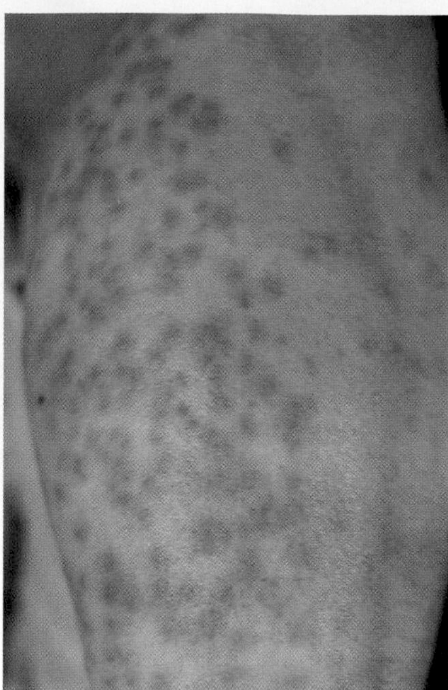

FIGURE 34–4. *Pseudomonas* folliculitis. (From Cohen J, Powderly WB: *Infectious diseases*, ed 2, St Louis, 2004, Mosby.)

otics, which tend to select for the more resistant strains of bacteria, such as *Pseudomonas.*

Ear Infections

External otitis is frequently caused by *P. aeruginosa,* with swimming an important risk factor **("swimmer's ear")**. This localized infection can be managed with topical antibiotics and drying agents. **Malignant external otitis** is a virulent form of disease seen primarily in persons with diabetes and elderly patients. It can invade the underlying tissues, can damage the cranial nerves and bones, and can be life threatening. Aggressive, antimicrobial and surgical intervention is required for patients with the latter disease. *P. aeruginosa* is also associated with **chronic otitis media.**

Eye Infections

Infections of the eye occur after initial trauma to the cornea (e.g., abrasion from contact lens, scratch on the eye surface) and then exposure to *P. aeruginosa* in contaminated water. **Corneal ulcers** develop and can progress to eye-threatening disease unless prompt treatment is instituted.

Bacteremia and Endocarditis

Bacteremia caused by *P. aeruginosa* is clinically indistinguishable from that caused by other gram-negative bacteria. However, the mortality rate in affected patients is higher with *P. aeruginosa* bacteremia because of (1) the predilection of the organism for immunocompromised patients and (2) the inherent virulence of *Pseudomonas.* Bacteremia occurs most often in patients with neutropenia, diabetes mellitus, extensive burns, and hematologic malignancies. Most bacteremias originate from infections of the lower respiratory tract, urinary tract, and skin and soft tissue (particularly burn wound infections). Although seen in a minority of bacteremic patients, characteristic skin lesions **(ecthyma gangrenosum)** may develop. The lesions manifest as erythematous vesicles that become hemorrhagic, necrotic, and ulcerated. Microscopic examination of the lesion shows abundant organisms, vascular destruction (which explains the hemorrhagic nature of the lesions), and an absence of neutrophils, as would be expected in neutropenic patients.

Pseudomonas **endocarditis** is most commonly observed in intravenous-drug abusers. These patients acquire the infection from the use of drug paraphernalia contaminated with the waterborne organisms. The tricuspid valve is often involved, and the infection is associated with a chronic course but with a more favorable prognosis than that in patients who have infections of the aortic or mitral valve.

Other Infections

P. aeruginosa is also the cause of a variety of other infections, including those localized in the gastrointestinal tract, central nervous system, and musculoskeletal system. The underlying conditions required for most infections are (1) the presence of the organism in a moist reservoir and (2) the circumvention or elimination of host defenses (e.g., cutaneous trauma, elimination of normal microbial flora as a result of antibiotic usage, neutropenia).

LABORATORY DIAGNOSIS

Culture

Because pseudomonads have simple nutritional requirements, they grow easily on common isolation media such as blood agar and MacConkey agar. They do require aerobic incubation (unless nitrate is available), so their growth in broth is generally confined to the broth-air interface, where the oxygen concentration is the highest.

Identification

The colonial morphology (e.g., colony size, hemolytic activity, pigmentation, odor; Figure 34–5) and the results of selected rapid biochemical tests (e.g., positive oxidase reaction) are sufficient for the preliminary identification of these isolates. For example, *P. aeruginosa* grows rapidly and

TABLE 34–2. Mechanisms of Antibiotic Resistance in *Pseudomonas aeruginosa*

Antibiotic	Resistance Mechanisms
β-Lactams	β-Lactamase hydrolysis; decreased permeability; altered binding proteins
Aminoglycosides	Enzymatic hydrolysis by acetylation, adenylation, or phosphorylation; decreased permeability; altered ribosomal target
Chloramphenicol	Enzymatic hydrolysis by acetyltransferase; decreased permeability
Fluoroquinolones	Altered target (DNA gyrase); decreased permeability

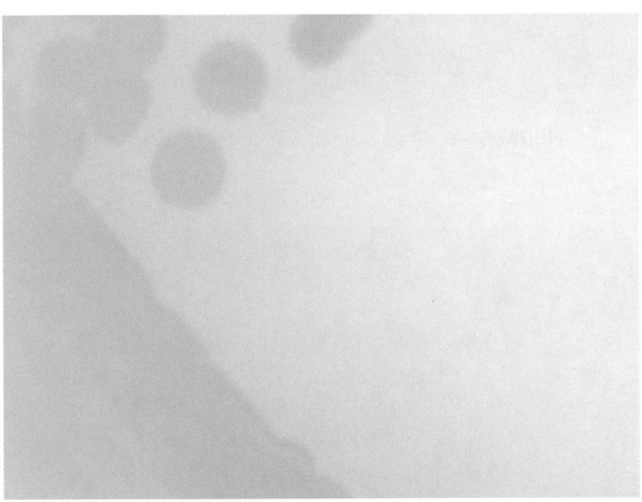

FIGURE 34–5. Colonial morphology of *Pseudomonas aeruginosa;* note the green pigmentation that results from the production of two water-soluble dyes: blue pyocyanin and yellow fluorescein.

has flat colonies with a spreading border, β-hemolysis, a green pigmentation caused by the production of the blue (pyocyanin) and yellow (fluorescein) pigments, and a characteristic sweet, grape-like odor. Although definitive identification of *P. aeruginosa* is relatively easy, an extensive battery of physiologic tests may be required to identify other pseudomonads.

TREATMENT, PREVENTION, AND CONTROL

The antimicrobial therapy for *Pseudomonas* infections is frustrating because (1) the bacteria are typically resistant to most antibiotics (Table 34–2) and (2) the infected patient with compromised host defenses cannot augment the antibiotic activity. Even susceptible organisms can become resistant during therapy by inducing the formation of antibiotic-inactivating enzymes (e.g., β-lactamases) or the mutation of the genes coding the outer membrane pore proteins or through the transfer of plasmid-mediated resistance from a resistant organism to a susceptible one. Furthermore, some groups of antibiotics are ineffective at certain sites of infection (e.g., aminoglycosides have poor activity in the acidic environment of an abscess). A combination of active antibiotics is generally required for therapy to be successful in patients with serious infections.

Attempts to eliminate *Pseudomonas* from the hospital environment are practically useless given the ubiquitous presence of the organism in water supplies. Effective infection-control practices should concentrate on preventing the contamination of sterile equipment, such as respiratory therapy and dialysis machines, and the cross-contamination of patients by medical personnel. The inappropriate use of broad-spectrum antibiotics should also be avoided because such use can suppress the normal microbial flora and permit the overgrowth of resistant pseudomonads.

Burkholderia

Four species formerly classified as *Pseudomonas* have been reclassified as members of the genus *Burkholderia.* It was subsequently appreciated that *B. cepacia* is a complex of nine species. However, because these species are nearly identical by phenotypic tests, the collection is commonly referred to as *B. cepacia* complex. *B. cepacia* complex and *Burkholderia pseudomallei* are important human pathogens (see Box 34–3); *Burkholderia gladioli* and *Burkholderia mallei* are only rarely associated with human disease.

Like *P. aeruginosa, B. cepacia* complex can colonize a variety of moist environmental surfaces and is commonly associated with nosocomial infections. Infections caused by this organism include the following: (1) respiratory tract infections in patients with cystic fibrosis or chronic granulomatous disease; (2) UTIs in catheterized patients; (3) septicemia, particularly in patients with contaminated intravascular catheters; and (4) other opportunistic infections.

With the exception of pulmonary infections, *B. cepacia* complex has a relatively low level of virulence, and infections with the organism do not commonly result in death. *B. cepacia* complex is susceptible to trimethoprim-sulfamethoxazole. Although the organism appears to be susceptible in vitro to piperacillin, to broad-spectrum cephalosporins, and to ciprofloxacin, the clinical response is generally poor.

B. pseudomallei is a saprophyte found in soil, water, and vegetation. It is endemic in Southeast Asia, India, Africa, and Australia. The organism causes opportunistic infections; however, such an infection **(melioidosis)** can occur in a previously healthy person as an acute suppurative infection or a chronic pulmonary infection. The disease can occur from a few days to many years after exposure. Thus, although *B. pseudomallei* is not found in the United States, latent disease can occur in U.S. residents who have traveled in endemic areas.

Melioidosis has protean manifestations. Most people exposed to *B. pseudomallei* remain **asymptomatic.** However, a localized, suppurative **cutaneous infection** accompanied by regional lymphadenitis, fever, and malaise can develop in some patients. This form of disease can resolve without incident or can progress rapidly to overwhelming sepsis. The third form of infection is **pulmonary disease,** which may range in severity from a mild bronchitis to necrotizing pneumonia. Cavitation can develop if appropriate antimicrobial therapy is not instituted. *B. pseudomallei* has been used in biologic weapons programs, so work with this organism is restricted to appropriately licensed laboratories, and the recovery from a patient justifies intervention by the public health department.

Isolation of *B. pseudomallei* for diagnostic purposes should be approached carefully because the organism is highly infectious. The combination of trimethoprim-sulfamethoxazole and a broad-spectrum cephalosporin is recommended for the treatment of systemic infections.

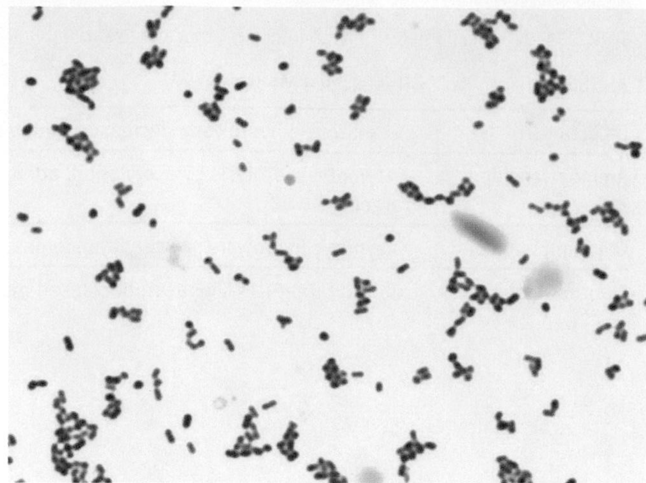

FIGURE 34–6. Gram stain of *Acinetobacter baumannii.*

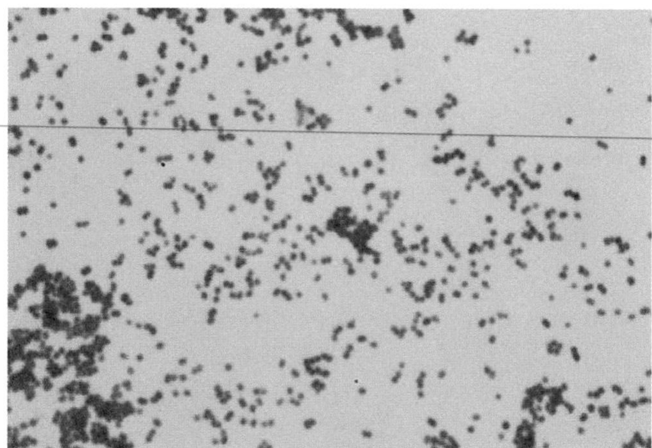

FIGURE 34–7. Gram stain of *Moraxella catarrhalis.*

Stenotrophomonas maltophilia

S. maltophilia was originally classified in the genus *Pseudomonas,* moved to the genus *Xanthomonas,* and then transferred to the genus *Stenotrophomonas.* Despite the confusion created by these taxonomic changes, the clinical importance of this opportunistic pathogen is well known. It is responsible for infections in debilitated patients with impaired host-defense mechanisms. Also, because *S. maltophilia* is resistant to most commonly used β-lactam and aminoglycoside antibiotics, patients receiving long-term antibiotic therapy are particularly at risk for acquiring infections with this organism.

The spectrum of nosocomial infections with *S. maltophilia* includes bacteremia, pneumonia, meningitis, wound infections, and UTIs (see Box 34–3). Hospital epidemics with this organism have been traced to contaminated disinfectant solutions, respiratory therapy or monitoring equipment, and ice machines.

Antimicrobial therapy is complicated because the organism is resistant to many commonly used drugs. Trimethoprim-sulfamethoxazole is the agent most active against the organism; good activity is also seen with chloramphenicol and ceftazidime.

Acinetobacter

Simply stated, the taxonomic classification of *Acinetobacter* is a bewildering mess. Without venturing into this morass, the genus can be subdivided into two groups: glucose-oxidizing species (*A. baumannii* is the most common) and glucose nonoxidizing species (*A. lwoffii* is the most common).

Acinetobacters are strictly aerobic, oxidase-negative, gram-negative, plump coccobacilli (Figure 34–6). They

CASE STUDY AND QUESTIONS

A 63-year-old man has been hospitalized for 21 days for the management of newly diagnosed leukemia. Three days after the patient entered the hospital, a urinary tract infection with Escherichia coli *developed. He was treated for 14 days with broad-spectrum antibiotics. On day 21 of his hospital stay the patient experienced fever and shaking chills. Within 24 hours he became hypotensive, and ecthymic skin lesions appeared. Despite aggressive therapy with antibiotics, the patient died. Multiple blood cultures were positive for* P. aeruginosa.

1. What factors put this man at increased risk for infection with *P. aeruginosa?*
2. What virulence factors possessed by the organism make it a particularly serious pathogen? What are the biologic effects of these factors?
3. What three mechanisms are responsible for the antibiotic resistance found in *P. aeruginosa?*
4. What diseases are caused by *B. cepacia* complex? *S. maltophilia? A. baumannii? M. catarrhalis?* What antibiotics can be used to treat these infections?

are ubiquitous saprophytes, recovered in nature and in the hospital. They survive on moist surfaces, including respiratory therapy equipment, and on dry surfaces, such as human skin (the latter feature is unusual for gram-negative rods). These bacteria are also part of the normal oropharyngeal flora of a small number of healthy people and can proliferate to large numbers during hospitalization.

Acinetobacters are opportunistic pathogens (see Box 34–3) that cause infections in the respiratory tract, urinary tract, and wounds; they also cause septicemia. Patients at risk for *Acinetobacter* infections are those receiving broad-spectrum antibiotics, recovering from surgery, or on respiratory ventilation. Treatment of *Acinetobacter* infections is problematic because these organisms, particularly *A. baumannii,* are often resistant to antibiotics. Specific therapy must be guided by in vitro susceptibility tests, but empirical therapy for serious infections should consist of a β-lactam antibiotic (e.g., ceftazidime, imipenem) and an aminoglycoside.

Moraxella

Like other genera discussed in this chapter, the genus *Moraxella* has been reorganized on the basis of nucleic acid analysis. Although the species classified in the genus continue to change, *M. catarrhalis* is the most important pathogen. *M. catarrhalis* is a strictly aerobic, oxidase-positive, gram-negative diplococci (Figure 34–7). This organism is a common cause of bronchitis and bronchopneumonia (in elderly patients with chronic pulmonary disease), sinusitis, and otitis (see Box 34–3). The latter two infections occur most commonly in previously healthy people. Most isolates produce β-lactamases and are resistant to penicillin; however, these bacteria are uniformly susceptible to most other antibiotics, including cephalosporins, erythromycin, tetracycline, trimethoprim-sulfamethoxazole, and the combination of penicillins with a β-lactamase inhibitor (e.g., clavulanic acid). Two other species of *Moraxella* colonize humans and are recovered with some frequency: *Moraxella osloensis* and *Moraxella nonliquefaciens.* Both species are found on the skin surface and mucosal membranes of the mouth and genitourinary tract. These species are rare causes of opportunistic infections.

Bibliography

Bergogne-Berezin E, Towner K: *Acinetobacter* spp. as nosocomial pathogens: Microbiological, clinical, and epidemiological features, *Clin Microbiol Rev* 9:148-165, 1996.

Berlau J et al: Distribution of *Acinetobacter* species on skin of healthy humans, *Eur J Clin Microbiol Infect Dis* 18:179-183, 1999.

Coenye T et al: Taxonomy and identification of the *Burkholderia cepacia* complex, *J Clin Microbiol* 39:3427-3436, 2001.

Dance DAB: Melioidosis: The tip of the iceberg, *Clin Microbiol Rev* 4:52-60, 1991.

Denton M, Kerr K: Microbiological and clinical aspects of infection associated with *Stenotrophomonas maltophilia, Clin Microbiol Rev* 11:57-80, 1998.

Forster D, Dashner F: *Acinetobacter* species as nosocomial pathogens, *Eur J Clin Microbiol Infect Dis* 17:73-77, 1998.

Govan J, Deretic V: Microbial pathogenesis in cystic fibrosis: Mucoid *Pseudomonas aeruginosa* and *Burkholderia cepacia, Microbiol Rev* 60:539-574, 1996.

Krueger K, Barbieri J: The family of bacterial ADP-ribosylating exotoxins, *Clin Microbiol Rev* 8:34-47, 1995.

Mendelson M et al: *Pseudomonas aeruginosa* bacteremia in patients with AIDS, *Clin Infect Dis* 18:886-895, 1994.

McGregor K et al: *Moraxella catarrhalis:* Clinical significance, antimicrobial susceptibility and BRO beta-lactamases, *Eur J Clin Microbiol Infect Dis* 17:219-234, 1998.

Muder R et al: Bacteremia due to *Stenotrophomonas (Xanthomonas) maltophilia:* A prospective, multicenter study of 91 episodes, *Clin Infect Dis* 22:508-512, 1996.

Palleroni NJ: Prokaryote taxonomy of the 20th century and the impact of studies on the genus *Pseudomonas:* A personal view, *Microbiol* 149:1-7, 2003.

Pier G: *Pseudomonas aeruginosa:* A key problem in cystic fibrosis, *ASM News* 64:339-347, 1998.

Wick MJ et al: Structure, function, and regulation of *Pseudomonas aeruginosa* exotoxin A, *Annu Rev Microbiol* 44:335-363, 1990.

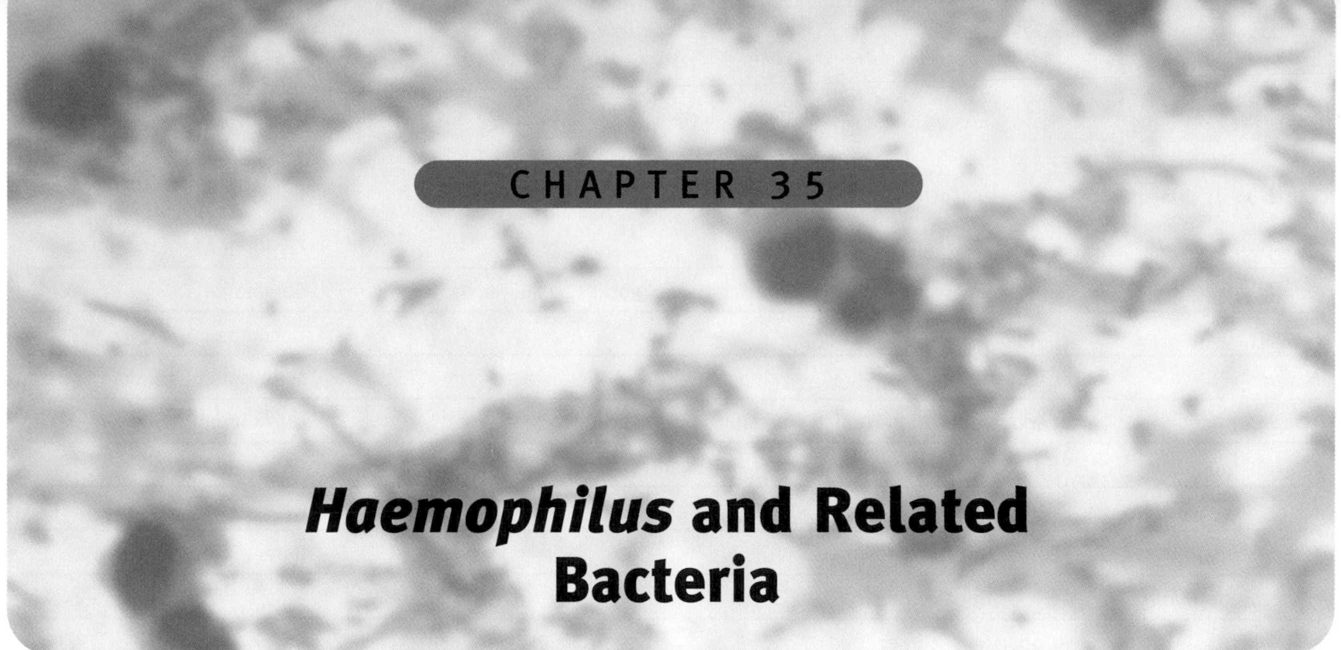

Haemophilus and Related Bacteria

The three most important genera in the family Pasteurellaceae are *Haemophilus, Actinobacillus,* and *Pasteurella.* The members of this family are small (0.2 to 0.3 × 1.0 to 2.0 μm), gram-negative, non–spore-forming, nonmotile, and aerobic or facultative anaerobic rods. Most have fastidious growth needs, requiring enriched media for isolation. Members of the genus *Haemophilus* are the most commonly isolated and significant human pathogens (Table 35–1).

Haemophilus

Haemophilae are small, sometimes pleomorphic, gram-negative rods present on the mucous membranes of humans (Figure 35–1; Box 35–1). *Haemophilus influenzae* is the species most commonly associated with disease, with infections most often reported in pediatric patients before the introduction of the *H. influenzae* type b (HIB) vaccine. *Haemophilus aegyptius* is an important cause of acute, purulent conjunctivitis. Taxonomically, *H. aegyptius* belongs in the species *H. influenzae* but has traditionally been separated. To make this classification more confusing, *H. influenzae* biogroup *aegyptius* is phenotypically related to *H. aegyptius* but is taxonomically distinct. Biogroup *aegyptius* is the etiologic agent of the fulminant pediatric disease **Brazilian purpuric fever.**

Although less frequently isolated, *Haemophilus ducreyi* is well recognized as the etiologic agent of the sexually transmitted disease **soft chancre,** or **chancroid.** It should be noted that, based on genomic analysis, *H. ducreyi* is a member of the family Pasteurellaceae but does not belong in the genus *Haemophilus.* Because it has not been reclassified into another genus, *H. ducreyi* will be discussed in this section. *Haemophilus aphrophilus* is an uncommon but important cause of endocarditis. The other members of the genus are commonly isolated in clinical specimens (e.g., *Haemophilus parainfluenzae* is the most common species in the mouth) but are rarely pathogenic, being responsible primarily for opportunistic infections.

PHYSIOLOGY AND STRUCTURE (BOX 35–2)

Most species of *Haemophilus* require media supplemented with the following growth-stimulating factors: (1) **hemin** (also called **X factor** for unknown factor), (2) **nicotinamide adenine dinucleotide** (NAD; also called **V factor** for "vitamin"), or (3) both. Although both factors are present in blood-enriched media, sheep blood agar must be gently heated to destroy the inhibitors of V factor. For this reason, heated blood ("chocolate") agar is used for the in vitro isolation of *Haemophilus.*

The cell wall structure of *Haemophilus* is typical of other gram-negative rods. Lipopolysaccharide with endotoxin activity is present in the cell wall, and strain-specific and species-specific proteins are found in the outer membrane. Analysis of these strain-specific proteins is valuable in epidemiologic investigations. The surface of many but not all strains of *H. influenzae* is covered with a **polysaccharide capsule,** and six antigenic serotypes (**a** through **f**) have been identified. Before the introduction of the HIB vaccine, *H. influenzae* serotype b was responsible for more than 95% of all invasive *Haemophilus* infections. After the introduction of the vaccine, most disease caused by this serotype disappeared. Currently, serotypes c and f and nonencapsulated *H. influenzae* are responsible for most *H. influenzae* disease.

In addition to the serologic differentiation of *H. influenzae,* the species is subdivided into eight biotypes (I through VIII) as determined by three biochemical reactions: indole production, urease activity, and ornithine decarboxylase activity. The separation of these biotypes is useful for epidemiologic purposes. Finally, *H. influenzae* has been subdivided into biogroups, which is useful for clinical pur-

TABLE 35–1. *Haemophilus* Species Associated with Human Disease

Species	Primary Diseases	Frequency
H. influenzae	Pneumonia, sinusitis, otitis, meningitis, epiglottitis, cellulitis, bacteremia	Common
H. aegyptius	Conjunctivitis	Uncommon
H. ducreyi	Chancroid	Uncommon (in United States)
H. aphrophilus	Endocarditis, opportunistic infections	Uncommon
H. parainfluenzae	Bacteremia, endocarditis, opportunistic infections	Rare
H. haemolyticus	Opportunistic infections	Rare
H. parahaemolyticus	Opportunistic infections	Rare
H. paraphrophilus	Opportunistic infections	Rare
H. segnis	Opportunistic infections	Rare

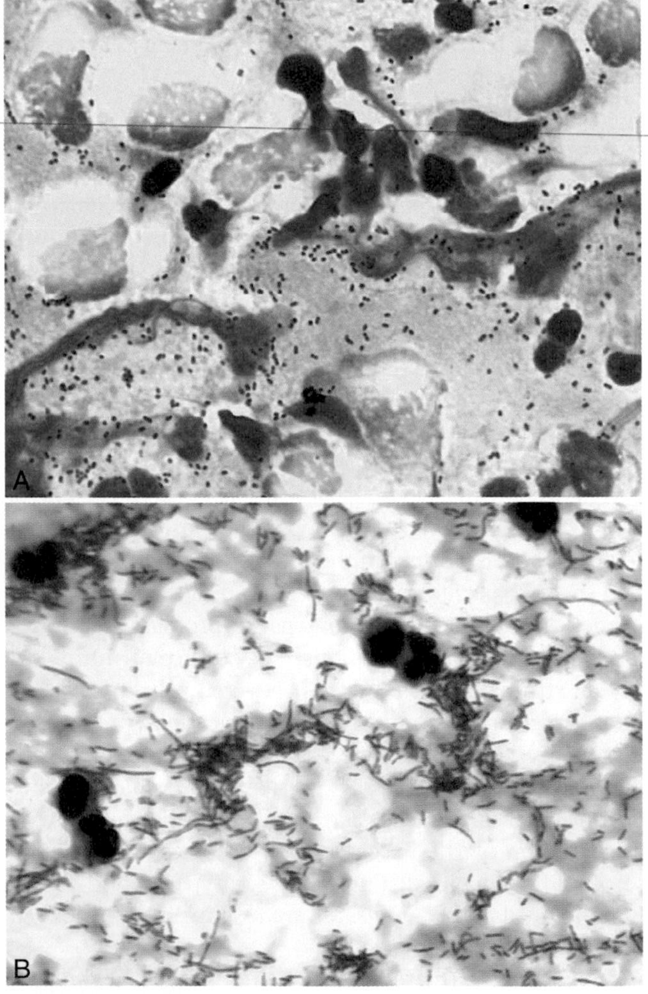

FIGURE 35–1. Gram stains of *Haemophilus influenzae.* **A,** Small coccobacilli forms seen in sputum from patient with pneumonia; **B,** thin, pleomorphic forms seen in 1-year-old, unvaccinated child in Africa with overwhelming meningitis.

BOX 35–1. Important Pasteurellaceae

Organism	Historical Derivation
Haemophilus	*haemo,* blood; *hilos,* lover ("blood lover"; requires blood for growth on agar media)
H. influenzae	Originally thought to be the cause of influenza
H. aegyptius	*aegyptius,* Egyptian (observed by R. Koch in 1883 in exudates from Egyptians with conjunctivitis)
H. ducreyi	Named after the bacteriologist Ducrey, who first isolated this organism)
H. aphrophilus	*aphros,* foam; *philos,* loving ("foam loving")
Actinobacillus	*actinis,* ray; *bacillus,* small staff or rod ("ray bacillus"; refers to the growth of filamentous forms [rays])
A. actinomycetemcomitans	*actino,* ray; *myces,* a fungus; *comitans,* accompanying ("accompanying an actinomycetes"; isolates are frequently associated with *Actinomyces*)
Pasteurella	Named after Louis Pasteur
P. multocida	*multus,* many; *cidus,* to kill ("many–killing"; pathogenic for many species of animals)
P. canis	*canis,* dogs (isolated from the mouths of dogs)

poses. *H. influenzae* biogroup *aegypticus* is important because it causes Brazilian purpuric fever. Although biogroup *aegyptius* and *H. influenzae* biotype III have identical biochemical profiles, they can be distinguished on the basis of (1) the nature of the clinical disease, (2) their in vitro growth properties, and (3) the outer membrane protein profiles.

BOX 35–2. Summary of *Haemophilus*

Physiology and Structure

Small, pleomorphic, gram-negative rods or coccobacilli
Facultative anaerobes, fermentative
Most species require X and/or V factor for growth
H. influenzae subdivided serologically (types a to f), biochemically (biotypes I to VIII), and clinically (biogroup *aegypticus*)

Virulence

H. influenzae type b is clinically most virulent (with PRP, [polyribitol phosphate] in capsule)
Haemophilus adhere to host cells via pili and nonpilus structures

Epidemiology

Noncapsular *Haemophilus* commonly colonized in humans; encapsulated *Haemophilus* species, particularly *H. influenzae* type b, are uncommon members of normal flora
Disease caused by *H. influenzae* type b was primarily a pediatric problem; eliminated in immunized populations
H. ducreyi disease is uncommon in the United States
With the exception of *H. ducreyi,* which is spread by sexual contact, most *Haemophilus* infections are caused by the patient's bacterial flora (endogenous infections)
Patients at greatest risk for disease are those with inadequate levels of protective antibodies, those with depleted complement, and those who have undergone splenectomy

Diseases

Refer to Table 35–1

Diagnosis

Microscopy is a sensitive test for detecting *H. influenzae* in cerebrospinal fluid (CSF), synovial fluid, and lower respiratory specimens
Culture is performed using chocolate agar
Antigen tests for *H. influenzae* type b are less useful following the introduction of *H. influenzae* type B (HIB) vaccine

Treatment, Prevention, and Control

Haemophilus infections are treated with broad-spectrum cephalosporins, azithromycin, or fluoroquinolones; many strains are resistant to ampicillin
Active immunization with conjugated PRP vaccines prevents most *H. influenzae* type b infections
Rifampin prophylaxis is used to eliminate carriage of *H. influenzae* in children at high risk for disease

In summary, *H. influenzae* is subdivided as follows: (1) serotypes a through f (determined by the presence of capsular antigens; type b the most important); (2) biotypes I through VIII (determined by biochemical properties); and (3) biogroups (biogroup *aegypticus* is the most important clinically).

PATHOGENESIS AND IMMUNITY

Haemophilus species, particularly *H. parainfluenzae* and nonencapsulated *H. influenzae,* colonize the upper respiratory tract in virtually all people within the first few months of life. These organisms can spread locally and cause disease in the ears (otitis media), sinuses (sinusitis), and lower respiratory tract (bronchitis, pneumonia). Disseminated disease, however, is relatively uncommon. In contrast, encapsulated *H. influenzae* (particularly serotype b [biotype I]) is uncommon in the upper respiratory tract or is present in only very small numbers but is a common cause of disease in unvaccinated children (i.e., meningitis, epiglottitis [obstructive laryngitis], cellulitis). Pili and nonpilus adhesins mediate colonization of the oropharynx with *H. influenzae.* Cell wall components of the bacteria (e.g., lipopolysaccharide and a low–molecular-weight glycopeptide) impair ciliary function, leading to damage of the respiratory epithelium. The bacteria can then be translocated across both epithelial and endothelial cells and can enter the blood. In the absence of specific opsonic antibodies directed against the polysaccharide capsule, high-grade bacteremia can develop, with dissemination to the meninges or other distal foci.

The major virulence factor in *H. influenzae* type b is the antiphagocytic polysaccharide capsule, which contains ribose, ribitol, and phosphate (commonly referred to as **polyribitol phosphate [PRP]**). Antibodies directed against the capsule greatly stimulate bacterial phagocytosis and complement-mediated bactericidal activity. These antibodies develop as a result of natural infection, vaccination with purified PRP, or the passive transfer of maternal antibodies. The severity of systemic disease is inversely related to the rate of clearance of bacteria from the blood. The risk of meningitis and epiglottitis is significantly greater in patients with no anti-PRP antibodies, those with depletion of complement, and those who have undergone splenectomy. The lipopolysaccharide lipid A component induces meningeal inflammation in an animal model and may be responsible for initiating this response in humans. Immunoglobulin (Ig)A1 proteases are produced by *H. influenzae* (both encapsulated and nonencapsulated strains) and may facilitate colonization of the organisms on mucosal surfaces by interfering with humoral immunity.

EPIDEMIOLOGY

Haemophilus species are present in almost all individuals, primarily colonizing the mucosal membranes of the respiratory tract. *H. parainfluenzae* constitutes 10% of the bacterial flora in saliva, and *Haemophilus aphrophilus*, *Haemophilus paraphrophilus*, and *Haemophilus segnis* occur predominantly on tooth surfaces. Most of the isolates of *H. influenzae* are nonencapsulated, with encapsulated strains detectable only in small numbers and only when highly selective culture methods are used. *H. influenzae* type b is the most common serotype that causes systemic disease; however, it is rarely isolated in healthy children (a fact that emphasizes the virulence of this bacterium). *Haemophilus* species can also be isolated in the gastrointestinal and genitourinary tracts but typically in relatively low numbers.

The epidemiology of *Haemophilus* disease has changed dramatically. Before the introduction of conjugated *H. influenzae* type b vaccines, an estimated 20,000 cases of invasive *H. influenzae* type b disease occurred annually in children younger than age 5 in the United States. The first polysaccharide vaccines for *H. influenzae* type b were not protective for children younger than 18 months (the population at greatest risk for disease), because there is a natural delay in the maturation of the immune response to polysaccharide antigens. Vaccines containing purified PRP antigens conjugated to protein carriers (i.e., diphtheria toxoid, tetanus toxoid, meningococcal outer membrane protein), however, were found to elicit a protective antibody response in infants 2 months and older. Since the introduction of the conjugated vaccine in December 1987, systemic disease in children younger than 5 years has been virtually eliminated in the United States, with only 32 cases reported in 2003. Most of the *H. influenzae* type b infections now occur in children who are not immune (because of incomplete vaccination or a poor response to the vaccine) and in elderly adults with waning immunity. In addition, invasive *H. influenzae* disease caused by other serotypes of encapsulated bacteria and by nonencapsulated strains has now become proportionally more common than that resulting from serotype b. It should be noted that the successful elimination of *H. influenzae* type b disease in the United States has not been seen in many developing countries where vaccination programs have been difficult to implement. Thus *H. influenzae* type b remains the most significant pediatric pathogen in many countries of the world. It is estimated that 3 million cases of serious disease and up to 700,000 fatalities occur in children each year worldwide. The epidemiology of disease caused by nonencapsulated *H. influenzae* and other *Haemophilus* species is distinct. Because it is common for people to be colonized with these species, invasive disease is relatively uncommon. Ear and sinus infections caused by these organisms are primarily pediatric diseases but can occur in adults. Pulmonary disease most commonly affects elderly people, particularly those with a history of underlying obstructive pulmonary disease or conditions predisposing to aspiration (e.g., alcoholism, altered mental state).

H. ducreyi is an important cause of genital ulcers (chancroid) in Africa and Asia but is less common in Europe and North America. The incidence of disease in the United States is cyclic. A peak incidence of more than 5000 cases was reported in 1988, which decreased to 54 cases in 2003. Despite this favorable trend, the Centers for Disease Control and Prevention have documented that the disease is significantly underreported, making the true incidence unknown.

CLINICAL DISEASES (BOX 35–3)

The clinical syndromes seen in patients with *H. influenzae* infections are represented in Figure 35–2. The diseases caused by all *Haemophilus* species are described in the following sections.

Meningitis

H. influenzae type b was the most common cause of pediatric meningitis, but this situation changed rapidly when the conjugated vaccines became widely used. Disease in nonimmune patients results from the bacteremic spread

BOX 35–3. Pasteurellaceae: Clinical Summaries

Haemophilus influenzae
Meningitis: A disease primarily of unimmunized children characterized by fever, severe headache, and systemic signs
Epiglottitis: A disease primarily of unimmunized children characterized by initial pharyngitis, fever, and difficulty breathing, and progressing to cellulitis and swelling of the supraglottic tissues, with obstruction of the airways possible
Pneumonia: Inflammation and consolidation of the lungs observed primarily in the elderly with underlying chronic pulmonary disease; typically caused by nontypeable strains

Haemophilus aegyptius
Conjunctivitis: An acute, purulent conjunctivitis ("pink eye")

Haemophilus ducreyi
Chancroid: Sexually transmitted disease characterized by a tender papule with an erythematous base that progresses to painful ulceration with associated lymphadenopathy

Haemophilus aphrophilus
Endocarditis: Responsible for subacute form of endocarditis in patients with underlying damage to the heart valve

Actinobacillus actinomycetemcomitans
Endocarditis: As with *H. aphrophilus*

Pasteurella multocida
Bite wound: Most common manifestation is infected cat or dog bite wound; particularly common with cat bites because the wounds are deep and difficult to disinfect

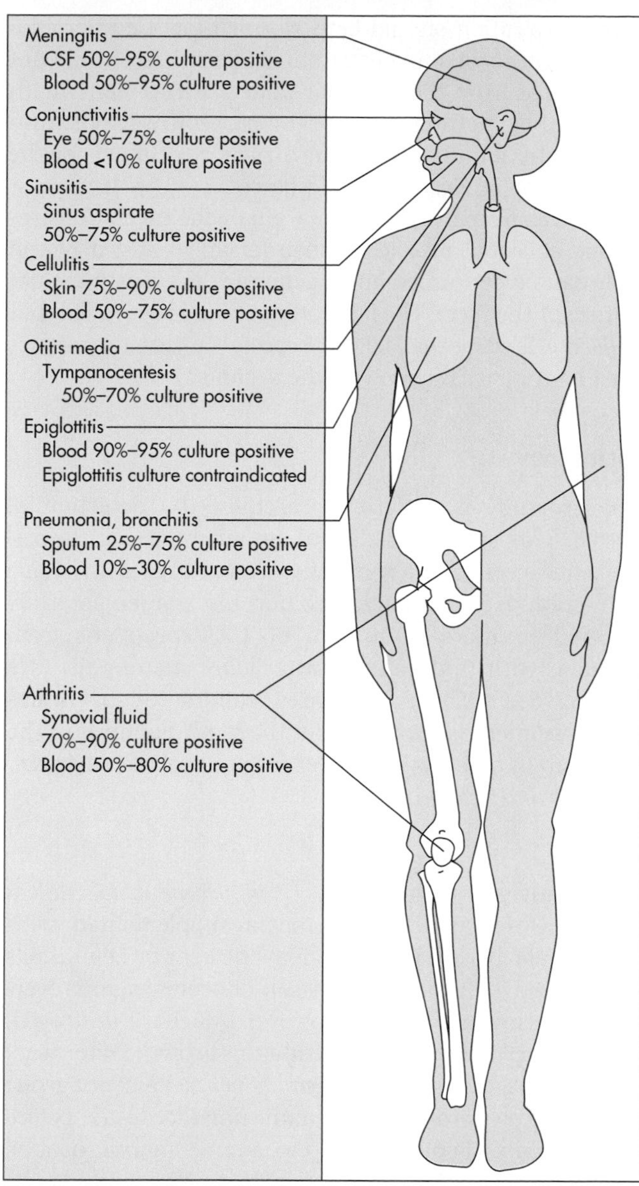

FIGURE 35–2. Infections caused by *Haemophilus influenzae.* With the advent of the conjugated vaccine, most infections in adults involve areas contiguous with the oropharynx (i.e., lower respiratory tract, sinuses, ears). Serious systemic infections (e.g., meningitis, epiglottitis) can occur in nonimmune patients. CSF, Cerebrospinal fluid.

of the organisms from the nasopharynx and cannot be differentiated clinically from other causes of bacterial meningitis. The initial presentation is a 1- to 3-day history of mild upper respiratory disease, after which the typical signs and symptoms of meningitis appear. Mortality is less than 10% in patients who receive prompt therapy, and carefully designed studies have documented a low incidence of serious neurologic sequelae (in contrast with the 50% incidence of severe residual damage in nonimmune children seen in initial studies). Person-to-person spread in a nonimmune population is well documented, so appropriate epidemiologic precautions must be used.

Epiglottitis

Epiglottitis, characterized by cellulitis and the swelling of the supraglottic tissues, represents a life-threatening emergency. Although epiglottitis is a pediatric disease, the peak incidence of this disease during the prevaccine era occurred in children 2 to 4 years of age; in contrast, the peak incidence of meningitis was seen in children 3 to 18 months of age. Children with epiglottitis have pharyngitis, fever, and difficulty breathing, which can progress rapidly to obstruction of the airway and death. Since the introduction of the vaccine, the incidence of this disease has also decreased dramatically in children and remains relatively rare in adults.

Cellulitis

Like meningitis and epiglottitis, cellulitis is a pediatric disease caused by *H. influenzae* that has largely been eliminated by vaccination. When it is observed, patients have fever and cellulitis characterized by the development of reddish-blue patches on the cheeks or periorbital areas. The diagnosis is strongly suggested by the typical clinical presentation, cellulitis proximal to the oral mucosa, and lack of documented vaccination in the child.

Arthritis

Before the advent of conjugated vaccines, the most common form of arthritis in children younger than 2 years was an infection of a single, large joint secondary to the bacteremic spread of *H. influenzae* type b. Disease does occur in older children and adults, but it is very uncommon and generally affects immunocompromised patients and patients with previously damaged joints.

Otitis, Sinusitis, and Lower Respiratory Tract Disease

Nonencapsulated strains of *H. influenzae* (primarily biotypes II and III) are opportunistic pathogens that can cause infections of the upper and lower airways. Most studies have shown that *H. influenzae* and *Streptococcus pneumoniae* are the two most common causes of acute and chronic otitis and sinusitis. Primary pneumonia is uncommon in children and adults who have normal pulmonary function. These organisms commonly colonize patients who have chronic pulmonary disease (including cystic fibrosis), and frequently are associated with exacerbation of bronchitis and frank pneumonia.

Conjunctivitis

H. aegyptius, also called the **Koch-Weeks bacillus** causes an acute, purulent conjunctivitis. This contagious organism is associated with epidemics, particularly during the warm months of the year.

Brazilian Purpuric Fever

As already mentioned, *H. influenzae* biogroup *aegyptius* (an organism that is different from *H. aegyptius;* see earlier section in this chapter) is the etiologic agent of Brazilian purpuric fever, a fulminant pediatric disease characterized by an initial conjunctivitis, followed a few days later by the acute onset of fever, vomiting, and abdominal pain. In untreated patients, petechiae, purpura, and shock culminating in death rapidly ensue. The pathogenesis of Brazilian purpuric fever and the specific virulence characteristics of the pathogen are poorly understood.

Chancroid

Chancroid is a sexually transmitted disease that is most commonly diagnosed in men, presumably because women can have asymptomatic or inapparent disease. Approximately 5 to 7 days after exposure, a tender papule with an erythematous base develops on the genitalia or perianal area. Within 2 days the lesion ulcerates and becomes painful, and inguinal lymphadenopathy is commonly present. Other causes of genital ulcers, such as syphilis and herpes simplex disease, must be excluded to diagnose chancroid.

Other Infections

Other species of *Haemophilus* can cause opportunistic infections, such as otitis media, conjunctivitis, sinusitis, meningitis, and dental abscesses. Some species that stick to tooth surfaces, such as *H. aphrophilus,* can spread from the mouth to the blood and then stick to a previously damaged heart valve or artificial valve, leading to subacute endocarditis. Subacute endocarditis caused by this organism is particularly difficult to diagnose with laboratory testing because the bacteria grow slowly in blood cultures.

LABORATORY DIAGNOSIS

Specimen Collection and Transport

It is necessary to obtain samples of cerebrospinal fluid (CSF) and blood to diagnose *Haemophilus* meningitis. Because there are approximately 10^7 bacteria per ml of CSF in patients with untreated meningitis, 1 to 2 ml of fluid is generally adequate for microscopy, culture, and antigen-detection tests. Microscopy and culture are less sensitive if the patient has been exposed to antibiotics before the CSF is collected. Blood cultures should also be performed for the diagnosis of epiglottitis, cellulitis, arthritis, or pneumonia. These cultures are less useful for the diagnosis of localized upper respiratory tract diseases (e.g., sinusitis, otitis). Culture of material obtained by direct needle aspiration should be performed for the microbiologic diagnosis of sinusitis or otitis. Specimens should not be collected from the posterior pharynx in patients with suspected epiglottitis, because the procedure may stimulate coughing and obstruct the airway. Specimens for the detection of *H. ducreyi* should be collected with a moistened swab from the base or margin of the ulcer. Cultures of pus collected by aspiration from an enlarged lymph node can be performed but is generally less sensitive than culture of the ulcer. The laboratory should be notified that *H. ducreyi* is suspected, because special culture techniques must be used for recovery of the organism.

Microscopy

If microscopy is performed carefully, the detection of *Haemophilus* species in clinical specimens is both sensitive and specific. Gram-negative rods ranging in shape from coccobacilli to long, pleomorphic filaments can be detected in more than 80% of CSF specimens from patients with untreated *Haemophilus* meningitis (see Figure 35–1). The microscopic examination of Gram-stain specimens is also useful for the rapid diagnosis of the organism in arthritis and lower respiratory tract disease.

Culture

It is relatively easy to isolate *H. influenzae* from clinical specimens inoculated onto media supplemented with appropriate growth factors. Chocolate agar or Levinthal's agar is used in most laboratories. If chocolate agar is overheated during preparation, however, V factor is destroyed, and *Haemophilus* species requiring this growth factor (e.g., *H. influenzae, H. aegyptius, H. parainfluenzae*) will not grow; thus each preparation of medium must be tested before use. The bacteria appear as 1- to 2-mm, smooth, opaque colonies after 24 hours of incubation. They can also be detected growing around colonies of *Staphylococcus aureus* on unheated blood agar (**satellite phenomenon;** Figure 35–3). The staphylococci provide the requisite growth factors by lysing the erythrocytes in the medium and releasing intracellular heme (X factor) and excreting NAD (V factor). The colonies of *H. influenzae* in these cultures are much smaller than they are on chocolate agar, however, because the V factor inhibitors present in blood are not inactivated.

The growth of *Haemophilus* in blood cultures is generally delayed, because most commercially prepared blood culture broths are not supplemented with optimum concentrations of X and V factors. Furthermore, the growth factors are released only when the blood cells lyse, but inhibitors of V factor present in the medium can delay recovery of the bacteria. Isolates of *H. influenzae* often grow better in anaerobically incubated blood cultures because under these conditions the organisms do not require X factor for growth.

H. aegyptius and *H. ducreyi* are fastidious and require specialized growth conditions. *H. aegyptius* grows best on chocolate agar supplemented with 1% IsoVitaleX (BBL Microbiology Systems, Cockeysville, Md.), with growth detected after incubation in a carbon dioxide atmosphere for 2 to 4 days. Culture of *H. ducreyi* is relatively insensitive (less than 85% of cultures yield organisms under optimal conditions) but reportedly is best on gonococcal (GC) agar supplemented with 1% to 2% hemoglobin, 5% fetal bovine serum, IsoViteleX enrichment, and vancomycin (3 μg/ml). Cultures should be incubated at 33°C in 5% to 10% carbon dioxide for 7 days or more. Because the media and incubation conditions are not used for other bacterial cultures, success in recovering *H. ducreyi* requires that the microbiologist look specifically for this organism.

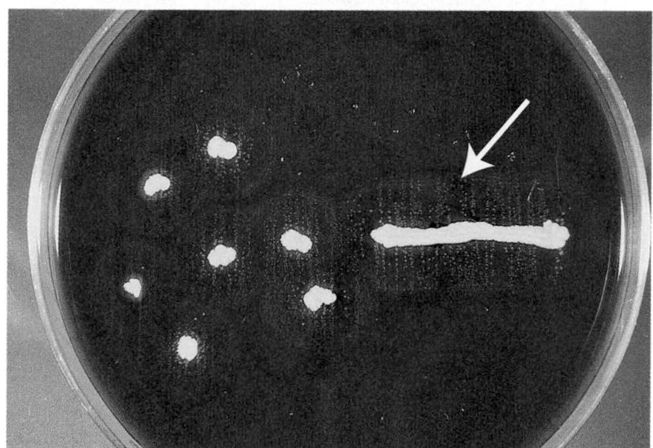

FIGURE 35–3. Satellite phenomenon. *Staphylococcus aureus* excretes nicotinamide adenine dinucleotide (NAD, or V factor) into the medium, providing a growth factor required for *H. influenzae* (small colonies surrounding *S. aureus* colonies).

Antigen Detection

The immunologic detection of *H. influenzae* antigen, specifically the PRP capsular antigen, is a rapid and sensitive way to diagnose *H. influenzae* type b disease. PRP can be detected with particle agglutination, which can detect less than 1 ng/ml of PRP in a clinical specimen. In this test, antibody-coated latex particles are mixed with the clinical specimen; agglutination occurs if PRP is present. Antigen can be detected in CSF and urine (in which the antigen is eliminated intact). However, this test has limited use because it can detect only *H. influenzae* type b, which is now uncommon in the United States. Other capsular serotypes and nonencapsulated strains do not give a positive reaction.

Identification

H. influenzae is readily identified by the demonstration of a requirement for both X and V factors and the specific biochemical properties summarized in Table 35–2. Further

TABLE 35–2. Differential Characteristics of Common Members of the Family Pasteurellaceae

Organism	Catalase	Growth Factor Requirement		Enhanced Growth with CO_2	Fermentation of:				
		X	V		Glucose	Sucrose	Lactose	Mannose	Xylose
Haemophilus									
H. influenzae	+	+	+	–	+	–	–	–	+
H. aegyptius	+	+	+	–	+	–	–	–	–
H. ducreyi	–	+	–	–	–	–	–	–	–
H. parainfluenzae	+/–	–	+	–	+	+	–	+	–
H. aphrophilus	–	–	–	+	+	+	+	+	–
Actinobacillus									
A. actinomycetemcomitans	+	–	–	+	+	–	–	+	+/–
Pasteurella									
P. multocida	+	–	–	–	+	+	–	+	+/–
P. canis	+	–	–	–	+	+/–	–	–	–

+, Positive reaction; –, negative reaction; +/–, variable reaction.

subgrouping of *H. influenzae* can be done with biotyping, electrophoretic characterization of the membrane protein antigens, and analysis of the strain-specific nucleic acid sequences.

TREATMENT, PREVENTION, AND CONTROL

Patients with systemic *H. influenzae* infections require prompt antimicrobial therapy, because the mortality rate in patients with untreated meningitis or epiglottitis approaches 100%. Serious infections are treated with broad-spectrum cephalosporins. Less severe infections such as sinusitis and otitis can be treated with ampicillin (if susceptible, approximately 30% of strains are resistant), an active cephalosporin, azithromycin, or a fluoroquinolone. Most isolates of *H. ducreyi* are susceptible to erythromycin, the drug recommended for treatment.

The primary approach to preventing *H. influenzae* type b disease is through active immunization with purified capsular PRP. As discussed previously, the use of conjugated vaccines has been remarkably successful in reducing the incidences of *H. influenzae* type b disease and colonization. Currently, it is recommended that children receive three doses of vaccine against *H. influenzae* type b disease before the age of 6 months, followed by booster doses.

Antibiotic chemoprophylaxis is used to eliminate the carriage of *H. influenzae* type b in children at high risk for disease (e.g., children younger than 2 years in a family or daycare center where systemic disease is documented). Rifampin prophylaxis has been used in these settings.

Actinobacillus

Actinobacillus species are small, facultatively anaerobic, gram-negative rods that grow slowly (generally requiring 2 to 3 days of incubation). *Actinobacillus actinomycetemcomitans* is the most important human pathogen, and the other species are rarely encountered (Table 35–3). By taxonomic rules, *A. actinomycetemcomitans* belongs in the genus *Haemophilus* but is traditionally included in the genus *Actinobacillus*.

Members of the genus *Actinobacillus* colonize the oropharynx of humans and animals and are responsible for periodontitis, endocarditis, bite wound infections, and opportunistic infections. *A. actinomycetemcomitans* is a relatively uncommon cause of subacute bacterial endocarditis. In patients in whom this disease occurs, however, there is usually preexisting valvular heart disease and evidence of oral disease (e.g., periodontitis, oral abscess, poor oral hygiene). The organism spreads from the oropharynx through the blood and adheres to the damaged heart valve. An interesting characteristic of *Actinobacillus* noted in vitro is that the bacteria are sticky, adhering to the surfaces of blood culture bottles and agar media in much the same way as they adhere to damaged heart valves. Virulent strains of *A. actinomycetemcomitans* produce a leukotoxin that induces pore formation in neutrophils and degranulation of lysosomes, with subsequent tissue inflammation.

Infections with *A. actinomycetemcomitans* are treated with cephalosporins, tetracyclines, or fluoroquinolones. Resistance to penicillins and macrolides is not uncommon.

Pasteurella

Pasteurella are small, facultatively anaerobic, fermentative coccobacilli (Figure 35–4) commonly found as commensals in the oropharynx of healthy animals. Most human infections result from animal contact (e.g., animal bites, scratches, shared food). *Pasteurella multocida* (the most common isolate) and *Pasteurella canis* are human pathogens; the other *Pasteurella* species are rarely associated with human infections (Table 35–4). The following three general forms of disease are reported: (1) localized cellulitis and lymphadenitis that occur after an animal bite or scratch (*P. multocida* from contact with cats or dogs; *P. canis* from dogs); (2) an exacerbation of chronic respiratory tract disease in patients with underlying pul-

TABLE 35–3. *Actinobacillus* Species Associated with Human Disease

Species	Primary Diseases	Frequency
A. actinomycetemcomitans	Periodontitis, endocarditis, bite wound infections	Common
A. equuli	Bite wound infections	Rare
A. hominis	Opportunistic infections (bacteremia, pneumonia)	Rare
A. lignieresii	Bite wound infections	Rare
A. ureae	Opportunistic infections (bacteremia, meningitis, pneumonia)	Rare

TABLE 35–4. Pasteurella Species Associated with Human Disease

Species	Primary Disease	Frequency
P. multocida	Bite wound infections, chronic pulmonary disease, bacteremia, meningitis	Common
P. canis	Bite wound infections	Uncommon
P. bettyae	Opportunistic infections (abscesses, bite wound infections, urogenital infections, bacteremia)	Rare
P. dagmatis	Bite wound infections	Rare
P. stomatis	Bite wound infections	Rare

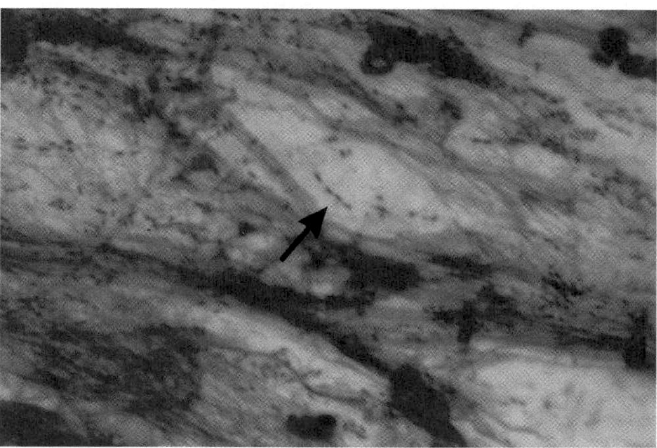

FIGURE 35–4. *Pasteurella multocida* in respiratory specimen from patient with pneumonia.

monary dysfunction (presumably related to colonization of the patient's oropharynx followed by the aspiration of oral secretions); and (3) a systemic infection in immunocompromised patients, particularly those with underlying hepatic disease.

P. multocida grows well on blood and chocolate agars but poorly on MacConkey agar and other media typically selective for gram-negative rods. After overnight incubation on blood agar, large, buttery colonies with a characteristic musty odor caused by the production of indole are present. They can be readily differentiated from other Pasteurellaceae, as indicated in Table 35–2. *P. multocida* is susceptible to a variety of antibiotics. Penicillin is the antibiotic of choice, and expanded spectrum cephalosporins, macrolides, tetracyclines, or fluoroquinolones are acceptable alternatives. Semisynthetic penicillins (e.g., oxacillin), first-generation cephalosporins, and aminoglycosides have poor activity.

CASE STUDY AND QUESTIONS

A 78-year-old man confined to a nursing home awoke with a severe headache and stiff neck. Because he had a high fever and signs of meningitis, the nursing home staff took him to a local emergency department. The CSF specimen was cloudy. Analysis revealed 400 white blood cells per mm^3 (95% polymorphonuclear neutrophils), a protein concentration of 75 mg/dl, and a glucose concentration of 20 mg/dl. Small gram-negative rods were seen on Gram stain of the CSF, and cultures of CSF and blood were positive for Haemophilus influenzae.

1. Discuss the epidemiology of *H. influenzae* meningitis, and compare it with the epidemiology of meningitis caused by *Streptococcus pneumoniae* and by *Neisseria meningitidis*.
2. Compare the biology of the *H. influenzae* strain that is likely to be the cause of this patient's disease with that of the strains that historically caused pediatric diseases (prior to vaccination).
3. What other diseases does this organism cause? What other *Haemophilus* species cause disease, and what are the diseases?
4. Why is chocolate agar needed for the isolation of *Haemophilus* organisms?
5. What diseases are caused by *Actinobacillus actinomycetemcomitans?* What is the source of this organism?
6. What diseases are caused by *Pasteurella multocida?* What is the source of this organism?

Bibliography

Albritton WL: Infections due to *Haemophilus* species other than *H. influenzae, Ann Rev Microbiol* 36:199-216, 1982.

Chen HI, Hulten K, Clarridge JE: Taxonomic subgroups of *Pasteurella multocida* correlate with clinical presentation, *J Clin Microbiol* 40:3438-3441, 2002.

Daum R et al: Epidemiology, pathogenesis, and prevention of *Haemophilus influenzae* disease, *J Infect Dis* 165(suppl):1-206, 1992.

Holst E et al: Characterization and distribution of *Pasteurella* species recovered from infected humans, *J Clin Microbiol* 30:2984-2987, 1992.

Kaplan AH et al: Infection due to *Actinobacillus actinomycetemcomitans:* 15 cases and review, *Rev Infect Dis* 11:46-63, 1989.

Killian M: *Haemophilus*. In Murray P et al, editors: *Manual of clinical microbiology*, ed 8, Washington, 2003, American Society of Microbiology.

Mortensen J, Giger O, Rodgers G: In vitro activity of oral antimicrobial agents against clinical isolates of *Pasteurella multocida, Diagn Microbiol Infect Dis* 30:99-102, 1998.

Peltola H: Worldwide *Haemophilus influenzae* type b disease at the beginning of the 21st century: Global analysis of the disease burden 25 years after the use of the polysaccharide vaccine and a decade after the advent of conjugates, *Clin Microbiol Rev* 13:302-317, 2000.

Talan D et al: Bacteriologic analysis of infected dog and cat bites, *N Engl J Med* 340:85-92, 1999.

Trees D, Morse S: Chancroid and *Haemophilus ducreyi:* An update, *Clin Microbiol Rev* 8:357-375, 1995.

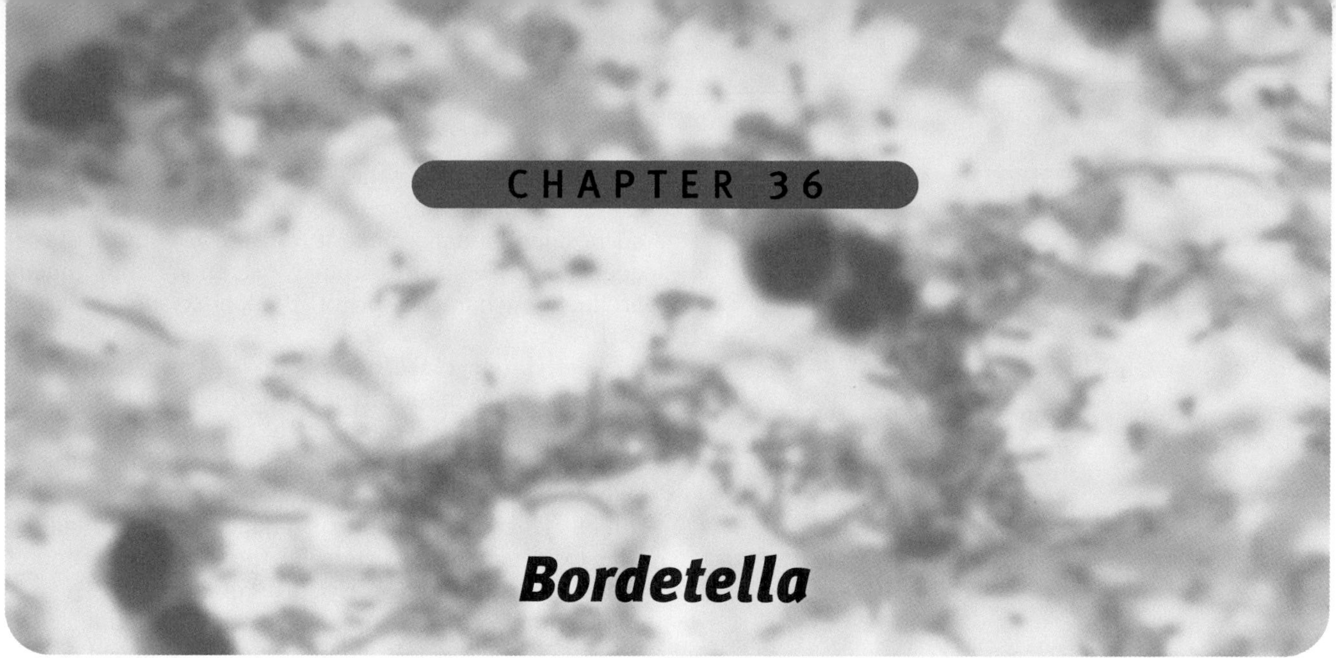

Bordetella

Bordetella is an extremely small (0.2 to 0.5 × 1 μm in diameter), strictly aerobic, gram-negative coccobacillus. Seven species are currently recognized, with three species responsible for human disease (Box 36–1): *Bordetella pertussis* (Box 36–2), the agent responsible for pertussis or whooping cough; *Bordetella parapertussis,* responsible for a milder form of pertussis; and *Bordetella bronchiseptica,* responsible for respiratory disease in dogs, swine, laboratory animals, and occasionally, pertussis-like symptoms in humans.

PHYSIOLOGY AND STRUCTURE

Bordetella species are differentiated on the basis of their growth characteristics, biochemical reactivity, and antigenic properties. Despite phenotypic differences, genetic studies have shown that the three species pathogenic for humans and a fourth species, *Bordetella holmesii,* are closely related or identical species, differing only in the expression of virulence genes. At this time, however, the species have not been reclassified and should be considered as distinct.

Bordetella species have simple nutritional requirements, but some species are highly susceptible to toxic substances and metabolites in common laboratory media. These species (particularly *B. pertussis*) require media supplemented with charcoal, starch, blood, or albumin to absorb these toxic substances. The organisms are nonmotile and oxidize amino acids, but they do not ferment carbohydrates.

PATHOGENESIS AND IMMUNITY

Infection with *B. pertussis* and the development of whooping cough require exposure to the organism, bacterial attachment to the ciliated epithelial cells of the respiratory tract, proliferation of the bacteria, and production of localized tissue damage and systemic toxicity. Attachment of the organisms to ciliated epithelial cells is mediated by protein adhesions (Table 36–1). **Pertactin** (also called **P69 protein** because the active form is 69 kDa in size) and **filamentous hemagglutinin** contain an Arg-Gly-Asp sequence (RGD motif) that promotes binding to sulfated glycoprotein integrins on the membranes of ciliated respiratory cells. These adhesins also bind to CR3, a glycoprotein receptor on the surface of macrophages. This interaction initiates the phagocytosis of the bacteria without initiating an oxidative burst, which is important in the intracellular survival and replication of the bacteria. This also protects *B. pertussis* from humoral antibodies. Similar proteins are also found in *B. parapertussis* and *B. bronchiseptica.* **Pertussis toxin** is a classic A-B toxin consisting of a toxic subunit (S1) and five binding subunits (S2 to S5; two S4 subunits are present in each toxin molecule). The S2 subunit binds to lactosylceramide, a glycolipid present on ciliated respiratory cells. The S3 subunit binds to receptors on phagocytic cells, leading to an increase in CR3 on the cell surface, which facilitates attachment mediated by the pertactin and filamentous hemagglutinin and subsequent bacterial phagocytosis. Another adhesin, **fimbria,** has been identified in *B. pertussis* and demonstrated to mediate the binding to cultured mammalian cells. The role of fimbriae in the attachment to ciliated cells in vivo is unknown; however, fimbriae and the other *B. pertussis* adhesins stimulate humoral immunity in vivo and are incorporated into acellular vaccines.

B. pertussis produces several toxins that mediate the localized and systemic manifestations of disease. The S1 portion of **pertussis toxin** has adenosine diphosphate (ADP)-ribosylating activity for the membrane surface G proteins (guanine nucleotide–binding regulatory proteins). These proteins regulate adenylate cyclase activity. Pertussis toxin inactivates $G_{i\alpha}$, the inhibitory protein that

BOX 36–1. Important *Bordetella* species

Organism	Historical Derivation
Bordetella	Named after Jules Bordet, who first isolated the organism responsible for pertussis
B. pertussis	*per,* very or severe; *tussis,* cough (a severe cough)
B. parapertussis	*para,* resembling (resembling pertussis)
B. bronchiseptica	*bronchus,* the trachea; *septicus,* septic (an infected bronchus)

BOX 36–2. Summary of *Bordetella pertussis*

Physiology and Structure

Very small gram-negative coccobacilli
Nonfermentative but can oxidize amino acids as an energy source
Strict aerobe
Growth in vitro requires prolonged incubation in media supplemented with charcoal, starch, blood or albumin

Virulence

Refer to Table 36–2

Epidemiology

Human reservoir host
Worldwide distribution
Children younger than 1 year at greatest risk for infection, but prevalence of disease is increasing in older children and adults
Nonvaccinated individuals at greatest risk for disease
Disease spread person-to-person by infectious aerosols

Diseases

Refer to Box 36–3
Pertussis characterized by three stages: catarrhal, paroxysmal, and convalescent
Most severe disease is in nonvaccinated individuals

Diagnosis

Microscopy is insensitive and nonspecific
Culture is specific but insensitive
Nucleic acid amplification tests are the most sensitive and specific tests
Detection of IgG or IgA can be used as a confirmatory test

Treatment, Prevention, and Control

Treatment with macrolide (i.e., erythromycin, azithromycin, clarithromycin) is effective in eradicating organisms and reducing length of infectious stage
Erythromycin has been used for prophylaxis, but the effectiveness is unknown
Acellular vaccines containing inactivated pertussis toxin and one or more other bacterial components are highly effective; administered in five doses (at ages 2, 4, 6, and 15 to 18 months, and between ages 4 and 6 years)

controls adenylate cyclase activity. The uncontrolled expression of the enzyme leads to an increase in cyclic adenosine monophosphate (cAMP) levels, and a subsequent increase in respiratory secretions and mucus production characteristic of the paroxysmal stage of pertussis.

Adenylate cyclase/hemolysin is a bifunctional toxin that is activated in the target mammalian cell by intracellular calmodulin and catalyzes the conversion of endogenous adenosine triphosphate (ATP) to cAMP in eukaryotic cells (as pertussis toxin does). Adenylate cyclase toxin also inhibits leukocyte chemotaxis, phagocytosis, and killing. This toxin may be important for the initial protection of the bacteria during the early stages of disease.

Dermonecrotic toxin is a heat-labile toxin that at low doses causes vasoconstriction of peripheral blood vessels in mice; this is accompanied by localized ischemia, the movement of leukocytes to extravascular spaces, and hemorrhage. At high doses this toxin causes fatal reactions in mice. The toxin probably is responsible for the localized tissue destruction in human infections, although further research is necessary to confirm this theory.

Tracheal cytotoxin is a low–molecular-weight cell wall peptidoglycan monomer that has a specific affinity for ciliated epithelial cells. At low concentrations, it causes ciliostasis (inhibition of cilia movement), and at the higher concentrations produced later in the infection, it causes extrusion of ciliated cells. Tracheal cytotoxin specifically interferes with deoxyribonucleic acid (DNA) synthesis, thereby impairing the regeneration of damaged cells. This process disrupts the normal clearance mechanisms in the respiratory tree and leads to the characteristic cough associated with pertussis. The toxin also stimulates the release of the cytokine interleukin-1 (IL-1), which leads to fever.

B. pertussis produces two distinct **lipopolysaccharides,** one with lipid A and the other with lipid X. Both lipopolysaccharide molecules can activate the alternate complement pathway and stimulate cytokine release. Their role in the disease process is unknown.

EPIDEMIOLOGY

B. pertussis is a human disease with no other recognized animal or environmental reservoir. Although the incidence of pertussis, with its associated morbidity and mortality, was reduced considerably after the introduction of effective vaccines in 1949, the disease is still endemic worldwide and affects more than 60 million people annually. Almost 12,000 new cases were reported in the United States in 2003 (Figure 36–1), but this is certainly an underestimation of the true incidence of disease. Historically, pertussis has been considered a pediatric disease, and certainly the majority of infections are found in

TABLE 36–1. Virulence Factors Associated with *Bordetella pertussis*

Virulence Factor	Biologic Effect
Adhesins	
Filamentous hemagglutinin	Binds to sulfated glycoproteins on ciliated cell membranes; binds to CR3 on surface of polymorphonuclear leukocytes and initiates phagocytosis
Pertactin (P69 protein)	As with filamentous hemagglutinin
Pertussis toxin	S2 subunit binds to glycolipid on surface of ciliated respiratory cells; S3 subunit binds to ganglioside on surface of phagocytic cells
Fimbriae	Bind to mammalian cells; role in disease is unknown but stimulate humoral immunity
Toxins	
Pertussis toxin	S1 subunit inactivates $G_{1\alpha}$, the membrane surface protein that controls adenylate cyclase activity; uncontrolled expression leads to increased cAMP levels; toxin inhibits phagocytic killing and monocyte migration
Adenylate cyclase/hemolysin toxin	Increases intracellular level of adenylate cyclase and inhibits phagocytic killing and monocyte migration
Dermonecrotic toxin	Causes dose-dependent skin lesions or fatal reactions in experimental animal model; role in disease is unknown
Tracheal cytotoxin	A peptidoglycan fragment that kills ciliated respiratory cells and stimulates the release of interleukin-1 (fever)
Lipopolysaccharide	Two distinct lipopolysaccharide molecules with either lipid A or lipid X; activates alternate complement pathway and stimulates cytokine release; role in disease is unknown

cAMP, Cyclic adenoside monophosphate.

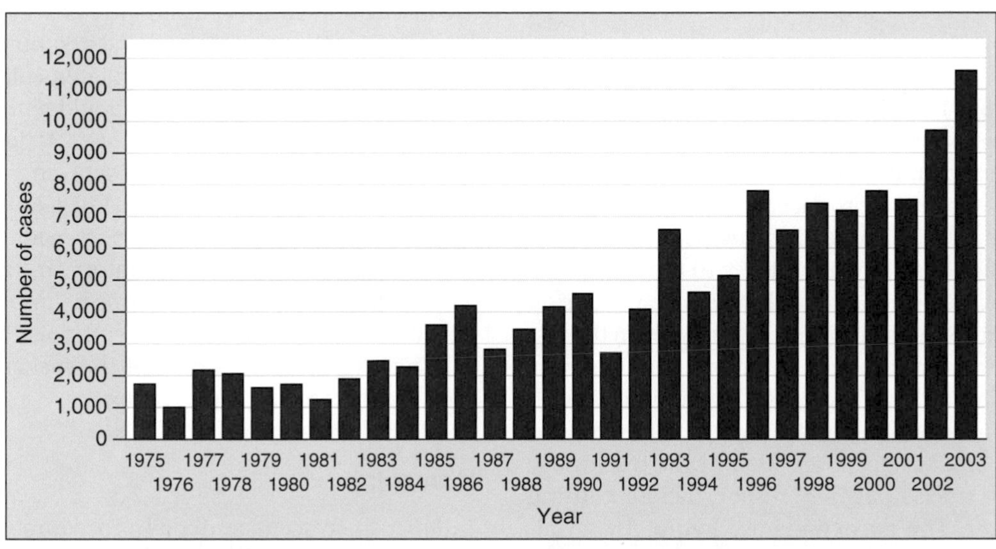

FIGURE 36–1. Incidence of pertussis in the United States from 1975 to 2003.

children younger than 1 year (Figure 36–2). However, in recent years there has been a dramatic increase in disease in older children and adults. This increase is attributed to waning immunity over time (even in vaccinated individuals) or the potential selection of bacterial strains not recognized by the current vaccines.

CLINICAL DISEASES (BOX 36–3)

Infection is initiated when infectious aerosols are inhaled and the bacteria become attached to and proliferate on ciliated epithelial cells. After a 7- to 10-day incubation period, the typical patient experiences the first of three

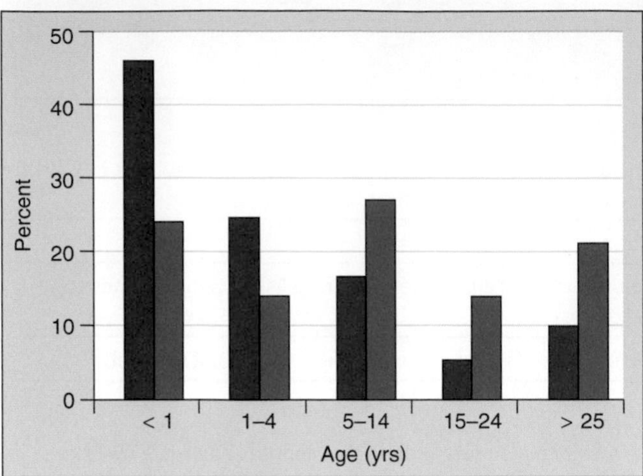

FIGURE 36–2. Age distribution for pertussis infections reported in 1988 *(red bars)* and 2002 *(blue bars).*

	Incubation	Catarrhal	Paroxysmal	Convalescent
Duration	7–10 days	1–2 weeks	2–4 weeks	3–4 weeks (or longer)
Symptoms	None	Rhinorrhea, malaise, fever, sneezing, anorexia	Repetitive cough with whoops, vomiting, leukocytosis	Diminished paroxysmal cough, development of secondary complications (pneumonia, seizures, encephalopathy)
Bacterial culture				

FIGURE 36–3. Clinical presentation of *Bordetella pertussis* disease.

BOX 36–3. *Bordetella* species: Clinical Summaries

Bordetella pertussis: After a 7 to 10 day incubation period, disease is characterized by the catarrhal stage (resembles the common cold), progressing to the paroxysmal stage (repetitive coughs followed by inspiratory whoops), then the convalescence stage (diminishing paroxysms and secondary complication)

Bordetella parapertussis: Produces a milder form of pertussis

Bordetella bronchiseptica: Primarily a respiratory disease of animals but can cause bronchopneumonia in humans

stages (Figure 36–3). The first stage, the **catarrhal stage,** resembles a common cold, with serous rhinorrhea, sneezing, malaise, anorexia, and low-grade fever. Because the peak number of bacteria is produced during this stage and the cause of the disease is not yet recognized, patients in the catarrhal stage pose the highest risk to their contacts. After 1 to 2 weeks, the **paroxysmal stage** begins. During this time, ciliated epithelial cells are extruded from the respiratory tract and the clearance of mucus is impaired. This stage is characterized by the classic whooping cough paroxysms (i.e., a series of repetitive coughs followed by an inspiratory whoop). Mucus production in the respiratory tract is common and is partially responsible for causing airway restriction. The paroxysms are frequently terminated with vomiting and exhaustion. A marked lymphocytosis is also prominent during this stage. Affected patients may experience as many as 40 to 50 paroxysms daily during the height of the illness. After 2 to 4 weeks, the disease enters the **convalescent stage;** at this time the paroxysms diminish in number and severity, but secondary complications can occur. This classic presentation of pertussis may not be seen in patients with partial immunity. Such patients may have a history of a chronic persistent cough with or without vomiting.

LABORATORY DIAGNOSIS

Specimen Collection and Transport

B. pertussis organisms are extremely sensitive to drying and do not survive unless care is taken during the collection and transport of the specimen to the laboratory. The optimal diagnostic specimen is a nasopharyngeal aspirate. Calcium alginate or Dacron fiber swabs must be used because cotton swabs contain fatty acids that are toxic to *B. pertussis.* Oropharyngeal swabs should not be used because sufficient numbers of ciliated epithelial cells are not collected. The specimen should either be directly inoculated onto freshly prepared isolation media (e.g., charcoal-horse blood agar, Bordet-Gengou medium) at the patient's bedside or be placed in a suitable transport medium (e.g., Regan-Lowe transport medium). Specimens cannot be delivered to the laboratory in traditional transport media because the organisms will not survive. Inoculated culture media must be kept moist because drying kills the organisms. A portion of the specimen can also be used for microscopic examination.

Microscopy

A direct fluorescent antibody procedure can be used to examine the specimens. In this method, the aspirated specimen is smeared onto a microscopic slide, air-dried and heat fixed, and then stained with fluorescein-labeled antibodies directed against *B. pertussis.* Antibodies against *B. parapertussis* should also be used to detect mild forms of pertussis caused by this organism. The direct fluorescent antibody test results are positive in slightly more than half of the patients with pertussis, but false-positive results can occur as a result of cross-reactions with other bacteria.

Culture

The sensitivity of culture is affected by patient factors (i.e., stage of illness, use of antibiotics), the quality of the specimen, transport conditions, and culture methods. The traditional use of Bordet-Gengou medium has been replaced by Regan-Lowe charcoal medium supplemented with glycerol, peptones, and horse blood. The media should be incubated in air at 35°C and in a humidified chamber. Prolonged incubation (e.g., 7 days) is necessary because the tiny colonies can be observed only after 3 or more days of incubation. Because the quality of the media dramatically affects the success of culture, laboratories that infrequently culture specimens for *Bordetella* should arrange for the state public health department to process these specimens. Despite use of optimized culture conditions, fewer than half the infected patients have positive cultures.

Nucleic Acid Amplification

The use of nucleic acid amplification methods such as polymerase chain reaction (PCR), in conjunction with culture, is the recommended diagnostic approach, replacing microscopy in many laboratories. Several studies have demonstrated a sensitivity of 80% to 100%. Although these tests have been restricted to "home-brew" procedures, it is anticipated that commercial tests (either for *Bordetella* only or for a panel of respiratory pathogens) will be offered in the near future.

Identification

B. pertussis organisms are identified by their characteristic microscopic and colonial morphology on selective media and their reactivity with a specific antiserum (either in an agglutination reaction or with the reagents used in the direct fluorescent antibody test). The reactions summarized in Table 36–2 can be used to differentiate *B. pertussis* and *B. parapertussis.*

Serology

It is difficult to interpret the results of serologic tests because microscopy and culture techniques are relatively insensitive standards by which to evaluate these results. Additionally, the Food and Drug Administration (FDA) has not approved any tests at this time. Enzyme-linked immunosorbent assay (ELISA) tests have been developed to detect immunoglobulin A (IgA), IgM, and IgG antibodies against filamentous hemagglutinin and pertussis toxin. Antibodies directed against pertussis toxin are specific for *B. pertussis;* however, filamentous hemagglutinin is present in both *B. pertussis* and *B. parapertussis.* A significant rise in antibody titer between acute serum and convalescent serum, or an initially high titer, is consistent with a recent infection.

TABLE 36–2. Differential Characteristics of Bordetella Species

Characteristics	*B. pertussis*	*B. parapertussis*	*B. bronchiseptica*
Oxidase	+	–	+
Urease	–	+	+
Motility	–	–	+
Growth on:			
Sheep blood agar	–	+	+
MacConkey agar	–	+/–	+

Modified from Murray P et al: *Manual of clinical microbiology,* ed 8, Washington, 2003, American Society for Microbiology.

TREATMENT, PREVENTION, AND CONTROL

The treatment for pertussis is primarily supportive, with nursing supervision during the paroxysmal and convalescent stages of the illness. Antibiotics can ameliorate the clinical course, but convalescence depends primarily on the rapidity and degree to which the layer of ciliated epithelial cells regenerates. Macrolides (i.e., erythromycin, azithromycin, clarithromycin) are effective in eradicating the organisms and can reduce the duration of infectivity; however, this effect has limited value because the illness is usually unrecognized during the peak of contagiousness. Strains resistant to erythromycin have been reported but are not widespread. Trimethoprim-sulfamethoxazole or fluoroquinolones can be used in patients unable to tolerate macrolides.

Whole-cell, inactivated vaccines for pertussis have been associated with unacceptable levels of complications and have been replaced with acellular vaccines in the United States. A number of acellular vaccines have been approved since 1996, all of which contain inactivated pertussis toxin and one or more other bacterial components (e.g., filamentous hemagglutinin, pertactin, fimbriae). It is currently recommended that the acellular pertussis vaccine be administered in combination with vaccines for diphtheria and tetanus (DTaP) to children at the ages of 2, 4, 6, and 15 to 18 months, with the fifth dose between the ages of 4 and 6 years. Although this vaccination approach provides a high level of protection, antigenic changes detected in pertussis toxin and pertactin may compromise the efficacy of these vaccines.

Because pertussis is highly contagious in a susceptible population and unrecognized infections in family members of a symptomatic patient can maintain disease in a community, erythromycin has been used for prophylaxis in select instances.

Other *Bordetella* Species

B. parapertussis is responsible for causing 10% to 20% of the cases of mild pertussis occurring annually in the United States. *B. bronchiseptica* causes respiratory disease primarily in animals but has been associated with human respiratory tract colonization and bronchopulmonary disease. Both organisms can be readily isolated on conventional laboratory media, and unlike *B. pertussis,* both have easily recognizable metabolic properties.

CASE STUDY AND QUESTIONS

A 5-year-old girl was brought to the local public health clinic because of a severe, intractable cough. During the previous 10 days, she had a persistent cold that had worsened. The cough developed the previous day and was so severe that vomiting frequently followed it. The child appeared exhausted from the coughing episodes. A blood cell count showed a marked leukocytosis with a predominance of lymphocytes. The examining physician suspected that the child had pertussis.

1. What laboratory tests can be performed to confirm the physician's clinical diagnosis? What specimens should be collected, and how should they be submitted to the laboratory?
2. What virulence factors are produced by *B. pertussis,* and what are their biologic effects? What is the natural progression and prognosis for this disease? How can it be prevented?

Bibliography

Carbonetti N et al: Pertussis toxin plays an early role in respiratory tract colonization by *Bordetella pertussis, Infect Immun* 71:6358-6366, 2003.

Cassiday P et al: Polymorphism in *Bordetella pertussis* pertactin and pertussis toxin virulence factors in the United States, 1935-1999, *J Infect Dis* 182:1402-1408, 2000.

Centers for Disease Control and Prevention: Pertussis: United States, *MMWR* 47:1–92, 1999.

Cherry J, Robbins J: Pertussis in adults: Epidemiology, signs, symptoms, and implications for vaccination, *Clin Infect Dis* 28(suppl 2), 1999.

Edwards K, Decker M: Acellular pertussis vaccines for infants, *N Engl J Med* 334:391-392, 1996 (editorial).

Guris D et al: Changing epidemiology of pertussis in the United States: Increasing reported incidence among adolescents and adults, 1990-1996, *Clin Infect Dis* 28:1230-1237, 1999.

He Q et al: Whooping cough caused by *Bordetella pertussis* and *Bordetella parapertussis* in an immunized population, *JAMA* 280:635-637, 1998.

Kerr J, Matthews R: *Bordetella pertussis* infection: Pathogenesis, diagnosis, management, and the role of protective immunity, *Eur J Clin Microbiol Infect Dis* 19:77-88, 2000.

Kirimanjeswara G, Mann P, Harvill E: Role of antibodies in immunity to *Bordetella* infections, *Infect Immun* 71:1719-1724, 2003.

Loeffelholz M et al: Comparison of PCR, culture, and direct fluorescent-antibody testing for detection of *Bordetella pertussis, J Clin Microbiol* 37:2872-2876, 1999.

Preziosi M, Halloran M: Effects of pertussis vaccination on disease: Vaccine efficacy in reducing clinical severity, *Clin Infect Dis* 37:772-779, 2003.

Tilley P et al: Detection of *Bordetella pertussis* in a clinical laboratory by culture, polymerase chain reaction, and direct fluorescent antibody staining: accuracy and cost. *Diagn Microbial Infect Dis* 37:17-23, 2000.

Woolfrey BF, Moody JA: Human infections associated with *Bordetella bronchiseptica, Clin Microbiol Rev* 4:243-255, 1991.

Wright S et al: Pertussis infection in adults with persistent cough, *JAMA* 273:1044-1046, 1996.

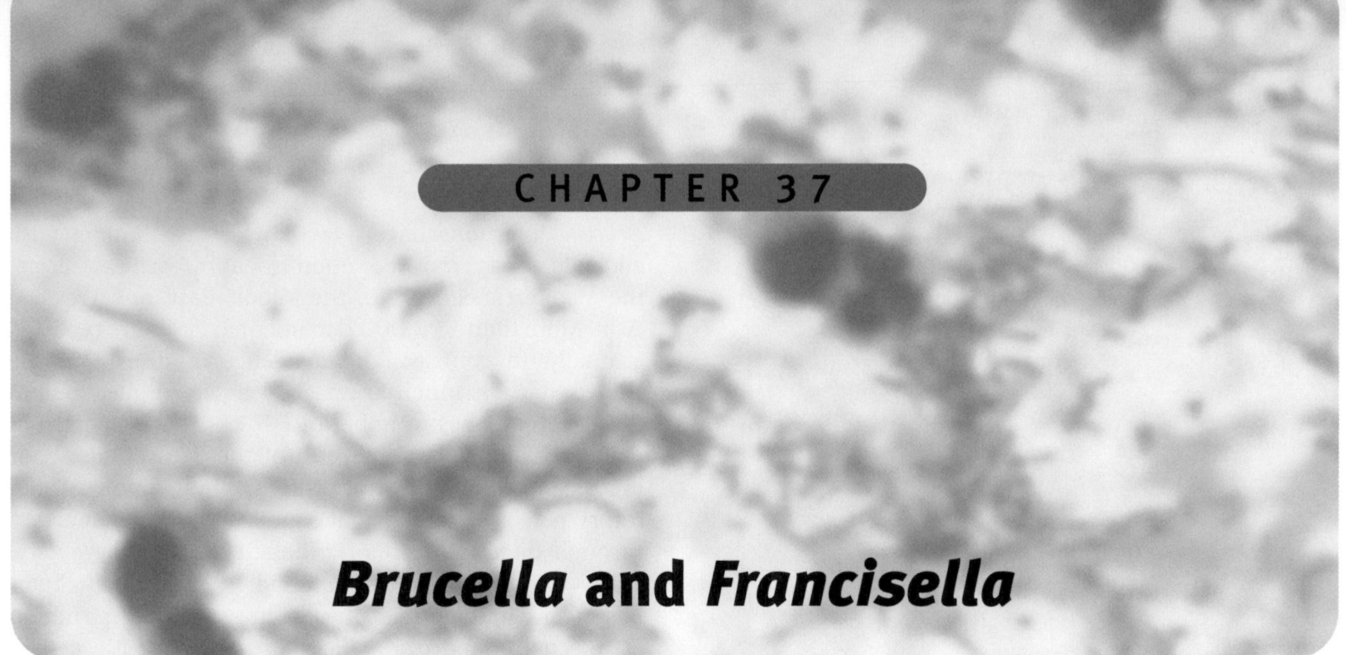

CHAPTER 37

Brucella and *Francisella*

Francisella and *Brucella* are important zoonotic pathogens that occasionally cause human disease. These organisms have also been pushed to the forefront as potential agents of bioterrorists. Although the organisms have some common properties (e.g., very small coccobacilli, fastidious and slow growth requirements, always pathogenic in humans), they are taxonomically unrelated. In the phylogenetic tree of bacterial life the α-proteobacteria occupy one limb and the γ-proteobacteria another. *Brucella* is a member of the α-proteobacteria group (with organisms such as *Rickettsia, Ehrlichia, Bartonella,* and other genera), and *Francisella* is a member of the γ-proteobacteria group (with many genera, including *Legionella, Pasteurella,* and *Pseudomonas*).

Brucella

Molecular studies of the genus *Brucella* demonstrate a close relationship among the strains and are consistent with a single genus; however, the genus has historically been subdivided into a number of species. Currently, there are six species of *Brucella,* with four species associated with human disease: *Brucella abortus, Brucella melitensis, Brucella suis,* and *Brucella canis* (Box 37–1). The diseases caused by members of this genus are characterized by a number of names based on the original microbiologists who isolated and described the organisms (e.g., Sir David Bruce **[brucellosis]**, Bernhard Bang **[Bang's disease]**), its clinical presentation **(undulant fever),** and the sites of recognized outbreaks (e.g., Malta fever, Mediterranean remittent fever, rock fever of Gibraltar, county fever of Constantinople, fever of Crete). However, the most commonly used term is **brucellosis,** which will be used in this chapter.

PHYSIOLOGY AND STRUCTURE (BOX 37–2)

Brucellae are small (0.5 × 0.6 to 1.5 μm), nonmotile, nonencapsulated, gram-negative coccobacilli. The organism grows slowly in culture (taking a week or more) and generally requires complex growth media; is strictly aerobic, with some strains requiring supplemental carbon dioxide for growth; and does not ferment carbohydrates.

Colonies can assume both smooth (translucent, homogeneous) and rough (opaque, granular, or sticky) forms, as determined by the O antigen of the cell wall lipopolysaccharide (LPS). Antisera to one form (e.g., smooth) do not cross-react with the other form (e.g., rough). *Brucella* species can be further characterized by the relative proportion of antigenic epitopes, referred to as A and M antigens, that reside on the O polysaccharide chain of the smooth LPS.

PATHOGENESIS AND IMMUNITY

Brucella does not produce a detectable exotoxin, and the endotoxin is less toxic than that produced by other gram-negative rods. Reversion of smooth strains to the rough morphology is associated with greatly reduced virulence, so the O chain of the smooth LPS is an important marker for virulence. *Brucella* is also an intracellular parasite of the reticuloendothelial system. After the initial exposure, the organisms are phagocytosed by macrophages and monocytes. In the acidic environment of the phagolysosome, essential virulence genes in the virB operon are induced and regulate intracellular replication. Phagocytosed bacteria are carried to the spleen, liver, bone marrow, lymph nodes, and kidneys. The bacteria secrete proteins that induce granuloma formation in these organs, and destructive changes in these and other tissues occur in patients with advanced disease.

BOX 37–1. Important Organisms

Organism	Historical Derivation
Brucella	Named after Sir David Bruce, who first recognized the organism as a cause of "undulant fever"
B. abortus	*abortus*, abortion or miscarriage (this organism is responsible for abortion in infected animals)
B. melitensis	*melitensis*, pertaining to the Island of Malta (Melita), where the first outbreak was recognized by Bruce
B. suis	*suis*, of the pig (a swine pathogen)
B. canis	*canis*, of the dog (a dog pathogen)
Francisella	Named after the American microbiologist Edward Francis, who first described tularemia
F. tularensis spp. *tularensis* (type A)	*tularensis*, pertaining to Tulare County, California, where the disease was first described
F. tularensis spp. *holarctica* (type B)	*holos*, whole; *arctos*, northern regions (reference to distribution in the arctic or northern regions)
F. tularensis spp. *mediaasiatica*	*media*, middle; *asiatica*, Asian (pertaining to middle Asia)
F. tularensis spp. *novicida*	*novus*, new; *cida*, to cut (a "new killer")
F. philomiragia	*philos*, loving; miragia, *mirage* ("loving of mirages," reference to presence in water)

EPIDEMIOLOGY

Brucella infections have a worldwide distribution, with endemic disease most common in Latin America, Africa, the Mediterranean basin, the Middle East, and Western Asia. More than 500,000 documented cases are reported annually. In contrast, the incidence of disease in the United States is much lower (104 reported infections in 2003). The highest number of U.S. cases are reported in California and Texas, and most of these infections occur in residents from Mexico or visitors to that country. Laboratory personnel are also at significant risk for infection through direct contact or inhalation of the organism. Disease in the animal population in the United States has been eliminated effectively through the destruction of infected animals and the vaccination of disease-free animals; thus infections in veterinarians, slaughterhouse workers, and farmers are much less common than before 1980.

Brucellosis in humans can be acquired by direct contact with the organism (e.g., a laboratory exposure), ingestion (e.g., consumption of contaminated food products), or inhalation. Of particular concern is the potential use of *Brucella* as a biologic weapon in which exposure would most likely be by inhalation.

Brucella causes mild or asymptomatic disease in the natural host: *B. abortus* infects cattle and American bison;

BOX 37–2. Summary of *Brucella*

Physiology and Structure

Very small gram-negative coccobacilli (0.5×0.6 to $1.5\ \mu m$)

Strict aerobe; nonfermenter

Requires complex media and prolonged incubation for in vitro growth

Virulence

Intracellular pathogen that is resistant to killing in serum and by phagocytes

Smooth colonies associated with virulence

Epidemiology

Animal reservoirs are goats and sheep *(Brucella melitensis);* cattle and American bison *(Brucella abortus);* swine, reindeer, and caribou *(Brucella suis);* and dogs, foxes, and coyotes *(Brucella canis)*

Infects tissues rich in erythritol (e.g., breast, uterus, placenta, epididymis)

Worldwide distribution, particularly in Latin America, Africa, the Mediterranean basin, Middle East, and Western Asia

Vaccination of herds has controlled disease in the United States; most disease in the United States is reported in California and Texas

No seasonal incidence

Individuals at greatest risk for disease are people who consume unpasteurized dairy products, people in direct contact with infected animals, and laboratory workers

Disease

Brucellosis (see Box 37–3)

Diagnosis

Microscopy is insensitive

Culture (blood, bone marrow, infected tissue if localized infection) is sensitive and specific if prolonged incubation is used (minimum of 3 days to 2 weeks)

Serology can be used to confirm the clinical diagnosis; fourfold increase in titer or single titer ≥1:160; high titers can persist for months to years; cross-reactive with other bacteria

Treatment, Prevention, and Control

Recommended treatment is doxycycline combined with rifampin for a minimum of 6 weeks for nonpregnant adults; trimethoprim-sulfamethoxazole for pregnant women and for children younger than 8 years

Human disease is controlled by eradication of the disease in the animal reservoir through vaccination and serologic monitoring of the animals for evidence of disease; pasteurization of dairy products; and use of proper safety techniques in clinical laboratories working with this organism

B. melitensis, goats and sheep; *B. suis,* swine, reindeer, and caribou; and *B. canis,* dogs, foxes, and coyotes (see Box 37–2). The organism has a predilection for infecting organs rich in erythritol, a sugar metabolized by many *Brucella* strains in preference to glucose. Animal (but not human) tissues, including breast, uterus, placenta, and epididymis, are rich in erythritol. The organisms thus localize in these tissues in nonhuman reservoirs and can cause sterility, abortions, or asymptomatic life-long carriage. Brucellae are shed in high numbers in milk, urine, and birth products. Human disease in the United States is most commonly caused by *B. melitensis* and results primarily from consumption of contaminated, unpasteurized milk and other dairy products.

CLINICAL DISEASES (Box 37–3)

The disease spectrum of **brucellosis** depends on the infecting organism. *B. abortus* and *B. canis* tend to produce mild disease with rare suppurative complications. In contrast, *B. suis* causes the formation of destructive lesions and has a prolonged course. *B. melitensis* also causes severe disease with a high incidence of serious complications because the organisms can multiply to high concentrations in phagocytic cells.

Acute disease develops in approximately half of the patients infected with *Brucella,* with symptoms first appearing up to 2 months after exposure. Initial symptoms are nonspecific and consist of malaise, chills, sweats, fatigue, weakness, myalgias, weight loss, arthralgias, and nonproductive cough. Almost all patients have fever, and this can be intermittent in untreated patients, hence the name **undulant fever.** Patients with advanced disease can have gastrointestinal tract symptoms (70% of patients), osteolytic lesions or joint effusions (20% to 60%), respiratory tract symptoms (25%), and less commonly, cutaneous, neurologic, or cardiovascular manifestations. Chronic infections can also develop in inadequately treated patients.

BOX 37–3. *Brucella* **and** *Francisella***: Clinical Summaries**

Brucella

Brucellosis: Initial nonspecific symptoms of malaise, chills, sweats, fatigue, myalgias, weight loss, arthralgias, and fever; can be intermittent (undulant fever); can progress to systemic involvement (gastrointestinal tract, bones or joints, respiratory tract, other organs)

Brucella melitensis: Severe, acute disease with complications common

Brucella abortus: Mild disease with suppurative complications

Brucella suis: Chronic, suppurative, destructive disease

Brucella canis: Mild disease with suppurative complications

Francisella

Ulceroglandular tularemia: Painful papule develops at the site of inoculation that progresses to ulceration; localized lymphadenopathy

Oculoglandular tularemia: Following inoculation into the eye (e.g., rubbing eye with a contaminated finger), painful conjunctivitis develops with regional lymphadenopathy

Pneumonic tularemia: Pneumonitis with signs of sepsis develops rapidly after exposure to contaminated aerosols; high mortality unless promptly diagnosed and treated

LABORATORY DIAGNOSIS

Specimen Collection

Several blood samples should be collected for culture and serologic testing. Bone marrow cultures and cultures of infected tissues may also be useful. To ensure safe handling of the specimen, the laboratory should be notified if brucellosis is suspected.

Microscopy

Brucella organisms are readily stained using conventional techniques, but their intracellular location and small size make them difficult to detect in clinical specimens. Currently, specific immunofluorescent antibody tests are not available.

Culture

Brucella organisms grow slowly during primary isolation. The organisms can grow on most enriched blood agars and occasionally on MacConkey agar; however, incubation for 3 or more days may be required. Blood cultures should be incubated for 2 weeks before they are considered negative. More extended incubation of blood cultures is now unnecessary with the use of automated culture systems.

Identification

Preliminary identification of *Brucella* is based on the isolate's microscopic and colonial morphology, positive oxidase and urease reactions, and reactivity with antibodies directed against *B. abortus* and *B. melitensis. B. melitensis, B. abortus,* and *B. suis* will react with antisera prepared against *B. abortus* or *B. melitensis* (illustrating the close relationship among these species). In contrast, *B. canis* is not reactive with either antisera. Identification at the genus level can also be accomplished by sequencing the 16S ribosomal ribonucleic acid (rRNA) gene. Because brucellosis is uncommon in the United States, most laboratories refer the organism to a state public health laboratory for definitive identification.

Serology

Subclinical brucellosis and many cases of acute and chronic diseases are identified by a specific antibody response in the infected patient. Antibodies are detected in virtually all patients. Immunoglobulin M (IgM) response is initially observed, after which both IgG and IgA antibodies are produced. Antibodies can persist for many months or years; thus a significant increase in the antibody titer is required to provide definitive serologic evidence of current disease. A presumptive diagnosis can be made if there is a fourfold increase in the titer or a single titer is greater than or equal to 1:160. High antibody titers (1:160 or more) are noted in 5% to 10% of the population living in endemic areas; thus serologic tests should be used to confirm the clinical diagnosis of brucellosis and not to form the basis of the diagnosis. The antigen used in the *Brucella* serum agglutination test (SAT) is from *B. abortus.* Antibodies directed against *B. melitensis* or *B. suis* cross-react with this antigen; however, there is no cross-reactivity with *B. canis.* The specific *B. canis* antigen must be used to diagnose infections with this organism. Antibodies directed against other genera of bacteria (e.g., some strains of *Escherichia, Salmonella, Vibrio, Yersinia, Stenotrophomonas,* and *Francisella*) are also reported to cross-react with the *B. abortus* antigen.

TREATMENT, PREVENTION, AND CONTROL

Tetracyclines, with doxycycline the preferred agent, are generally active against most strains of *Brucella;* however, because this is a bacteriostatic drug, relapse is common after an initially successful response. The World Health Organization currently recommends the combination of doxycycline with rifampin. Because the tetracyclines are toxic to young children and fetuses, doxycycline should be replaced with trimethoprim-sulfamethoxazole for pregnant women and for children younger than 8 years. Treatment must be continued for 6 weeks or longer for it to be successful. Fluoroquinolones, macrolides, penicillins, and cephalosporins are either ineffective or have unpredictable activity. Relapse of disease is caused by inadequate therapy and not the development of antibiotic resistance.

Control of human brucellosis is accomplished through control of the disease in livestock, as demonstrated in the United States. This requires systematic identification (by serologic testing) and elimination of infected herds and animal vaccination (currently with the rough strain of *B. abortus* strain RB51). The avoidance of unpasteurized dairy products, the observance of appropriate safety procedures in the clinical laboratory, and the wearing of protective clothing by abattoir workers are further ways to prevent brucellosis. The live-attenuated *B. abortus* and *B. melitensis* vaccines have been used successfully to prevent infection in animal herds. Vaccines have not been developed against *B. suis* or *B. canis,* and the existing vaccines cannot be used in humans because they produce symptomatic disease. The lack of an effective human vaccine is of concern because *Brucella* (as well as *Francisella*) could be used as an agent of bioterrorism.

Francisella tularensis

The genus *Francisella* consists of two species, *Francisella tularensis* and *Francisella philomiragia. F. tularensis* is the causative agent of **tularemia** (also called **glandular fever, rabbit fever, tick fever,** and **deer fly fever**) in animals and humans. *F. tularensis* is subdivided into four subspecies (see Box 37–1), of which subspecies *tularensis* (type A) is most important in the United States and subspecies *holarctica* is more important in Europe and Asia. *F. tularensis* ssp. *tularensis* is the most virulent member of the genus and will be the focus of this discussion. Subspecies *mediaasiatica* and ssp. *novicida* are rarely associated with human disease. *F. philomiragia* is also an uncommon, opportunistic pathogen that is associated with exposure to salt water. It has a particular predilection for patients with immunologic deficiencies (i.e., chronic granulomatous disease, myeloproliferative diseases). Because this pathogen is rarely isolated, it will not be discussed further in this chapter.

PHYSIOLOGY AND STRUCTURE (Box 37–4)

F. tularensis is a very small (0.2 × 0.2 to 0.7 μm), faintly staining, gram-negative coccobacillus (Figure 37–1). The organism is nonmotile, has a thin lipid capsule, and has fastidious growth requirements (i.e., most strains require cysteine for growth). It is strictly aerobic and requires 3 or more days before growth is detected in culture.

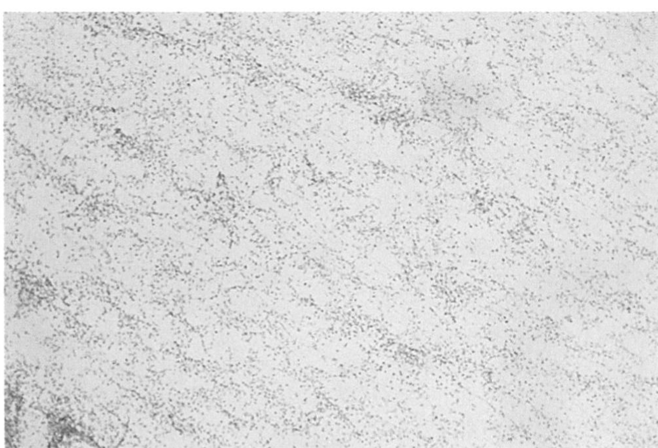

FIGURE 37–1. Gram stain of *Francisella tularensis* isolated in culture; note the extremely small coccobacilli.

BOX 37–4. Summary of *Francisella tularensis*

Physiology and Structure

Very small gram-negative coccobacilli (0.2 × 0.2 to 0.7 μm)
Strict aerobe; nonfermenter
Requires specialized media and prolonged incubation for growth in culture

Virulence

Antiphagocytic capsule
Intracellular pathogen resistant to killing in serum and by phagocytes

Epidemiology

Wild mammals, domestic animals, birds, fish, and blood-sucking arthropods are reservoirs; rabbits and hard ticks are most common hosts; humans are accidental hosts
Worldwide distribution; most common in United States in Oklahoma, Missouri, and Arkansas
Approximately 130 cases seen in United States, although the actual number may be much higher
The infectious dose is small when exposure is by arthropod, through skin, or by inhalation; large numbers of organisms must be ingested for infection by this route

Disease

Clinical symptoms and prognosis determined by route of infection: ulceroglandular, oculoglandular, glandular, typhoidal, oropharyngeal, gastrointestinal, pneumonic (see Box 37–3)

Diagnosis

Microscopy is insensitive
PCR-based nucleic acid amplification assays are under evaluation
Culture on cysteine-supplemented media (e.g., chocolate agar, BCYE agar) is sensitive and specific if prolonged incubation is used
Serology can be used to confirm the clinical diagnosis; fourfold increase in titer or single titer ≥1:160; high titers can persist for months to years; cross-reactive with *Brucella*

Treatment, Prevention, and Control

Because streptomycin is readily available, gentamicin is the antibiotic of choice; fluoroquinolones (e.g., ciprofloxacin) and doxycycline have good activity; penicillins and some cephalosporins are ineffective
Disease prevented by avoiding reservoirs and vectors of infection; clothing and gloves are protective
Live-attenuated vaccine available but rarely used in human disease

PATHOGENESIS AND IMMUNITY

F. tularensis is an intracellular parasite that can survive for prolonged periods in macrophages of the reticuloendothelial system because the organism inhibits phagosome-lysosome fusion. Pathogenic strains possess an antiphagocytic, polysaccharide-rich capsule, and loss of the capsule is associated with decreased virulence. The capsule protects the bacteria from complement-mediated killing during the bacteremia phase of disease. Like all gram-negative rods, this organism has endotoxin, but it is considerably less active than the endotoxin found in other gram-negative rods (e.g., *Escherichia coli*).

A strong, innate immune response with production of interferon-γ and tumor necrosis factor (TNF) are important for controlling bacterial replication in macrophages in the early phase of infection. Specific T-cell immunity is required for activation of macrophages for intracellular killing in the late stages of disease. Humoral immunity is less important for elimination of this facultative intracellular pathogen.

EPIDEMIOLOGY

Francisella is distributed throughout the Northern Hemisphere from the Artic Circle south to the approximate latitude 20 degrees north. Disease is not reported in southern regions (e.g., Central and South America, Australia). In the United States, disease is primarily observed in Oklahoma, Missouri, and Arkansas, although sporadic cases are reported in the majority of states. *F. tularensis* is found in a variety of wild animals, birds, and blood-sucking arthropods, with the most common endemic foci in rabbits, ticks, hares, voles, muskrats, and beavers. Human tularemia is acquired most often from the bite of an infected “hard-shell” tick (e.g., *Ixodes, Dermacentor, Amblyomma* spp.) or from contact with an infected animal or domestic pet (e.g., cat) that has caught an infected animal (e.g., rabbit). Hard-shell ticks feed on their host for hours or days, so careful questioning may elicit a history of tick exposure before the patient felt ill. Disease can also be acquired from the consumption of contaminated meat or water or from the inhalation of an infectious aerosol (most commonly in a laboratory or while dressing an infected animal). Infection with *F. tularensis* requires as few as 10 organisms when exposure is by an arthropod bite or contamination of unbroken skin, 50 organisms when inhaled, and 10^8 organisms when ingested.

The reported incidence of disease is low. In 2003, 129 cases were reported in the United States; however, the actual number of infections is likely to be much higher because tularemia is frequently unsuspected and is difficult to confirm by laboratory tests. Most of the infections occur during summer (when exposure to infected ticks is greatest) and winter (when hunters are exposed to infected rabbits) months. The incidence of disease increases dramatically when a relatively warm winter is followed by a wet summer, causing the tick population to proliferate. People at greatest risk for infection are hunters, laboratory personnel, and those exposed to ticks. In areas where the organism is endemic, it is said that if a rabbit is moving so slowly that it can be shot by a hunter or caught by a pet, the rabbit could be infected.

CLINICAL DISEASES (see BOX 37–3)

Disease caused by *F. tularensis* is subdivided into several forms based on the clinical presentation: **ulceroglandular** (cutaneous ulcer and swollen lymph node), **oculoglandular** (eye involvement and swollen cervical lymph nodes), glandular (primarily swollen lymph nodes with no other localized symptoms), **typhoidal** (systemic signs of sepsis), **pneumonic** (pulmonary symptoms), and **oropharyngeal** and **gastrointestinal** disease after ingestion of *F. tularensis*. Variations of these presentations are also common (e.g., pneumonic tularemia typically has systemic signs of sepsis).

Ulceroglandular tularemia is the most common manifestation. The skin lesion, which starts as a painful papule, develops at the site of the tick bite or direct inoculation of the organism into the skin (e.g., a laboratory accident). The papule then ulcerates and has a necrotic center and raised border. Localized lymphadenopathy and bacteremia are also typically present (although bacteremia may be difficult to document).

Oculoglandular tularemia (Figure 37–2) is a specialized form of the disease and results from direct contamination of the eye. The organism can be introduced into the eyes, for example, by contaminated fingers or through exposure to water or aerosols. Affected patients have a painful conjunctivitis and regional lymphadenopathy.

Pneumonic tularemia (Figure 37–3) results from inhalation of infectious aerosols and is associated with high morbidity and mortality unless the organism is recovered rapidly in blood cultures (it is generally difficult to detect in respiratory cultures). There is also concern that *F. tularensis* could be used as a biologic weapon. As such, creation of an infectious aerosol would be the most likely method of dispersal.

LABORATORY DIAGNOSIS

Specimen Collection

The collection and processing of specimens for the isolation of *F. tularensis* are hazardous for both the physician and the laboratory worker. The organism, by virtue of its small size, can penetrate through unbroken skin and the mucous membranes during collection of the sample, or it can be inhaled if aerosols are produced (a particular concern during processing of specimens in the laboratory). Although tularemia is rare, laboratory-acquired infections are disproportionately common. Gloves should be worn during collection of the specimen (e.g., aspiration of an ulcer or lymph node), and all laboratory work (both initial processing and identification tests) should be performed in a biohazard hood.

Microscopy

Detection of *F. tularensis* in Gram-stained aspirates from infected nodes or ulcers is almost always unsuccessful because the organism is extremely small and stains faintly (see Figure 37–1). A more sensitive and specific approach is direct staining of the clinical specimen with fluorescein-

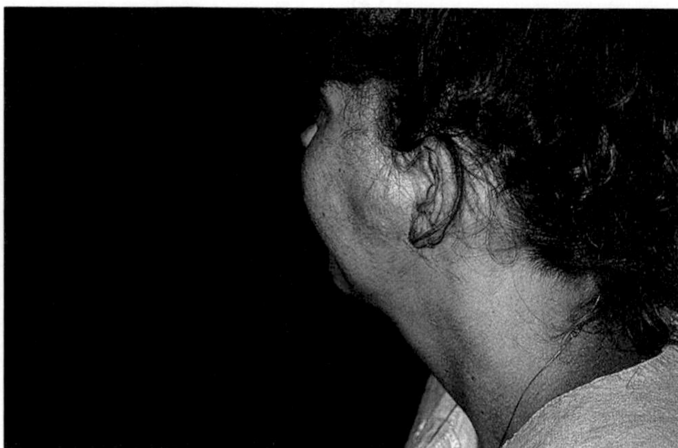

FIGURE 37–2. Patient with oculoglandular tularemia.

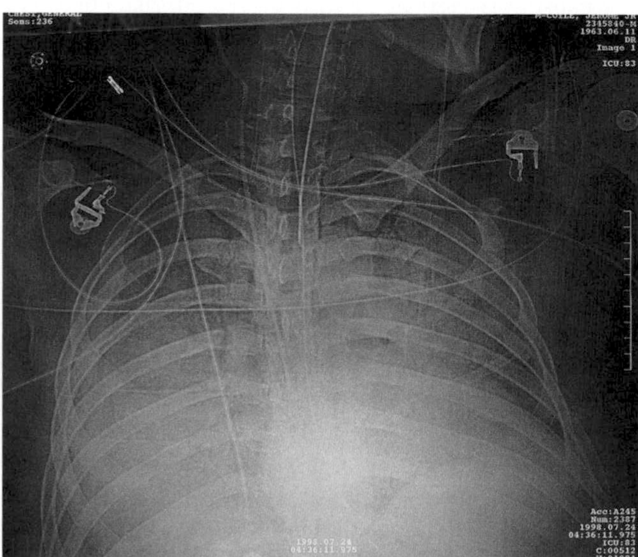

FIGURE 37–3. Chest radiograph of patient with pulmonary tularemia.

labeled antibodies directed against the organism. Antibody reagents against types A and B are available from the Centers for Disease Control and Prevention (CDC) and state public health facilities but are not available in most clinical laboratories.

Molecular Diagnostics

Polymerase chain reaction (PCR)-based assays are under development but are not widely available at this time. This may change rapidly with the increased interest in the development of diagnostic tests for this organism in the event of a bioterrorist attack.

Culture

It has been stated that *F. tularensis* cannot be reliably recovered on common laboratory media because the organism requires sulfhydryl-containing substances (e.g., cysteine) for growth. However, *F. tularensis* can grow on chocolate agar or buffered charcoal yeast extract (BCYE) agar, media supplemented with cysteine that are used in most laboratories. Thus it is usually not necessary for a laboratory to use specialized media such as cysteine blood agar or glucose cysteine agar. However, if infection with *F. tularensis* is suspected, the laboratory should be notified because *F. tularensis* grows slowly and may be overlooked if the cultures are not incubated for a prolonged period. Additionally, because this organism is highly infectious, special care is required for microbiologic testing. Blood cultures are generally negative for the organism unless the cultures are incubated for a week or longer. Cultures of respiratory specimens will be positive if appropriate selective media are used to suppress the more rapidly growing bacteria from the upper respiratory tract. *F. tularensis* also grows on the selective media used for *Legionella* (e.g., BCYE agar). Aspirates of lymph nodes or draining sinuses are usually positive if the cultures are incubated for 3 days or longer.

Identification

Preliminary identification of *F. tularensis* is based on the slow growth of very small gram-negative coccobacilli. Growth on chocolate agar but not blood agar (blood agar is not supplemented with cysteine) is also helpful. The identification is confirmed by demonstrating the reactivity of the bacteria with specific antiserum (i.e., agglutination of the organism with antibodies against *Francisella*). Further biochemical testing is not helpful and can be hazardous.

Serology

Tularemia is diagnosed in most patients by the finding of a fourfold or greater increase in the titer of antibodies during the illness or a single titer of 1:160 or greater. However, antibodies (including IgG, IgM, and IgA) can persist for many years, making it difficult to differentiate between past and current disease. Reagents that are currently available react with subspecies *tularensis* and *holarctica* but not the other subspecies or *F. philomiragia*. Antibodies directed against *Brucella* can cross-react with *Francisella*. Therefore the diagnosis of tularemia should not be based solely on serologic tests.

TREATMENT, PREVENTION, AND CONTROL

Streptomycin is the traditional antibiotic of choice for the treatment of all forms of tularemia; however, this antibiotic is not readily available and is associated with a high level of toxicity. Gentamicin is an acceptable alternative. The fluoroquinolones (e.g., ciprofloxacin) have good bactericidal activity in vitro and in a mouse animal model. Doxycycline is also bactericidal in the mouse model. *F. tularensis* strains produce β-lactamase, which renders penicillins and cephalosporins ineffective. The mortality rate is less than 1% if patients are treated promptly.

To prevent infection, people should avoid the reservoirs and vectors of infection (e.g., rabbits, ticks, biting insects), but this is often difficult. At a minimum, people should not handle ill-appearing rabbits and should wear gloves when skinning and eviscerating animals. Because the organism is present in the arthropod's feces and not saliva, the tick must feed for a prolonged time before the infection is transmitted. Prompt removal of the tick can therefore prevent infection. Wearing protective clothing and using insect repellents reduce the risk of exposure. Persons who have a high risk of exposure (e.g., exposure to an infectious aerosol) should be treated with prophylactic antibiotics. Live-attenuated vaccines are not completely effective in preventing disease but can lessen the severity of the disease. These are recommended for people at a significantly increased risk of exposure to the organism. Inactivated vaccines do not elicit protective cellular immunity.

CASE STUDY AND QUESTIONS

A 27-year-old man was mowing his field when he ran over two young rabbits. When he stopped his mower, he realized that two other rabbits were dead in the unmowed part of the lawn. He removed all the rabbits and buried them. Three days later he developed a fever, muscle aches, and a dry, nonproductive cough. Over the next 12 hours he got progressively sicker and was transported by his wife to the area hospital. Results of a chest x-ray showed infiltrates in both lung fields. Blood cultures and respiratory secretions were collected, and antibiotics were initiated. Blood cultures became positive with small gram-negative rods after 3 days of incubation, and the same organism grew from the respiratory specimen that was inoculated onto BCYE agar.

1. What test should be performed to confirm the tentative diagnosis of *Francisella tularensis*?
2. This infection was presumably acquired by inhalation of aerosolized contaminated blood. What are the most common sources of *F. tularensis* infections and the most common routes of exposure?
3. What are the different clinical manifestations of *F. tularensis*?

Bibliography

Boschiroli M et al: Brucellosis: A worldwide zoonosis, *Curr Opin Microbiol* 4:58-64, 2001.

Boschiroli M et al: The *Brucella suis* virB operon is induced intracellularly in macrophages, *PNAS* 99:1544-1549, 2002.

Capellan J, Fong I: Tularemia from a cat bite: Case report and review of feline-associated tularemia, *Clin Infect Dis* 16:472-475, 1993.

Chomel B et al: Changing trends in the epidemiology of human brucellosis in California from 1973 to 1992: A shift toward foodborne transmission, *J Infect Dis* 170:1216-1223, 1994.

Dennis D et al: Tularemia as a biological weapon: Medical and public health management, *JAMA* 285:2763-2773, 2001.

Feldman K et al: Outbreak of primary pneumonic tularemia on Martha's Vineyard, *N Engl J Med* 345:1601-1606, 2001.

Johansson A et al: Evaluation of PCR-based methods for discrimination of *Francisella* species and subspecies and development of a specific PCR that distinguishes the two major subspecies of *Francisella tularensis*, *J Clin Microbiol* 38:4180-4185, 2000.

Redklar R et al: Real time detection of *Brucella abortus, Brucella melitensis,* and *Brucella suis, Mol Cell Probes* 15:43-52, 2001.Yagupsky P: Detection of Brucellae in blood cultures, *J Clin Microbiol* 37:3437-3442, 1999.

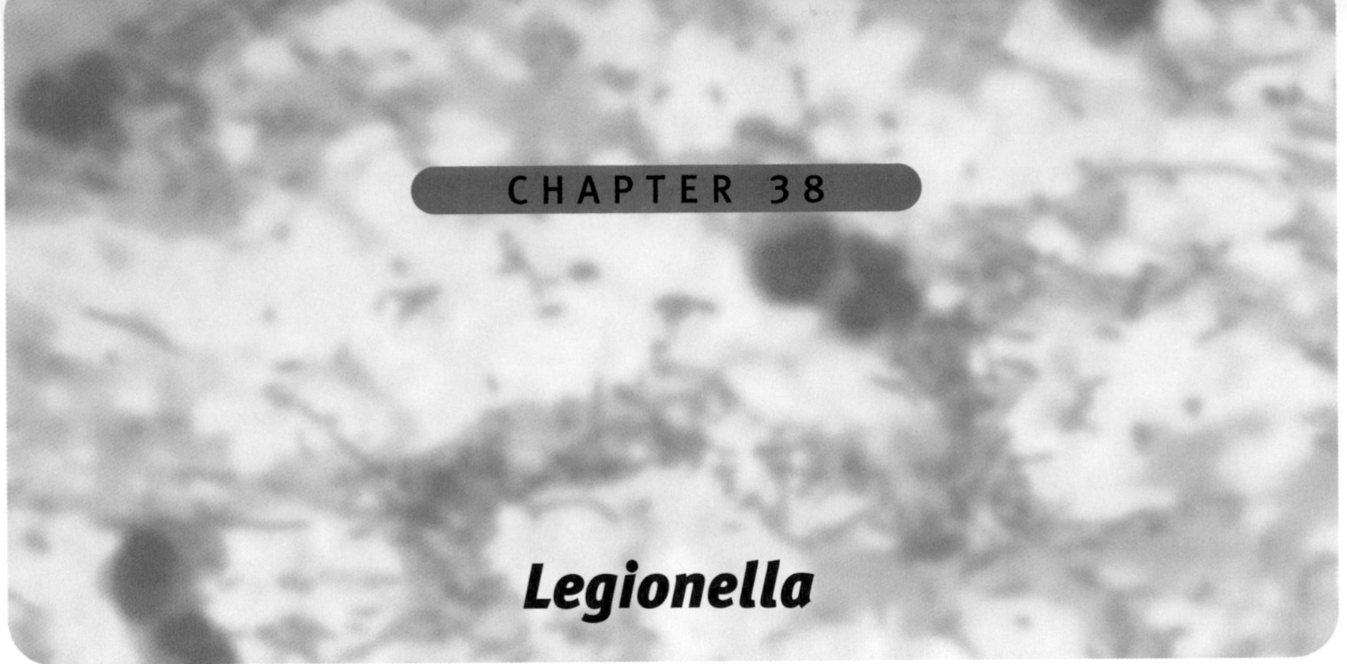

In the summer of 1976, public attention was focused on an outbreak of severe pneumonia that caused many deaths in American Legion members attending a convention in Philadelphia. After months of intensive investigations, a previously unknown gram-negative rod was isolated. Subsequent studies found this organism, named *Legionella pneumophila*, to be the cause of multiple epidemics and sporadic infections. The organism was not previously recognized, because it stains poorly with conventional dyes and does not grow on common laboratory media. Despite the initial problems with the isolation of *Legionella* organisms, it is now known to be a ubiquitous aquatic saprophyte.

Legionellaceae

Taxonomic studies have shown that the family Legionellaceae consists of one genus, *Legionella*, with 48 species and more than 70 serogroups. Approximately half of these species and serogroups have been implicated in human disease, with the others found in environmental sources. *L. pneumophila* is the cause of almost 85% of all infections; serotypes 1 and 6 are most commonly isolated (Figure 38–1).

PHYSIOLOGY AND STRUCTURE

Members of the genus *Legionella* are slender, pleomorphic, gram-negative rods measuring 0.3 to 0.9 × 2 μm in size (Box 38–1). The organisms characteristically appear as short coccobacilli in tissue but are very pleomorphic (up to 20 μm long) on artificial media (Figure 38–2). Legionellae in clinical specimens do not stain with common reagents but can be seen in tissues stained with Dieterle's silver stain. One species, *Legionella micdadei*, can also be stained with weak acid-fast stains, but the organism loses this property when grown in vitro.

Legionellae are obligatively aerobic and nutritionally fastidious. They require media supplemented with L-cysteine and iron for primary isolation. Growth of these bacteria on supplemented media but not on conventional blood agar media has been used as the basis for the preliminary identification of clinical isolates. The bacteria have developed multiple methods to acquire iron from their host cells or in vitro media, and loss of this ability is associated with loss of virulence. The organisms are nonfermentative and derive energy from the metabolism of amino acids. Most species are motile and catalase positive, liquefy gelatin, and do not reduce nitrate or hydrolyze urea.

PATHOGENESIS AND IMMUNITY

Respiratory tract disease caused by *Legionella* species develops in susceptible people who inhale infectious aerosols. Legionellae are facultative intracellular parasites that can multiply in alveolar macrophages, monocytes, and in nature in free-living amoebae. The replicative cycle is initiated by binding complement to an outer membrane porin protein and deposition of complement component C3b on the bacterial surface. This permits the bacteria to bind to CR3 complement receptors on mononuclear phagocytes, after which the organisms penetrate the cell through endocytosis. The bacteria are not killed in the cells through exposure to toxic superoxide, hydrogen peroxide, and hydroxyl radicals because phagolysosome fusion is inhibited. The organisms proliferate in their intracellular vacuole and produce proteolytic enzymes, phosphatase, lipase, and nuclease, which eventually kill the host cell when the vacuole is lysed. Immunity to disease is primarily cell mediated, with humoral immunity playing

BOX 38–1. Summary of *Legionella*

Physiology and Structure

Slender, pleomorphic, gram-negative rods
Stains poorly with common reagents
Nutritionally fastidious with requirement for L-cysteine and enhanced growth with iron salts
Nonfermentative

Virulence

Capable of replication in alveolar macrophages (and amoebae in nature)
Prevents phagolysosome fusion

Epidemiology

Capable of sporadic, epidemic, and nosocomial infections
Commonly found in natural bodies of water, cooling towers, condensers, and water systems (including hospital systems)
Estimated to be between 10,000 and 20,000 cases of infection in United States annually
Patients at high risk for symptomatic disease include patients with compromised pulmonary function and patients with decreased cellular immunity (particularly transplant patients)

Diseases

Legionnaires' disease
Pontiac fever

Diagnosis

Microscopy is insensitive
Culture on buffered charcoal yeast extract (BCYE) agar is the diagnostic test of choice
Antigen tests are sensitive for *L. pneumophila* serogroup 1 but have poor sensitivity for other serogroups and species
Seroconversion must be demonstrated; this can take as long as 6 months to develop; positive serology may persist for months
Nucleic acid amplification assays have a sensitivity and specificity approaching culture

Treatment, Control, and Prevention

Newer macrolides (e.g., azithromycin, clarithromycin) or fluoroquinolones (e.g., ciprofloxacin, levofloxacin) are the treatment of choice
Decrease environmental exposure to reduce risk of disease
For environmental sources associated with disease, treat with hyperchlorination, superheating, or copper-silver ionization

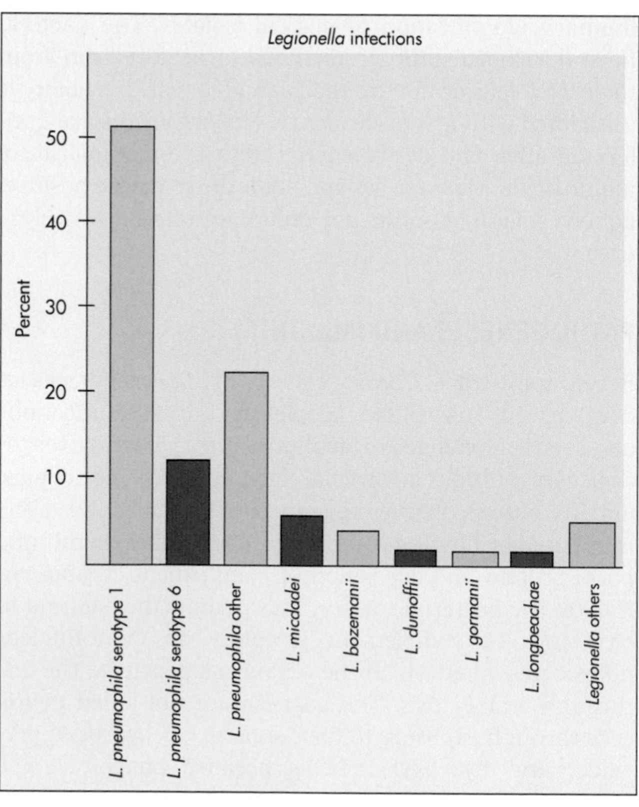

FIGURE 38–1. *Legionella* species associated with human disease.

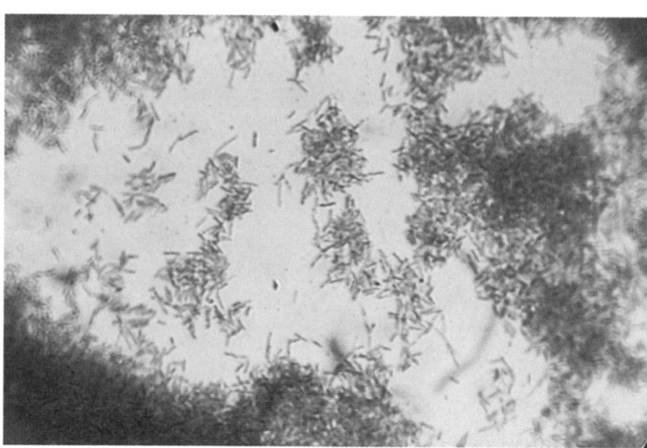

FIGURE 38–2. Gram stain of *Legionella pneumophila* grown on buffered charcoal yeast extract agar. Note the pleomorphic forms characteristic of *Legionella*. (Courtesy Dr. Janet Stout; Pittsburg, Pennsylvania.)

a minor role. The bacteria are not killed until sensitized T cells activate the parasitized macrophages.

EPIDEMIOLOGY

Sporadic and epidemic legionellosis has a worldwide distribution. The bacteria are commonly present in natural bodies of water, such as lakes and streams, as well as in air conditioning cooling towers and condensers and in water systems (e.g., showers, hot tubs). The organisms can survive in moist environments for a long time, at relatively high temperatures, and in the presence of disinfectants, such as chlorine. One reason for their survival is that the bacteria can parasitize amoebae in the water and replicate in this protected environment (similar to their replication in human macrophages). The bacteria also survive in biofilms that develop in the pipes of water systems.

The incidence of infections caused by *Legionella* species is unknown because disease is difficult to document. The number of reported cases has steadily risen during the past decade, with 1200 to 2200 cases reported annually. However, the Centers for Disease Control and Prevention (CDC) estimate that between 10,000 and 20,000 cases of Legionnaires' disease occur each year in the United States. Serologic studies have also shown that a significant proportion of the population has acquired immunity to this group of organisms. On the basis of these studies and the knowledge that legionellae are ubiquitous aquatic saprophytes, it is reasonable to conclude that contact with the organism and acquisition of immunity after an asymptomatic infection are common.

Although sporadic outbreaks of the disease occur throughout the year, most epidemics of the infection occur in late summer and autumn, presumably because the organism proliferates in water reservoirs during the warm months. Elderly persons are at greatest risk for disease because of their decreased cellular immunity and compromised pulmonary function. Almost 25% of reported cases are acquired in hospitals, presumably because of the predominance of high-risk patients. Person-to-person spread or an animal reservoir has not been demonstrated.

CLINICAL DISEASES

Asymptomatic *Legionella* infections are believed to be relatively common. Symptomatic infections primarily affect the lungs and present in one of two forms (Table 38–1): (1) an influenza-like illness (referred to as **Pontiac fever**) and (2) a severe form of pneumonia (i.e., **legionnaires' disease**).

Pontiac Fever

L. pneumophila was responsible for causing a self-limited, febrile illness in people working at the Pontiac, Michigan., Public Health Department in 1968. Fever, chills, myalgia, malaise, and headache but no clinical evidence of pneumonia are characteristic of the disease. The symptoms developed over 12 hours, persisted for 2 to 5 days, and then resolved spontaneously without antibiotic treatment and with minimal morbidity and no deaths. It is believed that the pathology of this disease is caused by a hypersensitivity reaction to the organism. Additional epidemics of **Pontiac fever** have been documented, and the attack rate has been high in the people exposed.

TABLE 38–1. Comparison of Diseases Caused by *Legionella*

	Legionnaires' Disease	Pontiac Fever
Epidemiology		
Presentation	Epidemic, sporadic	Epidemic
Attack rate (%)	<5	>90
Person-to-person spread	No	No
Underlying pulmonary disease	Yes	No
Time of onset	Epidemic disease in late summer or autumn; endemic disease throughout year	Throughout year
Clinical Manifestations		
Incubation period (days)	2–10	1–2
Pneumonia	Yes	No
Course	Requires antibiotic therapy	Self-limited
Mortality (%)	15–20; higher if diagnosis is delayed	<1

Legionnaires' Disease

Legionnaires' disease (legionellosis) is characteristically more severe and causes considerable morbidity, often leading to death unless therapy is initiated promptly. After an incubation period of 2 to 10 days, systemic signs of an acute illness appear abruptly (e.g., fever and chills, a dry, nonproductive cough, headache). Multiorgan disease involving the gastrointestinal tract, central nervous system, liver, and kidneys is common. The primary manifestation is pneumonia, with multilobar consolidation and inflammation and microabscesses in lung tissue observed on histopathologic studies. Pulmonary function steadily deteriorates in susceptible patients with untreated disease. The overall mortality rate is 15% to 20% but can be much higher in patients with severely depressed cell-mediated immunity (e.g., recipients of renal or cardiac transplants).

LABORATORY DIAGNOSIS

Since *Legionella* was first isolated, the laboratory diagnosis of infections caused by this organism has undergone a significant transition. Initial testing depended on microscopy, culture, and serology. Although culture remains the gold standard for diagnosis, microscopy and serology have been replaced by immunoassays for the detection of *Legionella*-specific antigens in urine and nucleic acid amplification assays.

Microscopy

Legionellae in clinical specimens stain poorly with Gram stain. Nonspecific staining methods, such as Dieterle's silver or Gimenez's stains, can be used to visualize the organisms but are of little value if the specimens are contaminated with normal oral bacteria. The most sensitive way of detecting legionellae microscopically in clinical specimens is to use the **direct fluorescent antibody (DFA)** test, in which fluorescein-labeled monoclonal or polyclonal antibodies directed against *Legionella* species are used. The test is specific, with false-positive reactions observed only rarely if monoclonal antibody preparations are used. However, the sensitivity of the DFA test is low (reported to range from 25% to 75%) because (1) the antibody preparations are serotype- or species-specific and (2) many organisms must be present for detection. The latter problem is a result of the relatively small size and predominantly intracellular location of the bacteria. The DFA test has been replaced by the urine antigen test in most laboratories. *L. micdadei* can stain weakly acid-fast when observed in clinical specimens. This property is lost when the organism is grown in culture.

Culture

Although legionellae were difficult to grow initially, commercially available media now make culture easy (test sensitivity, 80% to >90%). As mentioned earlier, legionellae require L-cysteine and iron salts (supplied in hemoglobin or ferric pyrophosphate) for primary isolation. The medium most commonly used for the isolation of legionellae is **buffered charcoal yeast extract (BCYE) agar**, although other supplemented media have been used. Antibiotics can be added to suppress the growth of rapidly growing, contaminating bacteria. Legionellae grow in air or 3% to 5% carbon dioxide at 35°C after 3 to 5 days. Their small (1 to 3 mm) colonies have a characteristic ground-glass appearance.

Urinary Antigen Tests

Enyzme-linked immunoassays (EIAs) are used to detected soluble *Legionella*-specific lipopolysaccharide antigens excreted in the urine of infected patients. The sensitivity of these assays for *L. pneumophila* serogroup 1 is relatively high (range, 60% to >90%), particularly with concentrated urines, but the sensitivity for other serogroups and *Legionella* species is low. A genus-specific lipoprotein associated with the cell surface has been identified in the urine of infected patients and may prove to be a more useful diagnostic target. Antigens persist in the urine of treated patients, with almost 50% of patients remaining positive at 1 month and 25% at 2 months. Persistence is particularly common with immunosuppressed patients, in which antigens can persist for up to 1 year.

Nucleic Acid Amplification Assays

Nucleic acid amplification (NAA) assays are highly specific and have a sensitivity approaching culture for the detection of *Legionella* species in respiratory secretions (i.e., bronchial alveolar lavage [BAL] fluid). Although these assays are not widely available, it is anticipated that they will be the diagnostic method of choice in the future. The presence of inhibitors in respiratory secretions may cause false-negative reactions, so all specimens should still be cultured. Additionally, culture has been demonstrated to be more sensitive than NAA assays for tissue specimens.

Serology

Legionellosis caused by *L. pneumophila* serogroup 1 is commonly diagnosed with the use of the **indirect fluorescent antibody (IFA)** test to measure a serologic response to infection. A fourfold or greater increase in the antibody titer (to a level of 1:128 or greater) is considered diagnostic. The response may be delayed. A significant increase in the titer can be detected in 25% to 40% of patients in the first week of disease; however, up to 6 months may be required before seroconversion is demonstrated for the remaining patients. Because high titers can persist for prolonged periods, a single, high-antibody titer cannot be used to define active disease. Additionally, although enzyme-linked immunosorbent assays (ELISAs) are commercially available, they have poor sensitivity and specificity when compared with the IFA tests and cannot be recommended.

Identification

It is easy to identify an isolate as *Legionella* from the findings of typical morphology and specific growth requirements. Legionellae appear as weakly staining, pleomorphic, thin, gram-negative rods. Their growth on BCYE agar but not on media without L-cysteine is presumptive evidence that the organism is *Legionella.* Specific staining with fluorescein-labeled antibodies can confirm the identity of the organisms. In contrast to the identification of the genus, species classification is problematic and generally relegated to reference laboratories. Although biochemical tests and the ability of rods to fluoresce under long-wave ultraviolet light are useful for differentiating species, the species can be identified definitively only through analysis of the major branched-chain fatty acids in the cell wall and deoxyribonucleic acid (DNA) homology.

TREATMENT, PREVENTION, AND CONTROL

In vitro susceptibility tests are not performed routinely with legionellae, because the organisms grow poorly on the media commonly used for these tests. Additionally, some antibiotics that appear active in vitro are ineffective in treating infections. One explanation is that these antibiotics cannot penetrate the macrophages where the legionellae survive and multiply. Accumulated clinical experience indicates that macrolides (e.g., azithromycin, clarithromycin) or fluoroquinolones (e.g., ciprofloxacin, levofloxacin) should be used to treat *Legionella* infections. Newer macrolide antiobiotics have replaced erythromycin. β-Lactam antibiotics are ineffective because most isolates produce β-lactamases, and these antibiotics do not penetrate macrophages. Specific therapy for Pontiac fever is generally unnecessary because it is a self-limited hypersensitivity disease.

Prevention of legionellosis requires identification of the environmental source of the organism and reduction of the microbial burden. Hyperchlorination of the water supply and the maintenance of elevated water temperatures have proved moderately successful. However, elimination of *Legionella* organisms from a water supply is often difficult or impossible to achieve. Because the organism has a low potential for causing disease, reducing the number of organisms in the water supply is often an adequate control measure. Hospitals with patients at high risk for disease should monitor their water supply on a regular basis for the presence of *Legionella* and their hospital population for disease. If hyperchlorination or superheating of the water does not eliminate disease (complete elimination of the organisms in the water supply is probably not possible), continuous copper-silver ionization of the water supply may be necessary.

CASE STUDY AND QUESTIONS

A 73-year-old man was admitted to the hospital because of breathing difficulties, chest pain, chills, and fever of several days' duration. He had been well until 1 week before admission, when he noted the onset of a persistent headache and a productive cough. The patient smoked two packs of cigarettes a day for more than 50 years and drank a six-pack of beer daily; he also had a history of bronchitis. Physical examination results revealed an elderly man in severe respiratory distress with a temperature of 39 °C, pulse of 120 beats/minute, respiratory rate of 36 breaths/minute, and blood pressure of 145/95 mm Hg. Chest radiograph revealed an infiltrate in the middle and lower lobes of the right lung. The white blood cell count was 14,000 cells/mm^3 (80% polymorphonuclear neutrophils). Gram stain of the sputum showed neutrophils but no bacteria, and routine bacterial cultures of sputum and blood were negative for organisms. Infection with Legionella pneumophila *was suspected.*

1. What laboratory tests can be used to confirm this diagnosis? Why were the routine culture and Gram-stained specimen negative for *Legionella* organisms?
2. How are *Legionella* species able to survive phagocytosis by the alveolar macrophages?
3. What environmental factors are implicated in the spread of *Legionella* infections? How can this risk be eliminated or minimized?

Bibliography

Edelstein P: Antimicrobial chemotherapy for Legionnaires disease: Time for a change, *Ann Intern Med* 129:328-330, 1998.

Fields BS, Benson RF, Besser RE: *Legionella* and Legionnaires' disease: 25 years of investigation, *Clin Microbiol Rev* 15:506-526, 2002.

Hayden RT et al: Direct detection of *Legionella* species from bronchoalveolar lavage and open lung biopsy specimens: Comparison of LightCycler PCR, in situ hybridization, direct fluorescence antigen detection, and culture, *J Clin Microbiol* 39:2618-2626, 2001.

Helbig JH et al: Clinical utility of urinary antigen detection for diagnosis of community-acquired, travel-associated, and nosocomial Legionnaires' disease, *J Clin Microbiol* 41:837-840, 2003.

Kim MJ et al: Characterization of a lipoprotein common to *Legionella* species as a urinary broad-spectrum antigen for diagnosis of Legionnaires disease, *J Clin Microbiol* 41:2974-2979, 2003.

Malan AK et al: Comparison of two commercial enzyme-linked immunosorbent assays with an immunofluorescence assay for detection of *Legionella pneumophila* types 1 to 6, *J Clin Microbiol* 41:3060-3063, 2003.

Schulin T et al: Susceptibilities of *Legionella* spp. to newer antimicrobials in vitro, *Antimicrob Agents Chemother* 42:1520-1523, 1998.

Sopena N et al: Factors related to persistence of *Legionella* urinary antigen excretion in patients with legionnaires' disease, *Eur J Clin Microbiol Infect Dis* 21:845-848, 2002.

Stout J, Yu V: Legionellosis, *N Engl J Med* 337:681-687, 1997.

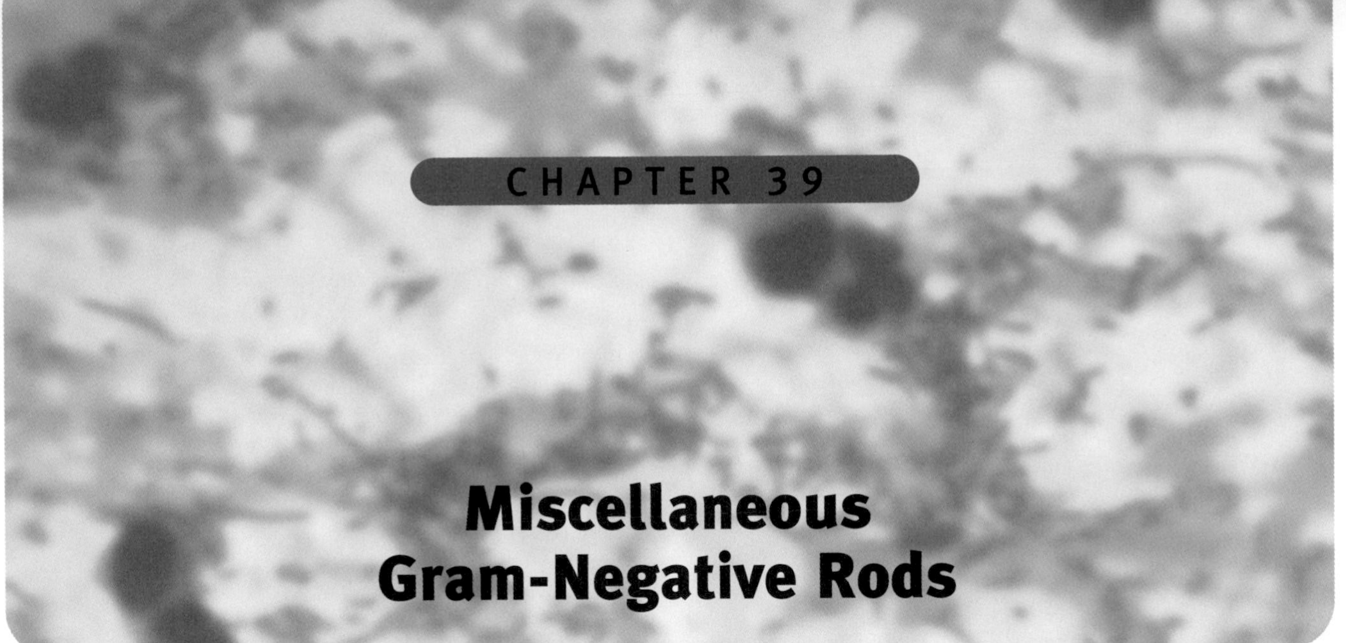

Miscellaneous Gram-Negative Rods

A few medically important gram-negative rods have not been discussed in the preceding chapters and are the subject of this chapter (Box 39–1).

Bartonella

As with many groups of bacteria studied in recent years, analysis of the 16S ribosomal ribonucleic acid (rRNA) gene has led to the reorganization of the genus *Bartonella.* Sixteen species are included in the genus; however, further genomic analysis has suggested that *Bartonella bacilliformis* is unrelated to many species currently included in this genus. Thus it is likely that further reorganization of the genus will occur. Members of the genus are short (0.3 to 0.5 × 1.0 to 1.7 μm), gram-negative, aerobic rods with fastidious growth requirements. Although the organisms can grow on enriched blood agar, prolonged incubation (1 to 6 weeks) in a humid (37°C) atmosphere supplemented with carbon dioxide is required for their initial recovery.

Members of the genus *Bartonella* are found in a variety of animal reservoirs and are typically present without evidence of disease. Insect vectors have also been shown or implicated in human infections. Because *Bartonella* organisms do not cause disease in other hosts, an animal model is not available for studying the pathogenesis of these infections.

B. bacilliformis, the original member of the genus, is responsible for bartonellosis, an acute febrile illness consisting of severe anemia **(Oroya fever),** followed by a chronic cutaneous form **(verruga).** Bartonellosis is restricted to Peru, Ecuador, and Colombia, the endemic regions of the sand fly vector *Phlebotomus.* After the bite of an infected sand fly, the bacteria enter the blood, multiply, and penetrate into erythrocytes. This process increases the fragility of the infected cells and facilitates their clearance by the reticuloendothelial system, leading to acute anemia. Myalgia, arthralgia, and headache are also common. This stage of illness ends with the development of humoral immunity. In the chronic stage of bartonellosis, 1- to 2-cm cutaneous nodules appear over the course of 1 to 2 months and may persist for months to years.

Bartonella quintana was originally described as the causative organism of **trench fever** (also called "5-day" fever; Box 39–2), a disease prevalent during World War I. Infection can vary from asymptomatic to a severe, debilitating illness. Typically, patients have severe headache, fever, weakness, and pain in the long bones (particularly the tibia). The fever can recur at 5-day intervals, hence the name of the disease. Although trench fever does not cause death, the illness can be very severe. No animal reservoir for this disease has been identified. Rather, the human body louse spreads disease from person-to-person.

More recently, *B. quintana* has been associated with **bacillary angiomatosis** (Figure 39–1), a vascular proliferative disorder seen primarily in immunocompromised patients (e.g., patients with human immunodeficiency virus [HIV]), as well as with subacute endocarditis in immunocompetent patients. Bacillary angiomatosis resulting from *B. quintana* primarily involves the skin, subcutaneous tissues, and bones (in contrast with disease caused by *Bartonella henselae*). As with trench fever, the vector of these diseases appears to be the human body louse, and disease is primarily restricted to the homeless population, in whom personal hygiene is substandard. The etiologic role of *B. quintana* and other *Bartonella* species in "culture-negative" endocarditis is supported by serologic studies.

B. henselae is also responsible for bacillary angiomatosis; however, it primarily involves the skin, lymph nodes, or liver and spleen **(peliosis hepatis).** The reasons for this differential tissue affinity are not known. Like *B. quantana,*

BOX 39–1. Miscellaneous Medically Important Gram-Negative Rods

Organism	Historical Derivation
Bartonella	*Bartonella*, named after Barton, who originally described *B. bacilliformis*
B. bacilliformis	*bacillus*, rod; *forma*, shape (rod-shaped)
B. henselae	*hensel*, named after D.M. Hensel, who worked with this organism
B. quintana	*quintana*, fifth (refers to 5-day fever)
Cardiobacterium hominis	*cardia*, heart; *bakterion*, small rod; *hominis*, of man (small rod of the hearts of men; refers to the predilection of this bacterium to cause endocarditis in humans)
Capnocytophaga	*capno*, smoke; *cytophaga*, eater (literally this means eater of smoke; refers to the requirement for carbon dioxide for growth)
Streptobacillus moniliformis	*streptos*, twisted or curved; *bacillus*, rod; *monile*, necklace; *forma*, shape (twisted, necklace-shaped bacillus; refers to the pleomorphic morphology of the bacteria)

BOX 39–2. Clinical Summaries

Bartonella quintana

Trench fever: Disease is characterized by severe headache, fever, weakness, and pain in the long bones; the fever recurs at 5-day intervals

Bacillary angiomatosis: Vascular proliferative disease in immunocompromised patients involving the skin, subcutaneous tissues, and bones

Subacute endocarditis: Mild but progressive infection of the endocardium

Bartonella henselae

Bacillary angiomatosis: Same as above, except primarily involving the skin, lymph nodes, or liver and spleen

Subacute endocarditis: Same as above

Cat-scratch disease: Chronic regional lymphadenopathy associated with cat scratch

Cardiobacterium hominis

Subacute endocarditis: Same as above

Capnocytophaga species

Opportunistic infections: Variety of infections including periodontitis, bacteremia, and endocarditis (from dysgonic fermenter 1 [DF-1] species); dog or cat bite wounds (from DF-2 species)

Streptobacillus moniliformis

Rat-bite fever: Irregular fever, headache, chills, myalgia, and arthralgia associated with rodent bite; pharyngitis and vomiting is associated with exposure to bacteria in food or water

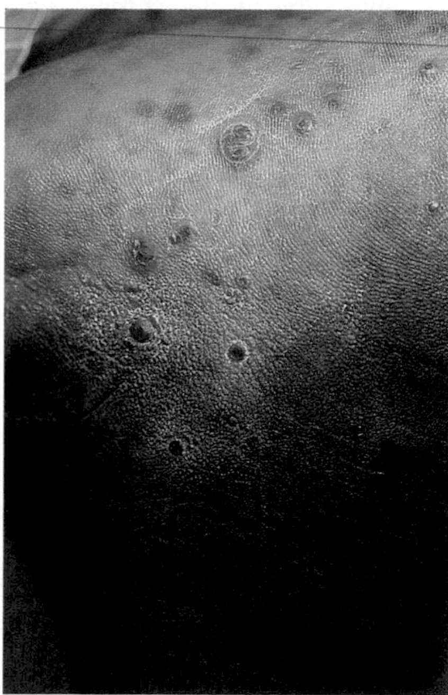

FIGURE 39–1. Skin lesions of bacillary angiomatosis caused by *Bartonella henselae.* (From Cohen J, Powderly WG: *Infectious diseases,* ed 2, St Louis, 2004, Mosby.)

B. henselae can cause subacute endocarditis. Finally, *B. henselae* is responsible for **cat-scratch disease.** The disease is acquired after exposure to cats (e.g., scratches, bites, contact with fleas). Typically, cat-scratch disease is a benign infection in children, characterized by chronic regional adenopathy of the lymph nodes draining the site of contact. Although rods can be seen in the lymph node tissues, culture is usually negative for organisms. A definitive diagnosis is based on the characteristic presentation and serologic evidence of a recent infection. Cultures are not useful because relatively few organisms are present in the tissues as a result of the vigorous cellular immune reaction in immunocompetent patients. In contrast, *B. henselae* can often be isolated from blood collected from immunocompromised patients with chronic bacteremia, if the cultures are incubated for 3 weeks or more (Figure 39–2).

Treatment of *Bartonella* infections is complicated because minimal information is available about the in vitro susceptibility of the organisms. Cat-scratch disease does not appear to respond to antimicrobial therapy. Trench fever, bacillary angiomatosis and peliosis hepatis, and endocarditis can be treated with gentamicin, either alone or with erythromycin. Broad-spectrum cephalosporins appear to be effective, and erythromycin or doxycycline has been used with initial success, but the bacteriostatic antibiotics are associated with a high rate of relapse. Penicillinase-resistant penicillins, first-generation cephalosporins, and clindamycin do not appear active in vitro. The incidence of *Bartonella* infections in HIV-infected patients has been reduced because these patients

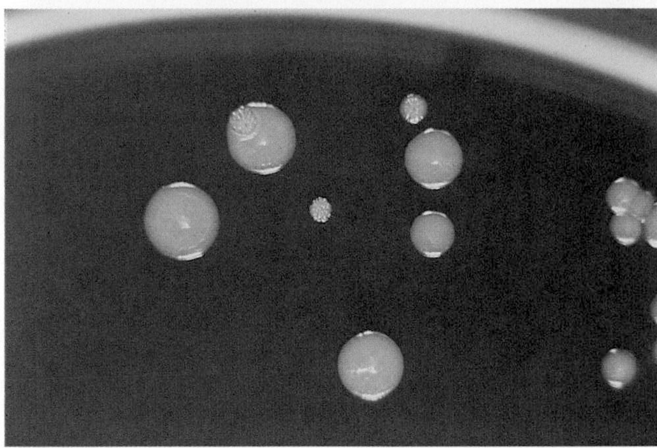

FIGURE 39–2. *B. henselae* growing on blood agar plates; note the two typical colonial morphologies (From Cohen J, Powderly WG: *Infectious diseases,* ed 2, St Louis, 2004, Mosby

are treated routinely with azithromycin or clarithromycin for prevention of *Mycobacterium avium* infections.

Cardiobacterium

Cardiobacterium hominis is named for the predilection of this bacterium to cause endocarditis in humans. These bacteria are nonmotile, facultatively anaerobic, and characteristically small (1 × 1 to 2 μm) pleomorphic, gram-negative or gram-variable rods. The bacteria are fermentative, indole and oxidase positive, and catalase negative. *C. hominis* is present in the upper respiratory tract of almost 70% of healthy people.

Although uncommon, endocarditis is the primary human disease caused by *C. hominis.* Many infections are likely to be unreported or undiagnosed because of the low virulence of this organism and its slow growth in vitro. Most patients with *C. hominis* endocarditis have preexisting heart disease and either have a history of oral disease or have undergone dental procedures before the clinical symptoms develop. The organisms are able to enter the blood from the oropharynx, adhere to the damaged heart tissue, and then slowly multiply. The course of disease is insidious and subacute; patients typically have symptoms (e.g., fatigue, malaise, and low-grade fever) for months before seeking medical care. Complications are rare, and complete recovery after appropriate antibiotic therapy is common.

The isolation of *C. hominis* from blood cultures confirms the diagnosis of endocarditis. The organism grows slowly in culture, requiring 1 to 2 weeks for growth to be detected. *C. hominis* appears in broth cultures as discrete clumps that can be easily overlooked. The organism requires enhanced carbon dioxide and humidity levels to grow on agar media, with pinpoint (1-mm) colonies seen on blood or chocolate agar plates after 3 days of incubation. The organism does not grow on MacConkey agar or other selective media commonly used for gram-negative rods. *C. hominis* can be readily identified from its growth properties, microscopic morphology, and reactivity in biochemical tests.

C. hominis is susceptible to many antibiotics, and most infections are treated successfully with penicillin or ampicillin for 2 to 6 weeks (although penicillin-resistant strains have been reported). *C. hominis* endocarditis in people with preexisting heart disease is prevented by the maintenance of good oral hygiene and the use of antibiotic prophylaxis at the time of dental procedures. Long-acting penicillin is effective prophylaxis, but erythromycin should not be used because *C. hominis* is commonly resistant to it.

Capnocytophaga

Members of the genus *Capnocytophaga* are filamentous, gram-negative rods capable of aerobic and anaerobic growth in the presence of carbon dioxide. The genus is subdivided into two groups: (1) dysgonic fermenter 1 (DF-1), with five species; and (2) dysgonic fermenter 2 (DF-2), with two species. DF-1 strains colonize the human oropharynx and are associated with periodontitis, bacteremia, and, rarely, endocarditis. DF-2 strains colonize the oral cavities of cats and dogs and are associated with bite wounds.

Overwhelming sepsis caused by *Capnocytophaga* can occur in patients who have undergone splenectomy or who have a compromised hepatic function (e.g., cirrhosis). Most *Capnocytophaga* infections can be treated with penicillins, cephalosporins, or fluoroquinolones; strains are typically resistant to the aminoglycosides.

Streptobacillus

Streptobacillus moniliformis, the causative agent of **rat-bite fever,** is a long, thin (0.1 to 0.5 × 1 to 5 μm), gram-negative rod that tends to stain poorly and to be more pleomorphic in older cultures. Granules, bulbous swellings resembling a string of beads, and extremely long filaments may be seen (Figure 39–3).

Streptobacillus is found in the nasopharynx of rats and other small rodents, as well as transiently in animals that feed on rodents (e.g., dogs, cats). Turkeys exposed to rats and mice, as well as contaminated water and milk, have also been implicated in *Streptobacillus* infections.

Human infections result from rodent bites (rat-bite fever) or consumption of contaminated food or water

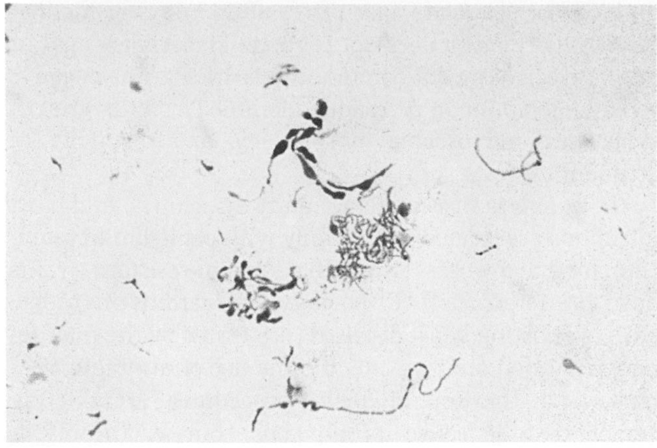

FIGURE 39–3. Gram stain of *Streptobacillus moniliformis;* note the pleomorphic forms and bulbous swellings.

(Haverhill fever). After a 2- to 10-day incubation period, the disease onset is abrupt, characterized by irregular fever, headache, chills, myalgia, and arthralgia. A maculopapular rash develops a few days later. Recurrent episodes of headache and arthralgia and complications, such as carditis, meningitis, or pneumonia, can occur in untreated patients. Vomiting and pharyngitis are characteristics of Haverhill fever (named after Haverhill, Mass., where the first epidemic was described).

Blood and joint fluid should be collected for the isolation of *S. moniliformis.* The organism can grow on enriched media supplemented with 15% blood, 20% horse or calf serum, or 5% ascitic fluid. *S. moniliformis* is slow growing, taking at least 3 days to be isolated. When grown in broth, it has the appearance of "puffballs"; small, round colonies are seen on agar, as are cell wall defective forms, with their typical fried-egg appearance. It is difficult to identify the organisms because they are relatively inactive, although acid is produced from glucose and other selected carbohydrates. The most reliable method for identifying isolates is sequencing the 16S rRNA gene. The serologic tests that can detect antibodies against *Streptobacillus* antigens are available in reference laboratories. A titer greater than or equal to 1:80 or a fourfold rise in the titer is considered diagnostic, although this test has not been standardized or carefully evaluated for cross-reactivity. *S. moniliformis* is susceptible to many antibiotics, including penicillin (not active against cell wall defective forms) and doxycycline.

CASE STUDY AND QUESTIONS

A previously healthy 12–year-old girl developed a slowly enlarging, swollen axillary lymph node. One week before the onset of disease, she had suffered a scratch while playing with a kitten. Her physician suspected the diagnosis of cat–scratch disease.

1. What is the most sensitive diagnostic test for confirming this diagnosis?
2. What infections are caused by *Bartonella quintana* and *Bartonella henselae?* How does the epidemiology of these infections differ?
3. What infection is caused by *Cardiobacterium? Streptobacillus?*

Bibliography

Agan BK, Dolan MJ: Laboratory diagnosis of Bartonella infections, *Clin Lab Med* 22:937-962, 2002.

Anderson B, Neuman M: *Bartonella* spp. as emerging human pathogens, *Clin Microbiol Rev* 10:203-219, 1997.

Koehler J et al: Molecular epidemiology of *Bartonella* infections in patients with bacillary angiomatosis-peliosis, *N Engl J Med* 337:1876-1883, 1997.

Koehler J et al: Prevalence of *Bartonella* infection among human immunodeficiency virus-infected patients with fever, *Clin Infect Dis* 37:550-666, 2003.

La Scola B, Raoult D: Culture of *Bartonella quintana* and *Bartonella henselae* from human samples: A 5-year experience (1993 to 1998), *J Clin Microbiol* 37:1899-1905, 1999.

Maurin M, Raoult D: *Bartonella (Rochalimaea) quintana* infections, *Clin Microbiol Rev* 9:273-292, 1996.

Metzkor-Cotter E et al: Long-term serological analysis and clinical follow-up of patients with cat scratch disease, *Clin Infect Dis* 37:1149-1154, 2003.

Resto-Ruiz S, Burgess A, Anderson B: The role of the host immune response in pathogenesis of *Bartonella henselae, DNA Cell Biol* 22:431-440, 2003.

Spach D et al: *Bartonella (Rochalimaea)* species as a cause of apparent "culture-negative" endocarditis, *Clin Infect Dis* 20:1044-1047, 1995.

Wormser GP, Bottone EJ: *Cardiobacterium hominis:* Review of microbiologic and clinical features, *Rev Infect Dis* 5:680-691, 1983.

Zeaiter Z et al: Phylogenetic classification of *Bartonella* species by comparing groEL sequences, *Intl J System Evol Microbiol* 52:165-171, 2002.

CHAPTER 40

Anaerobic, Spore-Forming, Gram-Positive Rods

Historically, the collection of all anaerobic, gram-positive rods capable of forming endospores was placed in the genus *Clostridium*. This genus was defined by four properties: (1) presence of endospores, (2) strict anaerobic metabolism, (3) inability to reduce sulfate to sulfite, and (4) gram-positive cell wall structure. Even with this broad classification scheme, some clinically significant members of the genus can be misclassified. Spores are only rarely demonstrated in some species (*Clostridium perfringens, Clostridium ramosum*), some species are aerotolerant and can grow on agar media exposed to air (e.g., *Clostridium tertium, Clostridium histolyticum*), and some clostridia consistently stain gram-negative (e.g., *C. ramosum, Clostridium clostridioforme*). The traditional method for classifying an isolate in the genus *Clostridium* was based on a combination of diagnostic tests, including the demonstration of spores, optimal growth in anaerobic conditions, a complex pattern of biochemical reactivity, and detection of characteristic volatile fatty acids by gas chromatography. With these methods, 177 species have been defined. Fortunately, most of the clinically important isolates fall within a few species (Table 40–1). It should not be surprising that the use of gene-sequencing techniques has led to the reorganization of this heterogeneous collection of organisms into a number of groups that should appropriately represent new genera. However, because the reclassification of these spore-forming anaerobes is still incomplete and not fully accepted, the conventional organization of these bacteria in the genus *Clostridium* is used in this chapter.

The organisms are ubiquitous in soil, water, and sewage and are part of the normal microbial flora in the gastrointestinal tracts of animals and humans. Most clostridia are harmless saprophytes, but some are well-recognized human pathogens with a clearly documented history of causing diseases, such as **tetanus** (*C. tetani*), **botulism** (*Clostridium botulinum, Clostridium baratii, Clostridium butyricum*), myonecrosis or **gas gangrene** (*C. perfringens, Clostridium novyi, Clostridium septicum, C. histolyticum*), and **antibiotic-associated diarrhea** and **colitis** (*Clostridium difficile*). The majority of infections seen today are skin and soft-tissue infections, food poisoning, and antibiotic-associated diarrhea and colitis. The remarkable capacity of clostridia to cause diseases is attributed to their (1) ability to survive adverse environmental conditions through spore formation; (2) rapid growth in a nutritionally enriched, oxygen-deprived environment, and (3) production of numerous histolytic toxins, enterotoxins, and neurotoxins. Six common or important human pathogens in the genus are discussed in this chapter (Box 40–1).

Clostridium Perfringens (Box 40–2)

PHYSIOLOGY AND STRUCTURE

C. perfringens can be associated with simple colonization or can cause life-threatening disease. *C. perfringens* is a large (0.6 to 2.4 × 1.3 to 19.0 μm), rectangular, gram-positive rod (Figure 40–1), with spores rarely observed either in vivo or after in vitro cultivation. This organism is one of the few nonmotile clostridia, but rapidly spreading growth on laboratory media (resembling the growth of motile organisms) is characteristic (Figure 40–2). The organism grows rapidly in tissues and in culture, is hemolytic, and is metabolically active, features that make possible its identification in the laboratory. The production of one or more major lethal toxins by *C. perfringens* (alpha [α], beta [β], epsilon [ε], and iota [ι] toxins) is used to subdivide isolates into five types (A through E; Table 40–2). Type A *C. perfringens* causes most of the human infections in the United States.

TABLE 40–1. Pathogenic Clostridia and Their Associated Human Diseases*

Species	Human Disease	Frequency
C. difficile	Antibiotic-associated diarrhea, pseudomembranous colitis	Common
C. perfringens	Soft-tissue infections (e.g., cellulitis, suppurative myositis, myonecrosis, gas gangrene), food poisoning, enteritis necroticans, septicemia	Common
C. septicum	Gas gangrene, septicemia	Uncommon
C. botulinum	Botulism	Uncommon
C. tetani	Tetanus	Uncommon
C. tertium	Opportunistic infections	Uncommon
C. baratii	Botulism	Rare
C. butyricum	Botulism	Rare
C. clostridioforme	Opportunistic infections	Rare
C. histolyticum	Gas gangrene	Rare
C. innocuum	Opportunistic infections	Rare
C. novyi	Gas gangrene	Rare
C. sordellii	Gas gangrene	Rare
C. sporogenes	Opportunistic infections	Rare

*Other clostridial species have been associated with human disease but primarily as opportunistic pathogens. Additionally, some species (e.g., *C. clostridioforme, C. innocuum, C. ramosum*) are commonly isolated but are rarely associated with disease.

BOX 40–1. Important Clostridia

Organism	Historical Derivation
Clostridium	*closter*, a spindle
C. botulinum	*botulus*, sausage (the first major outbreak was associated with insufficiently smoked sausage)
C. difficile	*difficile*, difficult (difficult to isolate and grow; refers to the extreme oxygen sensitivity of this organism)
C. perfringens	*perfringens*, breaking through (associated with highly invasive tissue necrosis)
C. septicum	*septicum*, putrefactive (associated with sepsis and a high mortality)
C. tertium	*tertium*, third (historically, the third most commonly isolated anaerobe from war wounds
C. tetani	*tetani*, related to tension (disease caused by this organism characterized by muscle spasms)

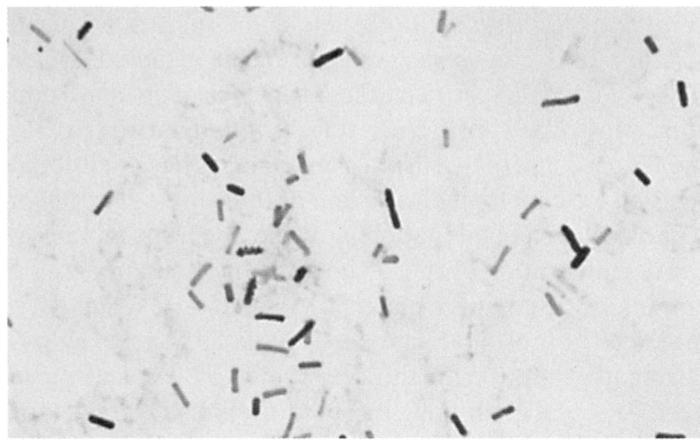

FIGURE 40–1. Gram stain of *Clostridium perfringens*.

PATHOGENESIS AND IMMUNITY

C. perfringens can cause a spectrum of diseases, from a self-limited gastroenteritis to an overwhelming destruction of tissue (e.g., clostridial myonecrosis) associated with a very high mortality, even in patients who receive early medical intervention. This pathogenic potential is attributed primarily to at least 12 toxins and enzymes produced by this organism (Table 40–3). **α-Toxin,** the most important toxin and the one produced by all five types of *C. perfringens*, is a lecithinase (phospholipase C, Figure 40–3) that lyses erythrocytes, platelets, leukocytes, and endothelial cells. This toxin mediates massive hemolysis, increased vascular permeability and bleeding (augmented by destruction of platelets), tissue destruction (as found in myonecrosis), hepatic toxicity, and myocardial dysfunction (bradycardia, hypotension). The largest quantities of α-toxin are produced by *C. perfringens* type A. **β-Toxin** is responsible for intestinal stasis, loss of mucosa with formation of the necrotic lesions, and progression to necrotizing enteritis **(enteritis necroticans, pig-bel). ε-Toxin,** a protoxin, is activated by trypsin and increases the

BOX 40–2. Summary of *Clostridium perfringens*

Physiology and Structure

Large, rectangular, gram-positive rods

Forms spores, but they are rarely seen in clinical specimens or culture

Replicates rapidly, so large, spreading colonies are seen within first day of culture; "double zone" of hemolysis on blood agar (produced by α-and θ-toxins)

Produces many toxins and hemolytic enzymes, so white blood cells and platelets are not seen in Gram-stained clinical specimens

Produces lecithinase (phospholipase C)

Subdivided into five types (A to E) on the basis of toxin production (refer to Table 40–2)

Virulence

Refer to Table 40–3

Epidemiology

Ubiquitous; present in soil, water, and intestinal tract of humans and animals

Type A is responsible for most human infections

Disease follows exogenous or endogenous exposure

Diseases

Refer to Box 40–3

Diagnosis

Characteristic forms seen on Gram stain

Grows rapidly in culture

Treatment, Prevention, and Control

Rapid treatment is essential for serious infections

Systemic infections require surgical débridement and high-dose penicillin therapy; antiserum against α-toxin not used today; the value of hyperbaric oxygen treatment is unproven

Treat with dêbridement and penicillin for localized infections

Symptomatic treatment for food poisoning

Proper wound care and judicious use of prophylactic antibiotics will prevent most infections

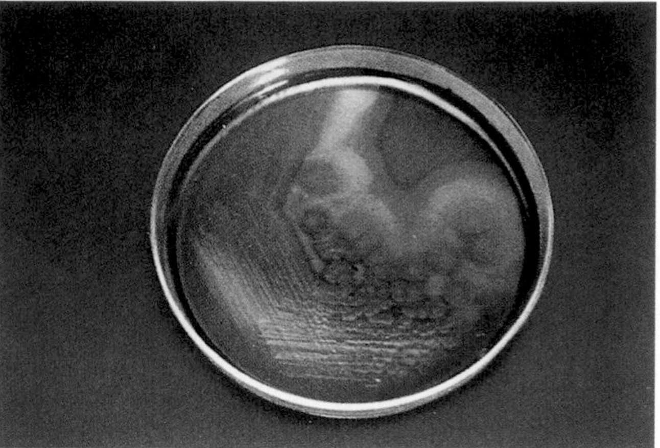

FIGURE 40–2. Growth of *Clostridium perfringens* on sheep blood agar. Note the flat, spreading colonies and the hemolytic activity of the organism. A presumptive identification of *C. perfringens* can be made by detection of a zone of complete hemolysis (caused by the θ-toxin) and a wider zone of partial hemolysis (caused by the α-toxin), combined with the characteristic microscopic morphology.

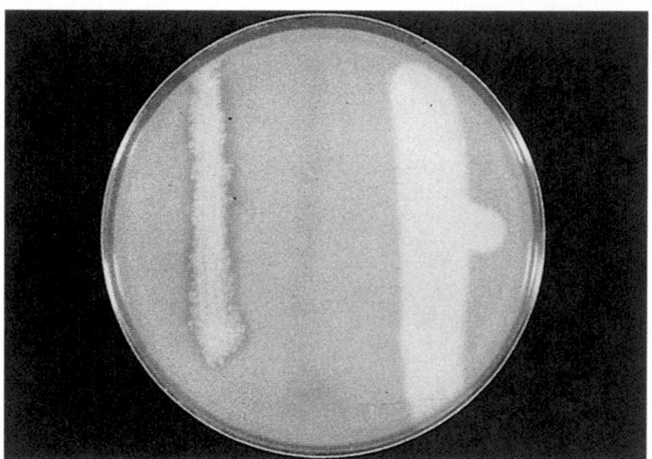

FIGURE 40–3. Growth of *Clostridium perfringens* on egg-yolk agar. The α-toxin (lecithinase) hydrolyzes phospholipids in serum and egg yolk, producing an opaque precipitate *(right)*. This precipitate is not observed when the organism is grown in the presence of antibodies against the toxin *(left)*. This reaction (Nagler's reaction) is characteristic of *C. perfringens*.

TABLE 40–2. Distribution of Lethal Toxins in *Clostridium perfringens* Types A to E

Type	Lethal Toxins			
	Alpha	Beta	Epsilon	Iota
A	+	–	–	–
B	+	+	+	–
C	+	+	–	–
D	+	–	+	–
E	+	–	–	+

vascular permeability of the gastrointestinal wall. **ι-Toxin,** the fourth major lethal toxin, is produced by type E *C. perfringens*. This toxin has necrotic activity and increases vascular permeability.

The *C. perfringens* **enterotoxin** is produced primarily by type A strains. The heat-labile toxin is susceptible to pronase. Exposure to trypsin enhances toxin activity threefold. The enterotoxin is produced during the phase transition from vegetative cells to spores and is released with the formed spores when the cells undergo the terminal stages of spore formation **(sporulation).** The alkaline conditions in the small intestine stimulate sporulation. The released enterotoxin binds to receptors on the brush

TABLE 40–3. Virulence Factors Associated with *Clostridium perfringens*

Virulence Factors	Biologic Activity
α-Toxin	Lethal toxin; phospholipase C (lecithinase); increases vascular permeability; hemolysin; produces necrotizing activity, as seen in myonecrosis
β-Toxin	Lethal toxin; necrotizing activity
ε-Toxin	Lethal toxin; permease
ι-Toxin	Lethal binary toxin; necrotizing activity; adenosine diphosphate (ADP) ribosylating
δ-Toxin	Hemolysin
θ-Toxin	Heat- and oxygen-labile hemolysin; cytolytic
κ-Toxin	Collagenase; gelatinase; necrotizing activity
λ-Toxin	Protease
μ-Toxin	Hyaluronidase
ν-Toxin	Deoxyribonuclease; hemolysin; necrotizing activity
Enterotoxin	Alters membrane permeability in ileum (cytotoxic, enterotoxic); superantigen
Neuraminidase	Alters cell surface ganglioside receptors; promotes capillary thrombosis

border membrane of the small intestine epithelium in the ileum (primarily) and jejunum but not duodenum. Insertion of the toxin into the cell membrane leads to altered membrane permeability and loss of fluids and ions. The enterotoxin also acts as a superantigen simulating T lymphocyte activity. Antibodies to enterotoxin, indicating previous exposure, are commonly found in adults but are not protective. The activities of the other toxins and enzymes of *C. perfringens* are summarized in Table 40–3.

EPIDEMIOLOGY

Type A *C. perfringens* commonly inhabits the intestinal tract of humans and animals and is widely distributed in nature, particularly in soil and water contaminated with feces (see Box 40–2). Spores are formed under adverse environmental conditions and can survive for prolonged periods. Strains of types B through E do not survive in soil but rather colonize the intestinal tracts of animals and occasionally humans. Type A *C. perfringens* is responsible for most human infections, including soft-tissue infections, food poisoning, and primary septicemia. Type C *C. perfringens* is responsible for one other important infection in humans—**enteritis necroticans**.

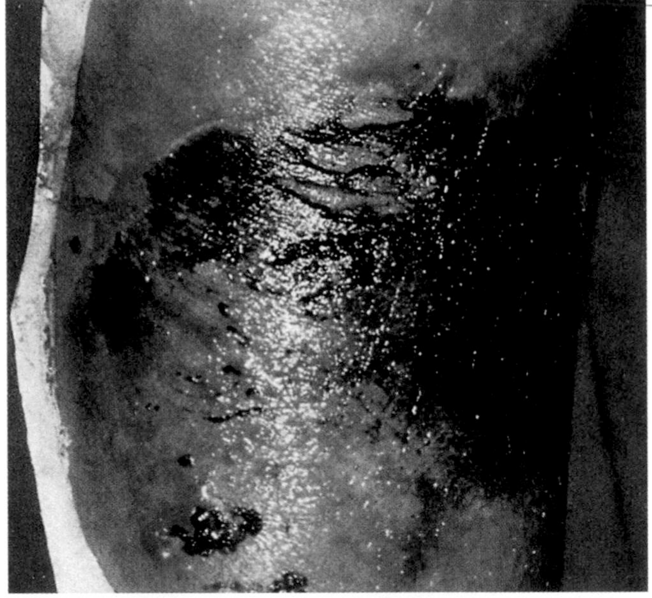

FIGURE 40–4. Clostridial cellulitis. Clostridia can be introduced into tissue during surgery or by a traumatic injury. This patient suffered a compound fracture of the tibia. Five days after the injury, the skin became discolored and bullae and necrosis developed. A serosanguineous exudate and subcutaneous gas were present, but there was no evidence of muscle necrosis. The patient had an uneventful recovery. (From Lambert H, Farrar W, editors: *Infectious diseases illustrated*, London, 1982, Gower.)

CLINICAL DISEASES (BOX 40–3)

Soft-Tissue Infections

Soft-tissue infections caused by *C. perfringens* are subdivided into (1) cellulitis, (2) fasciitis or suppurative myositis, and (3) myonecrosis or gas gangrene. Clostridial species can colonize wounds and skin with no clinical consequences. Indeed, most strains of *C. perfringens* and other clostridial species isolated in wound cultures are insignificant. However, these organisms can also initiate **cellulitis** (Figure 40–4) with gas formation in the soft tissue. This

BOX 40–3. Clostridia: Clinical Summaries

Clostridium perfringens
Soft-tissue infections
Cellulitis: Localized edema and erythema with gas formation in the soft tissue; generally nonpainful
Suppurative myositis: Accumulation of pus (suppuration) in the muscle planes without muscle necrosis or systemic symptoms
Myonecrosis: Painful, rapid destruction of muscle tissue; systemic spread with high mortality
Gastroenteritis
Food poisoning: Rapid onset of abdominal cramps and watery diarrhea with no fever, nausea, or vomiting; short, self-limited duration
Necrotizing enteritis: Acute, necrotizing destruction of jejunum with abdominal pain, vomiting, bloody diarrhea, and peritonitis

Clostridium tetani
Generalized tetanus: Generalized musculature spasms and involvement of the autonomic nervous system in severe disease (e.g., cardiac arrhythmias, fluctuations in blood pressure, profound sweating, dehydration)
Localized tetanus: Musculature spasms restricted to localized area of primary infection
Neonatal tetanus: Neonatal infection primarily involving the umbilical stump; very high mortality

Clostridium botulinum
Foodborne botulism: Initial presentation of blurred vision, dry mouth, constipation, and abdominal pain; progresses to bilateral descending weakness of the peripheral muscles with flaccid paralysis
Infant botulism: Initially nonspecific symptoms (e.g., constipation, weak cry, failure to thrieve) that progress to flaccid paralysis and respiratory arrest
Wound botulism: Clinical presentation same as with foodborne disease, although the incubation period is longer and fewer gastrointestinal symptoms
Inhalation botulism: Inhalation exposure to botulinum toxin would be expected to have a rapid onset of symptoms (flaccid paralysis, pulmonary failure) and high mortality

Clostridium difficile
Antibiotic-associated diarrhea: Acute diarrhea generally developing 5 to 10 days after initiation of antibiotic treatment (particularly clindamycin, penicillins, and cephalosporins); may be brief and self-limited or more protracted
Pseudomembranous colitis: Most severe form of *C. difficile* disease with profuse diarrhea, abdominal cramping, and fever; whitish plaques (pseudomembranes) over intact colonic tissue seen on colonoscopy

process can progress to **suppurative myositis** characterized by an accumulation of pus in the muscle planes, but muscle necrosis and systemic symptoms are absent.

Clostridial myonecrosis is a life-threatening disease that illustrates the full virulence potential of histotoxic clostridia. The onset of disease, characterized by intense pain, generally develops within a week after clostridia are introduced into tissue by trauma or surgery. The onset is followed rapidly by extensive muscle necrosis, shock, renal failure, and death, often within 2 days of initial onset. Macroscopic examination of muscle reveals devitalized necrotic tissue. Gas found in the tissue is caused by the metabolic activity of the rapidly dividing bacteria (hence the name **gas gangrene**). Microscopic examination reveals abundant rectangular, gram-positive rods in the absence of inflammatory cells (resulting from lysis by clostridial toxins). The clostridial toxins characteristically cause extensive hemolysis and bleeding. Clostridial myonecrosis is most commonly caused by *C. perfringens*, although other species (e.g., *C. septicum*, *C. histolyticum*, and *C. novyi*) can also produce this disease.

Food Poisoning

Clostridial food poisoning, a relatively common but underappreciated intoxication, is characterized by (1) a short incubation period (8 to 24 hours), (2) a clinical presentation that includes abdominal cramps and watery diarrhea but no fever, nausea, or vomiting, and (3) a clinical course lasting 24 to 48 hours. Disease results from the ingestion of meat products (e.g., beef, chicken, turkey) contaminated with large numbers (10^8 to 10^9 organisms) of enterotoxin-containing type A *C. perfringens*. Holding contaminated foods at temperatures below 60°C (46°C is optimal) allows spores that survived the cooking process to germinate and multiply to high numbers. The refrigeration of food after preparation prevents this bacterial growth. Alternatively, reheating of the food can destroy the heat-labile enterotoxin.

Necrotizing Enteritis

Necrotizing enteritis (also called **enteritis necroticans** or **pig-bel**) is a rare, acute necrotizing process in the jejunum characterized by acute abdominal pain, vomiting, bloody diarrhea, ulceration of the small intestine, and perforation of the intestinal wall, leading to peritonitis and shock. The mortality in patients with this infection approaches 50%. β-Toxin produced by *C. perfringens* type C is responsible for this disease. Necrotizing enteritis is most common in Papua New Guinea, with sporadic cases reported from other countries. It is associated with eating undercooked, contaminated pork with sweet potatoes, which contain a heat-resistant trypsin inhibitor. This inhibitor protects the β-toxin from inactivation by trypsin. Other risk factors for the disease are exposure to large numbers of organisms and malnutrition (with loss of the proteolytic activity that inactivates the toxin).

Septicemia

The isolation of *C. perfringens* or other clostridial species in blood cultures can be alarming. However, more than half of the isolates are clinically insignificant, representing a transient bacteremia or more likely contamination of the culture with clostridia colonizing the skin. The significance of an isolate must be viewed in light of other clinical findings. When *C. perfringens* is isolated in the blood from patients with significant infections (e.g., myonecrosis, necrotizing enteritis), the organism is typically associated with massive hemolysis.

LABORATORY DIAGNOSIS

The laboratory performs only a confirmatory role in the diagnosis of clostridial soft-tissue diseases because therapy must be initiated immediately. The microscopic detection of gram-positive rods in clinical specimens, usually in the absence of leukocytes, can be a very useful finding because these organisms have a characteristic morphology. It is also relatively simple to culture these anaerobes. *C. perfringens* can be detected on simple media after incubation for 1 day or less. Under appropriate conditions, *C. perfringens* divides every 8 to 10 minutes, so growth on agar media or in blood culture broths can be detected after incubation for only a few hours. The role of *C. perfringens* in food poisoning is documented by recovery of more than 10^5 organisms per gram of food or more than 10^6 bacteria per gram of feces collected within 1 day of the onset of disease. Immunoassays have also been developed for detection of the enterotoxin in fecal specimens, although culture or immunoassays are not commonly used in clinical labs for this diagnosis.

TREATMENT, PREVENTION, AND CONTROL

C. perfringens soft tissue infections, such as suppurative myositis and myonecrosis, must be treated aggressively with surgical débridement and high-dose penicillin therapy. Hyperbaric oxygen treatment has been used to manage these infections; however, the results are inconclusive. Treatment with antiserum against α-toxin also has not been successful and is no longer available. Despite all therapeutic efforts, the prognosis in patients with these diseases is poor, with reported mortality ranging from 40% to almost 100%. Less serious, localized soft tissue infections can be successfully treated with penicillin.

Antibiotic therapy for clostridial food poisoning is unnecessary because this is a self-limiting disease (i.e., the diarrhea washes the bacteria out of the intestines and the normal intestinal flora reestablishes itself).

Prevention and control of *C. perfringens* infections are difficult because the organisms are ubiquitous. Disease requires introduction of the organism into devitalized tissues and maintenance of an anaerobic environment favorable for bacterial growth. Thus proper wound care and the judicious use of prophylactic antibiotics can do much to prevent most infections.

Clostridium Tetani

PHYSIOLOGY AND STRUCTURE

C. tetani is a large (0.5 to 1.7 × 2.1 to 18.1 μm), motile, spore-forming rod. The organism produces round, terminal spores that give it the appearance of a drumstick (Figure 40–5). Unlike *C. perfringens, C. tetani* is difficult to grow because the organism is extremely sensitive to oxygen toxicity and, when growth is detected on agar media, it typically appears as a film over the surface of the agar rather than discrete colonies. The bacteria are proteolytic but unable to ferment carbohydrates.

PATHOGENESIS AND IMMUNITY

Although the vegetative cells of *C. tetani* die rapidly when exposed to oxygen, spore formation allows the organism to survive in the most adverse conditions. Of greater significance is the fact that *C. tetani* produces two toxins, an oxygen-labile hemolysin **(tetanolysin)** and a plasmid-

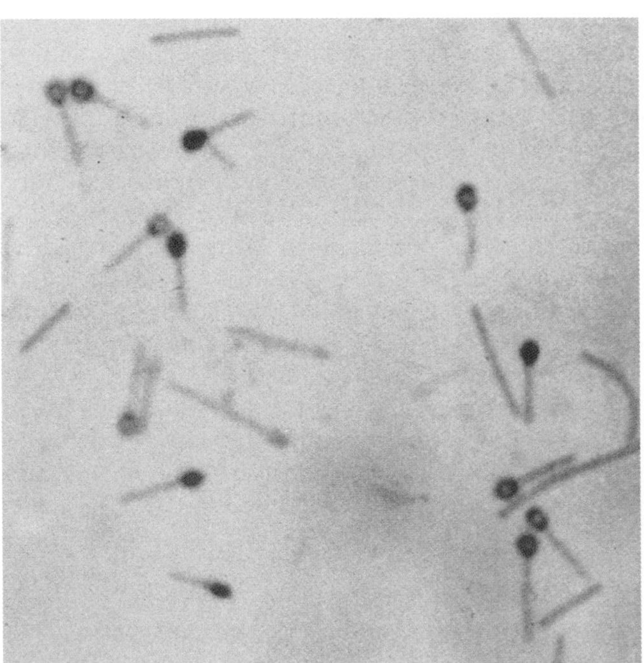

FIGURE 40–5. Gram stain of *Clostridium tetani.* Note the terminal spores.

encoded, heat-labile neurotoxin **(tetanospasmin).** The plasmid carrying the gene for tetanospasmin is nonconjugative, so a nontoxic *C. tetani* strain cannot be converted to a toxigenic strain. Tetanolysin is serologically related to streptolysin O and *C. perfringens* and *Listeria monocytogenes* hemolysins. The clinical significance of this enzyme is unknown, however, because it is inhibited by oxygen and serum cholesterol.

Tetanospasmin is produced during the stationary phase of growth, is released when the cell is lysed, and is responsible for the clinical manifestations of tetanus. Tetanospasmin (an A-B toxin) is synthesized as a single, 150,000-Da peptide that is cleaved into a light (A-chain) subunit and a heavy (B-chain) subunit by an endogenous protease when the cell releases the neurotoxin. A disulfide bond and noncovalent forces hold the two chains together. The carbohydrate-binding domain of the heavy (100,000-Da) chain, carboxyl-terminal portion, binds to specific sialic acid receptors (e.g., polysialogangliosides) and adjacent glycoproteins on the surface of motor neurons. The intact toxin molecules are internalized in endosomal vesicles and transported in the neuron axon to motor neuron soma located in the spinal cord. In this location the endosome becomes acidified, which results in a conformational change in the N-terminus domain of the heavy chain, which is followed by its insertion into the endosome membrane and passage of the toxin light chain into the cytosol of the cell. The light chain is a zinc endopeptidase that cleaves core proteins involved in the trafficking and release of neurotransmitters. Specifically, tetanospasmin inactivates proteins that regulate release of the inhibitory neurotransmitters glycine and gamma-aminobutryic acid (GABA). This leads to unregulated excitatory synaptic activity in the motor neurons resulting in **spastic paralysis.** The toxin binding is irreversible, so recovery depends on whether new axonal terminals form. For an excellent detailed description of the activities of the neurotoxins produced by *C. tetani* and *C. botulinum*, refer to the review by Lalli et al in the bibliography at the end of this chapter.

EPIDEMIOLOGY

C. tetani is ubiquitous. It is found in fertile soil and transiently colonizes the gastrointestinal tracts of many animals, including humans (Box 40–4). The vegetative forms of *C. tetani* are extremely susceptible to oxygen toxicity, but the organisms sporulate readily and can survive in nature for a long time. Disease is relatively rare in the United States because of the high incidence of vaccine-induced immunity. Fewer than 40 cases are reported annually, and the disease occurs primarily in elderly patients with waning immunity. However, tetanus is still responsible for many deaths in developing countries where vaccination is unavailable or medical practices are lax. It is estimated that more than 1 million cases occur worldwide, with a mortality rate ranging from 30% to 50%. At least half the deaths occur in neonates.

CLINICAL DISEASES (see Box 40–3)

The incubation period for tetanus varies from a few days to weeks. The duration of the incubation period is directly related to the distance of the primary wound infection from the central nervous system.

BOX 40–4. Summary of *Clostridium tetani*

Physiology and Structure

Gram-positive rods with prominent terminal spores (drumstick appearance)

Strict anaerobe (vegetative cells are extremely oxygen sensitive)

Difficult to isolate from clinical specimens

Virulence

Spore formation

Tetanospasmin (heat-labile neurotoxin; blocks release of neurotransmitters [i.e., gamma-aminobutyric acid, glycine] for inhibitory synapses)

Tetanolysin (heat-stable hemolysin of unknown significance)

Epidemiology

Ubiquitous; spores are found in most soils and can colonize gastrointestinal tract of humans and animals

Exposure to spores is common, but disease is uncommon, except in developing countries where there is poor access to vaccine and medical care

Risk is greatest for people with inadequate vaccine-induced immunity; disease does not induce immunity

Diseases

Refer to Box 40–3

Diagnosis

Diagnosis is based on clinical presentation

Microscopy and culture with poor sensitivity

Neither tetanus toxin nor antibodies are typically detected

Treatment, Prevention, and Control

Treatment requires débridement, antibiotic therapy (metronidazole), passive immunization with antitoxin globulin, and vaccination with tetanus toxoid

Prevention through use of vaccination, consisting of three doses of tetanus toxoid, followed by booster doses every 10 years

Generalized tetanus is the most common form. Involvement of the masseter muscles (trismus or lockjaw) is the presenting sign in most patients. The characteristic sardonic smile that results from the sustained contraction of the facial muscles is known as *risus sardonicus* (Figure 40–6). Other early signs are drooling, sweating, irritability, and persistent back spasms (*opisthotonos*) (Figure 40–7). The autonomic nervous system is involved in patients with more severe disease; the signs and symptoms include cardiac arrhythmias, fluctuations in blood pressure, profound sweating, and dehydration.

Another form of *C. tetani* disease is **localized tetanus**, in which the disease remains confined to the musculature at the site of primary infection. A variant is **cephalic tetanus**, in which the primary site of infection is the head. In contrast to the prognosis for patients with localized tetanus, the prognosis for patients with cephalic tetanus is very poor.

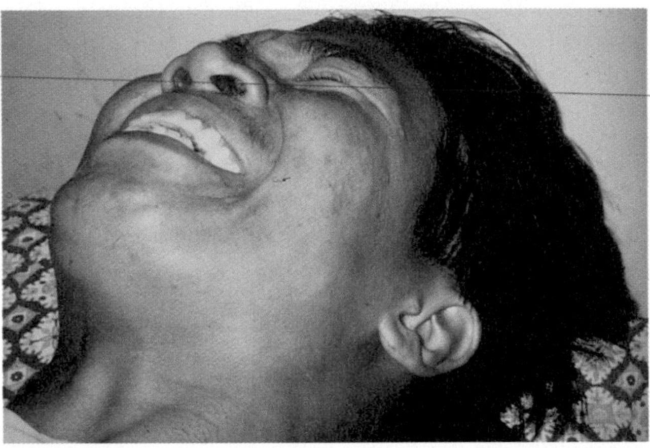

FIGURE 40–6. Facial spasm and risus sardonicus in a patient with tetanus. (From Cohen J, Powderly WG: *Infectious diseases*, ed 2, St Louis, 2004, Mosby).

Neonatal tetanus (tetanus neonatorum) is typically associated with an initial infection of the umbilical stump that progresses to become generalized. The mortality in infants exceeds 90%, and developmental defects are present in survivors. This is almost exclusively a disease in developing countries.

LABORATORY DIAGNOSIS

The diagnosis of tetanus, as with that of most other clostridial diseases, is made on the basis of the clinical presentation. The microscopic detection of *C. tetani* or recovery in culture is useful but frequently unsuccessful. Culture results are positive in only approximately 30% of patients with tetanus, because disease can be caused by relatively few organisms and the slow-growing bacteria are killed rapidly when exposed to air. Neither tetanus toxin nor antibodies to the toxin are detectable in the patient because the toxin is rapidly bound to motor neurons and internalized. If the organism is recovered in culture, production of toxin by the isolate can be confirmed with the tetanus antitoxin neutralization test in mice (a procedure performed only in Public Health reference laboratories).

TREATMENT, PREVENTION, AND CONTROL

The mortality associated with tetanus has steadily decreased during the past century, resulting in large part from the decreased incidence of tetanus in the United States. The highest mortality is in newborns and in patients in whom the incubation period is shorter than 1 week.

Treatment of tetanus requires débridement of the primary wound (which may appear innocuous), use of metronidazole, passive immunization with human

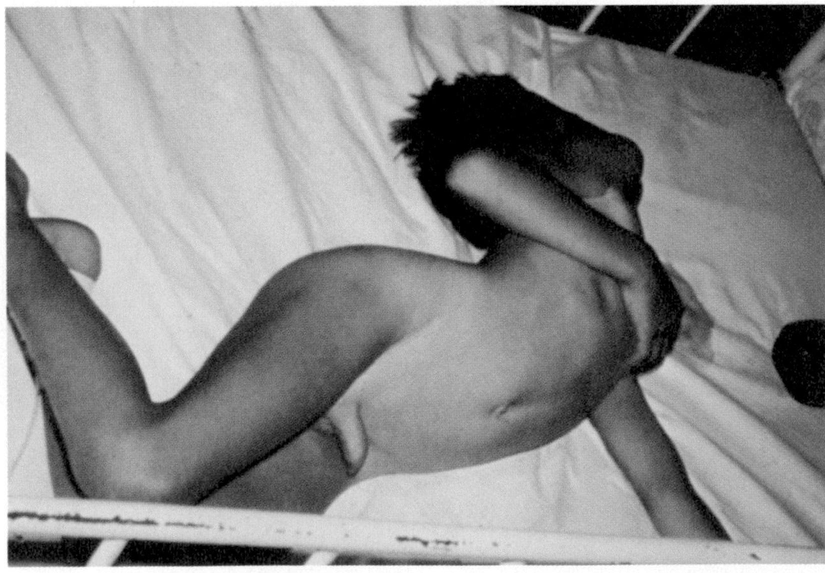

FIGURE 40–7. A child with tetanus and opisthotonos resulting from persistent spasms of the back muscles. (From Emond RT, Rowland HAK, Welsby P: *Colour atlas of infectious diseases*, ed 3, London, 1995, Wolfe.)

tetanus immunoglobulin, and vaccination with tetanus toxoid. Wound care and metronidazole therapy eliminate the vegetative bacteria that produce toxin, and the antitoxin antibodies work by binding free tetanospasmin molecules. Metronidazole and penicillin have equivalent activity against *C. tetani*; however, penicillin, like tetanospasmin, inhibits GABA activity and hence should not be used. Toxin bound to nerve endings is protected from antibodies. Thus the toxic effects must be controlled symptomatically until the normal regulation of synaptic transmission is restored. Vaccination with a series of three doses of tetanus toxoid, followed by booster doses every 10 years, is highly effective in preventing tetanus.

Clostridium Botulinum

PHYSIOLOGY AND STRUCTURE

C. botulinum, the etiologic agent of botulism, is a heterogeneous group of large (0.6 to 1.4 × 3.0 to 20.2 μm), fastidious, spore-forming, anaerobic rods. These bacteria are subdivided into four groups based on phenotypic and genetic properties, and certainly represent four separate species that have been historically classified within a single species. Seven antigenically distinct botulinum toxins (A to G) have been described; human disease is associated with types A, B, E, and F. Toxin production is associated with specific groups (Table 40–4). Other species of clostridia produce botulinum toxins, including *C. butyricum* (type E toxin), *C. baratii* (type F toxin), and *Clostridium argentinense* (type G toxin). Human disease has only rarely been associated with *C. butyricum* and *C. baratii*, and not definitively demonstrated with *C. argentinense*.

PATHOGENESIS AND IMMUNITY

Like tetanus toxin, *C. botulinum* toxin is a 150,000-Da progenitor protein (A-B toxin) consisting of a small subunit (light or A chain) with zinc-endopeptidase activity and a large, nontoxic subunit (B or heavy chain). In contrast with the tetanus neurotoxin, the *C. botulinum* toxin is complexed with nontoxic proteins that protect the neurotoxin during passage through the digestive tract (this is unnecessary for tetanus neurotoxin). The carboxyl-terminal portion of the botulinum heavy chain binds specific sialic acid receptors and glycoproteins (different from those targeted by tetanospasmin) on the surface of motor neurons and stimulates endocytosis of the toxin molecule. Also in contrast with tetanospasmin, the botulinum neurotoxin remains at the neuromuscular junction. Acidification of the endosome stimulates N-terminal, heavy chain mediated release of the light chain. The botulinum endopeptidase then inactivates the proteins that regulate release of acetylcholine, blocking neurotransmission at peripheral cholinergic synapses. Because acetylcholine is required for excitation of muscle, the resulting clinical presentation of botulism is a **flaccid paralysis.** As with tetanus, recovery of function after botulism requires regeneration of the nerve endings.

TABLE 40–4. *Clostridium botulinum* Classification and Toxin Production

Group	Neurotoxin Type	Phenotypic Properties
I	A, B, F	Proteolytic, saccharolytic
II	B, E, F	Nonproteolytic, saccharolytic
III	C, D	Weakly proteolytic, saccharolytic
IV	G	Weakly proteolytic, asaccharolytic

EPIDEMIOLOGY

C. botulinum is commonly isolated in soil and water samples throughout the world (Box 40–5). In the United States, type A strains are found mainly in neutral or alkaline soil west of the Mississippi River; type B strains are found primarily in the eastern part of the country in rich, organic soil; and type E strains are found only in wet soil. Although *C. botulinum* is commonly found in soil, disease is uncommon in the United States.

The following four forms of botulism have been identified: (1) classic or foodborne botulism, (2) infant botulism, (3) wound botulism, and (4) inhalation botulism. In the United States, fewer than 30 cases of **foodborne botulism** are seen annually; most are associated with the consumption of home-canned foods (types A and B toxins) and occasionally with the consumption of preserved fish (type E toxin). The food may not appear spoiled, but even a small taste can cause full-blown clinical disease. **Infant botulism** is more common (although fewer than 100 cases are reported annually) and has been associated with the consumption of foods (particularly honey) contaminated with botulinum spores. The incidence of **wound botulism** is unknown, but the disease is very rare. **Inhalation botulism** is a major concern in this era of bioterrorism. Botulinum toxin has been concentrated for purposes of aerosolization as a biologic weapon. When administered in this manner, inhalation disease has a rapid onset and potentially high mortality.

CLINICAL DISEASES (BOX 40–3)

Foodborne Botulism

Patients with foodborne botulism typically become weak and dizzy 1 to 2 days after consuming the contaminated

BOX 40–5. Summary of *Clostridium botulinum*

Physiology and Structure
Gram-positive, spore-forming rod
Strict anaerobe (vegetative cells extremely oxygen-sensitive)
Fastidious growth requirements
Can produce one of seven distinct botulinum toxins (A to G)
Strains associated with human disease produce lipase, digest milk proteins, hydrolyze gelatin, and ferment glucose

Virulence
Spore formation
Botulinum toxin (prevents release of neurotransmitter acetylcholine)
Binary toxin

Epidemiology
Ubiquitous; *C. botulinum* spores are found in soil worldwide
Human diseases associated with toxins A, B, E, and F
Relatively few cases of botulism in the United States
Infant botulism more common than other forms

Diseases
Refer to Box 40–3

Diagnosis
Botulism confirmed by isolating the organism or detecting the toxin in food products or the patient's feces or serum

Treatment, Prevention, and Control
Treatment involves administration of metronidazole or penicillin, trivalent botulinum antitoxin, and ventilatory support
Spore germination in foods prevented by maintaining food in an acid pH, by high sugar content (e.g., fruit preserves), or by storing the foods at 4°C or colder
Toxin is heat-labile and therefore can be destroyed by heating of food for 10 minutes at 60° to 100°C
Infant botulism is associated with consumption of contaminated foods (particularly honey). Infants younger than 1 year should not be given honey or foods containing it

food. The initial signs include blurred vision with fixed, dilated pupils, dry mouth (indicative of the anticholinergic effects of the toxin), constipation, and abdominal pain. Fever is absent. Bilateral descending weakness of the peripheral muscles develops in patients with progressive disease (flaccid paralysis), and death is most commonly attributed to respiratory paralysis. Patients maintain a clear sensorium throughout the disease. Despite aggressive management of the patient's condition, the disease may continue to progress, because the neurotoxin is irreversibly bound and inhibits the release of excitatory neurotransmitters for a prolonged period. Complete recovery in patients often requires many months to years, or until the affected nerve endings regrow. Mortality in patients with foodborne botulism, which once approached 70%, has been reduced to 10% through the use of better supportive care, particularly in the management of respiratory complications.

Infant Botulism

Infant botulism was first recognized in 1976 and is now the most common form of botulism in the United States. In contrast with foodborne botulism, this disease is caused by neurotoxin produced in vivo by *C. botulinum* colonizing the gastrointestinal tracts of infants. Although adults are exposed to the organism in their diet, *C. botulinum* cannot survive and proliferate in their intestines. In the absence of competitive bowel microbes, however, the organism can become established in the gastrointestinal tracts of infants. The disease typically affects infants younger than 1 year (most between 1 and 6 months), and the symptoms are initially nonspecific (e.g., constipation, weak cry, or "failure to thrive"). Progressive disease with flaccid paralysis and respiratory arrest can develop; however, mortality in documented cases of infant botulism is very low (1% to 2%). Some infant deaths attributed to other conditions (e.g., sudden infant death syndrome) may actually be caused by botulism.

Wound Botulism

As the name implies, wound botulism develops from toxin production by *C. botulinum* in contaminated wounds. Although the symptoms of disease are identical to those of foodborne disease, the incubation period is generally longer (4 days or more), and the gastrointestinal tract symptoms are less prominent.

LABORATORY DIAGNOSIS

The clinical diagnosis of botulism is confirmed if the organism is isolated or toxin activity is demonstrated. Toxin activity is most likely to be found early in the disease. An attempt should be made to culture *C. botulinum* from the feces of patients with foodborne disease and from the implicated food if it is available. No single test for foodborne botulism has sensitivity greater than 60%. In contrast, toxin is detected in the serum of more than 90% of infants with botulism.

Isolation of *C. botulinum* from specimens contaminated with other organisms can be improved by heating the specimen for 10 minutes at 80°C to kill all non-clostridial cells. Culture of the heated specimen on nutritionally enriched anaerobic media allows the heat-resistant *C. botulinum* spores to germinate. The strains of *C. botulinum* associated with human botulism are characterized by lipase production (appears as an iridescent film on colonies grown on egg-yolk agar) and the ability to digest milk proteins, hydrolyze gelatin, and ferment glucose.

Demonstration of toxin production (typically performed at Public Health laboratories) must be done with a mouse bioassay. This procedure consists of the preparation of two aliquots of the isolate, mixing of one aliquot with antitoxin, and intraperitoneal inoculation of each aliquot into mice. If the antitoxin treatment protects the mice, toxin activity is confirmed. Samples of the implicated food, stool specimen, and patient's serum should also be tested for toxin activity.

The diagnosis of infant botulism is supported if (1) *C. botulinum* is isolated from feces or (2) toxin activity is detected in feces or serum. The organism can be isolated from stool cultures in virtually all patients, because carriage of the organism may persist for many months, even after a baby has recovered. Wound botulism is confirmed by isolation of the organism from the wound or by detection of toxin activity in wound exudate or serum.

TREATMENT, PREVENTION, AND CONTROL

Patients with botulism require the following treatment measures: (1) adequate ventilatory support; (2) elimination of the organism from the gastrointestinal tract, through the judicious use of gastric lavage and metronidazole or penicillin therapy; and (3) the use of trivalent botulinum antitoxin versus toxins A, B, and E to bind toxin circulating in the bloodstream. Ventilatory support is extremely important in reducing mortality. Protective levels of antibodies do not develop after disease, so patients are susceptible to multiple infections.

Disease is prevented by destroying the spores in food (virtually impossible for practical reasons), preventing spore germination (by maintaining the food in an acid pH or storage at 4°C or colder), or destroying the preformed toxin (all botulinum toxins are inactivated by heating at 60°C to 100°C for 10 minutes). Infant botulism has been associated with the consumption of honey contaminated with *C. botulinum* spores, so children younger than 1 year should not eat honey.

Clostridium Difficile

Until the mid-1970s the clinical importance of *C. difficile* was not appreciated. This organism was infrequently isolated in fecal cultures and its role in human disease was unknown. Systematic studies now clearly show, however, that toxin-producing *C. difficile* is responsible for antibiotic-associated gastrointestinal diseases (Box 40–6), ranging from a relatively benign, self-limited diarrhea to severe, life-threatening pseudomembranous colitis (Figures 40–8 and 40–9).

C. difficile produces two toxins (Table 40–5), an **enterotoxin** (toxin A) and a **cytotoxin** (toxin B). The enterotoxin is chemotactic for neutrophils, stimulating the infiltration of polymorphonuclear neutrophils into the ileum with release of cytokines. Toxin A also produces a cytopathic effect, resulting in disruption of the tight cell-cell junction, increased permeability of the intestinal wall, and subsequent diarrhea. The cytotoxin causes actin to depolymerize, with the resultant destruction of the cellular cytoskeleton both in vivo and in vitro. Although both toxins appear to interact synergistically in the pathogene-

BOX 40–6. Summary of *Clostridium difficile*

Physiology and Structure
Gram-positive, spore-forming rod
Strict anaerobe (vegetative cells are extremely oxygen sensitive)

Virulence
Refer to Table 40–4

Epidemiology
The organism is ubiquitous
Colonizes the intestines of a small proportion of healthy individuals (<5%)
Exposure to antibiotics is associated with overgrowth of *C. difficile* and subsequent disease (endogenous infection)
Spores can be detected in hospital rooms of infected patients (particularly around beds and in the bathrooms); these can be an exogenous source of infection

Diseases
Refer to Box 40–3

Diagnosis
C. difficile disease is confirmed by detecting the cytotoxin or enterotoxin in the patient's feces

Treatment, Prevention, and Control
The implicated antibiotic should be discontinued
Treatment with metronidazole or vancomycin should be used in severe disease
Relapse is common because antibiotics do not kill spores; a second course of therapy with the same antibiotic is usually successful
The hospital room should be carefully cleaned after the infected patient is discharged

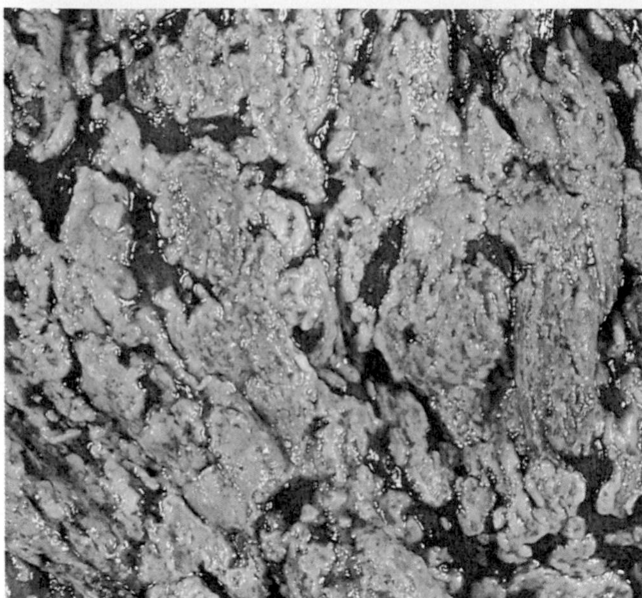

FIGURE 40–8. Antibiotic-associated colitis: gross section of the lumen of the colon. Note the white plaques of fibrin, mucus, and inflammatory cells overlying the normal red intestinal mucosa.

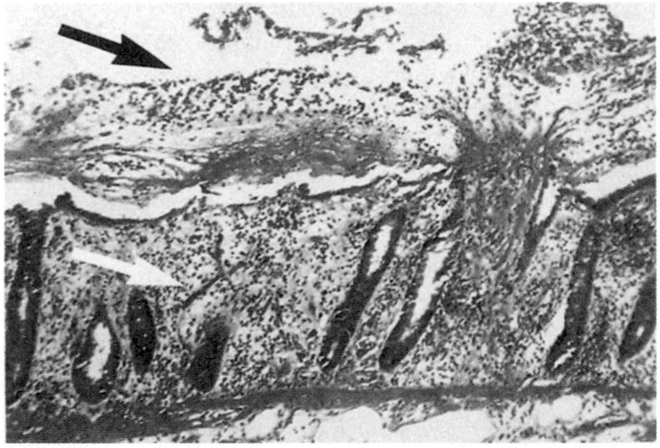

FIGURE 40–9. Antibiotic-associated colitis caused by *Clostridium difficile.* A histologic section of colon shows an intense inflammatory response, with the characteristic "plaque" *(black arrow)* overlying the intact intestinal mucosa *(white arrow).* (Hematoxylin and eosin stain.) (From Lambert HP, Farrar WE, editors: *Infectious diseases illustrated,* London, 1982, Gower.)

sis of disease, enterotoxin A-negative isolates can still produce disease. Additionally, production of one or both toxins does not appear to be sufficient alone for disease (e.g., carriage of *C. difficile* and high levels of toxins are common in young children while disease is rare). Bacterial "surface layer proteins" (SLPs) are important for the binding of *C. difficile* to the intestinal epithelium, leading to localized production of toxins and subsequent tissue damage. Other *C. difficile* virulence factors are summarized in Table 40–5.

TABLE 40–5. Virulence Factors Associated with *Clostridium difficile*

Virulence Factor	Biologic Activity
Enterotoxin (toxin A)	Produces chemotaxis; induces cytokine production with hypersecretion of fluid; produces hemorrhagic necrosis
Cytotoxin (toxin B)	Induces depolymerization of actin with loss of cellular cytoskeleton
Adhesin factor	Mediates binding to human colonic cells
Hyaluronidase	Produces hydrolytic activity
Spore formation	Permits organism's survival for months in hospital environment

C. difficile is part of the normal intestinal flora in a small number of healthy people and hospitalized patients. The disease develops in people taking antibiotics, because the drugs alter the normal enteric flora, either permitting the overgrowth of these relatively resistant organisms or making the patient more susceptible to the exogenous acquisition of *C. difficile.* The disease occurs if the organisms proliferate in the colon and produce their toxins.

The diagnosis of *C. difficile* infection is confirmed by demonstration of the enterotoxin or cytotoxin in a stool specimen from a patient with compatible clinical symptoms. Isolation of the organism in stool culture documents colonization but not disease. The enterotoxin and cytotoxin can be detected with a number of commercial immunoassays. These assays vary tremendously in sensitivity and specificity, so care must be used in selecting the appropriate test, and a negative test result does not exclude the diagnosis. The cytotoxin can also be detected by an in vivo cytotoxicity assay using tissue culture cells and specific neutralizing antibodies for the cytotoxin; however, this assay is technically cumbersome and requires 1 to 2 days before results are available. Most laboratories have replaced the cytotoxicity assay with immunoassay methods.

Discontinuation of the implicated antibiotic (e.g., ampicillin, clindamycin) is generally sufficient to alleviate mild disease. However, specific therapy with metronidazole or vancomycin is necessary for the management of severe diarrhea or colitis. Relapses may occur in as many as 20% to 30% of patients after the completion of therapy, because only the vegetative forms of *C. difficile* are killed by the antibiotics; the spores are resistant. A second course of treatment with the same antibiotic is frequently successful. It is difficult to prevent the disease, because the organism commonly exists in hospitals, particularly in areas adjacent to infected patients (e.g., beds, bathrooms). The spores of *C. difficile* are difficult to eliminate unless thorough housekeeping measures are used. Thus the organism can contaminate an environment for many months and can be a major source of nosocomial outbreaks of *C. difficile* disease.

Other Clostridial Species

Many other clostridia have been associated with clinically significant disease. Their virulence is a result of their ability to survive exposure to oxygen by forming spores and producing many diverse toxins and enzymes. The virulence factors produced by some of the more important clostridia are summarized in Table 40–6. *C. septicum* (Figure 40–10) is a particularly important pathogen because it is a cause of nontraumatic myonecrosis and often exists in patients with occult colon cancer, acute leukemia, or diabetes. If the integrity of the bowel mucosa is compromised and the patient's body is less able to mount an effective response to the organism, *C. septicum* can spread into tissue and rapidly proliferate there. Most patients have a fulminant course, dying within 1 to 2 days after initial presentation. *C. tertium* is another important clostridia that is commonly isolated in soil samples. It has primarily been associated with traumatic wound infections (e.g., war wounds, a fall producing a soil-contaminated wound). This organism can pose a diagnostic challenge because it can grow on aerobically incubated agar media. The correct identification can be made once spores are observed and it is determined that the organism grows better anaerobically.

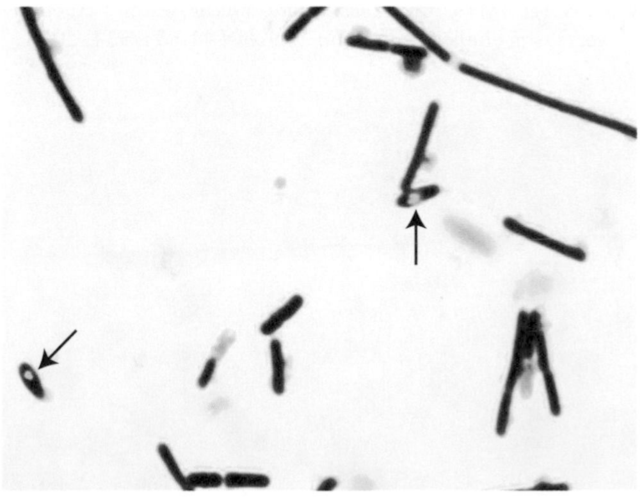

FIGURE 40–10. *Clostridium septicum:* Note the spores *(arrows)* within the rods.

TABLE 40–6. Virulence Factors Associated with Other Clostridial Species

Species and Their Virulence Factors	Biologic Activity
C. septicum	
α-Toxin	Necrotizing, hemolytic toxin
β-Toxin	Heat-stable deoxyribonuclease
γ-Toxin	Hyaluronidase
δ-Toxin	Oxygen-labile hemolysin
Neuraminidase	Alters cell membrane glycoproteins
C. sordellii	
Lecithinase	Phospholipase C
Hemolysin	Oxygen-labile hemolytic activity
Fibrinolysin	Tissue destruction
Lethal β-toxin	Necrotic enterotoxin activity
Hemorrhagic toxin	Hemorrhagic cytotoxin activity
C. histolyticum	
α-Toxin	Necrotizing (not hemolytic) toxin
β-Toxin	Collagenase
γ-Toxin	Protease
δ-Toxin	Elastase
ε-Toxin	Oxygen-labile hemolysin
C. novyi	
α-Toxin	Necrotizing toxin
β-Toxin	Lecithinase; necrotizing, hemolytic toxin
γ-Toxin	Lecithinase; necrotizing, hemolytic toxin
δ-Toxin	Oxygen-labile hemolysin
ε-Toxin	Lipase
ζ-Toxin	Hemolysin
η-Toxin	Tropomyosinase (degrades muscle proteins myosin and tropomyosin)
θ-Toxin	Lecithinase
C. baratii	
Botulinum toxin	Neurotoxin
C. butyricum	
Botulinum toxin	Neurotoxin

CASE STUDY AND QUESTIONS

A 61-year-old woman with left-sided face pain came to the emergency department of a local hospital. She was unable to open her mouth because of facial muscle spasms and had been unable to eat for 4 days because of severe pain in her jaw. Her attending physician had noted trismus and risus sardonicus.

The patient reported that 1 week before presentation, she had incurred a puncture wound to her toe while walking in her garden. She had cleaned the wound and removed small pieces of wood from it, but she had not sought medical attention. Although she had received tetanus immunizations as a child, she had not had a booster vaccination since she was 15 years old. The presumptive diagnosis of tetanus was made.

1. How should this diagnosis be confirmed?
2. What is the recommended procedure for treating this patient? Should management wait until the laboratory results are available? What is the long-term prognosis for this patient?
3. Compare the mode of action of the toxins produced by *C. tetani* and *C. botulinum*.
4. What virulence factors are produced by *C. perfringens*?
5. *C. perfringens* causes what diseases?
6. *C. difficile* causes what diseases? Why is it difficult to manage infections caused by this organism?

Biography

Bongaerts G, Lyerly D: Role of toxins A and B in the pathogenesis of *Clostridium difficile* disease, *Microb Pathog* 17:1-12, 1994.

Boone J, Carman R: *Clostridium perfringens*: Food poisoning and antibiotic-associated diarrhea, *Clin Microbiol Newsletter* 19:65-67, 1997.

Bryant A et al: Clostridial gas gangrene. I and II, *J Infect Dis* 182:799-807, 808-815, 2000.

Calabi E et al: Binding of *Clostridium difficile* surface layer proteins to gastrointestinal tissues, *Infect Immun* 70:5770-5778, 2002.

Gergen P et al: A population-based serologic survey of immunity to tetanus in the United States, *N Engl J Med* 332:761-766, 1995.

Johnson EA: *Clostridium botulinum* and *Clostridium tetani*. In *Topley & Wilson's microbiology and microbial infections: Bacteriology*, ed 10, vol 1, London, 2005, Hodder Arnold (in press).

Kelly C, LaMont JT: *Clostridium difficile* infection, *Annu Rev Med* 49:375-390, 1998.

Lalli G et al: The journey of tetanus and botulinum neurotoxins in neurons, *Trends Microbiol* 11:431-437, 2003.

Midura T: Update: Infant botulism, *Clin Microbiol Rev* 9:119-125, 1996.

Shapiro R, Hatheway C, Swerdlow D: Botulism in the United States: A clinical and epidemiologic review, *Ann Intern Med* 129:221-228, 1998.

Stevens DL, Bryant AE: The role of clostridial toxins in the pathogenesis of gas gangrene, *Clin Infect Dis* 35(suppl1):S93-100, 2002.

Stevens DL et al: Spontaneous, nontraumatic gangrene due to *Clostridium septicum*, *Rev Infect Dis* 12:286-296, 1990.

Wilkins TD, Lyerly DM: *Clostridium difficile* testing: After 20 years, still challenging, *J Clin Microbiol* 41:531-534, 2003.

CHAPTER 41

Anaerobic, Non–Spore-Forming, Gram-Positive Bacteria

The anaerobic gram-positive cocci and non–spore-forming rods are a heterogeneous group of bacteria that characteristically colonize the skin and mucosal surfaces. These organisms are opportunistic pathogens, typically responsible for endogenous infections and usually recovered in mixtures of aerobic and anaerobic bacteria. Additionally, most of these anaerobes have fastidious nutritional requirements and grow slowly on laboratory media. Thus the isolation and identification of individual strains are difficult and often time consuming. Fortunately, the appropriate management and treatment of most infections with these organisms can be based on the knowledge that a mixture of aerobic and anaerobic organisms is present in the clinical specimen and does not require the isolation and identification of the individual organisms.

Anaerobic Gram-Positive Cocci (Box 41–1)

In the fourth edition of this textbook, all clinically significant anaerobic cocci were included in the genus *Peptostreptococcus*. Unfortunately, it was recognized that these organisms were organized in a single genus based primarily on their Gram stain morphology and inability to grow aerobically. More sophisticated methods have since been used to reclassify many of these species into new genera. The most common isolates are listed in Table 41–1. Although some anaerobic cocci are more virulent than others and some are associated with specific diseases, biochemical separation of the different genera is generally unnecessary and knowledge that an anaerobic coccus is associated with an infection is typically sufficient.

The anaerobic gram-positive cocci normally colonize the oral cavity, gastrointestinal tract, genitourinary tract, and skin. They produce infections when they spread from these sites to normally sterile sites. For example, bacteria colonizing the upper airways can cause sinusitis and pleuropulmonary infections; bacteria in the intestines can cause intraabdominal infections; bacteria in the genitourinary tract can cause endometritis, pelvic abscesses, and salpingitis; bacteria on the skin can cause cellulitis and soft-tissue infections; and bacteria that invade the blood can produce infections in bones and solid organs (Figure 41–1).

Laboratory confirmation of infections with anaerobic cocci is complicated by the following three factors: (1) care must be taken to prevent contamination of the clinical specimen with the anaerobic cocci that normally colonize the mucosal surface; (2) the collected specimen must be transported in an oxygen-free container to prevent loss of the organisms; and (3) specimens should be cultured on nutritionally enriched media for a prolonged period (i.e., 5 to 7 days).

Additionally, some species of staphylococci and streptococci grow initially in an anaerobic atmosphere only and may be mistaken for anaerobic cocci. However, these organisms eventually grow well in air supplemented with 10% carbon dioxide (CO_2), so they cannot be classified as anaerobes.

Anaerobic cocci are usually susceptible to penicillin, metronidazole, imipenem, and chloramphenicol. They have intermediate susceptibility to broad-spectrum cephalosporins, clindamycin, erythromycin, and the tetracyclines, and are resistant to the aminoglycosides (as are all anaerobes). Specific therapy is generally indicated in monomicrobic infections; however, because most infections with these organisms are polymicrobic, broad-spectrum therapy against aerobic and anaerobic bacteria is usually selected.

BOX 41–1. Important Anaerobic Gram-Positive Bacteria

Organism	Historical Derivation
Anaerobic Cocci	
Anaerococcus	*an*, without; *aer*, air; *coccus*, berry or coccus (anaerobic coccus)
Finegoldia	Named after the American microbiologist S. Finegold
Micromonas	*micro*, tiny; *monas*, cell (tiny cell)
Peptostreptococcus	*pepto*, cook or digest (the digesting streptococcus)
Schleiferella	Named after the German microbiologist K.H. Schleifer
Anaerobic Rods	
Actinomyces	*aktinos*, ray; *mykes*, fungus (ray fungus referring to the radial arrangement of filaments in granules)
Bifidobacterium	*bifidus*, cleft; *bakterion*, small rod (a small clefted or bifurcated rod)
Eubacterium	*eu*, good or beneficial (a beneficial rod; that is, a rod normally present)
Lactobacillus	*lacto*, milk (milk bacillus; organism originally recovered in milk; also, lactic acid is the primary metabolic product of fermentation)
Mobiluncus	*mobilis*, capable of movement or being active; *uncus*, hook (motile, curved rod)
Propionibacterium propionicum	propionic acid (propionic acid is the primary metabolic product of fermentation)

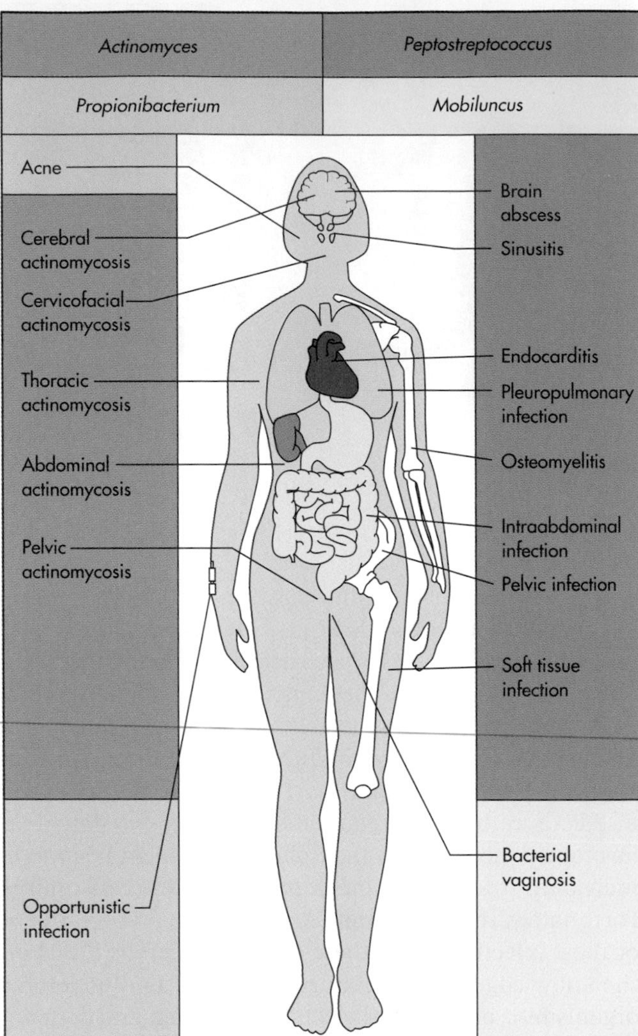

FIGURE 41–1. Diseases associated with anaerobic cocci, *Actinomyces, Propionibacterium,* and *Mobiluncus,* which are all anaerobic, non–spore-forming, gram-positive rods.

TABLE 41–1. New Classification of Selected Anaerobic Cocci Formerly in the Genus *Peptostreptococcus*

Former Classification	New Classification
P. anaerobius	Unchanged
P. asaccharolyticus	*Schleiferella asaccharolytica*
P. magnus	*Finegoldia magna*
P. micros	*Micromonas micros*
P. prevotii	*Anaerococcus prevotii*

Anaerobic, Non–Spore-Forming, Gram-Positive Rods (see Box 41–1)

The non–spore-forming, gram-positive rods are a diverse collection of facultatively anaerobic or strictly anaerobic bacteria that colonize the skin and mucosal surfaces (Table 41–2). *Actinomyces, Mobiluncus, Lactobacillus,* and *Propionibacterium* are well-recognized opportunistic pathogens, whereas members of the genera *Bifidobacterium* and *Eubacterium* can be isolated in clinical specimens but rarely cause human disease.

TABLE 41–2. Anaerobic, Non–Spore-Forming, Gram-Positive Rods

Anaerobic Rods	Human Disease
Actinomyces spp.	Actinomycosis (cervicofacial, thoracic, abdominal, pelvic, central nervous system)
Propionibacterium spp.	Acne, lacrimal canaliculitis, opportunistic infections
Mobiluncus spp.	Bacterial vaginosis, opportunistic infections
Lactobacillus spp.	Endocarditis, opportunistic infections
Eubacterium spp.	Opportunistic infections
Bifidobacterium spp.	Opportunistic infections

Actinomyces

PHYSIOLOGY AND STRUCTURE

Actinomyces organisms are facultatively anaerobic or strictly anaerobic, gram-positive rods. They are not acid-fast (in contrast to the morphologically similar *Nocardia* species), they grow slowly in culture, and they tend to produce chronic, slowly developing infections. They typically develop delicate filamentous forms or hyphae (resembling fungi) in clinical specimens or when isolated in culture (Figure 41–2). However, these organisms are true bacteria in that they lack mitochondria and a nuclear membrane, reproduce by fission, and are inhibited by penicillin but not antifungal antibiotics. Numerous species have been described; *Actinomyces israelii, Actinomyces meyeri, Actinomyces naeslundii, Actinomyces odontolyticus,* and *Actinomyces viscosus* are responsible for most human infections. Only *A. meyeri* is a strict anaerobe. The other species grow best in anaerobic conditions but can grow aerobically.

PATHOGENESIS AND IMMUNITY

Actinomyces organisms colonize the upper respiratory, gastrointestinal, and female genital tracts. These bacteria are not normally present on the skin surface. The organisms have a low virulence potential and cause disease only when the normal mucosal barriers are disrupted by trauma, surgery, or infection.

Disease caused by actinomyces is termed **actinomycosis** (in keeping with the original idea that these organisms were fungi or "mycoses"). Actinomycosis is characterized by the development of chronic granulomatous lesions that become suppurative and form abscesses connected by sinus tracts. Macroscopic colonies of organisms resembling grains of sand can frequently be seen in the abscesses and sinus tracts. These colonies, called **sulfur granules** because they appear yellow or orange, are masses of filamentous organisms bound together by calcium phosphate (Figure 41–3). The areas of suppuration are surrounded by fibrosing granulation tissue, which gives the surface overlying the involved tissues a hard or woody consistency.

EPIDEMIOLOGY

Actinomycosis is an endogenous infection with no evidence of person-to-person spread or disease originating from an external source, such as soil or water. Disease is classified according to the organ systems involved. Cervicofacial infections are seen in patients who have poor oral hygiene or have undergone an invasive dental procedure or oral trauma. In these patients, the actinomyces that are present in the mouth invade into the diseased tissue and initiate the infectious process.

Patients with thoracic infections generally have a history of aspiration, with the disease becoming established in the lungs and then spreading to adjoining tissues. Abdominal infections most commonly occur in patients who have undergone gastrointestinal surgery or have suffered trauma to the bowel. Pelvic infection can be a secondary manifestation of abdominal actinomycosis or may be a primary infection in a woman with an intrauterine device (Figure 41–4). Central nervous system infections usually represent hematogenous spread from another infected tissue, such as the lungs.

CLINICAL DISEASES

Most cases of actinomycosis are the **cervicofacial** type (Figure 41–5). The disease may occur as an acute, pyogenic infection or, more commonly, as a slowly evolving, relatively painless process. The finding of tissue swelling

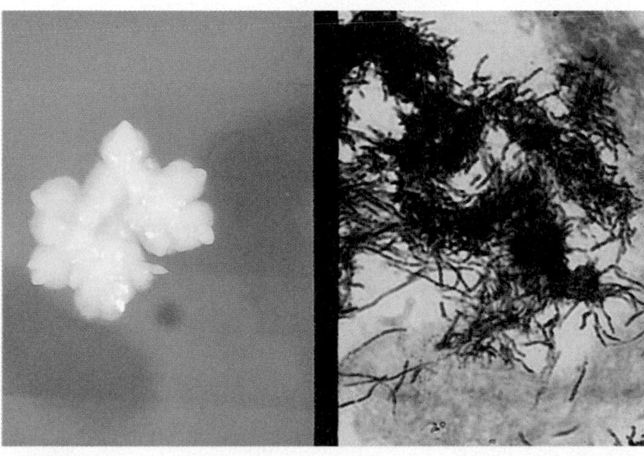

FIGURE 41–2. Macroscopic colony *(left)* and Gram stain *(right)* of *Actinomyces.*

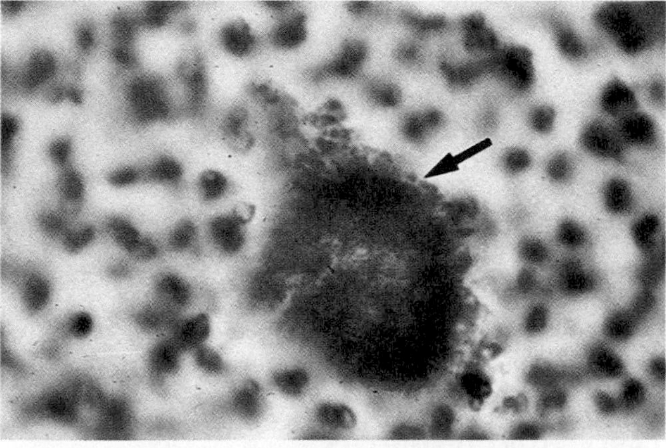

FIGURE 41–3. Sulfur granule collected from the sinus tract in a patient with actinomycosis. Delicate filamentous rods *(arrow)* are seen at the periphery of the crushed granule.

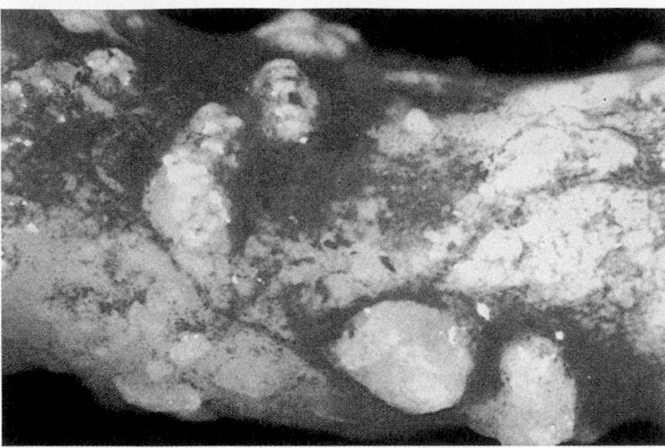

FIGURE 41–4. *Actinomyces* species can colonize the surface of foreign bodies, such as this intrauterine device, leading to the development of pelvic actinomycosis. (From Smith E: In Lambert H, Farrar W, editors: *Infectious diseases illustrated,* London, 1982, Gower.)

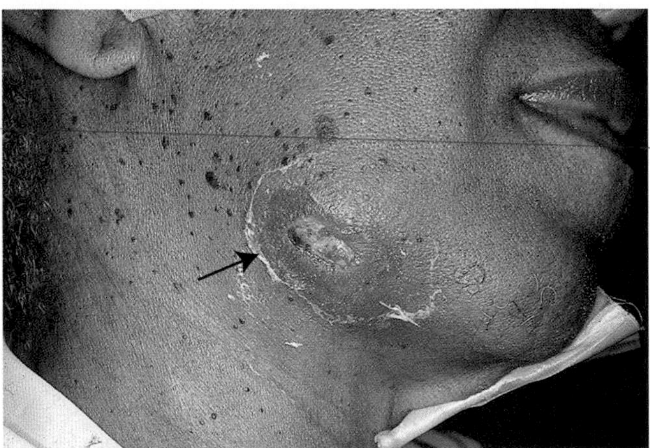

FIGURE 41–5. This patient is suffering from cervicofacial actinomycosis. Note the draining sinus tract.

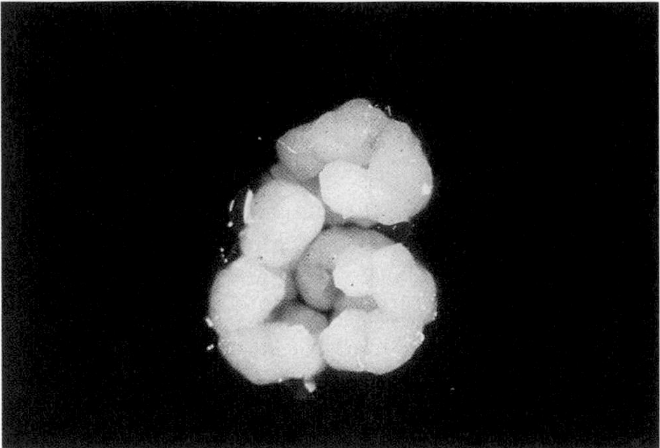

FIGURE 41–6. Molar tooth appearance of *Actinomyces israelii* after incubation for 1 week. This colonial morphology serves as a reminder that the bacteria are normally found in the mouth.

with fibrosis and scarring, as well as draining sinus tracts along the angle of the jaw and neck, should alert the physician to the possibility of actinomycosis. Symptoms of **thoracic actinomycosis** are nonspecific. Abscesses may form in the lung tissue early in the disease and then spread into adjoining tissues as the disease progresses. **Abdominal actinomycosis** can spread throughout the abdomen, potentially involving virtually every organ system. **Pelvic actinomycosis** can occur as a relatively benign form of vaginitis or, more commonly, there can be extensive tissue destruction, including the development of tuboovarian abscesses or ureteral obstruction. The most common manifestation of **central nervous system actinomycosis** is a solitary brain abscess, but meningitis, subdural empyema, and epidural abscess are also seen.

LABORATORY DIAGNOSIS

Laboratory confirmation of actinomycosis is often difficult. Care must be used during collection of clinical specimens that they not become contaminated with actinomyces that are part of the normal bacterial population on mucosal surfaces. The significance of actinomyces isolated from contaminated specimens cannot be determined. Because the organisms are concentrated in sulfur granules and are sparse in involved tissues, a large amount of tissue or pus should be collected. If sulfur granules are detected in a sinus tract or in tissue, the granule should be crushed between two glass slides, stained, and examined microscopically. Thin, gram-positive, branching rods can be seen along the periphery of the granules.

Actinomyces are fastidious and grow slowly under anaerobic conditions; it can take 2 weeks or more for the organisms to be isolated. Colonies appear white and have a domed surface that can become irregular after incubation for a week or more, resembling the top of a molar (Figure 41–6). The individual species of actinomyces can be differentiated by biochemical tests; however, this process can be time consuming. Generally, it is necessary to determine only that the isolate is a member of the genus *Actinomyces*.

Recovery of actinomyces in blood cultures should be evaluated carefully. Most isolates represent transient, insignificant bacteremia from the oropharynx or gastrointestinal tract. If the isolate is clinically significant, evidence of tissue pathology should be obtained.

TREATMENT, PREVENTION, AND CONTROL

Treatment for actinomycosis involves the combination of surgical débridement of the involved tissues and the prolonged administration of antibiotics. Actinomyces are uniformly susceptible to penicillin (considered the antibiotic of choice), erythromycin, and clindamycin. Most species are resistant to metronidazole, and the tetracyclines have variable activity. An undrained focus should be suspected in patients with infections that do not appear to respond to prolonged therapy (e.g., 4 to 12 months). The clinical response is generally good even in patients who have suffered extensive tissue destruction. Maintenance of good oral hygiene and the use of appropriate antibiotic prophylaxis when the mouth or gastrointestinal tract is penetrated can lower the risk of these infections.

Propionibacterium

Propionibacteria are small gram-positive rods often arranged in short chains or clumps (Figure 41–7). They are commonly found on the skin (in contrast with the actinomyces), conjunctiva, external ear, and in the oropharynx and female genital tract. The organisms are anaerobic or aerotolerant, nonmotile, catalase positive, and capable of fermenting carbohydrates, producing propionic acid as their major by-product (hence the name). The two most commonly isolated species are *Propionibacterium acnes* and *Propionibacterium propionicus*.

P. acnes is responsible for two types of infections: (1) acne (as the name implies) in teenagers and young adults and (2) opportunistic infections in patients with prosthetic devices (e.g., artificial heart valves or joints) or intravascular lines (e.g., catheters, cerebrospinal fluid shunts). Propionibacteria are also commonly isolated in blood cultures, but this finding usually represents contamination with bacteria on the skin at the phlebotomy site.

The central role of *P. acnes* in acne is to stimulate an inflammatory response. Production of a low–molecular-weight peptide by the bacteria residing in sebaceous follicles attracts leukocytes. The bacteria are phagocytized and, after release of bacterial hydrolytic enzymes (lipases, proteases, neuraminidase, and hyaluronidase), stimulate a localized inflammatory response. When injected into experimental animals, *P. propionicus* causes lacrimal canaliculitis (inflammation of the tear duct) and abscesses.

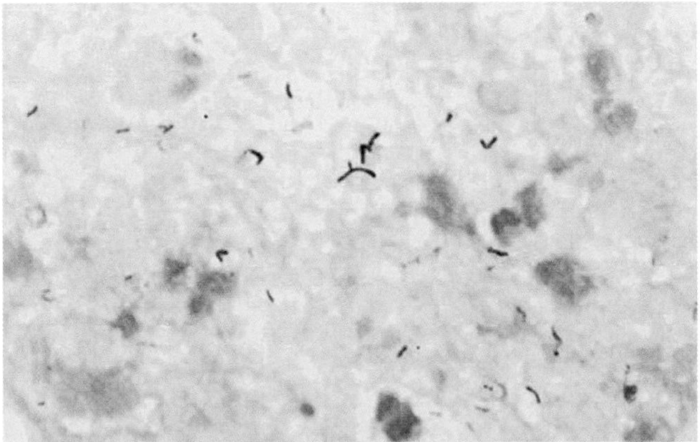

FIGURE 41–7. Gram stain of *Propionibacterium* in a blood culture.

Propionibacteria can grow on most common media, although it may take 2 to 5 days for growth to appear. Care must be taken to avoid contamination of the specimen with the organisms normally found on the skin. The significance of the recovery of an isolate must also be interpreted in light of the clinical presentation (e.g., a catheter or other foreign body can serve as a focus for these opportunistic pathogens).

Acne is unrelated to the effectiveness of skin cleansing because the lesion develops within the sebaceous follicles. For this reason, acne is managed primarily through the topical application of benzoyl peroxide and antibiotics. Antibiotics such as erythromycin and clindamycin have proved effective for treatment.

Mobiluncus

Members of the genus *Mobiluncus* are obligate anaerobic, gram-variable or gram-negative, curved rods with tapered ends. Despite their appearance in Gram-stained specimens (Figure 41–8), they are classified as gram-positive rods because they (1) have a gram-positive cell wall, (2) lack endotoxin, and (3) are susceptible to vancomycin, clindamycin, erythromycin, and ampicillin but resistant to colistin. The organisms are fastidious, growing slowly even on enriched media supplemented with rabbit or horse serum.

Two species, *Mobiluncus curtisii* and *Mobiluncus mulieris*, have been identified in humans. The organisms colonize the genital tract in low numbers but are abundant in women with **bacterial vaginosis** (vaginitis). Their microscopic appearance is a useful marker for this disease, but the precise role of these organisms in the pathogenesis of bacterial vaginosis is unclear.

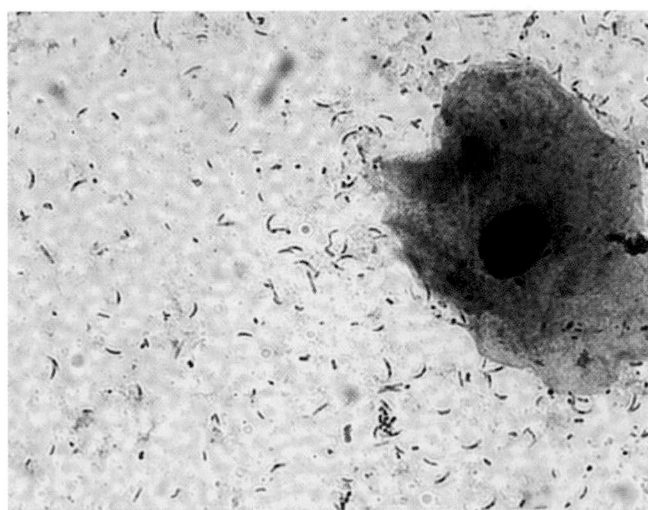

FIGURE 41–8. Gram stain of *Mobiluncus*. The cells are curved and have pointed ends.

Lactobacillus

Lactobacillus species are facultatively anaerobic or strictly anaerobic rods. They are found as part of the normal flora of the mouth, stomach, intestines, and genitourinary tract. The organisms are most commonly isolated in urine specimens and blood cultures. Because lactobacilli are the most common organism in the urethra, their recovery in urine cultures usually is a result of contamination of the specimen, even when large numbers of the organisms are present. The reason lactobacilli rarely cause infections of the urinary tract is their inability to grow in urine. Invasion into blood occurs in one of the following three settings: (1) transient bacteremia from a genitourinary source (e.g., after childbirth or a gynecologic procedure), (2) endocarditis, and (3) opportunistic septicemia in an immunocompromised patient.

Treatment of endocarditis and opportunistic infections is difficult because lactobacilli are resistant to vancomycin (an antibiotic commonly active against gram-positive bacteria) and are inhibited but not killed by other antibiotics. A combination of penicillin with an aminoglycoside is required for bactericidal activity.

Bifidobacterium and *Eubacterium*

Bifidobacterium and *Eubacterium* species are commonly found in the oropharynx, large intestine, and vagina. These bacteria can be isolated in clinical specimens but have a very low virulence potential and usually represent clinically insignificant contaminants. Confirmation of their etiologic role in an infection requires their repeated isolation in large numbers from multiple specimens and the absence of other pathogenic organisms.

CASE STUDY AND QUESTIONS

A 41-year-old man entered the university hospital for the treatment of a chronically draining wound in his jaw. The patient had undergone extraction of many teeth 3 months before admission and had poor oral hygiene and fetid breath at the time of admission. Multiple pustular nodules were observed overlying the carious teeth, and some nodules had ruptured. The drainage material consisted of serosanguineous fluid containing small, hard granules.

1. The diagnosis of actinomycosis is considered. How would you collect and transport specimens for confirmation of this diagnosis? What diagnostic tests can be performed?
2. Describe the epidemiology of actinomycosis. What is the risk factor for this patient?
3. What diseases does *Propionibacterium* cause? What is the most common source of this organism?

Bibliography

Antonio M, Hawes S, Hillier S: The identification of vaginal *Lactobacillus* species and the demographic and microbiologic characteristics of women colonized by these species, *J Infect Dis* 180:1950-1956, 1999.

Antony S, Stratton C, Dummer S: *Lactobacillus* bacteremia: Description of the clinical course in adult patients without endocarditis, *Clin Infect Dis* 23:773-778, 1996.

Brook I, Frazier EH: Infections caused by *Propionibacterium* species, *Rev Infect Dis* 3:819-822, 1991.

Fruchart C et al: *Lactobacillus* species as emerging pathogens in neutropenic patients, *Eur J Clin Microbiol Infect Dis* 16:681-684, 1997.

Hofstad T: Current taxonomy of medically important nonsporing anaerobes, *Rev Infect Dis* 12(suppl):122-126, 1990.

Hollick G: Isolation and identification of aerobic actinomycetes, *Clin Microbiol Newsletter* 17:25-29, 1995.

Murdoch D: Gram-positive anaerobic cocci, *Clin Microbiol Rev* 11:81-120, 1998.

Pulverer G, Schutt-Gerowitt H, Schaal KP. Human cervicofacial Actinomycoses: Microbiological data for 1997 cases, *Clin Infect Dis* 37:490-497, 2003.

Smego RA: Actinomycosis of the central nervous system, *Rev Infect Dis* 9:855-865, 1987.

Spiegel CA: Bacterial vaginosis, *Clin Microbiol Rev* 4:485-502, 1991.

Stackebrandt E, Rainey F, Ward-Rainey N: Proposal for a new hierarchic classification system, *Actinobacteria classis* nov., *Int J Syst Bacteriol* 47:479-491, 1997.

Tiveljung A, Forsum U, Monstein H-J: Classification of the genus *Mobiluncus* based on comparative partial 16S rRNA gene analysis, *Int J Syst Bacteriol* 46:332-336, 1996.

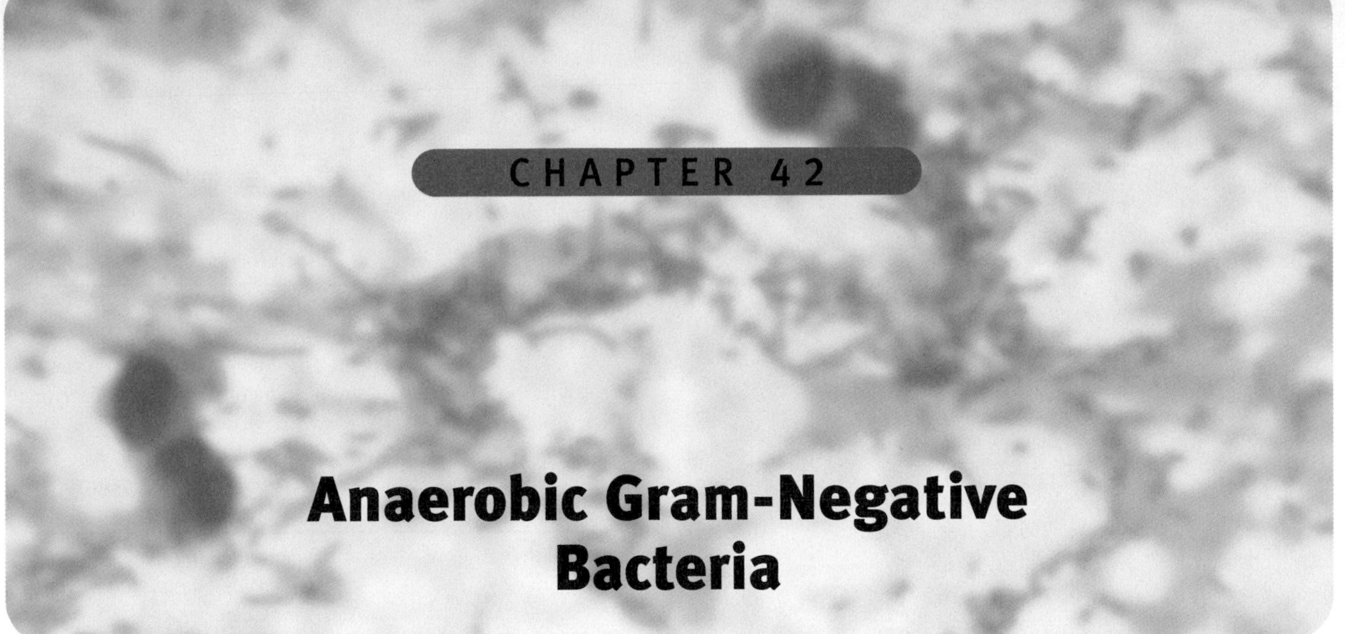

Anaerobic Gram-Negative Bacteria

With each edition of this textbook, the number of genera of anaerobic gram-negative rods and gram-negative cocci has expanded. Many new genera represent reclassification of well-known organisms, and some represent newly discovered bacteria. The most important gram-negative anaerobes that colonize the human upper respiratory, gastrointestinal, and genitourinary tracts are the rods in the genera *Bacteroides, Fusobacterium, Porphyromonas,* and *Prevotella* and the cocci in the genus *Veillonella* (Box 42–1). Anaerobes are the predominant bacteria at each of these sites, outnumbering aerobic bacteria tenfold to 1000-fold. The diversity of species is also great, with as many as 500 different species of bacteria estimated to colonize the periodontal pocket, many of which are anaerobes. Despite the abundance and diversity of these bacteria, most infections are caused by relatively few species (Table 42–1). Among these pathogens, the most important is *Bacteroides fragilis,* the prototypical endogenous anaerobic pathogen.

Physiology and Structure

At one time the genus *Bacteroides* consisted of almost 50 species, but many of these species have been transferred to new genera. A characteristic common to the current species remaining in the genus *Bacteroides* is that their growth is stimulated by 20% bile. In contrast, bile-susceptible species were reclassified into other genera, such as *Porphyromonas* (pigmented, asaccharolytic rods) and *Prevotella* (pigmented and nonpigmented, saccharolytic rods).

B. fragilis, the most important member of this genus, is pleomorphic in size and shape and resembles a mixed population of organisms in a casually examined Gram stain (Figure 42–1). Other gram-negative rods can be very small (e.g., *Prevotella* species) or elongated (e.g., *Fusobacterium;* Figure 42–2). Most gram-negative anaerobes respond weakly to Gram stain, so stained specimens must be carefully examined. Although *Bacteroides* species grow rapidly in culture, the other anaerobic gram-negative rods are fastidious, and cultures may have to be incubated for 3 days or longer before the bacteria can be detected.

Bacteroides have a typical gram-negative cell wall structure, which can be surrounded by a polysaccharide capsule. A major component of the cell wall is a surface lipopolysaccharide (LPS). In contrast to the LPS molecules in *Fusobacterium* and the aerobic gram-negative rods, however, the *Bacteroides* glycolipid has little or no endotoxin activity. This is because the lipid A component of LPS lacks phosphate groups on the glucosamine residues and the number of fatty acids linked to the amino sugars is reduced; both factors are correlated with the loss of pyrogenic activity.

The anaerobic gram-negative cocci are rarely isolated in clinical specimens, except when present as contaminants. Members of the genus *Veillonella* are the predominant anaerobes in the oropharynx, but they represent less than 1% of all anaerobes isolated in clinical specimens. The other anaerobic cocci are rarely isolated.

Pathogenesis and Immunity

Despite the variety of anaerobic species that colonize the human body, relatively few are responsible for causing disease. For example, *Bacteroides distasonis* and *Bacteroides thetaiotaomicron* are the predominant species of *Bacteroides* found in the gastrointestinal tract; however, the majority of intraabdominal infections are associated with

BOX 42–1. Important Gram-Negative Anaerobes

Organism	Historical Derivation
Bacteroides	*bacter,* staff or rod; *idus,* shape (rod shaped)
B. fragilis	*fragilis,* fragile (related to fragile colonies)
B. thetaiotaomicron	from the Greek letters theta, iota, omicron
B. distasonis	*distasonis,* Distaso (named after A. Distaso, a Romanian bacteriologist)
Fusobacterium	*fusus,* a spindle; *bakterion,* a small rod (a small, spindle-shaped rod)
F. nucleatum	*nucleatum,* having a kernel or nucleated (refers to the "flecked" or ground-glass appearance of colonies)
F. necrophorum	*necros,* dead; *phorum,* bearing (necrosis producing)
Porphyromonas	*porphyreos,* purple; *monas,* unit (pigmented rods)
P. asaccharolytica	*a,* not; *sacchar,* sugar; *lyticus,* able to loosen (not digesting sugar; asaccharolytic)
P. gingivalis	*gingivalis,* of the gums
Prevotella	*Prevotella,* named after the French microbiologist A.R. Prevot, a pioneer in anaerobic microbiology
P. intermedia	*intermedius,* intermediate (formerly classified as one of three subspecies of *Bacteroides melaninogenicus:* ssp. *melaninogenicus,* ssp. *intermedius,* and ssp. *asaccharolyticus*)
P. melaninogenica	*melas,* black; *genicus,* producing (producing a black color or colony)
P. bivia	*bivius,* having two ways (pertaining to the saccharolytic and proteolytic activities of the species)
P. disiens	*disiens,* going in two ways (saccharolytic and proteolytic activities)
Veillonella parvula	*Veillonella,* named after A. Veillon, the French bacteriologist who isolated the type species; *parvula,* very small (refers to the size of the cocci—not the bacteriologist!)

TABLE 42–1. Predominant Anaerobic Gram-Negative Bacteria Responsible for Human Disease

Infection	Bacteria
Head and neck	*Bacteroides ureolyticus* *Fusobacterium nucleatum* *Fusobacterium necrophorum* *Porphyromonas asaccharolytica* *Porphyromonas gingivalis* *Prevotella intermedia* *Prevotella melaninogenica* *Veillonella parvula*
Intraabdominal	*Bacteroides fragilis* *Bacteroides thetaiotaomicron* *P. melaninogenica*
Gynecologic	*B. fragilis* *Prevotella bivia* *Prevotella disiens*
Skin and soft tissue	*B. fragilis*
Bacteremia	*B. fragilis* *B. thetaiotaomicron* *Fusobacterium* spp.

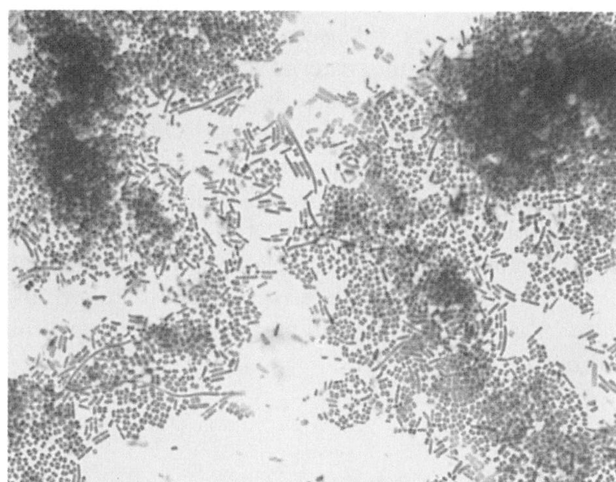

FIGURE 42–1. *Bacteroides fragilis.* Organisms appear as faintly staining, pleomorphic, gram-negative rods.

B. fragilis, an organism that is a minor member of the gastrointestinal flora. The enhanced virulence of this and other pathogenic anaerobes is attributed to a variety of virulence factors that facilitate adherence of the organisms to host tissues, protection from the host immune response, and tissue destruction (Table 42–2).

ADHESINS

B. fragilis and *Prevotella melaninogenica* strains can adhere to peritoneal surfaces more effectively than other anaerobes because their surface is covered with a polysaccharide capsule. *B. fragilis* and other *Bacteroides* species and *Porphyromonas gingivalis* can adhere to epithelial cells and extracellular molecules (e.g., fibrinogen, fibronectin, lactoferrin) by means of fimbriae. The fimbriae of *P. gingivalis* are also important for inducing expression of proinflammatory cytokines, such as tumor necrosis factor-α (TNF-α) and interleukin-1β (IL-1β).

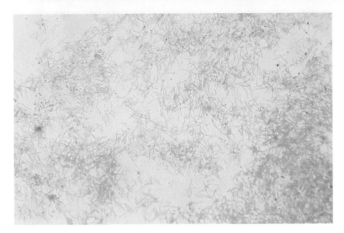

FIGURE 42–2. *Fusobacterium nucleatum.* Organisms are thin, faintly staining, and elongated with tapered ends (e.g., fusiform).

PROTECTION AGAINST PHAGOCYTOSIS

The capsular polysaccharide of these organisms is antiphagocytic like other bacterial capsules. In addition, the short-chain fatty acids (e.g., succinic acid) produced during anaerobic metabolism inhibit phagocytosis and intracellular killing. Finally, proteases are produced by some *Porphyromonas* and *Prevotella* species that degrade immunoglobulins.

PROTECTION AGAINST OXYGEN TOXICITY

Generally, anaerobes capable of causing disease can tolerate exposure to oxygen. Catalase and superoxide dismutase, which inactivate hydrogen peroxide and the superoxide free radicals (O_2^-), respectively, are present in many pathogenic strains.

TISSUE DESTRUCTION

A variety of cytotoxic enzymes have been associated with gram-negative anaerobes. Many of these enzymes are found in both virulent and avirulent isolates. Nonetheless, the ability of these organisms to cause tissue destruction, inactivate immunoglobulins, and resist oxygen toxicity (superoxide dismutase) most likely plays an important role in the pathogenesis of anaerobic infections.

TOXIN PRODUCTION

Strains of enterotoxigenic *B. fragilis* that cause diarrheal disease produce a heat-labile zinc metalloprotease toxin (*B. fragilis* toxin [BFT]). This toxin causes morphologic changes of the intestinal epithelium via F-actin rearrangement, with the resultant stimulation of chloride secretion and fluid loss.

TABLE 42–2. Virulence Factors in Anaerobic Gram-Negative Rods

Virulence Factor	Bacteria
Adhesins	
Capsule	*Bacteroides fragilis, Prevotella melaninogenica*
Fimbriae	*B. fragilis, Porphyromonas gingivalis*
Hemagglutinin	*P. gingivalis*
Lectin	*Fusobacterium nucleatum*
Resistant to Oxygen Toxicity	
Superoxide dismutase	Many species
Catalase	Many species
Antiphagocytic	
Capsule	*B. fragilis, P. melaninogenica*
Immunoglobulin (Ig)A, IgM, IgG proteases	*Porphyromonas* spp., *Prevotella* spp.
Lipopolysaccharide	*Fusobacterium* sp.
Succinic acid	Many species
Tissue Destruction	
Phospholipase C	*Fusobacterium necrophorum*
Hemolysins	Many species
Proteases	Many species
Collagenase	Many species
Fibrinolysin	Many species
Neuraminidase	Many species
Heparinase	Many species
Chondroitin sulfatase	Many species
Glucuronidases	Many species
N-Acetylglucosaminidase	Many species
Volatile fatty acids	Many species
Toxin	
Enterotoxigenic toxin	*B. fragilis*

Modified from Duerden B: *Clin Infect Dis* 18(suppl 4):S253-S259, 1994; and Lorber B: *Bacteroides, Prevotella, Porphyromonas,* and *Fusobacterium* species. In *Mandell, Douglas and Bennett's principles and practice of infectious diseases,* ed 6, New York, 2005, Churchill Livingstone.

Epidemiology

As already stated, anaerobic gram-negative cocci and rods colonize the human body in large numbers. Their numerous important functions at these sites include stabilizing the resident bacterial flora, preventing colonization by pathogenic organisms from exogenous sources, and aiding in the digestion of food. These normal protective organisms produce serious disease when they move from their endogenous homes to normally sterile sites (i.e., the same as is described for gram-positive, non–spore-forming anaerobes in Chapter 41). Thus the organisms in the resident flora are able to spread by trauma or disease from the normally colonized mucosal surfaces to sterile tissues or fluids.

As expected, these endogenous infections are characterized by the presence of a polymicrobial mixture of organisms. It is important to realize, however, that the mixture of organisms present on healthy mucosal surfaces differs from the mixture in diseased tissues. The difference relates to the virulence potential of pathogenic organisms and their ability to increase from existing in relatively small numbers on mucosal surfaces to being the predominant organisms at the site of infection. For example, *B. fragilis* is commonly associated with pleuropulmonary, intraabdominal, and genital infections. However, the organism constitutes less than 1% of the colonic flora and is rarely isolated from the oropharynx or genital tract of healthy people unless highly selective techniques are used.

Clinical Diseases

RESPIRATORY TRACT INFECTIONS

Nearly half of the chronic infections of the sinuses and ears and virtually all periodontal infections involve mixtures of gram-negative anaerobes, with *Prevotella, Porphyromonas, Fusobacterium,* and non-*fragilis Bacteroides* most commonly isolated. Anaerobes are less commonly associated with infections of the lower respiratory tract unless there is a history of aspiration of oral secretions.

BRAIN ABSCESS

Anaerobic infections of the brain are typically associated with a history of chronic sinusitis or otitis. Such history is confirmed by radiologic evidence of direct extension into the brain. A less common cause of such infections is bacteremic spread from a pulmonary source. In this case, multiple abscesses are present. The most common anaerobes in these polymicrobial infections are species of *Prevotella, Porphyromonas,* and *Fusobacterium* (as well as *Peptostreptococcus* and other anaerobic and aerobic cocci).

INTRAABDOMINAL INFECTIONS

Despite the diverse population of bacteria that colonize the gastrointestinal tract, relatively few species are associated with intraabdominal infections. Anaerobes are recovered in virtually all of these infections, with *B. fragilis* the most common organism (Figure 42–3). Other important anaerobes are *B. thetaiotaomicron* and *P. melaninogenica,* as well as the anaerobic and aerobic gram-positive cocci.

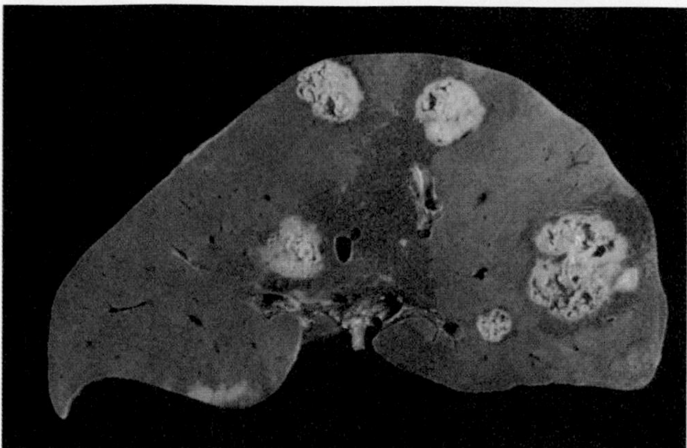

FIGURE 42–3. Liver abscesses caused by *Bacteroides fragilis.*

GYNECOLOGIC INFECTIONS

Mixtures of anaerobes are often responsible for causing infections of the female genital tract (e.g., pelvic inflammatory disease, abscesses, endometritis, surgical wound infections). Although a variety of anaerobes can be isolated in patients with these infections, *Prevotella bivia* and *Prevotella disiens* are the most important; *B. fragilis* is commonly responsible for abscess formation.

SKIN AND SOFT-TISSUE INFECTIONS

Although anaerobic gram-negative bacteria are not part of the normal flora of the skin (in contrast to *Peptostreptococcus* and *Propionibacterium* organisms), they can be introduced by a bite or through contamination of a traumatized surface. In some cases, the organisms may simply colonize a wound without producing disease; in other cases, colonization may quickly progress to life-threatening disease, such as myonecrosis (Figure 42–4). *B. fragilis* is the organism most commonly associated with significant disease.

BACTEREMIA

Anaerobes were at one time responsible for more than 20% of all clinically significant cases of bacteremia; however, these organisms now cause 1% to 3% of such infections. The reduced incidence of disease is not completely understood but probably can be attributed to the widespread use of broad-spectrum antibiotics. *B. fragilis* is the anaerobe most commonly isolated in blood cultures.

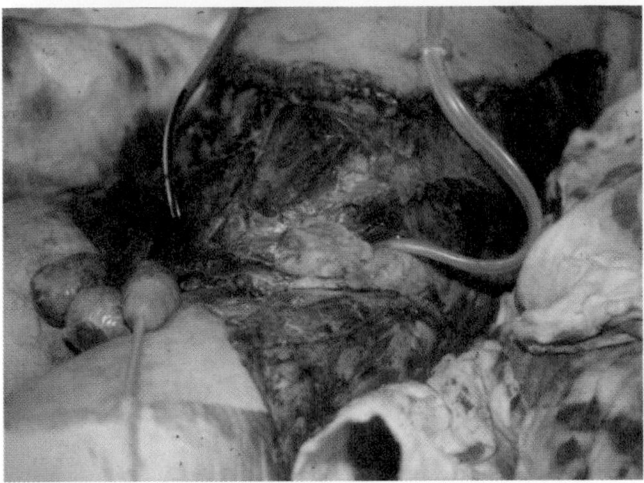

FIGURE 42–4. Synergistic polymicrobial infection involving *Bacteroides fragilis* and other anaerobes. The infection started at the scrotum and rapidly spread up the trunk and down the thighs, with extensive myonecrosis.

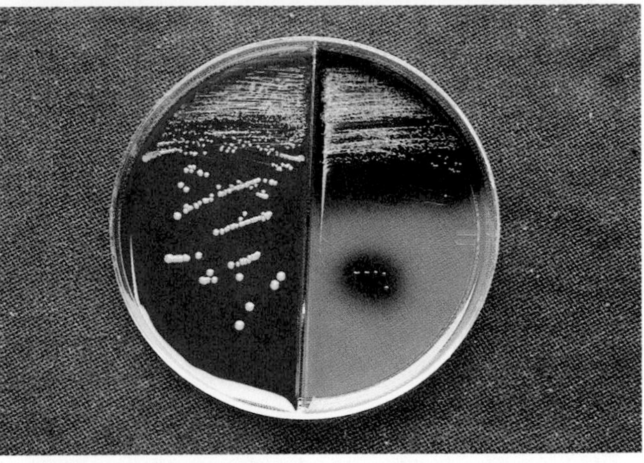

FIGURE 42–5. Growth of *Bacteroides fragilis* on *Bacteroides* bile-esculin agar. Most aerobic and anaerobic bacteria are inhibited by bile and gentamicin in this medium, whereas the *B. fragilis* group of organisms is stimulated by bile, resistant to gentamicin, and able to hydrolyze esculin, producing a black precipitate.

GASTROENTERITIS

Strains of enterotoxin-producing *B. fragilis* can produce a self-limited watery diarrhea. The majority of infections have been observed in children younger than 5 years of age, although disease has also been reported in adults.

Laboratory Diagnosis

MICROSCOPY

Microscopic examination of specimens from patients with suspected anaerobic infections can be useful. Although the bacteria may stain faintly and irregularly, the finding of pleomorphic, gram-negative rods can serve as useful preliminary information.

CULTURE

Specimens should be collected and transported to the laboratory in an oxygen-free system, promptly inoculated onto specific media for the recovery of anaerobes, and incubated in an anaerobic environment. Because most anaerobic infections are endogenous, it is important to collect specimens so that they are not contaminated with the normal bacterial population present on the adjacent mucosal surface. Specimens should also be kept in a moist environment, because drying causes significant bacterial loss.

Most *Bacteroides* grow rapidly and should be detected within 2 days; however, other gram-negative anaerobes may have to be incubated longer. In addition, it is sometimes difficult to recover all clinically significant bacteria because of the different organisms present in polymicrobial infections. The use of selective media, such as media supplemented with bile, has facilitated the recovery of most important anaerobes (Figure 42–5). Additionally, lysed-blood–enriched media stimulates pigment production in organisms such as *Porphyromonas* and *Prevotella* (Figure 42–6).

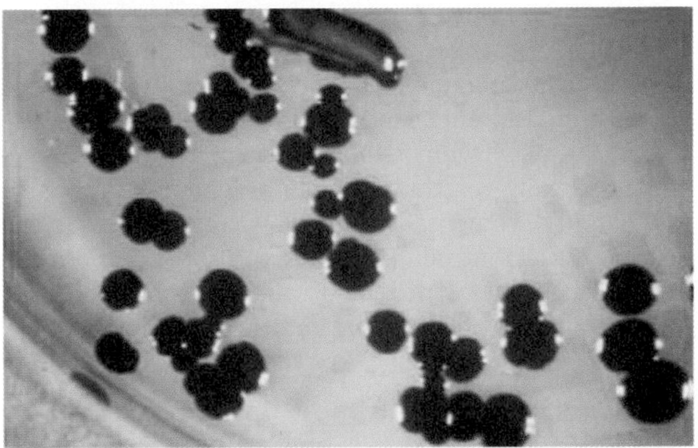

FIGURE 42–6. Growth of *Prevotella* on lysed blood agar. Note the black pigmentation of the colonies.

BIOCHEMICAL IDENTIFICATION

The preliminary identification of the *B. fragilis* group can be made from (1) Gram stain and colonial morphology, (2) resistance to kanamycin, vancomycin, and colistin, and (3) stimulated growth in 20% bile. The definitive identification of this group and other gram-negative anaerobes is made with the use of commercially prepared biochemical systems that measure the activity of preformed enzymes. Gas chromatography has occasionally proved to be a useful, simple technique for detecting metabolic byproducts (short-chain fatty acids) and can be used to supplement biochemical testing.

Treatment, Prevention, and Control

Antibiotic therapy combined with surgical intervention is the main approach for managing serious anaerobic infections. Virtually all members of the *B. fragilis* group, many *Prevotella* and *Porphyromonas* species, and some *Fusobacterium* isolates produce β-lactamases. This enzyme renders the bacteria resistant to penicillin and many cephalosporins. Antibiotics with the best activity against gram-negative anaerobic rods are metronidazole, carbapenems (e.g., imipenem), and β-lactam-β-lactamase inhibitors (e.g., piperacillin-tazobactam). Clindamycin resistance in *Bacteroides*, which is plasmid mediated, has become more prevalent; an average of 20% to 25% of the isolates in the United States are now resistant.

Because *Bacteroides* species constitute an important part of the normal microbial flora, and because infections result from the endogenous spread of the organisms, disease is virtually impossible to control. It is important to recognize, however, that disruption of the natural barriers around the mucosal surfaces by diagnostic or surgical procedures can introduce these organisms into normally sterile sites. If the barriers are invaded, prophylactic treatment with antibiotics may be indicated.

CASE STUDY AND QUESTIONS

A 65-year-old man entered the emergency department of a local hospital. He appeared to be acutely ill, with abdominal tenderness and a temperature of 40°C. The patient was taken to surgery because appendicitis was suspected. A ruptured appendix surrounded by approximately 20 ml of foul-smelling pus was found at laparotomy. The pus was drained and submitted for aerobic and anaerobic bacterial culture analysis. Postoperatively, the patient was started on antibiotic therapy. Gram stain of the specimen revealed a polymicrobial mixture of organisms, and culture was positive for B. fragilis, Escherichia coli, *and* Enterococcus faecalis.

1. Which organism or organisms are responsible for causing the abscess formation? What virulence factors are responsible for causing abscess formation?
2. *B. fragilis* causes infections at what other body sites?
3. What antibiotics should be selected to manage this polymicrobial infection?
4. What other anaerobic gram-negative rods are important causes of human disease?

Bibliography

Aldridge KE et al: Bacteremia due to *Bacteroides fragilis* group: Distribution of species, β-lactamase production, and antimicrobial susceptibility patterns, *Antimicrob Agents Chemother* 47:148-156, 2003.

Aldridge KE, O'Brien M: In vitro susceptibilities of the *Bacteroides fragilis* group species: Change in isolation rates significantly affects overall susceptibility data, *J Clin Microbiol* 40:4349-4352, 2002.

Bjornson AB: Role of humoral factors in host resistance to the *Bacteroides fragilis* group, *Rev Infect Dis* 12:S161-S168, 1990.

Duerden B: Virulence factors in anaerobes, *Clin Infect Dis* 18(suppl 4):S253-S259, 1994.

Finegold SM, Baron EJ, Wexler HM: *A clinical guide to anaerobic infections*, Belmont, Calif, 1992, Star.

Jousimies-Somer H et al: *Bacteroides, Porphyromonas, Prevotella, Fusobacterium*, and other anaerobic gram-negative bacteria. In Murray P et al, editors: *Manual of clinical microbiology*, ed 8, Washington, 2003, American Society for Microbiology.

Jousimies-Somer H, Summanen P: Recent taxonomic changes and terminology update of clinically significant anaerobic gram-negative bacteria (excluding Spirochetes), *Clin Infect Dis* 35(suppl 1):S17-S21, 2002

Lindberg AA et al: Structure-activity relationships in lipopolysaccharides of *Bacteroides fragilis*, *Rev Infect Dis* 12:S133-S140, 1990.

Tessier F et al: Antigenic relationships among *Bacteroides* species studied by rocket-line immunoelectrophoresis, *Int J Syst Bacteriol* 43:191-195, 1993.

Wu S et al: Diversity of the metalloprotease toxin produced by enterotoxigenic *Bacteroides fragilis*, *Infect Immun* 70:2463-2471, 2002.

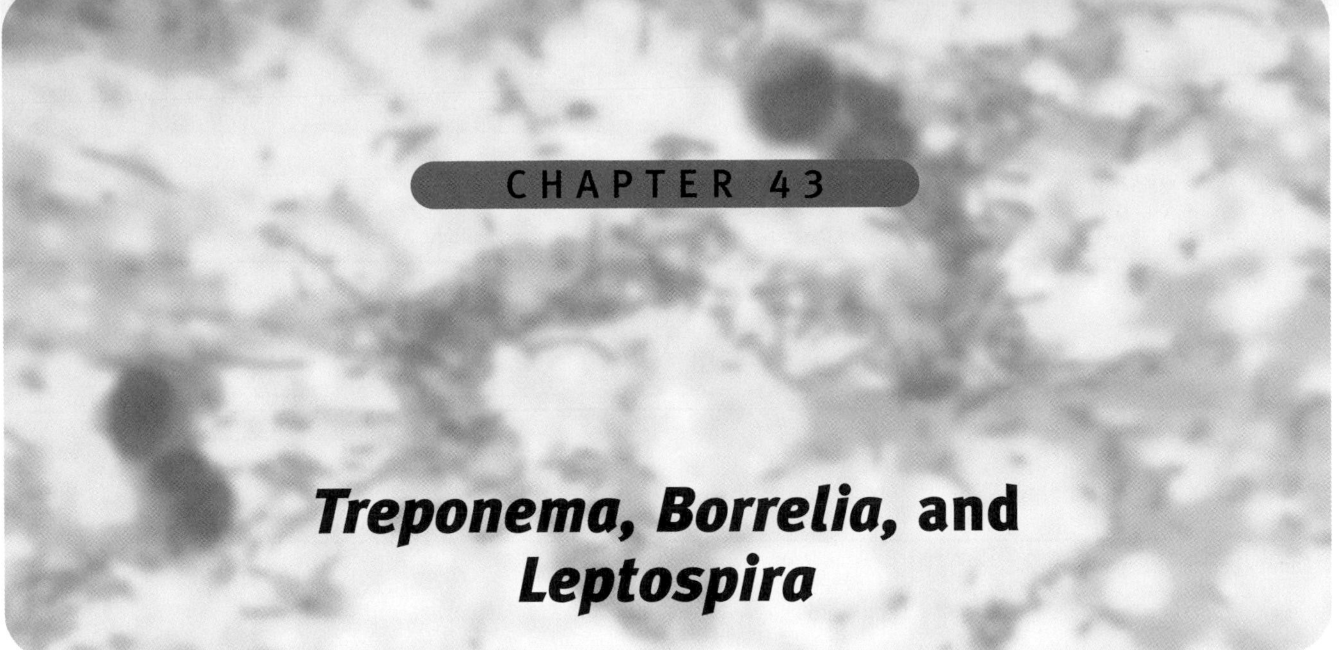

Treponema, Borrelia, and *Leptospira*

The bacteria in the order Spirochaetales have been grouped together on the basis of their common morphologic properties. These spirochetes are thin, helical (0.1 to 0.5 × 5 to 20 μm), gram-negative bacteria. The order Spirochaetales is subdivided into three families and 13 genera, of which three (*Treponema, Borrelia,* and *Leptospira*) are responsible for human disease (Table 43–1, Box 43–1).

Treponema (Box 43–2)

The two treponemal species that cause human disease are *Treponema pallidum* (with three subspecies) and *Treponema carateum.* All are morphologically identical, produce the same serologic response in humans, and are susceptible to penicillin. The organisms are distinguished by their epidemiologic characteristics and clinical presentation. *T. pallidum* subspecies *pallidum* (referred to as *T. pallidum* in this chapter) is the etiologic agent of the venereal disease **syphilis;** *T. pallidum* subspecies *endemicum* causes endemic syphilis **(bejel);** *T. pallidum* subspecies *pertenue* causes **yaws;** and *T. carateum* causes **pinta.** Bejel, yaws, and pinta are nonvenereal diseases. Syphilis is discussed initially; the other treponemal diseases are discussed at the end of the section.

PHYSIOLOGY AND STRUCTURE

T. pallidum and related pathogenic treponemes are thin, tightly coiled spirochetes (0.1 to 0.2 × 6 to 20 μm) with pointed, straight ends. Three periplasmic flagellae are inserted at each end. These spirochetes do not grow in cell-free cultures. Limited growth of the organisms has been achieved in cultured rabbit epithelial cells, but replication is slow (doubling time is 30 hours) and can be maintained for only a few generations. The spirochetes were once considered strict anaerobes; however, it is now known that they can use glucose oxidatively.

The spirochetes are too thin to be seen with light microscopy in specimens stained with Gram or Giemsa stain. However, motile forms can be visualized by darkfield illumination or by staining with specific antitreponemal antibodies labeled with fluorescent dyes.

PATHOGENESIS AND IMMUNITY

The inability to grow *T. pallidum* to high concentrations in vitro has limited detection of specific virulence factors in this organism. However, several investigators have now cloned *T. pallidum* genes in *Escherichia coli* and isolated the protein products. Several gene products have been associated specifically with virulent strains, although their role in pathogenesis remains to be delineated. The outer membrane proteins are associated with adherence to the surface of host cells, and virulent spirochetes produce hyaluronidase, which may facilitate perivascular infiltration. Virulent spirochetes are also coated with host cell fibronectin, which can protect against phagocytosis.

The tissue destruction and lesions observed in syphilis are primarily the consequence of the patient's immune response to infection. The clinical course of syphilis evolves through three phases. The initial or **primary phase** is characterized by one or more skin lesions **(chancres)** at the site where the spirochete penetrated (Figure 43–1). Although spirochetes are disseminated in the blood soon after infection, the chancre represents the primary site of initial replication. Histologic examination of the lesion reveals endarteritis and periarteritis (characteristic of syphilitic lesions at all stages) and infiltration of the ulcer with polymorphonuclear leukocytes and macrophages. Phagocytic cells ingest spirochetes, but the

TABLE 43–1. Medically Important Genera in the Order Spirochaetales

Spirochaetales	Human Disease	Etiologic Agent
Family Spirochaetaceae		
Genus *Borrelia*	Epidemic relapsing fever	*Borrelia recurrentis*
	Endemic relapsing fever	Many *Borrelia* species
	Lyme borreliosis	*Borrelia burgdorferi, Borrelia garinii, Borrelia afzelii*
Genus *Treponema*	Syphilis	*Treponema pallidum* ssp. *pallidum*
	Bejel	*T. pallidum* ssp. *endemicum*
	Yaws	*T. pallidum* ssp. *pertenue*
	Pinta	*Treponema carateum*
Family Leptospiraceae		
Genus *Leptospira*	Leptospirosis	*Leptospira* spp.

BOX 43–1. Important Spirochetes

Organism	Historical Derivation
Treponema	***trepo,*** turn; ***nema,*** a thread (a turning thread; refers to the morphology of the bacteria)
T. pallidum	***pallidum,*** pale (refers to the fact these organisms are not stained with traditional dyes
T. carateum	***carate,*** name of a South American disease, pinta
Borrelia	Named after A. Borrel
B. recurrentis	***recurrens,*** recurring (reference to relapsing fever)
B. hermsii	***hermsii,*** of hermsi (named after the tick vector, *Ornithodoros hermsii*)
B. burgdorferi	Named after W. Burgdorfer
Leptospira	***lepto,*** thin; ***spira,*** a coil (a thin coil; refers to the morphology of the bacteria)

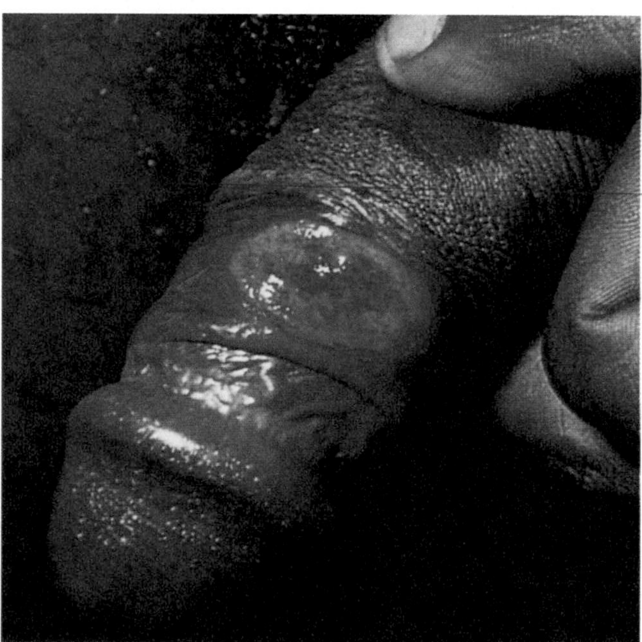

FIGURE 43–1. Primary chancre of the penile shaft. Typically the lesion is painless unless secondary bacterial infection is present. Large numbers of spirochetes are present in the lesion. (From Morse S et al: *Atlas of sexually transmitted diseases and AIDS*, St Louis, 2003, Mosby.)

organisms often survive. In the **secondary phase**, the clinical signs of disseminated disease appear, with prominent skin lesions dispersed over the entire body surface (Figure 43–2). Spontaneous remission may occur after the primary or secondary stages, or the disease may progress to the **late phase** of disease, in which virtually all tissues may be involved. Each stage represents localized multiplication of the spirochete and tissue destruction. Although replication is slow, numerous organisms are present in the initial chancre, as well as in the secondary lesions, making the patient highly infectious at these stages.

EPIDEMIOLOGY

Syphilis is found worldwide and is the third most common sexually transmitted bacterial disease in the United States (after *Chlamydia* and *Neisseria gonorrhoeae* infections). The incidence of disease has decreased since the advent of penicillin therapy in the early 1940s, although periodic increases have been observed that correspond to changes in sexual practices (e.g., use of birth control pills in the 1960s, gay bath houses in the 1970s, increased prostitution related to crack cocaine use in the 1990s). More than 34,000 cases of syphilis were reported in the United States in 2003. However, numerous infections remain unreported, thus contributing to an underestimation of the true incidence of this disease.

Natural syphilis is exclusive to humans and has no other known natural hosts. *T. pallidum* is extremely labile, unable to survive exposure to drying or disinfectants. Thus, syphilis cannot be spread through contact with

BOX 43–2. Summary of *Treponema*

Physiology and Structure

Thin, coiled spirochete (0.1 to 0.2 × 6 to 20 μm)
Cannot be seen with Gram or Giemsa stains; observed by dark-field microscopy
Cannot be grown in vitro except in selected cultured cells

Virulence Factors

Outer membrane proteins promote adherence to host cells
Hyaluronidase may facilitate perivascular infiltration
Coating of fibronectin protects against phagocytosis
Tissue destruction primarily results from host's immune response to infection

Epidemiology

Humans are the only natural host
Venereal syphilis transmitted by sexual contact or congenitally; patients at risk include sexually active adolescents and adults, and children born of mothers with active disease
Other *Treponema* infections transmitted by contact of mucous membranes with infectious lesions; congenital infections are rare; patients at risk are children or adults in contact with infectious lesions
Venereal syphilis occurs worldwide; endemic syphilis (bejel) occurs in desert and temperate regions of North Africa, Middle East, and northern Australia; yaws occurs in tropical and desert regions of Africa, South America, and Indonesia; pinta occurs in tropical areas of Central and South America
No seasonal incidence

Diseases

Venereal syphilis (*Treponema pallidum* ssp. *pallidum*)
Endemic syphilis or bejel (*T. pallidum* ssp. *endemicum*)
Yaws (*T. pallidum* ssp. *pertenue*)
Pinta (*Treponema carateum*)

Diagnosis

Microscopy (dark-field or DFA) and serology (refer to Table 43–2)

Treatment, Prevention, and Control

Penicillin is drug of choice; tetracycline or doxycycline is administered if the patient is allergic to penicillin
Safe sex practices should be emphasized, and sexual partners of infected patients should be treated
Endemic syphilis, yaws, and pinta can be eliminated through organized public health measures (treatment, education); however, these efforts have been inconsistently applied

inanimate objects, such as toilet seats. The most common route of spread is by direct sexual contact. The disease can also be acquired congenitally or by transfusion with contaminated blood. Syphilis is not highly contagious; the risk of contracting the disease after a single sexual contact is estimated to be 30%. However, contagiousness is influenced by the stage of disease in the infectious person. As mentioned previously, the spirochetes cannot survive on dry skin surfaces. Thus, *T. pallidum* is transferred primarily during the early stages of disease, when many organisms are present in moist, cutaneous or mucosal lesions. During the early stages of disease, the patient becomes bacteremic and, if the disease is untreated, bacteremia can persist for as long as 8 years. Congenital transmission from mother to fetus can occur at any time during this period. After 8 years, the disease can remain active, but bacteremia is not believed to occur.

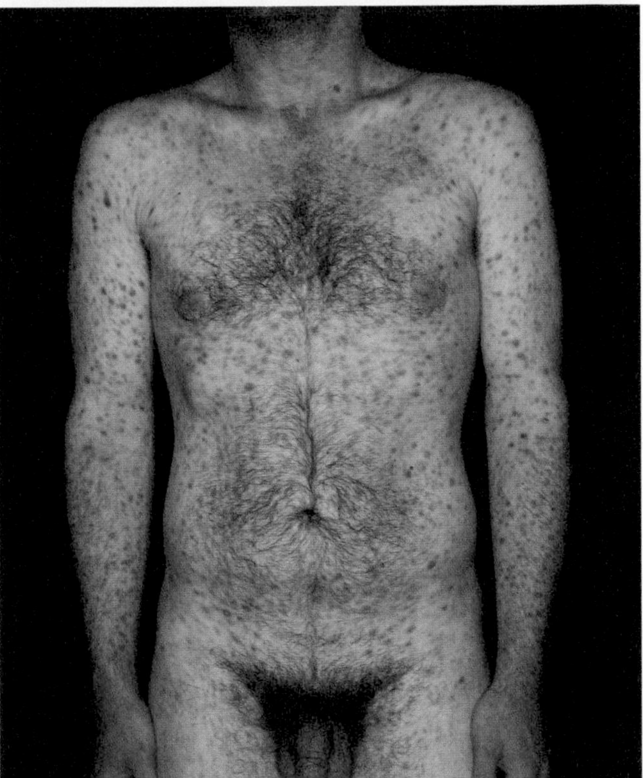

FIGURE 43–2. Disseminated rash in secondary syphilis. (From Habif TP: *Clinical dermatology: A color guide to diagnosis and therapy,* St Louis, 1996, Mosby.)

With the advent of effective antimicrobial therapy, the incidence of late (tertiary) syphilis has markedly decreased. Although antibiotic therapy has led to a decrease in the length of infectivity in infected persons, the incidence of primary and secondary syphilis has remained high because of sexual practices, particularly prostitution to support drug habits. The incidence of congenital syphilis corresponds to the pattern of syphilis in women of childbearing age. It should be noted that when active genital lesions are present, the patient is at greater risk for transmitting and acquiring human immunodeficiency virus (HIV).

CLINICAL DISEASES (FIGURE 43–3)

Primary Syphilis

As already noted, the initial syphilitic chancre develops at the site where the spirochete is inoculated. The lesion

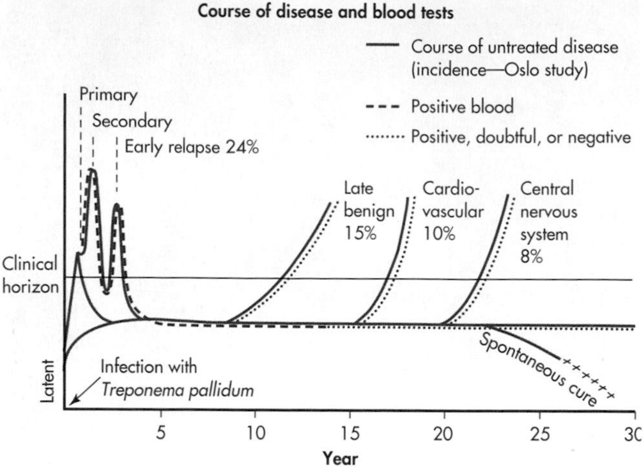

FIGURE 43–3. The natural history of untreated acquired syphilis was carefully chronicled at the University of Oslo (Norway). (Modified from Morgan H: *South Med J* 26:18-22, 1933; incidence data from Clark E, Danbolt N: *J Chron Dis* 2:311-344, 1955.)

TABLE 43–2. Diagnostic Tests for Syphilis

Diagnostic Test	Method or Examination
Microscopy	Dark-field Direct fluorescent antibody staining
Culture	Not available
Serology	Nontreponemal tests Venereal Disease Research Laboratory (VDRL) test Rapid plasma reagin (RPR) test Unheated serum reagin (USR) test Toluidine red unheated serum test (TRUST) Treponemal tests Fluorescent treponemal antibody-absorption (FTA-ABS) *Treponema pallidum* particle agglutination (TP-PA) test Enzyme immunoassay (EIA)

starts as a papule but then erodes to become a **painless ulcer** with raised borders (see Figure 43–1). In most patients, a painless regional lymphadenopathy develops 1 to 2 weeks after the appearance of the chancre, which represents a local focus for the proliferation of spirochetes. Abundant spirochetes are present in the chancre and can be disseminated throughout the patient by way of the lymphatic system and blood. The fact that this ulcer heals spontaneously within 2 months gives the patient a false sense of relief.

Secondary Syphilis

The clinical evidence of disseminated disease marks the second stage of syphilis. In this stage, patients typically experience a flulike syndrome with sore throat, headache, fever, myalgias (muscle aches), anorexia, lymphadenopathy (swollen lymph nodes), and a generalized mucocutaneous rash (see Figure 43–2). The flulike syndrome and lymphadenopathy generally appear first and then are followed a few days later by the disseminated skin rash. The rash can be variable (macular, papular, pustular), cover the entire skin surface (including the palms and soles), and may resolve slowly over a period of weeks to months. As with the primary chancre, the rash in secondary syphilis is highly infectious. The rash and symptoms gradually resolve spontaneously, and the patient enters the latent or clinically inactive stage of disease.

Tertiary (Late) Syphilis

A small proportion of cases can progress to the tertiary stage of syphilis. The diffuse, chronic inflammation characteristic of late syphilis can cause a devastating destruction of virtually any organ or tissue (e.g., arteritis, dementia, blindness). Granulomatous lesions **(gummas)** may be found in bone, skin, and other tissues. The nomenclature of late syphilis reflects the organs of primary involvement (e.g., neurosyphilis, cardiovascular syphilis). An increased incidence of neurosyphilis despite adequate therapy for early syphilis has been documented in patients with acquired immune deficiency syndrome (AIDS).

Congenital Syphilis

In utero infections can lead to serious fetal disease, resulting in latent infections, multiorgan malformations, or death of the fetus. Most infected infants are born without clinical evidence of the disease, but rhinitis then develops and is followed by a widespread desquamating maculopapular rash. Teeth and bone malformation, blindness, deafness, and cardiovascular syphilis are common in untreated infants who survive the initial phase of disease.

LABORATORY DIAGNOSIS (TABLE 43–2)

Microscopy

The diagnosis of primary, secondary, or congenital syphilis can be made rapidly by dark-field examination of the exudate from skin lesions (Figure 43–4). However, the test is reliable only when an experienced microscopist immediately examines the clinical material with actively motile spirochetes. The spirochetes do not survive transport to the laboratory, and tissue debris can be mistaken for spirochetes. Material collected from oral and rectal

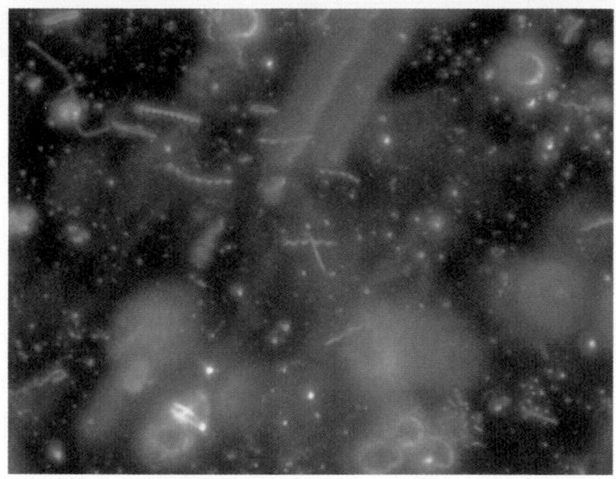

FIGURE 43–4. *Treponema pallidum* in a dark-field microscopy study. (From Peters W, Gilles HM: *A color atlas of tropical medicine and parasitology,* ed 4, London, 1995, Wolfe.)

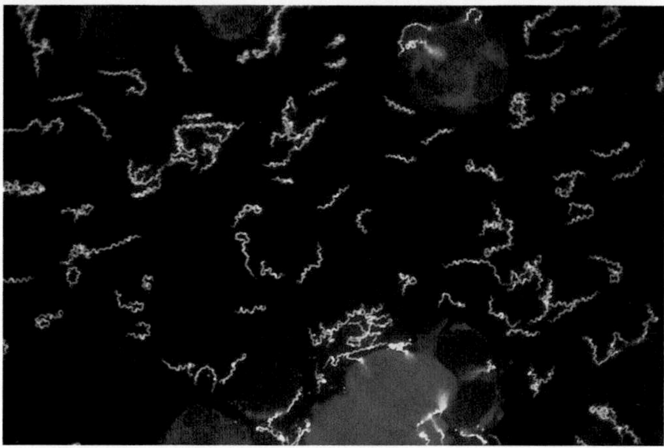

FIGURE 43–5. *Treponema pallidum* in the direct fluorescent antibody test for *T.a pallidum.* (From Morse S et al: *Atlas of sexually transmitted diseases and AIDS,* St Louis, 2003, Mosby.)

TABLE 43–3. Sensitivity and Specificity of Serologic Tests for Syphilis

Test	Sensitivity (%)				Specificity (%)
	Primary	Secondary	Latent	Late	
Nontreponemal					
VDRL	78 (74–87)	100	95 (88–100)	71 (37–94)	98 (96–99)
RPR	86 (77–100)	100	98 (95–100)	73	98 (93–99)
USR	80 (72–88)	100	95 (88–100)		99
TRUST	85 (77–86)	100	98 (95–100)		99 (98–99)
Treponemal					
FTA-ABS	84 (70–100)	100	100	96	97 (94–100)
TP-PA	88 (86–100)	100	100		96 (95–100)

FTA-APS, Flourescent treponemal antibody-absorption; RPR, rapid plasma reagin; TP-PA, *T. pallidum* particle agglutination; TRUST, toluidine red unheated serum test; USR, unheated serum reagin; VDRL, Venereal Disease Research Laboratory.

lesions should not be examined because nonpathogenic spirochetes can contaminate the specimen. A more useful test for detecting *T. pallidum* is the direct fluorescent antibody test. Fluorescein-labeled antitreponemal antibodies are used to stain the bacteria (Figure 43–5). The test is specific for pathogenic treponemes, so oral and rectal specimens can be examined. Nonmotile spirochetes will also stain, therefore specimens do not need to be examined immediately after collection. Histologic stains have also been used to demonstrate treponemes in tissue specimens. Silver stains are the most commonly used stains.

Culture

Efforts to culture *T. pallidum* in vitro should not be attempted because the organism does not grow in artificial cultures.

Serology

Syphilis is diagnosed in most patients on the basis of serologic tests. The two general types of tests used are biologically nonspecific (nontreponemal) tests and specific treponemal tests (Table 43–3).

Nontreponemal tests measure immunoglobulin (Ig)G and IgM antibodies (also called **reaginic antibodies**) developed against lipids released from damaged cells during the early stage of disease and present on the cell surface of treponemes. The antigen used for the nontreponemal tests is **cardiolipin,** which is derived from beef heart. The two tests used most commonly are the **Venereal Disease Research Laboratory (VDRL) test** and the **Rapid Plasma Reagin (RPR) test.** Both tests measure the flocculation of cardiolipin antigen by the patient's serum. Both tests can be performed rapidly, although complement in serum must be inactivated for

30 minutes before the VDRL test can be performed. Only the VDRL test should be used to test cerebrospinal fluid (CSF) from patients with suspected neurosyphilis.

Treponemal tests are specific antibody tests used to confirm positive reactions with the VDRL or RPR tests. The treponemal test results can also be positive before the nontreponemal test results become positive in early syphilis, or they can remain positive when the nonspecific test results revert to negative in some patients who have late syphilis. The tests most commonly used are the **fluorescent treponemal antibody-absorption (FTA-ABS) test** and ***Treponema pallidum* particle agglutination (TP-PA) test**. The FTA-ABS test is an indirect fluorescent antibody test. *T. pallidum* immobilized on glass slides is used as the antigen. The slide is overlayed with the patient's serum, which has been mixed with an extract of nonpathogenic treponemes. The fluorescein-labeled antihuman antibodies are then added to detect the presence of specific antibodies in the patient's serum. The TP-PA test is a microtiter agglutination test. Gelatin particles sensitized with *T. pallidum* antigens are mixed with dilutions of the patient's serum. If antibodies are present, the particles agglutinate. A variety of specific **enzyme immunoassays (EIAs)** have been developed recently and appear to have sensitivities and specificities similar to the FTA-ABS and TP-PA tests.

Because positive reactions with the nontreponemal tests develop late during the first phase of disease, the serologic findings are negative in many patients who initially have chancres. However, serologic results are positive within 3 months in all patients and remain positive in untreated patients with secondary syphilis. The antibody titers decrease slowly in patients with untreated syphilis, and serologic results are negative in approximately 25% to 30% of patients with late syphilis. Although the results of treponemal tests generally remain positive for the life of the person who has syphilis, a negative test is unreliable in patients with AIDS.

Successful treatment of primary or secondary syphilis and to a lesser extent, late syphilis, leads to reduced titers measured in the VDRL and RPR tests. Thus, these tests can be used to monitor the effectiveness of therapy, although seroreversion is slowed in patients in an advanced stage of disease, those with high initial titers, and those who have previously had syphilis. The treponemal tests are influenced less by therapy than the VDRL and RPR tests are, with seroconversion observed in less than 25% of patients successfully treated during the primary stage of the disease.

The specificity of the nontreponemal tests is at least 98%. However, transient false-positive reactions are seen in patients with acute febrile diseases, after immunizations, and in pregnant women. Long-term false-positive reactions occur most often in patients with chronic autoimmune diseases or infections that involve the liver or that cause extensive tissue destruction. The specificity of the treponemal tests is 97% to 99%, with most false-positive reactions observed in patients with elevated immunoglobin levels and autoimmune diseases (Box 43–3). Many of the false-positive reactions can be resolved using the Western blot assay, which may become the preferred confirmatory test.

BOX 43–3. Conditions Associated with False-Positive Serologic Test Results

Nontreponemal Tests	Treponemal Tests
Viral infection	Pyoderma
Rheumatoid arthritis	Skin neoplasm
Systemic lupus erythematosus	Acne vulgaris
Acute or chronic illness	Mycoses
Pregnancy	Crural ulceration
Recent immunization	Rheumatoid arthritis
Drug addiction	Psoriasis
Leprosy	Systemic lupus erythematosus
Malaria	Pregnancy
	Drug addiction
	Herpes genitalis

Positive serologic test results in infants of infected mothers can represent a passive transfer of antibodies or a specific immunologic response to infection. These two possibilities are distinguished by measuring the antibody titers in the sera of the infant during a 6-month period. The antibody titers in noninfected infants decrease to undetectable levels within 3 months of birth but remain elevated in infants who have congenital syphilis.

TREATMENT, PREVENTION, AND CONTROL

Penicillin is the drug of choice for treating *T. pallidum* infections. Long-acting benzathine penicillin is used for the early stages of syphilis, and penicillin G is recommended for congenital and late syphilis. Tetracycline and doxycycline can be used as alternative antibiotics for patients allergic to penicillin. Only penicillin can be used for the treatment of neurosyphilis; thus, penicillin-allergic patients must undergo desensitization. This is also true for pregnant women, who should not be treated with the tetracyclines.

Because protective vaccines are not available, syphilis can be controlled only through the practice of safe-sex techniques and adequate contact and treatment of the sex partners of patients who have been documented with infection. The control of syphilis and other venereal diseases has been complicated by an increase in prostitution among drug abusers.

Other Treponemes

Three other nonvenereal treponemal diseases are important: bejel, yaws, and pinta. These diseases are primarily observed in impoverished children. *T. pallidum* subspecies *endemicum* is responsible for **bejel,** also called **endemic syphilis.** Disease is spread person to person by the use of contaminated eating utensils. The initial oral lesions are rarely observed, but secondary lesions include oral papules and mucosal patches. Gummas of the skin, bones, and nasopharynx are late manifestations. The disease is present in Africa, Asia, and Australia.

T. pertenue is the etiologic agent of **yaws,** a granulomatous disease in which patients have skin lesions early in the disease (Figure 43–6) and then late destructive lesions of the skin, lymph nodes, and bones. The disease is present in primitive tropical areas of South America, Central Africa, and Southeast Asia and is spread by direct contact with infected skin lesions.

T. carateum is responsible for causing **pinta,** a disease that primarily affects the skin. Small pruritic papules develop on the skin surface after a 1- to 3-week incubation period. These lesions enlarge and persist for months to years before resolving. Disseminated, recurrent, hypopigmented lesions can develop over years, resulting in scarring and disfigurement. Pinta is present in Central and South America and is spread by direct contact with infected lesions.

Bejel, yaws, and pinta are diagnosed by their typical clinical manifestation in an endemic area. The diagnoses of yaws and pinta are confirmed by the detection of spirochetes in skin lesions by dark-field microscopy, but this test cannot be used to detect spirochetes in patients with the oral lesions of bejel. The results of serologic tests for syphilis are also positive.

Penicillin, tetracycline, and chloramphenicol have been used to treat these diseases. The diseases are controlled through the treatment of infected people and the elimination of person-to-person spread.

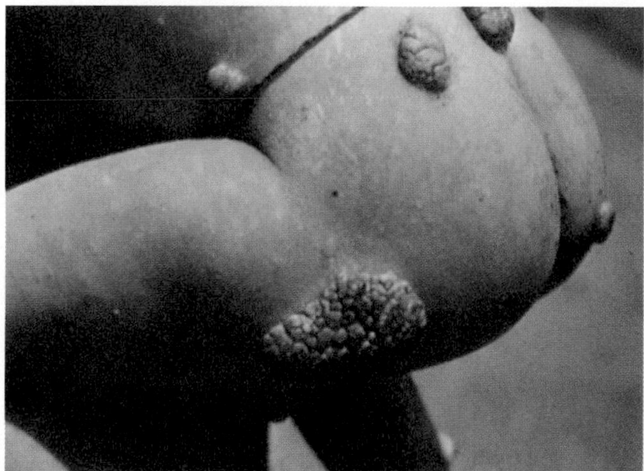

FIGURE 43–6. The elevated papillomatous nodules characteristic of early yaws are widely distributed and painless. They contain numerous spirochetes, which are easily seen on dark-field microscopy studies. (From Peters W, Gilles HM: *A color atlas of tropical medicine and parasitology,* ed 4, London, 1995, Wolfe.)

Borrelia (Box 43–4)

Members of the genus *Borrelia* cause two important human diseases: relapsing fever and Lyme disease. Relapsing fever is a febrile illness characterized by recurrent episodes of fever and septicemia separated by afebrile periods. Two forms of the disease are recognized. *Borrelia recurrentis* is the etiologic agent of **epidemic** or **louse-borne relapsing fever** and is spread person-to-person by the human body **louse** (*Pediculus humanus*). **Endemic relapsing fever** is caused by as many as 15 species of borreliae and is spread by infected **soft ticks** of the genus *Ornithodoros.*

The history of **Lyme disease** began in 1977, when an unusual cluster of children with arthritis was noted in Lyme, Conn. Five years later, W. Burgdorfer discovered the spirochete responsible for this disease. Lyme disease is a tick-borne disease with protean manifestations, including dermatologic, rheumatologic, neurologic, and cardiac abnormalities. Initially it was believed that all cases of Lyme disease (or Lyme borreliosis) were caused by one organism, *B. burgdorferi.* However, subsequent studies have determined that a complex of at least 10 *Borrelia* species is responsible for Lyme disease in animals and humans. Three species (i.e., *B. burgdorferi, Borrelia garinii, Borrelia afzelii*) cause human disease, with *B. burgdorferi* found in the United States and Europe and *B. garinii* and *B. afzelii* found in Europe and Japan. This chapter focuses on *B. burgdorferi* infections.

PHYSIOLOGY AND STRUCTURE

Members of the genus *Borrelia* are weakly staining, gram-negative spirochetes. They tend to be larger than other spirochetes (0.2 to 0.5 × 8 to 30 μm), stain well with aniline dyes (e.g., Giemsa or Wright stain), and can be easily seen by light microscopy in smears of peripheral blood from patients with relapsing fever (Figure 43–7) but not those with Lyme disease. From seven to 20 periplasmic flagella (depending on the species) are present between the periplasmic cylinder and the outer envelope and are responsible for the organism's twisting motility (Figure 43–8). Borreliae are microaerophilic and have complex nutritional needs (i.e., requiring N-acetylglucosamine and long-chain saturated and unsaturated fatty acids). The species that have been successfully cultured have generation times of 18 hours or longer. Because culture is generally unsuccessful, diagnosis of diseases caused by borreliae is by microscopy (relapsing fever) or serology (Lyme disease).

BOX 43–4. Summary of *Borrelia*

Physiology and Structure

Spirochetes measure 0.2 to 0.5 × 8 to 30 μm

Can be seen when stained with aniline dyes (e.g., Giemsa, Wright stains)

Can grow in culture, but bacteria are microaerophilic and have complex nutritional requirements

Virulence Factors

Borrelia species responsible for relapsing fever are able to undergo antigenic shift and escape immune clearance; periodic febrile and afebrile periods result from antigenic variation

Immune reactivity against the Lyme disease agents may be responsible for the clinical disease

Epidemiology

Epidemic relapsing fever: transmitted person-to-person; reservoir—humans; vector—human body louse

Endemic relapsing fever: transmitted from rodents to humans; reservoirs—rodents, small mammals, and soft ticks; vector—soft ticks

Individuals at risk for relapsing fever include people exposed to lice (epidemic disease) in crowded or unsanitary conditions and people exposed to ticks (endemic disease) in rural areas

Epidemic relapsing fever occurs in Ethiopia, Rwanda, and the Andean foothills

Endemic relapsing fever has worldwide distribution and is in the western part of the United States

Lyme disease: transmitted by hard ticks from mice to humans; reservoir—mice, deer, ticks; vectors include *Ixodes scapularis* in eastern and midwestern United States, *Ixodes pacificus* in the western United States, *Ixodes ricinus* in Europe, and *Ixodes persulcatus* in Eastern Europe and Asia

Individuals at risk for Lyme disease include people exposed to ticks in areas of high endemicity

Lyme disease has worldwide distribution

Seasonal incidence corresponds to feeding patterns of vectors; most cases of Lyme disease in the United States occur in late spring and early summer (feeding pattern of nymph stage of ticks)

Diseases

Epidemic relapsing fever: etiologic agent is *Borrelia recurrentis*

Endemic relapsing fever: many *Borrelia* species are responsible

Lyme disease: *Borrelia burgdorferi* causes disease in the United States and Europe; *Borrelia garinii* and *Borrelia afzelii* cause disease in Europe and Asia

Diagnosis

Refer to Box 43–5

Treatment, Prevention, and Control

For relapsing fever, treatment is with tetracycline or erythromycin

For early localized or disseminated Lyme disease, treatment is with amoxicillin, tetracycline, cefuroxime; late manifestations are treated with intravenous penicillin or ceftriaxone

Exposure to the insect vector can be decreased by using insecticides and applying insect repellents to clothing and by wearing protective clothing that reduces exposure of skin to insects

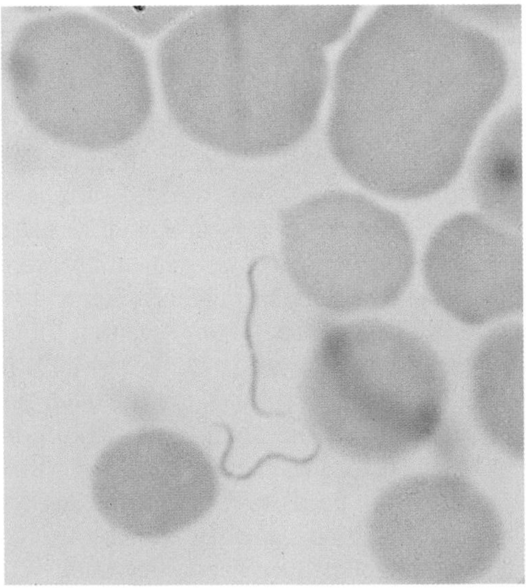

FIGURE 43–7. *Borrelia* organisms are present in the blood of this patient with endemic relapsing fever (Giemsa stain).

PATHOGENESIS AND IMMUNITY

After a person is exposed to infected arthropods, borreliae spread in the blood to many organs. Members of the genus do not produce recognized toxins and are removed rapidly when a specific antibody response is mounted. The periodic febrile and afebrile cycles of relapsing fever stem from the ability of the borreliae to undergo antigenic variation. When specific IgM antibodies are formed, agglutination with complement-mediated lysis occurs, and the borreliae are cleared rapidly from the blood. However, organisms residing in internal tissues can alter their serotype-specific outer envelope proteins through gene rearrangement and emerge as antigenically novel organisms. The clinical manifestations of relapsing fever are in part a response to the release of endotoxin by the organisms.

B. burgdorferi organisms are present in low numbers in the skin when erythema migrans develops. This has been shown by culture of the organism from skin lesions or detection of bacterial nucleic acids by polymerase chain

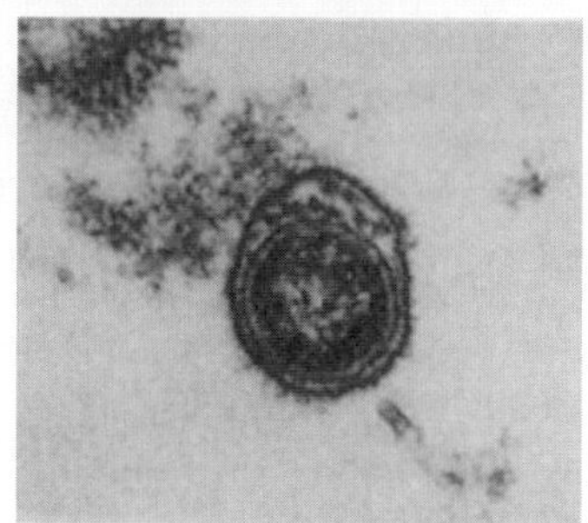

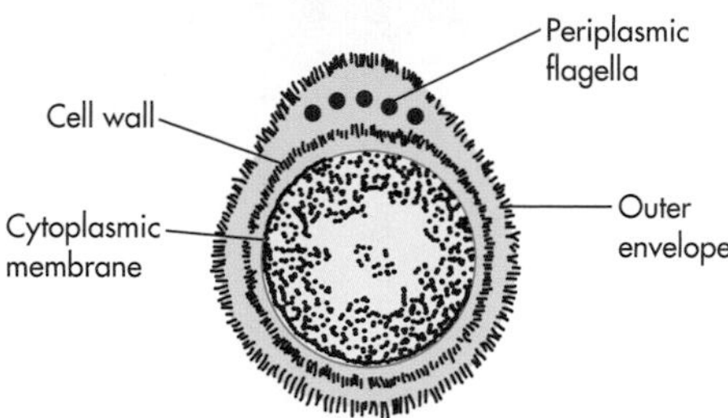

FIGURE 43–8. Electron micrograph and drawing of a cross-section through *Borrelia burgdorferi*, the agent that causes Lyme borreliosis. The protoplasmic core of the bacterium is enclosed in a cytoplasmic membrane and conventional cell wall. This in turn is surrounded by an outer envelope, or sheath. Between the protoplasmic core and outer sheath are periplasmic flagella (also called *axial fibrils*), which are anchored at either end of the bacterium and wrap around the protoplasmic core. (From Steere AC et al: *N Engl J Med* 308:733-740, 1983.)

reaction (PCR) amplification. Spirochetes are infrequently isolated from clinical material late in the disease. It is not known whether the viable organisms cause these late manifestations of disease or whether they represent immunologic cross-reactivity to *Borrelia* antigens. Although the immune response to the organism is depressed at the time that skin lesions initially develop, antibodies develop over months to years and are responsible for producing the complement-mediated clearance of the borreliae.

EPIDEMIOLOGY

As previously mentioned, the etiologic agent of louse-borne epidemic relapsing fever is *B. recurrentis*, the vector is the human body louse, and humans are the only reservoir (Figure 43–9). Lice become infected after feeding on an infected person. The organisms are ingested, pass through the wall of the gut, and multiply in hemolymph. Disseminated disease is not believed to occur in lice; thus human infection occurs when the lice are crushed during feeding. Because infected lice do not survive for more than a few months, maintenance of the disease requires crowded, unsanitary conditions (e.g., wars, natural disasters) that permit frequent human contact with infected lice. Although epidemics of louse-borne relapsing fever swept from Eastern to Western Europe in the past century, disease now appears to be restricted to Ethiopia, Rwanda, and the Andean foothills.

Infection	Reservoir	Vector
Relapsing fever Epidemic (louse-borne)	Humans	Body louse
Relapsing fever Endemic (tick-borne)	Rodents, soft-shelled ticks	Soft-shelled tick
Lyme disease	Rodents, deer, domestic pets, hard-shelled ticks	Hard-shelled tick

FIGURE 43–9. Epidemiology of *Borrelia* infections.

Several features distinguish endemic relapsing fever from epidemic disease. Tick-borne endemic relapsing fever is a zoonotic disease, with rodents, small mammals, and soft ticks (*Ornithodoros* species) the main reservoirs and many species of *Borrelia* responsible for the disease. Unlike the louse-borne infections, the borreliae that cause endemic disease produce a disseminated infection in ticks. Additionally, the arthropods can survive and maintain an endemic reservoir of infection by transovarian transmission. Furthermore, ticks can survive for months between feedings. A history of a tick bite may also not be elicited because soft ticks are primarily nocturnal feeders and remain attached for only a few minutes. The ticks contaminate the bite wound with borreliae present in saliva or feces. Tick-borne disease is found worldwide, corresponding to the distribution of the *Ornithodoros* tick. In the United States, disease is primarily found in the western states.

Despite the relatively recent recognition of Lyme disease in the United States, retrospective studies have shown that the disease was present for many years in this and other countries. Lyme disease has been described on six continents, in at least 20 countries, and in 49 U.S. states. The incidence of disease has risen dramatically between 1982 (when 497 cases were reported) and 2003 (when 21,273 cases were reported). Lyme disease is the leading vector-borne disease in the United States. The three principal foci of infection in the United States are the Northeast (Massachusetts to Maryland), the upper Midwest (Minnesota and Wisconsin), and the Pacific West (California and Oregon). Hard ticks are the major vectors of Lyme disease: *Ixodes scapularis* in the Northeast and Midwest and *Ixodes pacificus* on the West Coast. *Ixodes ricinus* is the major tick vector in Europe, and *Ixodes persulcatus* is the major tick vector in Eastern Europe and Asia. The major reservoir hosts in the United States are the white-footed mouse and the white-tailed deer. The white-footed mouse is the primary host of larval and nymph forms of *Ixodes* species, and the adult *Ixodes* species infest the white-tailed deer. Because the nymph stage causes more than 90% of the cases of documented disease, the mouse host is more relevant for human disease.

Ixodes larvae become infected when they feed on the mouse reservoir. The larva molts to a nymph in late spring and takes a second blood meal; in this case, humans can be accidental hosts. Although the borreliae are transmitted in the tick's saliva during a prolonged period of feeding (48 hours or more), most patients do not remember having had a specific tick bite because the nymph is the size of a poppy seed. The nymphs mature into adults in the late summer and take a third feeding. Although the white-tailed deer is the natural host, humans can also be infected at this stage. Most infected patients are identified in May to August, although disease can be encountered throughout the year.

CLINICAL DISEASES

Relapsing Fever

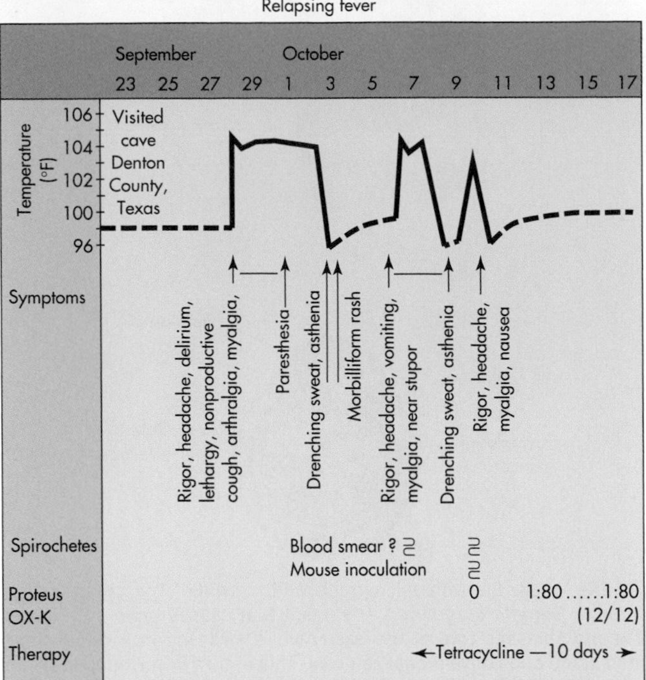

FIGURE 43–10. The clinical evolution of tick-borne relapsing fever in a 14-year-old boy. The initial febrile episode is typically the most severe. Subsequent episodes tend to be shorter and less intense. Although nonspecific reactivity with *Proteus* OX-K antigens is often observed, the specific diagnosis is made on the basis of the observation of borreliae in peripheral blood smears. These are positive for organisms only during the febrile periods. (Modified from Southern PM, Sanford J: *Medicine* 48:129-149, 1969.)

The clinical presentations of epidemic louse-borne and endemic tick-borne relapsing fever are essentially the same, although a small, pruritic eschar may develop at the site of the tick bite (Figure 43–10). After a 1-week incubation period, the disease is heralded by the abrupt onset of shaking chills, fever, muscle aches, and headache. Splenomegaly and hepatomegaly are common. These symptoms correspond to the bacteremic phase of the disease and resolve after 3 to 7 days, when the borreliae are cleared from the blood. Bacteremia and fever return after a 1-week afebrile period. The clinical symptoms are generally milder and last a shorter time during this and subsequent febrile episodes. A single relapse is characteristic of epidemic louse-borne disease, and repeated relapses are common in endemic tick-borne disease. The clinical course and outcome of epidemic relapsing fever tend to be more severe than they are in those with endemic disease, but this may be related to the patients' underlying poor state of health. Mortality with endemic disease is less than 5% but can be as high as 40% in louse-borne epidemic disease. Deaths are caused by cardiac failure, hepatic necrosis, or cerebral hemorrhage.

BOX 43–5. Definition of Lyme Disease

Clinical Case Definition

Either of the following:

Erythema migrans (~5 cm in diameter)

At least one late manifestation (i.e., musculoskeletal, nervous system, or cardiovascular involvement) and laboratory confirmation of infection

Laboratory Criteria for Diagnosis

At least one of the following:

Isolation of *Borrelia burgdorferi*

Demonstration of diagnostic levels of immunoglobulin (Ig)M or IgG antibodies to the spirochetes

Significant increase in antibody titer between acute and convalescent serum samples

Lyme Disease

Clinical diagnosis of Lyme disease is complicated by the varied manifestations of disease caused by *B. burgdorferi* and other *Borrelia* species, as well as the lack of reliable diagnostic tests. The clinical and laboratory definitions of Lyme disease that are recommended by the Centers for Disease Control and Prevention (CDC) are summarized in Box 43–5. The following is paragraph is a description of Lyme disease in the United States. The frequency of the skin lesions and late manifestations differ in disease observed in other countries.

Lyme disease begins as an early localized infection, progresses to an early disseminated stage, and, if untreated, can progress to a late manifestation stage. After an incubation period of 3 to 30 days, one or more skin lesions typically develop at the site of the tick bite. The

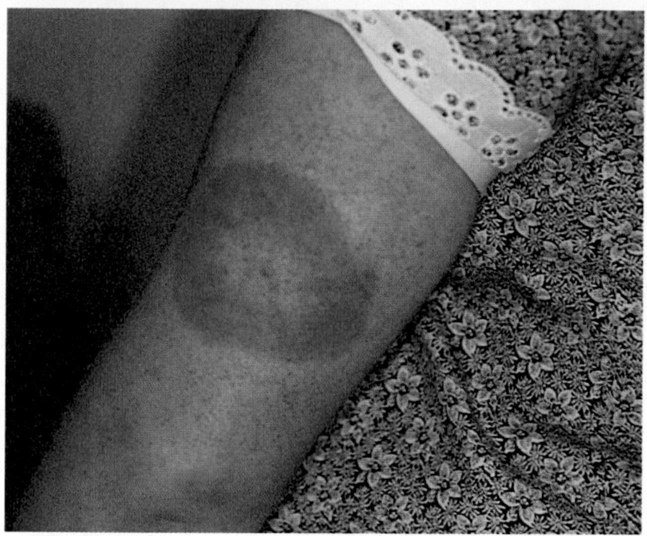

FIGURE 43–11. Erythema migrans rash on the arm of a patient with Lyme borreliosis.

lesion **(erythema migrans)** begins as a small macule or papule and then enlarges over the next few weeks, ultimately covering an area ranging from 5 cm to more than 50 cm in diameter (Figure 43–11). The lesion typically has a flat, red border and central clearing as it develops; however, erythema, vesicle formation, and central necrosis can also be seen. The lesion fades and disappears within weeks, although new transient lesions may subsequently appear. Other early signs and symptoms of Lyme disease include malaise, severe fatigue, headache, fever, chills, musculoskeletal pains, myalgias, and lymphadenopathy. These symptoms last for an average of 4 weeks.

Hematogenous dissemination will occur in untreated patients within days to weeks of the primary infection. This stage is characterized by systemic signs of disease (e.g., severe fatigue, headache, fever, malaise), arthralgia, myalgia, erythematous skins lesions, cardiac dysfunction (e.g., heart block, myopericarditis, congestive heart failure), and neurologic signs (e.g., facial palsy, meningitis, encephalitis).

Late-stage manifestations of Lyme disease in the United States typically develop months to years after the initial infection, when they present as arthritis. The arthritis can involve one or more joints intermittently. Chronic skin involvement with discoloration and swelling (acrodermatitis chronica atrophicans [ACA]; Figure 43–12) is more common in Lyme disease seen in Europe.

LABORATORY DIAGNOSIS

Microscopy

Because of their relatively large size, borreliae that cause relapsing fever can be seen during the febrile period on Giemsa- or Wright-stained preparation of blood. This is the most sensitive method for diagnosing relapsing fever, with smears positive for organisms in more than 70% of patients. Inoculating a mouse with blood from infected patients and then examining the mouse's blood for the presence of borreliae after 1 to 10 days can improve the sensitivity of the test. Microscopic examination of blood or tissues from patients with Lyme disease is not recommended because *B. burgdorferi* is rarely seen in clinical specimens.

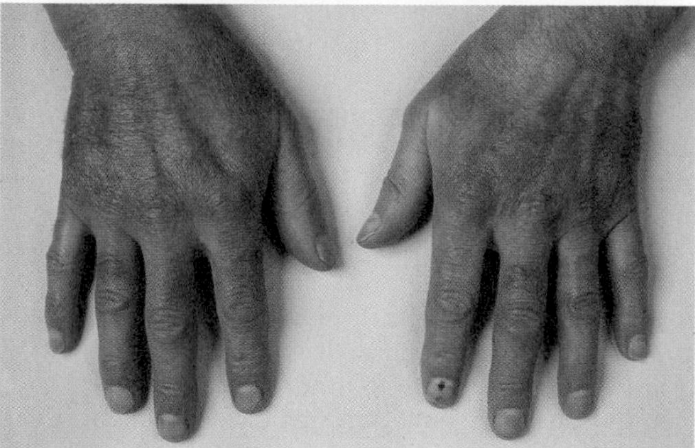

FIGURE 43–12. Acrodermatitis chronica atrophicans. Bluish-red skin lesions characteristic of late, disseminated manifestions of Lyme borreliosis. (From Cohen J, Powderly W: *Infectious diseases,* ed 2, St Louis, 2004, Mosby.)

Culture

Some borreliae, including *B. recurrentis* and *Borrelia hermsii* (a common cause of endemic relapsing fever in the United States), can be cultured in vitro on specialized media. The cultures are rarely performed in most clinical laboratories, however, because the media are not readily available and the organisms grow slowly on them. There has been limited success with the culture of *B. burgdorferi,* although isolation of the organism has been improved through the use of specialized media. However, the sensitivity of culture is low for all specimens except the initial skin lesion, which is pathognomonic, thus making culture rarely necessary.

Molecular Diagnosis

Nucleic acid amplification techniques for the diagnosis of Lyme disease have a sensitivity generally lower than culture. This reflects the fact that relatively few organisms are present in the tissues and body fluids of patients with Lyme disease.

Serology

Serologic tests are not useful in the diagnosis of relapsing fever, because the borreliae that cause this condition undergo antigenic phase variation. In contrast, serologic testing is an important diagnostic test for patients with suspected Lyme disease. The tests most commonly used are the **immunofluorescence assay (IFA)** and **enzyme-linked immunosorbent assay (ELISA)**. ELISA using purified or recombinant antigens is preferred because it is more sensitive and specific for all stages of Lyme disease. Unfortunately, all serologic tests are relatively insensitive during the early acute stage of disease. IgM antibodies appear 2 to 4 weeks after the onset of erythema migrans in untreated patients; the levels peak after 6 to 8 weeks of illness and then decline to a normal range after 4 to 6 months. The IgM level may remain elevated in some patients with a persistent infection. The IgG antibodies appear later. Their levels peak after 4 to 6 months of illness and persist during the late manifestations of the disease. Thus, most patients with late complications of Lyme disease have detectable antibodies to *B. burgdorferi*, although the antibody level may be ablated in patients treated with antibiotics. Detection of antibodies in CSF is strong evidence for neuroborreliosis.

Although cross-reactions are uncommon, positive serologic results must be interpreted carefully, particularly if the titers are low (Box 43–6). Most false-positive reactions occur in patients with syphilis. These false results can be excluded by performing a nontreponemal test for syphilis; the result is negative in patients with Lyme disease.

Western blot analysis has been used to confirm the specificity of a positive ELISA reaction. In the early phase of Lyme disease, IgM antibodies develop against a limited number of surface proteins: p21 (OspC), p35, and flagella proteins p37 (FlaA) and p41 (FlaB). IgG antibodies develop first against OspC, p37, and p41, then against additional antigens (e.g., p39, p58) in the early disseminated stage of disease, and finally against a wide spectrum of *Borrelia* antigens in the late stage of disease.

Antigenic heterogeneity in *B. burgdorferi* and other *Borrelia* species that cause Lyme disease affects the test sensitivity. The magnitude of this problem in the United States is unknown, but it should be significant in Europe and Asia, where many *Borrelia* species are found to cause Lyme disease. At present, serologic tests should be considered confirmatory and should not be performed in the absence of an appropriate history and clinical symptoms of Lyme disease.

BOX 43–6. Bacteria and Diseases Associated with Cross-Reactions in Serologic Tests for Lyme Borreliosis

Treponema pallidum
Oral spirochetes
Other *Borrelia* species
Juvenile rheumatoid arthritis
Rheumatoid arthritis
Systemic lupus erythematosus
Infectious mononucleosis
Subacute bacterial endocarditis

TREATMENT, PREVENTION, AND CONTROL

Relapsing fever has been treated most effectively with tetracycline or erythromycin. Tetracycline is the drug of choice but is contraindicated for pregnant women and young children. A Jarisch-Herxheimer reaction (shocklike profile with rigors, leukopenia, an increase in temperature, and a decrease in blood pressure) can occur in patients within a few hours after therapy is started and must be carefully managed. This reaction corresponds to the rapid killing of borreliae and the possible release of toxic products, such as endotoxin.

The early manifestations of Lyme disease are managed effectively with orally administered amoxicillin, doxycycline, or cefuroxime. Antibiotic treatment lessens the likelihood and the severity of late complications. Despite this intervention, Lyme arthritis and other complications occur in a small number of patients. Ceftriaxone, doxycycline, or amoxicillin has been used for the treatment of these manifestations. Patients with neurologic and musculoskeletal disease typically require prolonged treatment with intravenous penicillin G or ceftriaxone, and relapses may necessitate re-treatment.

Prevention of tick-borne *Borrelia* diseases includes avoiding ticks and their natural habitats; wearing protective clothing, such as long pants tucked into socks; and applying insect repellents. Rodent control is also important in the prevention of endemic relapsing fever. Epidemic louse-borne disease is controlled through the use of delousing sprays and improvements in hygienic conditions.

Vaccines are not available for relapsing fever. A recombinant vaccine directed against the OspA antigen of *B. burgdorferi* was licensed for use in the United States but was recently removed from the market. Other recombinant vaccines are under development.

Leptospira (Box 43–7)

The taxonomy of the genus *Leptospira* is a source of great confusion. Traditionally, the genus has been grouped by phenotypic properties, serologic relationships, and pathogenicity. Pathogenic strains were placed in the species *Leptospira interrogans*, and nonpathogenic strains were placed in the species *Leptospira biflexa*. Each of the two species contained many serovars (i.e., serologically distinct groups). However, this classification is not consistent

BOX 43–7. Summary of *Leptospira*

Physiology and Structure

Complex taxonomy with many species and many serovars
Thin, coiled spirochetes (0.1 × 6 to 20 μm); one or both ends hook shaped
Obligate aerobe; slow growth in culture

Virulence Factors

Direct invasion and replication in tissues
Immune complex glomerulonephritis

Epidemiology

U.S. reservoirs: rodents (particularly rats), dogs, farm animals, and wild animals
Humans: accidental end-stage host
Organism can penetrate the skin through minor breaks in the epidermis
People are infected with leptospires through exposure to water contaminated with urine from an infected animal or handling of tissues from an infected animal
People at risk are those exposed to urine-contaminated streams, rivers, and standing water; occupational exposure to infected animals for farmers, meat handlers, and veterinarians
Infection is rare in the United States but has worldwide distribution
Disease is more common during warm months (recreational exposure)

Diseases

Mild, viruslike syndrome
Systemic leptospirosis with aseptic meningitis
Overwhelming disease (Weil's disease) with vascular collapse, thrombocytopenia, hemorrhage, and hepatic and renal dysfunction

Diagnosis

Microscopy not useful
Culture blood or CSF in the first 7-10 days of illness; urine after the first week
Serology using the MAT is relatively sensitive and specific but not widely available; ELISA tests are less accurate but can be used to screen patients

Treatment, Prevention, and Control

Treatment with penicillin or doxycycline
Doxycycline but not penicillin is used for prophylaxis
Herds and domestic pets should be vaccinated
Rats should be controlled

*CSF, Cerebrospinal fluid; ELISA, enzyme-linked immunosorbent assay; MAT, microscopic agglutination test.

with nucleic acid analysis, which supports subdividing the genus into three genera with 17 species. To avoid confusion, leptospires will be referred to as pathogenic (for humans) and nonpathogenic without reference to either specific species or serovars.

PHYSIOLOGY AND STRUCTURE

Leptospires are thin, coiled spirochetes (0.1 × 6.0 to 20.0 μm) with a hook at one or both pointed ends (Figure 43–13). Motility is by means of two periplasmic flagella extending the length of the bacteria and anchored at opposite ends. Leptospires are obligate aerobes with optimum growth at 28° to 30°C in media supplemented with vitamins (i.e., B_2, B_{12}), long-chain fatty acids, and ammonium salts. The practical significance of this is that these organisms can be cultured from clinical specimens collected from infected patients.

PATHOGENESIS AND IMMUNITY

Pathogenic leptospires can cause subclinical infection, a mild influenza-like febrile illness, or severe systemic disease **(Weil's disease),** with renal and hepatic failure, extensive vasculitis, myocarditis, and death. The number of infecting organisms, the host's immunologic defenses, and the virulence of the infecting strain influence the severity of the disease.

Because leptospires are thin and highly motile, they can penetrate intact mucous membranes or skin through small cuts or abrasions. They can then spread in the blood to all tissues, including the central nervous system. *L. interrogans* multiply rapidly and damage the endothelium of small blood vessels, resulting in the major clinical manifestations of disease (e.g., meningitis, hepatic and renal dysfunction, hemorrhage). Organisms can be found in blood and CSF early in the disease and in urine during the later stages. Clearance of leptospires occurs when humoral immunity develops. However, some clinical manifestations may stem from immunologic reactions with

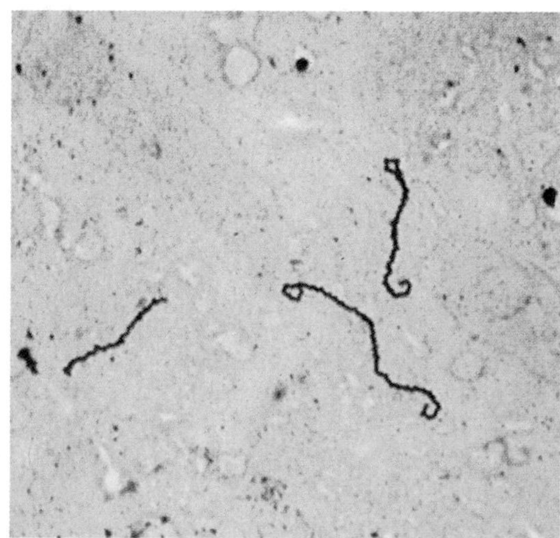

FIGURE 43–13. Silver staining of leptospires grown in culture. Notice the tightly coiled body with hooked ends. (From Emond R, Rowland H: *Color atlas of infectious diseases,* ed 3, London, 1995, Wolfe.)

the organisms. For example, meningitis develops after the organisms have been removed from the CSF and immune complexes have been detected in renal lesions.

EPIDEMIOLOGY

Leptospirosis has a worldwide distribution. From 100 to 200 human infections occur in the United States each year, with more than half the cases reported in Hawaii. However, the incidence of disease is significantly underestimated because most infections are mild and misdiagnosed as a "viral syndrome" or viral aseptic meningitis. Because many states failed to report this disease to the public health service, mandatory reporting was discontinued in 1995. Thus the true prevalence of this disease cannot be determined.

Leptospires infect two types of hosts: reservoir hosts and incidental hosts. Endemic, chronic infections are established in **reservoir hosts**, which serve as a permanent reservoir for maintaining the bacteria. Different species and serovars of leptospires are associated with specific reservoir hosts (important for epidemiologic investigations). The most common reservoirs are rodents and other small mammals. Leptospires usually cause asymptomatic infections in their reservoir host, in which the spirochetes colonize the renal tubules and are shed in urine in large numbers. Streams, rivers, standing water, and moist soil can be contaminated with urine from infected animals, with organisms surviving for as long as 6 weeks in such sites. Contaminated water or direct exposure to infected animals can serve as a source for infection in **incidental hosts** (e.g., dogs, farm animals, humans). Most human infections result from recreational exposure to contaminated water (e.g., lakes) or occupational exposure to infected animals (farmers, slaughterhouse workers, veterinarians). Most human infections occur during the warm months, when recreational exposure is greatest. Person-to-person spread has not been documented. By definition, chronic carriage is not established in incidental hosts.

CLINICAL DISEASES

Most human infections with leptospires are clinically inapparent and detected only through the demonstration of specific antibodies. Symptomatic infections develop after a 1- to 2-week incubation period and in two phases. The initial phase is similar to an influenza-like illness with fever and myalgia (muscle pain). During this phase, the patient is bacteremic with the leptospires, and the organisms can frequently be isolated in CSF, even though no meningeal symptoms are present. The fever and myalgia may remit after 1 week, or the patient may progress to the second phase, which is characterized by sudden onset of headache, myalgia, chills, abdominal pain, and conjunctival suffusion (i.e., reddening of the eye). Severe disease can progress to vascular collapse, thrombocytopenia, hemorrhage, and hepatic and renal dysfunction.

Leptospirosis confined to the central nervous system can be mistaken for viral aseptic meningitis because the course of the disease is generally uncomplicated and has a very low mortality rate. Culture of CSF is usually negative at this stage. In contrast, the icteric form of generalized disease (approximately 10% of all symptomatic infections) is more severe and is associated with a mortality approaching 10% to 15%. Although hepatic involvement with jaundice (termed **icteric disease** or Weil's disease) is striking in patients with severe leptospirosis, hepatic necrosis is not seen and surviving patients do not suffer permanent hepatic damage. Similarly, most patients recover full renal function.

Congenital leptospirosis can also occur. This disease is characterized by the sudden onset of headache, fever, myalgias, and a diffuse rash.

LABORATORY DIAGNOSIS

Microscopy

Because leptospires are thin, they are at the limit of the resolving power of a light microscope and thus cannot be seen easily by conventional light microscopy. Neither Gram stain nor silver stain is reliable in the detection of leptospires. Dark-field microscopy is also relatively insensitive, capable of yielding nonspecific findings. Although leptospires can be seen in blood specimens early in the disease, protein filaments from erythrocytes can be easily mistaken for organisms. Fluorescein-labeled antibody preparations have been used to stain leptospires but are not available in most clinical laboratories.

Culture

Leptospires can be cultured on specially formulated media (e.g., Fletcher, EMJH, or Tween 80–albumin). They grow slowly (generation time, 6 to 16 hours), requiring incubation at 28° to 30°C for as long as 4 months; however, most cultures are positive within 2 weeks. Consistent with the two phases of illness, leptospires are present in blood or CSF during the first 10 days of infection and in urine after the first week and for as long as 3 months. Because the concentration of organisms in blood, CSF, and urine may be low, several specimens should be collected if leptospirosis is suspected. In addition, inhibitors present in blood and urine may delay or prevent recovery of leptospires. In contrast with most blood cultures, only 1 to 2 drops of blood are inoculated into the culture medium. Likewise, urine must be treated to neutralize the pH and concentrated by centrifugation. A few drops of the sediment are then inoculated into the culture medium.

Growth of the bacteria in culture is detected by dark-field microscopy.

Nucleic Acid Probes

Preliminary work with the detection of leptospires using nucleic acid probes has had limited success. Techniques using nucleic acid amplification (e.g., PCR) are more sensitive than culture. Unfortunately, this technique is not expected to become widely available.

Serology

Because of the need for specialized media and prolonged incubation, most laboratories do not attempt to culture leptospires and thus rely on serologic techniques. The reference method for all serologic tests is the **microscopic agglutination test (MAT).** This test measures the ability of the patient's serum to agglutinate live leptospires. Because the test is directed against specific serotypes, it is necessary to use pools of leptospiral antigens. In this test, serial dilutions of the patient's serum are mixed with the test antigens and then examined microscopically for agglutination. Agglutinins appear in the blood of untreated patients during the second week of illness, although this response may be delayed for as long as several months. Infected patients have a titer of at least 1:200 (i.e., agglutinins are detected in a 1:200 dilution of the patient's serum), and it may be 1:25,000 or higher. Patients treated with antibiotics may have a diminished antibody response or nondiagnostic titers. Agglutinating antibodies are detectable for many years after the acute illness; thus their presence may represent either a blunted antibody response in a treated patient with acute disease or residual antibodies in a person with a distant, unrecognized infection with leptospires. Because the microscopic agglutination test uses live organisms, it is performed only in reference laboratories. Alternative tests such as indirect hemagglutination, slide agglutination, and ELISA are less sensitive and specific. These tests can be used to screen a patient, but positive reactions must be confirmed with the MAT or preferably culture. Serologic cross-reactions occur with other spirochetal infections (i.e., syphilis, relapsing fever, Lyme disease) and legionellosis.

TREATMENT, PREVENTION, AND CONTROL

Leptospirosis is usually not fatal, particularly in the absence of icteric disease. Patients should be treated with either intravenously administered penicillin or doxycycline. Doxycycline but not penicillin can be used to prevent disease in persons exposed to infected animals or water contaminated with urine. It is difficult to eradicate leptospirosis, because the disease is widespread in wild and domestic animals. However, vaccination of livestock and pets has proved successful in reducing the incidence of disease in these populations and therefore subsequent human exposure. Rodent control is also effective in eliminating leptospirosis in communities.

CASE STUDY AND QUESTIONS

An 18-year-old woman complained of knee pain that started 2 weeks previously. Three months earlier, soon after vacationing in Connecticut, she noticed a circular area of redness on her lower leg; it was approximately 10 cm in diameter. During the next 2 weeks, the area enlarged and the border became more clearly demarcated; however, the rash gradually disappeared. A few days after the rash disappeared, the woman experienced the onset of headaches, an inability to concentrate, and nausea. These symptoms also gradually abated. The pain in her knee developed approximately 1 month after these symptoms disappeared. On examination of the knee, mild tenderness and pain were elicited. A small amount of serous fluid was aspirated from the joint, and it had an elevated white blood cell count. Antibodies to Borrelia burgdorferi were present in the patient's serum (titers of 1:32 and 1:1024 for IgM and IgG, respectively), confirming the clinical diagnosis of Lyme arthritis.

1. What are the initial and late manifestations of Lyme disease?
2. What are the limitations of the following diagnostic tests for Lyme disease: microscopy, culture, and serology? How do these compare with the diagnostic tests for other relapsing fevers?
3. Name two examples each of nontreponemal and treponemal tests for syphilis. What reactions to those tests would you expect in patients with primary, secondary, and late syphilis?
4. What are the reservoir and vectors for syphilis, epidemic and endemic relapsing fever, Lyme disease, and leptospirosis?
5. What diagnostic tests can be used for the diagnosis of leptospirosis?

Bibliography

Antal GM, Lukehart SA, Meheus AZ: The endemic treponematoses, *Microbes Infect* 4:83-94, 2002.

Balmelli T, Piffaretti J: Analysis of the genetic polymorphism of *Borrelia burgdorferi sensu lato* by multilocus enzyme electrophoresis, *Int J Syst Bacteriol* 46:167-172, 1996.

Barbour AG, Hayes SF: Biology of *Borrelia* species, *Microbiol Rev* 50:381-400, 1986.

Butler T et al: Infection with *Borrelia recurrentis:* Pathogenesis of fever and petechiae, *J Infect Dis* 140:665-672, 1979.

Centers for Disease Control and Prevention: Surveillance for Lyme disease—United States, 1992-1998, *MMWR* 49:1-12, 2000.

Centers for Disease Control and Prevention: *Sexually transmitted disease surveillance 2002 supplement, syphilis surveillance report*, Atlanta, 2004, U.S. Department of Health and Human Services.

Cutler S et al: *Borrelia recurrentis* characterization and comparison with relapsing fever, Lyme-associated, and other *Borrelia* spp., *Int J Syst Bacteriol* 47:958-968, 1997.

Gardner P: Lyme disease vaccines, *Ann Intern Med* 129:583-585, 1998 (editorial).

Johnson B et al: Serodiagnosis of Lyme disease: Accuracy of a two-step approach using a flagella-based ELISA and immunoblotting, *J Infect Dis* 174:346-353, 1996.

Larsen S, Steiner B, Rudolph A: Laboratory diagnosis and interpretation of tests for syphilis, *Clin Microbiol Rev* 8:1-21, 1995.

Levitt PN: Leptospirosis, *Clin Microbiol Rev* 14:296-326, 2001.

Mouritsen C et al: Polymerase chain reaction detection of Lyme disease: Correlation with clinical manifestations and serologic responses, *Am J Clin Pathol* 105:647-654, 1996.

Ras N et al: Phylogenesis of relapsing fever *Borrelia* spp., *Int J Syst Bacteriol* 46:859-865, 1996.

Romanowski B et al: Serologic response to treatment of infectious syphilis, *Ann Intern Med* 114:1005-1009, 1991.

Southern PM, Sanford JP: Relapsing fever: A clinical and microbiological review, *Medicine* 48:129-149, 1969.

Spach D et al: Tick-borne diseases in the United States, *N Engl J Med* 329:936-947, 1993.

Steigbigel R, Benach J: Immunization against Lyme Disease—an important first step, *N Engl J Med* 339:263-264, 1998.

Tugwell P et al: Guidelines for laboratory evaluation in the diagnosis of Lyme disease, I and II, *Ann Intern Med* 127:1106-1123, 1997.

Van Dam A et al: Different genospecies of *Borrelia burgdorferi* are associated with distinct clinical manifestations of Lyme borreliosis, *Clin Infect Dis* 17:708-717, 1993.

Vinetz J et al: Sporadic urban leptospirosis, *Ann Intern Med* 125:794-798, 1996.

Wang G et al: Molecular typing of *Borrelia burgdorferi sensu lata:* Taxonomic, epidemiological, and clinical implications, *Clin Microbiol Rev* 12:633-653, 1999.

Wormser G et al: Practice guidelines for the treatment of Lyme disease, *Clin Infect Dis* 31(S1):1-14, 2000.

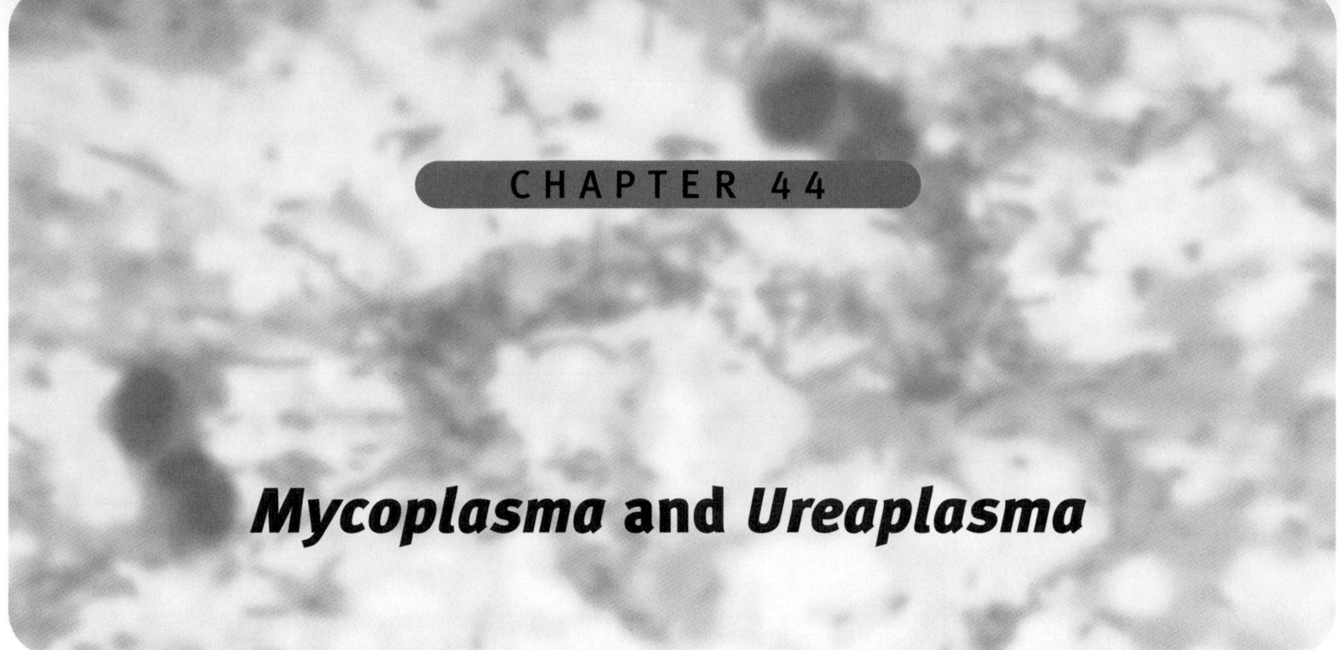

Mycoplasma and *Ureaplasma*

The class of organisms Mollicutes is subdivided into five families with almost 200 species. Sixteen species colonize humans and five species are associated with human disease (Table 44–1). The most important species is *Mycoplasma pneumoniae* (also called **Eaton's agent** after the investigator who originally isolated it). *M. pneumoniae* causes respiratory tract diseases, such as tracheobronchitis and pneumonia (Box 44–1). Other commonly isolated pathogens include *Mycoplasma hominis, Mycoplasma genitalium,* and *Ureaplasma urealyticum,* which cause genitourinary tract diseases. These and other mycoplasmas that colonize humans have been associated with a variety of maladies (e.g., infertility, spontaneous abortion, vaginitis, cervicitis, epididymitis, prostatitis); however, their etiologic role in these diseases remains incompletely defined.

Physiology and Structure

Mycoplasma and *Ureaplasma* organisms are the smallest free-living bacteria (Table 44–2). They are unique among bacteria because they do not have a cell wall and their cell membrane contains **sterols.** In contrast, other cell wall–deficient bacteria (called **L forms**) do not have sterols in their cell membrane and can form cell walls under the appropriate growth conditions. The absence of the cell wall renders the mycoplasmas resistant to penicillins, cephalosporins, vancomycin, and other antibiotics that interfere with synthesis of the cell wall.

The mycoplasmas form pleomorphic filaments with an average diameter of 0.1 to 0.3 µm, and many can pass through the 0.45-µm filters used to remove bacteria from solutions. For these reasons, the mycoplasmas were originally thought to be viruses. However, the organisms divide by binary fission (typical of all bacteria), grow on artificial cell-free media, and contain both ribonucleic acid (RNA) and deoxyribonucleic acid (DNA). Mycoplasmas are facultatively anaerobic (except *M. pneumoniae,* which is a strict aerobe) and require exogenous sterols supplied by animal serum added to the growth medium. The mycoplasmas grow slowly, with a generation time of 1 to 6 hours, and most form small colonies that have a fried-egg appearance (Figure 44–1). *M. pneumoniae* is an exception in this respect as well, because its colonies do not have a thin halo and have been described as "mulberry shaped." Colonies of *Ureaplasma* are extremely small, measuring 10 to 50 mm in diameter.

Because the Mycoplasmataceae do not have a cell wall, the major antigenic determinants are membrane glycolipids and proteins. These antigens cross-react with human tissues and other bacteria.

Pathogenesis and Immunity

M. pneumoniae is an extracellular pathogen that adheres to the respiratory epithelium by means of a specialized terminal protein attachment factor. This adhesin protein, called **P1,** interacts specifically with sialated glycoprotein receptors at the base of cilia on the epithelial cell surface (and on the surface of erythrocytes). Ciliostasis then occurs, after which first the cilia, then the ciliated epithelial cells, are destroyed. The loss of these cells interferes with the normal clearance of the upper airways and permits the lower respiratory tract to become contaminated with microbes and mechanically irritated. This process is responsible for the persistent cough present in patients with symptomatic disease. *M. pneumoniae* functions as a superantigen, stimulating inflammatory cells to migrate to the site of infection and release cytokines, initially tumor necrosis factor-α (TNF-α) and interleukin-1

TABLE 44–1. Mycoplasmataceae Isolated in Humans

Organism	Site	Disease
Mycoplasma pneumoniae	Respiratory tract	Upper respiratory tract disease; atypical pneumonia; tracheobronchitis; rarely, extrapulmonary manifestations (cardiac, neurologic, dermatologic)
Mycoplasma hominis	Respiratory tract, genitourinary tract	Pyelonephritis; pelvic inflammatory disease; postpartum fever
Mycoplasma genitalium	Genitourinary tract	Urethritis
Mycoplasma fermentans	Respiratory tract, genitourinary tract	Influenza-like illness; pneumonia
Ureaplasma urealyticum	Respiratory tract, genitourinary tract	Urethritis

TABLE 44–2. Properties of *Mycoplasma* and *Ureaplasma*

Properties	Characteristics
Cell size	0.1–0.3 μm
Cell wall	Absent
Growth	
Atmosphere	Facultatively anaerobic*
Nutritional requirement	Sterols
Nutritional supplements	Vitamins, amino acids, nucleic acid precursors
Other	Cell-free growth
Replication	Binary fission
Generation time	1–6 hrs
Antibiotic susceptibility	
Penicillins	Resistant
Cephalosporins	Resistant
Tetracyclines	Susceptible
Erythromycin	Susceptible†

**Mycoplasma pneumoniae* is an obligate aerobe.
†*Mycoplasma hominis* is resistant.

(IL-1) and later, IL-6. This process contributes to both the clearance of the bacteria and the observed disease.

BOX 44–1. Summary of *Mycoplasma pneumoniae*

Physiology and Structure

The smallest free-living bacterium; able to pass through 0.45-μm pore filters
Absence of cell wall and a cell membrane containing sterols are unique among bacteria
Slow rate of growth (generation time, 1 to 6 hours); strict aerobe

Virulence

P1 adhesin protein binds to base of cilia on epithelial cells, leading to eventual loss of ciliated epithelial cells
Acts as superantigen, stimulating migration of inflammatory cells and release of cytokines
Worldwide disease with no seasonal incidence (in contrast to disease caused by most respiratory pathogens)
Primarily infects children between ages 5 and 15 years, but all populations susceptible to disease
Transmitted by inhalation of aerosolized droplet
Strict human pathogen

Diseases

Upper respiratory infections
Lower respiratory infections, including tracheobronchitis and bronchopneumonia

Diagnosis

Refer to Table 44–3

Treatment, Control, and Prevention

Drug of choice is erythromycin, newer fluoroquinolones, or tetracycline
Immunity to reinfection is not lifelong, and vaccines have proved ineffective

Epidemiology

Pneumonia caused by *M. pneumoniae* occurs worldwide throughout the year, with no consistent increase in seasonal activity. However, because pneumonia caused by other infectious agents (e.g., *Streptococcus pneumoniae*, viruses) is more common during the cold months, *M. pneumoniae* disease is proportionally more common during the summer and fall. Epidemic disease occurs every 4 to 8 years. Disease is most common in school-age children and young adults (ages 5 to 15 years). Disease was once believed to be uncommon in older adults; however, studies have now demonstrated that all age groups are susceptible to infections with this organism.

It has been estimated that 2 million cases of *M. pneumoniae* pneumonia and 100,000 pneumonia-related

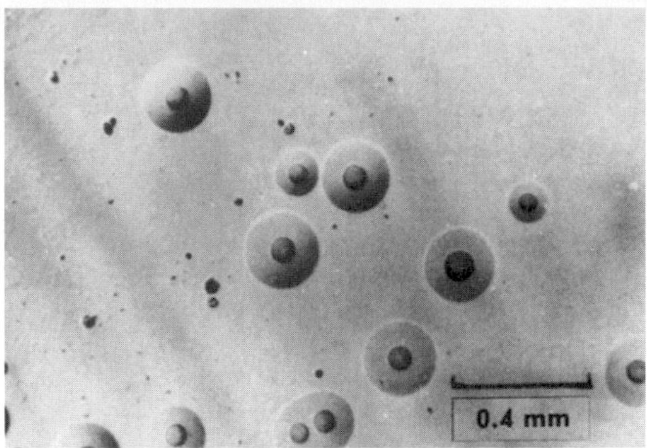

FIGURE 44–1. Fried-egg appearance of colonies of mycoplasmas. All mycoplasmas except *Mycoplasma pneumoniae* typically show this morphology. *M. pneumoniae* has a strict aerobic atmosphere requirement. It is one of the slowest growing mycoplasmas, appearing as homogeneous granular colonies after incubation for 1 week or longer. The other mycoplasmas generally grow within 1 to 4 days. (From Razin S, Oliver O: *J Gen Microbiol* 24:225-237, 1961.)

hospitalizations occur annually in the United States. However, *M. pneumoniae* disease is not a reportable disease and reliable diagnostic tests are not readily available, so the true incidence is not known.

Nasal secretions spread *M. pneumoniae* infection. Close contact is necessary for transmission, and the infection usually occurs among classmates or family members. The attack rate is higher in children than in adults (overall average, approximately 60%), presumably because most adults are partially immune from previous exposure. The incubation period and time of infectivity are prolonged; thus, disease can persist for months among classmates or family members.

Infants, particularly females, are colonized with *M. hominis*, *M. genitalium*, and *Ureaplasma* species at birth, with *Ureaplasma* organisms being isolated most often. Although carriage of these mycoplasmas usually does not persist, a small proportion of prepubertal children remains colonized. The incidence of genital mycoplasmas rises after puberty, corresponding to sexual activity. Approximately 15% of sexually active men and women are colonized with *M. hominis*, and 45% to 75% are colonized with *Ureaplasma*. The incidence of carriage in adults who are sexually inactive is no greater than that in prepubertal children.

Clinical Diseases

Infection with *M. pneumoniae* typically produces mild **upper respiratory tract disease.** Low-grade fever, malaise, headache, and a dry, nonproductive cough develop 2 to 3 weeks after exposure. Symptoms gradually worsen over the next few days and can persist for 2 weeks or longer. More severe disease with lower respiratory tract symptoms occurs in less than 10% of patients. **Tracheobronchitis,** in which the bronchial passages primarily become infiltrated with lymphocytes and plasma cells, can occur. Pneumonia (referred to as primary **atypical pneumonia** or walking pneumonia) can also develop, with a patchy bronchopneumonia seen on chest radiographs that is typically more impressive than the physical findings. Myalgias and gastrointestinal tract symptoms are uncommon. Secondary complications include otitis media, erythema multiforme **(Stevens-Johnson syndrome),** hemolytic anemia, myocarditis, pericarditis, and neurologic abnormalities. The disease resolves slowly. Secondary infections can occur because immunity is incomplete.

The role of other mycoplasmas in human disease is less clearly defined. *M. genitalium* and *U. urealyticum* can cause **nongonococcal urethritis,** and *M. hominis* has been implicated as a cause of **pyelonephritis, pelvic inflammatory disease,** and **postpartum fever.** The evidence implicating the organisms in these diseases is based on (1) recovery of the bacteria from specimens from infected patients, (2) a serologic response to the organism, (3) clinical improvement after treatment with specific antibiotics, (4) demonstration of disease in animal models, or (5) a combination of these findings. It is common, however, for the genitourinary tract to be colonized with these organisms, and their presence can mask a more important pathogen.

Laboratory Diagnosis

The diagnostic tests for *M. pneumoniae* infections are summarized in Table 44–3.

MICROSCOPY

Microscopy is of no diagnostic value. Mycoplasmas stain poorly because they have no cell wall.

CULTURE

Unlike other mycoplasmas, *M. pneumoniae* is a strict aerobe. These mycoplasmas can be isolated from throat washings, bronchial washings, or expectorated sputum. Washings are more reliable than sputum specimens, because most infected patients have a dry, nonproductive cough and do not produce sputum. The specimen should be inoculated into special media supplemented with serum (provides sterols), yeast extract (for nucleic acid precursors), glucose, a pH indicator, and penicillin (to inhibit other bacteria). The organisms grow slowly in culture, with a generation time of 6 hours.

TABLE 44–3. Diagnostic Tests for *Mycoplasma pneumoniae* Infections

Test	Assessment
Microscopy	Test is not useful because organisms do not have a cell wall and do not stain with conventional reagents
Culture	Test is slow (2 to 6 weeks before positive diagnosis) and insensitive; it is not available in most laboratories
Molecular diagnosis	PCR-based amplification assays with excellent sensitivity; specificity is not well defined; expected to be the diagnostic test of choice when assays become more widely available
Serology	
Complement fixation	Antibody titers vs. glycolipid antigens peak in 4 weeks and persist for 6–12 months; poor sensitivity and specificity
Enzyme immunoassays	Multiple assays available with varying sensitivity and specificity; assays directed vs. P1 adhesin protein may be most specific
Cold agglutinin	Sensitivity approximately 65%; specificity poor with cross-reactions with other respiratory pathogens (e.g., Epstein-Barr virus, cytomegalovirus, adenovirus); test commonly used but not recommended

PCR, Polymerase chain reaction.

Although a positive culture result is definitive evidence of disease, it is relatively insensitive. In one well-designed study, 36% of the isolates were detected within 2 weeks, whereas detection of the remaining isolates required prolonged incubation (as long as 6 weeks). In another study, only 64% of cultures from patients with serologic evidence of an acute *Mycoplasma* infection had positive results. Growth of the organisms in culture is indicated by the metabolism of glucose with a corresponding pH change.

Colonies of *M. pneumoniae* are small and have a homogeneous granular appearance ("mulberry shaped"), unlike the fried-egg morphology of other mycoplasmas. Identification of isolates can be confirmed by inhibition of their growth with specific antisera. Because this organism is difficult to grow and results are typically not available for many weeks, however, most laboratories do not perform cultures.

M. hominis is a facultative anaerobe that grows within 1 to 4 days and metabolizes arginine but not glucose. The colonies have a typical, large fried-egg appearance (see Figure 44–1). Inhibition of their growth with specific antisera is used to differentiate them from other genital mycoplasmas. *Ureaplasma* requires urea for growth but is inhibited by the higher alkalinity resulting from the metabolism of urea. Thus the growth medium must be supplemented with urea and be highly buffered. Even if these steps are taken, ureaplasmas die rapidly after initial isolation.

MOLECULAR DIAGNOSIS

Polymerase chain reaction (PCR)-based assays have been developed for all pathogenic *Mycoplasma* and *Ureaplasma* species. The tests have excellent sensitivity, but the specificity is not well defined; that is, these assays may cross-react with avirulent species that colonize humans. In addition, commercial PCR assays are not available at this time.

SEROLOGY

Serologic tests are available only for *M. pneumoniae.* Detection of antibodies directed against *M. pneumoniae* by complement fixation is the traditional serologic reference standard. However, the test has poor sensitivity and antibodies directed against the target glycolipid antigen are also elicited by other *Mycoplasma* species and by host tissues. A number of enzyme immunoassays for the detection of immunoglobulin M (IgM) and IgG antibodies are available. The format and target antigens vary among the tests, so they cannot be considered equivalent. Assays using the P1 adhesin protein may be the most specific but may lack sensitivity compared with whole cell assays. Further comparison of these kits is required.

It is also possible to measure nonspecific reactions to the outer membrane glycolipids of *M. pneumoniae.* The most useful of these reactions is the production of **cold agglutinins** (e.g., IgM antibodies that bind the I antigen on the surface of human erythrocytes at 4°C). The cold agglutinin assay is positive in approximately 65% of patients with *M. pneumoniae* infections, particularly those who are symptomatic, and is often positive at the time the patient presents with symptoms. Because this test is not specific for *M. pneumoniae,* cross-reactions are observed in patients with respiratory tract diseases caused by other organisms (e.g., Epstein-Barr virus, cytomegalovirus, adenovirus). A strongly reactive cold agglutinin titer of at least 1 : 128 or a significant increase in the titer constitutes presumptive evidence of *Mycoplasma* disease.

Treatment, Prevention, and Control

Erythromycin, tetracycline (or doxycycline), and newer fluoroquinolones (e.g., gatifloxacin, moxifloxacin) are equally effective in treating *M. pneumoniae* infections, although the tetracyclines and fluoroquinolones are reserved for use in adults. Tetracyclines have the advantage of also being active against most other mycoplasmas and chlamydia, a common cause of nongonococcal urethritis. Erythromycin is used to treat *Ureaplasma* infections, because these organisms are resistant to tetracycline. Unlike the other mycoplasmas, *M. hominis* is resistant to erythromycin and occasionally to the tetracyclines. Clindamycin has been used to treat infections caused by these resistant strains.

The prevention of *Mycoplasma* disease is problematic. *M. pneumoniae* infections are spread by close contact; thus the isolation of infected people could theoretically reduce the risk of infection. Isolation is impractical, however, because patients are typically infectious for a prolonged period, even while receiving appropriate antibiotics. Inactivated vaccines and attenuated live vaccines have also proved disappointing. The protective immunity conferred by infection has been low. Infections with *M. hominis, M. genitalium,* and *Ureaplasma* are transmitted by sexual contact. Therefore these diseases can be prevented by avoidance of sexual activity or the use of proper barrier precautions.

CASE STUDY AND QUESTIONS

Increased lethargy, headache, cough, a low-grade fever, and chills and sweats at night developed in a 21-year-old university student. When she was seen at the student health center, she had a nonproductive cough and shortness of breath on exertion. Her pulse rate was 95 beats/min, and her respiratory rate was 28 breaths/min. Her pharynx was erythematous; scattered rhonchi and rales but no consolidation were noted on auscultation. Results of a chest radiograph showed patchy infiltrates. A Gram stain of sputum revealed many white blood cells but no organisms. The antibody titer for a Mycoplasma complement fixation test performed on a specimen collected at admission was 1:8; the titer for a specimen collected a week later was 1:32. The patient was treated with erythromycin, to which her disease responded slowly during the next 2 weeks.

1. If cultures were performed, what would be the best specimen? When would the results be available? What are the sensitivity and specificity of culture in a patient infected with *M. pneumoniae?*
2. How do *Mycoplasma* species differ from other bacteria?
3. Describe the epidemiology of *M. pneumoniae* infections. What aspects of this case are characteristic of such infections?
4. What other mycoplasmas cause human disease? What diseases do they cause?

Bibliography

Cole B, Sawitzke A: Mycoplasmas, superantigens and autoimmune arthritis. In Henderson B et al, editors: *Mechanisms and models in rheumatoid arthritis,* San Diego, 1996, Academic Press.

Kenny GE et al: Diagnosis of *Mycoplasma pneumoniae* pneumonia: Sensitivities and specificities of serology with lipid antigen and isolation of the organism on soy peptone medium for identification of infections, *J Clin Microbiol* 28:2087-2093, 1990.

Lo S: New understandings of mycoplasmal infections and diseases, *Clin Microbiol Newsletter* 17:169-173, 1995.

Loens K et al: Molecular diagnosis of *Mycoplasma pneumoniae* respiratory tract infections, *J Clin Microbiol* 41:4915-4923, 2003.

Luby JP: Pneumonia caused by *Mycoplasma pneumoniae* infection, *Clin Chest Med* 12:237-244, 1991.

Maniloff J et al, editors: *Mycoplasmas: Molecular biology and pathogenesis,* Washington, 1992, American Society for Microbiology.

McMahon DK et al: Extragenital *Mycoplasma hominis* infections in adults, *Am J Med* 89:275-281, 1990.

Templeton KE et al: Comparison and evaluation of real-time PCR, real-time nucleic acid sequence-based amplification, conventional PCR, and serology for diagnosis of *Mycoplasma pneumoniae, J Clin Microbiol* 41:4366-4371, 2003.

Waites K et al: Laboratory diagnosis of mycoplasmal and ureaplasmal infections, *Clin Microbiol Newsletter* 18:105-112, 1996.

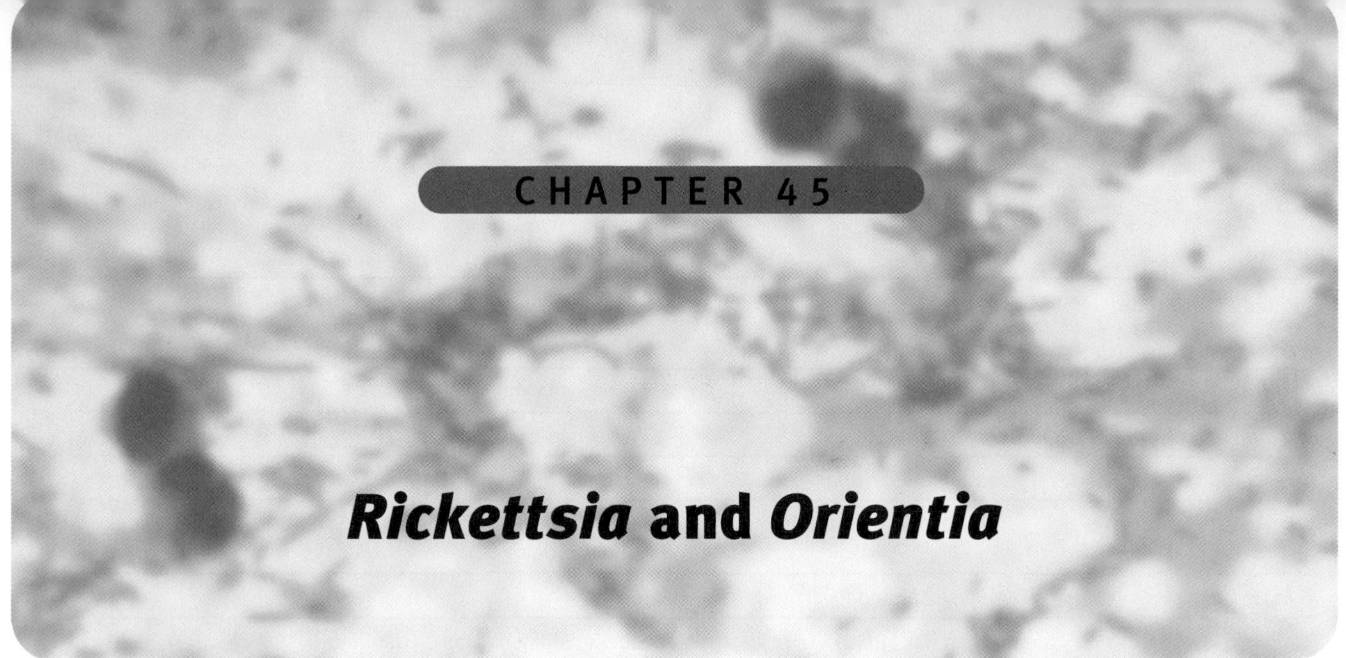

Rickettsia and *Orientia*

Rickettsia (named after Howard Ricketts), *Ehrlichia* (named after Paul Ehrlich), and *Coxiella* (named after Harold Cox) were historically classified in a single family, Rickettsiaceae, based on the observation that they were obligate intracellular, aerobic, gram-negative rods. Analysis of their deoxyribonucleic acid (DNA) sequences revealed that this classification was invalid. Furthermore, it was observed that *Rickettsia* should be subdivided into two genera (*Rickettsia* and *Orientia*) and *Ehrlichia* into two genera (*Ehrlichia* and *Anaplasma*). *Rickettsia* and *Orientia* are discussed in this chapter and the other intracellular organisms are discussed in Chapter 46.

The organisms of the family Rickettsiaceae were originally thought to be viruses because they were small (0.3×1 to 2 µm), stained poorly with the Gram stain, and grew only in the cytoplasm of eukaryotic cells. Nevertheless, these organisms have the following characteristics of bacteria: (1) structurally similar to gram-negative rods; (2) contain DNA, ribonucleic acid (RNA), and enzymes for the Krebs cycle and ribosomes for protein synthesis; (3) multiply by binary fission; and (4) are inhibited by antibiotics (e.g., tetracycline, chloramphenicol). The pathogenic species of *Rickettsia* and *Orientia* are maintained in animal and arthropod reservoirs and are transmitted by arthropod vectors (e.g., ticks, mites, lice, fleas). Humans are accidental hosts. *Rickettsia* species are subdivided into the spotted fever group and the typhus group. The most common species that cause human disease are summarized in Table 45–1 and Figure 45–1.

Many species of rickettsiae are maintained in their arthropod hosts by transovarian transmission. The exception to this rule is *Rickettsia prowazekii*, which kills its host, the human body louse. The distribution of rickettsial diseases is determined by the distribution of the arthropod host/vector. Most infections with tick vectors (e.g., spotted fevers) have a restricted geographic distribution, whereas rickettsial infections with other vectors, such as lice *(R. prowazekii)*, fleas *(Rickettsia typhi)*, and mites *(Rickettsia akari, Orientia tsutsugamushi)*, have worldwide distribution.

Physiology and Structure

The cell wall structures of *Rickettsia* and *Orientia* are typical of gram-negative rods, with a peptidoglycan layer and lipopolysaccharide (LPS). However, the peptidoglycan layer is minimal (stains poorly with the Gram stain) and the LPS has only weak endotoxin activity. *Orientia* lacks both the peptidoglycan layer and LPS. The organisms are seen best with Giemsa or Gimenez stains (Figure 45–2). The bacteria do not have flagella and are surrounded by a loosely adherent slime layer. *Rickettsia* and *Orientia* are strict intracellular parasites found free in the cytoplasm of infected cells.

The bacteria enter eukaryotic cells by stimulating phagocytosis. After engulfment, *Rickettsia* and *Orientia* degrade the phagosome membrane by producing a phospholipase and must be released into the cytoplasm or the organism will not survive. Multiplication in the host cell by binary fission is slow (generation time, 9 to 12 hours). *Orientia* and the spotted fever group of *Rickettsia* grow in the cytoplasm and nucleus of infected cells and are continually released from cells through long, cytoplasmic projections. In contrast, the typhus group accumulates in the cell cytoplasm until the cell membranes lyse, signaling cell death and bacterial release. It is believed that the fundamental difference is caused by intracellular motility—the spotted fever group is able to polymerize host cell acitin, whereas the typhus group lacks the required gene. Once these bacteria are released from the host cell, they are unstable and die quickly.

TABLE 45–1. Distribution of *Rickettsia* and *Orientia* Species Associated with Human Disease

Organism	Human Disease	Distribution
Spotted Fever Group		
R. rickettsii	Rocky Mountain spotted fever	Western hemisphere
R. africae	African tick bite fever	Eastern and southern Africa
R. akari	Rickettsialpox	Worldwide
R. australis	Australian tick typhus	Australia
R. conorii	Mediterranean spotted fever	Mediterranean countries, Black Sea, Africa, India, Georgia, Russia southwest Asia
R. japonica	Japanese spotted fever	Japan
R. sibirica	Siberian tick typhus	Siberia, Mongolia, northern China
Typhus group		
R. prowazekii	Epidemic typhus Recrudescent typhus Sporadic typhus	Worldwide Worldwide United States
R. typhi	Endemic (murine) typhus	Worldwide
Scrub typhus group		
O. tsutsugamushi	Scrub typhus	Asia, Oceania

Disease	Organism	Vector	Reservoir
Rocky Mountain spotted fever	*R. rickettsii*	Tick-borne 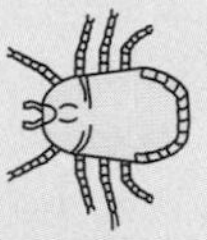	Ticks, wild rodents
Rickettsialpox	*R. akari*	Mite-borne 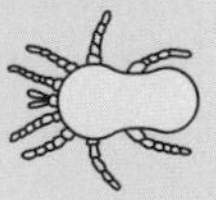	Mites, wild rodents
Scrub typhus	*O. tsutsugamushi*		Mites (chiggers), wild rodents
Epidemic typhus	*R. prowazekii*	Louse-borne 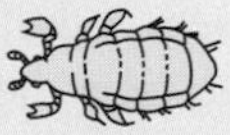	Humans, squirrel fleas, flying squirrels
Murine endemic typhus	*R. typhi*	Flea-borne 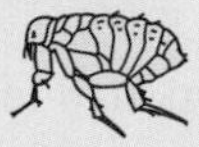	Wild rodents

FIGURE 45–1. Epidemiology of common *Rickettsia* and *Orientia* infections.

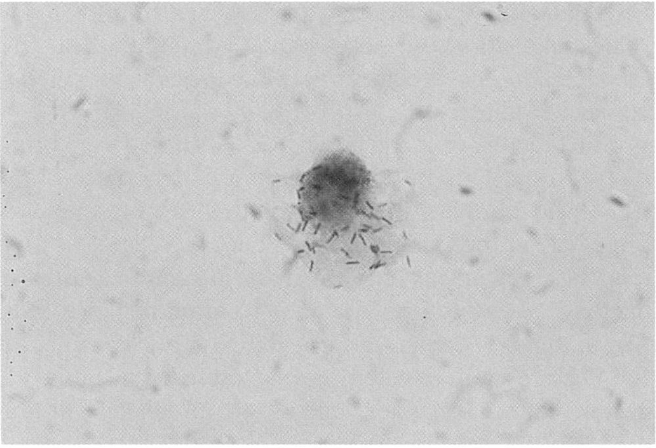

FIGURE 45–2. Gimenez stain of tissue culture cells infected with spotted fever group *Rickettsia.* (From Cohen J, Powderly WG: *Infectious diseases,* ed 2, St Louis, 2004, Mosby.)

The genomes of *R. prowazekii* and *Rickettsia conorii* have been sequenced, providing information about the parasitic nature of these bacteria. The bacteria are capable of protein synthesis and can produce adenosine triphosphate (ATP) by means of the tricarboxylic acid cycle. It appears that the bacteria are energy parasites that use the host cell ATP as long as it is available. *R. prowazekii,* the best-studied species, has a parasitic enzyme (ATP/ADP [adenosine diphosphate] translocase) that facilitates transfer of ATP from the host cell. The bacteria depend on their host cell for many functions: glycolysis, sugar nucleotide, and the pentose phosphate pathway for energy metabolism; purine and pyrimidine ribonucleotide biosynthesis enzymes and amino acid biosynthetic pathways for biosynthesis functions.

Rickettsia rickettsii (Box 45–1)

PATHOGENESIS AND IMMUNITY

The most common rickettsiae causing human disease in the United States is *R. rickettsii*, the agent responsible for **Rocky Mountain spotted fever.** There is no evidence that *R. rickettsii* produces toxins or that the host's immune response is responsible for the pathologic manifestations of Rocky Mountain spotted fever. The primary clinical manifestations appear to result from the replication of bacteria in endothelial cells, with subsequent damage to the cells and leakage of the blood vessels. Hypovolemia and hypoproteinemia caused by the loss of plasma into tissues can lead to reduced perfusion of various organs and organ failure. The host immune response to infection is based on cytokine-mediated intracellular killing and clearance by cytotoxic CD8 lymphocytes. Antibody response to rickettsial outer membrane proteins may also be important.

BOX 45–1. Summary of *Rickettsia rickettsii*

Physiology and Structure

Small, intracellular bacteria
Stain poorly with Gram stain; best with Giemsa or Gimenez stains
Replication occurs in cytoplasm and nucleus of infected cells

Virulence

Intracellular growth protects the bacteria from immune clearance
Replicates in endothelial cells with resulting vasculitis

Epidemiology

R. rickettsii is most common rickettsial pathogen in United States
Hard ticks are the primary reservoirs and vectors
Transmission requires prolonged contact (24 to 48 hours)
Distribution in Western hemisphere; in United States, infection is most common in southeast Atlantic and south central states
Disease is most common April through October

Disease

Rocky Mountain spotted fever

Diagnosis

DFA, MIF, and PCR tests used most commonly for detection of the genus; Western blot assay used to differentiate species

Treatment, Prevention, and Control

Doxycycline is the drug of choice; alternative antibiotics include fluoroquinolones
People should avoid tick-infected areas, wear protective clothing, and use effective insecticides
People should remove attached ticks immediately
No vaccine is currently available

*DFA, Direct fluorescent antibody, MIF, microimmunofluorescence, PCR, polymerase chain reaction.

EPIDEMIOLOGY

Approximately 500 to 1000 documented cases of Rocky Mountain spotted fever are reported annually in the United States. Although the disease was first described in Idaho and later in Montana, most cases today are seen in the southeastern Atlantic and south central states. The reason for this shift is not known, but it could be a result of changes in the tick population or changes in the proportion of infected ticks in the specific areas. The principal reservoir and vector for *R. rickettsii* are infected **hard ticks:** the wood tick *(Dermacentor andersoni)* in Rocky Mountain states and the dog tick *(Dermacentor variabilis)* in the southeastern states and the West Coast. Other tick reservoirs include *Rhipicephalus sanguineus* in Mexico, and *Amblyomma cajennense* in Central and South America. It is not clear whether the Lone Star tick *(Amblyomma americanum)* in the south central states is a reservoir. The rickettsiae are maintained in the tick population by transovarian transmission. Mammals such as wild rodents can also serve as reservoirs, but this source is considered uncommon for tick-to-human infections.

Rickettsial infections are spread to humans by the adult ticks when they feed. More than 90% of all infections occur from April through October, corresponding to the period of greatest tick activity. To become infected, a person must be exposed to the tick for a lengthy period (e.g., 24 to 48 hours). The dormant avirulent rickettsiae are activated by the warm blood meal, then must be released from the tick salivary glands to penetrate into the blood of the human host.

CLINICAL DISEASES

Clinically, symptomatic disease develops 2 to 14 days (average, 7 days) after the tick bite (Table 45–2). The patient may not recall the painless tick bite. The onset of disease is heralded by high fever, chills, headache, and myalgias. A rash may develop after 3 or more days and can evolve from macular to petechial form. It initially involves the extremities and then spreads to the trunk. The palms and soles can also be involved. Complications of Rocky Mountain spotted fever include gastrointestinal symptoms, respiratory failure, encephalitis, and renal failure. Complications increase and the prognosis is worse when the characteristic rash does not develop or develops late in the disease, because the diagnosis is delayed.

TABLE 45-2. Clinical Course of Human Diseases Caused by *Rickettsia* and *Orientia* Species

Disease	Average Incubation Period (days)	Clinical Presentation	Rash	Eschar	Mortality without Treatment (%)
Rocky Mountain spotted fever	7	Abrupt onset; fever, chills, headache, myalgias	>90%; macular; centripetal spread	No	20–40
Rickettsialpox	9–14	Abrupt onset; fever, headache, chills, myalgias, photophobia	100%; papulovesicular; generalized	Yes	low
Epidemic typhus	8	Abrupt onset; fever, headache, chills, myalgias, arthralgia	40%–80%; macular; centrifugal spread	No	20
Endemic typhus	7–14	Gradual onset; fever, headache, myalgias, cough	50%; maculopapular rash on trunk	No	low
Scrub typhus	10–12	Abrupt onset; fever, headache, myalgias	<50%; maculopapular rash; centrifugal	No	1–15

LABORATORY DIAGNOSIS

Culture

Rickettsiae can be isolated in tissue culture or embryonated eggs. Reference laboratories that routinely work with these bacteria report bacterial recovery is relatively easy using traditional shell vial culture assay systems. However, microscopy, serologic procedures, and polymerase chain reaction (PCR)-based assays are the techniques used in most diagnostic laboratories and are probably less hazardous than working with live cultures.

Microscopy

Although rickettsiae stain poorly with Gram stain, they can be stained with Giemsa or Gimenez stains. Specific fluorescein-labeled antibodies can also be used to stain the intracellular bacteria in biopsy tissue specimens. This direct detection of rickettsial antigens is a rapid, specific method for confirming the clinical diagnosis of Rocky Mountain spotted fever.

Serology

Although the **Weil-Felix test** (which involves the differential agglutination of *Proteus* antigens) has been used historically for the diagnosis of rickettsial infections, it is no longer recommended, because it is insensitive and nonspecific. The test most commonly used for detecting rickettsial antibodies is microimmunofluorescence (MIF). The test detects antibodies directed against outer membrane proteins (species-specific) and the LPS antigen. Because the LPS antigen is shared among rickettsial species, the Western blot immunoassay must be performed to define the individual species. Cross-reactions with other genera (e.g., *Legionella*) are observed.

Molecular Diagnosis

A number of reference laboratories have developed PCR-based assays directed against a variety of gene targets (e.g., gene sequences for outer membrane proteins, 17-kDa lipoprotein, 16S ribosomal RNA [rRNA]). These assays are not species-specific, so further testing is required to identify the species.

TREATMENT, PREVENTION, AND CONTROL

Rickettsiae are susceptible to tetracyclines (e.g., doxycycline) and fluoroquinolones (e.g., ciprofloxacin). Chloramphenicol has activity in vitro against rickettsiae, but use for treatment of infections is associated with a higher incidence of relapse compared with doxycycline. The prompt diagnosis and institution of appropriate therapy usually result in a satisfactory prognosis; unfortunately, this scenario may not occur if key clinical signs (e.g., rash) develop late or not at all. In addition, the serologic findings often are not available until 2 to 4 weeks after the onset of disease, also delaying the start of treatment. The morbidity and mortality are high if the diagnosis or specific therapy is delayed.

There is no vaccine for Rocky Mountain spotted fever. Thus, avoidance of tick-infested areas, the use of protective clothing and insect repellents, and the prompt removal of attached ticks are the best preventive measures. It is virtually impossible to eliminate the tick reservoir, because the ticks can survive for as long as 4 years without feeding.

Other Spotted Fever Rickettsiae

At least six other rickettsial species in the spotted fever group cause human disease (see Table 45–1). *R. akari*, the agent responsible for causing **rickettsialpox**, is occasionally isolated in the United States. Infections with *R. akari* are maintained in the rodent population through the bite of mouse ectoparasites (e.g., mites) and in mites by transovarian transmission. Humans become accidental hosts when bitten by infected mites. The other rickettsiae in the spotted fever group are transmitted by ticks.

Clinical infection with *R. akari* is biphasic. First, a papule develops at the site where the mite has bitten the host. The papule appears approximately 1 week after the bite and quickly progresses to ulceration and then eschar formation. During this period, the rickettsiae spread systemically. After an incubation period of 7 to 24 days (average, 9 to 14 days), the second phase of the disease develops abruptly, with high fever, severe headache, chills, sweats, myalgias, and photophobia. A generalized papulovesicular rash forms within 2 to 3 days. A poxlike progression of the rash is then seen, in which vesicles form and then crust over. Despite the appearance of the disseminated rash, rickettsialpox is usually mild and uncomplicated, and complete healing is seen within 2 to 3 weeks without treatment. Specific therapy with doxycycline or chloramphenicol speeds the process.

BOX 45–2. Summary of *Rickettsia prowazekii*

Physiology and Structure
Small, intracellular bacteria
Stain poorly with Gram stain; best with Giemsa or Gimenez stains
Replicate in cytoplasm of infected cells

Virulence
Intracellular growth protects the bacteria from immune clearance
Replicates in endothelial cells with resulting vasculitis

Epidemiology
Humans are the primary reservoir, with person-to-person transmission by louse vector
It is believed that sporadic disease is spread from squirrels to humans via squirrel fleas
Recrudescent disease can develop years after initial infection
People at greatest risk are those living in crowded, unsanitary conditions
Disease is worldwide, with most infections in Central and South America and Africa
Sporadic disease is seen in the eastern United States

Diseases
Epidemic typhus (louse-borne typhus)
Recrudescent typhus (Brill-Zinsser disease)
Sporadic typhus

Diagnosis
The MIF test is the test of choice

Treatment, Prevention, and Control
Doxycycline is the drug of choice
Controlled through improvements in living conditions and reduction of the lice population through use of insecticides
Inactivated vaccine is available for high-risk populations

*MIF, Microimmunofluorescence.

Rickettsia prowazekii (Box 45–2)

EPIDEMIOLOGY

R. prowazekii is the etiologic agent of **epidemic typhus,** also called **louse-borne typhus,** and the principal vector is the human body louse, *Pediculus humanus*. Unlike with most other rickettsial diseases, humans are the primary reservoir of typhus. Epidemic typhus occurs among people living in crowded, unsanitary conditions that favor the spread of body lice—conditions such as those that arise during wars, famines, and natural disasters. Lice die from their infection within 2 to 3 weeks, preventing the transovarian transmission of *R. prowazekii*. The disease is present in Central and South America, Africa, and less commonly in the United States.

The incidence of the disease in the United States is unknown because it is not classified as a disease reportable to public health departments. Sporadic disease in the United States is primarily restricted to rural areas of the eastern states. It occurs in this area because flying squirrels, as well as squirrel fleas and lice, are infected with *R. prowazekii*. Squirrel lice do not feed on humans, but the fleas are less discriminating and may be responsible for transmitting the *Rickettsia* from squirrels to humans. Epidemiologic and serologic evidence supports this hypothesis, but such transmission has not been documented.

Recrudescent disease with *R. prowazekii* **(Brill-Zinsser disease)** can occur in people years after their initial infection. Such people in the United States are primarily Eastern European immigrants who were exposed to epidemic typhus during World War II.

CLINICAL DISEASES

In one study of epidemic typhus in Africa, clinical disease was found to develop after a 2- to 30-day incubation period (average, 8 days). Most of the patients initially had nonspecific symptoms; then within 1 to 3 days, high fever, severe headache, chills, myalgias, arthralgia, and anorexia developed. Less than 40% of the patients had a petechial or macular rash, but darkly pigmented skin can obscure the rash. Complications of epidemic typhus include myocarditis and central nervous system dysfunction; a mortality rate as high as 66% has been reported in some epidemics. This high mortality rate undoubtedly stems from the poor general health, nutrition, and hygiene of the population together with the lack of antibiotic therapy and proper supportive medical care. In patients with uncomplicated disease, the body temperature returns to normal within 2 weeks, but complete convalescence may take 3 months or longer.

As noted earlier, reactivation or recrudescent epidemic typhus (Brill-Zinsser disease) can occur years after the initial disease. However, the course is generally milder than that of epidemic typhus, and the convalescence is shorter.

LABORATORY DIAGNOSIS

The MIF test is the diagnostic method of choice for documenting disease with *R. prowazekii.*

TREATMENT, PREVENTION, AND CONTROL

Tetracyclines and chloramphenicol are highly effective in the treatment of epidemic typhus. However, antibiotic treatment must be combined with effective louse-control measures for the management of an epidemic. A formaldehyde-inactivated typhus vaccine is available, and its use is recommended in high-risk populations.

Rickettsia typhi

EPIDEMIOLOGY

Endemic or murine typhus is caused by *R. typhi.* Disease is distributed worldwide primarily in warm, humid areas. In the United States, 50 to 100 cases are reported annually with most cases in the Gulf states (especially Texas) and southern California. Endemic disease continues to be reported in people living in the temperate and subtropical coastal areas of Africa, Asia, Australia, Europe, and South America. Rodents are the primary reservoir, and the rat flea *(Xenopsylla cheopis)* is the principal vector. However, the cat flea *(Ctenocephalides felis),* which infests cats, opossums, raccoons, and skunks, is considered an important vector for disease in the United States. Most cases occur during the warm months.

CLINICAL DISEASE

The incubation period for *R. typhi* disease is 7 to 14 days. The symptoms appear abruptly, with fever, severe headache, chills, myalgias, and nausea most common. A rash develops in approximately half of infected patients, most commonly late in the illness. It is typically restricted to the chest and abdomen. The course of disease is generally uncomplicated, lasting less than 3 weeks even in untreated patients.

LABORATORY DIAGNOSIS

A *R.* typhi–specific indirect fluorescent assay (IFA) test is used to confirm the diagnosis of murine typhus. A fourfold increase in the titer or a single titer of at least 1:128 is diagnostic. Significant titers are usually detectable within 1 to 2 weeks of the onset of disease.

TREATMENT, PREVENTION, AND CONTROL

Tetracycline, doxycycline, or chloramphenicol is effective in the treatment of murine typhus, and patients respond promptly to these agents. It is difficult to control or prevent endemic typhus because the reservoir and vector are widely distributed. Any such efforts should be directed at controlling the rodent reservoir. An effective vaccine is not available.

Orientia tsutsugamushi

O. tsutsugamushi, formerly classified with the *Rickettsia,* is the etiologic agent for **scrub typhus,** a disease transmitted to humans by mites (chiggers, red mites). The reservoir is the mite population, in which the bacteria are transmitted by transovarian means. Infection is also present in the rodent population, which can serve as a reservoir for mite infections. Because mites feed only once during their life span, rodents are not believed to be an important reservoir for human disease. Scrub typhus is present in people living in eastern Asia, Australia, and Japan and other western Pacific islands. It can also be imported into the United States.

O. tsutsugamushi disease develops suddenly after a 6- to 18-day incubation period (average, 10 to 12 days), with severe headache, fever, and myalgias. A macular to papular rash develops on the trunk in less than half of patients and spreads centrifugally to the extremities. Generalized lymphadenopathy, splenomegaly, central nervous system complications, and heart failure can occur. Fever in untreated patients disappears after 2 to 3 weeks, whereas fever in patients who receive appropriate treatment with tetracycline, doxycycline, or chloramphenicol respond promptly. No vaccine is available, so the disease is prevented by avoidance of exposure to chiggers (i.e., the wearing of protective clothing, the use of insect repellents).

CASE STUDY AND QUESTIONS

A 24-year-old man living in North Carolina came to the local emergency department because of fever, arthralgias, myalgias, and malaise. He was well until 4 days before admission, when he developed a fever reaching 40°C, chills, severe headache, and muscle aches. Physical examination revealed a critically ill man with a temperature of 39.7°C, pulse of 110 beats/min, respiratory rate of 28 breaths/min, blood pressure of 100/60 mm Hg, and a rash over his extremities, including his palms and soles. The patient recalled having had numerous tick bites 10 days before the onset of symptoms. Rocky Mountain spotted fever was considered in the diagnosis, and serologic tests for Rickettsia species confirmed this diagnosis.

1. What antibiotics can be used to treat this infection? Which antibiotics should not be used?
2. Which rickettsiae are associated with the following vectors: ticks, lice, mites, fleas?
3. Why is use of the Gram stain inappropriate for the diagnosis of rickettsial infections?

Bibliography

Archibald L, Sexton D: Long-term sequelae of Rocky Mountain spotted fever, *Clin Infect Dis* 20:1122-1125, 1995.

Dumler JS: Laboratory diagnosis of human rickettsial and ehrlichial infections, *Clin Microbiol Newsletter* 18:57-61, 1996.

La Scola B, Raoult D: Minireview: Laboratory diagnosis of rickettsioses: Current approaches to diagnosis of old and new rickettsial diseases, *J Clin Microbiol* 35:2715-2727, 1997.

Raoult D, Dumler JS: Rickettsia and Orientia, *Topley and Wilson's microbiology and microbial infections,* ed 10, London, 2005, Holder-Arnold.

Raoult D, Roux V: Rickettsioses as paradigms of new or emerging infectious diseases, *Clin Microbiol Rev* 10:694-719, 1997.

Rolain J et al: In vitro susceptibilities of 27 rickettsiae to 13 antimicrobials, *Antimicrob Agents Chemother* 42:1537-1541, 1998.

Spach D et al: Tick-borne diseases in the United States, *N Engl J Med* 329:936-947, 1993.

Walker DH: *Biology of rickettsial diseases,* Boca Raton, Fla, 1988, CRC Press.

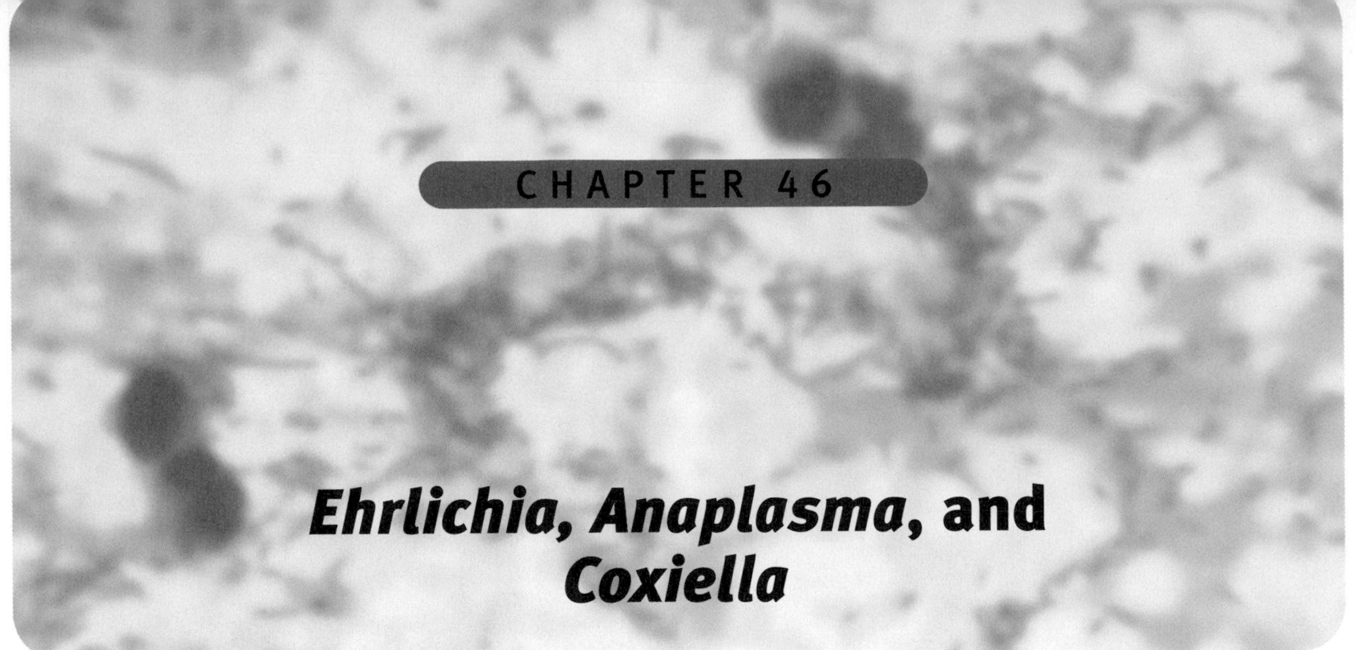

CHAPTER 46

Ehrlichia, *Anaplasma*, and *Coxiella*

In 2001, the taxonomy of the order Rickettsiales was reorganized, with four genera placed in the family Anaplasmataceae: *Anaplasma*, *Ehrlichia*, *Neorickettsia*, and *Wolbachia*. Important common properties of these genera are (1) survival within a cytoplasmic vacuole in the infected arthropod or mammalian cell, and (2) infection of hematopoietic cells. Most human pathogens in this family reside in the genera *Anaplasma* and *Ehrlichia* and will be the focus of this chapter (Box 46–1). *Coxiella* is an intracellular pathogen that was historically classified with the *Rickettsia*. Although it is now recognized that *Coxiella* is not closely related to the Rickettsiales, it will also be discussed in this chapter.

Ehrlichia and *Anaplasma* (Box 46–2)

PHYSIOLOGY AND STRUCTURE

The genera *Ehrlichia* and *Anaplasma* consist of intracellular bacteria that parasitize mononuclear or granulocytic phagocytes but not erythrocytes. The bacteria are small (0.2 to 0.4 μm) and stain poorly with the Gram stain. In contrast with *Rickettsia* and *Orientia*, *Ehrlichia* and *Anaplasma* remain in the phagocytic vacuole after entry into the host cell. Fusion with lysosomes is prevented because expression of appropriate receptors on the phagocytic vacuole surface is interrupted. Thus the bacteria can multiple by binary fission in the phagosome without exposure to the hydrolytic lysosome enzymes. The replicating bacteria assemble into membrane-enclosed masses called **morulae** (Figure 46–1). Observation of cells with morulae can be diagnostic. Information about the metabolism of *Ehrlichia* and *Anaplasma* is more limited than with *Rickettsia*. However, complete genomic sequencing of these bacteria will be completed in the near future, which will make it possible to determine parasitic relationship between the bacteria and their host cells.

The cell wall structure of *Ehrlichia* and *Anaplasma* is similar to that of gram-negative bacteria; however, peptidoglycan and lipopolysaccharide (LPS) are not present. A number of protein antigens are shared among species in these genera, as well as with species of other genera. For this reason, cross-reactive antibodies are commonly observed in serologic assays.

PATHOGENESIS AND IMMUNITY

The intracellular location of the organisms protects them from the host's antibody response. However, bacterial stimulation of interferon-γ (IFN-γ) production is believed to play an important role in activating macrophages that act either directly on infected cells or on antibody-opsonized bacteria during their extracellular phase.

EPIDEMIOLOGY (TABLE 46–1)

The first reported infection in the United States with these *Rickettsia*-like organisms was in 1986. *Ehrlichia canis* was believed initially to be responsible for the newly named disease, **human monocytic ehrlichiosis;** however, a new species, *Ehrlichia chaffeensis*, was recognized as the etiologic agent. Between 1987 and 2005, more than 1500 cases were reported. The prevalence of this disease is underestimated because serologic studies have shown that antibodies to *E. chaffeensis* are at least as common as antibodies to *Rickettsia rickettsii*, which has a similar geographic distribution. Disease is found predominantly in the southeastern, mid-Atlantic, Midwestern, and south central areas of the United States (e.g., Arkansas, Georgia, Missouri, Oklahoma, South Carolina, and Texas). This area corresponds to the geographic distribution of *Amblyomma americanum* (Lone Star tick), the primary vector

BOX 46–1. *Ehrlichia, Anaplasma,* and *Coxiella*

Organism	Historical Derivation
Ehrlichia	Named after Paul Ehrlich
E. chaffeensis	First isolated in an Army reservist at Fort Chaffee, Ark.
E. ewingii	Named after William Ewing
Anaplasma	*An,* without; *plasma,* anything formed (a thing without form; referring to the intracytoplasmic inclusions)
A. phagocytophilum	*phago,* to eat; *kytos,* a vessel or enclosure; *philein,* to love (found in phagocytes)
Coxiella burnetii	Named after Harold Cox and F.M. Burnet

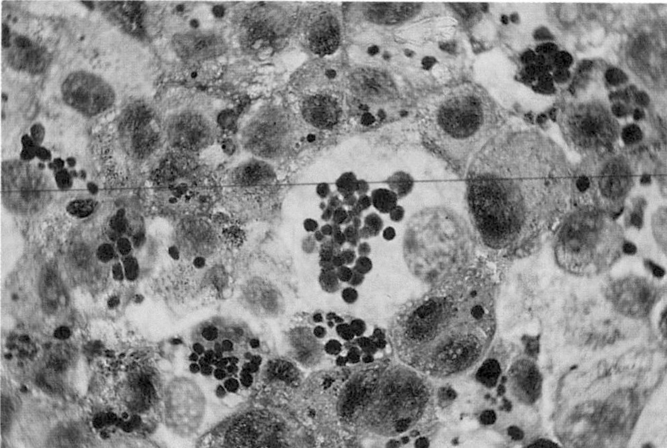

FIGURE 46–1. Multiple morulae of *Ehrlichia canis* in DH82 tissue culture cells. (From Cohen J, Powderly WG: *Infectious diseases*, ed 2, St Louis, 2004, Mosby.)

responsible for transmitting the organism, and of white-tailed deer, an important reservoir for *E. chaffeensis.* Transovarian transmission of *Anaplasma* and *Ehrlichia* in ticks is inefficient (in contrast with *Rickettsia* and *Orientia*), so these bacteria must be maintained in reservoir vertebrate hosts. Other animals that can serve as hosts include domestic dogs, foxes, coyotes, wolves, raccoons, opossums, goats, and mice.

Granulocytic ehrlichiosis is caused by two bacteria —*Ehrlichia ewingii* and *Anaplasma phagocytophilum. E. ewingii* has a geographic distribution similar to *E. chaffeensis* because they share the same tick vector *(Amblyomma americanum)* and reservoir hosts. The frequency with which it is associated with human disease is unknown because serologic response to this organism cross-reacts with antibodies against *E. chaffeensis.* Disease caused by *A. phagocytophilum* is found primarily in the northern and central Midwestern states and northeast and central Atlantic states. The reservoirs are small mammals (e.g., white-footed mouse, chipmunks, voles), and the vectors are *Ixodes* ticks. More than 90% of all disease caused by *Ehrlichia* and *Anaplasma* in the United States occurs between mid-April and late October.

BOX 46–2. Summary of *Ehrlichia* and *Anaplasma*

Physiology and Structure

Small, intracellular bacteria
Stain poorly with Gram stain; best with Giemsa or Gimenez stains
Replicates in phagosome of infected cells

Virulence

Intracellular growth protects bacteria from immune clearance
Able to prevent fusion of phagosome with lysosome of monocytes or granulocytes
Initiates inflammatory response that contributes to pathology

Epidemiology

Depending on the species of *Ehrlichia,* important reservoirs are white-tailed deer, white-footed mouse, chipmunks, voles, and canines
Ticks are important vectors, but transovarian transmission in inefficient
Disease in United States is most common in the Atlantic states; northern, central, and southern Midwest states; and northern California
People at greatest risk are those exposed to ticks in the endemic areas
Disease is most common from April to October

Diseases

Human monocytic ehrlichiosis
Human anaplasmosis (formerly called human granulocytic ehrlichiosis)

Diagnosis

Microscopy of limited value
Serology and DNA probe tests are methods of choice

Treatment, Prevention, and Control

Doxycycline is the drug of choice; rifampin is an acceptable alternative
Prevention involves avoidance of tick-infested areas, use of protective clothing and insect repellents, and prompt removal of embedded ticks
Vaccines are not available

CLINICAL DISEASES

Human Monocytic Ehrlichiosis

Human monocytic ehrlichiosis is caused by *E. chaffeensis* following infection of blood monocytes and mononuclear phagocytes in tissues and organs. Approximately 1 to 3 weeks after a tick bite, patients develop a flulike illness with fever, headache, and myalgias. Gas-

TABLE 46–1. Epidemiology of *Ehrlichia*, *Anaplasma*, and *Coxiella*

Species	Disease	Invertebrate Vector	Vertebrate Hosts	Geographic Distribution
Anaplasma phagocytophilum	Human anaplasmosis (formerly human granulocytic ehrlichiosis	Ticks (*Ixodes*)	Humans, horses, dogs, ruminants, llamas	North and South America, Europe, Asia, Africa
Ehrlichia chaffeensis	Human monocytic ehrlichiosis	Ticks (*Amblyomma*)	Humans, dogs	United States (southeast, south central states), Asia (?)
Ehrlichia ewingii	Canine granulocytic ehrlichiosis	Ticks (*Amblyomma*)	Dogs, humans	United States (southeast, south central states)
Coxiella burnetii	Q fever	Not significant in humans	Many, including arthropods, fish, birds, rodents, marsupials, livestock	Worldwide (relatively uncommon in United States)

trointestinal symptoms develop in fewer than half the infected patients, and a late-onset rash develops in 30% to 40% of patients (more common in children than in adults). Leukopenia, thrombocytopenia, and elevated serum transaminases develop in the majority of patients and can range from mild to severe. Although mortality is low (2% to 3%), more than half the infected patients require hospitalization and experience a prolonged recovery period. The pathology of this infection is disproportionate to the number of infected cells or microbial burden present in tissue. It is believed that *E. chaffeensis* disturbs mononuclear phagocytic function and the regulation of the inflammatory response. Thus the immune response both eliminates the pathogen and produces much of the tissue damage.

Canine Granulocytic Ehrlichiosis

E. ewingii primarily causes disease in canines, with humans the accidental hosts. Because there is serologic cross-reactivity between *E. ewingii* and *E. chaffeensis*, the incidence of infections with this organism is likely to be underestimated. The clinical presentation is similar to that of *E. chaffeensis*, with fever, headaches, and myalgias. Leukopenia, thrombocytopenia, and elevated serum transaminases are also seen.

Human Anaplasmosis

Human anaplasmosis, formerly called human granulocytic ehrlichiosis, is caused by *A. phagocytophilum*. Bone marrow myeloid cells (i.e., neutrophils) are primarily infected. The disease presents as a flulike illness, with fever, headache, and myalgias; gastrointestinal symptoms are present in fewer than half the patients; and a skin rash is observed in less than 10% of the patients. Leukopenia, thrombocytopenia, and serum transaminase elevation are observed in the majority of patients. More than half the infected patients require hospitalization, and severe complications are common. Despite the potential severity of this disease, mortality is less than 1%. As with *E. chaffeensis* infections, the pathology of this disease appears related to macrophage activation.

LABORATORY DIAGNOSIS

Microscopy is of limited value for diagnosing infections. Giemsa-stained preparations of peripheral blood should be performed, because detection of intracellular organisms **(morulae)** is diagnostic. However, morulae are detected in less than 10% of patients with monocytic ehrlichiosis and in 20% to 80% of patients with granulocytic ehrlichiosis and anaplasmosis. Likewise, although *Ehrlichia* have been cultured in vitro in established cell lines, this procedure is not performed in most clinical laboratories. The most common methods for confirming the clinical diagnosis of ehrlichiosis are deoxyribonucleic acid (DNA) amplification tests and serology. Species-specific DNA amplification tests are available in some reference laboratories and can provide a sensitive, specific diagnostic test for acute disease. An increase in the antibody titer is typically observed 3 to 6 weeks after the initial presentation, so these tests are primarily confirmatory. *E. chaffeensis* and *E. ewingii* are closely related and are not distinguished serologically. The specificity of the serology tests is compromised by cross-reactions with organisms responsible for Rocky Mountain spotted fever, Q fever, Lyme disease, brucellosis, and Epstein-Barr virus infections.

TREATMENT, PREVENTION, AND CONTROL

Patients with suspected ehrlichiosis should be treated with doxycycline. Therapy should not be delayed to wait for laboratory confirmation of the disease. Rifampin has been used to treat pregnant women (in whom the tetracyclines are contraindicated). Both doxycycline and rifampin are bactericidal in vitro. The fluoroquinolones are bacteriostatic in vitro, and resistance has been detected in some *Ehrlichia* species, so use of these drugs is contraindicated. Penicillins, cephalosporins, chloramphenicol, aminoglycosides, and macrolides are ineffective. Infection is prevented by avoidance of tick-infested areas, wearing of protective clothing, and use of insect repellents. Embedded ticks should be removed promptly. Vaccines are not available.

Coxiella burnetii

Coxiella were originally classified with *Rickettsia* because they stain weakly with the Gram stain, grow intracellularly in eukaryotic cells, and are associated with arthropods (e.g., ticks). However, it is now recognized that these bacteria are more closely related to *Legionella* and *Francisella*. The disease caused by *Coxiella* is **Q fever,** which may be asymptomatic in humans and develops either acutely or as a chronic infection.

PHYSIOLOGY AND STRUCTURE

C. burnetii is a small, pleomorphic coccobacillus (0.2 to 0.7 μm) that is an obligate intracellular pathogen. Intracellular multiplication is initiated after the bacteria are phagocytized and the phagosome fuses to form a phagolysosome. The acidic environment activates the bacterial metabolic machinery. The small replicating cells will mature to large-cell variants, which then evolve to stable spores. These spores can survive in nature for many months.

PATHOGENESIS AND IMMUNITY

Understanding of the pathogenesis of Q fever is limited because most infections are self-limited and there is no animal model for the chronic disease. Human infection usually occurs after the inhalation of airborne particles from a contaminated environmental source rather than from the bite of an arthropod vector (despite the fact that more than 40 species of ticks are infected with *C. burnetii*). *Coxiella* proliferate in the respiratory tract and then disseminate to other organs. Pneumonia and granulomatous hepatitis develop in patients with severe, acute infections, whereas most chronic infections manifest as endocarditis.

An important characteristic of *Coxiella* infections is the ability to undergo **antigenic variation** in expression of the cell wall LPS antigen. The highly infectious form of the bacteria possesses LPS with a complex carbohydrate **(phase I antigen)** that blocks antibody interaction with surface proteins. After cultivation of the bacterium, the phase I antigen gene undergoes a deletion mutation, producing the **phase II antigen.** This antigenic change exposes the surface proteins to antibodies. Antibody response to these antigens in disease is a useful marker for acute and chronic diseases. Acute disease is characterized by antibodies against the exposed phase II antigen, whereas high antibody titers against the phase I and II antigens are detected in patients with chronic infections. The high antibody titers observed in patients with chronic disease lead to the formation of immune complexes and are responsible for producing some of the signs and symptoms of this disease. Thus humoral immunity contributes to the pathologic manifestations of the disease and clinical improvement is associated with cellular immunity.

EPIDEMIOLOGY (see TABLE 46–1)

C. burnetii is extremely stable in harsh environmental conditions and can survive in soil for months to years. The range of hosts for *C. burnetii* is wide, with infections being found in mammals, birds, and numerous different genera of ticks (Box 46–3). Farm animals such as sheep, cattle, and goats, and recently infected cats, dogs, and rabbits, are the primary reservoirs for human disease. Ticks are an important vector for disease in animals but not in humans. The bacteria can reach high concentrations in the placenta of infected livestock. Dried placentas left on the ground after parturition and feces, urine, and tick feces can contaminate soil, which in turn can serve as a focus for infection if these bacteria become airborne and are inhaled. *C. burnetii* is also excreted in milk, so people who consume contaminated unpasteurized milk can become infected.

Q fever has a worldwide distribution. Although only 20 to 30 cases are reported annually in the United States, this figure is certainly an underestimation of the actual prevalence of the disease. Infection is common in livestock in the United States; however, actual disease in livestock is rare. Human exposure, particularly for ranchers, veterinarians, and food handlers, is frequent, and experimental studies have shown that the infectious dose of *C. burnetii* is small. Thus most human infections are mild or asymptomatic. This finding is confirmed by serologic studies, which have shown that more than half of all patients with detectable antibodies do not have a history of disease. Infections also go undiagnosed because *C. burnetii* is often not considered in patients who have symptomatic disease.

CLINICAL DISEASES

C. burnetii infection can present in an acute or a chronic fashion. Acute disease is characterized by a long incubation period (average, 20 days), followed by the sudden onset of severe headache, high fever, chills, and myalgias. Respiratory symptoms are generally mild, mimicking the

BOX 46-3. Summary of *Coxiella*

Physiology and Structure
Small, intracellular bacteria
Stain poorly with Gram stain; best with Giemsa or Gimenez stains
Replicate in phagolysosome of infected cells
Capable of phase transition with phase I (infectious) and phase II lipopolysaccharide antigens

Virulence
Intracellular growth protects the bacteria from immune clearance
Able to replicate in acidic environment of fused phagosomes and lysosomes
Phase I forms are protected from antibody interaction with bacterial surface proteins
Extracellular form extremely stable; can survive in nature for a prolonged period

Epidemiology
Many reservoirs, including mammals, birds, and ticks
Most human infections associated with contact with infected cattle, sheep, goats, dogs, and cats
Most disease acquired through inhalation; possible disease from consumption of contaminated milk; ticks are not an important vector for human disease
Worldwide distribution, although disease in the United States is relatively uncommon
No seasonal incidence

Diseases
Acute diseases include influenza-like syndrome, atypical pneumonia, hepatitis, pericarditis, myocarditis, meningoencephalitis
Chronic diseases include endocarditis, hepatitis, pulmonary disease, and infection of pregnant women

Diagnosis
Detection of antibody response to phase I and phase II antigens is test of choice

Treatment, Prevention, and Control
Tetracyclines are the drugs of choice for acute infections; rifampin combined with either doxycycline or trimethoprim-sulfamethoxazole is used to treat chronic infections
Phase I antigen vaccines are protective and safe if administered in a single dose before the animal or human has been exposed to *Coxiella*

"atypical pneumonia" caused by *Mycoplasma* species (see Chapter 44) and *Chlamydia* organisms (see Chapter 47), but can be severe. Hepatosplenomegaly is present in approximately half of patients. Histologically diffuse granulomas are seen in the livers of most patients who have acute Q fever.

The most common presentation of chronic Q fever is **subacute endocarditis**, generally on a prosthetic or previously damaged heart valve. The incubation period for chronic Q fever can be months to years, and the presentation is insidious. Unfortunately, chronic disease frequently progresses in an unrelenting fashion, and the prognosis is poor.

LABORATORY DIAGNOSIS

At present, Q fever can be diagnosed by culture (not commonly performed), polymerase chain reaction (PCR), or by specific serologic tests. Nucleic acid amplification techniques such as PCR have been developed in reference laboratories and demonstrated to be more sensitive than culture and highly specific tests. Sensitivity is best with tissue samples and less reliable with serum. In areas where *C. burnetii* infections are common, PCR is the method of choice for a rapid diagnosis.

Currently, serology is the most commonly used diagnostic test. As previously mentioned, *C. burnetii* undergoes phase variation characterized by the development of phase I and II antigens. The phase I antigens are only weakly antigenic. A variety of methods have been used to measure antibody production: the microagglutionation test, complement fixation test, indirect immunofluorescent-antibody (IFA) test, and enzyme-linked immunosorbent assay (ELISA). IFA is the test of choice, although ELISA is used in many laboratories and appears to be more sensitive. Cross-reactions occur with *Bartonella* (which can cause a similar disease), so all serologic tests should include an assay for both organisms. In acute Q fever, immunoglobulin (Ig)M and IgG antibodies are developed primarily against phase II antigens. A diagnosis of chronic Q fever is confirmed by the demonstration of antibodies against both phase I and II antigens, with the titers to the phase I antigen typically higher.

TREATMENT, PREVENTION, AND CONTROL

In vitro susceptibility tests have not proved useful for predicting clinical efficacy. For this reason, treatment of acute and chronic *C. burnetii* infections is guided by clinical experience. Currently, it is recommended that acute infections be treated with a tetracycline (e.g., doxycycline). Chronic disease should be treated for a prolonged period with a bactericidal combination of drugs, such as rifampin and either doxycycline or trimethoprim-sulfamethoxazole. The difficulty in the treatment of patients with these infections is that antibiotic activity is suboptimal against the bacteria replicating in intracellular, acidic vacuoles.

Inactivated whole-cell vaccines and partially purified antigen vaccines for Q fever have been developed, and the vaccines prepared from phase I organisms have been shown to provide the best protection. Vaccination of animal herds appears efficacious unless the animals have been previously infected naturally. Vaccination does not eradicate *Coxiella* in infected animals or decrease asymptomatic shedding. Likewise, vaccination of humans with phase I vaccines is protective if the vaccinees are uninfected. Vaccination of previously infected individuals is contraindicated because immune stimulation can lead to an increase in adverse reactions. For this reason, a single-dose vaccine with no booster immunizations is recommended.

CASE STUDY AND QUESTIONS

A 46-year-old man went to his physician with a 2-month history of weight loss (15 lbs), night sweats, and a low-grade fever. Results of a chest examination revealed a new heart murmur. The physician suspected his patient had subacute endocarditis, and three sets of blood cultures were collected. After 1 week of incubation, the cultures remained negative.

1. What diagnostic test(s) should be performed to determine if this patient has endocarditis caused by *Coxiella burnetii?*
2. If this diagnosis is confirmed, how did the patient most likely acquire his infection?
3. How should this infection be treated?

Bibliography

Bakken J et al: Human granulocytic ehrlichiosis in the upper Midwest United States: A new species emerging? *JAMA* 272:212-218, 1994.

Dumler JS: Laboratory diagnosis of human rickettsial and ehrlichial infections, *Clin Microbiol Newsletter* 18:57-61, 1996.

Dumler JS, Bakken JS: Human ehrlichiosis: Newly recognized infections transmitted by ticks, *Annu Rev Med* 49:201-213, 1998.

Fournier P, Marrie T, Raoult D: Minireview: Diagnosis of Q fever, *J Clin Microbiol* 36:1823-1834, 1998.

Magnarelli L, Dumler J: Ehrlichioses: Emerging infectious diseases in tick-infected areas, *Clin Microbiol Newsletter* 18:81-83, 1996.

Maurin M, Raoult D: Q fever, *Clin Microbiol Rev* 12:518-553, 1999.

Schaffner W, Standaert S: Ehrlichiosis—in pursuit of an emerging infection, *N Engl J Med* 334:262-263, 1996 (editorial).

Spach D et al: Tick-borne diseases in the United States, *N Engl J Med* 329:936-947, 1993.

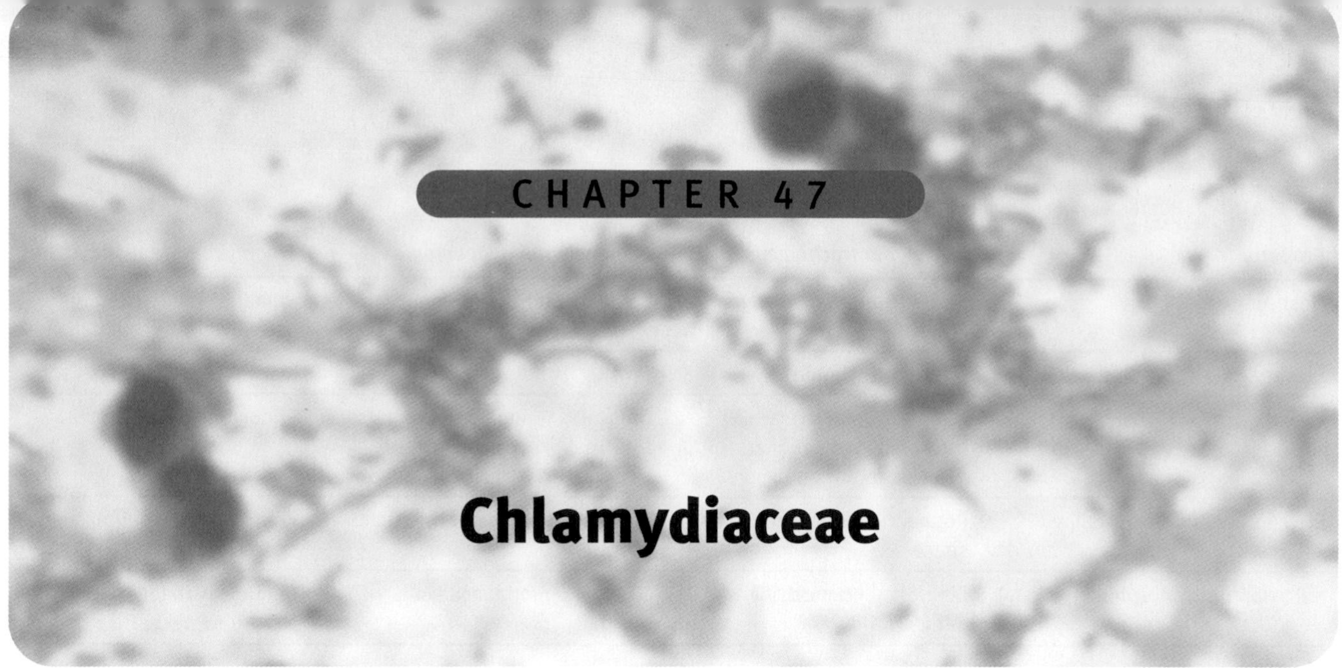

CHAPTER 47

Chlamydiaceae

In 1999 the taxonomy of the family Chlamydiaceae was revised extensively on the basis of genomic studies of these organisms (Box 47–1). Previously, the family consisted of one genus, *Chlamydia*, with four species. Now the family has been divided into two genera, *Chlamydia* and *Chlamydophila*. *Chlamydia trachomatis* was retained in the genus *Chlamydia*, but *Chlamydia psittaci* and *Chlamydia pneumoniae* were transferred into the new genus, *Chlamydophila* (Box 47–2). Other species have been placed into the two genera, but they are uncommon human pathogens and are not discussed in this chapter.

The Chlamydiaceae were once considered viruses because they are small enough to pass through 0.45-μm filters and are obligate intracellular parasites. However, the organisms have the following properties of bacteria: (1) possess inner and outer membranes similar to those of gram-negative bacteria; (2) contain both deoxyribonucleic acid (DNA) and ribonucleic acid (RNA); (3) possess prokaryotic ribosomes; (4) synthesize their own proteins, nucleic acids, and lipids; and (5) are susceptible to numerous antibacterial antibiotics.

Unlike other bacteria, the Chlamydiaceae have a unique developmental cycle, forming metabolically inactive infectious forms **(elementary bodies [EBs])** and metabolically active, noninfectious forms **(reticulate bodies [RBs]).** Properties that differentiate the three important human pathogens in this family are summarized in Table 47–1.

Family Chlamydiaceae

PHYSIOLOGY AND STRUCTURE

Much like a spore, EBs are resistant to many harsh environmental factors. Although these bacteria lack the rigid peptidoglycan layer found in most other bacteria, their outer membrane proteins are extensively cross-linked by disulfide bonds between cysteine residues. The bacteria do not replicate in the EB form, but they are infectious in this form; that is, they can bind to receptors on host cells and stimulate uptake by the infected cell. The precise nature of this binding has not yet been defined. The RBs are the metabolically active, replicating chlamydial form. Because the extensive cross-linked proteins are absent in RBs, this form is osmotically fragile; however, RBs are protected by their intracellular location.

Other important structural components of Chlamydiaceae are a genus-specific lipopolysaccharide (LPS) that can be detected in a complement fixation (CF) test and species- and strain-specific outer membrane proteins.

The Chlamydiaceae replicate by means of a unique growth cycle that occurs within susceptible host cells (Figure 47–1). The cycle is initiated when the small (300 to 400 nm), infectious EBs become attached to the microvilli of susceptible cells, followed by active penetration into the host cell. After they are internalized, the bacteria remain within cytoplasmic phagosomes, where the replicative cycle proceeds. The fusion of cellular lysosomes with the EB-containing phagosome and subsequent intracellular killing is inhibited. Phagolysosomal fusion is prevented if the outer membrane is intact. If the outer membrane is damaged or the bacteria are inactivated by heat or coated with antibodies, phagolysosomal fusion occurs with subsequent bacterial killing.

Within 6 to 8 hours after entering the cell, the EBs reorganize into the larger (800 to 1000 nm), metabolically active RBs. RBs are able to synthesize their own DNA, RNA, and protein. The Chlamydiaceae are **energy parasites** because they use host cell adenosine triphosphate for their energy requirements. Some strains may also depend on the host to provide specific amino acids. The RBs replicate by binary fission, which continues for the next 18 to

TABLE 47–1. Differentiation of Chlamydiaceae That Cause Human Disease

Property	*Chlamydia trachomatis*	*Chlamydophila pneumoniae*	*Chlamydophila psittaci*
Host range	Primarily human pathogen	Primarily human pathogen	Primarily animal pathogen; occasionally infects humans
Biovars	LGV and trachoma	TWAR	Many
Diseases	LGV Trachoma: ocular trachoma, oculogenital disease, infant pneumonia	Bronchitis, pneumonia, sinusitis, pharyngitis, coronary artery disease (?)	Pneumonia (psittacosis)
Elementary body morphology	Round, narrow periplasmic space	Pear-shaped, large periplasmic space	Round, narrow periplasmic space
Inclusion body morphology	Single, round inclusion per cell	Multiple uniform inclusions per cell	Multiple, variably sized inclusions per cell
Plasmid DNA	Yes	No	Yes
Iodine-staining glycogen in inclusions	Yes	No	No
Susceptibility to sulfonamides	Yes	No	No

DNA, Deoxyribonucleic acid; LGV, lymphogranuloma venereum.

BOX 47–1. Revised Classification of the Family Chlamydiaceae

Genus *Chlamydia*	Genus *Chlamydophila*
C. trachomatis	*C. pneumoniae*
C. muridarum	*C. psittaci*
C. suis	*C. pecorum*
	C. abortus
	C. caviae
	C. felis

BOX 47–2. Important Chlamydiaceae

Organism	Historical Derivation
Chlamydia	*chlamydis,* a cloak
C. trachomatis	*trachomatis,* of trachoma or rough (the disease trachoma is characterized by granulations on the conjunctival surfaces that lead to chronic inflammation and blindness)
Chlamydophila	*chlamydis,* a cloak; phila, dear (dear to the cloak; related to *Chlamydia*)
C. pneumoniae	*pneumoniae,* pneumonia
C. psittaci	*psittacus,* a parrot (disease associated with birds)

24 hours. Histologic stains can readily detect the phagosome with accumulated RBs, called an **inclusion.** Approximately 18 to 24 hours after infection, the RBs begin reorganizing into the smaller EBs, and between 48 and 72 hours the cell ruptures and then releases the infective EBs.

TABLE 47–2. Clinical Spectrum of *Chlamydia trachomatis* Infections

Serovars	Site of Infection
A, B, Ba, C	Primarily conjunctiva
D–K	Primarily urogenital tract
L1, L2, L2a, L3	Inguinal lymph nodes

Chlamydia trachomatis (Box 47–3)

C. trachomatis has a limited host range with infections restricted to humans (Box 47–4). The species has been subdivided into three biovars, **trachoma, LGV (lymphogranuloma venereum),** and mouse pneumonitis. The biovars (Table 47–2) have been further divided into serotypes (commonly called serologic variants, or **serovars**) on the basis of antigenic differences in the major outer membrane protein (MOMP). Specific serovars are associated with specific disease. LGV is associated with serovars L1 to L3; endemic trachoma is associated with serovars A to C; urethritis, epididymitis, proctitis, conjunctivitis, cervicitis, endometritis, salpingitis, perihepatitis, and Reiter's syndrome are associated with serovars D to K.

PATHOGENESIS AND IMMUNITY

The range of cells that *C. trachomatis* can infect is limited. Receptors for EBs are primarily restricted to nonciliated columnar, cuboidal, and transitional epithelial cells,

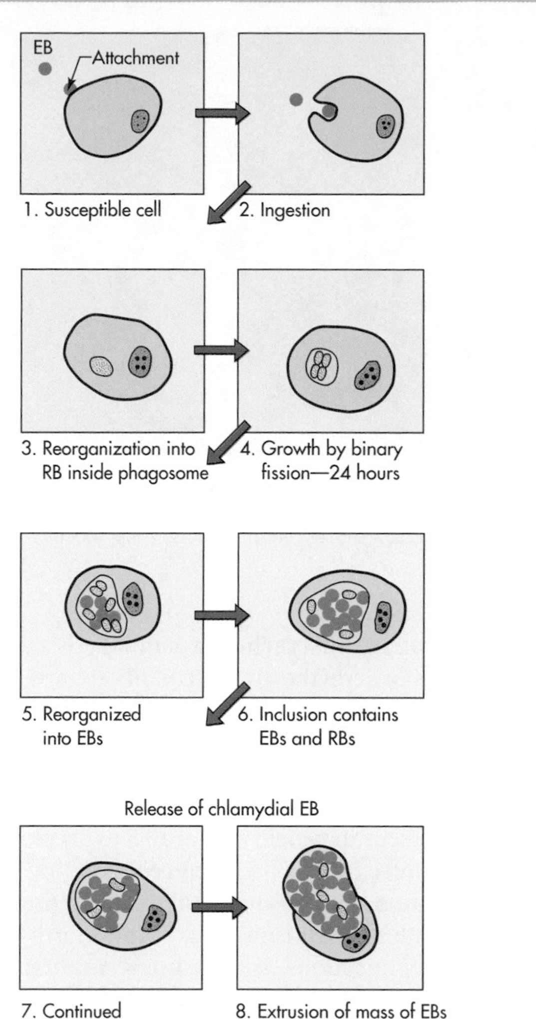

FIGURE 47–1. The growth cycle of *Chlamydia trachomatis.* (Redrawn from Batteiger B, Jones R: *Infect Dis Clin North Am* 1:55-81, 1987.)

which are found on the mucous membranes of the urethra, endocervix, endometrium, fallopian tubes, anorectum, respiratory tract, and conjunctivae. The LGV biovar replicates in mononuclear phagocytes present in the lymphatic system. The clinical manifestations of chlamydial infections are caused by (1) the direct destruction of cells during replication and (2) the host inflammatory response.

Chlamydiae gain access through minute abrasions or lacerations. In LGV the lesions form in the lymph nodes, draining the site of primary infection (Figure 47–2). Granuloma formation is characteristic. The lesions may become necrotic, attract polymorphonuclear leukocytes, and cause the inflammatory process to spread to surrounding tissues. Subsequent rupture of the lymph node leads to formation of abscesses or sinus tracts. Infection with non-LGV serovars of *C. trachomatis* stimulates a severe inflammatory response consisting of neutrophils, lymphocytes, and plasma cells. True lymphoid follicles with germinal centers eventually are induced.

Infection does not confer long-lasting immunity. Rather, reinfection characteristically induces a vigorous inflammatory response with subsequent tissue damage. This response produces the vision loss in patients with chronic ocular infections, and scarring with sterility and sexual dysfunction in patients with genital infections.

BOX 47–3. Summary of *Chlamydia trachomatis*

Physiology and Structure

Small, gram-negative rods with no peptidoglycan layer in cell wall
Strict intracellular parasite of humans
Two distinct forms: infectious elementary bodies and noninfectious reticulate bodies
Lipopolysaccharide antigen shared by *Chlamydia* and *Chlamydophila* species
Major outer membrane proteins are species specific
Two biovars associated with human disease: trachoma (with 15 serovars) and lymphogranuloma venereum (LGV; four serovars)
Infects nonciliated columnar, cuboidal, and transitional epithelial cells

Virulence

Intracellular replication
Prevents fusion of phagosome with cellular lysosomes
Pathologic effects of trachoma caused by repeated infections

Epidemiology

Most common sexually transmitted bacteria in United States
Ocular trachoma worldwide (most common in Middle East, North Africa, India), with blindness developing in 7 to 9 million patients
LGV highly prevalent in Africa, Asia, and South America

Diseases

Refer to Box 47–4

Diagnosis

Culture is highly specific but is relatively insensitive
Antigen tests (DFA, ELISA) are relatively insensitive.
Molecular amplification tests are the most sensitive and specific tests currently available

Treatment, Prevention, and Control

Treat LGV with tetracyclines, macrolides, or sulfisoxazole
Treat ocular or genital infections with azithromycin or doxycycline
Treat newborn conjunctivitis or pneumonia with erythromycin
Safe sex practices and prompt treatment of patient and sexual partners help control infections

*DFA, Direct fluorescent antibody; ELISA, enzyme-linked immunosorbent assay.

BOX 47–4. Chlamydiaceae: Clinical Summaries

Chlamydia trachomatis

Trachoma: Chronic, inflammatory granulomatous process of eye surface, leading to corneal ulceration, scarring, pannus formation, and blindness

Adult inclusion conjunctivitis: Acute process with mucopurulent discharge, dermatitis, corneal infiltrates, and corneal vascularization in chronic disease

Neonatal conjunctivitis: Acute process characterized by a mucopurulent discharge

Infant pneumonia: After a 2- to –3-week incubation period, the infant develops rhinitis, followed by bronchitis with a characteristic dry cough

Urogenital infections: Acute process involving the genitourinary tract with characteristic mucopurulent discharge; asymptomatic infections common in women

Lymphogranuloma venereum: A painless ulcer develops at the site of infection that spontaneously heals, followed by inflammation and swelling of lymph nodes draining the area, then progression to systemic symptoms

Chlamydophila pneumoniae

Respiratory infections: Can range from asymptomatic or mild disease to severe, atypical pneumonia requiring hospitalization

Atherosclerosis: *C. pneumoniae* has been associated with inflammatory plaques in blood vessels; the etiologic role in this disease is controversial

Chlamydophila psittaci

Respiratory infections: Can range from asymptomatic colonization to severe bronchopneumonia with localized infiltration of inflammatory cells, necrosis, and hemorrhage

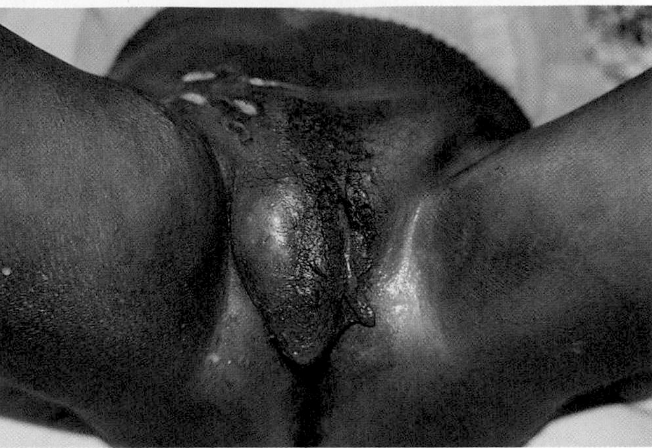

FIGURE 47–2. Patient with lymphogranuloma venereum causing unilateral vulvar lymphedema and inguinal buboes. (From Cohen J, Powderly W: *Infectious diseases,* ed 2, St Louis, 2004, Mosby.)

EPIDEMIOLOGY

C. trachomatis is found worldwide and causes trachoma (chronic keratoconjunctivitis), oculogenital disease, pneumonia, and LGV. An estimated 500 million people worldwide are infected with the biovar trachoma, 7 to 9 million of whom are blinded as a result.

Trachoma is endemic in the Middle East, North Africa, and India. Infections occur predominantly in children, who are the chief reservoir of *C. trachomatis* in endemic areas. The incidence of infection is lower in older children and adolescents; however, the incidence of blindness continues to rise through adulthood as the disease progresses. Trachoma is transmitted eye-to-eye by droplet, hands, contaminated clothing, and eye-seeking flies, which transmit ocular discharges from the eyes of infected children to the eyes of uninfected children. Because a high percentage of children in endemic areas harbor *C. trachomatis* in their respiratory and gastrointestinal tracts, the pathogen may also be transmitted by respiratory droplet or through fecal contamination. Trachoma generally is endemic in communities where the living conditions are crowded, sanitation is poor, and the personal hygiene of the people is poor—all risk factors that promote the transmission of infections.

Most cases of *C. trachomatis* **adult inclusion conjunctivitis** occur in people who are 18 to 30 years of age, and genital infection probably precedes eye involvement. Autoinoculation and oral-genital contact are believed to be the routes of transmission. A third form of *C. trachomatis* eye infections is **newborn inclusion conjunctivitis,** an infection acquired during passage of the infant through an infected birth canal. *C. trachomatis* conjunctivitis develops in approximately 25% of infants whose mothers have active genital infections.

Pulmonary infection with *C. trachomatis* also occurs in newborns. A diffuse **interstitial pneumonia** develops in 10% to 20% of infants exposed to the pathogen at birth.

C. trachomatis is thought to be the most common **sexually transmitted bacterial disease** in the United States. In 2003, 877,478 infections were reported in the United States. However, this figure is believed to be an underestimate because most infected patients either do not seek medical treatment or are treated without a specific diagnosis. It is estimated that 2.8 million Americans are infected each year and as many as 50 million new infections occur annually worldwide. Most genital tract infections are caused by serotypes D through K.

LGV is a chronic sexually transmitted disease caused by *C. trachomatis* serotypes L1, L2, L2a, and L3. It occurs sporadically in North America, Australia, and Europe but is highly prevalent in Africa, Asia, and South America. In the United States, 200 to 500 cases have been reported annually during the past decade, with male homosexuals being the major reservoir of disease. Acute LGV is seen more frequently in men, primarily because symptomatic infection is less common in women.

CLINICAL DISEASES

Trachoma

Trachoma is a chronic disease caused by serovars A, B, Ba, and C. Initially, patients have a follicular conjunctivitis with diffuse inflammation that involves the entire conjunctiva. The conjunctivae become scarred as the disease progresses, causing the patient's eyelids to turn inward. The turned-in eyelashes abrade the cornea, eventually resulting in corneal ulceration, scarring, pannus formation (invasion of vessels into the cornea), and loss of vision. It is common for trachoma to recur after apparent healing, most likely a result of subclinical infections that have been documented in children in endemic areas and in immigrants to the United States who acquired trachoma during childhood in their native countries.

Adult Inclusion Conjunctivitis

An acute follicular conjunctivitis caused by the *C. trachomatis* strains associated with genital infections (serovars A, B, Ba, D to K) has been documented in sexually active adults. The infection is characterized by mucopurulent discharge, keratitis, corneal infiltrates, and occasionally some corneal vascularization. Corneal scarring has been observed in patients with chronic infection.

Neonatal Conjunctivitis

Eye infections can also develop in infants exposed to *C. trachomatis* at birth. After an incubation of 5 to 12 days, the infant's eyelids swell, hyperemia occurs, and copious purulent discharge appears. Untreated infections may run a course as long as 12 months, during which time conjunctival scarring and corneal vascularization occur. Infants who are untreated or are treated with topical therapy only are at risk for *C. trachomatis* pneumonia.

Infant Pneumonia

The incubation period for infant pneumonia is variable, but the onset generally occurs 2 to 3 weeks after birth. Rhinitis is initially observed in such infants, after which a distinctive staccato cough develops. The child remains afebrile throughout the clinical illness, which can last for several weeks. Radiographic signs of infection can persist for months.

Ocular Lymphogranuloma Venereum

The LGV serotypes of *C. trachomatis* have been implicated in Parinaud's oculoglandular conjunctivitis, a conjunctival inflammation associated with preauricular, submandibular, and cervical lymphadenopathy.

Urogenital Infections

Most genital tract infections in women are asymptomatic (as many as 80%) but can nevertheless become symptomatic. The clinical manifestations include bartholinitis, cervicitis, endometritis, perihepatitis, salpingitis, and urethritis. Chlamydial infection may be overlooked in asymptomatic patients. A mucopurulent discharge (Figure 47–3) and hypertrophic ectopy are seen in patients with symptomatic infection, whose specimens generally yield more organisms on cultures than specimens from patients with asymptomatic infections. Urethritis caused by *C. trachomatis* may occur with or without a concurrent cervical infection.

As previously mentioned, most *C. trachomatis* genital infections in men are symptomatic; however, as many as 25% of chlamydial infections in men may be asymptomatic (Figure 47–4). Approximately 35% to 50% of cases of nongonococcal urethritis are caused by *C. trachomatis;* dual infections with both *C. trachomatis* and *Neisseria gonorrhoeae* are not uncommon. Symptoms of the chlamydial infection develop after successful treatment of the gonorrhea, because the incubation period is longer and the use of β-lactam antibiotics to treat gonorrhea would be ineffective against *C. trachomatis*. Although there is less purulent exudate in patients with chlamydial urethral infections, such infections cannot be differentiated reliably from gonorrhea, so specific diagnostic tests for both organisms should be performed.

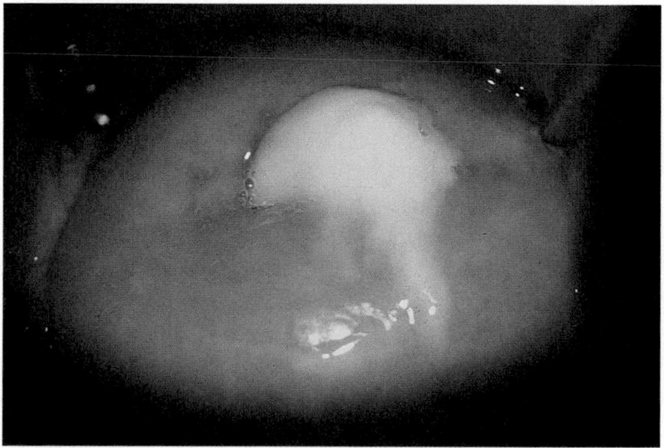

FIGURE 47–3. Mucopurulent cervicitis caused by *Chlamydia trachomatis.* ((From Cohen J, Powderly W: *Infectious diseases,* ed 2, St Louis, 2004, Mosby. Photo by J. Paavonen.)

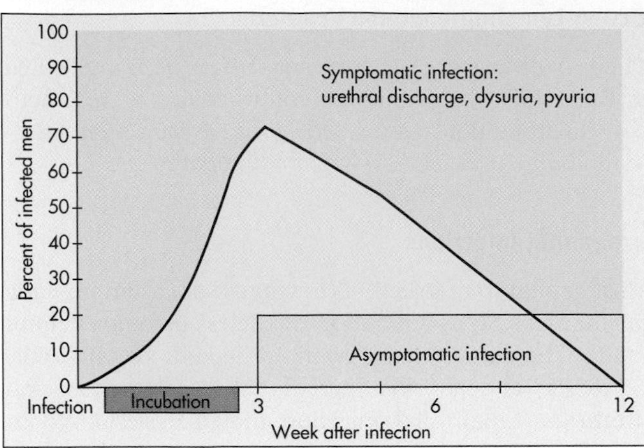

FIGURE 47–4. Time course of untreated chlamydial urethritis in men.

It is believed that **Reiter's syndrome** (urethritis, conjunctivitis, polyarthritis, and mucocutaneous lesions) is initiated by genital infection with *C. trachomatis*. Although chlamydiae have not been isolated from the synovial fluid of such patients, EBs have been observed in synovial fluid or tissue specimens from men with sexually acquired reactive arthritis. The disease usually occurs in young white men. Approximately 50% to 65% of patients with Reiter's syndrome have a chlamydial genital infection at the onset of arthritis, and serologic studies indicate that more than 80% of men with Reiter's syndrome have evidence of a preceding or concurrent infection with *C. trachomatis*.

Lymphogranuloma Venereum

After an incubation of 1 to 4 weeks, a primary lesion appears at the site of infection (e.g., penis, urethra, glans, scrotum, vaginal wall, cervix, vulva) in patients with LGV. The lesion (either a papule or an ulcer) is often overlooked, however, because it is small, painless, and inconspicuous and heals rapidly. The absence of pain differentiates these ulcers from those observed in syphilis and herpes simplex virus infections. The patient may experience fever, headache, and myalgia when the lesion is present.

The second stage of infection is marked by inflammation and swelling of the lymph nodes draining the site of initial infection. The inguinal nodes are most commonly involved, becoming painful, fluctuant **buboes** that gradually enlarge and can rupture, forming draining fistulas. Systemic manifestations include fever, chills, anorexia, headache, meningismus, myalgias, and arthralgia.

Proctitis is common in women with LGV, resulting from lymphatic spread from the cervix or the vagina. Proctitis develops in men after anal intercourse or as the result of lymphatic spread from the urethra. Untreated LGV may resolve at this stage or may progress to a chronic ulcerative phase, in which genital ulcers, fistulas, strictures, or genital elephantiasis develop.

LABORATORY DIAGNOSIS

C. trachomatis infection can be diagnosed (1) on the basis of cytologic, serologic, or culture findings, (2) through the direct detection of antigen in clinical specimens, and (3) through the use of molecular probes. The sensitivity of each method depends on the patient population examined, the site where the specimen is obtained, and the nature of the disease. For example, symptomatic infections are generally easier to diagnose than asymptomatic infections, because more chlamydiae are present in the specimen from a patient with symptoms. The quality of the specimen is also important. Because chlamydiae are obligate intracellular bacteria, specimens must be obtained from the involved site (e.g., urethra, cervix, rectum, oropharynx, conjunctiva). A specimen of pus or a urethral exudate is inadequate. Chlamydiae infect columnar or squamocolumnar cells; therefore, endocervical and not vaginal specimens should be collected. It has been estimated that 30% of the specimens submitted for study in patients with suspected *Chlamydia* infection are inappropriate.

Cytology

Examination of Giemsa-stained cell scrapings for the presence of inclusions was the first method used for the diagnosis of *C. trachomatis* infection. However, this method is insensitive and is not recommended. Likewise, Papanicolaou's staining of cervical material has been found to be an insensitive and nonspecific method.

Culture

The isolation of *C. trachomatis* in cell culture remains the most specific method of diagnosing *C. trachomatis* infections (Figure 47–5). The bacteria infect a restricted range of cell lines in vitro (e.g., HeLa, McCoy, HEp-2, and others), similar to the narrow range of cells they infect in vivo. The sensitivity of culture is compromised if inadequate specimens are used and if chlamydial viability has been lost during transport of the specimen. It has been estimated that the sensitivity of the findings yielded by a single endocervical specimen may be only 70% to 85%.

Antigen Detection

Two general approaches have been used to detect chlamydial antigens in clinical specimens, direct immunofluorescence staining with fluorescein-conjugated monoclonal antibodies (Figure 47–6) and enzyme-linked

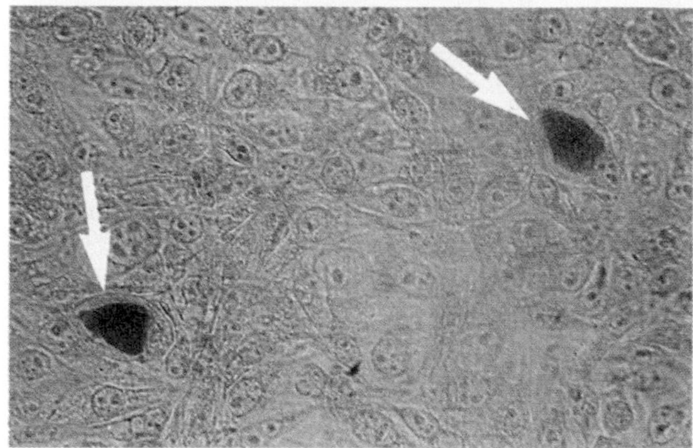

FIGURE 47–5. *Chlamydia trachomatis* is grown in cell cultures and detected by staining inclusion bodies (*arrows*) with either iodine or specific fluorescein-labeled antibodies.

FIGURE 47–6. Fluorescent-stained elementary bodies in a clinical sample. (From Hart T, Shears P: *Color atlas of medical microbiology,* London, 2000, Mosby-Wolfe.)

immunosorbent assays. In both assays, antibodies are used that have been prepared against either the chlamydial MOMP or the cell wall LPS. Because antigenic determinants on LPS may be shared with other bacteria, particularly those in fecal specimens, antibody tests that target the LPS antigen are less specific. The sensitivity of each assay method has been reported to vary enormously, but neither is considered as sensitive as culture, particularly if male urethral specimens or specimens from asymptomatic patients are used. The latter pose a problem because they may contain relatively few chlamydiae.

Nucleic Acid Probes

Different nucleic acid probe tests are currently available. The tests measure for the presence of a species-specific sequence of 16S ribosomal RNA. The advantage of these tests is that the nucleic acid does not have to be amplified, making the tests rapid and relatively inexpensive. However, these tests are relatively insensitive for the detection of small numbers of chlamydiae. For this reason, a number of molecular diagnostic tests have been developed that first amplify a specific sequence of genetic information and then detect it with species-specific probes.

A number of nucleic acid amplification tests (NAATs) are now commercially available for chlamydia testing, including (1) polymerase chain reaction (PCR), (2) ligase chain reaction, (3) transcription-mediated amplification, and (4) strand displacement amplification. NAATs are highly sensitive (generally reported to be 90% to 98% sensitive) and, if properly monitored, are very specific. First-voided urine from a patient with urethritis can be used. Care must be used to monitor for the presence of inhibitors (e.g., urine) to the amplification reaction and to prevent cross-contamination of specimens. Despite these cautions, NAATs are currently considered the tests of choice for the laboratory diagnosis of genital *C. trachomatis* infection.

Serology

Serologic testing is of limited value in the diagnosis of *C. trachomatis* urogenital infections in adults, because antibody titers can persist for a prolonged period. Thus the test cannot differentiate between current and past infections. Demonstration of a significant increase in antibody levels can be useful; however, this increase may not be demonstrated for a month or longer, particularly in patients who receive antibiotic treatment. Testing for immunoglobulin (Ig)M antibodies is also usually not helpful because adolescents and adults often do not produce these antibodies. An exception is the detection of IgM antibodies in infants with chlamydial pneumonitis.

Additionally, antibody tests for the diagnosis of LGV can be helpful. Infected patients produce a vigorous antibody response that can be detected by complement fixation, microimmunofluorescence (MIF), or enzyme immunoassay (EIA). The CF test is directed against the genus-specific LPS antigen. Thus a positive result (i.e., fourfold increase in titer or a single titer $\geq 1:256$) is highly suggestive of LGV. Confirmation is determined by the MIF test, which is directed against species- and serovar-specific antigens (the chlamydial MOMPs). Like the CF test, EIAs are genus specific. The advantage of these tests is that they are less technically cumbersome. However, the results must be confirmed by MIF.

TREATMENT, PREVENTION, AND CONTROL

It is recommended that patients with LGV be treated with a tetracycline (e.g., doxycycline) for 21 days. Treatment with a macrolide (e.g., erythromycin, azithromycin) or sulfisoxazole is recommended for children younger than 9 years, pregnant women, and patients unable to tolerate tetracyclines. Ocular and genital infections in adults should be treated with one dose of azithromycin or doxycycline for 7 days. Newborn conjunctivitis and pneumonia should be treated with erythromycin for 10 to 14 days. The effectiveness of tetracyclines, macrolides, and fluoroquinolones is unknown because resistance to all of these antibiotics has not been observed.

It is difficult to prevent *C. trachomatis* infections because the population with endemic disease commonly has limited access to medical care. The blindness associated with advanced stages of trachoma can be prevented only by prompt treatment of early disease and the prevention of reexposure. Although treatment can be successful in individuals living in areas where the disease is endemic, it is difficult to eradicate the disease within a population and to prevent reinfections unless sanitary conditions are improved. *Chlamydia* conjunctivitis and genital infections are prevented through the use of safe sex practices and the prompt treatment of symptomatic patients and their sexual partners.

Chlamydophila pneumoniae

C. pneumoniae was first isolated from the conjunctiva of a child in Taiwan. It was initially considered a psittacosis strain because the morphology of the inclusions produced in cell culture was similar. However, it was subsequently shown that the Taiwan isolate (TW-183) was related serologically to a pharyngeal isolate, designated AR-39, and was unrelated to psittacosis strains. This new organism was initially called TWAR, then classified as *Chlamydia pneumoniae*, and, finally, placed in the new genus *Chlamydophila*. Only a single serotype (TWAR) has been identified. Respiratory secretions transmit infection; no animal reservoir has been identified.

C. pneumoniae is a human pathogen. It is an important cause of bronchitis, pneumonia, and sinusitis, infections being transmitted person to person by respiratory secretions. Infection is believed to be common (an estimated 200,000 to 300,000 cases of *C. pneumoniae* pneumonia occur annually), and most common in adults. More than 50% of people have serologic evidence of past infections. Most *C. pneumoniae* infections are asymptomatic or mild, causing a persistent cough and malaise; most patients do not require hospitalization. More severe respiratory tract infections typically involve a single lobe of the lungs. These infections cannot be differentiated from other atypical pneumonias, such as those caused by *Mycoplasma pneumoniae*, *Legionella pneumophila*, and respiratory viruses.

The role of *C. pneumoniae* in the pathogenesis of atherosclerosis remains to be defined. It is known that *C. pneumoniae* can infect and grow in smooth muscle cells, endothelial cells of the coronary artery, and macrophages. The organism has also been demonstrated in biopsy specimens of atherosclerotic lesions by means of culture, PCR amplification, immunohistologic staining, electron microscopy, and in situ hybridization. Thus the association of *C. pneumoniae* with atherosclerotic lesions is clear. What is not clear is the role of the organism in the development of atherosclerosis. The disease is believed to result from an inflammatory response to chronic infection; however, this remains to be proven.

Diagnosis of *C. pneumoniae* infections is difficult. The organisms do not grow in the cell lines used for the isolation of *C. trachomatis*, and although *C. pneumoniae* will grow in the HEp-2 cell line, this cell line is not used in most clinical laboratories. Detection of *C. pneumoniae* by NAATs has been successful, and these tests appear to be the most sensitive diagnostic methods available. However, NAATs are not used in most laboratories at this time. CF or MIF tests can be used to make a serologic diagnosis. Because the CF test reacts with *Chlamydia* and *Chlamydophila*, it is not specific for *C. pneumoniae* infection. The MIF test uses *C. pneumoniae* EBs as antigen, so it is specific.

Macrolides (erythromycin, azithromycin, clarithromycin), tetracyclines (tetracycline, doxycycline), or levofloxacin administered for 10 to 14 days has been used to treat infections. Control of exposure to *C. pneumoniae* is likely to be difficult because the bacterium is ubiquitous.

Chlamydophila psittaci

C. psittaci is the cause of psittacosis (parrot fever), which can be transmitted to humans. The disease was first observed in parrots, thus the name **psittacosis** (*psittakos* is the Greek word for parrot). In reality, however, the natural reservoir of *C. psittaci* is virtually any species of bird, and the disease has been referred to more appropriately as **ornithosis** (derived from the Greek word *ornithos*, for bird). Other animals such as sheep, cows, and goats, as well as humans, can become infected. The organism is present in the blood, tissues, feces, and feathers of infected birds that may appear either ill or healthy.

Infection occurs by means of the respiratory tract, after which the bacteria spread to the reticuloendothelial cells of the liver and spleen. The organisms multiply in these sites, producing focal necrosis. The lung and other organs are then seeded as the result of hematogenous spread, which causes a predominantly lymphocytic inflammatory response in the alveolar and interstitial spaces. Edema, thickening of the alveolar wall, infiltration of macrophages, necrosis, and occasionally hemorrhage occur at these sites. Mucous plugs develop in the bronchioles, causing cyanosis and anoxia.

Fewer than 50 cases of the disease are reported annually in the United States, with most infections in adults. This number certainly is an underestimation of the true prevalence of disease, however, because (1) human infections may be asymptomatic or mild, (2) exposure to an infected bird may not be suspected, (3) convalescent serum may not be collected so that the clinical diagnosis can be confirmed, and (4) antibiotic therapy may blunt the antibody response. Furthermore, because of the serologic cross-reactions with *C. pneumoniae*, specific estimates of the prevalence of disease will remain unreliable until a definitive diagnostic test is developed.

The bacterium is usually transmitted to humans through the inhalation of dried bird excrement, urine, or respiratory secretions. Most infections result from exposure to psittacine birds (e.g., parrots, parakeets, macaws, cockatiels). Person-to-person transmission is rare. Veterinarians, zookeepers, pet shop workers, and employees of poultry-processing plants are at increased risk for this infection.

The illness develops after an incubation of 5 to 14 days and usually manifests as headache, high fever, chills, malaise, and myalgias (Figure 47–7). Pulmonary signs include a nonproductive cough, rales, and consolidation. Central nervous system involvement is common, usually consisting of headache, but encephalitis, convulsions, coma, and death may occur in severe, untreated cases. Patients may suffer gastrointestinal tract symptoms, such as nausea, vomiting, and diarrhea. Other systemic symptoms include carditis, hepatomegaly, splenomegaly, and follicular keratoconjunctivitis.

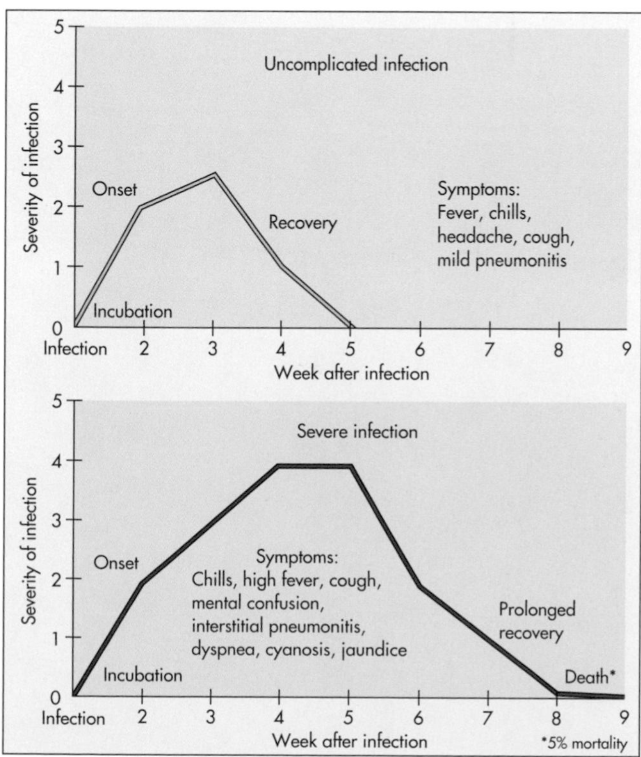

FIGURE 47–7. Time course of *Chlamydophila psittaci* infection.

Psittacosis is usually diagnosed on the basis of serologic findings. A fourfold increase in titer, shown by the CF testing of paired acute and convalescent phase sera, is suggestive of *C. psittaci* infection, but the species-specific MIF test must be performed to confirm the diagnosis. *C. psittaci* can be isolated in cell culture (e.g., with L cells) after 5 to 10 days of incubation, although this procedure is rarely performed in clinical laboratories.

Infections can be treated successfully with tetracyclines or macrolides. Person-to-person transmission occurs rarely, so isolation of the patient and prophylactic treatment of contacts are not necessary. Psittacosis can be prevented only through the control of infections in domestic and imported pet birds. Such control can be achieved by treating birds with chlortetracycline hydrochloride for 45 days. No vaccine currently exists for this disease.

CASE STUDY AND QUESTIONS

A 22-year-old man came to the emergency department with a history of urethral pain and purulent discharge that developed after he had sexual contact with a prostitute. Gram stain of the discharge revealed abundant gram-negative diplococci resembling Neisseria gonorrhoeae. The patient was treated with penicillin and sent home. Two days later, the patient returned to the emergency room with a complaint of persistent, watery urethral discharge. Abundant white blood cells but no organisms were observed on Gram stain of the discharge. Culture of the discharge was negative for N. gonorrhoeae but positive for C. trachomatis.

1. Why is penicillin ineffective against *Chlamydia?* What antibiotic can be used to treat this patient?
2. Describe the growth cycle of *Chlamydia*. What structural features make the EBs and RBs well suited for their environment?
3. Describe the differences among the three species in the family Chlamydiaceae that cause human disease.
4. *C. trachomatis, C. pneumoniae,* and *C. psittaci* each cause respiratory tract infections. Describe the patient population most commonly infected and the epidemiology of these infections.

Bibliography

Black C: Current methods of laboratory diagnosis of *Chlamydia trachomatis* infections, *Clin Microbiol Rev* 10:160-184, 1997.

Boman J, Gaydos C, Quinn T: Minireview: Molecular diagnosis of *Chlamydia pneumoniae* infection, *J Clin Microbiol* 37:3791-3799, 1999.

Boman J, Hammerschlag MR: *Chlamydia pneumoniae* and atherosclerosis: Critical assessment of diagnostic methods and relevance to treatment studies, *Clin Microbiol Rev* 15:1-20, 2002.

Centers for Disease Control and Prevention: Screening tests to detect *Chlamydia trachomatis* and *Neisseria gonorrhoeae* infections—2002, *MMWR* 51(RR-15):1-38, 2002.

Everett K, Bush R, Andersen A: Emended description of the order Chlamydiales, proposal of Parachlamydiaceae fam. nov. and Simkaniaceae fam. nov., each containing one monotypic genus, revised taxonomy of the family Chlamydiaceae, including a new genus and five new species, and standards for the identification of organisms, *Int J System Bacteriol* 49:415-440, 1999.

Morre S et al: Urogenital *Chlamydia trachomatis* serovars in men and women with a symptomatic or asymptomatic infection: An association with clinical manifestations? *J Clin Microbiol* 38:2292-2296, 2000.

Ngeh J, Anand V, Gupta S: *Chlamydia pneumoniae* and atherosclerosis—what we know and what we don't know, *Clin Microbiol Infect* 8:2-13, 2002.

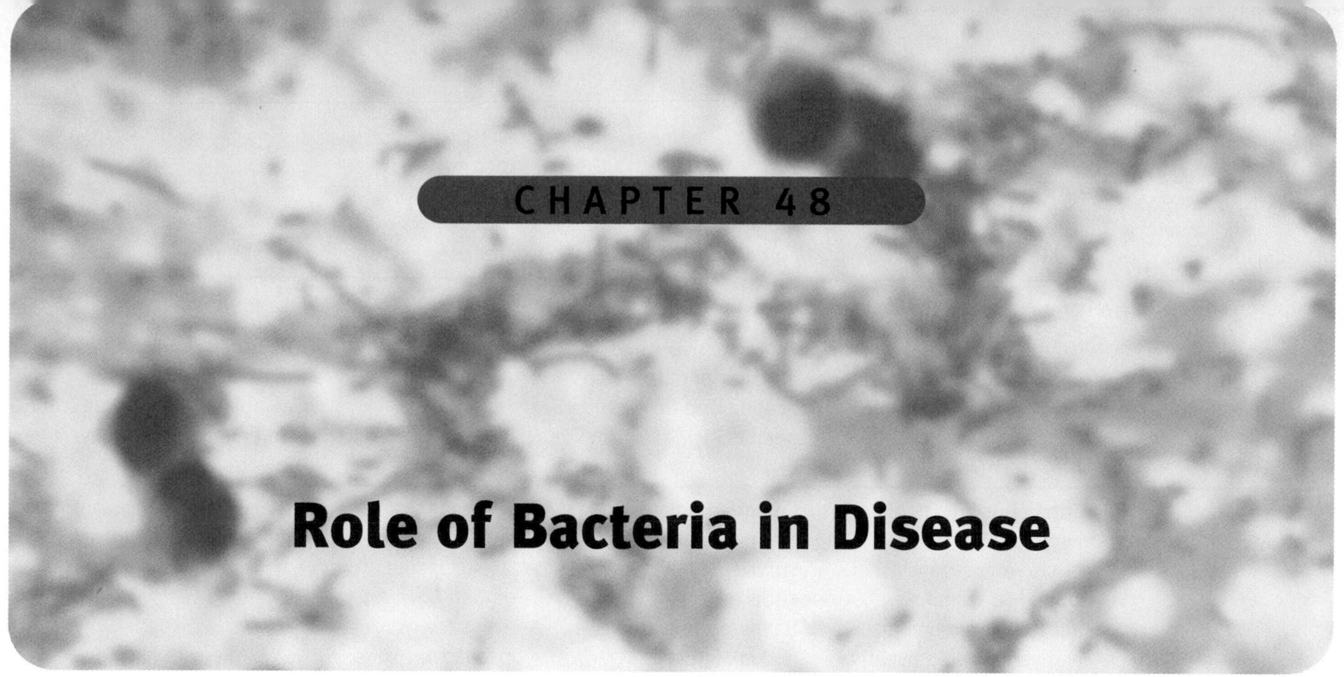

Role of Bacteria in Disease

This chapter summarizes material presented in chapters 22 to 47. The preceding chapters have focused on individual organisms and the diseases they cause. We believe this is an important process in understanding how individual organisms produce disease. However, when a patient develops an infection, a physician approaches diagnosis by assessing the clinical presentation and constructing a list of organism that are most likely to cause the disease. The etiology in some diseases can be attributed to a single organism (e.g., tetanus—*Clostridium tetani*). More commonly, however, multiple organisms can produce a disease syndrome. The clinical management of infections is therefore predicated on the ability to develop an acute differential diagnosis; that is, it is critical to know which organisms are most commonly associated with a particular infectious process (e.g., bacteremia, pneumonia, gastroenteritis) or an epidemiologic situation (e.g., foodborne or waterborne diseases, arthropod-associated infections).

The development of an infection depends on the complex interactions of (1) the host's susceptibility to infection, (2) the organism's virulence potential, and (3) the opportunity for interaction between host and organism. It is impossible to summarize in a single chapter the complex interactions that lead to the development of disease in each organ system. That is the domain of texts in infectious disease. Rather, this chapter is intended to serve as a very broad overview of the bacteria commonly associated with infections at specific body sites and with specific clinical manifestations (Tables 48–1 to 48–5). Because many factors influence the relative frequency with which specific organisms cause disease (e.g., age, underlying disease, epidemiologic factors, host immunity), no attempt is made to define all the factors associated with disease caused by specific organisms. That material is provided, in part, in the preceding chapters and in comprehensive infectious disease texts cited in this chapter and in the preceding chapters. Furthermore, the roles of fungi, viruses, and parasites are not considered here but rather in the subsequent sections of this book.

Bibliography

Braunwald E et al, editors *Harrison's principles of internal medicine*, ed 15, New York, 2001, McGraw-Hill.

Cohen J, Powderly WG: *Infectious Diseases*, ed 2, St Louis, 2004, Mosby.

Mandell GL, Bennett JE, Dolin R, editors: *Principles and practice of infectious diseases*, ed 6, New York, 2005, Churchill Livingstone.

Murray P, Shea Y: *Pocket guide to clinical microbiology*, ed 3, Washington, 2004, American Society for Microbiology.

Murray PR et al, editors: *Manual of clinical microbiology*, ed 8, Washington, 2003, American Society for Microbiology.

TABLE 48–1. Overview of Selected Bacterial Pathogens

Organism	Clinical Features	Epidemiologic Features	Virulence Factors	Treatment
Aerobic and Facultatively Anaerobic Gram-Positive Cocci				
Enterococcus faecalis and *faecium*	Bacteremia, intraabdominal abscess, urinary tract infection, endocarditis	Elderly patients and patients who have been hospitalized for extended periods	Relatively avirulent	Penicillin/ampicillin/ piperacillin or vancomycin; combined with gentamicin for endocarditis or severe infection
Staphylococcus aureus	Cutaneous infections: impetigo, folliculitis, furuncles, carbuncles, wound; disseminated infections: pneumonia, empyema, osteomyelitis, septic arthritis; toxin-mediated infections: toxic shock syndrome, scalded skin syndrome, food poisoning	Colonize human skin and mucosal surfaces; survive on environmental surfaces; able to grow at temperature extremes and in high salt concentrations	Possess thick peptidoglycan layer, capsule, protein A, various toxins (cytotoxins, exfoliative toxins, enterotoxins, toxic shock syndrome toxin, Panton Valentine (PV) leukocidin) and hydrolytic enzymes	Nafcillin; vancomycin (for methicillin-resistant strains)
Staphylococcus, coagulase negative	Opportunistic pathogen causing infections on foreign bodies (e.g., catheters, shunts, prosthetic joints and heart valves); urinary tract infections (e.g., *S. saprophyticus*)	Colonize human skin and mucosal surfaces; survive on environmental surfaces; able to grow at temperature extremes	Possess thick peptidoglycan layer and loose polysaccharide slime layer; *S. saprophyticus* produces high concentrations of urease	Nafcillin; vancomycin (for methicillin-resistant strains)
Streptococcus pyogenes (group A)	Suppurative infections: pharyngitis, scarlet fever, sinusitis, skin and soft-tissue infection (impetigo, erysipelas, cellulitis, necrotizing fasciitis), toxic shock–like syndrome; nonsuppurative infections: rheumatic fever; glomerulonephritis	Diverse populations	Capsule, M protein, M-like protein, F protein, pyrogenic exotoxins, streptolysin S and O, streptokinase, deoxyribonuclease (DNase); C5a peptidase	Penicillin, macrolides, cephalosporins, clindamycin, vancomycin; surgical débridement for necrotizing fasciitis
Streptococcus agalactiae (group B)	Neonatal disease (early onset, late onset; bacteremia, pneumonia, meningitis); urinary tract infections, bacteremia, pneumonia	Neonates; pregnant women; patients with diabetes, cancer, or alcoholism	Similar to group A but no capsule	Penicillin, macrolides, cephalosporins, clindamycin, vancomycin; penicillin and aminoglycoside for serious infections
Other β-hemolytic streptococci	Pharyngitis, otitis, sinusitis, skin and soft-tissue infection, impetigo, erysipelas, cellulitis, necrotizing fasciitis	Diverse populations	Similar to group A *Streptococcus*	Penicillin (drug of choice), macrolides, cephalosporins, clindamycin, vancomycin; surgical débridement for necrotizing fasciitis

TABLE 48–1. Overview of Selected Bacterial Pathogens—*cont'd*

Organism	Clinical Features	Epidemiologic Features	Virulence Factors	Treatment
Streptococcus bovis	Bacteremia, endocarditis	Older patients with colon cancer	Relatively avirulent	Penicillin
Viridans streptococci	Abscess formation; septicemia in neutropenic patients; subacute endocarditis; odontogenic infections; dental caries	Patients with abnormal heart valves	Relatively avirulent	Penicillin; penicillin combined with aminoglycoside
Streptococcus pneumoniae	Pneumonia and other respiratory tract infections; meningitis; spontaneous bacterial peritonitis, endocarditis, septic arthritis; bacteremia	Diverse: neonates, children, adults with chronic diseases, elderly persons	Polysaccharide capsule; teichoic acid; immunoglobulin (Ig)A proteases; pneumolysin O	Penicillin; levofloxacin, cephalosporins, clindamycin
Aerobic or Facultatively Anaerobic Gram-Positive Rods				
Bacillus anthracis	Cutaneous anthrax, inhalation anthrax, gastrointestinal anthrax	Animal workers; microbiologic accidents; bioterrorism; eating contaminated meat	Capsule; edema toxin; lethal toxin; spore formation	Fluoroquinolones (ciprofloxacin); penicillin, doxycycline, erythromycin, or chloramphenicol as alternative therapy
Bacillus cereus	Gastroenteritis, ocular infections, bacteremia	Contaminated food; traumatic eye injury with introduction of soil; injection drug use	Heat-stable and heat-labile toxins, necrotic toxin	Fluoroquinolones, vancomycin
Corynebacterium diphtheriae	Diphtheria: respiratory, cutaneous	Spread by respiratory droplets to unimmunized individuals	Diphtheria toxin	Neutralizing exotoxin; penicillin or erythromycin to eliminate organism and terminate toxin production; immunization with diphtheria toxoid
Corynebacterium jeikeium	Septicemia, endocarditis; wound infections; foreign body infections	Immunocompromised patients at increased risk	Unknown	Vancomycin
Corynebacterium urealyticum	Urinary tract infections, including pyelonephritis with calculi; septicemia; endocarditis; wound infections	Risk factors include immunosuppression, underlying genitourinary disorders, antecedent urologic procedures, prior antibiotic therapy	Urease production	Vancomycin
Erysipelothrix rhusiopathiae	Erysipeloid (painful, pruritic inflammatory skin lesion)	Occupational disease of butchers, meat processors, farmers, poultry workers, fish handlers, and veterinarians	Unknown	Penicillin; cephalosporins, fluoroquinolones, erythromycin, or clindamycin as alternative therapy

TABLE 48–1. Overview of Selected Bacterial Pathogens—*cont'd*

Organism	Clinical Features	Epidemiologic Features	Virulence Factors	Treatment
Listeria monocytogenes	Early onset neonatal disease (granulomatosis infantiseptica); late-onset neonatal disease (meningitis with septicemia); flulike illness in adults; bacteremia or disseminated disease in pregnant women or patients with cell-mediated immune defects	Immunocompromised hosts, elderly persons, neonates, pregnant women; ingestion of contaminated food	Listeriolysin O; internalins; intracellular survival and growth; intracellular motility; growth at 4°C	Ampicillin (alone or in combination with gentamicin)
Mycobacteria				
Mycobacterium avium complex	Localize pulmonary disease; disseminated disease with multiorgan involvement	Localized disease in patients with chronic pulmonary disease; disseminated disease in AIDS and other immunocompromised patients	Intracellular replication	Clarithromycin or azithromycin combined with rifabutin or ethambutol
Mycobacterium leprae	Leprosy: range from tuberculoid form to lepromatous form	Close contact with infected individual most likely responsible for spread	Ability to survive and replicate in macrophages	Dapson and rifampicin for tuberculoid form; add clofazimine for lepromatous form
Mycobacterium tuberculosis	Tuberculosis: pulmonary, extrapulmonary	All ages with HIV-infected patients at greatest risk for active disease	Ability to survive and replicate in macrophages	Multidrug therapy with isoniazid, rifampin, ethambutol, and pyrazinamide
Nocardia species	Bronchopulmonary disease; primary or secondary cutaneous infections; brain abscesses	Opportunistic pathogen in immunocompetent patients with chronic pulmonary disease or immunocompromised patients with T-cell deficiencies	Intracellular survival and growth; catalase and superoxide dismustase	Sulfonamides; amikacin, carbapenems, or broad-spectrum cephalosporins as alternative therapy if active
Rhodococcus equi	Bronchopulmonary disease (lung abscesses); opportunistic infections in immunocompetent patients	Pathogen most commonly found in immunocompromised patients (e.g., AIDS patients, transplant recipients)	Intracellular survival and growth	Combination therapy with vancomycin, carbapenems, aminoglycosides, ciprofloxacin, rifampin, and/or erythromycin
Aerobic Gram-Negative Cocci				
Neisseria gonorrhoeae	Gonorrhoea, pelvic inflammatory disease, arthritis	Sexual transmission, asymptomatic carriage	Pili, adhesins, IgA protease, transferring-binding proteins, antigenic variation	Ceftriaxone, ciprofloxacin; cefoxitin plus doxycycline

TABLE 48–1. Overview of Selected Bacterial Pathogens—*cont'd*

Organism	Clinical Features	Epidemiologic Features	Virulence Factors	Treatment
Neisseria meningitidis	Meningitis, bacteremia (meningococcemia)	Carrier state, aerosol transmission, most common in children and young adults	Polysaccharide capsule, endotoxin, pili, adhesins, IgA protease, transferring-binding proteins	Ceftriaxone, penicillin, chloramphenicol
Aerobic and Facultatively Anaerobic Gram-Negative Rods				
Acinetobacter	Pneumonia, septicemia, opportunistic infections	Nosocomial infections	Unknown	Imipenem or ceftazidime combined with aminoglycoside for serious infections
Aeromonas	Wound infections; gastroenteritis	Healthy and immunocompromised patients	Unknown	Ciprofloxacin; trimethoprim-sulfamethoxazole, gentamicin, or amikacin as alternative therapy
Bartonella henselae	Bacillary angiomatosis; subacute endocarditis; cat scratch disease (CSD)	Healthy (endocarditis, CSD) and immunocompromised patients (BA)	Unknown	Gentamicin alone or with erythromycin; broad-spectrum cephalosporins used as alternative therapy; CSD does not response to antibiotic therapy
Bartonella quintana	Trench fever (TF); bacillary angiomatosis (BA)	Healthy (TF) or immunocompromised patients (BA)	Unknown	As with *B. henselae*
Bordetella pertussis, Bordetella parapertussis	Pertussis (whooping cough)	Aerosol transmission; severe diseases in infants, milder in adults	Pertussis toxin, adenylate cyclase toxin, adhesins, tracheal cytotoxin	Supportive therapy, erythromycin (or other macrolides) to decrease infectivity and prophylaxis for contacts
Brucella	Brucellosis	Exposure to infected goats, sheep, cattle, or other animals; bioterrorism	Ability to persist and replicate in macrophages	Doxycycline plus rifampin or gentamicin; trimethoprim-sulfamethoxazole
Burkholderia cepacia complex	Pulmonary infections; opportunistic infections	Compromised individuals, especially cystic fibrosis and chronic granulomatous disease patients	Unknown	Trimethoprim-sulfamethoxazole; piperacillin, ceftazidime, or ciprofloxacin as alternative therapy if trimethoprim-sulfamethoxazole resistant
Burkholderia pseudomallei	Meliodosis (asymptomatic to severe pulmonary disease)	Opportunistic pathogen	Unknown	Trimethoprim-sulfamethoxazole combined with ceftazidime

TABLE 48–1. Overview of Selected Bacterial Pathogens—*cont'd*

Organism	Clinical Features	Epidemiologic Features	Virulence Factors	Treatment
Campylobacter jejuni, Campylobacter coli, Campylobacter upsaliensis	Gastroenteritis	Zoonotic infection following ingestion of contaminated food, milk, or water	Factors regulating adherence and invasion into intestinal mucosa	Self-limited; severe infections treated with erythromycin; tetracycline or fluoroquinolones used as alterative therapy
Camplyobacter fetus	Septicemia; meningitis; gastroenteritis; spontaneous abortion	Infects elderly, immunocompromised patients	Unknown	Aminoglycosides, carbapenems, chloramphenicol
Cardiobacterium hominis	Subacute endocarditis	Opportunistic pathogen in patients with previously damaged heart valve	Unknown	Penicillin or ampicillin
Eikenella corrodens	Subacute endocarditis; wound infections	Human bite wounds; opportunistic pathogen in patients with previously damaged heart valve	Unknown	Penicillin, cephalosporins, tetracycline, or fluoroquinolones
Escherichia coli—enteropathogenic (EPEC)	Watery diarrhea and vomiting	Infants in developing countries	Bundle-forming pili, attaching and effacing	Unknown
E. coli—enterohemorrhagic (EHEC)	Watery diarrhea, hemorrhagic colitis, hemolytic uremic syndrome	Foodborne, waterborne outbreaks in developed countries	Shiga toxins, attaching and effacing	Antibiotics contraindicated
E. coli—enterotoxigenic (ETEC)	Watery diarrhea	Childhood diarrhea in developing countries, travelers' diarrhea	Pili, heat-labile and heat-stable enterotoxins	Ciprofloxacin shortens course (high level of resistance)
E. coli—enteroaggregative (EAEC)	Diarrhea with mucus	Childhood diarrhea	Pili, cytotoxins	Fluoroquinolones in AIDS patients
E. coli—enteroinvasive (EIEC)	Watery diarrhea, hemorrhagic colitis	Childhood diarrhea in developing countries	Invasion and destruction of colonic epithelial cells	Antibiotics reduce duration of disease and infectivity
E. coli—uropathogenic	Cystitis, pyelonephritis	Sexually active women	Adhesins (P pili, AAF/I, AAF/III, Dr), hemolysin, pathogenicity islands	Trimethoprim-sulfamethoxazole, fluoroquinolones
E. coli—meningitis associated	Acute meningitis	Neonates	K1 capsule, S fimbriae, cellular invasion	Extended-spectrum cephalosporins
Francisella tularensis	Tularemia: ulceroglandular, oculoglandular, pneumonic	Tick bites; skinning infected animals (rabbits); bioterrorism	Capsule	Streptomycin, gentamicin; fluoroquinolones

TABLE 48–1. Overview of Selected Bacterial Pathogens—*cont'd*

Organism	Clinical Features	Epidemiologic Features	Virulence Factors	Treatment
Haemophilus influenzae	Encapsulated type b strains: meningitis, septicemia, cellulitis, epiglottitis; unencapsulated strains: otitis media, sinusitis, bronchitis, pneumonia	Aerosol transmission in young, unimmunized children; spread from upper respiratory tract in elderly patients with chronic respiratory disease	Polysaccharide capsule, pili, adhesins, IgA protease	Broad-spectrum cephalosporin, azithromycin, or fluoroquinolone; many strains resistant to ampicillin
Helicobacter pylori	Gastritis, peptic, and duodenal ulcers; gastric adenocarcinoma	Infections common particularly in people in low socioeconomic class or in developing countries	Urease; heat-shock protein; acid-inhibitory protein adhesins; mucinase; phospholipases; vacuolating cytotoxin; other factors	Multidrug therapy: tetracycline, metronidazole, bismuth, and omeprazole
Kingella kingae	Subacute endocarditis	Opportunistic pathogen in patients with previously damaged heart valve	Unknown	β-Lactam with β-lactamase inhibitor, cephalosporins, macrolides, tetracycline, fluoroquinolones
Klebsiella pneumoniae	Pneumonia, urinary tract infections	Nosocomial infections; alcoholism	Capsule	Cephalosporins, fluoroquinolones
Legionella pneumophila	Legionnaires' disease (pneumonia), Pontiac fever (flulike illness)	Waterborne; elderly and immunocompromised patients	C3b adhesin, cytotoxins, evasion of phagolysosome fusion	Macrolides (erythromycin, azithromycin, clarithromycin); fluoroquinolones (ciprofloxacin, levofloxacin) used as alternative therapy
Moraxella catarrhalis	Ear, eye, and respiratory infections	Children; patients with compromised pulmonary system	Unknown	Cephalosporins; amoxicillin/clavulanic acid
Proteus	Urinary tract infections, wound infections	Structural abnormality in urinary tract	Urease, swarming motility	Amoxicillin, trimethoprim-sulfamethoxazole, cephalosporins, fluoroquinolones
Pseudomonas aeruginosa	Pulmonary; primary skin infection; urinary tract infection; ear or eye infections; bacteremia	Nosocomial infections	Capsule; exotoxin A; ExoS; phospholipase C; elastase	Combination therapy generally required (e.g., aminoglycoside with extended-spectrum cephalosporins, piperacillin-tazobactam, or carbapenem)
Salmonella enterica	Diarrhea, enteric fever (serovar *Typhi*)	Contaminated food; immunocompromised patients at higher risk for bacteremia	Type III secretion system; epithelial cell invasion; survival in macrophages	May prolong carrier state in simple diarrhea treatment; fluoroquinolones for enteric fever
Serratia, Enterobacter	Pneumonia, urinary tract infections, wound infections	Nosocomial infections	Unknown	Carbapenems; piperacillin-tazobactam

TABLE 48–1. Overview of Selected Bacterial Pathogens—*cont'd*

Organism	Clinical Features	Epidemiologic Features	Virulence Factors	Treatment
Shigella	Bacillary dysentery	Contaminated food or water; person-to-person spread	Type III secretion system; intracellular spread; induction of macrophage apoptosis	Ampicillin; trimethoprim-sulfamethoxazole; fluoroquinolones
Stenotrophomonas maltophilia	Wide variety of local and systemic infections	Nosocomial infections	Unknown	Trimethoprim-sulfamethoxazole
Streptobacillus moniliformis	Rat-bite fever; Haverhill fever	Bite of rat or other small rodents; ingestion of contaminated food or water	Unknown	Penicillin, doxycycline
Vibrio cholerae	Severe watery diarrhea	Children and adults in developing countries	Cholera toxin; toxin-co-regulated pilus (TCP); other toxins; neuraminidase	Rehydration; doxycycline, trimethoprim-sulfamethoxazole, or furazolidone shortens course
Vibrio parahaemolyticus	Watery diarrhea	Seafood-borne outbreaks	Hemolysin/ enterotoxin oxin	Rehydration
Vibrio vulnificus	Wound infections; primary septicemia	Compromised individuals with preexisting hepatic or chronic diseases	Capsule; numerous degradative enzymes	Minocycline combined with a fluoroquinolone or cefotaxime; débridement
Anaerobes				
Actinomyces	Actinomycosis: cervicofacial, thoracic, abdominal, pelvic, central nervous system	Colonizes human mucosal surface (oropharynx, intestine, vagina)	Unknown	Penicillin; alternative drugs include erythromycin, clindamycin
Bacteroides fragilis	Polymicrobial infections of abdomen, female genital tract, cutaneous and soft tissues	Normal inhabitant of gastrointestinal tract	Polysaccharide capsule; short-chain fatty acids; catalase; superoxide dismutase; hydrolytic enzymes	Metronidazole
Clostridium botulinum	Botulism: foodborne, infant, wound	Found in environment (e.g., soil, water, sewage) and gastrointestinal tract of animals and humans	Spores; botulinum toxin blocks release of neurotransmitter acetylcholine	Ventilatory support; use of trivalent botulinum antitoxin
Clostridium difficile	Antibiotic-associated diarrhea; pseudomembraneous colitis	Colonized human gastrointestinal tract and female genital tract; contaminates hospital environment; prior antibiotic use	Spores; enterotoxin; cytotoxin	Discontinue implicated antibiotic; metronidazole

TABLE 48–1. Overview of Selected Bacterial Pathogens—*cont'd*

Organism	Clinical Features	Epidemiologic Features	Virulence Factors	Treatment
Clostridium perfringens	Soft-tissue infections: cellulitis, fasciitis, myonecrosis; food poisoning; septicemia	Found in environment (e.g., soil, water, sewage) and gastrointestinal tract of animals and humans	Spores; production of many toxins and hemolytic enzymes	Surgical intervention and penicillin
Clostridium tetani	Tetanus: generalized, localized, neonatal	Found in environment (e.g., soil, water, sewage) and gastrointestinal tract of animals and humans	Spores; tetanospasmin blocks release of neurotransmitters for inhibitory synapses	Clean wound; passive immunization; vaccination with tetanus toxoid
Propionibacterium acne	Acne; opportunistic infections (e.g., of prosthetic devices)	Colonize human skin and mucosal surfaces	Opportunistic pathogen of relatively low virulence	Acne treated with benzoyl peroxide plus clindamycin or erythromycin
Anaplasma, Ehrlichia, Rickettsia, Coxiella, Mycoplasma, Chlamydia,* and *Chlamydophila				
Anaplasma phagocytophilum	Anaplasmosis (granulocytic ehrlichiosis)	Transmission by tick bite (*Ixodes*)	Intracellular survival and growth; oxidant-mediated cell injury	Doxycycline; rifampin used as alternative therapy
Chlamydophila pneumoniae	Pneumonia; cardiovascular disease (?)	Children, young adults	Unknown	Macrolides; fluoroquinolones; tetracyclines
Chlamydophila psittaci	Pneumonia	Exposure to birds and their secretions	Unknown	Macrolides; tetracyclines
Chlamydia trachomatis	Trachoma; neonatal conjunctivitis and pneumonia; urethritis; cervicitis; salpingitis; lymphogranuloma venereum	Trachoma in developing countries; exposure to infected secretions during birth or sexual activities	Unknown	Tetracyclines; macrolides; fluoroquinolones
Coxiella burnetii	Q fever: acute (fever, headache, chills, myalgias, granulomatous hepatitis) and chronic (endocarditis, hepatic dysfunction)	Persons exposed to infected livestock; primarily acquired by inhalation; relatively uncommon in United States	Intracellular survival and replication; formation of endospore-like structures that enhance survival in the environment; formation of immune complexes in chronic disease	Doxycycline; rifampin with trimethoprim-sulfamethoxazole
Ehrlichia chaffeensis	Monocytic ehrlichiosis	Transmission by tick bite (*Amblyomma*)	Intracellular survival and replication; oxidant-mediated cell injury	Doxycycline; rifampin used as alternative therapy

TABLE 48–1. Overview of Selected Bacterial Pathogens—*cont'd*

Organism	Clinical Features	Epidemiologic Features	Virulence Factors	Treatment
Mycoplasma pneumoniae	Atypical pneumonia	Symptomatic disease more common in children than adults; severe disease in patients with hypogammaglobulinemia	P1 adhesin protein	Macrolides; tetracycline; fluoroquinolones
Rickettsia rickettsii	Rocky Mountain spotted fever	Most prevalent in hikers and other individuals who spend a lot of time outdoors; transmission by tick bite (Dermacentor in United States)	Intracellular and rapid cell-to-cell spread; oxidant-mediated cell injury	Doxycycline; fluoroquinolones used as alternative therapy
Spirochetes				
Borrelia burgdorferi	Lyme disease: erythema migrans; cardiac, neurologic, or rheumatologic abnormalities	Transmission by ticks (*Ixodes*)	Surface-binding proteins	Oral penicillin; tetracyclines; ceftriaxone
Borrelia recurrentis	Epidemic relapsing fever	Transmission by human body louse; no animal host	Antigenic variation during infection causes relapses	Tetracyclines; erythromycin; chloramphenicol; penicillin
Borrelia species	Endemic relapsing fever	Transmission by tick bite (Ornithodoros); rodent and small mammal reservoir	Antigenic variation during infection causes relapses	Tetracyclines; erythromycin; chloramphenicol; penicillin
Leptospira interrogans	Leptospirosis: mild, viral-like illness to severe multiorgan illness (Weil's disease)	Transmission by exposure to infected urine or tissues of rodents, dogs, farm animals, wild animals	Direct invasion through skin and replication in tissues; immune complex glomerulonephritis	Penicillin; doxycycline; vaccination of pets and herds
Treponema pallidum	Syphilis: primary, secondary, tertiary, congenital	Transmission congenitally or through sexual activity	Adherence to host cells; hyaluronidase; antiphagocytic coat; tissue destruction primarily mediated by host immune response	Penicillin; tetracyclines; erythromycin

TABLE 48–2. Summary of Bacteria Associated with Human Disease

System Affected	Pathogens
Upper Respiratory Infections	
Pharyngitis	Groups A and C *Streptococcus, Arcanobacterium haemolyticum, Chlamydophila pneumoniae, Neisseria gonorrhoeae, Corynebacterium diphtheriae, Corynebacterium ulcerans, Mycoplasma pneumoniae*
Sinusitis	*Streptococcus pneumoniae, Haemophilus influenzae,* mixed anaerobes and aerobes, *Staphylococcus aureus, Moraxella catarrhalis,* group A *Streptococcus, Chlamydophila pneumoniae, Pseudomonas aeruginosa* and other gram-negative rods
Epiglottitis	*Haemophilus influenzae, Streptococcus pneumoniae, Staphylococcus aureus*
Ear Infections	
Otitis externa	*Pseudomonas aeruginosa, Staphylococcus aureus,* group A *Streptococcus*
Otitis media	*Streptococcus pneumoniae, Haemophilus influenzae, Moraxella catarrhalis, Staphylococcus aureus,* group A *Streptococcus,* mixed anaerobes and aerobes
Eye Infections	
Conjunctivitis	*Streptococcus pneumoniae,* group B *Streptococcus,* viridans *Streptococcus, Staphylococcus aureus, Moraxella catarrhalis, Haemophilus aegyptius, Neisseria gonorrhoeae, Pseudomonas aeruginosa, Corynebacterium* species, *Francisella tularensis, Chlamydia trachomatis*
Keratitis	*Staphylococcus aureus,* coagulase-negative *Staphylococcus, Streptococcus pneumoniae,* viridans *Streptococcus,* group A *Streptococcus, Pseudomonas aeruginosa, Proteus mirabilis* and other Enterobacteriaceae, *Bacillus* species, *Clostridium perfringens, Neisseria gonorrhoeae*
Endophthalmitis	*Staphylococcus aureus,* coagulase-negative *Staphylococcus, Pseudomonas aeruginosa, Bacillus* species, *Propionibacterium* species, *Corynebacterium* species
Pleuropulmonary and Bronchial Infections	
Bronchitis	*Bordetella pertussis, Mycoplasma pneumoniae, Chlamydophila pneumoniae, Moraxella catarrhalis, Haemophilus influenzae, Streptococcus pneumoniae*
Empyema	*Staphylococcus aureus, Streptococcus pneumoniae,* group A *Streptococcus, Bacteroides fragilis, Klebsiella pneumoniae* and other Enterobacteriaceae, *Actinomyces* species, *Nocardia* species, *Mycobacterium tuberculosis* and other species
Pneumonia	*Streptococcus pneumoniae, Staphylococcus aureus, Haemophilus influenzae, Neisseria meningitidis, Mycoplasma pneumoniae, Chlamydia trachomatis, Chlamydophila pneumoniae, Chlamydophila psittaci, Klebsiella pneumoniae* and other Enterobacteriaceae, *Pseudomonas aeruginosa, Burkholderia* species, *Legionella* species, *Francisella tularensis, Bacteroides fragilis, Nocardia* species, *Rhodococcus equi, Mycobacterium tuberculosis* and other species, *Coxiella burnetii, Rickettsia rickettsii,* and many other species
Urinary Tract Infections	
Cystitis and pyelonephritis	*Escherichia coli, Proteus mirabilis,* other Enterobacteriaceae, *Pseudomonas aeruginosa, Staphylococcus aureus, Staphylococcus epidermidis, Staphylococcus saprophyticus,* group B *Streptococcus, Enterococcus* species, *Aerococcus urinae, Mycobacterium tuberculosis*
Renal calculi	*Proteus* species, *Morganella morganii, Klebsiella pneumoniae, Corynebacterium urealyticum, Staphylococcus saprophyticus, Ureaplasma urealyticum*

TABLE 48–2. Summary of Bacteria Associated with Human Disease—*cont'd*

System Affected	Pathogens
Renal abscess	*Staphylococcus aureus,* mixed anaerobes and aerobes
Prostatitis	*Escherichia coli, Klebsiella pneumoniae,* other Enterobacteriaceae, *Enterococcus* species, *Neisseria gonorrhoeae, Mycobacterium tuberculosis* and other species
Intraabdominal Infections	
Peritonitis	*Escherichia coli, Klebsiella pneumoniae,* other Enterobacteriaceae, *Pseudomonas aeruginosa, Streptococcus pneumoniae, Staphylococcus aureus, Enterococcus* species, *Bacteroides fragilis* and other species, *Fusobacterium* species, *Clostridium* species, *Peptostreptococcus* species, *Neisseria gonorrhoeae, Chlamydia trachomatis, Mycobacterium tuberculosis*
Dialysis-associated peritonitis	Coagulase-negative *Staphylococcus, Staphylococcus aureus, Streptococcus* species, *Corynebacterium* species, *Propionibacterium* species, *Escherichia coli* and other Enterobacteriaceae, *Pseudomonas aeruginosa, Acinetobacter* species
Visceral abscesses	*Escherichia coli* and other Enterobacteriaceae, *Enterococcus* species, *Staphylococcus aureus, Bacteroides fragilis, Fusobacterium* species, *Actinomyces* species, mixed anaerobic and aerobic infections, *Yersinia enterocolitica, Mycobacterium tuberculosis* and other species
Cardiovascular Infections	
Endocarditis	Viridans *Streptococcus, Streptococcus pneumoniae, Abiotrophia* species, *Staphylococcus aureus,* coagulase-negative *Staphylococcus, Rothia mucilaginosa, Enterococcus* species, HACEK organisms, *Bartonella* species, *Coxiella burnetii, Brucella* species, *Erysipelothrix rhusiopathiae,* Enterobacteriaceae, *Pseudomonas aeruginosa, Corynebacterium* species, *Propionibacterium* species
Myocarditis	*Corynebacterium diphtheriae, Clostridium perfringens,* group A *Streptococcus, Borrelia burgdorferi, Neisseria meningitidis, Staphylococcus aureus, Mycoplasma pneumoniae, Chlamydophila pneumoniae, Chlamydophila psittaci, Rickettsia rickettsii, Orientia tsutsugamushi*
Pericarditis	*Streptococcus pneumoniae, Staphylococcus aureus, Neisseria gonorrhoeae, Neisseria meningitidis, Mycoplasma pneumoniae, Mycobacterium tuberculosis* and other species
Sepsis	
General sepsis	*Staphylococcus aureus,* coagulase-negative *Staphylococcus, Streptococcus pneumoniae* and other species, *Enterococcus* species, *Escherichia coli, Klebsiella* species, *Enterobacter* species, *Proteus mirabilis,* other Enterobacteriaceae, *Pseudomonas aeruginosa,* many other bacteria
Transfusion-associated sepsis	*Yersinia enterocolitica,* coagulase-negative *Staphylococcus, Staphylococcus aureus, Pseudomonas fluorescens* group, *Salmonella* species, other Enterobacteriaceae, *Campylobacter jejuni* and other species, *Treponema pallidum, Bacillus cereus* and other species, *Borrelia* species
Septic thrombophlebitis	*Staphylococcus aureus, Klebsiella* species, *Enterobacter* species, *Pseudomonas aeruginosa, Bacteroides* species, *Fusobacterium* species
Central Nervous System Infections	
Meningitis	Group B *Streptococcus, Streptococcus pneumoniae, Neisseria meningitidis, Listeria monocytogenes, Haemophilus influenzae, Escherichia coli,* other Enterobacteriaceae, *Staphylococcus aureus,* coagulase-negative *Staphylococcus, Propionibacterium* species, *Nocardia* species, *Mycobacterium tuberculosis* and other species, *Borrelia burgdorferi, Leptospira* species, *Treponema pallidum, Brucella* species

TABLE 48–2. Summary of Bacteria Associated with Human Disease—*cont'd*

System Affected	Pathogens
Encephalitis	*Listeria monocytogenes, Treponema pallidum, Leptospira* species, *Actinomyces* species, *Nocardia* species, *Borrelia* species, *Rickettsia rickettsii, Coxiella burnetii, Mycoplasma pneumoniae, Mycobacterium tuberculosis* and other species
Brain abscess	*Staphylococcus aureus,* Enterobacteriaceae, *Pseudomonas aeruginosa,* viridans *Streptococcus, Bacteroides* species, *Prevotella* species, *Porphyromonas* species, *Fusobacterium* species, *Peptostreptococcus* species, other anaerobic cocci, *Actinomyces* species, *Clostridium perfringens, Listeria monocytogenes, Nocardia* species, *Rhodococcus equi, Mycobacterium tuberculosis* and other species
Subdural empyema	*Staphylococcus aureus, Streptococcus pneumoniae,* group B *Streptococcus, Neisseria meningitidis,* mixed anaerobes and aerobes
Skin and Soft-Tissue Infections	
Impetigo	Group A *Streptococcus, Staphylococcus aureus*
Folliculitis	*Staphylococcus aureus, Pseudomonas aeruginosa*
Furuncles and carbuncles	*Staphylococcus aureus*
Paronychia	*Staphylococcus aureus,* group A *Streptococcus,* Pseudomonas aeruginosa
Erysipelas	Group A *Streptococcus*
Cellulitis	Group A *Streptococcus, Staphylococcus aureus, Haemophilus influenzae,* many other bacteria
Necrotizing cellulitis and fasciitis	Group A *Streptococcus, Clostridium perfringens* and other species, *Bacteroides fragilis,* other anaerobes, Enterobacteriaceae, *Pseudomonas aeruginosa*
Bacillary angiomatosis	*Bartonella henselae, Bartonella quintana*
Infections of burns	*Pseudomonas aeruginosa, Enterobacter* species, *Enterococcus* species, *Staphylococcus aureus,* group A *Streptococcus,* many other bacteria
Bite wounds	*Eikenella corrodens, Pasteurella multocida, Pasteurella canis, Staphylococcus aureus,* group A *Streptococcus,* mixed anaerobes and aerobes, many gram-negative rods
Surgical wounds	*Staphylococcus aureus,* coagulase-negative *Staphylococcus,* groups A and B streptococci, *Clostridium perfringens, Corynebacterium* species, many other bacteria
Traumatic wounds	*Bacillus* species, *Staphylococcus aureus,* group A *Streptococcus,* many gram-negative rods, rapid-growing mycobacteria
Gastrointestinal Infections	
Gastritis	*Helicobacter pylori*
Gastroenteritis	*Campylobacter jejuni* and other species, *Salmonella* species, *Shigella* species, *Vibrio cholerae, Vibrio parahaemolyticus,* other *Vibrio* species, *Yersinia enterocolitica, Escherichia coli* (ETEC, EIEC, EHEC, EPEC, others), *Edwardsiella tarda, Bacillus cereus, Pseudomonas aeruginosa, Aeromonas* species, *Plesiomonas shigelloides, Bacteroides fragilis, Clostridium botulinum, Clostridium perfringens, Clostridium difficile*
Food intoxication	*Staphylococcus aureus, Bacillus cereus, Clostridium botulinum, Clostridium perfringens*
Proctitis	*Neisseria gonorrhoeae, Chlamydia trachomatis, Treponema pallidum*
Bone and Joint Infections	
Osteomyelitis	*Staphylococcus aureus,* β-hemolytic *Streptococcus, Streptococcus pneumoniae, Escherichia coli, Salmonella* species and other Enterobacteriaceae, *Pseudomonas aeruginosa, Mycobacterium tuberculosis* and other species, many less common bacteria

TABLE 48–2. Summary of Bacteria Associated with Human Disease—*cont'd*

System Affected	Pathogens
Arthritis	*Staphylococcus aureus, Neisseria gonorrhoeae, Streptococcus pneumoniae, Salmonella* species, *Pasteurella multocida, Mycobacterium* species
Prosthetic-associated infections	*Staphylococcus aureus,* coagulase-negative *Staphylococcus,* group A *Streptococcus,* viridans *Streptococcus, Corynebacterium* species, *Propionibacterium* species, *Peptostreptococcus* species, other anaerobic cocci
Genital Infections	
Genital ulcers	*Treponema pallidum, Haemophilus ducreyi, Chlamydia trachomatis, Francisella tularensis, Klebsiella granulomatis, Mycobacterium tuberculosis*
Urethritis	*Neisseria gonorrhoeae, Chlamydia trachomatis, Ureaplasma urealyticum*
Vaginitis	*Mobiluncus* species, *Gardnerella vaginalis, Mycoplasma hominis*
Cervicitis	*Neisseria gonorrhoeae, Neisseria meningitidis, Chlamydia trachomatis,* group B *Streptococcus, Mycobacterium tuberculosis, Actinomyces* species
Granulomatous Infections	
General	*Mycobacterium tuberculosis* and other species, *Nocardia* species, *Brucella* species, *Francisella tularensis, Listeria monocytogenes, Burkholderia pseudomallei, Actinomyces* species, *Bartonella henselae, Tropheryma whippelii, Chlamydia trachomatis, Coxiella burnetii, Treponema pallidum, Treponema carateum*

EHEC, Enterohemorrhagic *E. coli;* EIEC, enteroinvasive *E. coli;* EPEC, enteropathogenic *E. coli;* ETEC, enterotoxic *E. coli;* HACEK organisms, *Haemophilus influenzae, Actinobacillus actinomycetemcomitans, Cardiobacterium hominis, Eikenella corrodens*, and *Kingella kingae.*

TABLE 48–3. Selected Bacteria Associated with Foodborne Diseases

Organism	Implicated Food(s)
Aeromonas species	Meats, produce, dairy products
Bacillus cereus	Fried rice, meats, vegetables
Brucella species	Unpasteurized dairy products, meat
Campylobacter species	Poultry, unpasteurized dairy products
Clostridium botulinum	Vegetables, fruits, fish, honey
Clostridium perfringens	Beef, poultry, pork, gravy
Escherichia coli	
Enterohemorrhagic	Beef, unpasteurized milk, fruit juices
Enterotoxigenic	Lettuce, fruits, vegetables
Enteroinvasive	Lettuce, fruit, vegetables
Francisella tularensis	Rabbit meat
Listeria monocytogenes	Unpasteurized dairy products, coleslaw, poultry, cold cut meats
Plesiomonas shigelloides	Seafood
Salmonella species	Poultry, unpasteurized dairy products
Shigella species	Eggs, lettuce
Staphylococcus aureus	Ham, poultry, egg dishes, pastries
Streptococcus, group A	Egg dishes
Vibrio cholerae	Shellfish
Vibrio parahaemolyticus	Shellfish
Yersinia enterocolitica	Unpasteurized dairy products, pork

TABLE 48–4. Selected Bacteria Associated with Waterborne Diseases

Organism	Disease
Aeromonas species	Gastroenteritis, wound infections, septicemia
Campylobacter species	Gastroenteritis
Francisella tularensis	Tularemia
Legionella species	Respiratory disease
Leptospira species	Systemic disease
Mycobacterium marinum	Cutaneous infection
Plesiomonas shigelloides	Gastroenteritis
Pseudomonas species	Dermatitis
Salmonella species	Gastroenteritis
Shigella species	Gastroenteritis
Vibrio species	Gastroenteritis, wound infection, septicemia
Yersinia enterocolitica	Gastroenteritis

TABLE 48–5. Arthropod-Associated Diseases

Arthropod	Organism	Disease
Tick	*Anaplasma phagocytophilum*	Human anaplasmosis (formerly called human granulocytic ehrlichiosis)
	Borrelia burgdorferi	Lyme disease
	Borrelia garinii	Lyme disease
	Borrelia afzelii	Lyme disease
	Borrelia, other species	Endemic relapsing fever
	Coxiella burnetii	Q fever
	Ehrlichia chaffeensis	Human monocytic ehrlichiosis
	Ehrlichia ewingii	Canine (human) granulocytic ehrlichiosis
	Francisella tularensis	Tularemia
	Rickettsia rickettsii	Rocky Mountain spotted fever
	Rickettsia africae	African tick bite fever
	Rickettsia australis	Australian tick typhus
	Rickettsia conorii	Mediterranean spotted fever
	Rickettsia japonica	Japanese spotted fever
	Rickettsia sibirica	Siberian tick typhus
Flea	*Rickettsia prowazekii*	Sporadic typhus
	Rickettsia typhi	Murine typhus
	Yersinia pestis	Plague
Lice	*Bartonella quintana*	Trench fever
	Borrelia recurrentis	Epidemic relapsing fever
	Rickettsia prowazekii	Epidemic typhus
Mite	*Rickettsia akari*	Rickettsialpox
	Orientia tsutsugamushi	Scrub typhus
Sandfly	*Bartonella bacilliformis*	Bartonellosis (Carrión's disease)

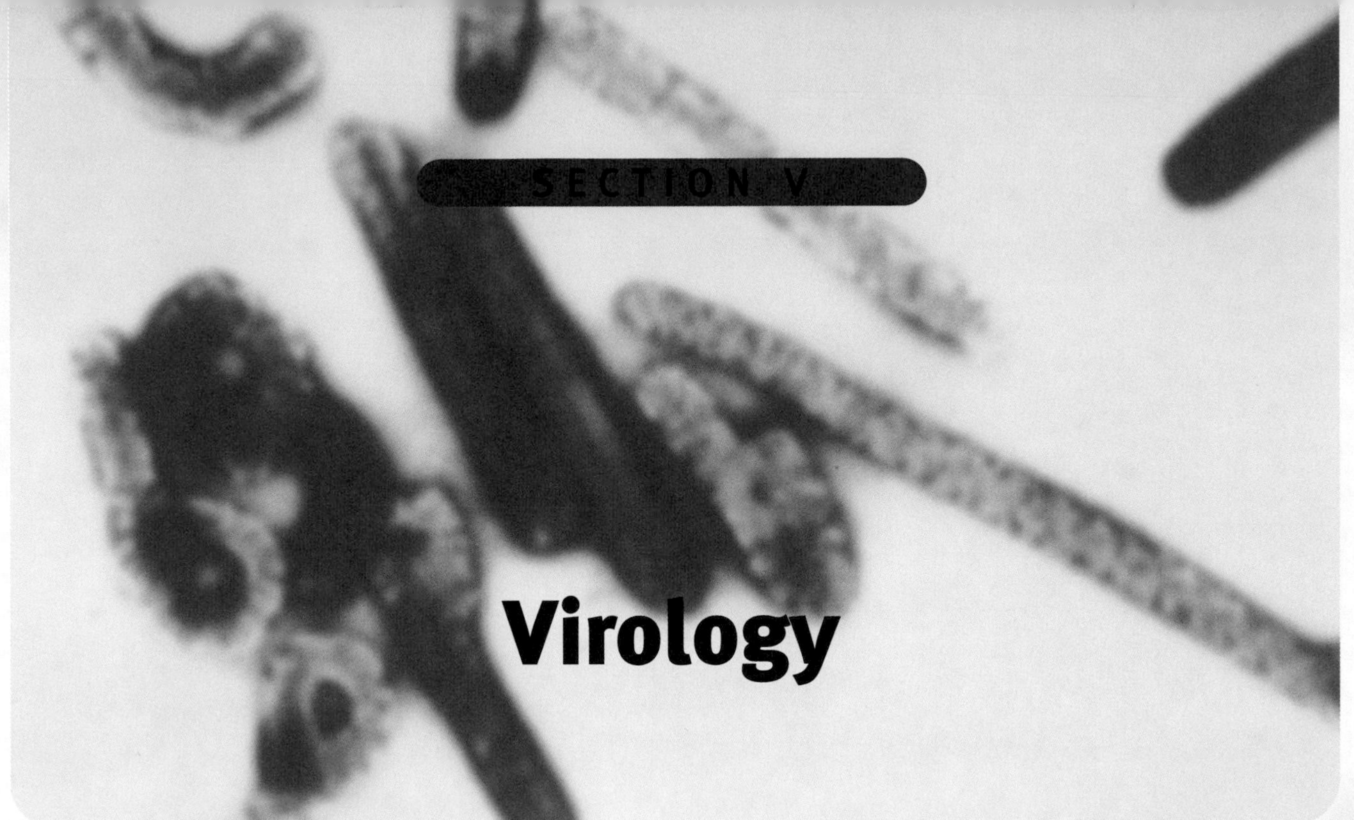

SECTION V

Virology

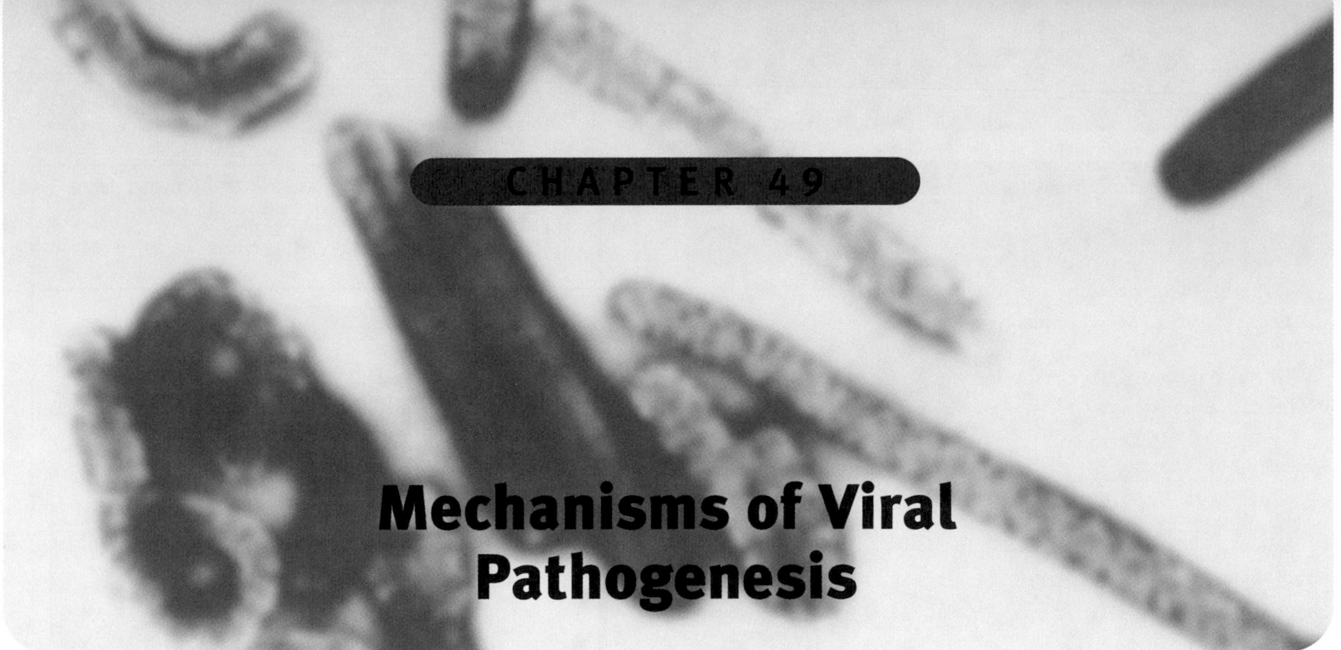

Mechanisms of Viral Pathogenesis

Viruses cause disease after they break through the natural protective barriers of the body, evade immune control, and either kill cells of an important tissue (e.g., brain) or trigger a destructive immune and inflammatory response. The outcome of a viral infection is determined by the nature of the virus-host interaction and the host's response to the infection (Box 49–1). The immune response is the best treatment, but it often contributes to the pathogenesis of a viral infection. The tissue targeted by the virus affects the nature of the disease and its symptoms. Viral and host factors govern the severity of the disease; they include the strain of virus, the inoculum size, and the general health of the infected person. The ability of the infected person's immune response to control the infection determines the severity and duration of the disease.

A particular disease may be caused by several viruses that have a common tissue **tropism** (preference), such as hepatitis, liver; common cold, upper respiratory tract; encephalitis, central nervous system. On the other hand, a particular virus may cause several different diseases or no observable symptoms. For example, herpes simplex virus (HSV) type 1 (HSV-1) can cause gingivostomatitis, pharyngitis, herpes labialis (cold sores), genital herpes, encephalitis, or keratoconjunctivitis, depending on the affected tissue, or it can cause no disease at all. Although normally benign, this virus can be life threatening in a newborn or an immunocompromised person.

Many viruses encode activities **(virulence factors)** that promote the efficiency of viral replication, viral transmission, the access and binding of the virus to target tissue, or the escape of the virus from host defenses and immune resolution (see Chapter 14). These activities may not be essential for viral growth in tissue culture but are necessary for the pathogenicity or the survival of the virus in the host. Loss of these virulence factors results in **attenuation** of the virus. Many live-virus vaccines are attenuated virus strains.

The discussion in this chapter focuses on viral disease at the cellular level (cytopathogenesis), the host level (mechanisms of disease), and the population level (epidemiology and control). The antiviral immune response is discussed here and in Chapter 14.

Basic Steps in Viral Disease

Viral disease in the body progresses through defined steps, just like viral replication in the cell (Figure 49–1*A*). These steps are noted in Box 49–2.

The incubation period may proceed without symptoms **(asymptomatic)** or may produce nonspecific early symptoms, termed the **prodrome.** The symptoms of the disease are caused by tissue damage and systemic effects caused by the virus and possibly the immune system. These symptoms may continue through the **convalescence** while the body repairs the damage. The individual usually develops a memory immune response for future protection against a similar challenge with this virus.

Infection of the Target Tissue

The virus gains **entry into the body** through breaks in the skin or through the mucoepithelial membranes that line the orifices of the body (eyes, respiratory tract, mouth, genitalia, and gastrointestinal tract). The skin is an excellent barrier to infection, and tears, mucus, ciliated epithelium, stomach acid, bile, and immunoglobulin A protect the orifices. *Inhalation is probably the most common route of viral infection.*

BOX 49–1. Determinants of Viral Disease

Nature of the Disease
Target tissue
Portal of entry of virus
Access of virus to target tissue
Tissue tropism of virus
Permissiveness of cells for viral replication
Viral pathogen (strain)

Severity of Disease
Cytopathic ability of virus
Immune status
Competence of the immune system
Prior immunity to the virus
Immunopathology
Virus inoculum size
Length of time before resolution of infection
General health of the person
Nutrition
Other diseases influencing immune status
Genetic makeup of the person
Age

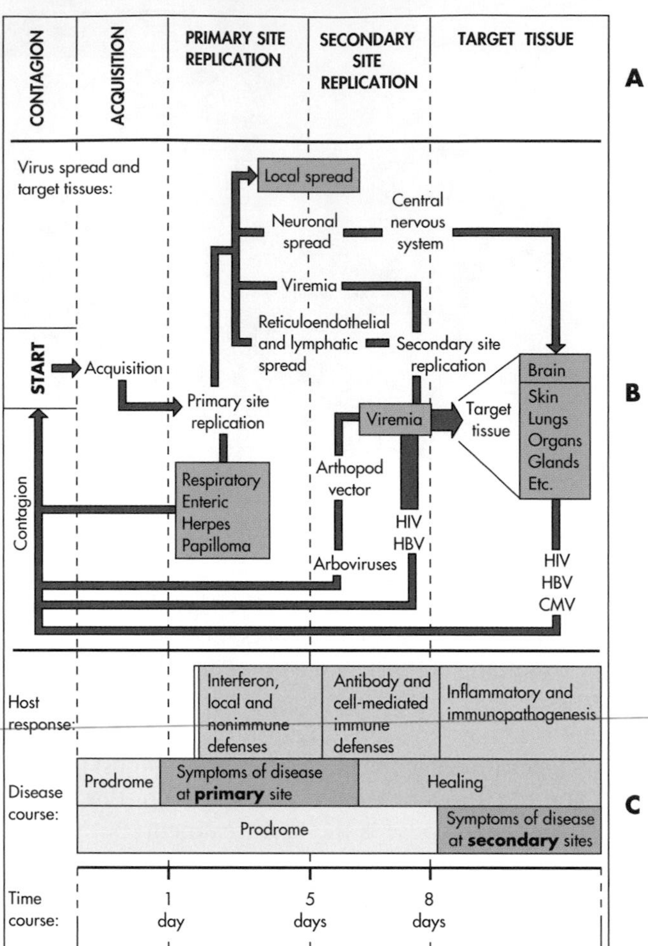

FIGURE 49–1. A, The stages of viral infection. The virus is released from one person, is acquired by another, replicates, and initiates a primary infection at the site of acquisition. Depending on the virus, it may then spread to other body sites and finally to a target tissue characteristic of the disease. **B,** The cycle starts with acquisition, as indicated, and proceeds until the release of new virus. The thickness of the arrow denotes the degree to which the original virus inoculum is amplified on replication. The boxes indicate a site or cause of symptoms. **C,** Time course of viral infection. The time course of symptoms and the immune response correlate with the stage of viral infection and depend on whether the virus causes symptoms at the primary site or only after dissemination to another (secondary) site. CMV, Cytomegalovirus; HBV, hepatitis B virus; HIV, human immunodeficiency virus.

On entry into the body, the virus replicates in cells that express viral receptors and have the appropriate biosynthetic machinery. Many viruses initiate infection in the oral mucosa or upper respiratory tract. Disease signs may accompany viral replication at the primary site. The virus may replicate and remain at the primary site, may disseminate to other tissues via the bloodstream or the mononuclear phagocyte and lymphatic system, or may disseminate through neurons (Figure 49–1*B*).

The bloodstream and the lymphatic system are the predominant means of viral transfer in the body. The virus may gain access to them after tissue damage, by means of phagocytosis, or on transport past the mucoepithelial cells of the oropharynx, gastrointestinal tract, vagina, or anus. Several enteric viruses (picornaviruses and reoviruses) bind to receptors on M cells, which translocate the virus to the underlying Peyer's patches of the lymphatic system.

The transport of virus in the blood is termed **viremia.** The virus may either be free in the plasma or be cell associated in lymphocytes or macrophages. Viruses taken up by phagocytic macrophages may be inactivated, may replicate, or may be delivered to other tissues by way of the mononuclear phagocyte system. Replication of a virus in macrophages, the endothelial lining of blood vessels, or the liver can cause the infection to be amplified and initiate the development of a **secondary viremia.** In many cases, a secondary viremia precedes delivery of the virus to the **target tissue** (e.g., liver, brain, skin) and the manifestation of symptoms.

Viruses can gain access to the central nervous system or brain (1) from the bloodstream (e.g., arboencephalitis viruses), (2) from infected meninges or cerebrospinal fluid, (3) by means of the migration of infected macrophages, or (4) the infection of peripheral and sensory (olfactory) neurons. Viruses in the blood may infect and disrupt the endothelial cell lining and exit the blood vessels or traverse the blood-brain barrier to infect the central nervous system. The meninges are accessible to many of the viruses spread by viremia, which may also provide access to neurons. Herpes simplex, varicella-zoster, and rabies viruses initially infect mucoepithelium, skin, or muscle, and then the peripheral innervating neuron, which transports the virus to the central nervous system or brain.

BOX 49–2. Progression of Viral Disease

1. **Acquisition** (entry into the body).
2. **Initiation of infection** at a primary site.
3. An **incubation period,** when the virus is amplified and may spread to a secondary site.
4. Replication in the **target tissue,** which causes the characteristic disease signs.
5. **Immune responses** that limit and contribute (immunopathogenesis) to the disease.
6. Virus production in a tissue that releases the virus to other people for **contagion.**
7. **Resolution** or **persistent infection/chronic disease.**

Viral Pathogenesis

CYTOPATHOGENESIS

The three potential outcomes of a viral infection of a cell are as follows (Box 49–3 and Table 49–1):

1. Failed infection **(abortive infection).**
2. Cell death **(lytic infection).**
3. Infection without cell death **(persistent infection).**

Viral mutants, which cause abortive infections, do not multiply and therefore disappear. Persistent infections may be (1) **chronic** (nonlytic, productive), (2) **latent** (limited viral macromolecular but no virus synthesis), (3) **recurrent**, or (4) **transforming** (immortalizing).

The nature of the infection is determined by the characteristics of the virus and the target cell. A **nonpermissive cell** does not allow replication of a particular type or strain of virus. A **permissive cell** provides the biosynthetic machinery (e.g., transcription factors, posttranslational processing enzymes) to support the complete replicative cycle of the virus. Replication of the virus in a **semipermissive cell** may be very inefficient, or the cell may support some but not all the steps in viral replication.

Replication of the virus can initiate changes in cells that lead to cytolysis or to alterations in the cell's appearance, functional properties, or antigenicity. The effects on the cell may result from viral takeover of macromolecular synthesis, the accumulation of viral proteins or particles, or a modification or disruption of cellular structures (Table 49–2).

Lytic Infections

Lytic infection results when virus replication kills the target cell. Some viruses prevent cellular growth and repair by inhibiting the synthesis of cellular macromolecules or by producing degradative enzymes and toxic proteins. For example, HSV and other viruses produce proteins that inhibit the synthesis of cellular

BOX 49–3. Determinants of Viral Pathogenesis

Interaction of Virus with Target Tissue
Access of virus to target tissue
Stability of virus in the body
  Temperature
  Acid and bile of the gastrointestinal tract
Ability to cross skin or mucous epithelial cells (e.g., cross the gastrointestinal tract into the bloodstream)
Ability to establish viremia
Ability to spread through the reticuloendothelial system
Target tissue
  Specificity of viral attachment proteins
  Tissue-specific expression of receptors

Cytopathologic Activity of the Virus
Efficiency of viral replication in the cell
  Optimum temperature for replication
  Permissiveness of cell for replication
Cytotoxic viral proteins
Inhibition of cell's macromolecular synthesis
Accumulation of viral proteins and structures (inclusion bodies)
Altered cell metabolism (e.g., cell immortalization)

Host Protective Responses
Antigen-nonspecific antiviral responses
  Interferon
  Natural killer cells and macrophages
Antigen-specific immune responses
  T-cell responses
  Antibody responses
Viral mechanisms of escape of immune responses

Immunopathology
Interferon: Flulike systemic symptoms
T-cell responses: Delayed-type hypersensitivity
Antibody: Complement, antibody-dependent cellular cytotoxicity, immune complexes
Other inflammatory responses

TABLE 49–1. Types of Viral Infections at the Cellular Level

Type	Virus Production	Fate of Cell
Abortive	–	No effect
Cytolytic	+	Death
Persistent		
Productive	+	Senescence
Latent	–	No effect
Transforming		
DNA viruses	–	Immortalization
RNA viruses	+	Immortalization

TABLE 49–2. Mechanisms of Viral Cytopathogenesis

Mechanism	Examples
Inhibition of cellular protein synthesis	Polioviruses, herpes simplex virus, togaviruses, poxviruses
Inhibition and degradation of cellular DNA	Herpesviruses
Alteration of cell membrane structure	Enveloped viruses
Glycoprotein insertion	All enveloped viruses
Syncytia formation	Herpes simplex virus, varicella-zoster virus, paramyxoviruses, human immunodeficiency virus
Disruption of cytoskeleton	Nonenveloped viruses (accumulation), herpes simplex virus
Permeability	Togaviruses, herpesviruses
Inclusion bodies	
Negri bodies (intracytoplasmic)	Rabies
Owl's eye (intranuclear)	Cytomegalovirus
Cowdry type A (intranuclear)	Herpes simplex virus, subacute sclerosing panencephalitis (measles) virus
Intranuclear basophilic	Adenoviruses
Intracytoplasmic acidophilic	Poxviruses
Perinuclear cytoplasmic acidophilic	Reoviruses
Toxicity of virion components	Adenovirus fibers, reovirus NSP4 protein

deoxyribonucleic acid (DNA) and messenger RNA (mRNA) and synthesize other proteins that degrade host DNA to provide substrates for viral genome replication. Cellular protein synthesis may be actively blocked (e.g., poliovirus inhibits translation of 5′-capped cellular mRNA) or passively blocked (e.g., through the production of much viral mRNA that successfully competes for ribosomes) (see Chapter 6).

Replication of the virus and the accumulation of viral components and progeny within the cell can disrupt the structure and function of the cell or disrupt lysosomes, causing autolysis. The expression of viral antigens on the cell surface and disruption of the cytoskeleton can change cell-to-cell interactions and the cell's appearance, making the cell a target for immune cytolysis.

Cell surface expression of the glycoproteins of some paramyxoviruses, herpesviruses, and retroviruses triggers the fusion of neighboring cells into multinucleated giant cells called **syncytia.** Cell-to-cell fusion may occur in the absence of new protein synthesis (fusion from without), as occurs in infections with Sendai virus and other paramyxoviruses, or may require new protein synthesis (fusion from within), as occurs in infection with HSV. Syncytia formation allows the virus to spread from cell to cell and escape antibody detection. Syncytia may be fragile and susceptible to lysis. The syncytia that occurs in infection with human immunodeficiency virus (HIV) also causes death of the cells.

Virus infection or cytolytic immune responses may induce **apoptosis** in the infected cell. Apoptosis is a preset cascade of events that, when triggered, leads to cellular suicide. This process may facilitate release of the virus from the cell, but it also limits the amount of virus that is produced by destroying the viral "factory." As a result, *many viruses (e.g., herpesviruses, adenoviruses, hepatitis C virus) encode methods for inhibiting apoptosis.* The cell can also limit virus production by phosphorylating eIF2α (elongation initiation factor 2 alpha) to prevent the assembly of ribosomes on mRNA, which shuts down protein synthesis. This protection can be triggered by the large amount of protein synthesis required for virus production or a response to interferon-α (INF-α) or interferon-β (INF-β) and a double-stranded RNA replicative intermediate. Herpesviruses and some other viruses prevent this by inhibiting the phosphorylating enzyme (protein kinase R) or by activating a cellular protein phosphatase to remove the phosphate on eIF2α.

Some viral infections cause characteristic changes in the appearance and properties of the target cells. For example, chromosomal aberrations and degradation may occur and can be detected with histologic staining (e.g., marginated chromatin ringing the nuclear membrane in HSV-infected and adenovirus-infected cells). In addition, new, stainable structures called **inclusion bodies** may appear within the nucleus or cytoplasm. These structures may result from virus-induced changes in the membrane or chromosomal structure or may represent the sites of viral replication or accumulations of viral capsids. Because the nature and location of these inclusion bodies are characteristic of particular viral infections, the presence of such bodies facilitates laboratory diagnosis (see Table 49–2). Viral infection may also cause vacuolization, or rounding of the cells, and other nonspecific histologic changes are indicative of sick cells.

Nonlytic Infections

A **persistent infection** occurs in an infected cell that is not killed by the virus. Some viruses cause a persistent productive infection because the virus is released gently from the cell through exocytosis or through budding (enveloped viruses) from the plasma membrane.

A **latent infection** may result from DNA virus infection of a cell that restricts or lacks the machinery for transcribing all the viral genes. The specific transcription factors required by such a virus may be expressed only in specific tissues, in growing but not resting cells, or after hormone or cytokine induction. For example, HSV establishes a latent infection in neurons that lack the nuclear factors required to transcribe the immediate early viral genes, but stress and other stimuli can activate the cells to allow viral replication.

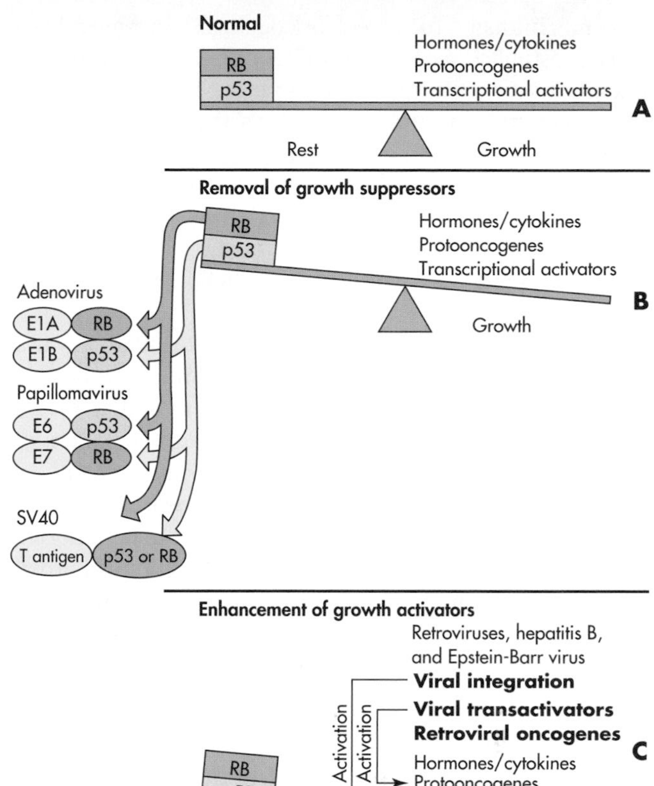

FIGURE 49–2. Mechanisms of viral transformation and immortalization. Cell growth is controlled (**A**) by the maintenance of a balance in the external and internal growth activators (accelerators) and by growth suppressors, such as p53 and the RB gene product (brakes). Oncogenic viruses alter the balance by removing the brakes (**B**) or by enhancing the effects of the accelerators (**C**). RB, Retinoblastoma.

Oncogenic Viruses

Some DNA viruses and retroviruses establish persistent infections that can also stimulate uncontrolled cell growth, causing the **transformation** or **immortalization** of the cell (Figure 49–2). Characteristics of transformed cells include continued growth without senescence, alterations in cell morphology and metabolism, increased cell growth rate and sugar transport, loss of cell-contact inhibition of growth, and ability to grow in a suspension or pileup into foci when grown in a semisolid agar.

Different **oncogenic** viruses have different mechanisms for immortalizing cells. Viruses immortalize cells by (1) activating or providing growth-stimulating genes, (2) removing the inherent braking mechanisms that limit DNA synthesis and cell growth, or (3) preventing apoptosis. Immortalization by DNA viruses occurs in semipermissive cells, which express only select viral genes but do not produce virus. The synthesis of viral DNA, late mRNA, late proteins, or virus leads to cell death, which precludes immortalization. Several oncogenic DNA viruses integrate into the host cell chromosome. Papillomavirus, SV40 virus, and adenovirus encode proteins that bind and inactivate cell growth-regulatory proteins, such as p53 and the retinoblastoma gene product, thus releasing the brakes on cell growth. Loss of p53 also makes the cell more susceptible to mutation. Epstein-Barr virus immortalizes B cells by stimulating cell growth (as a B-cell mitogen) and by inducing expression of the cell's *bcl-2* oncogene, which prevents programmed cell death (apoptosis).

Retroviruses (RNA viruses) use two approaches to oncogenesis. Some oncoviruses encode **oncogene** proteins (e.g., *sis, ras, src, mos, myc, jun, fos*), which are almost identical to the cellular proteins involved in cellular growth control (e.g., components of a growth-factor signal cascade [receptors, G proteins, protein kinases], or growth-regulating transcription factors). The overproduction or altered function of these oncogene products stimulates cell growth. These oncogenic viruses *rapidly* cause tumors to form. *However, no human retrovirus of this type has been identified.*

Human T-cell lymphotropic virus type 1 (HTLV-1), the only human oncogenic retrovirus identified, uses more subtle mechanisms of leukemogenesis. It encodes a protein **(tax)** that **transactivates** gene expression, including genes for growth-stimulating cytokines (e.g., interleukin-2). This constitutes the second approach to oncogenesis. The integration of HTLV-1 near a cellular growth-stimulating gene can also cause the gene to be activated by the strong viral enhancer and promoter sequences encoded at each end of the viral genome (LTR sequences). *HTLV-1–associated leukemias* ***develop slowly,*** *occurring 20 to 30 years after infection.* Retroviruses continue to produce virus in immortalized or transformed cells.

Some viruses may initiate tumor formation indirectly. Hepatitis B virus (HBV) and hepatitis C virus (HCV) may have mechanisms for direct oncogenesis; however, both viruses establish persistent infections that require significant tissue repair. Stimulation of liver cell growth and repair may promote mutations that lead to tumor formation. Human herpesvirus 8 (HHV8) promotes the development of Kaposi's sarcoma by means of growth-promoting cytokines encoded by the virus; this disease occurs most often in immunosuppressed patients, such as those with acquired immune deficiency syndrome (AIDS).

Viral transformation is the first step but is generally not sufficient to cause oncogenesis and tumor formation. Instead, over time, immortalized cells are more likely than normal cells to accumulate other mutations or chromosomal rearrangements that promote development of tumor cells. Immortalized cells may also be more susceptible to cofactors and tumor promoters (e.g., phorbol esters, butyrate) that enhance tumor formation. Approximately 15% of human cancers can be related to oncogenic viruses such as HTLV-1, HBV and HCV, papillomaviruses 16 and 18, HHV8, and Epstein-Barr virus. HSV-2 may be a cofactor for human cervical cancer.

HOST DEFENSES AGAINST VIRAL INFECTION

The skin is the best barrier to infection, but openings in the skin, whether natural orifices (e.g., mouth, eyes, nose, ears, anus) or a result of trauma such as abrasion or puncture, provide pathogens with access to the body. The natural openings have basic protections that, in addition to skin, are part of **the natural barriers of the body** (e.g., mucus, ciliated epithelium, gastric acid, tears, bile). After the virus penetrates the natural barriers, it activates the **antigen-nonspecific (innate) immune defenses** (e.g., fever, interferon, macrophages, dendritic cells, natural killer [NK] cells), which attempt to limit and control local viral replication and spread. Double-stranded RNA, which is the replicative intermediate of RNA viruses and which is produced during many DNA virus infections, is an excellent inducer of interferon production and an activator of the antiviral response within the infected cell. Some viral glycoproteins, viral DNA, RNA, and the double-stranded RNA may activate innate cellular responses through interaction with Toll-Like Receptors (TLRs). **Antigen-specific immune responses** (e.g., antibodies, helper T [TH] cells) are the last to be activated and can be divided into (1) early local responses **(TH1)**, (2) later systemic-antibody responses **(TH2)**, and (3) **immune memory.** Interferon and cytotoxic T-cell responses may have evolved primarily as antiviral defense mechanisms.

The ultimate goal of the host response is to eliminate the virus and the cells harboring or replicating the virus ***(resolution)****. The immune response is the best, and in most cases the only, means of controlling a viral infection. Both humoral and cellular immune responses are important for antiviral immunity.* A detailed description of the antiviral immune response is presented in Chapter 14.

A viral infection resolves when all infectious virus and virus-infected cells are cleared from the body. The innate responses stimulated by viral components and interferon are often sufficient to limit infection and promote resolution. **Antibody** *is effective against extracellular virus* and may be sufficient to *control cytolytic viruses,* because the virion factory within the infected cell is eliminated by viral replication. *Antibody is essential to control virus spread to target tissue by viremia.* **Cell-mediated immunity** *is required for lysis of the target cell for the setting* **noncytolytic infections** *(e.g., hepatitis A virus) and infections caused by* **enveloped viruses.**

Most viruses have mechanisms for evading or inhibiting immune responses to extend their existence in the host. These mechanisms include preventing interferon action, changing virus antigens, spreading by cell-to cell transmission to escape antibody, and suppressing antigen presentation and lymphocyte function. Failure to resolve the infection may lead to persistent infection, chronic disease, or death of the patient.

Prior immunity, caused by memory B and T cells, may not prevent the initial stages of infection but in most cases does prevent disease progression. On rechallenge, serum antibody can prevent viremic spread of the virus, and secondary responses develop much more rapidly and are more effective than primary responses; this is the basis for the development of vaccine programs.

Many viruses, especially the larger viruses, have the means to escape one or more aspects of immune control (See Table 14–4). By preventing the consequences of the antiviral state induced by INF-α and INF-β, herpes simplex viral protein synthesis and replication can continue. Inhibition of major histocompatibility complex I expression by cytomegalovirus and adenoviruses prevents T-cell killing of the infected cell. Antigenic variation over the course of several years (antigenic shift and drift) by influenza or during the lifetime of the infected individual by HIV limits the antiviral efficacy of antibody.

IMMUNOPATHOLOGY

The hypersensitivity and inflammatory reactions initiated by antiviral immunity can be the major cause of the pathologic manifestations and symptoms of viral disease (Table 49–3). Early responses to the virus and viral infection, such as interferon and cytokines, and activation of the C3 component of complement by the alternative pathway can initiate local inflammatory and systemic responses. For example, interferon and cytokines stimulate the **flulike systemic symptoms** that are usually associated with *respiratory viral infections and viremias* (e.g., fever, runny nose, malaise, headache). These symptoms often precede **(prodrome)** the characteristic symptoms of

TABLE 49–3. Viral Immunopathogenesis

Immunopathogenesis	Immune Mediators	Examples
Flulike symptoms	Interferon, cytokines	Respiratory viruses, arboviruses (viremia- inducing viruses)
Delayed-type hypersensitivity and inflammation	T cells, macrophages, and polymorphonuclear leukocytes	Enveloped viruses
Immune complex disease	Antibody, complement	Hepatitis B virus, rubella
Hemorrhagic disease	T cell, antibody, complement	Yellow fever, dengue, Lassa fever, Ebola viruses
Postinfection cytolysis	T cells	Enveloped viruses (e.g., postmeasles encephalitis)
Immunosuppression	—	Human immunodeficiency virus, cytomegalovirus, measles virus, influenza virus

the viral infection, during the viremic stage. Later, immune complexes and complement activation (classic pathway), CD4 T-cell–induced delayed-type hypersensitivity, and CD8 cytolytic T-cell action may induce tissue damage. These actions often promote neutrophil infiltration and more cell damage.

The inflammatory response initiated by cell-mediated immunity is difficult to control and damages tissue. *Infections by enveloped viruses in particular induce cell-mediated immune responses that usually produce more extensive immunopathologic conditions.* For example, the classic symptoms of measles and mumps result from the T-cell–induced inflammatory and hypersensitivity responses rather than from cytopathologic effects of the virus. The presence of large amounts of antigen in blood during viremias or chronic infections (e.g., HBV infection) can initiate the **classic type III immune complex hypersensitivity reactions. Immune complexes** containing virus or viral antigen can activate the complement system, triggering inflammatory responses and tissue destruction. These immune complexes often accumulate in the kidney and cause renal problems.

In the case of dengue and measles viruses, partial immunity to a related or inactivated virus can result in a more severe host response and disease on subsequent challenge with a related or virulent virus. This is because antigen-specific T-cell and antibody responses are enhanced and induce significant inflammatory and hypersensitivity damage to infected endothelial cells *(dengue hemorrhagic fever)* or skin and the lung *(atypical measles)*. In addition, a non-neutralizing antibody can facilitate the uptake of dengue and yellow fever viruses into macrophages through Fc receptors, where they can replicate.

Children generally have a less active cell-mediated immune response (e.g., NK cells) than adults and therefore usually have milder symptoms during infections by some viruses (e.g., measles, mumps, Epstein-Barr, and varicella-zoster viruses). However, in the case of hepatitis B virus, mild or no symptoms correlate with an inability to resolve the infection, resulting in chronic disease.

VIRAL DISEASE

The relative **susceptibility** of a person and the **severity** of the disease depend on the following factors:

1. The nature of the exposure.
2. The immune status, age, and general health of the person.
3. The viral dose.
4. The genetics of the virus and the host.

Once the host is infected, however, the host's immune status and competence are probably the major factors that determine whether a viral infection causes a life-threatening disease, a benign lesion, or no symptoms at all.

The stages of viral disease are shown in Figure 49–1*C*. During the **incubation period,** the virus is replicating but has not reached the target tissue or induced sufficient damage to cause the disease. *The incubation period is relatively short if the primary site of infection is the target tissue and produces the characteristic symptoms of the disease. Viruses that must spread to other sites and be amplified before reaching the target tissue have longer incubation periods.* Nonspecific or flulike symptoms may precede the characteristic symptoms during the **prodome.** The incubation periods for many common viral infections are listed in Table 49–4. Specific viral diseases are discussed in subsequent chapters and reviewed in Chapter 68.

The nature and severity of the symptoms of a viral disease are related to the function of the infected target tissue (e.g., liver, hepatitis; brain, encephalitis) and the extent of the immunopathologic responses triggered by the infection. **Inapparent infections** result if (1) the infected tissue is undamaged, (2) the infection is controlled before the virus reaches its target tissue, (3) the target tissue is expendable, (4) the damaged tissue is rapidly repaired, or (5) the extent of damage is below a

TABLE 49–4. Incubation Periods of Common Viral Infections

Disease	Incubation Period (days)*
Influenza	1–2
Common cold	1–3
Bronchiolitis, croup	3–5
Acute respiratory disease (adenoviruses)	5–7
Dengue	5–8
Herpes simplex	5–8
Enteroviruses	6–12
Poliomyelitis	5–20
Measles	9–12
Smallpox	12–14
Chickenpox	13–17
Mumps	16–20
Rubella	17–20
Mononucleosis	30–50
Hepatitis A	15–40
Hepatitis B	50–150
Rabies	30–100
Papilloma (warts)	50–150
Human immunodeficiency virus (acquired immune deficiency syndrome)	1–10 years

Modified from White DO, Fenner F: *Medical virology,* ed 3, New York, 1986, Academic.

*Until first appearance of prodromal symptoms. Diagnostic signs (e.g., rash, paralysis) may not appear until 2 to 4 days later.

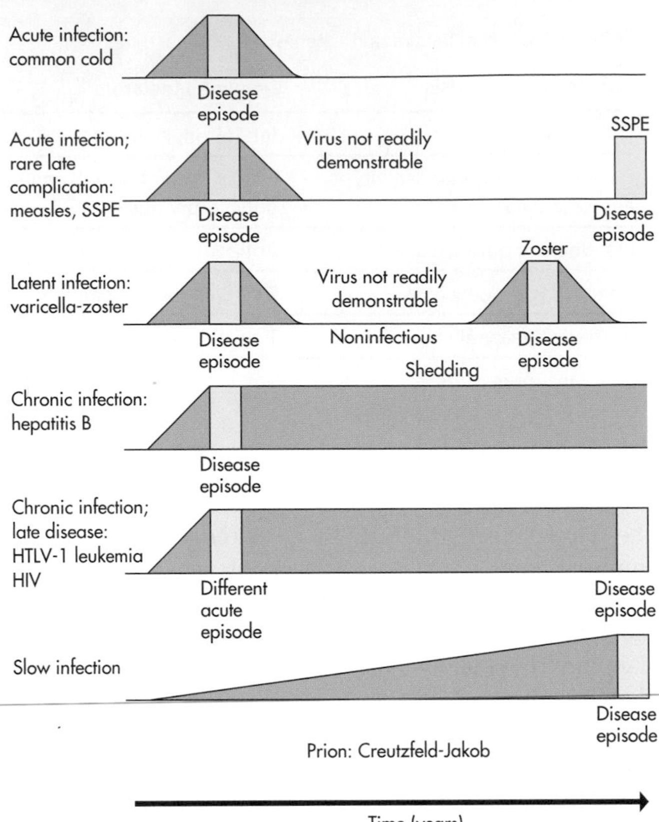

FIGURE 49–3. Acute infection and various types of persistent infection, as illustrated by the diseases indicated in the column at the left. Blue represents presence of virus; green indicates episode of disease. SSPE, Subacute sclerosing panencephalitis. (Modified from White DO, Fenner FJ: *Medical virology,* ed 3, New York, 1986, Academic.)

functional threshold for that particular tissue. For example, many infections of the brain are inapparent or are below the threshold of severe loss of function, but encephalitis results if the loss of function becomes significant. However, *asymptomatic infections are major sources of contagion.* Despite the lack of symptoms, virus-specific antibody will be produced. For example, although 97% of adults have antibody (seropositive) to varicella-zoster virus, less than half remember having had chickenpox.

Viral infections may cause **acute** or **chronic disease (persistent infection).** The ability and speed with which a person's immune system controls and resolves a viral infection usually determine whether acute or chronic disease ensues, as well as the severity of the symptoms (Figure 49–3). The acute episode of a persistent infection may be asymptomatic (JC polyomavirus) or may, later in life, cause symptoms that are similar to (varicella and zoster) or different from (HIV) those of the acute disease. **Slow viruses** have long incubation periods, during which sufficient virus or tissue destruction accumulates before a rapid progression of symptoms.

Epidemiology

Epidemiology studies the spread of disease through a population. Infection of a population is similar to infection of a person in that the virus must spread through the population and is controlled by immunization of the population (Box 49–4). To endure, viruses must continue to infect new, immunologically naïve, susceptible hosts.

EXPOSURE

People are exposed to viruses throughout their lives. However, some situations, vocations, lifestyles, and living

BOX 49–4. Viral Epidemiology*

Mechanisms of Viral Transmission[†]
Aerosols
Food, water
Fomites (e.g., tissues, clothes)
Direct contact with secretions (e.g., saliva, semen)
Sexual contact, birth
Blood transfusion or organ transplant
Zoonoses (animals, insects [arboviruses])

Disease and Viral Factors That Promote Transmission
Stability of virion in response to the environment (e.g., drying, detergents, temperature)
Replication and secretion of virus into transmissible aerosols and secretions (e.g., saliva, semen)
Asymptomatic transmission
Transience or ineffectiveness of immune response to control reinfection or recurrence

Risk Factors
Age
Health
Immune status
Occupation: Contact with agent or vector
Travel history
Lifestyle
Children in daycare centers
Sexual activity

Critical Community Size
Seronegative, susceptible people

Geography and Season
Presence of cofactors or vectors in the environment
Habitat and season for arthropod vectors (mosquitoes)
School session: Close proximity and crowding
Home-heating season

Modes of Control
Quarantine
Elimination of the vector
Immunization
Vaccination
Treatment

*Infection of a population instead of a person.
[†]See also Table 49–5.

arrangements increase the likelihood that a person will come in contact with certain viruses. In contrast, many viruses are ubiquitous. Exposure to HSV-1, HHV6, varicella-zoster virus, parvovirus B19, Epstein-Barr virus, and many respiratory and enteric viruses can be detected in most young children or by early adulthood by the presence of antibodies to the virus.

Poor hygiene and crowded living, school, and job conditions promote exposure to respiratory and enteric viruses. Daycare centers are consistent sources of viral infections, especially viruses spread by the respiratory and fecal-oral routes. Travel, summer camp, and vocations that bring people in contact with a virus vector (e.g., mosquitoes) put them at particular risk for infection by arboviruses and other zoonoses. Sexual promiscuity also promotes the spread and acquisition of several viruses. Health care workers, such as physicians, dentists, nurses, and technicians, are frequently exposed to respiratory and other viruses but are uniquely at risk for acquiring viruses from contaminated blood (HBV, HIV) or vesicle fluid (HSV).

TRANSMISSION OF VIRUSES

Viruses are transmitted by direct contact (including sexual contact), injection with contaminated fluids or blood, the transplantation of organs, and the respiratory and fecal-oral routes (Table 49–5). *The route of transmission depends on the source of the virus (the tissue site of viral replication and secretion) and the ability of the virus to endure the hazards and barriers of the environment and the body en route to the target tissue.* For example, viruses that replicate in the respiratory tract (e.g., influenza A virus) are released in aerosol droplets, whereas enteric viruses (e.g., picornaviruses and reoviruses) are passed by the fecal-oral route. Cytomegalovirus is transmitted in most bodily secretions because it infects mucoepithelial, secretory, and other cells found in the skin, secretory glands, lungs, liver, and other organs.

The presence or absence of an envelope is the major structural determinant of the mode of viral transmission. **Nonenveloped viruses** (naked capsid viruses) can withstand drying, the effects of detergents, and extremes of pH and temperature, whereas enveloped viruses generally cannot. Specifically, most nonenveloped viruses can withstand the acidic environment of the stomach and the detergent-like bile of the intestines and mild disinfection and insufficient sewage treatment. These viruses are generally transmitted by the respiratory and fecal-oral routes and can often be acquired from contaminated objects, termed **fomites.** For example, hepatitis A virus, a picornavirus, is a nonenveloped virus that is transmitted by the fecal-oral route and acquired from contaminated water, shellfish, and food. Rhinoviruses and many other nonenveloped viruses can be spread by contact with fomites such as handkerchiefs and toys.

Unlike the sturdy nonenveloped viruses, **enveloped viruses** are comparatively fragile. They require an intact envelope for infectivity. These viruses must remain wet and are spread (1) in respiratory droplets, blood, mucus, saliva, and semen; (2) by injection; or (3) in organ

TABLE 49–5. Viral Transmission

Mode	Examples
Respiratory transmission	Paramyxoviruses, influenza viruses, picornaviruses, rhinoviruses, varicella-zoster virus, B19 virus
Fecal-oral transmission	Picornaviruses, rotavirus, reovirus, noroviruses, adenovirus
Contact (lesions, saliva, fomites)	Herpes simplex virus, rhinoviruses, poxviruses, adenovirus
Zoonoses (animals, insects)	Togaviruses (alpha), flaviviruses, bunyaviruses, orbiviruses, arenaviruses, hantaviruses, rabies virus, influenza A virus, orf (pox)
Transmission via blood	Human immunodeficiency virus, HTLV-1, hepatitis B virus, hepatitis C virus, hepatitis delta virus, cytomegalovirus
Sexual contact	Blood-borne viruses, herpes simplex virus, human papillomavirus, molluscum contagiosum
Maternal-neonatal transmission	Rubella virus, cytomegalovirus, B19 virus, echovirus, herpes simplex virus, varicella-zoster virus
Genetic	Prions, retroviruses

HTLV-1, Human T-cell lymphotrophic virus type 1.

transplants. Most enveloped viruses are also labile in response to acid and detergents, a feature that precludes their being transmitted by the fecal-oral route. Exceptions are HBV and coronaviruses.

Animals can also act as **vectors** that spread viral disease to other animals and humans and even to other locales. They can also be **reservoirs** for the virus, which maintain and amplify the virus in the environment. Viral diseases that are shared by animals or insects and humans are called **zoonoses.** For example, raccoons, foxes, bats, dogs, and cats are vectors for the rabies virus. Arthropods, including mosquitoes, ticks, and sandflies, can act as vectors for togaviruses, flaviviruses, bunyaviruses, and reoviruses. These viruses are often referred to as **arboviruses** because they are *ar*thropod *bo*rne. A more detailed discussion of arboviruses is presented in Chapter 63. Most arboviruses have a very broad host range, capable of replicating in specific insects, birds, amphibians, and mammals, in addition to humans. Also, the arboviruses must establish a viremia in the animal reservoir so that the insect can acquire the virus during its blood meal.

Other factors that can promote the transmission of viruses are the potential for asymptomatic infection, crowded living conditions, certain occupations, certain lifestyles, daycare centers, and travel. With regard to the first of these conditions, many viruses (e.g., HIV, varicella-zoster virus) are released before symptoms appear, making it difficult to restrict transmission. Viruses that cause persistent productive infections (e.g., cytomegalovirus, HIV) are a particular problem because the infected person is a continual source of virus that can be spread to immunologically naïve people. Viruses with many different serotypes (rhinoviruses), or viruses capable of changing their antigenicity (influenza and HIV), also readily find immunologically naïve populations.

MAINTENANCE OF A VIRUS IN THE POPULATION

The persistence of a virus in a community depends on the availability of a critical number of immunologically naïve (seronegative), susceptible people. The efficiency of virus transmission determines the size of the susceptible population necessary for maintenance of the virus in the population. Immunization, produced by natural means or by vaccination, is the best way of reducing the number of such susceptible people.

AGE

A person's age is an important factor in determining his or her susceptibility to viral infections. Infants, children, adults, and elderly persons are susceptible to different viruses and have different symptomatic responses to the infection. These differences may result from variations in body size, recuperative abilities, and, most important, immune status in people in these age groups. Differences in lifestyles, habits, school environments, and job settings at different ages also determine when people are exposed to viruses.

Infants and children acquire a series of respiratory and exanthematous viral diseases at first exposure, because they are immunologically naïve. Infants are especially prone to more serious presentations of paramyxovirus respiratory infections and gastroenteritis, because of their small size and physiologic requirements (e.g., nutrients, water, electrolytes). However, children generally do not mount as severe an immunopathologic response as adults, and some diseases (herpesviruses) are more benign in children.

Elderly persons are especially susceptible to new viral infections and the reactivation of latent viruses. Because they are less able to initiate a new immune response, repair damaged tissue, and recover, elderly persons are therefore more susceptible to complications after infection and outbreaks of the new strains of the influenza A and B viruses. Elderly persons are also more prone to zoster (shingles), a recurrence of varicella-zoster virus, as a result of a decline in this specific immune response with age.

IMMUNE STATUS

The competence of a person's immune response and his or her immune history determine how quickly and efficiently the infection is resolved and can also determine the severity of the symptoms. The rechallenge of a person with prior immunity usually results in asymptomatic or mild disease without transmission. People who are in an immunosuppressed state as a result of AIDS, cancer, or immunosuppressive therapy are at greater risk of suffering more serious disease on primary infection (measles, vaccinia) and are more prone to suffer recurrences of infections with latent viruses (e.g., herpesviruses, papovaviruses).

OTHER HOST FACTORS

A person's general health plays an important role in determining the competence and nature of his or her immune response and ability to repair diseased tissue. Poor nutrition can compromise a person's immune system and decrease his or her tissue regenerative capacity. Immunosuppressive diseases and therapies may allow viral replication or recurrence to proceed unchecked. A person's genetic makeup also plays an important role in determining the response of his or her immune system to viral infection. Specifically, genetic differences in immune response genes, genes for viral receptors, and other genetic loci affect the person's susceptibility to a viral infection and the severity of disease.

GEOGRAPHIC AND SEASONAL CONSIDERATIONS

The geographic distribution of a virus is usually determined by whether the requisite cofactors or vectors are present or whether there is an immunologically naïve, susceptible population. For example, many of the arboviruses are limited to the ecologic niche of their arthropod vectors. Extensive global transportation is eliminating many of the geographically determined restrictions to virus distribution.

Seasonal differences in the occurrence of viral disease correspond with behaviors that promote the spread of the virus. For example, respiratory viruses are more prevalent in the winter because crowding facilitates the spread of such viruses and the temperature and humidity conditions stabilize them. Enteric viruses, on the other hand, are more prevalent during the summer, possibly because hygiene is more lax during this season. The seasonal differences in arboviral diseases reflect the life cycle of the arthropod vector or its reservoir (e.g., birds).

OUTBREAKS, EPIDEMICS, AND PANDEMICS

Outbreaks of a viral infection often result from the introduction of a virus (e.g., hepatitis A) into a new location. The outbreak originates from a **common source** (e.g., food preparation) and often can be stopped once the source is identified. **Epidemics** occur over a larger geographic area and generally result from the introduction of a new strain of virus into an immunologically naïve population. **Pandemics** are worldwide epidemics, usually resulting from the introduction of a new virus (e.g., HIV). Pandemics of influenza A used to occur approximately every 10 years as the result of the introduction of new strains of the virus.

Control of Viral Spread

The spread of a virus can be controlled by quarantine, good hygiene, changes in lifestyle, elimination of the vector, or immunization of the population. **Quarantine** was once the only means of limiting epidemics of viral infections and is most effective for limiting the spread of viruses that always cause symptomatic disease (e.g., smallpox). It is now used especially in hospitals to limit the **nosocomial spread** of viruses, especially to high-risk patients (e.g., immunosuppressed people). The proper sanitation of contaminated items and disinfection of the water supply are means of limiting the spread of enteric viruses. Changes in lifestyle have made a difference in the spread of sexually transmitted viruses such as HIV, HBV, and HSV. Elimination of an arthropod or its ecologic niche (e.g., drainage of the swamps it inhabits) has proved effective for controlling arboviruses.

The best way to limit viral spread, however, is to immunize the population. Immunization, whether produced by natural infection or by vaccination, protects the person and reduces the size of the immunologically naïve, susceptible population necessary to promote the spread and maintenance of the virus.

QUESTIONS

1. What are the routes by which viruses gain entry into the body? For each route, list the barriers to infection and a virus that infects by it.
2. Describe or draw the disease path of a virus that is transmitted by an aerosol and causes lesions on the skin (similar to varicella).
3. Identify the structures that elicit a protective antibody response to adenovirus, influenza A virus, poliovirus, and rabies virus.
4. Describe the major roles of each of the following in promoting resolution of a viral infection: interferon, macrophage, natural killer cells, CD4 T cells, CD8 T cells, and antibody.
5. Why are interferon-α and interferon-β produced before interferon-γ?
6. How does the nucleoprotein of influenza virus become an antigen for cytolytic CD8 T cells?
7. What events occur during the prodromal periods of a respiratory virus disease (e.g., parainfluenza virus) and encephalitis (e.g., St. Louis encephalitis virus)?
8. List the viral characteristics (structure, replication, target tissue) that would promote transmission by the fecal-oral route, by arthropods, by fomites, by mother's milk, and by sexual activity.
9. What are the different mechanisms by which oncogenic viruses immortalize cells? Describe them.

Bibliography

Belshe RB: *Textbook of human virology,* ed 2, St Louis, 1991, Mosby.

Cann AJ: *Principles of molecular virology,* San Diego, 2001, Academic Press.

Cohen J, Powderly WG, editors: *Infectious diseases,* ed 2, St Louis, 2004, Mosby.

Ellner PD, Neu HC: *Understanding infectious disease,* St Louis, 1992, Mosby.

Emond RT, Welsby PD, Rowland HAK: *Color atlas of infectious diseases,* ed 4, St Louis, 2003, Mosby.

Evans AS, Kaslow RA: *Viral infections of humans. Epidemiology and control,* ed 4, New York, 1997, Plenum.

Flint SJ et al: *Principles of virology: Molecular biology, pathogenesis and control of animal viruses,* ed 2, Washington, 2003, American Society for Microbiology Press.

Gorbach SL et al: *Infectious diseases,* Philadelphia, 1997, WB Saunders.

Hart CA, Broadhead RL: *Color atlas of pediatric infectious diseases,* St Louis, 1992, Mosby.

Hart CA, Shears P: *Color atlas of medical microbiology,* London, 2004, Mosby.

Katz SL, Gershon AA, Hotez PJ: *Krugman's infectious diseases of children,* ed 10, St Louis, 1998, Mosby.

Knipe DM, Howley PM, editors: *Fields virology,* ed 4, New York, 2001, Lippincott-Williams and Wilkins.

Mandell GL, Bennet JE, Dolin R, editors: *Principles and practice of infectious diseases,* ed 6, Philadelphia, 2005, Churchill Livingstone.

Mims CA et al: *Medical microbiology,* ed 3, Edinburgh, 2004, Mosby.

Mims CA, White DO: *Viral pathogenesis and immunology,* Oxford, England, 1984, Blackwell.

Richman DD et al: *Clinical virology,* New York, 1997, Churchill Livingstone.

Shulman ST et al: *The biologic and clinical basis of infectious diseases,* ed 5, Philadelphia, 1997, WB Saunders.

Stark GR et al: How cells respond to interferons, *Ann Rev Biochem* 67:227-264, 1998.

Strauss JH, Strauss EG: *Viruses and human disease,* San Diego, 2002, Academic Press.

White DO, Fenner FJ: *Medical virology,* ed 4, San Diego, 1994, Academic Press.

Zuckerman AJ, Banatvala JE, Pattison JR: *Principles and practice of clinical virology,* Chichester, NY, 2000, Wiley.

Websites

Centers for Disease Control Health Topics A to Z: Available at www.cdc.gov/health/diseases.htm

National Center for Infectious Disease, Infectious disease information: Available at www.cdc.gov/ncidod/diseases/index.htm

National Center for Infectious Disease: Traveler's health: Available at www.cdc.gov/travel/diseases.htm

National Foundation for Infectious Diseases, fact sheets on diseases: Available at www.nfid.org/factsheets/Default.html

Virology on the Internet and specific viruses: Available at www.virology.net/garryfavwebindex.html

Virus diseases: Karolinska Library: www.mic.ki.se/Diseases/C02.html#C02.081.343

World Health Organization: Diseases and vaccines: Available at www.who.int/vaccines-diseases/index.html

World Health Organization: Infectious diseases: www.who.int/health-topics/idindex.htm

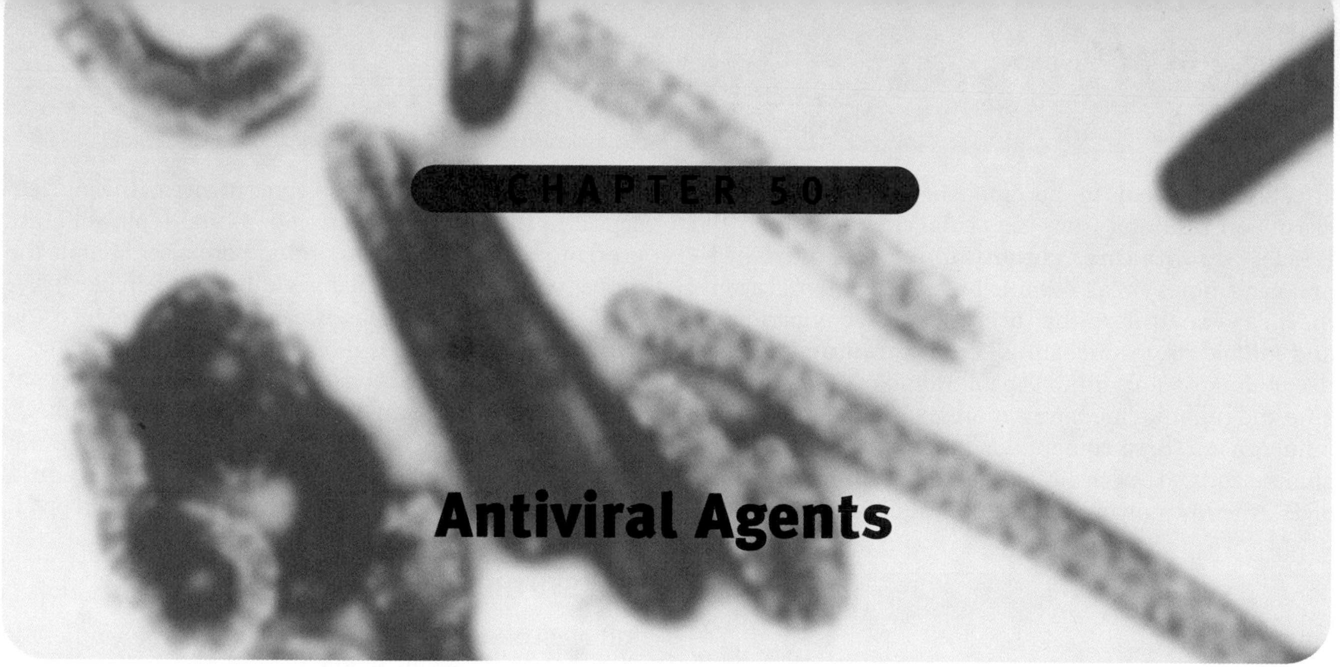

CHAPTER 50

Antiviral Agents

Unlike bacteria, viruses are obligate intracellular parasites that use the host cell's biosynthetic machinery and enzymes for replication (see Chapter 6). Hence it is more difficult to inhibit viral replication without also being toxic to the host. Most antiviral drugs are targeted toward viral-encoded enzymes or structures of the virus that are important for replication. Most of these compounds are classic biochemical inhibitors of viral-encoded enzymes. Some antiviral drugs are actually stimulators of host innate immune protective responses.

Unlike antibacterial drugs, the activity of most antiviral drugs is limited to a specific family of viruses. Antiviral drugs are available for viruses that cause significant morbidity and mortality, which also provide reasonable targets for drug action (Box 50–1). As has occurred with antibacterial drugs, however, resistance to antiviral drugs is becoming more of a problem because of the high rate of mutation for viruses and the long-term treatment of some patients, especially those who are immunocompromised (e.g., patients with the acquired immune deficiency syndrome [AIDS]).

Targets for Antiviral Drugs

The different targets for antiviral drugs (e.g., structures, enzymes, or processes important or essential for virus production) are discussed with respect to the steps of the viral replication cycle that they inhibit. These targets and their respective antiviral agents are listed in Table 50–1 (see also Figure 6–10).

VIRION DISRUPTION

Enveloped viruses are susceptible to certain lipid and detergent-like molecules that disperse or disrupt the envelope membrane, thereby preventing acquisition of the virus. Nonoxynol-9, a detergent-like component in birth control jellies, can inactivate herpes simplex virus (HSV) and human immunodeficiency virus (HIV) and prevent sexual acquisition of the virus. Rhinoviruses are susceptible to acid, and citric acid can be incorporated into facial tissues as means of blocking virus transmission.

ATTACHMENT

The first step in viral replication is mediated by the interaction of a viral attachment protein with its cell surface receptor. This interaction can be blocked by **neutralizing antibodies,** which bind and coat the virion, or by **receptor antagonists.** The administration of specific antibodies **(passive immunization)** is the oldest form of antiviral therapy. Receptor antagonists include peptide or sugar analogues of the cell receptor or the viral attachment protein that competitively block the interaction of the virus with the cell. Specific peptides of HIV glycoprotein gp120 or its receptor, the CD4 molecule of T cells, block infection and are being investigated for their clinical potential. Acidic polysaccharides, such as heparan and dextran sulfate, interfere with viral binding and have been suggested for the treatment of infection with HIV, HSV, and other viruses.

PENETRATION AND UNCOATING

Penetration and uncoating of the virus are required to deliver the viral genome into the cytoplasm of the host cell. Arildone, disoxaril, **pleconaril,** and other **methylisoxazole** compounds block uncoating of picornaviruses by fitting into a cleft in the receptor-binding canyon of the capsid and preventing disassembly of the capsid. For viruses that enter through endocytic vesicles, uncoating may be triggered by conformational changes in attachment proteins that promote fusion or by membrane disruption resulting from the acidic environment of the vesicle. **Amantadine, rimantadine,** and other hydrophobic amines (weak organic bases) are antiviral agents that can neutralize the pH of these compartments and inhibit virion uncoating. **Tromantadine,** a derivative of amantadine, inhibits penetration of HSV. Amantadine and rimantadine have a more specific activity against influenza A. These compounds bind to and block the H^+ channel formed by the viral M_2 protein. Without the influx of H^+, the M_1 matrix proteins do not dissociate from the nucleocapsid (uncoating), so movement of the nucleocapsid to the nucleus, transcription, and replication are prevented. Blockage of this proton pore also disrupts the proper processing of the hemagglutinin protein late in the replication cycle. In the absence of a functional M_2 proton pore, the hemagglutinin inopportunely changes its conformation into its "fusion form" and is inactivated as it traverses the normally acidic Golgi environment. Penetration and uncoating of HIV are blocked by a 33-amino—acid peptide, T20, **(enfuvirtide [Fuzeon]),** which inhibits the action of the viral fusion protein gp41.

BOX 50–1. Viruses Treatable with Antiviral Drugs

- Herpes simplex virus
- Varicella-zoster virus
- Cytomegalovirus
- Human immunodeficiency virus
- Influenza A and B viruses
- Respiratory syncytial virus
- Hepatitis B and C viruses
- Papillomavirus
- Picornavirus

RNA SYNTHESIS

Although messenger ribonucleic acid (mRNA) synthesis is essential for the production of virus, it is not a good target for antiviral drugs. It would be difficult to inhibit viral mRNA synthesis without affecting cellular mRNA synthesis. Deoxyribonucleic acid (DNA) viruses use the host cell's transcriptases for mRNA synthesis. The RNA polymerases encoded by RNA viruses may not be sufficiently different from host cell transcriptases to selectively inhibit this activity, and the high rate at which RNA viruses

TABLE 50–1. Examples of Targets for Antiviral Drugs

Replication Step or Target	Agent	Targeted Virus*
Attachment	Peptide analogues of attachment protein	Human immunodeficiency virus (HIV) (gp 120/CD4 receptor)
	Neutralizing antibodies	Most viruses
	Heparan and Dextran sulfate	HIV; herpes simplex virus (HSV)
Penetration and uncoating	Amantadine, rimantadine	Influenza A virus
	Tromantadine	HSV
	Arildone, disoxaril, pleconaril	Picornaviruses
Transcription	Interferon	Hepatitis A, B, and C viruses; papillomavirus
	Antisense oligonucleotides	Papillomavirus
Protein synthesis	Interferon	Hepatitis A, B, and C viruses; papillomavirus
DNA replication (polymerase)	Nucleoside analogues	Herpesviruses; HIV; hepatitis B virus, poxviruses, etc.
	Phosphonoformate, phosphonoacetic acid	Herpesviruses
Nucleoside biosynthesis	Ribavirin	Respiratory syncytial virus; Lassa fever virus
Nucleoside scavenging (thymidine kinase)	Nucleoside analogues	HSV; varicella-zoster virus
Glycoprotein processing	—	HIV
Assembly (protease)	Hydrophobic substrate analogues	HIV
Virion integrity	Nonoxynol-9	HIV; HSV

*Therapies may not have received approval for human use.

mutate results in the generation of many drug-resistant strains. **Guanidine** and 2-hydroxybenzylbenzimidine are two compounds that can block picornavirus RNA synthesis by binding to the 2C picornavirus protein, which is essential for RNA synthesis. **Ribavirin** resembles riboguanosine and inhibits nucleoside biosynthesis, mRNA capping, and other processes (cellular and viral) important to the replication of many viruses.

The proper processing (splicing) and translation of viral mRNA can be inhibited by interferon and antisense oligonucleotides. **Isatin-β-thiosemicarbazone** induces mRNA degradation in poxvirus-infected cells and was used as a treatment for smallpox. Viral infection of an **interferon**-treated cell triggers a cascade of biochemical events that block viral replication. Specifically, the degradation of viral and cellular mRNA is enhanced, and ribosomal assembly is blocked, preventing protein synthesis and viral replication. Interferon is described further in Chapter 14. Interferon and artificial interferon inducers **(Ampligen, poly rI:rC)** have been approved for clinical use (papilloma, hepatitis B and C) or are in clinical trials.

GENOME REPLICATION

The viral **DNA polymerases** of the herpesviruses and the **reverse transcriptases** of HIV and hepatitis B virus *are the prime targets for most antiviral drugs, because they are essential for virus replication and are different from host enzymes.* Most antiviral drugs are **nucleoside analogues,** which are nucleosides with modifications of the base, sugar, or both (Figure 50–1). Before being used by the polymerase, the nucleoside analogues must be phosphorylated to the triphosphate form by viral enzymes (e.g., HSV thymidine kinase), cellular enzymes, or both. For example, the thymidine kinase of HSV and varicella-zoster virus (VZV) applies the first phosphate to **acyclovir (ACV),** and the cellular enzymes apply the rest. HSV mutants lacking thymidine kinase activity are resistant to ACV. Cellular enzymes phosphorylate **azidothymidine (AZT)** and many other nucleoside analogues.

Nucleoside analogues selectively inhibit viral polymerases because these enzymes are less accurate than host cell enzymes. The binding of a nucleoside analogue with modifications of the base, sugar, or both, is several hundred times better than the host cell enzyme. These drugs either *prevent chain elongation,* as a result of the absence of a 3′-hydroxyl on the sugar, or *alter recognition and base pairing,* as a result of a base modification (see Figure 50–1). Antiviral drugs that cause termination of the DNA chain by means of modified nucleoside sugar residues include ACV, ganciclovir (GCV), valacyclovir, penciclovir, famciclovir, adefovir, cidofovir, adenosine arabinoside (vidarabine, ara-A), zidovudine (AZT), lamivudine (3TC), dideoxycytidine, and dideoxyinosine. Antiviral drugs that become incorporated into the viral genome and cause errors in replication (mutation) and transcription (inactive mRNA and proteins) because of modified nucleoside bases include **5-iododeoxyuridine (idoxuridine)** and **trifluorothymidine (trifluridine).** The rapid rate and large extent of nucleotide incorporation during viral replication make DNA virus replication especially susceptible to these drugs. A variety of other nucleoside analogues are also being developed as antiviral drugs.

Pyrophosphate analogues resembling the by-product of the polymerase reaction, such as **phosphonoformic acid (foscarnet, PFA)** and **phosphonacetic acid,** are classic inhibitors of the herpesvirus polymerases. **Nevirapine, delavirdine,** and other non–nucleoside reverse transcriptase inhibitors bind to sites on the enzyme other than the substrate site as noncompetitive inhibitors of the enzyme.

Deoxyribonucleotide scavenging enzymes (e.g., the thymidine kinase and ribonucleoside reductase of the herpesviruses) are also enzyme targets of antiviral drugs. Inhibition of these enzymes reduces the levels of deoxyribonucleotides necessary for the replication of the DNA virus genome preventing virus replication.

PROTEIN SYNTHESIS

Although bacterial protein synthesis is the target for several antibacterial compounds, viral protein synthesis is a poor target for antiviral drugs. The virus uses host cell ribosomes and synthetic mechanisms for replication, so selective inhibition is not possible. **Interferon-α (INF-α)** and **interferon-β (INF-β)** stop a virus by promoting the inhibition of most protein synthesis in the infected cell. Inhibition of the post-translational modification of proteins, such as the proteolysis of a viral polyprotein, glycoprotein processing (castanospermine, deoxynojirimycin), or phosphorylation (D609 xanthate), can inhibit virus replication. Agents that inhibit the glycoprotein processing of HIV or HSV block viral release and inhibit glycoprotein functions, such as attachment and fusion, thereby preventing both the production and the spread of the virus.

VIRION ASSEMBLY AND RELEASE

The **HIV protease** is unique and *essential* to the assembly of virions and the production of infectious virions. Computer-assisted molecular modeling was used to design inhibitors of the HIV protease, such as **saquinavir, ritonavir,** and **indinavir,** by modeling inhibitors that would fit into the active site of the enzyme. The enzyme structures were defined by x-ray crystallographic and molecular biologic studies. Proteases of other viruses are also targets for antiviral drugs.

The **neuraminidase of influenza** has also become a target for antiviral drugs. **Zanamivir (Relenza)** and

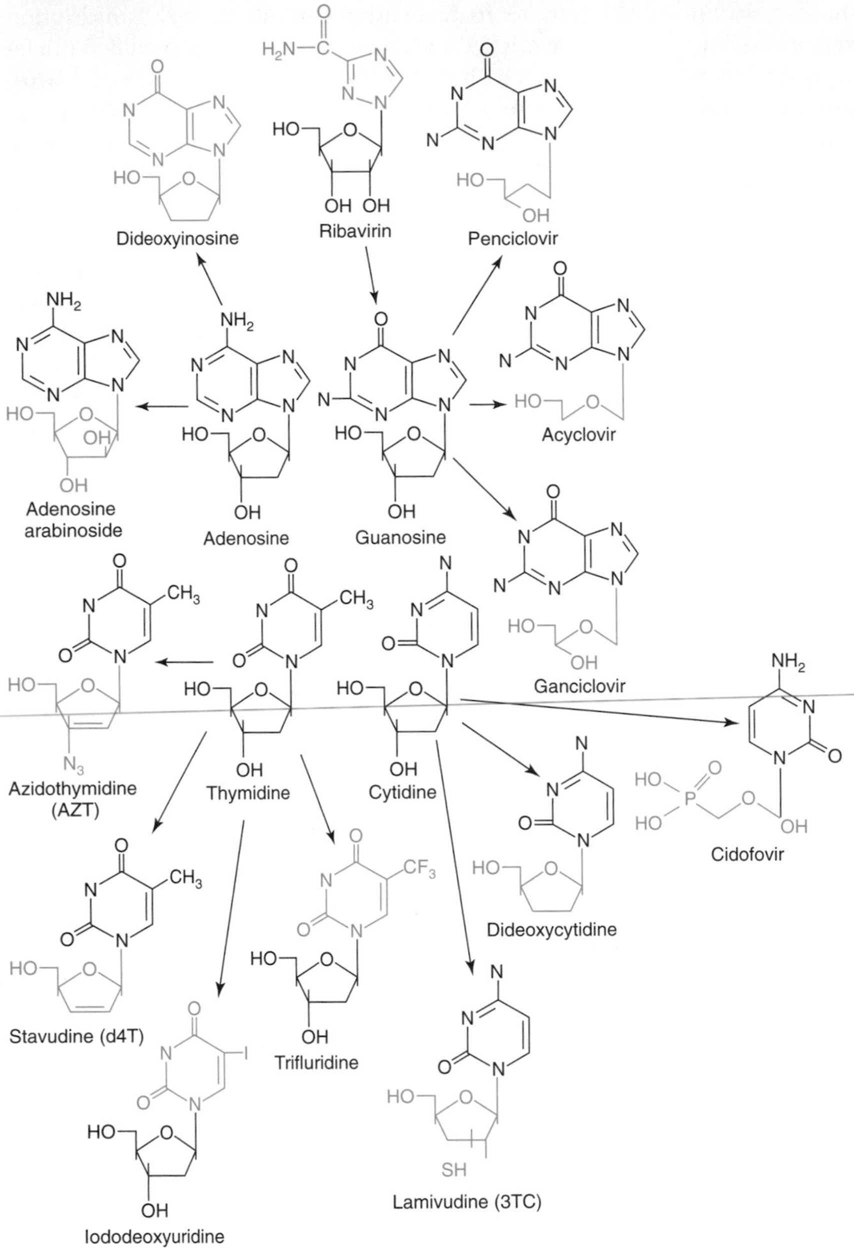

FIGURE 50–1. Structure of the most common nucleoside analogues that are antiviral drugs. The chemical distinctions between the natural deoxynucleoside and the antiviral drug analogues are highlighted. Arrows indicate related drugs. Valacyclovir (*not shown*) is the l-valyl ester of acyclovir. Famciclovir (*not shown*) is the diacetyl 6-deoxyanalogue of penciclovir. Both of these drugs are metabolized to the active drug in the liver or intestinal wall.

oseltamivir (Tamiflu) act as enzyme inhibitors and, unlike amantadine and rimantadine, can inhibit influenza A and B. Amantadine and rimantadine also inhibit release of influenza A.

STIMULATORS OF HOST INNATE IMMUNE PROTECTIVE RESPONSES

The best antiviral agents are those of the host's innate and immune antiviral response. Stimulation or supplemenation of the natural response is an effective approach to limit or treat viral infections. Innate responses of dendritic cells, macrophages, and other cells can be stimulated by **imiquimod, resiquimod, and CpG oligodeoxynucleotides,** which bind to Toll-Like Receptors to stimulate release of protective (Th1) cytokines and activation of natural killer cells and subsequent cell-mediated immune responses. **Interferon** and interferon inducers, including mismatched polynucleotides and double-stranded RNA (e.g., **Ampligen, poly rI:rC**), facilitate the treatment of chronic diseases of hepatitis C and papillomaviruses. **Antibodies,** acquired naturally or by passive immunization (see Chapter 15), prevent both the acquisition and the spread of the virus. For example, passive immunization is administered after exposure to rabies and hepatitis A and hepatitis B viruses.

Nucleoside Analogues

Most of the antiviral drugs approved by the U.S. Food and Drug Administration (FDA) (Table 50–2) are nucleoside analogues that inhibit viral polymerases. These drugs are generally activated by phosphorylation by cellular or viral kinases. Selective inhibition of viral replication occurs because (1) a drug can bind better to viral rather than cellular DNA polymerases or (2) a drug will be used more extensively than in uninfected cells because of the more rapid synthesis of DNA in the infected cells.

ACYCLOVIR AND VALACYCLOVIR, PENCICLOVIR AND FAMCICLOVIR

Acyclovir (acycloguanosine) and its valyl derivative, valacyclovir, differ only in pharmacologic considerations. Acyclovir differs from the nucleoside guanosine by having an acyclic (hydroxyethoxymethyl) side chain instead of a ribose or deoxyribose sugar. ACV has selective action against HSV and VZV, the herpesviruses that encode a thymidine kinase (Figure 50–2). The viral thymidine kinase activates the drug by phosphorylation, and host

TABLE 50–2. Some Antiviral Drug Therapies Approved by the U. S. Food and Drug Administration

Virus	Antiviral Drug	Trade Name
Herpes simplex and varicella-zoster viruses	Acyclovir*	Zovirax
	Valacyclovir*	Valtrex
	Penciclovir	Denavir
	Famciclovir*	Famvir
	Iododeoxyuridine (idoxuridine)[†]	Stoxil
	Trifluridine	Viroptic
Cytomegalovirus	Ganciclovir	Cytovene
	Valganciclovir	Valcyte
	Cidofovir	Vistide
	Phosphonoformate (foscarnet)	Foscavir
Human immunodeficiency virus		
Nucleoside analogue reverse transcriptase inhibitors	Azidothymidine (zidovudine)	Retrovir
	Dideoxyinosine (didanosine)	Videx
	Dideoxycytidine (zalcitabine)	Hivid
	Stavudine (d4T)	Zerit
	Lamivudine (3TC)	Epivir
Non-nucleoside reverse transcriptase inhibitors	Nevirapine	Viramune
	Delaviridine	Rescriptor
Protease inhibitors	Saquinavir	Invirase
	Ritanavir	Norvir
	Indinavir	Crixivan
	Nelfinavir	Viracept
Fusion inhibitor	Enfuvirtide	Fuzeon
Influenza A virus	Amantadine	Symmetrel
	Rimantadine	Flumadine
Influenza A and B viruses	Zanamivir	Relenza
	Oseltamivir	Tamiflu
Hepatitis B virus	Lamivudine	Epivir
	Adefovir dipivoxil	Hepsera
Hepatitis C virus	Interferon-α + ribavirin	
Papillomavirus	Interferon-α	
Respiratory syncytial virus, Lassa virus	Ribavirin	Virazole
Picornaviruses	Pleconaril	

*Also active against varicella-zoster virus.
[†]Topical use only.

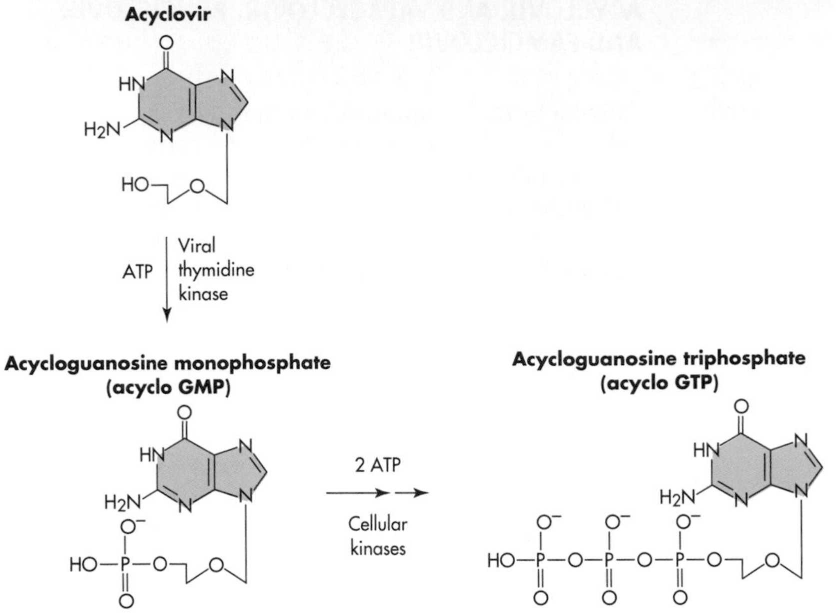

Acyclovir

Viral thymidine kinase

ATP

Acycloguanosine monophosphate (acyclo GMP)

2 ATP

Cellular kinases

Acycloguanosine triphosphate (acyclo GTP)

FIGURE 50–2. Activation of ACV (acycloguanosine) in herpes simplex virus–infected cells. ACV is converted to acycloguanosine monophosphate (acyclo GMP) by herpes-specific viral thymidine kinase, then to acycloguanosine triphosphate (acyclo GTP) by cellular kinases.

cell enzymes complete the progression to the diphosphate form and, finally, to the triphosphate form. Because there is no initial phosphorylation in uninfected cells, there is no active drug to inhibit cellular DNA synthesis or to cause toxicity. The ACV triphosphate competes with the guanosine triphosphate to inhibit the polymerase and cause termination of the growing viral DNA chain, because there is no 3′-hydroxyl group on the ACV molecule to allow chain elongation. This inactivates the DNA polymerase. The minimal toxicity of ACV is also a result of a 100-fold or greater use by the viral DNA polymerase than by cellular DNA polymerases. **Resistance to acyclovir** develops by mutation of either the thymidine kinase, so that activation of ACV cannot occur, or the DNA polymerase, to prevent ACV binding.

ACV is effective against all HSV infections, including encephalitis, disseminated herpes, and other serious herpes diseases. The fact that it is not toxic to uninfected cells allows its use as a prophylactic treatment to prevent recurrent outbreaks, especially in immunosuppressed people. A recurrent episode may be prevented if it is treated before the onset of inflammatory responses. ACV inhibits the replication of HSV but cannot resolve the latent HSV infection.

ACV can also be used for the treatment of VZV infection, although higher doses are required. VZV is less sensitive to the agent because ACV is phosphorylated less efficiently by the VZV thymidine kinase. **Valacyclovir,** the valyl ester derivative of ACV, is more efficiently absorbed after oral administration and rapidly converted into ACV, increasing the bioavailability of ACV for the treatment of HSV and serious VZV.

Penciclovir inhibits HSV and VZV in the same way that ACV does but is concentrated and persists in the infected cells to a greater extent than ACV. Penciclovir also has some activity against the Epstein-Barr virus and cytomegalovirus (CMV). **Famciclovir** is a prodrug derivative of penciclovir that is well absorbed orally and then is converted to penciclovir in the liver or intestinal lining. Resistance to penciclovir and famciclovir develops in the same manner as that to acyclovir.

GANCICLOVIR

Ganciclovir (dihydroxypropoxymethyl guanine) differs from ACV in having a single hydroxymethyl group in the acyclic side chain (see Figure 50–1). The remarkable result of this addition is that it confers considerable activity against CMV. CMV does not encode a thymidine kinase, but a viral-encoded protein kinase phosphorylates GCV. Once activated by phosphorylation, GCV inhibits all herpesvirus DNA polymerases. The viral DNA polymerases have nearly 30 times greater affinity for the drug than the cellular DNA polymerase. Similar to acyclovir, a valyl ester of GCV **(valganciclovir)** was developed to improve the pharmacologic properties of ganciclovir.

GCV is effective in the treatment of CMV retinitis and shows some efficacy in the treatment of CMV esophagitis, colitis, and pneumonia in patients with AIDS. The potential for bone marrow toxicity limits its use to the treatment of CMV infections in patients with AIDS.

Interestingly, this potential toxicity has been used as the basis for the development of an antitumor therapy. In one application, an HSV thymidine kinase gene was incorporated into the cells of a brain tumor, with the use of a retrovirus vector. The retrovirus replicated only in the growing cells of the tumor, and the thymidine kinase was expressed only in the tumor cells, making the tumor cells susceptible to GCV.

CIDOFOVIR AND ADEFOVIR

Cidofovir and **adefovir** are both nucleoside analogues that contain a phosphate attached to the sugar analogue. This obviates the need for the more difficult initial phosphorylation to become a nucleotide. Compounds with this type of sugar analogue are substrates for DNA polymerases or reverse transcriptases and have an expanded spectrum of susceptible viruses. Cidofovir, a cytidine analogue, is effective against all of the herpesviruses, polyomavirus, papillomavirus, adenovirus, and poxvirus polymerases and has been approved for treatment of CMV disease. Adefovir and adefovir dipivoxil (a diester prodrug) are analogues of adenosine and are approved for treatment of hepatitis B virus.

AZIDOTHYMIDINE

Originally developed as an anticancer drug, **azidothymidine** was the first useful therapy for HIV infection. AZT (Retrovir), a nucleoside analogue of thymidine, inhibits the reverse transcriptase of HIV (see Figure 50–1). Like other nucleosides, AZT must be phosphorylated by host cell enzymes. It lacks the 3′-hydroxyl necessary for DNA chain elongation and prevents complementary DNA synthesis. The selective therapeutic effect of AZT stems from the 100-fold lower sensitivity of the host cell DNA polymerase in comparison with the HIV reverse transcriptase.

Continuous oral AZT treatment is administered to HIV-infected people with depleted CD4 T-cell counts to prevent progression of disease. AZT treatment of pregnant HIV-infected women can reduce the likelihood of or prevent transmission of the virus to the baby. Side effects of AZT range from nausea to life-threatening bone marrow toxicity.

The high error rate of the HIV polymerase creates extensive mutations and promotes the development of antiviral-drug—resistant strains. This problem is being addressed by the administration of multiple-drug therapy as initial therapy (highly active antiretroviral therapy [HAART]). It is more difficult for the HIV to develop resistance to multiple drugs with multiple target enzymes. Multiple-drug—resistant HIV strains are likely to be much weaker than the parent strains.

DIDEOXYINOSINE, DIDEOXYCYTIDINE, STAVUDINE, AND LAMIVUDINE

Several other nucleoside analogues have been approved as anti-HIV agents. **Dideoxyinosine** (didanosine) is a nucleoside analogue that is converted to dideoxyadenosine triphosphate (see Figure 50–1). Like AZT, dideoxyinosine, **dideoxycytidine,** and **stavudine** (d4T) lack a 3′-hydroxyl group. The modified sugar attached to **lamivudine** (2′-deoxy-3′-thiacytidine [3TC]) also inhibits the HIV reverse transcriptase by preventing DNA chain elongation and HIV replication. These drugs are available for the treatment of AIDS that is unresponsive to AZT therapy, or they can be given in combination with AZT. Lamivudine is also active on the reverse transcriptase—like polymerase of hepatitis B virus.

RIBAVIRIN

Ribavirin is an analogue of the nucleoside guanosine (see Figure 50–1) but differs from guanosine in that its base ring is incomplete and open. Like other nucleoside analogues, ribavirin must be phosphorylated. The drug is active in vitro against a broad range of viruses.

Ribavirin monophosphate resembles guanosine monophosphate and inhibits nucleoside biosynthesis, mRNA capping, and other processes important to the replication of many viruses. Ribavirin depletes the cellular stores of guanine by inhibiting inosine monophosphate dehydrogenase, an enzyme important in the synthetic pathway of guanosine. It also prevents the synthesis of the mRNA 5′ cap by interfering with the guanylation and methylation of the nucleic acid base. In addition, ribavirin triphosphate inhibits RNA polymerases and promotes hypermutation of the viral genome. Its multiple sites of action may explain the lack of ribavirin-resistant mutants of respiratory syncytial virus and influenza A virus.

Ribavirin is administered in an aerosol to children with severe respiratory syncytial virus bronchopneumonia and, potentially, to adults with severe influenza or measles. The drug may be effective for the treatment of influenza B, as well as Lassa, Rift Valley, Crimean-Congo, Korean, and Argentine hemorrhagic fevers, for which it is administered orally or intravenously. Ribavirin is also active against hepatitis C virus, especially in combination with INF-α.

OTHER NUCLEOSIDE ANALOGUES

Idoxuridine, trifluorothymidine (see Figure 50–1), and **fluorouracil** are analogues of thymidine. These drugs either (1) inhibit the biosynthesis of thymidine, a nucleotide essential for DNA synthesis, or (2) replace thymidine and become incorporated into the viral DNA. These actions inhibit further synthesis of the virus or cause extensive misreading of the genome, leading to mutation and inactivation of the virus. These drugs target cells in which extensive DNA replication is taking place, such as those infected with HSV, and spare nongrowing cells from harm.

Idoxuridine was the first anti-HSV drug approved for human use but has been replaced by trifluridine and other more effective, less toxic agents. Fluorouracil is an antineoplastic drug that kills rapidly growing cells but has also been used for the topical treatment of warts caused by human papillomaviruses.

Adenine arabinoside was the principal anti-HSV drug until ACV was introduced. Ara-A is a purine nucleoside analogue identical in structure to adenosine, except that arabinose is substituted for ribose as the sugar moiety (see Figure 50–1). This agent is phosphorylated by cellular enzymes (especially adenosine kinase), even in uninfected cells, and thus has a greater potential for causing toxicity than ACV. The viral enzyme is 6 to 12 times more sensitive than the cellular enzyme. Resistance can develop as a result of a mutation of the viral DNA polymerase.

Many other nucleoside analogues that have antiviral activity are being investigated for clinical use against the herpesviruses, hepatitis B virus, and HIV. These compounds include modified pyrimidines such as bromovinyldeoxyuridine with a modified base, fluoroiodoaracytosine with a modified base and a 2-fluoro arabinose sugar instead of ribose, and 2-fluoromethylarauridine with the same modified sugar as fluoroiodoaracytosine. Researchers have also developed purine analogues that lack or have alternate sugar residues attached to the nucleoside base, similar in concept to ACV.

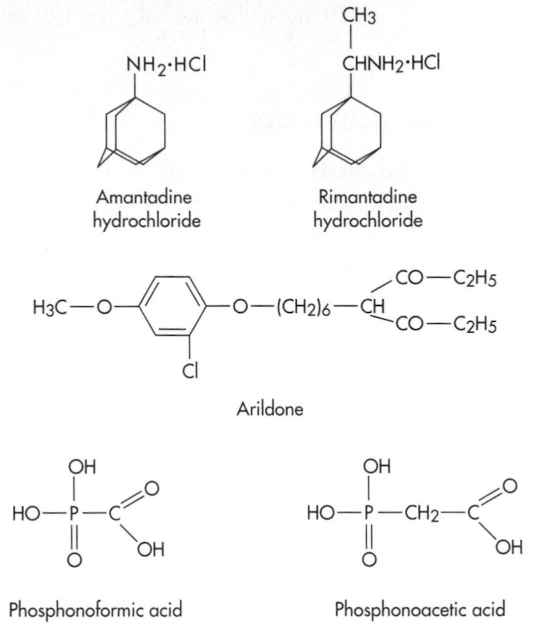

Non-Nucleoside Polymerase Inhibitors

Foscarnet (PFA) and the related phosphonoacetic acid (PAA) are simple compounds that resemble pyrophosphate (Figure 50–3). These drugs inhibit viral replication by binding to the pyrophosphate-binding site of the DNA polymerase to block nucleotide binding. PFA and PAA do not inhibit cellular polymerases at pharmacologic concentrations, but they can cause renal and other problems because of their ability to chelate divalent metal ions (e.g., calcium) and become incorporated into bone. PFA inhibits the DNA polymerase of all herpesviruses and the HIV reverse transcriptase without having to be phosphorylated by nucleoside kinases (e.g., thymidine kinase). PFA has been approved for the treatment of CMV retinitis in patients with AIDS.

Nevirapine, delavirdine, efavirenz, and other non-nucleoside reverse transcriptase inhibitors bind to sites on the enzyme different from the substrate. Because these drugs' mechanisms of action differ from those of the nucleoside analogues, the mechanism of HIV resistance to the agents is also different. As a result, these drugs are very useful in combination with nucleoside analogues for the treatment of HIV infection.

FIGURE 50–3. Structures of non-nucleoside antiviral drugs.

Protease Inhibitors

The unique structure of the HIV protease and its essential role in the production of a functional virion has made this enzyme a good target for antiviral drugs. **Saquinavir, indinavir, ritonavir, nelfinavir, amprenavir,** and other agents work by slipping into the hydrophobic active site of the enzyme to inhibit its action. As occurs with the other anti-HIV drugs, drug-resistant strains arise through mutation of the protease. The combination of a protease inhibitor with AZT and a second nucleoside analogue can reduce blood levels of HIV to undetectable levels. Development of resistance to a "cocktail" of anti-HIV drugs is also less likely than that to a single drug.

Anti-Influenza Drugs

Amantadine and **rimantadine** are amphipathic amine compounds with clinical efficacy against the influenza A virus but not the influenza B or other viruses (see Figure 50–3). These drugs have several effects on influenza A replication. Both compounds are acidotrophic and concentrate in and buffer the contents of the endosomal vesicles involved in the uptake of the influenza virus. This effect can inhibit the acid-mediated change in conformation in the hemagglutinin protein that promotes the fusion of the viral envelope with cell membranes. However, the specificity for influenza A is a result of its ability to bind to and block the proton channel formed by the M_2 matrix protein of the influenza A virus. Resistance is the result of an altered M_2 matrix or hemagglutinin protein.

Amantadine and rimantadine may be useful in ameliorating an influenza A infection if either agent is taken within 48 hours of exposure. They are also useful as a prophylactic treatment in lieu of vaccination. In addition, amantadine is an alternative therapy for Parkinson's disease. The principal toxic effect is on the central nervous system, with patients experiencing nervousness, irritability, and insomnia.

Zanamivir (Relenza) and **oseltamivir (Tamiflu)** inhibit influenza A and B as enzyme inhibitors of the neuraminidase of influenza. Without the neuraminidase, the hemagglutinin of the virus binds to sialic acid on other viral particles, forming clumps and preventing virus release. These drugs reduce the length of illness if taken within the first 48 hours of infection.

Immunomodulators

Genetically engineered forms of INF-α have been approved for human use. Interferons work by binding to cell surface receptors and initiating a cellular antiviral response. In addition, interferons stimulate the immune response and promote the immune clearance of viral infection.

INF-α is active against many viral infections, including hepatitis A, B, and C, HSV, papillomavirus, and rhinovirus. It has been approved for the treatment of condyloma acuminatum (genital warts, a presentation of papillomavirus) and hepatitis C (especially with ribavirin). Natural interferon causes the influenza-like symptoms observed during many viremic and respiratory tract infections, and the synthetic agent has similar side effects during treatment. Interferon is discussed further in Chapter 14.

Imiquimod, a Toll-Like Receptor ligand, stimulates innate responses to attack the virus infection. This therapeutic approach can activate local protective responses against papillomas, which generally escape immune control.

QUESTIONS

1. List the steps in viral replication that are poor targets for antiviral drugs. Why?
2. Which viruses can be treated with an antiviral drug? Distinguish the viruses treatable with an antiviral nucleoside analogue.
3. A mutation in the gene for which enzymes or proteins would confer resistance to the following antiviral drugs: ACV, ara-A, phosphonoformate, amantadine, AZT?
4. A patient has been exposed to influenza A virus and is in his third day of symptoms. He has heard that an anti-influenza drug is available and requests therapy. You tell him that therapy is not appropriate. To what therapeutic agents is the patient referring, and why did you decline to use the treatment?

Bibliography

Cohen J, Powderly WG, editors: *Infectious diseases,* ed 2, St Louis, 2004, Mosby.

De Clercq, E: In search of a selective antiviral chemotherapy, *Clin Microbiol Rev* 10:674-693, 1997.

Evans AS, Kaslow RA: *Viral infections of humans: Epidemiology and control,* ed 4, New York, 1997, Plenum Medical Books. Wilkins.

Flint SJ et al: *Principles of virology: Molecular biology, pathogenesis and control of animal viruses,* ed 2, Washington, 2003, American Society for Microbiology Press. Galasso GJ, Whitley RJ, Merigan TC: *Antiviral agents and human viral diseases,* ed 4, Philadelphia, 1997, Lippincott-Raven.

Hodinka RL: What clinicians need to know about antiviral drugs and viral resistance, *Infect Dis Clin North Am* 11:945-967.

Knipe DM, Howley PM, editors: *Virology,* ed 4, New York, 2001, Lippincott-Williams and Wilkins.

Richman DD, Whitley RJ, Hayden FG: *Clinical virology,* New York, 1997, Churchill Livingstone.

Specter S, Hodinka RL, Young SA: *Clinical virology manual,* ed 3, Washington, 2000, ASM Press.

Strauss JM, Strauss EG: *Viruses and human diseases,* San Diego, 2002, Academic Press.

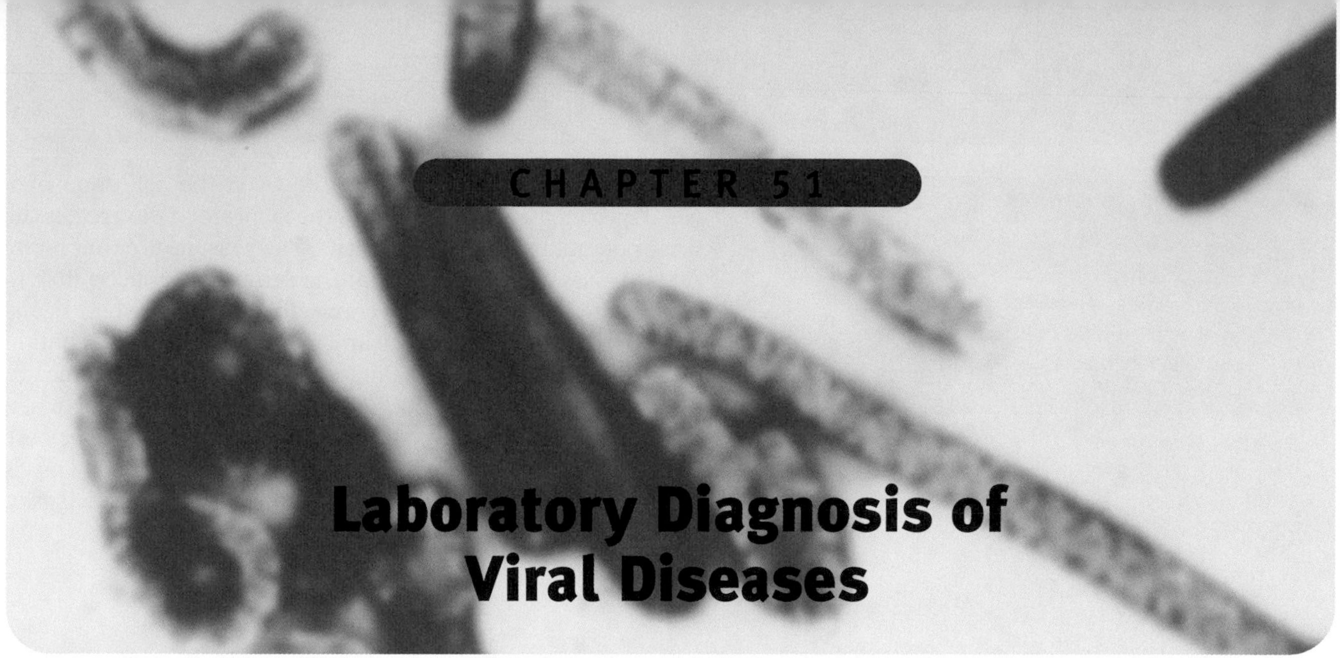

Laboratory Diagnosis of Viral Diseases

There have been many new developments in laboratory viral diagnosis that are more sensitive and provide more rapid viral identification from clinical samples. These include better antibody reagents for direct analysis of samples and molecular genetic techniques for direct identification of viral genomes. Often, isolation of the organism is unnecessary and avoided to minimize the risk to laboratory and other personnel. The quicker turnaround allows a more rapid choice of the appropriate antiviral therapy.

The patient's history and symptoms provide the first clues to the diagnosis of a viral infection, often by excluding other types of infection (e.g., bacterial, fungal). Viral laboratory studies are performed to (1) confirm the diagnosis by identifying the viral agent of infection, (2) determine appropriate antiviral therapy, (3) define the course of the disease, (4) monitor the disease epidemiologically, and (5) educate physicians and patients.

The laboratory methods accomplish the following results:

1. Description of virus-induced **cytopathologic effects (CPEs)** on cells.
2. Electron microscopic detection of viral particles.
3. Isolation and growth of the virus.
4. Detection of viral components (e.g., proteins, enzymes, genomes).
5. Evaluation of the patient's immune response to the virus **(serology).**

The molecular and immunologic techniques used for many of these procedures are described in Chapters 17 and 18. Viruses, viral antigens, viral genomes, and CPEs can be detected by means of direct analysis of clinical specimens or after growth of the virus on tissue culture cells in the laboratory (Box 51–1).

Specimen Collection

The patient's symptoms and travel history, the season of the year, and a presumptive diagnosis help determine the appropriate procedures to be used to identify a viral agent (Table 51–1). For example, specimens of cerebrospinal fluid and urine are appropriate in a patient who has symptoms of central nervous system disease after parotitis, because the mumps virus that can cause such disease can be isolated in these specimens. A focal encephalitis with a temporal lobe localization preceded by headaches and disorientation suggests herpes simplex virus (HSV) infection, for which cerebrospinal fluid is analyzed for viral deoxyribonucleic acid (DNA) sequences by polymerase chain reaction (PCR) amplification. The development of meningitis symptoms during the summer indicates an enterovirus etiology, in which case cerebrospinal fluid, throat swab, and stool specimens should be collected for PCR analysis and possible virus isolation.

The selection of the appropriate specimen for viral culture is often complicated because several viruses may cause the same clinical disease. For example, many agents can cause aseptic meningitis, so it may be necessary to obtain several types of specimens to identify the causal virus.

Specimens should be collected early in the acute phase of infection, before the virus ceases to be shed. For example, respiratory viruses may be shed for only 3 to 7 days, and shedding may lapse before the symptoms cease. HSV and varicella-zoster virus (VZV) may not be recoverable from lesions more than 5 days after the onset of symptoms. It may be possible to isolate an enterovirus from the cerebrospinal fluid for only 2 to 3 days after the onset of the central nervous system manifestations. In addition, antibody produced in response to the infection may block the detection of virus.

BOX 51–1. Laboratory Procedures for Diagnosing Viral Infections

Cytologic examination
Electron microscopy
Virus isolation and growth
Detection of viral proteins (antigens and enzymes)
Detection of viral genomes
Serology

The shorter the interval between the collection of a specimen and its delivery to the laboratory, the greater the potential for isolating a virus. The reasons are that many viruses are labile and that the samples are susceptible to bacterial and fungal overgrowth. Viruses are best transported and stored on ice and in special media that contain antibiotics and proteins, such as serum albumin or gelatin. Significant losses in infectious titers occur when enveloped viruses (e.g., HSV, VZV, influenza virus) are kept at room temperature or frozen at −20°C. This is not a risk for nonenveloped viruses (e.g., adenoviruses, enteroviruses).

TABLE 51–1. Specimens for Viral Diagnosis

Common Pathogenic Viruses	Specimens for Culture	Comments
Respiratory Tract		
Adenovirus; influenza virus; enterovirus (picornavirus); rhinovirus; paramyxovirus; rubella virus; HSV	Nasal washing, throat swab, nasal swab, sputum	Enterovirus is also shed in stool
Gastrointestinal Tract		
Reovirus; rotavirus; adenovirus; Norwalk virus, calicivirus	Stool, rectal swab	Samples are analyzed by electron microscopy and antigen detection (ELISA); viruses are not cultured
Maculopapular Rash		
Adenovirus; enterovirus (picornavirus)	Throat swab, rectal swab	—
Rubella virus; measles virus	Urine	—
Vesicular Rash		
Coxsackievirus; echovirus; HSV; VZV	Vesicle fluid, scraping, or swab, enterovirus in stool	Initial diagnosis of HSV and VZV can be obtained from vesicle scraping (Tzanck smear)
Central Nervous System (Aseptic Meningitis, Encephalitis)		
Enterovirus (picornavirus)	Stool	PCR
Arboviruses (e.g., togaviruses, bunyavirus)	Rarely cultured	Diagnosis is by serologic tests
Rabies virus	Tissue, saliva, brain biopsy	Diagnosis is by immunofluorescence analysis for antigen
HSV; CMV; mumps virus; measles virus	Cerebrospinal fluid	PCR, virus isolation, and antigen are assayed
Urinary Tract		
Adenovirus; CMV	Urine	CMV may be shed without apparent disease
Blood		
HIV; human T-cell leukemia virus; hepatitis B, C, and D viruses	Blood	Serologic antigen or antibody detection (ELISA), PCR, and RT-PCR are performed

Data from Cherneskey MA et al: *Cumitech 15: Laboratory diagnosis of viral infections,* Washington, 1982, American Society for Microbiology; and from Hsiung GD: *Diagnostic virology,* New Haven, Conn, 1982, Yale University Press.

CMV, Cytomegalovirus; ELISA, enzyme-linked immunosorbent assay; HIV, human immunodeficiency virus; HSV, herpes simplex virus; PCR, polymerase chain reaction; RT-PCR, reverse transcriptase PCR; VZV, varicella-zoster virus.

Cytology

The cytologic examination of specimens provides a rapid initial diagnosis for viral infections that produce a characteristic CPE. Characteristic CPEs in the tissue sample or in cell culture include changes in cell morphology, cell lysis, vacuolation, syncytia (Figure 51–1), and inclusion bodies. **Syncytia** are multinucleated giant cells formed by viral fusion of individual cells. Paramyxoviruses, HSV, VZV, and HIV promote syncytia formation. **Inclusion bodies** constitute either histologic changes in the cells caused by viral components or virus-induced changes in cell structures. For example, nuclear, owl's-eye inclusion bodies found in the cells of tissues with cytomegalovirus (CMV) (see Figure 54–17) or in the sediment of urine from patients with the infection are readily identifiable. Cowdry type A inclusions in single cells or in large syncytia (multiple cells fused together) are a characteristic finding in cells infected with HSV or VZV (Figure 51–2). Rabies may be detected through the finding of Negri bodies (rabies virus inclusions) in brain tissue (Figure 51–3).

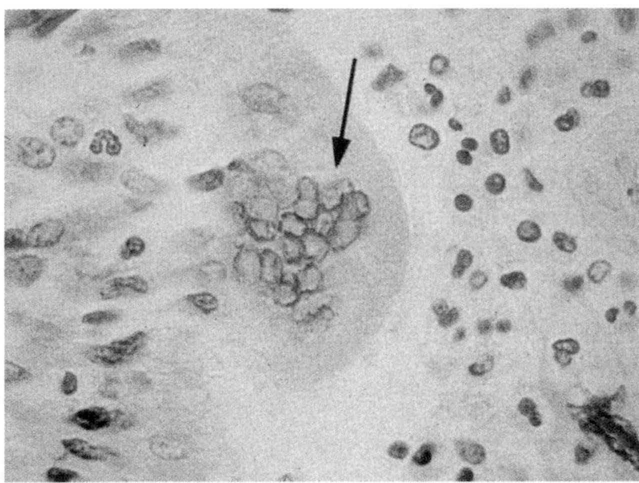

FIGURE 51–1. Syncytium formation by measles virus. Multinucleated giant cell (*arrow*) visible in a histologic section of lung biopsy tissue from a measles virus–induced giant cell pneumonia in an immunocompromised child. (From Hart C, Broadhead RL: *A color atlas of pediatric infectious diseases,* London, 1992, Wolfe.)

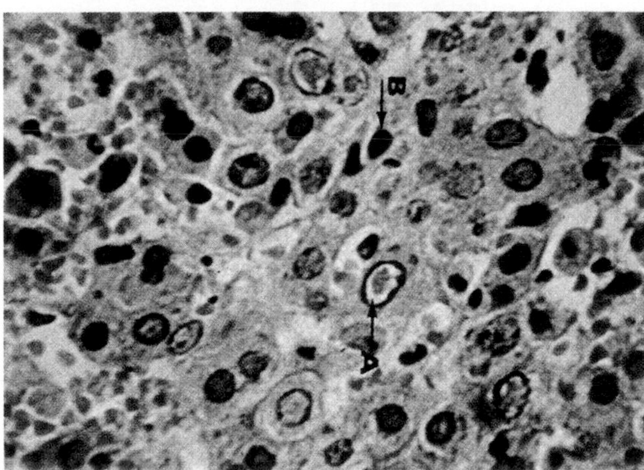

FIGURE 51–2. HSV-induced CPE. A biopsy specimen of an HSV-infected liver shows an eosinophilic Cowdry type A intranuclear inclusion body (*A*) surrounded by a halo and a ring of marginated chromatin at the nuclear membrane. An infected cell (*B*) exhibits a smaller condensed nucleus (pyknotic). CPE, Cytopathologic effect; HSV, herpes simplex virus. (Courtesy Dr. J.I. Pugh, St. Albans; from Emond RT, Rowland HAK: *A color atlas of infectious diseases,* ed 3, London, 1995, Mosby.)

Often the cytologic specimens will be examined for specific viral antigens by immunofluorescence or viral genomes by PCR for a rapid, definitive identification. These tests are specific for individual viruses and must be chosen based on the differential diagnosis. These methods are discussed in the following paragraphs.

Electron Microscopy

Electron microscopy is not a standard clinical laboratory technique, but it can be used to detect and identify some

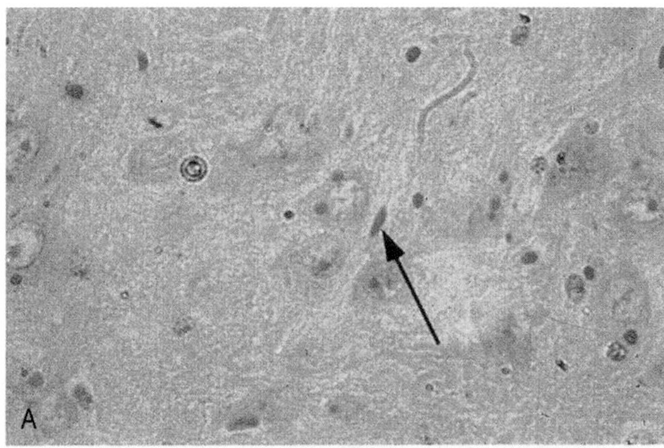

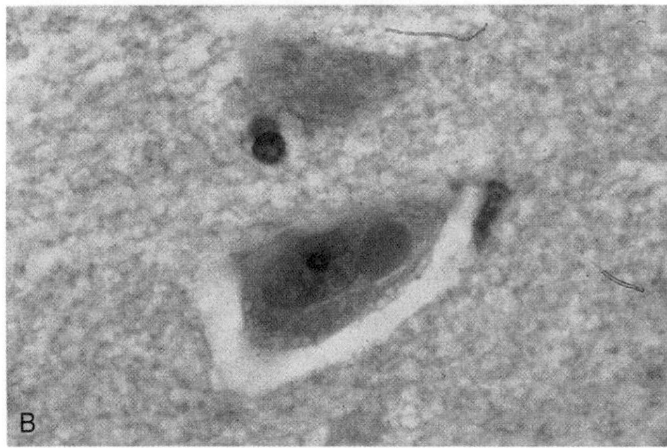

FIGURE 51–3. Negri bodies caused by rabies. **A,** A section of brain from a patient with rabies shows Negri bodies (*arrow*). **B,** Higher magnification from another biopsy specimen. (**A** from Hart C, Broadhead RL: *A color atlas of pediatric infectious diseases,* London, 1992, Wolfe.)

viruses if sufficient viral particles are present. The addition of virus-specific antibody to a sample can cause viral particles to clump, thereby facilitating the detection and simultaneous identification of the virus (immunoelectron microscopy). This method is useful for the detection of enteric viruses, such as rotavirus, that are produced in abundance and have a characteristic morphology. Appropriately processed tissue from a biopsy or clinical specimen can also be examined for the presence of viral structures.

Viral Isolation and Growth

A virus can be grown in tissue culture, embryonated eggs, and experimental animals (Box 51–2). Although embryonated eggs are still used for the growth of virus for some vaccines (e.g., influenza), they have been replaced by cell cultures for routine virus isolation in clinical laboratories. Experimental animals are rarely used in clinical laboratories for the purpose of isolating viruses.

CELL CULTURE

Specific types of tissue culture cells are used to grow viruses. **Primary cell cultures** are obtained by dissociating specific animal organs with trypsin or collagenase. The cells yielded by this method are then grown as monolayers (fibroblast or epithelial) or in suspension (lymphocyte) in artificial media supplemented with bovine serum or another source of growth factors. Primary cells can be dissociated with trypsin, diluted and allowed to grow into new monolayers (*passed*) to become secondary cell cultures. **Diploid cell lines** are cultures of a single cell type that are capable of being passed a large but finite number of times before they senesce, or undergo a significant change in their characteristics. **Tumor cell lines** and **immortalized cell lines,** which are initiated from patient tumors and by viruses or chemicals, respectively, consist of single cell types that can be passed continuously without senescing.

Primary monkey kidney cells are excellent for the recovery of influenza viruses, paramyxoviruses, many enteroviruses, and some adenoviruses. Human fetal diploid cells, which are generally fibroblastic cells, support the growth of a broad spectrum of viruses (e.g., HSV, VZV, CMV, adenoviruses, picornaviruses). HEp-2 cells, a continuous line of epithelial cells derived from a human cancer, are excellent for the recovery of respiratory syncytial virus, adenoviruses, and HSV. Many clinically significant viruses can be recovered in at least one of these cell cultures.

BOX 51–2. Systems for the Propagation of Viruses

- People
- Animals: Cows (e.g., Jenner's cowpox vaccine), chickens, mice, rats, suckling mice
- Embryonated eggs
- Organ culture
- Tissue culture
    - Primary
    - Diploid cell line
    - Tumor or immortalized cell line

VIRAL DETECTION

A virus can be detected and initially identified through observation of the virus-induced CPE in the cell monolayer (Box 51–3; Figure 51–4) or by immunofluorescence or genome analysis of the infected cell culture. For example, a single virus infects, spreads, and kills surrounding cells **(plaque).** The type of cell culture, the characteristics of the CPE, and the rapidity of viral growth can be used to initially identify many clinically important viruses. This approach to identifying viruses is similar to that used in the identification of bacteria, which is based

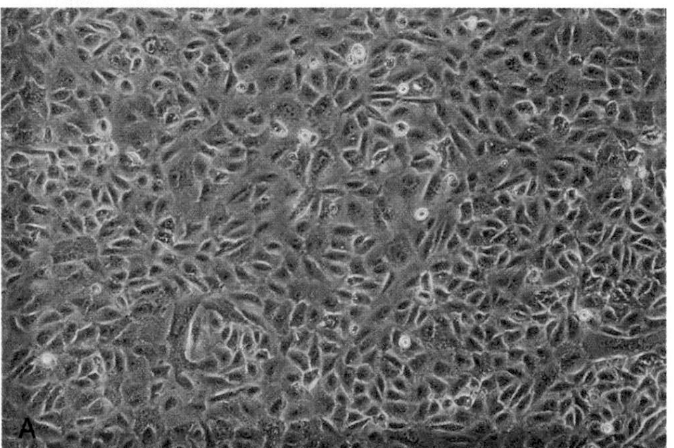

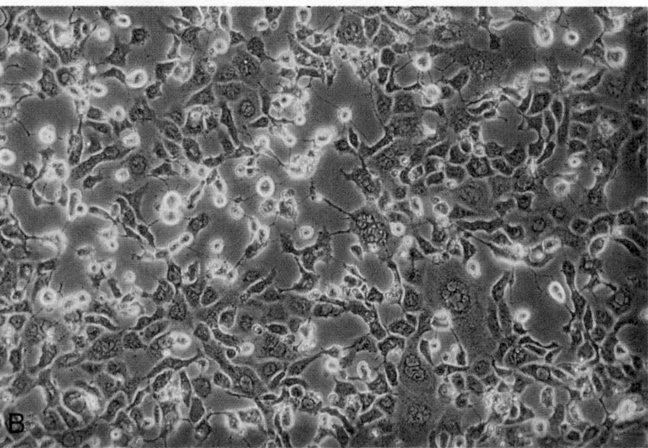

FIGURE 51–4. CPE of HSV infection. **A,** Uninfected Vero cells, an African green monkey kidney cell line. **B,** HSV-1–infected Vero cells showing rounded cells, multinucleated cells, and loss of the monolayer.

BOX 51–3. Viral Cytopathologic Effects

Cell death
- Cell rounding
- Degeneration
- Aggregation
- Loss of attachments to culture dish

Characteristic histologic changes: Inclusion bodies in the nucleus or cytoplasm, margination of chromatin

Syncytia: Multinucleated giant cells caused by virus-induced cell-cell fusion

Cell surface changes
- Viral antigen expression
- Hemadsorption (hemagglutinin expression)

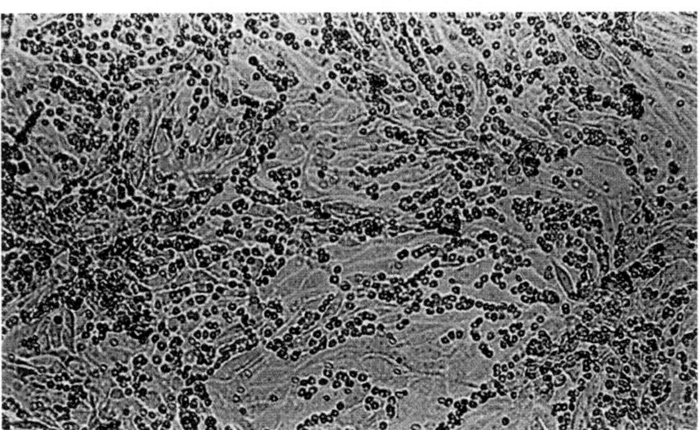

FIGURE 51–5. Hemadsorption of erythrocytes to cells infected with influenza viruses, mumps virus, parainfluenza viruses, or togaviruses. These viruses express a hemagglutinin on their surfaces, which bind erythrocytes of selected animal species.

on the growth and morphology of colonies on selective differential media.

Some viruses grow slowly or not at all or do not readily cause a CPE in cell lines typically used in clinical virology laboratories. Some cause diseases that are hazardous to personnel. These viruses are most frequently diagnosed on the basis of serologic findings or through the detection of viral genomes or antigens.

Characteristic viral properties can also be used to identify viruses that do not have a classic CPE. For example, the rubella virus may not cause a CPE, but it does prevent (interfere with) the replication of picornaviruses in a process known as **heterologous interference,** which can be used to identify the rubella virus. Cells infected with the influenza virus, parainfluenza virus, mumps virus, and togavirus express a viral glycoprotein (hemagglutinin) that binds erythrocytes of defined animal species to the infected cell surface **(hemadsorption)** (Figure 51–5). When released into the cell culture medium, such viruses can be detected from the agglutination of erythrocytes, a process termed **hemagglutination.** The strain of virus can then be identified from the specific antibody that blocks the hemagglutination, a process called **hemagglutination inhibition (HI).** An innovative approach to detection of herpes simplex virus infection uses genetically modified tissue culture cells that express the β-galactosidase gene and can be stained blue when infected with HSV (enzyme-linked virus inducible system).

One can quantitate a virus by determining the greatest dilution that retains the following properties **(titer):**

1. **Tissue culture dose (TCD_{50}):** Titer of virus that causes cytopathologic effects in half the tissue culture cells.
2. **Lethal dose (LD_{50}):** Titer of virus that kills 50% of a set of test animals.
3. **Infectious dose (ID_{50}):** Titer of virus that initiates a detectable symptom, antibody, or other response in 50% of a set of test animals.

The number of infectious viruses can also be evaluated with a count of the plaques produced by tenfold dilutions of sample **(plaque-forming units).** The ratio of viral particles (from electron microscopy) to plaque-forming units is always greater than one because numerous defective viral particles are produced during viral replication.

INTERPRETATION OF CULTURE RESULTS

In general the detection of any virus in host tissues, cerebrospinal fluid, blood, or vesicular fluid can be considered a highly significant finding. However, viral shedding may also be induced by an underlying condition (e.g., another infection, an immunosuppressed state, stress) and may therefore be unrelated to the disease symptoms. Certain viruses can be intermittently shed without causing symptoms in the affected person for periods ranging from weeks (enteroviruses in feces) to many months or years (HSV or CMV in the oropharynx and vagina; adenoviruses in the oropharynx and intestinal tract). Also, virus may not be isolated from a sample if the sample is improperly handled, contains neutralizing antibody, or is acquired before or after viral shedding.

Detection of Viral Proteins

Enzymes and other proteins are produced during viral replication and can be detected by biochemical, immunologic, and molecular biologic means (Box 51–4). The viral proteins can be separated by electrophoresis, and their patterns used to identify and distinguish different viruses. For example, the electrophoretically separated HSV-infected cell proteins and virion proteins exhibit different

BOX 51–4. Assays for Viral Proteins and Nucleic Acids

Proteins
Protein patterns (electrophoresis)
Enzyme activities (e.g., reverse transcriptase)
Hemagglutination and hemadsorption
Antigen detection (e.g., direct and indirect immunofluorescence, enzyme-linked immunosorbent assay, Western blot)

Nucleic Acids
Restriction endonuclease cleavage patterns
Size of RNA for segmented RNA viruses (electrophoresis)
DNA genome hybridization in situ (cytochemistry)
Southern, Northern, and dot blots
PCR (DNA)
Reverse transcriptase polymerase chain reaction (RNA)
Real-time PCR
Branched-chain DNA and related tests (DNA, RNA)

PCR, Polymerase chain reaction.

patterns for different types and strains of HSV-1 and HSV-2.

The detection and assay of characteristic enzymes or activities can identify and quantitate specific viruses. For example, the presence of reverse transcriptase in serum or cell culture indicates the presence of a retrovirus. Similarly, hemagglutination or hemadsorption can be used to easily assay the hemagglutinin produced by the influenza virus.

Antibodies can be used as sensitive and specific tools to detect, identify, and quantitate the virus and viral antigen in clinical specimens or cell cultures (immunohistochemistry). Specifically, monoclonal or monospecific antibodies are useful for distinguishing among viral strains and mutants. Viral antigens on the cell surface or within the cell can be detected by **immunofluorescence** and enzyme immunoassay (EIA) (see Figures 18–2 and 18–3). Virus or antigen released from infected cells can be detected by **enzyme-linked immunosorbent assay (ELISA),** radioimmunoassay (RIA), and **latex agglutination (LA)** (see Chapter 18 for definitions). Tests for specific viral agents are commercially available.

The detection of CMV and other viruses can be enhanced through the use of a combination of cell culture and immunologic means. In this method the clinical sample is centrifuged onto cells grown on a coverslip on the bottom of a **shell vial** (glass tube). This step increases the efficiency and accelerates the progression of infection of the cells on the coverslip. The cells can then be analyzed with immunofluorescence **(direct fluorescence)** or EIA for early viral antigens, which are detectable within 24 hours, instead of the 7 to 14 days it takes for a CPE to become evident.

Detection of Viral Genetic Material

The genome structure and genetic sequence are major distinguishing characteristics of the family, type, and strain of virus (see Box 51–4). The electrophoretic patterns of ribonucleic acid (RNA) (influenza, reovirus) or restriction endonuclease fragment lengths from DNA viral genomes are like genetic fingerprints for these viruses. Different strains of HSV-1 and HSV-2 can be distinguished in this way by restriction fragment length polymorphism. Newer methods for viral genome detection use sequence-specific genetic probes and PCR-like DNA amplification approaches, which allow more rapid analysis with a minimum of risk from infectious virus.

DNA probes with sequences complementary to specific regions of a viral genome can be used, like antibodies, as sensitive and specific tools for detecting a virus. These probes can detect the virus even in the absence of viral replication. DNA probe analysis is especially useful for detecting slowly replicating or nonproductive viruses, such as CMV and human papillomavirus, for which there is no CPE, or the viral antigen cannot be detected using immunologic tests (see Figure 17–3). Specific viral genetic sequences in fixed, permeabilized tissue biopsy specimens can be detected by **in situ hybridization.**

Viral genomes can also be detected in clinical samples with the use of **dot blot** or **Southern blot analysis.** For the latter method, the viral genome or electrophoretically separated restriction endonuclease cleavage fragments of the genome are blotted onto nitrocellulose filters and then detected on the filter by their hybridization to DNA probes. Electrophoretically separated viral RNA (**Northern blot**–RNA:DNA probe hybridization) blotted onto a nitrocellulose filter can be detected in a similar manner. The DNA probes are detected with autoradiography or with fluorescent or EIA-like methods. Many viral probes and kits for detecting viruses are now commercially available.

Detection of viral genomes by **PCR, reverse transcriptase PCR (RT-PCR),** and related assays are becoming the primary tool for detection and identification of several viruses for many laboratories. Use of the appropriate primers for PCR can promote a millionfold amplification of a target sequence in a few hours. This technique is especially useful for detecting latent and integrated sequences of viruses, such as retroviruses, herpesviruses, papillomaviruses, and other papovaviruses, as well as evidence of viruses present in low concentrations and viruses that are difficult or too dangerous to isolate in cell culture. RT-PCR uses the retroviral reverse transcriptase to convert viral RNA to DNA and allow PCR amplification of the viral nucleic acid sequences. This approach was very useful for identifying and distinguishing the Hantaviruses that caused the outbreak in New Mexico in 1993.

Quantification of the amount of HIV within a patient (virus load) can be determined by **real-time PCR.** The concentration of HIV genome in a blood sample is proportional to the rate of PCR amplification of the genomic DNA.

PCR is the prototype for several other genome amplification techniques. **Transcription-based amplification** uses reverse transcriptase and viral sequence specific primers to make a complementary DNA (cDNA) that also has a sequence recognized by the DNA-dependent RNA polymerase from the T7 bacteriophage. An RNAse H digests the RNA, and the DNA is transcribed to RNA by the T7 RNA polymerase. The new RNA sequences are then cycled back into the reaction to amplify the relevant sequence. Unlike PCR, these reactions do not require special equipment.

Some other genome amplification and detection approaches are similar in concept to ELISA. These approaches use immobilized DNA sequences complementary to the relevant viral genomic sequence to capture the viral genome. This is followed by the binding of another complementary sequence that contains a detection system. The cDNA sequence may be attached to an extensively **branched chain of DNA** in which each of the branches elicits a reaction that amplifies the signal to detectable levels. Another variation of the theme uses an antibody that recognizes DNA-RNA complexes to capture viral DNA-RNA probe hybrids in the well of a plate, followed by an enzyme-labeled antibody and ELISA methods to detect the presence of the genome. Like ELISA, these methods can be automated and set up to analyze a panel of viruses.

Viral Serology

The humoral immune response provides a history of a patient's infections. Serologic studies are used for the identification of viruses that are difficult to isolate and grow in cell culture, as well as viruses that cause diseases of long duration (see Box 18–2). Serology can be used to identify the virus and its strain or serotype, whether it is acute or chronic disease, and determine whether it is a primary infection or a reinfection. The antibody type and titer and the nature of the antigenic targets provide serologic data about a viral infection. The detection of **virus-specific immunoglobulin (Ig)M antibody,** which is present during the first 2 or 3 weeks of a primary infection, generally indicates a recent primary infection. **Seroconversion** is indicated by at least a fourfold increase in the antibody titer between the serum obtained during the acute phase of disease and that obtained at least 2 to 3 weeks later, during the convalescent phase. Reinfection or recurrence later in life causes an anamnestic (secondary or booster) response. Antibody titers may remain high in patients who suffer frequent recurrence of a disease (e.g., herpesviruses).

Because of the inherent imprecision of serologic assays based on twofold serial dilutions, a fourfold increase in the antibody titer between acute and convalescent sera is required to indicate seroconversion. For example, samples with 512 and 1023 units of antibody would both give a signal on a 512-fold dilution but not on a 1024-fold dilution, and the titers of both would be reported as 512. On the other hand, samples with 1020 and 1030 units are not significantly different but would be reported as titers of 512 and 1024, respectively.

The course of a chronic infection can also be determined from a serologic profile. Specifically, the presence of antibodies to several key viral antigens and their titers can be used to identify the stage of disease caused by certain viruses. This approach is especially useful for the diagnosis of viral diseases with slow courses (e.g., hepatitis B, infectious mononucleosis caused by Epstein-Barr virus). In general the first antibodies to be detected are directed against the antigens most available to the immune system (e.g., expressed on the virion or infected-cell surfaces). Later in the infection, when the infecting virus or the cellular immune response has lysed the cells, antibodies directed against the intracellular viral proteins and enzymes are detected. For example, antibodies to the envelope and capsid antigens of Epstein-Barr virus are detected first. Then, during convalescence, antibodies to nuclear antigens, such as the Epstein-Barr virus nuclear antigen, are detected.

A serologic battery or panel consisting of assays for several viruses may be used for the diagnosis of certain diseases. Local epidemiologic factors, the time of year, and patient factors such as immunocompetence, travel history, and age influence the choice of virus assays to be included in a panel. For example, HSV and the viruses of mumps, western and eastern equine encephalitides, and St. Louis and Califronia encephalitides might be included in a panel of tests for central nervous system diseases.

SEROLOGIC TEST METHODS

The serologic tests used in virology are listed in Box 18–1 and described further in Chapter 18. **Neutralization** and **HI tests** assay antibody on the basis of its recognition of and binding to virus. The antibody coating of the virus blocks its binding to indicator cells (Figure 51–6). Neutralization involves inhibition by the antibody of infection and cytopathologic effects of the virus in tissue culture cells. A neutralization antibody response is virus and strain specific. The response often develops with the onset of symptoms and persists for long periods. HI is used for the identification of viruses that can selectively agglutinate erythrocytes of various animal species (e.g., chicken, guinea pig, human). Antibody in serum prevents a standardized amount of virus from binding to and agglutinating erythrocytes.

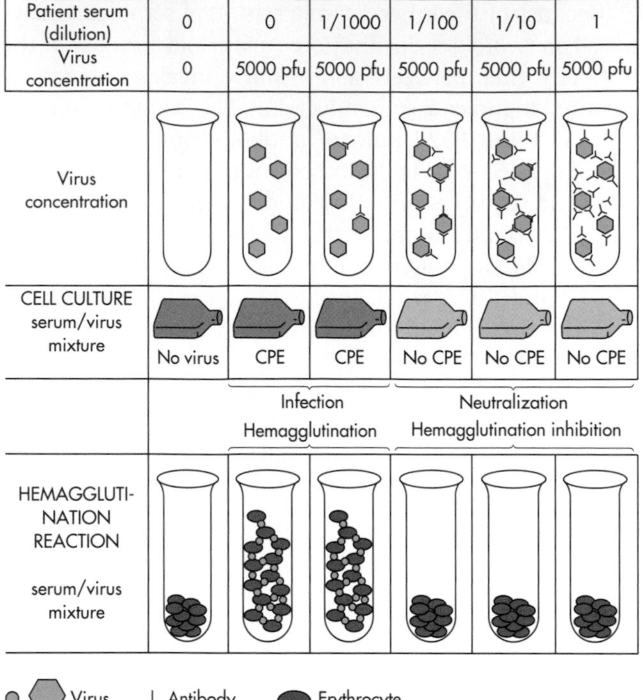

FIGURE 51–6. Neutralization, hemagglutination, and hemagglutination inhibition assays. In the assay shown, tenfold dilutions of serum were incubated with virus. Aliquots of the mixture were then added to cell cultures or erythrocytes. In the absence of antibody, the virus infected the monolayer (indicated by CPE) and caused hemagglutination (i.e., formed a gel-like suspension of erythrocytes). In the presence of the antibody, infection was blocked (neutralization), and hemagglutination was inhibited, allowing the erythrocytes to pellet. The titer of antibody in the serum was 100. pfu, Plaque-forming units.

The indirect fluorescent antibody test and solid-phase immunoassays such as **LA, ELISA,** and **RIA** are commonly used to detect and quantitate viral antigen and antiviral antibody. The ELISA test is used to screen the blood supply to exclude individuals who are seropositive for hepatitis B and C viruses and HIV. Western blot analysis has become very important to confirm seroconversion and hence infection with HIV. The ability of the patient antibody to recognize specific viral proteins separated by electrophoresis, transferred (blotted) onto a filter paper (e.g., nitrocellulose, nylon), and visualized with an enzyme-conjugated antihuman antibody confirms the ELISA-indicated diagnosis of HIV infection (Figure 51–7).

LIMITATIONS OF SEROLOGIC METHODS

The presence of an antiviral antibody indicates previous infection but is not sufficient to indicate when the infection occurred. The finding of virus-specific IgM, a fourfold increase in the antibody titer between acute and convalescent sera, or specific antibody profiles is indicative of recent infection. False-positive or false-negative test results may confuse the diagnosis. In addition, patient antibody may be bound with viral antigen (as occurs in patients with hepatitis B) in immune complexes, thereby preventing antibody detection. Serologic cross-reactions between different viruses may also confuse the identity of the infecting agent (e.g., parainfluenza and mumps express related antigens). Conversely, the antibody used in the assay may be too specific (many monoclonal antibodies) and may not recognize other viruses from the same family, giving a false-negative result (e.g., rhinovirus). A good understanding of the clinical symptoms and a knowledge of the limitations and potential problems with serologic assays aid the diagnosis.

QUESTIONS

1. Brain tissue is obtained at autopsy from a person who died of rabies. What procedures could be used to confirm the presence of rabies virus–infected cells in the brain tissue?
2. A cervical Papanicolaou smear is taken from a woman with a vaginal papilloma (wart). Certain types of papilloma have been associated with cervical carcinoma. What method or methods would be used to detect and identify the type of papilloma in the cervical smear?
3. A legal case would be settled by identification of the source of an HSV infection. Serum and viral isolates are obtained from the infected person and two contacts. What methods could be used to determine whether the person is infected with HSV-1 or HSV-2? What methods could be used to compare the type and strain of HSV obtained from each of the three people?
4. A 50-year-old man experiences flulike symptoms. The figure below shows results of hemagglutination inhibition (HI) tests on serum specimens collected when the disease manifested (*acute*) and 3 weeks later. The HI data for the current strain of influenza A (H3N2) are presented at top right. Filled circles indicate hemagglutination. Is the patient infected with the current strain of influenza A?

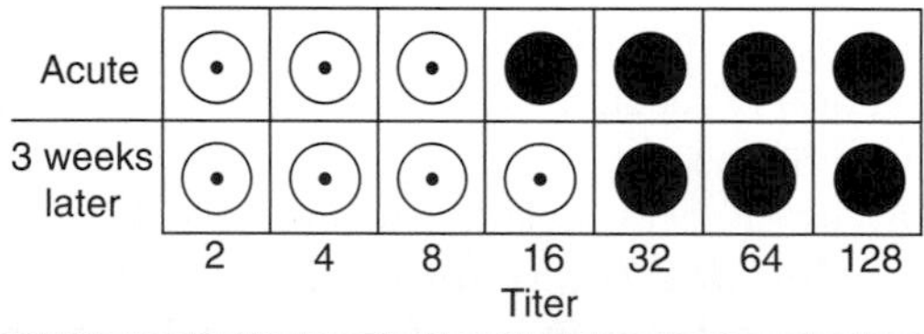

5. A policeman accidentally sticks his finger with a drug addict's syringe needle. He is concerned that he may be infected with HIV. Samples are taken from the policeman a month later for analysis. What assays would be appropriate to determine whether the man is infected with the virus? In this case it may be too early to detect an antibody response to the virus. What procedures would be appropriate to assay for virus or viral components?

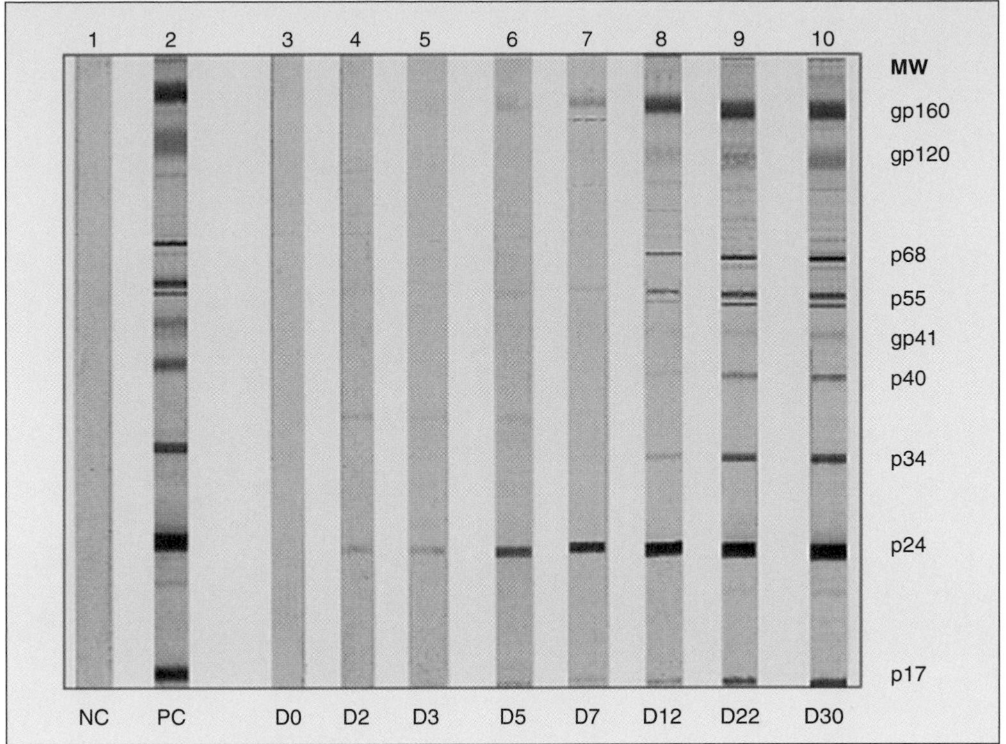

FIGURE 51–7. Western blot analysis of HIV antigens and antibody. HIV protein antigens are separated by electrophoresis and blotted onto nitrocellulose paper strips. The strip is incubated with patient antibody, washed to remove the unbound antibody, and then reacted with enzyme-conjugated antihuman antibody and chromophoric substrate. Serum from an HIV-infected person binds and identifies the major antigenic proteins of HIV. This data demonstrates the seroconversion of one HIV-infected individual with sera collected on day 0 (D0) to day 30 (D30) compared to a known positive control (PC) and negative control (NC). (From Kuritzkes DR: Diagnostic tests for HIV infection and resistance assays. In Cohen J, Powderly WG: *Infectious diseases,* ed 2, St Louis, 2004, Mosby.)

Bibliography

Cohen J, Powderly WG, editors: *Infectious diseases,* ed 2, St Louis, 2004, Mosby.

Flint SJ et al: *Principles of virology: Molecular biology, pathogenesis and control of animal viruses,* ed 2, Washington, 2003, American Society for Microbiology Press.

Forbes BA, Weissfeld AS, Sahm DF: *Baily and Scott's diagnostic microbiology,* ed 11, St Louis, 2002, Mosby.

Hsiung GD: *Diagnostic virology,* ed 3, New Haven, Conn, 1982, Yale.

Knipe DM, Howley PM, editors: *Fields virology,* ed 4, New York, 2001, Lippincott-Williams and Wilkins.

Lennette EH, editor: *Laboratory diagnosis of viral infections,* ed 3, New York, 1999, Marcel Dekker.

Menegus MA: Diagnostic virology. In Belshe RB, editor: *Textbook of human virology,* ed 2, St Louis, 1991, Mosby.

Specter S et al: *Clinical virology manual,* ed 3, Washington, 2000, ASM Press.

Strauss JM, Strauss EG: *Viruses and human disease,* San Diego, 2002, Academic Press.

Website

Viruses in cell culture: Available at www.uct.ac.za/depts/mmi/stannard/linda.html

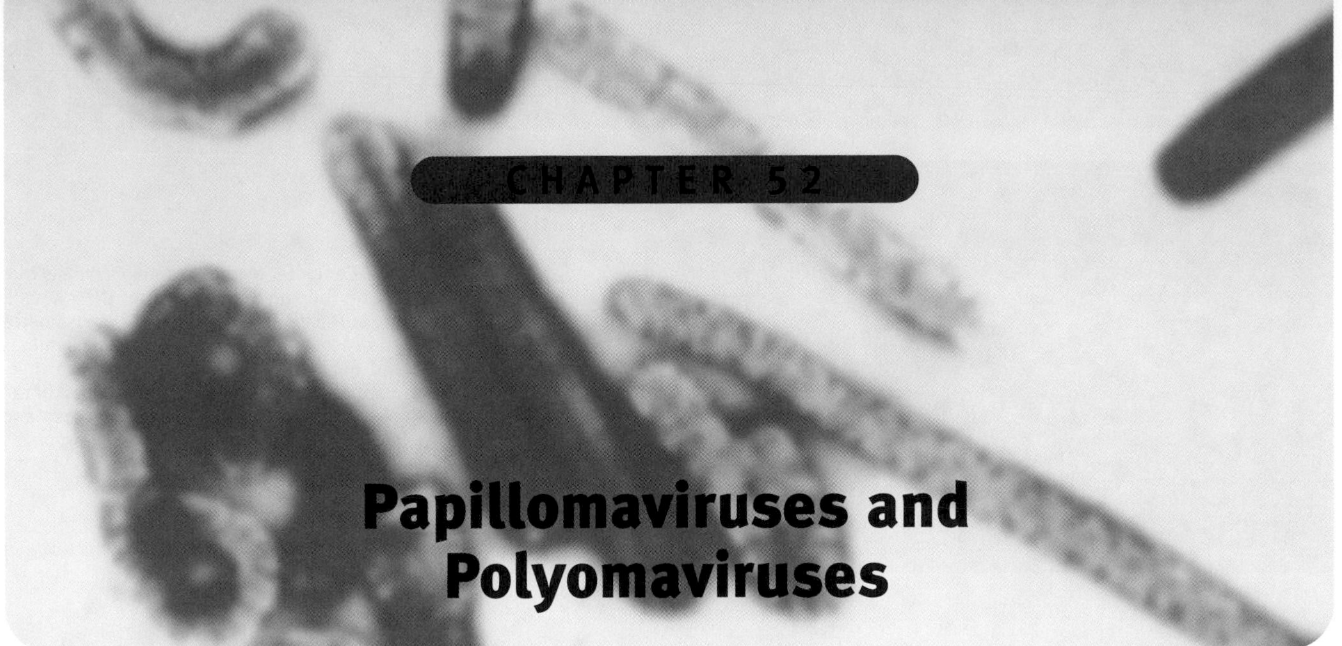

Papillomaviruses and Polyomaviruses

What used to be called the papovavirus family (Papovaviridae) has been divided into two families, Papillomaviridae and Polyomaviridae (Table 52–1). These viruses are capable of causing lytic, chronic, latent, and transforming infections, depending on the host cell. Human papillomaviruses (HPVs) cause **warts**, and several genotypes are associated with human cancer (e.g., **cervical carcinoma**). BK and JC viruses, members of the Polyomaviridae, usually cause asymptomatic infection but are associated with renal disease and **progressive multifocal leukoencephalopathy (PML)**, respectively, in immunosuppressed people. Simian virus 40 **(SV40)** is the prototype polyomavirus.

The papillomaviruses and polyomaviruses are small, nonenveloped, icosahedral capsid viruses with double-stranded circular deoxyribonucleic acid (DNA) genomes (Box 52–1). They encode proteins that promote cell growth. The promotion of cell growth facilitates lytic viral replication in a permissive cell type but *may oncogenically transform a cell that is nonpermissive.* The polyomaviruses, especially SV40, have been studied extensively as model oncogenic viruses.

Human Papillomaviruses

STRUCTURE AND REPLICATION

Classification of the HPVs is based on DNA sequence homology. At least 100 types have been identified and classified into 16 (A through P) groups. HPV can be distinguished further as **cutaneous HPV** or **mucosal HPV**, on the basis of the susceptible tissue. Within the mucosal HPV, there is a group associated with cervical cancer. Viruses in similar groups frequently cause similar types of warts.

The **icosahedral capsid** of HPV is 50 to 55 nm in diameter and consists of two structural proteins forming 72 capsomeres (Figure 52–1). The HPV genome is **circular** and has approximately 8000 base pairs. The HPV DNA encodes seven or eight early genes (E1 to E8), depending on the virus, and two late or structural genes (L1 and L2). An upstream regulatory region contains the control sequences for transcription, the shared *N*-terminal sequence for the early proteins, and the origin of replication. All the genes are located on one strand (the plus strand) (Figure 52–2).

HPV replication is controlled by the host cell's transcriptional machinery as determined by the differentiation of the skin or mucosal epithelium. The virus accesses the basal cell layer through breaks in the skin. The early genes of the virus stimulate cell growth, which facilitates replication of the viral genome by the host cell DNA polymerase when the cells divide. The virus–induced increase in cell number causes the basal and the prickle cell layer (stratum spinosum) to thicken (wart or papilloma). As the basal cell differentiates, the specific nuclear factors expressed in the different layers and types of skin and mucosa promote transcription of different viral genes. Expression of the viral genes correlates with the expression of specific keratins. The late genes encoding the structural proteins are expressed only in the terminally differentiated upper layer, and the virus assembles in the nucleus. Using the maturation of the skin cell, the virus works its way through the layers of the skin to be shed with the dead cells of the upper layer.

PATHOGENESIS

Papillomaviruses infect and replicate in the squamous epithelium of skin **(warts)** and mucous membranes **(genital, oral,** and **conjunctival papillomas)** to induce epithelial proliferation. The HPV types are very tissue spe-

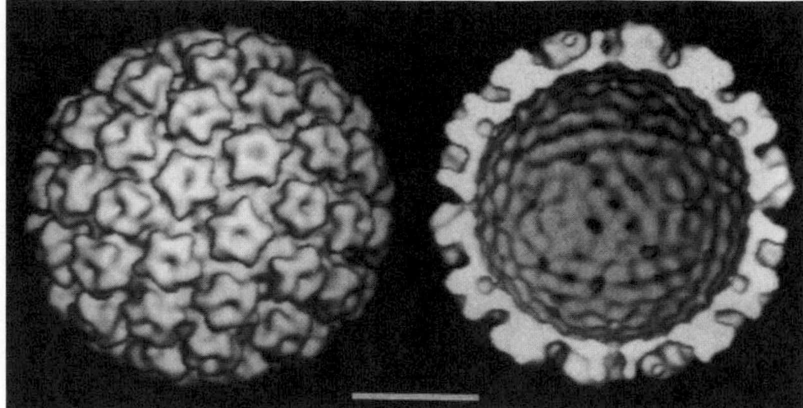

FIGURE 52–1. Computer reconstruction of cryoelectron micrographs of (human papillomavirus [HPV]). *Left,* View of the surface of HPV shows 72 capsomeres arranged in an icosadeltahedron. All the capsomeres (pentons and hexons) appear to form a regular five-point–star shape. *Right,* Computer cross-section of the capsid shows the interaction of the capsomeres and channels in the capsid. (From Baker TS et al: *Biophys J* 60:1445–1456, 1991.)

TABLE 52–1. Human Papillomaviruses and Polyomaviruses and Their Diseases

Virus	Disease
Papillomavirus	Warts
Polyomavirus	
BK virus	Renal disease*
JC virus	Progressive multifocal leukoencephalopathy*

*Disease occurs in immunosuppressed patients.

BOX 52–1. Unique Properties of Polyomaviruses and Papillomaviruses

Small icosahedral capsid virion.

Double-stranded circular DNA genome is replicated and assembled in the nucleus.

Papillomavirus: **HPV** types 1 to 58+ (as determined by genotype; types defined by DNA homology, tissue tropism, and association with oncogenesis).

Polyomavirus: SV40, **JC virus,** and **BK virus.**

Viruses have defined tissue tropisms determined by receptor interactions and the transcriptional machinery of the cell.

Viruses encode proteins that promote cell growth by binding to the cellular growth-suppressor proteins p53 and p105RB (p105 retinoblastoma gene product). Polyoma T antigen binds to p105RB and p53. **Papilloma E6 binds to p53, and E7 binds to p105RB.**

Viruses can cause lytic infections in permissive cells but cause abortive, persistent, or latent infections or **immortalize (transform)** nonpermissive cells.

cific, causing different disease presentations. The wart develops as a result of virus stimulation of cell growth and thickening of the basal and prickle layers (stratum spinosum), as well as the stratum granulosum. **Koilocytes,** characteristic of papillomavirus infection, are enlarged keratinocytes with clear haloes around shrunken nuclei. It usually takes 3 to 4 months for the wart to develop. The

Genome is a double-stranded circular molecule.

E1 protein binds DNA at ori and promotes viral DNA replication and has helicase activity (like T antigen of SV 40). E2 protein binds DNA, helps E1, and activates viral mRNA synthesis.

E5 oncoprotein that activates the EGF receptor to promote growth. E4 disrupts cytokeratins to promote release. E6 and E7 of HPV-16 and HPV-18 can become immortalizing genes; HPV-16 is associated with human cervical cancer.

L1 and L2 gene products are late structural (capsid) proteins.

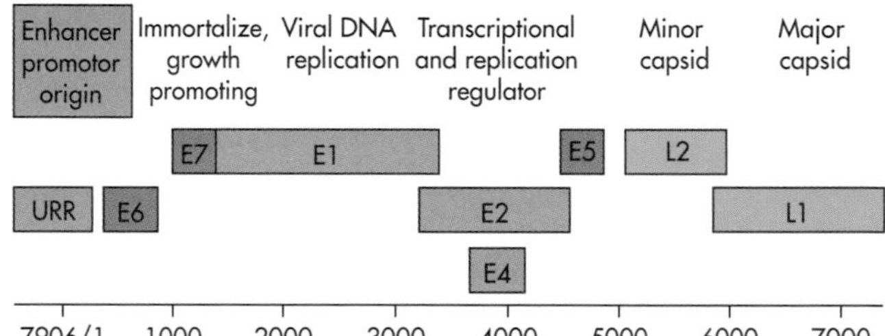

FIGURE 52–2. Genome of human papillomavirus type 16 (HPV-16). DNA is normally a double-stranded circular molecule, but it is shown here in a linear form. E6, Oncogene protein that binds p53 and promotes its degradation; E7, oncogene protein that binds p105RB (p105 retinoblastoma gene product); L1, major capsid protein; L2, minor capsid protein; rep ori, origin of replication; URR, upstream regulatory region. (Courtesy Tom Broker, Baltimore.)

viral infection remains local and generally regresses spontaneously but can recur (Figure 52–3). The HPV pathogenic mechanisms are summarized in Box 52–2.

Innate and cell-mediated immunity are important for control and resolution of HPV infections. HPV can suppress or hide from protective immune responses. In addition to very low levels of antigen expression (except in the "near-dead" terminally differentiated skin cell), the keratinocyte is an immunologically privileged site for

BOX 52–2. Disease Mechanisms of Papillomaviruses and Polyomaviruses

Papillomaviruses

Virus is acquired by **close contact** and infects the epithelial cells of the skin or mucous membranes.
Tissue tropism and disease presentation depend on the papillomavirus type.
Virus persists in the basal layer and then produces virus in terminally differentiated keratinocytes.
Viruses cause benign outgrowth of cells into **warts.**
HPV infection is hidden from immune responses and persists.
Warts resolve spontaneously, possibly as a result of immune response.
Certain types are associated with **dysplasia** that may become **cancerous** with the action of cofactors.
DNA of specific HPV types is present (integrated) in the tumor cell chromosomes.

Polyomaviruses (JC and BK Viruses)

Virus is probably acquired through the respiratory route and spread by viremia to the kidneys early in life.
Infections are **asymptomatic.**
Virus establishes **persistent** and **latent** infection in organs such as the kidneys and lungs.
In **immunocompromised** people, JC virus is activated, spreads to the brain, and causes progressive multifocal leukoencephalopathy **(PML),** a conventional slow virus disease.
In PML, JC virus partially transforms astrocytes and kills oligodendrocytes, causing characteristic lesions and sites of demyelination.
BK virus is ubiquitous but is not associated with serious disease.

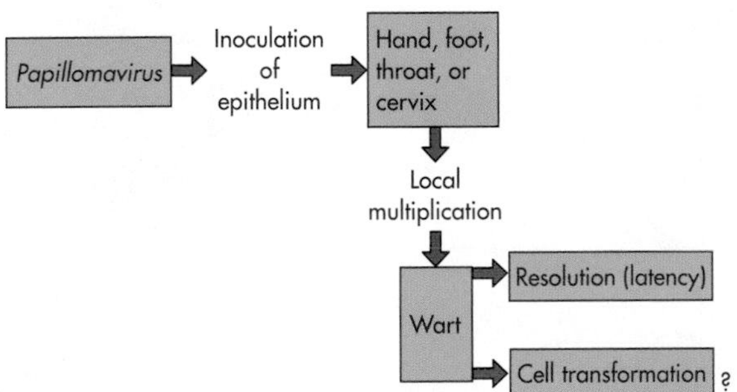

FIGURE 52–3. Progression of human papillomavirus infection.

replication. Inflammatory responses are required to activate protective cytolytic responses and promote resolution of warts. Immunosuppressed persons have recurrences and more severe presentations of papillomavirus and other papovavirus infections.

The oncogenic potential of HPV has been extensively studied. Viral DNA is found in benign and malignant tumors, especially mucosal papillomas. HPV-16 and HPV-18 cause cervical papillomas and dysplasia, and *at least 85% of cervical carcinomas contain integrated HPV-DNA.* Breaking of the circular genome within the E1 or E2 genes to promote integration often causes these genes to be inactivated, thereby preventing viral replication without preventing the expression of other HPV genes, including the E6 and E7 genes. The E6 and E7 proteins of HPV-16 and HPV-18 have been identified as **oncogenes** because they bind and inactivate the cellular growth–suppressor (transformation-suppressor) proteins, p53 and p105 retinoblastoma gene product (p105RB). E6 binds the p53 protein and targets it for degradation, and E7 binds and inactivates p105RB. Without these brakes on cell growth, the cell is more susceptible to mutation, chromosomal aberrations, or the action of a cofactor and thereby develops into cancer.

BOX 52–3. Epidemiology of Polyomaviruses–and Papillomaviruses

Disease/Viral Factors

Capsid virus is resistant to inactivation.
Virus persists in host.
Asymptomatic shedding is likely.

Transmission

Papillomavirus: **Direct contact, sexual contact** (sexually transmitted disease) for certain virus types, or passage through infected birth canal for laryngeal papillomas (types 6 and 11).
Polyomavirus: Inhalation of infectious aerosols.

Who Is at Risk?

Papillomavirus: Warts are common; sexually active people are at risk for infection with HPV types correlated with oral and genital cancers.
Polyomavirus: Ubiquitous; immunocompromised people at risk for progressive multifocal leukoencephalopathy.

Geography/Season

Viruses are found worldwide.
There is no seasonal incidence.

Modes of Control

There are no modes of control.

EPIDEMIOLOGY

HPV resists inactivation and can be transmitted on fomites, such as the surfaces of countertops or furniture, bathroom floors, and towels (Box 52–3). Asymptomatic shedding may promote transmission. HPV infection is acquired (1) by direct contact through small breaks in the skin or mucosa, (2) during sexual intercourse, or (3) while an infant is passing through an infected birth canal.

Common, plantar, and flat warts are most common in children and young adults. Laryngeal papillomas occur in young children and middle-aged adults.

Human papillomavirus is possibly the most prevalent sexually transmitted infection in the world, with certain HPV types common among sexually active people. At least 20 million people in the United States are infected with HPV, with approximately 5.5 million new genital cases per year. HPV is present in 99.7% of all cervical cancers. HPV-16, HPV-18, HPV-31, and HPV-45 are high-risk and HPV-6 and HPV-11 are low-risk HPV types for cervical carcinoma, the second leading cause of cancer death in women (approximately 12,200 cases and 4100 deaths per year in the United States). Approximately 5% of all Pap smears contain HPV-infected cells. Approximately 10% of women infected with the high-risk HPV types will develop cervical **dysplasia,** a precancerous state. Multiple sexual partners, smoking, a family history of cervical cancer, and immunosuppresion are the major risk factors for infection and progression to cancer.

CLINICAL SYNDROMES

The clinical syndromes and the HPV types that cause them are summarized in Table 52–2.

TABLE 52–2. Clinical Syndromes Associated with Papillomaviruses

Syndrome	HPV Types	
	Common	Uncommon
Cutaneous Syndromes		
Skin warts		
Plantar wart	1	2, 4
Common wart	2, 4	1, 7, 26, 29
Flat wart	3, 10	27, 28, 41
Epidermodysplasia verruciformis	5, 8, 17, 20, 36	9, 12, 14, 15, 19, 21-25, 38, 46
Mucosal Syndromes		
Benign head and neck tumors		
Laryngeal papilloma	6, 11	—
Oral papilloma	6, 11	2, 16
Conjunctival papilloma	11	—
Anogenital warts		
Condyloma acuminatum	6, 11	1, 2, 10, 16, 30, 44, 45
Cervical intraepithelial neoplasia, cancer	16, 18	11, 31, 33, 35, 42–44

Modified from Balows A et al: *Laboratory diagnosis of infectious diseases: Principles and practice,* vol 2, New York, 1988, Springer-Verlag.

Warts

A **wart** is a benign, self–limited proliferation of skin that regresses with time. Most people with HPV infection have the common types of the virus (HPV-1 through HPV-4), which infect keratinized surfaces, usually on the hands and feet (Figure 52–4). Initial infection occurs in childhood or early adolescence. The incubation period before a wart develops may be as long as 3 to 4 months. The appearance of the wart (dome shaped, flat, or plantar) depends on the HPV type and the infected site.

Benign Head and Neck Tumors

Single oral papillomas are the most benign epithelial tumors of the oral cavity. They are pedunculated with a fibrovascular stalk, and their surface usually has a rough, papillary appearance. They can occur in people of any age group, are usually solitary, and rarely recur after surgical excision. **Laryngeal papillomas** are commonly associated with HPV-6 and HPV-11 and are the most common benign epithelial tumors of the larynx. Laryngeal papillomatosis can be life threatening in children because the papillomas may obstruct the airway. Occasionally,

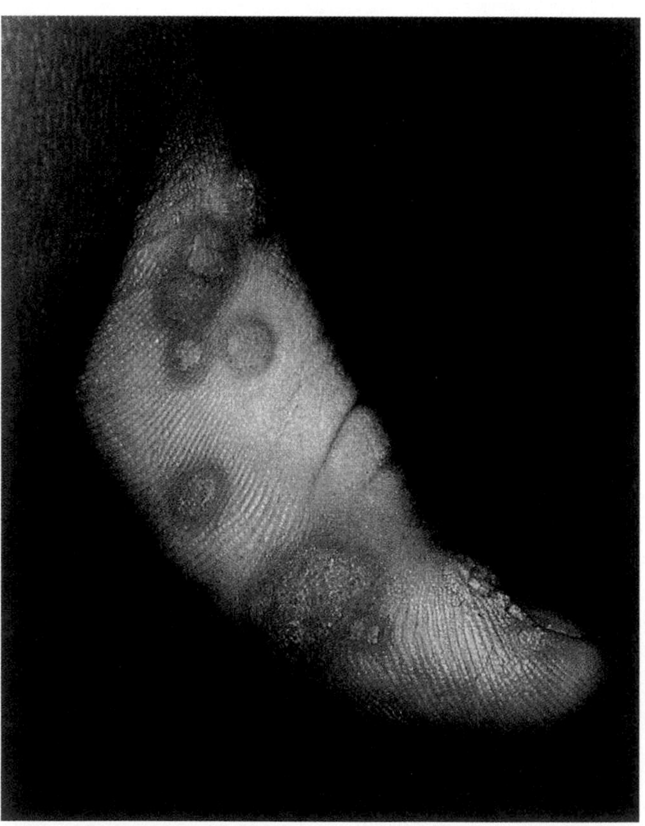

FIGURE 52–4. Common warts with thrombosed vessels *(black dots).* (From Habif TP: *Clinical dermatology: A color guide to diagnosis and therapy,* St Louis, 1985, Mosby.)

papillomas may be found further down in the trachea and into the bronchi.

Anogenital Warts

Genital warts **(condylomata acuminata)** occur almost exclusively on the squamous epithelium of the external genitalia and perianal areas. Approximately 90% are caused by HPV-6 and HPV-11. Anogenital lesions infected with these types of HPV rarely become malignant in otherwise healthy people.

Cervical Dysplasia and Neoplasia

HPV infection of the genital tract is now recognized as a common sexually transmitted disease. Infection is usually asymptomatic but may result in slight itching. Genital warts may appear like soft, flesh-colored warts that are flat, raised, and sometimes cauliflower shaped. The warts can appear within weeks or months of sexual contact with an infected person. Cytologic changes indicating HPV infection **(koilocytotic cells)** are detected in **Papanicolaou-stained cervical smears** (Pap smears) (Figure 52–5). Infection of the female genital tract by HPV types 16, 18, 31, and 45 and, rarely, by other types of HPV, is associated with intraepithelial cervical neoplasia and cancer. The first neoplastic changes noted on light microscopy are termed **dysplasia.** Approximately 40% to 70% of the mild dysplasias spontaneously regress.

Cervical cancer is thought to develop through a continuum of progressive cellular changes, from mild (cervical intraepithelial neoplasia [CIN I]) to moderate neoplasia (CIN II) to severe neoplasia or carcinoma in situ. This sequence of events can occur over 1 to 4 years. Routine and regular Pap smears can prevent or promote early treatment and cure of cervical cancer.

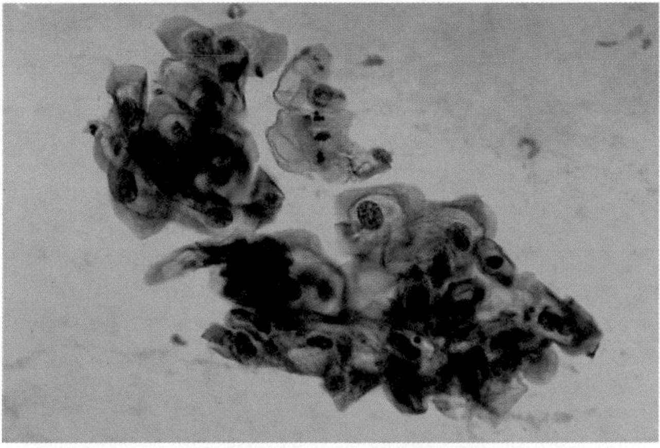

FIGURE 52–5. Papanicolaou stain of the exfoliated cervicovaginal squamous epithelial cells showing the perinuclear cytoplasmic vacuolization, termed *koilocytosis* (vacuolated cytoplasm), which is characteristic of human papillomavirus infection. (400× magnification)

LABORATORY DIAGNOSIS

A wart can be confirmed microscopically on the basis of its characteristic histologic appearance, which consists of hyperplasia of the **prickle cells** and an excess production of keratin **(hyperkeratosis)** (Figure 52–6). Papillomavirus infection can be detected in Pap smears by the presence of koilocytotic (vacuolated cytoplasm) squamous epithelial cells, which are rounded and occur in clumps (Table 52–3; see Figure 52–5). **DNA molecular probes** and the **polymerase chain reaction (PCR)** from cervical swabs and tissue specimens are the methods of choice for establishing the diagnosis and typing of the HPV infection. Papillomaviruses do not grow in cell cultures, and tests for HPV antibodies are rarely used except in research surveys.

TREATMENT, PREVENTION, AND CONTROL

Warts spontaneously regress, but the regression may take many months to years. Warts are removed because of pain and discomfort, for cosmetic reasons, and to prevent spread to other parts of the body or to other people. They are removed through the use of surgical cryotherapy, electrocautery, or chemical means (e.g., 10% to 25% solution of podophilin), although recurrences are common. Surgery may be necessary for the removal of laryngeal papillomas.

Stimulators of innate and inflammatory responses, such as **imiquimod** (Aldara), **interferon,** and even stripping off duct tape, can promote more rapid healing. Topical or intralesional delivery of **cidofovir** can treat warts by selectively killing the HPV–infected cells. A new HPV vaccine consisting of the capsid protein assembled

TABLE 52–3. Laboratory Diagnosis of Papillomavirus Infections

Test	Detects
Cytology	Koilocytotic cells
In situ DNA probe analysis*	Viral nucleic acid
Polymerase chain reaction*	Viral nucleic acid
Southern blot hybridization	Viral nucleic acid
Immunofluorescent and immunoperoxidase staining	Viral structural antigens
Electron microscopy	Virus
Culture	Not useful

*Method of choice.

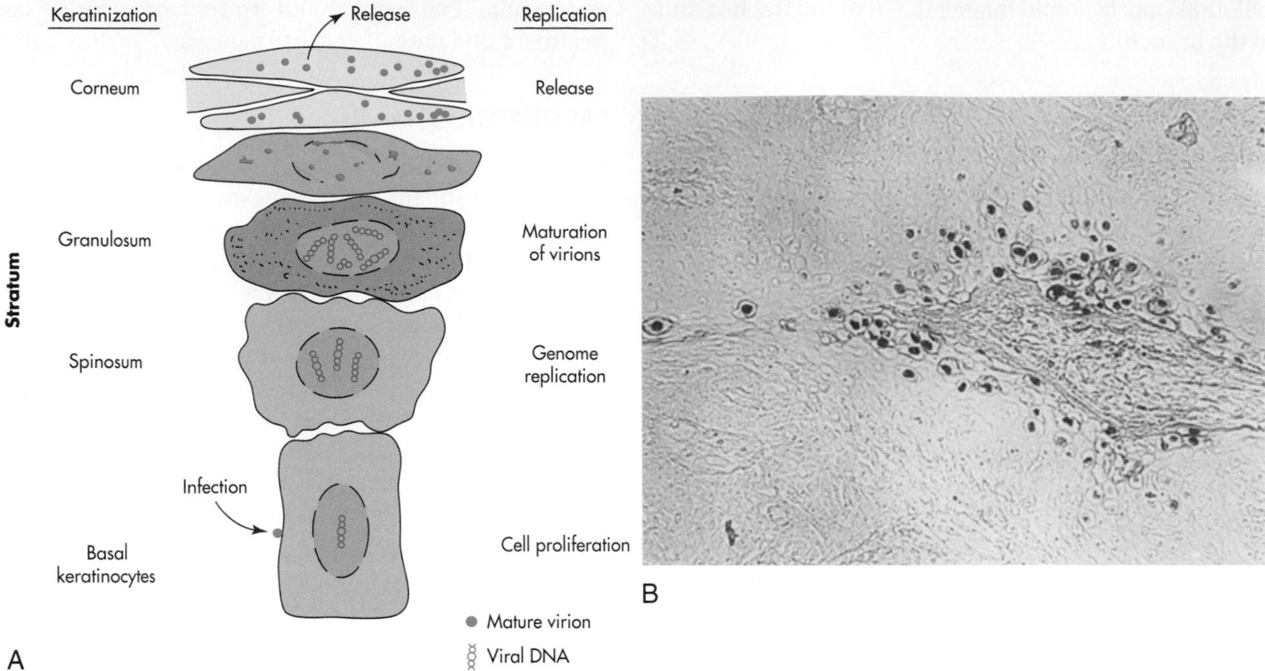

FIGURE 52–6. A, Comparison of normal skin and a papilloma (wart). Human papillomavirus (HPV) infection promotes the outgrowth of the basal layer, increasing the number of prickle cells (acanthosis). These changes cause the skin to thicken and promote the production of keratin (hyperkeratosis), thereby causing epithelial spikes to form (papillomatosis). Virus is produced in the granular cells close to the final keratin layer. **B,** DNA probe analysis of an HPV-6–induced anogenital condyloma. A biotin-labeled DNA probe was localized by horseradish peroxidase–conjugated avidin conversion of a substrate to a chromogen precipitate. Dark staining is seen over the nuclei of koilocytotic cells. (**B** from Belshe RB, editor: *Textbook of human virology,* ed 2, St Louis, 1991, Mosby.)

into virus–like particles has promise for preventing infection. The vaccine would be administered to presexually active girls.

At present, the best way to prevent transmission of warts is to avoid coming in direct contact with infected tissue. Proper precautions (e.g., the use of condoms) can prevent the sexual transmission of HPV.

BOX 52–4. Polyomavirus Proteins

Early

Large T: Regulation of early and late messenger RNA transcription; DNA replication; cell growth promotion and transformation
Small t: Viral DNA replication

Late

VP1: Major capsid protein and viral attachment protein
VP2: Minor capsid protein
VP3: Minor capsid protein

Polyomaviridae

The human polyomaviruses (**BK** and **JC viruses**) are ubiquitous but usually do not cause disease. They are difficult to grow in cell culture. SV40, a simian polyomavirus, and murine polyomaviruses in particular have been studied extensively as models of tumor–causing viruses but have not been associated with any human disease.

STRUCTURE AND REPLICATION

The polyomaviruses are smaller (45 nm in diameter), contain less nucleic acid (5000 base pairs), and are less complex than the papillomaviruses (see Box 52–1). The genomes of BK virus, JC virus, and SV40 are closely related and are divided into early, late, and noncoding regions (Figure 52–7). The early region on one-strand codes for nonstructural **T (transformation) proteins** (including **large T and small t antigens**), and the late region, which is on the other strand, codes for **three viral capsid proteins (VP1, VP2,** and **VP3)** (Box 52–4). The noncoding region contains the origin of DNA replication and transcriptional control sequences for both early and late genes.

After the virus enters a cell, the DNA is uncoated and delivered to the nucleus. The early genes encode the large T and small t antigens, proteins that promote cell growth. Viral replication requires the transcriptional and DNA replication machinery provided by a growing cell. The

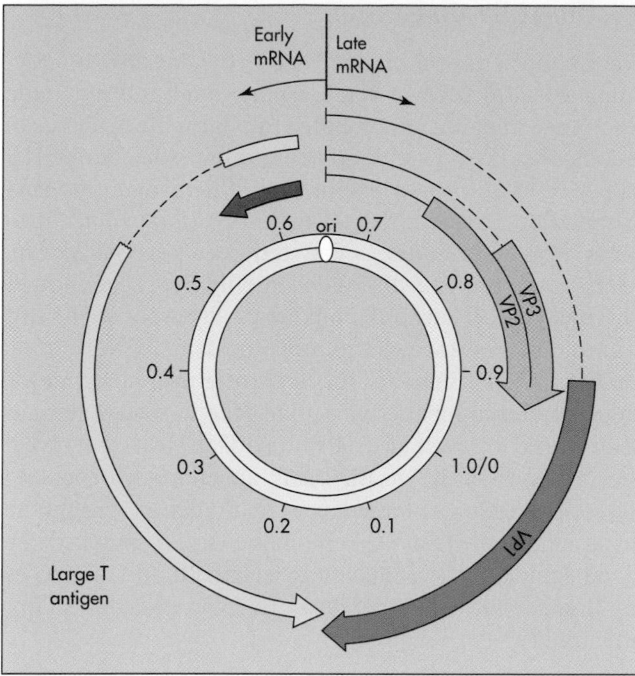

FIGURE 52–7. Genome of the SV40 virus. The genome is a prototype of other polyomaviruses and contains early, late, and noncoding regions. The noncoding region contains the start sequence for the early and late genes and for DNA replication *(ori)*. The individual early and late messenger RNAs are processed from the larger nested transcripts. (Redrawn from Butel JS, Jarvis DL: *Biochem Biophys Acta* 865:171–195, 1986.)

large T antigens of SV40 and BK and JC viruses have several functions. For example, the T antigen of SV40 binds to DNA and controls early and late gene transcription, as well as viral DNA replication. In addition, the T antigen binds to and inactivates the two major cellular growth–suppressor proteins, p53 and p105RB, promoting cell growth.

Like replication of the HPVs, replication of polyomavirus is highly dependent on host cell factors. Permissive cells allow the transcription of late viral messenger ribonucleic acid (mRNA) and viral replication, which results in cell death. Some nonpermissive cells, however, allow only the early genes, including T antigen, to be expressed, promoting cell growth and potentially leading to oncogenic transformation of the cell.

The polyomavirus genome is used very efficiently. The noncoding region of the genome contains the initiation sites for the early and late mRNAs and the origin of DNA replication. The three late proteins are produced from mRNAs, which have the same initiation site, and then are processed into three unique mRNAs.

The circular viral DNA is maintained and replicated bidirectionally, similar to the way in which a bacterial plasmid is maintained and replicated. DNA replication precedes late mRNA transcription and protein synthesis. The virus is assembled in the nucleus, and virus is released by cell lysis.

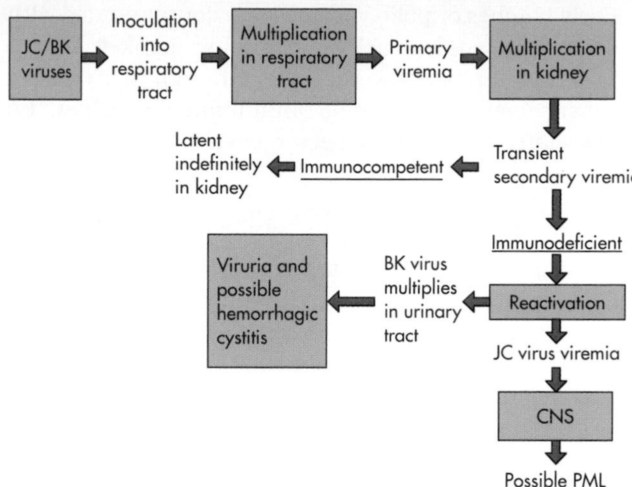

FIGURE 52–8. Mechanisms of spread of polyomaviruses within the body. PML, Progressive multifocal leukoencephalopathy.

PATHOGENESIS

Each polyomavirus is limited to specific hosts and cell types within that host. For example, JC and BK viruses are human viruses that probably enter the respiratory tract, after which they infect lymphocytes and then the kidney with a minimal cytopathologic effect. The BK virus establishes latent infection in the kidney, and the JC virus establishes infection in the kidneys, in B cells, and in monocyte-lineage cells. Replication is blocked in immunocompetent persons.

In immunocompromised patients, such as those with the acquired immune deficiency syndrome (AIDS), reactivation of the virus in the kidney leads to viral shedding in the urine and potentially severe urinary tract infections (BK virus) or viremia and central nervous system infection (JC virus) (Figure 52–8). JC virus crosses the blood–brain barrier by replicating in the endothelial cells of capillaries. An abortive infection of astrocytes results in partial transformation, yielding enlarged cells with abnormal nuclei resembling glioblastomas. Productive lytic infections of oligodendrocytes cause demyelination (see Box 52–3). Although SV40 and BK and JC viruses can cause tumors in hamsters, these viruses are not associated with any human tumors.

EPIDEMIOLOGY

Polyomavirus infections are ubiquitous, and most people are infected with both the JC and BK viruses by the age of 15 years (see Box 52–3). Respiratory transmission is the probable mode of spread. Latent infections can be reactivated in people whose immune systems are suppressed as a result of AIDS, organ transplantation, or pregnancy. Approximately 10% of people with AIDS develop PML, and the disease is fatal in approximately 90% of all cases.

Early batches of polio vaccine were contaminated with SV40 that was undetected in the primary monkey cell cultures used to prepare the vaccine. Although many people were vaccinated with the contaminated vaccines, no SV40-related tumors have been reported.

CLINICAL SYNDROMES (BOX 52–5)

Primary infection is almost always asymptomatic. The BK and JC viruses are activated in immunocompromised patients, as indicated by the presence of virus in the urine of as many as 40% of these patients. The viruses are also reactivated during pregnancy, but no effects on the fetus have been noted.

The ureteral stenosis observed in renal transplant recipients appears to be associated with BK virus, as is the hemorrhagic cystitis observed in bone marrow transplant recipients. PML is a subacute demyelinating disease caused by the **JC virus** that occurs in immunocompromised patients, including those with AIDS. Although rare, PML's incidence is increasing because of the increased numbers of people with AIDS. As the name implies, patients may have multiple neurologic symptoms unattributable to a single anatomic lesion. Speech, vision, coordination, mentation, or a combination of these functions is impaired, followed by paralysis of the arms and legs and, finally, death. People who are diagnosed with PML live 1 to 4 months, and most die within 2 years.

LABORATORY DIAGNOSIS

The diagnosis of PML is confirmed by the presence of PCR-amplified viral DNA in cerebrospinal fluid and magnetic resonance imaging or computed tomographic evidence of lesions. Histologic examination of brain tissue obtained by biopsy or at autopsy will show foci of demyelination surrounded by oligodendrocytes with inclusions adjacent to areas of demyelination. The term *leukoencephalopathy* refers to the presence of lesions in only the white matter. There is little, if any, inflammatory cell response. In situ immunofluorescence, immunoperoxidase, DNA probe analysis, and PCR analysis of cerebrospinal fluid, urine, or biopsy material for the particular genetic sequences can also be used to detect virus. Urine cytologic tests can reveal the presence of JC or BK virus infection by revealing the existence of enlarged cells with dense, basophilic intranuclear inclusions resembling those induced by cytomegalovirus. It is difficult to isolate BK and JC viruses in tissue cultures; therefore this procedure is not attempted.

TREATMENT, PREVENTION, AND CONTROL

No specific treatment for polyomavirus infection is available, other than to decrease the immunosuppression responsible for allowing the polyomavirus to be reactivated and symptoms to occur. The ubiquitous nature of polyomaviruses and the lack of understanding of their modes of transmission make it unlikely that the primary infection can be prevented.

BOX 52–5. Clinical Summaries

Wart: A 22-year-old patient develops a conical, flesh-colored, hard, scaly round area (papule) over the index finger. It has a rough surface and is nontender. Otherwise the patient is healthy and has no other complaints. The wart was treated topically on a daily basis with salicylic acid to kill the cells harboring the virus and remove the wart.

Cervical papilloma: On cervical examination, a large, flat papule was observed that turned white with application of 4% acetic acid. The Pap smear from this 25-year-old sexually active woman had koilocytotic cells.

Cervical carcinoma: A 32-year-old woman presents for her routine Pap smear, which shows evidence of abnormal cells. A biopsy shows squamous cell carcinoma. PCR analysis of cellular DNA yields HPV-16 DNA.

Progressive multifocal leukoencephalopathy: A 42-year-old AIDS patient has become forgetful and has difficulty speaking, seeing, and keeping his balance, which is suggestive of lesions in many sites in the brain. The condition progresses to paralysis and death. Autopsy shows foci of demyelination with oligodendrocytes containing inclusion bodies only in the white matter.

PCR, Polymerase chain reaction.

CASE STUDY AND QUESTIONS

A 25-year-old carpenter notices the appearance of several hyperkeratotic papules (warts) on the palm side of his index finger. They do not change in size and cause him only minimal discomfort. After a year, they spontaneously disappear.

1. Will this virus infection spread to other body sites?
2. After its disappearance, is the infection likely to be completely resolved or to persist in the host?
3. What viral, cellular, and host conditions regulate the replication of this virus and other HPVs?
4. How would the papillomavirus type causing this infection be identified?
5. Is it likely that this type of HPV is associated with human cancer? If not, which types are associated with cancers, and which cancers are they?

Bibliography

Arthur RR et al: Association of BK viruria with hemorrhagic cystitis in recipients of bone marrow transplants, *N Engl J Med* 315:230-234, 1986.

Cohen J, Powderly WG, editors: *Infectious diseases*, ed 2, St Louis, 2004, Mosby.

Crum CP, Barber S, Roche JK: Pathobiology of papillomavirus-related cervical diseases, *Clin Microbiol Rev* 4:270-285, 1991.

Flint SJ et al: *Principles of virology: Molecular biology, pathogenesis and control of animal viruses*, ed 2, Washington, 2003, American Society for Microbiology Press.

Frazer IH et al: Potential strategies utilised by papillomavirus to evade host immunity, *Immunol Rev* 168:131-42, 1999.

Gorbach SL, Bartlett JG, Blacklow NR, editors: *Infectious diseases*, ed 2, Philadelphia, 1997, WB Saunders.

Howley PM: Role of the human papillomaviruses in human cancer, *Cancer Res* 51(suppl 18):5019S-5022S, 1991.

Hseuh C, Reyes CV: Progressive multifocal leukoencephalopathy, *Am Fam Physician* 37:129-132, 1988.

Knipe DM, Howley PM, editors: *Fields virology*, ed 4, New York, 2001, Lippincott–Williams and Wilkins.

Major EO et al: Pathogenesis and molecular biology of progressive multifocal leukoencephalopathy, *Clin Microbiol Rev* 5:49-73, 1992.

Mandell GL, Bennet JE, Dolin R, editors: *Principles and practice of infectious diseases*, ed 6, Philadelphia, 2004, Churchill Livingstone

Miller DM, Brodell RT: Human papillomavirus infection: Treatment options for warts, *Am Fam Physician* 53:135-143, 1996.

Morrison EA: Natural history of cervical infection with human papillomavirus, *Clin Infect Dis* 18:172-180, 1994.

Strauss JM, Strauss EG: *Viruses and human disease*, San Diego, 2002, Academic Press.

White DO, Fenner FJ: *Medical virology*, ed 4, New York, 1994, Academic Press.

zür–Hausen H: Viruses in human cancers, *Science* 254:1167-1173, 1991.

zür–Hausen H: Human pathogenic papillomaviruses, *Curr Top Microbiol Immunol* 186:1-274, 1994.

Websites

Human papillomavirus: Centers for Disease Control and Prevention, Division of Sexually Transmitted Diseases: Available at www.cdc.gov/std/HPV/

Papillomavirus: NIAID fact sheet: Available at www.niaid.nih.gov/factsheets/stdhpv.htm

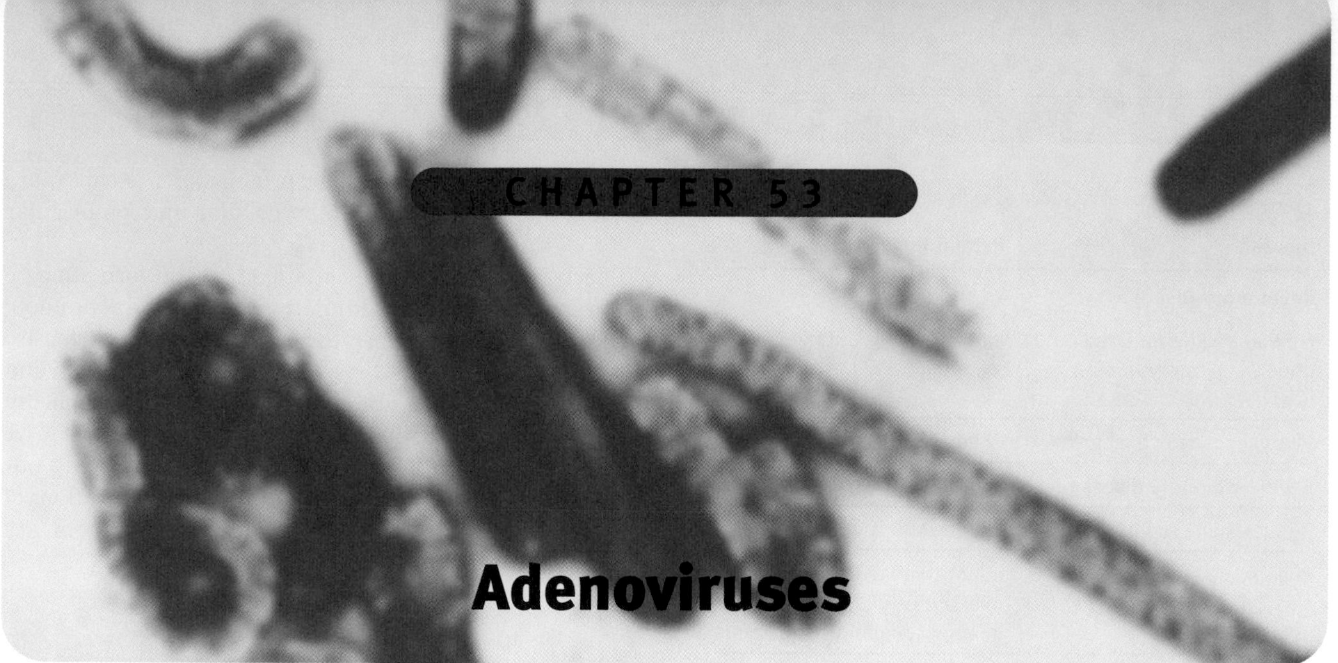

Adenoviruses

Adenoviruses were first isolated in 1953 in a human adenoid cell culture. Since then, approximately 100 serotypes have been recognized, at least 47 of which infect humans. All human serotypes are included in a single genus within the family Adenoviridae. On the basis of the findings from deoxyribonucleic acid (DNA) homology studies and the hemagglutination patterns, all of the 49 serotypes have been classified into six subgroups (A through F) (Table 53–1). The viruses in each subgroup share many properties.

The first human adenoviruses to be identified, numbered 1 to 7, are the most common. Common disorders caused by the adenoviruses include **respiratory tract infection, conjunctivitis (pinkeye), hemorrhagic cystitis,** and **gastroenteritis.** Several adenoviruses have oncogenic potential in animals and for this reason have been extensively studied by molecular biologists. These studies have elucidated many viral and eukaryotic cellular processes. For example, analysis of the gene for the adenovirus hexon protein led to the discovery of introns and the splicing of eukaryotic messenger ribonucleic acid (mRNA). Adenovirus is also being used to deliver DNA for gene replacement therapy (e.g., cystic fibrosis).

Structure and Replication

Adenoviruses are double-stranded DNA viruses with a genome of approximately 36,000 base pairs, large enough to encode 30 to 40 genes. The adenovirus genome is a **linear, double-stranded DNA** with a **terminal protein** (molecular mass, 55 kDa) covalently attached at each 5′ end. The virions are **nonenveloped icosadeltahedrons** with a diameter of 70 to 90 nm (Figure 53–1 and Box 53–1). The capsid comprises 240 capsomeres, which consist of hexons and pentons. The 12 pentons, which are located at each of the vertices, have a penton base and a fiber. The **fiber** contains the **viral attachment proteins** and can act as a hemagglutinin. The penton base and fiber are toxic to cells. The pentons and fibers also carry type-specific antigens.

The core complex within the capsid includes viral DNA and at least two major proteins. There are at least 11 polypeptides in the adenovirus virion, nine of which have an identified structural function (Table 53–2).

A map of the adenovirus genome shows the locations of the viral genes (Figure 53–2). The genes are transcribed from both DNA strands and in both directions at different times during the replication cycle. Genes for related functions are clustered together. Most of the RNA transcribed from the adenovirus genome is processed into several individual mRNAs in the nucleus. Early proteins promote cell growth and include a **DNA polymerase** that is involved in the replication of the genome. Adenovirus also encodes proteins that suppress host immune and inflammatory responses. Late proteins, which are synthesized after the onset of viral DNA replication, are primarily components of the capsid.

The replication of adenoviruses has been studied extensively in HeLa cell cultures. One virus cycle takes approximately 32 to 36 hours and produces 10,000 virions. Adenovirus binding to the cell surface occurs in two steps. The viral fiber proteins interact with a glycoprotein member of the immunoglobulin superfamily of proteins (approximately 100,000 fiber receptors are present on each cell). This same receptor is used by many Coxsackie B viruses, which give it the name, Coxsackie adenovirus receptor. Some adenoviruses use the class I major histocompatibility complex (MHC I) molecule as a receptor. Then the penton base interacts with an α_v integrin to promote internalization by receptor-mediated endocytosis in a clathrin-coated vesicle. The virus lyses the endosomal vesicle, and the capsid delivers the DNA genome to the

TABLE 53–1. Illnesses Associated with Adenoviruses

Disease	Patient Population
Respiratory Diseases	
Febrile, undifferentiated upper respiratory tract infection	Infants, young children
Pharyngoconjunctival fever	Children, adults
Acute respiratory disease	Military recruits
Pertussis-like syndrome	Infants, young children
Pneumonia	Infants, young children; military recruits; immunocompromised patients
Other Diseases	
Acute hemorrhagic cystitis	Children; bone marrow transplant recipients
Epidemic keratoconjunctivitis	Any age; renal transplant recipients
Gastroenteritis	Infants, young children
Hepatitis	Liver transplant recipients; other immunocompromised patients
Meningoencephalitis	Children; immunocompromised patients

nucleus. The penton and fiber proteins of the capsid are toxic to the cell and can inhibit cellular macromolecular synthesis.

Early transcriptional events lead to the formation of gene products that can stimulate cell growth and promote viral DNA replication. As is the case for the papovaviruses, several adenovirus mRNAs use the same promoter and initial sequences but are produced through the splicing out of different introns. Transcription of the early E1 gene, processing of the primary transcript (splicing out of introns to yield three mRNAs), and translation of the immediate early **E1A transactivator** protein are

BOX 53–1. Unique Features of Adenovirus

Naked icosadeltahedral capsid has **fibers** (viral attachment proteins) at vertices.

Linear double-stranded genome has 5′ terminal proteins.

Synthesis of viral DNA polymerase activates switch from early to late genes.

Virus encodes proteins to promote messenger RNA and DNA synthesis, including its own **DNA polymerase.**

Human adenoviruses are grouped A through F by DNA homologies and by serotype (more than 42 types).

Serotype is mainly a result of differences in the penton base and fiber protein, which determine the nature of tissue tropism and disease.

Virus causes **lytic, persistent,** and **latent** infections in humans, and some strains can **immortalize certain animal cells.**

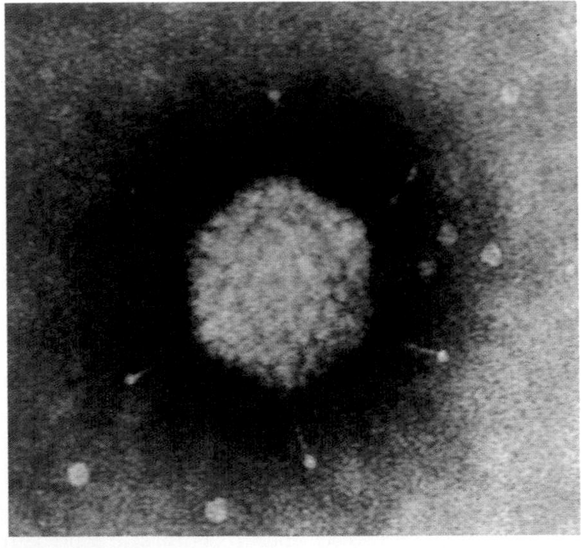

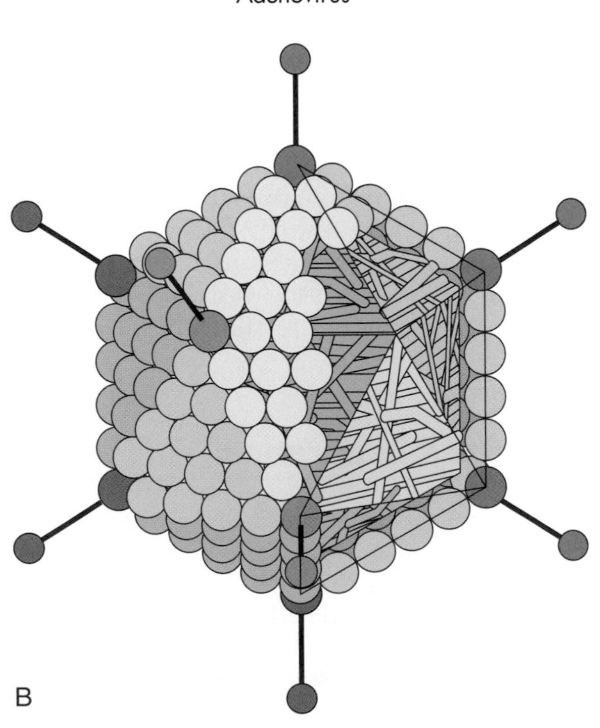

FIGURE 53–1. **A,** Electron micrograph of adenovirus virion with fibers. **B,** Model of adenovirus virion with fibers. (**A** from Valentine RC, Pereira HG: *J Mol Biol* 13:13–20, 1965; **B** from Armstrong D, Cohen J: *Infectious diseases,* St Louis, 1999, Mosby.)

TABLE 53–2. Major Adenovirus Proteins

Gene	Number	Molecular Mass (kDa₂)	Function
E1A*			Activates viral gene transcription Binds cellular growth suppressor: p105RB promotes transformation Deregulates cell growth Inhibits activation of interferon response elements
E1B			Binds cellular growth suppressor: p53 promotes transformation Blocks apoptosis
E2			Activates some promoters Terminal protein on DNA DNA polymerase
E3			Prevents tumor necrosis factor-α (TFN-α) inflammation
E4			Limits viral cytopathologic effect
VA RNAs			Inhibit interferon response
Capsid			
	II	120	Contains family antigen and some serotyping antigens
	III	85	Penton base protein Toxic to tissue culture cells
	IV	62	Fiber Responsible for attachment and hemagglutination; contains some serotyping antigens
	VI	24	Hexon-associated proteins
	VIII	13	Penton-associated proteins
	IX	12	
	IIIa	66	
Core			
	V	48	Core protein 1: DNA-binding protein
	VII	18	Core protein 2: DNA-binding protein

E, Early; RB, retinoblastoma gene product; VA, virus associated.
*Early genes encode several messenger RNA and proteins by alternative splicing patterns.

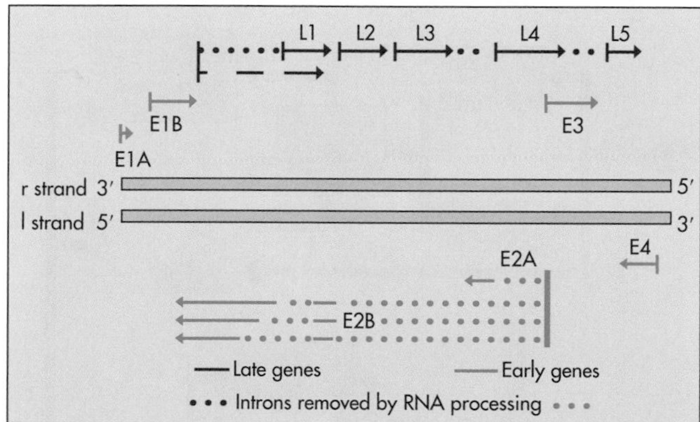

FIGURE 53–2. Simplified genome map of adenovirus type 2. Genes are transcribed from both strands (l and r) in opposite directions. The early genomes are transcribed from four promoter sequences and generate several messenger RNAs. Alternative splicing patterns of primary RNA transcripts produce the full repertoire of viral proteins. The splicing pattern for only the E2 transcript is shown as an example. All of the late genes are transcribed from one promoter sequence. E, Early protein; L, late protein. (Modified from Jawetz E et al, editors: *Review of medical microbiology,* ed 17, Norwalk, Conn, 1987, Appleton & Lange.)

required for transcription of the early proteins. The early proteins include more DNA-binding proteins, the DNA polymerase, and proteins to help the virus escape the immune response. The **E1A** protein is also an oncogene, and together with the **E1B** protein, can stimulate cell growth by binding to the cellular growth–suppressor proteins **p105RB** (p105RB retinoblastoma gene product) (E1A) and **p53** (E1B). In permissive cells, stimulation of cell division facilitates transcription and replication of the genome with cell death resulting from virus replication. In nonpermissive cells, the virus establishes latency and the genome remains in the nucleus. For rodent cells, the E1A and E1B may promote cell growth without cell death and therefore oncogenically transform the cell.

Viral DNA replication occurs in the nucleus and is mediated by the viral encoded DNA polymerase. The polymerase uses the 55-kDa viral protein (terminal protein) with an attached cytosine monophosphate as a primer to replicate both strands of the DNA. The terminal protein remains attached to the DNA.

Late gene transcription starts after DNA replication. Most of the individual late mRNAs are generated from a large (83% of the genome) primary RNA transcript encoded by the right strand of the genome, which is processed into individual mRNAs.

Capsid proteins are produced in the cytoplasm and then transported to the nucleus for viral assembly. Empty procapsids first assemble, and then the viral DNA and core proteins enter the capsid through an opening at one of the vertices. The replication and assembly process are inefficient and prone to error, producing only one infectious unit per 11 to 2300 particles. DNA, protein, and numerous defective particles accumulate in nuclear inclusion bodies. The virus remains in the cell and is released when the cell degenerates and lyses.

Pathogenesis and Immunity

Adenoviruses are capable of causing lytic (e.g., mucoepithelial cells), latent (e.g., lymphoid and adenoid cells), and transforming (hamster, not human) infections. These viruses infect epithelial cells lining the oropharynx, as well as the respiratory and enteric organs (Box 53–2). The viral fiber proteins determine the target cell specificity. The toxic activity of the penton base protein can result in inhibition of cellular mRNA transport and protein synthesis, cell rounding, and tissue damage.

The histologic hallmark of adenovirus infection is a dense, central intranuclear inclusion within an infected epithelial cell that consists of viral DNA and protein (Figure 53–3). These inclusions may resemble those seen in cells infected with cytomegalovirus, but adenovirus does not cause cellular enlargement (cytomegaly). Mononuclear cell infiltrates and epithelial cell necrosis are seen at the site of infection.

Viremia may occur after local replication of the virus, with subsequent spread to visceral organs (Figure 53–4). This dissemination is more likely to occur in immunocompromised patients than in immunocompetent people.

BOX 53–2. Disease Mechanisms of Adenoviruses

Virus is spread by **aerosol, close contact,** or **fecal-oral** means to establish pharyngeal infection. Fingers spread virus to eyes.

Virus infects **mucoepithelial cells** in the respiratory tract, gastrointestinal tract, and conjunctiva or cornea, causing cell damage directly.

Disease is determined by the tissue tropism of the specific group or serotype of the virus strain.

Virus **persists** in lymphoid tissue (e.g., tonsils, adenoids, Peyer's patches).

Antibody is important for prophylaxis and resolution.

The virus has a propensity to become **latent and persist** in lymphoid and other tissue, such as adenoids, tonsils, and Peyer's patches, and can be reactivated in immunosuppressed patients or patients who have been infected with other agents. Although certain adenoviruses (groups A and B) are **oncogenic in certain rodents,** adenovirus transformation of human cells has not been observed.

Antibody is important for resolving lytic adenovirus infections and protects the person from reinfection with the same serotype but not other serotypes. Cell–mediated immunity is important in limiting virus outgrowth, as borne out by the fact that immunosuppressed people suffer more serious and recurrent disease. Adenoviruses have several mechanisms to evade host defenses to help them persist in the host. They encode small virus-associated RNAs (VA RNA) that prevent the activation of

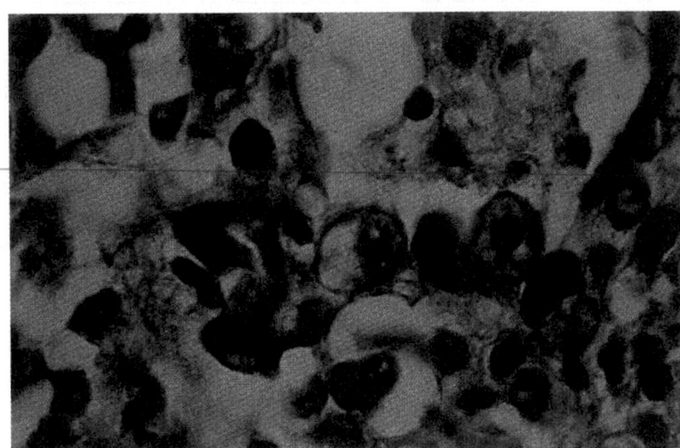

FIGURE 53–3. Histologic appearance of adenovirus-infected cells. Inefficient assembly of virions yields dark basophilic nuclear inclusion bodies containing DNA, proteins, and capsids.

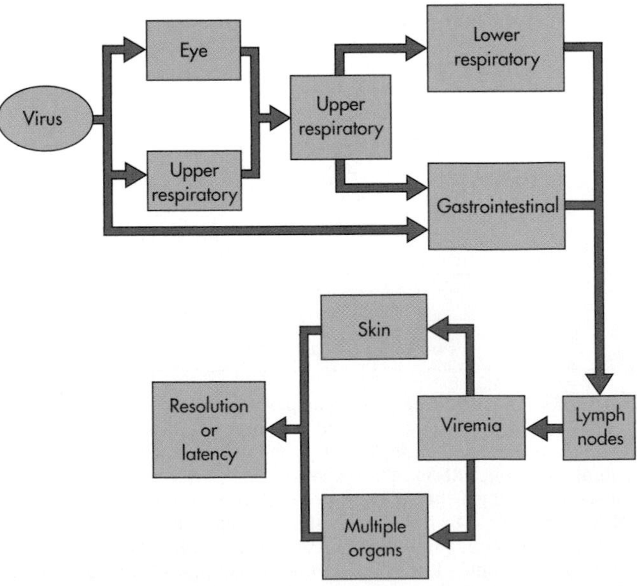

FIGURE 53–4. Mechanism of adenovirus spread within the body.

the interferon-induced protein kinase R mediated inhibition of viral protein synthesis. The viral E3 and E1A proteins block apoptosis induced by cellular responses to the virus or by T cell or cytokine (e.g., TNF-α) actions. Some strains of adenoviruses can inhibit CD8(+) cytotoxic T-cell action by preventing proper expression of MHC I molecules and therefore antigen presentation.

Epidemiology

Adenovirus virions resist drying, detergents, gastrointestinal tract secretions (acid, protease, and bile), and even mild chlorine treatment (Box 53–3). These virions can therefore be spread by the fecal-oral route, by fingers, by fomites (including towels and medical instruments), and in poorly chlorinated swimming pools.

The human adenoviruses are spread mainly by respiratory or fecal-oral contact from human to human, with no apparent animal reservoirs for the virus. Close interaction among people, as occurs in classrooms and military barracks, promotes spread of the virus. Adenoviruses may be shed intermittently and over long periods from the pharynx and especially in feces. Most infections are asymptomatic, a feature that greatly facilitates their spread in the community.

Adenoviruses 1 through 7 are the most prevalent serotypes. From 5% to 10% of cases of pediatric respiratory tract disease are caused by adenovirus types 1, 2, 5, and 6, and the infected children shed virus for months after infection. Serotypes 4 and 7 seem especially able to spread among military recruits because of their close proximity and rigorous lifestyle.

BOX 53–3. Epidemiology of Adenoviruses

Disease/Viral Factors

Capsid virus is resistant to inactivation by gastrointestinal tract and drying.

Disease symptoms may resemble those of other respiratory virus infections.

Virus may cause asymptomatic shedding.

Transmission

Direct contact via respiratory droplets and fecal matter, on hands, on fomites (e.g., towels, contaminated medical instruments), close contact, and inadequately chlorinated swimming pools.

Who Is at Risk?

Children younger than 14 years of age.

People in crowded areas (e.g., daycare centers, military training camps, swimming clubs).

Geography/Season

Virus is found worldwide.

There is no seasonal incidence.

Modes of Control

Live vaccine for serotypes 4 and 7 is available for military use.

Clinical Syndromes (Box 53–4)

Adenoviruses primarily infect children and less commonly infect adults. Disease from reactivated virus occurs in immunocompromised children and adults. Several distinct clinical syndromes are associated with adenovirus infection (see Table 53–1). The time course of adenovirus respiratory infection is shown in Figure 53–5.

ACUTE FEBRILE PHARYNGITIS AND PHARYNGOCONJUNCTIVAL FEVER

Adenovirus causes **pharyngitis,** which is often accompanied by **conjunctivitis (pinkeye)** and **pharyngoconjunctival fever.** Pharyngitis alone occurs in young children, particularly those younger than 3 years, and may mimic streptococcal infection. Affected patients have mild, flulike symptoms (including nasal congestion, cough, coryza, malaise, fever, chills, myalgia, and headache) that may last 3 to 5 days. Pharyngoconjunctival fever occurs more often in outbreaks involving older children.

ACUTE RESPIRATORY DISEASE

Acute respiratory disease is a syndrome consisting of fever, cough, pharyngitis, and cervical adenitis. It is usually caused by adenovirus serotypes 4 and 7. The high incidence of infection of military recruits stimulated the development and use of a vaccine for these serotypes.

OTHER RESPIRATORY TRACT DISEASES

Adenoviruses cause coldlike symptoms, laryngitis, croup, and bronchiolitis. They can also cause a pertussis-like illness in children and adults that consists of a prolonged clinical course and true viral pneumonia.

BOX 53–4. Clinical Summaries

Pharyngoconjunctival fever: A 7-year-old student develops sudden onset of red eyes, sore throat, and a fever of 38.9°C (102°F). Several children in the local elementary school have similar symptoms.

Gastroenteritis: An infant has diarrhea and is vomiting. Adenovirus serotype 41 was identified by polymerase chain reaction analysis of stool for epidemiologic reasons.

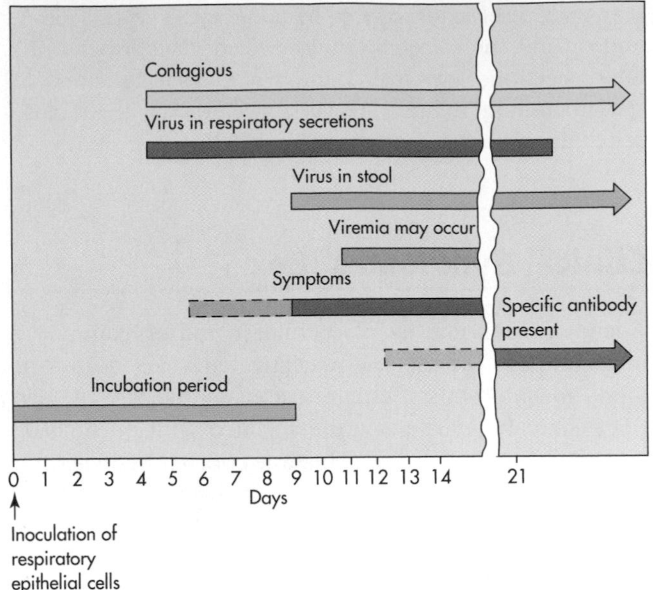

FIGURE 53–5. Time course of adenovirus respiratory infection.

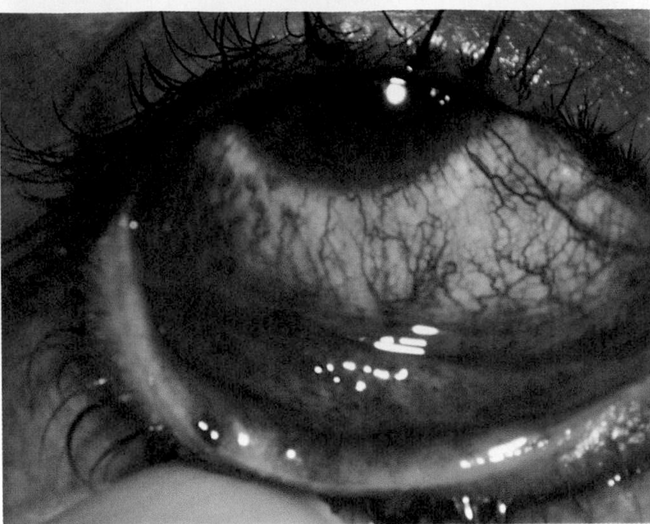

FIGURE 53–6. Conjunctivitis caused by adenovirus.

CONJUNCTIVITIS AND EPIDEMIC KERATOCONJUNCTIVITIS

Adenoviruses cause a follicular conjunctivitis in which the mucosa of the palpebral conjunctiva becomes pebbled or nodular and both conjunctivae (palpebral and bulbar) become inflamed (Figure 53–6). Such conjunctivitis may occur sporadically or in outbreaks that can be traced to a common source. Swimming pool conjunctivitis is a familiar example of a common-source adenovirus infection. Epidemic keratoconjunctivitis may be an occupational hazard for industrial workers. The most striking such epidemic occurred in people working in the naval shipyards of Pearl Harbor in Hawaii, where it caused more than 10,000 cases during 1941 and 1942. Irritation of the eye by a foreign body, dust, debris, and the like is a risk factor for the acquisition of this infection.

GASTROENTERITIS AND DIARRHEA

Adenovirus is a major cause of acute viral gastroenteritis; 15% of the cases of gastroenteritis in hospitalized patients are caused by this virus. Adenovirus serotypes 40 to 42 have been grouped as enteric adenoviruses (group F) and appear to be responsible for episodes of diarrhea in infants. These enteric adenoviruses do not replicate in the same tissue culture cells as other adenoviruses and rarely cause fever or respiratory tract symptoms.

OTHER MANIFESTATIONS

Adenovirus has also been associated with a pertussis-like illness, intussusception in young children, acute hemorrhagic cystitis with dysuria and hematuria in young boys, musculoskeletal disorders, and genital and skin infections.

SYSTEMIC INFECTION IN IMMUNOCOMPROMISED PATIENTS

Immunocompromised patients are at risk for serious adenovirus infections, although not as much as they are for infections caused by herpesviruses. Adenoviral disease in immunocompromised patients includes pneumonia and hepatitis. Infection can originate from exogenous or endogenous (reactivation) sources.

Laboratory Diagnosis

For the results of virus isolation to be significant, the isolate should be obtained from a site or secretion relevant to the disease symptoms. The presence of adenovirus in the throat of a patient with pharyngitis is usually diagnostic if laboratory findings eliminate other common causes of pharyngitis, such as *Streptococcus pyogenes*.

Direct analysis of the clinical sample without virus isolation can be used for rapid detection and identification of adenoviruses. Immunoassays, including fluorescent antibody and enzyme-linked immunosorbent assays, and genome assays, including different variations of the polymerase chain reaction and DNA probe analysis, can be used to detect, type, and group the virus in clinical samples and tissue cultures. These approaches must be used for enteric adenovirus serotypes 40 to 42, which do not grow readily in available cell cultures. Serologic testing is rarely used except for epidemiologic purposes or

CASE STUDY AND QUESTIONS

A 7-year-old boy attending summer camp complains of sore throat, headache, cough, red eyes, and tiredness and is sent to the infirmary. His temperature is 40°C. Within hours, other campers and counselors visit the infirmary with similar symptoms. Symptoms last for 5 to 7 days. All the patients have gone swimming in the camp pond. More than 50% of the people in the camp complain of symptoms similar to those in the initial case. The Public Health Department identifies the agent as adenovirus serotype 3.

1. Toward which adenovirus syndrome do the symptoms point?
2. An outbreak as large as this indicates a common source of infection. What was the most likely source or sources? What were the most likely routes by which the virus was spread?
3. What physical properties of the virus facilitate its transmission?
4. What precautions should the camp owners take to prevent other outbreaks?
5. What sample or samples would have been used by the Public Health Department to identify the infectious agent, and what tests would be required to diagnose the infection?

to confirm the significance of a fecal or upper respiratory tract isolate by identifying its serotype.

The isolation of most adenovirus types is best accomplished in cell cultures derived from epithelial cells (e.g., primary human embryonic kidney cells, continuous [transformed] lines such as HeLa and human epidermal carcinoma cells). Within 2 to 20 days, the virus causes a lytic infection with characteristic inclusion bodies. Recovery of virus from cell culture requires an average of 6 days. The characteristic intranuclear inclusions can be seen in infected tissue during histologic examination. However, such inclusions are rare and must be distinguished from those produced by cytomegalovirus.

Treatment, Prevention, and Control

There is no approved treatment for adenovirus infection. Live oral vaccines have been used to prevent infections with adenovirus types 4 and 7 in military recruits but are not used in civilian populations.

Gene Replacement Therapy

Adenoviruses have been used and are being considered for more applications of gene delivery for correction of several human diseases, including immune deficiencies (e.g., adenosine deaminase deficiency), cystic fibrosis, lysosomal storage diseases, and even cancer. The virus is inactivated by deletion or mutation of the E1 and other viral genes (e.g., E2, E4). The appropriate gene is inserted into the genome, replacing this DNA, and is controlled by an appropriate promoter. The resultant virus vector must be grown in a cell that expresses the missing viral functions (E1, E4) and can complement the deficiency to allow production of virus. Adenovirus types 4 and 7 have been used most extensively since attenuated (vaccine) strains have been developed. Despite the genetically engineered attenuation, these viruses still can cause serious disease in people.

Bibliography

Balows A, Hausler WJ Jr, Lennette EH, editors: *Laboratory diagnosis of infectious diseases: Principles and practice*, vol 2, New York, 1988, Springer-Verlag.

Belshe RB, editor: *Textbook on human virology*, ed 2, St Louis, 1991, Mosby.

Benihoud K, Yeh P, Perricaudet M: Adenovirus vectors for gene delivery, *Curr Opin Biotechnol* 10:440-447, 1999.

Cohen J, Powderly WG, editors: *Infectious diseases*, ed 2, St Louis, 2004, Mosby.

Doerfleur W, Böhm P, editors: Adenoviruses: Model and vectors in virus-host interactions, *Curr Top Microbiol Immunol*, 272-273, 2003.

Flint SJ et al: *Principles of virology: Molecular biology, pathogenesis and control of animal viruses*, ed 2, Washington, 2003, American Society for Microbiology.

Ginsberg HS: *The adenoviruses*, New York, 1984, Plenum.

Gorbach SL, Bartlett JG, Blacklow NR, editors: *Infectious diseases*, ed 2, Philadelphia, 1997, WB Saunders.

Knipe DM, Howley PM, editors: *Fields virology*, ed 4, New York, 2001, Lippincott-Williams and Wilkins.

Mandell GL, Bennet JE, Dolin R, editors: *Principles and practice of infectious diseases*, ed 6, Philadelphia, 2004, Churchill Livingstone.

Robbins PD, Ghivizzani SC: Viral vectors for gene therapy, *Pharmacol Ther* 80:35-47, 1998.

Strauss JH, Strauss EG: *Viruses and human disease*, San Diego, 2002, Academic Press.

White DO, Fenner FJ: *Medical virology*, ed 4, New York, 1994, Academic Press.

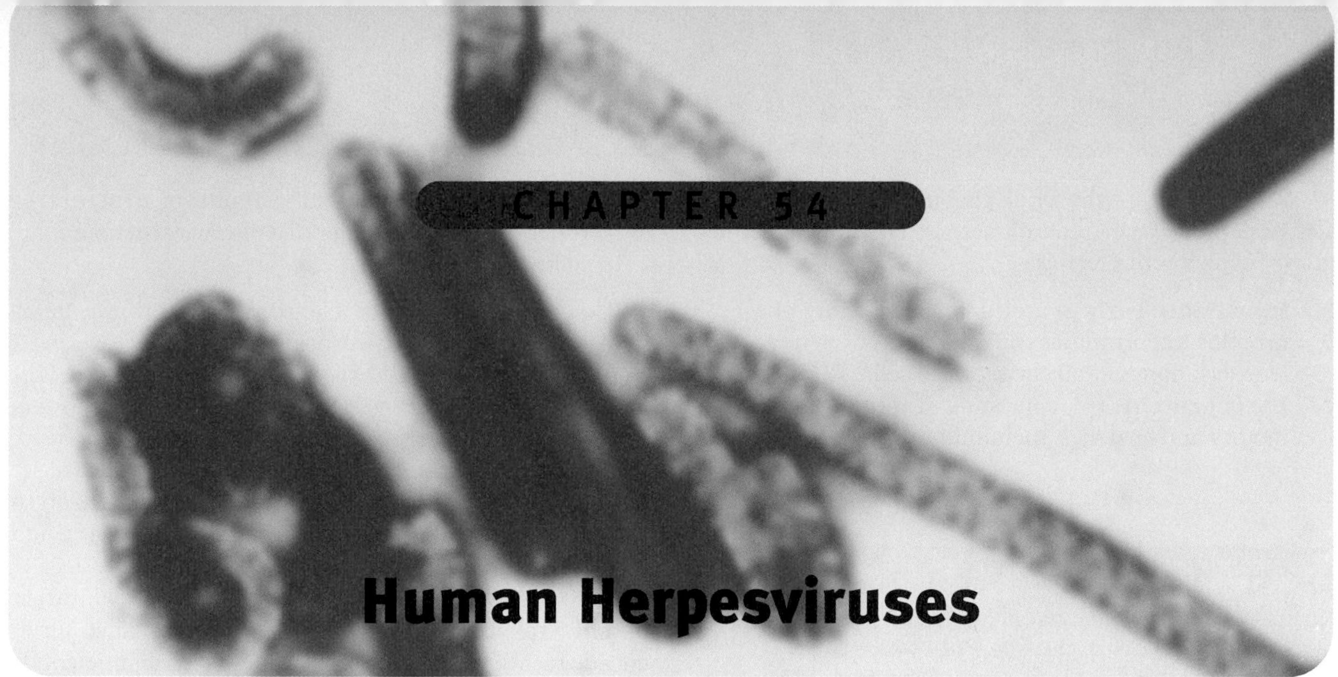

Human Herpesviruses

The herpesviruses are an important group of large deoxyribonucleic acid (DNA) enveloped viruses with the following features in common: virion morphology, basic mode of replication, and capacity to establish latent and recurrent infections. Cell-mediated immunity is important for controlling infection with these viruses and causing symptoms. Herpesviruses encode proteins and enzymes that facilitate the replication and interaction of the virus with the host. The herpesviruses can cause lytic, persistent, latent/recurrent, and, in the case of Epstein-Barr virus (EBV), immortalizing infections (Box 54–1).

The human herpesviruses are grouped into three subfamilies on the basis of differences in viral characteristics (genome structure, tissue tropism, cytopathologic effect, and site of latent infection), as well as the pathogenesis of the disease and disease manifestation (Table 54–1). The human herpesviruses are herpes simplex viruses types 1 and 2 (HSV-1 and HSV-2), varicella-zoster virus (VZV), Epstein-Barr virus, cytomegalovirus (CMV), human herpesviruses 6 and 7 (HHV6 and HHV7), and the more recently discovered human herpesvirus 8 (HHV8), associated with Kaposi's sarcoma.

Herpesvirus infections are common, and the viruses are **ubiquitous.** Although these viruses usually cause benign disease, especially in children, they can also cause significant morbidity and mortality, especially in immunosuppressed people. Fortunately, the herpesviruses encode targets for antiviral agents. The U.S. Food and Drug Administration (FDA) approved a live-virus vaccine for VZV.

Structure of Herpesviruses

The herpesviruses are **large, enveloped** viruses that contain **double-stranded DNA.** The virion is approximately 150 nm in diameter and has the characteristic morphology shown in Figure 54–1. The DNA core is surrounded by an **icosadeltahedral capsid** containing 162 capsomeres. This capsid is enclosed by a glycoprotein-containing envelope. Herpesviruses encode several glycoproteins for viral attachment, fusion, and for escaping immune control. The space between the envelope and the capsid, called the tegument, contains viral proteins and enzymes that help initiate replication. As enveloped viruses, the herpesviruses are sensitive to acid, solvents, detergents, and drying.

Herpesviral genomes are linear, double-stranded DNA, but they differ in size and gene orientation (Figure 54–2). Direct or inverted repeat sequences bracket unique regions of the genome (unique long [U_L], unique short [U_S]), allowing circularization and recombination within the genome. Recombination among inverted repeats of HSV, CMV, and VZV allows large portions of the genome to switch the orientation of their U_L and U_S gene segments, with respect to each other, to form isomeric genomes.

Herpesvirus Replication

Herpesvirus replication is initiated by the interaction of viral glycoproteins with cell surface receptors (see Figure 6–12). The tropism of some herpesviruses (e.g., EBV) is restricted as a result of the tissue-specific expression of their receptors. The nucleocapsid is then released into the cytoplasm through fusion of the envelope with the plasma membrane. Enzymes and transcription factors are carried into the cell in the tegument of the virion. The nucleocapsid docks with the nuclear membrane and delivers the genome into the nucleus, where the genome is transcribed and replicated.

Transcription of the viral genome and viral protein synthesis proceeds in a coordinated and regulated manner in the following three phases:

1. **Immediate early proteins (α),** consisting of proteins important for the regulation of gene transcription and takeover of the cell.
2. **Early proteins (β),** consisting of more transcription factors and enzymes, including the DNA polymerase.
3. **Late proteins (γ),** consisting mainly of structural proteins, which are generated after viral genome replication has begun.

BOX 54–1. Unique Features of Herpesviruses

Herpesviruses have large, enveloped icosadeltahedral capsids containing **double-stranded DNA genomes.**
Herpesviruses encode many proteins that manipulate the host cell and immune response.
Herpesviruses encode enzymes **(DNA polymerase)** that promote viral DNA replication and that are good targets for **antiviral drugs.**
DNA replication and capsid assembly occurs in the nucleus.
Virus is released by exocytosis, cell lysis, and through cell-cell bridges.
Herpesviruses can cause **lytic, persistent, latent,** and, for Epstein-Barr virus, **immortalizing infections.**
Herpesviruses are ubiquitous.
Cell-mediated immunity is required for control.

The viral genome is transcribed by the cellular DNA–dependent ribonucleic acid (RNA) polymerase *and is regulated by viral-encoded and cellular nuclear factors. The interplay of these factors determines whether the proteins necessary for a lytic, persistent, or latent infection are produced.* Cells that promote latent infection transcribe a special set of viral genes without genome replication. Progression to early and late gene expression results in cell death and lytic infection.

The viral-encoded DNA polymerase, which is a target of antiviral drugs, replicates the viral genome. Viral-encoded scavenging enzymes provide deoxyribonucleotide substrates for the polymerase. These and other viral enzymes facilitate replication of the virus in nongrowing cells that lack sufficient deoxyribonucleotides and enzymes for viral DNA synthesis (e.g., neurons).

Empty procapsids assemble in the nucleus, are filled with DNA, acquire an envelope at the nuclear or Golgi membrane, and exit the cell by exocytosis or by lysis of the cell. Transcription, protein synthesis, glycoprotein processing, and exocytotic release from the cell are performed by cellular machinery. The replication of HSV is discussed in more detail as the prototype of the herpesviruses.

TABLE 54–1. Properties Distinguishing the Herpesviruses

Subfamily	Virus	Primary Target Cell	Site of Latency	Means of Spread
Alphaherpesvirinae				
Human herpesvirus 1	Herpes simplex type 1	Mucoepithelial cells	Neuron	Close contact
Human herpesvirus 2	Herpes simplex type 2	Mucoepithelial cells	Neuron	Close contact (sexually transmitted disease)
Human herpesvirus 3	Varicella-zoster virus	Mucoepithelial cells	Neuron	Respiratory and close contact
Gammaherpesvirinae				
Human herpesvirus 4	Epstein-Barr virus	B cells and epithelial cells	B cell	Saliva (kissing disease)
Human herpesvirus 8	Kaposi's sarcoma–related virus	Lymphocyte and other cells	B cell	Close contact (sexual), saliva?
Betaherpesvirinae				
Human herpesvirus 5	Cytomegalovirus	Monocyte, lymphocyte, and epithelial cells	Monocyte, lymphocyte, and ?	Close contact, transfusions, tissue transplant, and congenital
Human herpesvirus 6	Herpes lymphotropic virus	T cells and ?	T cells and ?	Respiratory and close contact?
Human herpesvirus 7	Human herpesvirus 7	T cells and ?	T cells and ?	?

? indicates that other cells may also be the primary target or site of latency.

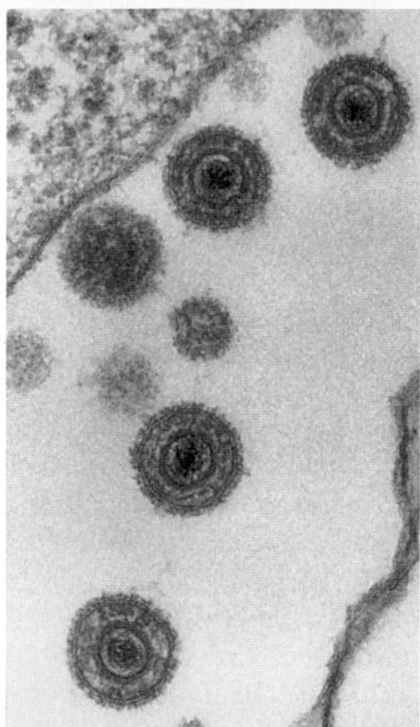

A

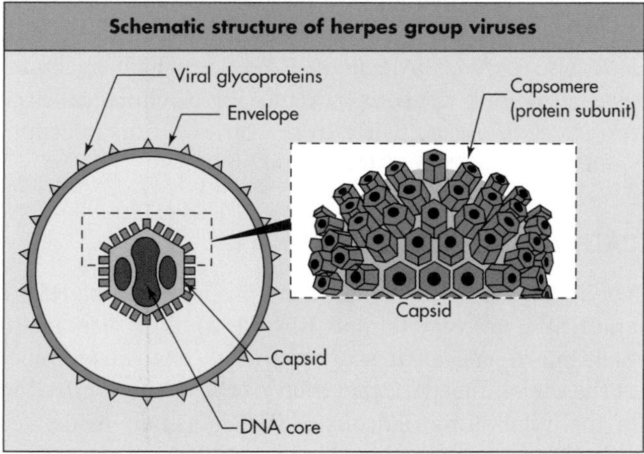

B

FIGURE 54–1. Electron micrograph **(A)** and general structure **(B)** of the herpesviruses. The DNA genome of the herpesvirus in the core is surrounded by an icosadeltahedral capsid and an envelope. Glycoproteins are inserted into the envelope. (**A** from Armstrong D, Cohen J: *Infectious diseases,* St Louis, 1999, Mosby.)

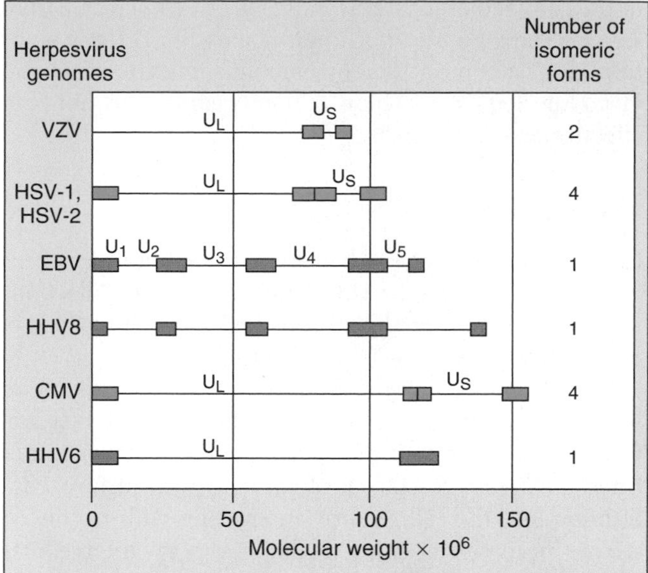

FIGURE 54–2. Herpesvirus genomes. The genomes of the herpesvirus are doubled-stranded DNA. The length and complexity of the genome differ for each virus. Inverted repeats in herpes simplex virus (HSV), varicella-zoster virus (VZV), and cytomegalovirus (CMV) allow the genome to recombine with itself to form isomers. Large genetic repeat sequences are boxed. The genomes of HSV and CMV have two sections, the unique long (U_L) and the unique short (U_S), each of which is bracketed by two sets of inverted repeats of DNA. The inverted repeats facilitate the replication of the genome but also allow the U_L and U_S regions to invert independently of each other to yield four different genomic configurations, or isomers. VZV has only one set of inverted repeats and can form two isomers. Epstein-Barr virus (EBV) exists in only one configuration, with several unique regions surrounded by direct repeats. Purple bars indicate direct repeat DNA sequences; green bars indicate inverted repeated DNA sequences. HHV6, Human herpesvirus 6; HHV8, human herpesvirus 8.

Herpes Simplex Virus

HSV was the first human herpesvirus to be recognized. The name "herpes" is derived from a Greek word meaning to creep. "Cold sores" were described in antiquity, and their viral etiology was established in 1919.

The two types of herpes simplex virus, HSV-1 and HSV-2, share many characteristics, including DNA homology, antigenic determinants, tissue tropism, and disease symptoms. However, they can still be distinguished by subtle but significant differences in these properties.

STRUCTURE

The HSV genome is large enough to encode approximately 80 proteins. Only half of the proteins are required for viral replication; the others facilitate the HSV's interaction with different host cells and the immune response. The HSV genome encodes enzymes, including a DNA-dependent DNA polymerase and scavenging enzymes, such as deoxyribonuclease, thymidine kinase, ribonucleotide reductase, and protease. Ribonucleotide reductase converts ribonucleotides to deoxyribonucleotides, and thymidine kinase phosphorylates the deoxyribonucleosides to provide substrates for replication of the viral genome. The substrate specificities of these enzymes and the DNA polymerase differ significantly from those of their cellular analogues and thus represent potentially good targets for antiviral chemotherapy.

HSV encodes at least 10 glycoproteins that serve as viral attachment proteins (gB, gC, gD, gH), fusion proteins (gB), structural proteins, immune escape proteins (gC, gE, gI), and other functions. For example, the C3 component of the complement system binds to gC and is depleted from serum. The Fc portion of immunoglobulin G (IgG) binds to a gE/gI complex, thereby camouflaging the virus and virus-infected cells. These actions reduce the antiviral effectiveness of antibody.

REPLICATION

HSV can infect most types of human cells and even cells of other species. The virus generally causes lytic infections of fibroblasts and epithelial cells and latent infections of neurons (see Figure 6–12 for diagram).

HSV-1 binds quickly and efficiently to cells through an initial interaction with heparan sulfate, a proteoglycan, found on the outside of many cell types, and then a tighter interaction with receptor proteins at the cell surface. Penetration into the cell requires interaction with nectin-1α (HveC [herpesvirus entry mediator C]), an intercellular adhesion molecule that is a member of the immunoglobulin protein family and similar to the poliovirus receptor. Nectin-1α is found on most cells and neurons. Another receptor is HveA, a member of the tumor necrosis factor receptor family, which is expressed on activated T cells, neurons, and other cells. HSV penetrates the host cell by fusion of its envelope with the cell surface membrane. On fusion the virion releases its capsid into the cytoplasm, along with a protein that promotes the initiation of viral gene transcription, a viral-encoded protein kinase, and cytotoxic proteins. The capsid docks with a nuclear pore and delivers the genome into the nucleus.

The **immediate early gene products** include DNA-binding proteins, which stimulate DNA synthesis and promote the transcription of the early viral genes. During a latent infection of neurons, the only region of the genome to be transcribed generates the **latency-associated transcripts (LATs)**, but these RNAs are not translated into protein.

The **early proteins** include the DNA-dependent DNA polymerase and a thymidine kinase. As catalytic proteins, relatively few copies of these enzymes are required to promote replication. Other early proteins inhibit the production and initiate the degradation of cellular messenger RNA (mRNA) and DNA. Expression of the early and late genes generally leads to cell death.

The genome is replicated as soon as the polymerase is synthesized. Circular, end-to-end concatameric forms of the genome are made initially. Later in the infection, the DNA is replicated by a rolling circle mechanism to produce a linear string of genomes that, in concept, resembles a roll of toilet paper. The concatamers are cleaved into individual genomes as the DNA is sucked into a procapsid.

Genome replication triggers transcription of the late genes from which structural and other proteins are encoded. Many copies of the structural proteins are required. The capsid proteins are then transported to the nucleus, where they are assembled into empty procapsids and filled with DNA. DNA-containing capsids associate with viral protein disrupted nuclear membranes and bud into and then out of the endoplasmic reticulum into the cytoplasm. The viral glycoproteins are synthesized and processed like cellular glycoproteins. Tegument proteins associate with the viral capsid in the cytoplasm, and then the capsid buds into a portion of the trans-Golgi network to acquire their glycoprotein-containing envelope. The virus is released by exocytosis or cell lysis. Virus can also spread between cells through intracellular bridges, which allows the virus to escape antibody detection. Virus-induced syncytia formation also spreads the infection.

HSV infection of neurons may result in virus replication or establishment of latency, depending on which viral genes the neuron is capable of transcribing. Transcription of the LAT and no other viral gene will result in latency. If the cell can transcribe the immediate early genes of the virus, virus will replicate. As for other alphaherpesviruses, HSV encodes a thymidine kinase (scavenging enzyme) to facilitate replication in nondividing cells, like neurons. HSV also encodes a protein, ICP34.5, which facilitates virus growth in neurons by removing a cellular block to protein synthesis activated in response to virus infection, similar to the action of interferon alpha.

PATHOGENESIS AND IMMUNITY

The mechanisms involved in the pathogenesis of HSV-1 and HSV-2 are very similar (Box 54–2). Both viruses initially infect, replicate in mucoepithelial cells, cause disease at the site of infection, and then establish latent infection of the innervating neurons. HSV-1 is usually associated with infections above the waist, and HSV-2 with infections below the waist (Figure 54–3), consistent with the means of spread for these viruses. HSV-1 and HSV-2 also differ in growth characteristics and antigenicity, and HSV-2 has a greater potential to cause viremia with associated systemic flulike symptoms.

BOX 54–2. Disease Mechanisms for Herpes Simplex Viruses

- Disease is initiated by direct contact and depends on infected tissue (e.g., oral, genital, brain).
- Virus causes direct cytopathologic effects.
- Virus avoids antibody by cell-to-cell spread (syncytia).
- Virus establishes latency in neurons (hides from immune response).
- Virus is reactivated from latency by stress or immune suppression.
- Cell-mediated immunity is *required* for resolution with limited role for antibody.
- Cell-mediated immunopathologic effects contribute to symptoms.

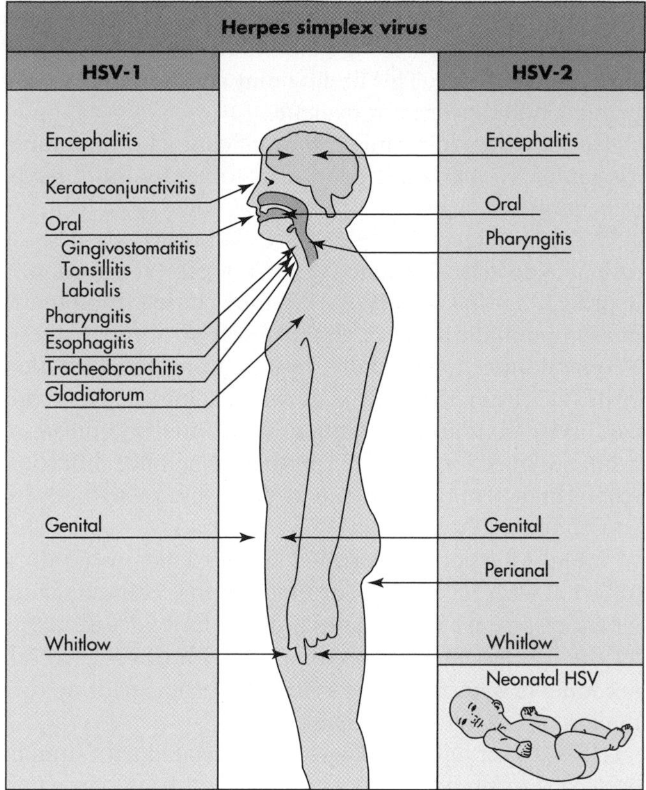

FIGURE 54–3. Disease syndromes of herpes simplex virus (HSV). HSV-1 and HSV-2 can infect the same tissues and cause similar diseases but have a predilection for the sites and diseases indicated.

HSV can cause **lytic** infections of most cells, persistent infections of lymphocytes and macrophages, and **latent** infection of neurons. Cytolysis generally results from the virus-induced inhibition of cellular macromolecular synthesis, the degradation of host cell DNA, membrane permeation, cytoskeletal disruption, and senescence of the cell. In addition, changes in the nuclear structure and margination of the chromatin occur, and **Cowdry type A acidophilic intranuclear inclusion bodies** are produced. Many strains of HSV also initiate **syncytia** formation. In tissue culture, HSV rapidly kills cells.

HSV initiates infection through mucosal membranes or breaks in the skin. The virus replicates in the cells at the base of the lesion and infects the innervating neuron, traveling by retrograde transport to the ganglion (the trigeminal ganglia for oral HSV and the sacral ganglia for genital HSV). The virus then returns to the initial site of infection and may be inapparent or may produce **vesicular lesions.** The vesicle fluid contains infectious virions. Tissue damage is caused by a combination of viral pathology and immunopathology. The lesion generally heals without producing a scar.

Innate protections including interferon and natural killer cells may be sufficient to limit the initial progression of the infection. T-helper 1 *(TH1)-associated and cytotoxic killer T-cell responses are required to kill infected cells and resolve the current disease.* The immunopathologic effects of the cell-mediated and inflammatory responses are also a major cause of the symptoms. Antibody directed against the glycoproteins of the virus neutralizes extracellular virus, limiting its spread, but is not sufficient to resolve the infection. In the absence of functional cell-mediated immunity, HSV infection is more severe and may disseminate to the vital organs and the brain.

BOX 54–3. Triggers of HSV Recurrences

UV-B radiation (skiing, tanning)
Fever (hence the name "fever blister")
Emotional stress (e.g. final examinations, big date)
Physical stress (irritation)
Menstruation
Foods: Spicy, acidic, allergies
Immunosuppression
- Transient (stress related)
- Chemotherapy, radiotherapy
- Human immunodeficiency virus

HSV has several ways to escape host protective responses. The virus blocks the interferon-induced inhibition of viral protein synthesis and encodes a protein to plug the transporter associated with processing (TAP) channel, preventing delivery of peptides into the endoplasmic reticulum (ER), which blocks their association with class I major histocompatibility complex (MHC I) molecules and prevents CD8 T-cell recognition of infected cells. The virus can escape antibody neutralization and clearance by direct cell-to-cell spread and by going into hiding during latent infection of the neuron. In addition, the virion and virus-infected cells express antibody (Fc) and complement receptors that weaken these humoral defenses.

Latent infection occurs in neurons and results in no detectable damage. A **recurrence** can be activated by various stimuli (e.g., stress, trauma, fever, sunlight [ultraviolet B]) (Box 54–3). These events trigger virus replication in an individual nerve cell within the bundle and allow the virus to travel back down the nerve to cause lesions to develop at the same dermatome and location each time. The stress triggers reactivation by promoting replication of the virus in the nerve, by transiently depressing cell-mediated immunity, or by inducing both processes. The virus can be reactivated despite the presence of antibody. However, recurrent infections are generally less severe, more localized, and of shorter duration than the primary episodes because of the nature of the spread and the existence of memory immune responses.

EPIDEMIOLOGY

Because HSV can establish latency with the potential for asymptomatic recurrence, the infected person is a lifelong

BOX 54–4. Epidemiology of Herpes Simplex Virus (HSV)

Disease/Viral Factors

Virus causes lifelong infection.
Recurrent disease is source of contagion.
Virus may cause asymptomatic shedding.

Transmission

Virus is transmitted in saliva, in vaginal secretions, and by contact with lesion fluid (mixing and matching of mucous membranes).
Virus is transmitted orally and sexually and by placement into eyes and breaks in skin.
HSV-1 is generally transmitted orally; HSV-2 is generally transmitted sexually.

Who Is at Risk?

Children and sexually active people: At risk for classic presentations of HSV-1 and HSV-2, respectively.
Physicians, nurses, dentists, and others in contact with oral and genital secretions: At risk for infections of fingers (herpetic whitlow).
Immunocompromised people and neonates: At risk for disseminated, life-threatening disease.

Geography/Season

Virus is found worldwide.
There is no seasonal incidence.

Modes of Control

Antiviral drugs are available.
No vaccine is available.
Health care workers should wear gloves to prevent herpetic whitlow.
People with active genital lesions should refrain from intercourse until lesions are completely reepithelialized.

source of contagion (Box 54–4). As an enveloped virus, HSV is transmitted in secretions and by close contact. The virus is very labile and is readily inactivated by drying, detergents, and the conditions of the gastrointestinal tract. Although HSV can infect animal cells, HSV infection is exclusively a human disease.

HSV is transmitted in vesicle fluid, saliva, and vaginal secretions (the **"mixing and matching of mucous membranes"**). The site of infection, and hence the disease, is determined primarily by which mucous membranes are mixed. Both types of HSV can cause oral and genital lesions.

HSV-1 is usually spread by oral contact (kissing) or through the sharing of drinking glasses, toothbrushes, or other saliva-contaminated items. HSV-1 infection of the fingers or body can result from mouth-to-skin contact, with the virus entering through a break in the skin. Autoinoculation may also cause infection of the eyes.

HSV-1 infection is common. More than 90% of people living in underdeveloped areas have the antibody to HSV-1 by 2 years of age. This finding may result from crowded living conditions or poor hygiene.

HSV-2 is spread mainly by sexual contact or autoinoculation or from an infected mother to her infant at birth. Depending on a person's sexual practices and hygiene, HSV-2 may infect the genitalia, anorectal tissues, or oropharynx. The incidence of HSV-1 genital infection is approaching that of HSV-2. HSV may cause symptomatic or asymptomatic primary genital infection or recurrences. Neonatal infection usually results from the excretion of HSV-2 from the cervix during vaginal delivery but can occur from an ascending in utero infection during a primary infection of the mother. Neonatal infection results in disseminated and neurologic disease with severe consequences.

Initial infection with HSV-2 occurs later in life than infection with HSV-1 and correlates with increased sexual activity. The current statistics indicate that 22% of adults in the United States are infected with HSV-2, which amounts to approximately 45 million people with up to 1 million newly infected people per year.

HSV-2 is seroepidemiologically associated with human cervical cancer, possibly as a cofactor with human papillomavirus or another infectious agent. Partial inactivation of the HSV-2 genome with ultraviolet light allows the virus to immortalize cells in tissue culture.

CLINICAL SYNDROMES

HSV-1 and HSV-2 are common human pathogens that can cause painful but benign manifestations and recurrent disease. In the classic manifestation, the lesion is a clear vesicle on an erythematous base ("dewdrop on a rose petal") and then progresses to pustular lesions, ulcers, and crusted lesions (Figure 54–4). However, **both viruses can cause significant morbidity and mortality on infection of the eye or brain and on disseminated infection of an immunosuppressed person or a neonate.**

Oral herpes can be caused by HSV-1 or HSV-2. Primary herpetic gingivostomatitis in toddlers and children is almost always caused by HSV-1, whereas young adults may be infected with HSV-1 or HSV-2. The lesions begin as clear vesicles that rapidly ulcerate. These whitish areas may be widely distributed throughout the mouth, involving the palate, pharynx, gingivae, buccal mucosa, and tongue (Figure 54–5). Many other conditions (e.g., coxsackie virus, canker sores, acne) may resemble oral HSV lesions.

People may experience recurrent mucocutaneous HSV infection **(cold sores, fever blisters)** (Figure 54–6), even though they never had clinically apparent primary infection. The lesions usually occur at the corners of the mouth or next to the lips. Recurrent facial herpes infections are

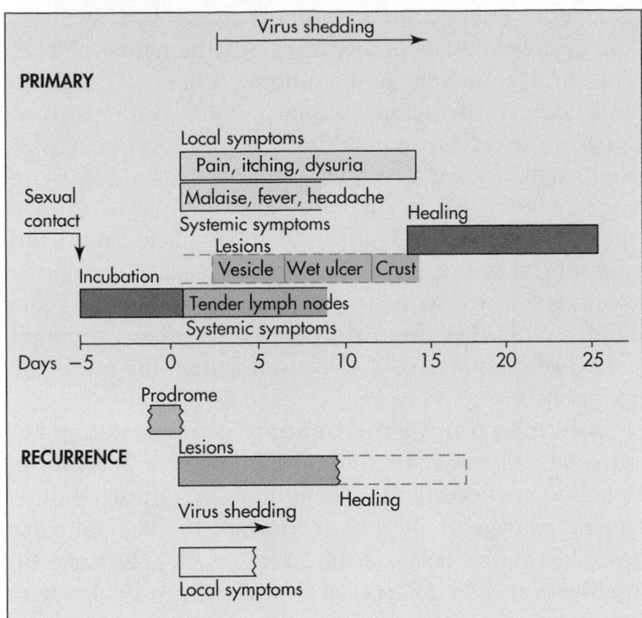

FIGURE 54–4. Clinical course of genital herpes infection. The time course and symptoms of primary and recurrent genital infection with herpes simplex virus type 2 (HSV-2) are compared. *Top,* Primary infection; *bottom,* recurrent disease. (Data from Corey L et al: *Ann Intern Med* 98:958-973, 1983.)

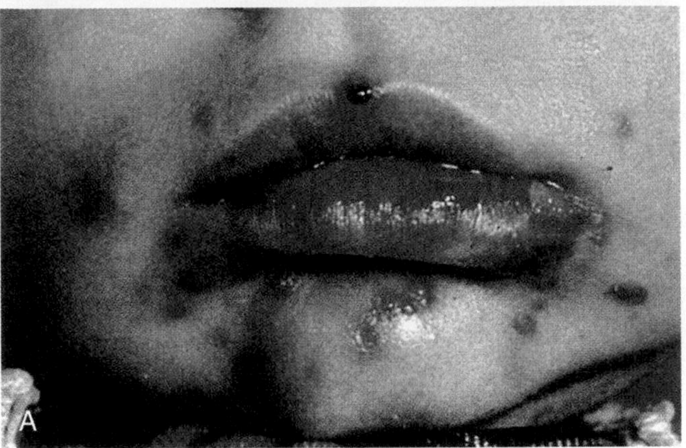

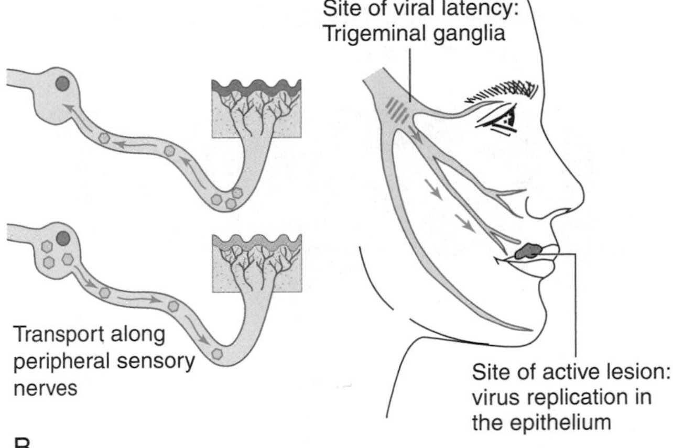

FIGURE 54–5. A, Primary herpes gingivostomatitis. *B,* Herpes simplex virus establishes latent infection and can recur from the trigeminal ganglia. (**A** from Hart CA, Broadhead RL: *A color atlas of pediatric infectious diseases,* London, 1992, Wolfe; **B** modified from Straus SE: Herpes simplex virus and its relatives. In Schaechter M, Eisenstein BI, Medoff G, editors: *Mechanisms of microbial disease,* ed 2, Baltimore, 1993, Williams & Wilkins.)

generally activated from the trigeminal ganglia. As noted earlier, the symptoms of a recurrent episode are less severe, more localized, and of shorter duration than those of a primary episode. **Herpes pharyngitis** is becoming a prevalent diagnosis in young adults with sore throats. Severe HSV stomatitis, resembling a primary gingivostomatitis, may occur in immunosuppressed patients.

Herpetic keratitis is almost always limited to one eye. It can cause recurrent disease, leading to permanent scarring, corneal damage, and blindness.

Herpetic whitlow is an infection of the finger, and **herpes gladiatorum** is an infection of the body. The virus establishes infection through cuts or abrasions in the skin. Herpetic whitlow often occurs in nurses or physicians who attend patients with HSV infections, in thumb-sucking children (Figure 54–7), and in people who have genital HSV infections. Herpes gladiatorum is often acquired during wrestling or rugby.

Eczema herpeticum is acquired by children with active eczema. The underlying disease promotes the spread of the infection along the skin and potentially to the adrenal glands, liver, and other organs.

Genital herpes is usually caused by HSV-2 but can also be caused by HSV-1 (responsible for at least 10% of genital infections). In male patients, the lesions typically develop on the glans or shaft of the penis and occasionally in the urethra. In female patients, the lesions may be seen on the vulva, vagina, cervix, perianal area, or inner thigh and are frequently accompanied by itching and a mucoid

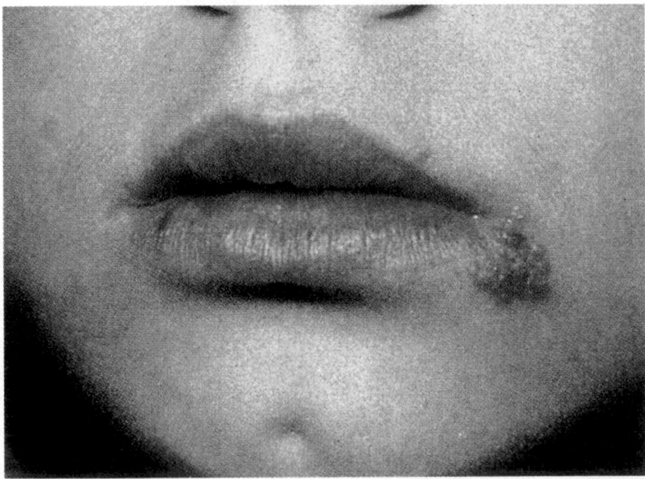

FIGURE 54–6. Cold sore of recurrent herpes labialis. It is less severe than that of primary disease. (From Hart CA, Broadhead RL: *A color atlas of pediatric infectious diseases,* London, 1992, Wolfe.)

vaginal discharge. The lesions are usually painful. In patients of both sexes a primary infection may be accompanied by fever, malaise, myalgia, and inguinal adenitis, which are symptoms related to a transient viremia. HSV proctitis is a painful disease in which the lesions are found in the lower rectum and anus. The symptoms and time course of primary and recurrent genital herpes are compared in Figure 54–4.

Recurrent genital HSV disease is shorter in duration and less severe than the primary episode. In approximately 50% of patients, recurrences are preceded by a characteristic prodrome of burning or tingling in the area in which the lesions eventually erupt. Episodes of recurrence may be as frequent as every 2 to 3 weeks or may be infrequent. Unfortunately, any infected person may shed virus asymptomatically. Such individuals may be important vectors for spread of this virus.

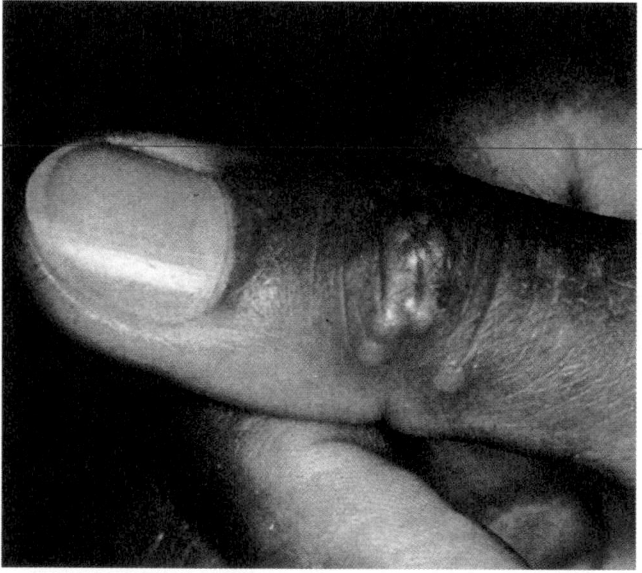

FIGURE 54–7. Herpetic whitlow. (From Emond RTD, Rowland HAK: *A color atlas of infectious diseases,* ed 3, London, 1995, Mosby.)

Herpes encephalitis is usually caused by HSV-1. The lesions are generally limited to one of the temporal lobes. The viral pathology and immunopathology cause the destruction of the temporal lobe and give rise to erythrocytes in the cerebrospinal fluid, seizures, focal neurologic abnormalities, and other characteristics of viral encephalitis. HSV is the most common viral cause of sporadic encephalitis and results in significant morbidity and mortality, even in patients who receive appropriate treatment. The disease occurs at all ages and at any time of the year. **HSV meningitis** is most often a complication of genital HSV-2 infection; symptoms resolve by themselves.

HSV infection in the neonate is a devastating and often fatal disease caused most often by HSV-2. It may be acquired in utero but more commonly is contracted either during passage of the infant through the vaginal canal (possibly at the baby's scalp monitor site), because the mother is shedding herpesvirus at the time of delivery, or postnatally from family members or hospital personnel. The baby initially appears septic, and vesicular lesions may be present. Because the cell-mediated immune response is not yet developed in the neonate, HSV disseminates to the liver, lung, and other organs, as well as to the central nervous system (CNS). Progression of the infection to the CNS results in death, mental retardation, or neurologic disability, even with treatment.

LABORATORY DIAGNOSIS

Direct Analysis of Clinical Sample

Characteristic cytopathologic effects (CPEs) can be identified in a **Tzanck smear** (a scraping of the base of a lesion), Papanicolaou (Pap) smear, or biopsy specimen (Table 54–2). CPEs include syncytia, "ballooning" cytoplasm, and Cowdry type A intranuclear inclusions (see Figure 51–2). A definitive diagnosis can be made by

TABLE 54–2. Laboratory Diagnosis of Herpes Simplex Virus (HSV) Infections

Approach	Test/Comment
Direct microscopic examination of cells from base of lesion	**Tzanck smear** shows **multinucleated giant cells** and **Cowdry type A inclusion bodies.**
Cell culture	HSV replicates and causes identifiable cytopathologic effect in most cell cultures.
Assay of tissue biopsy, smear, cerebrospinal fluid, or vesicular fluid for HSV antigen or genome	Enzyme immunoassay, immunofluorescent stain, in situ DNA probe analysis, and polymerase chain reaction (PCR).
HSV type distinction (HSV-1 vs. HSV-2)	Type-specific antibody, DNA maps of restriction enzyme fragments, sodium dodecyl sulfate–gel protein patterns, DNA probe analysis, and PCR.
Serology	Serology is not useful except for epidemiology.

demonstrating viral antigen (using immunofluorescence or the immunoperoxidase method) or DNA (using in situ hybridization or polymerase chain reaction [PCR]) in the tissue sample or vesicle fluid. PCR analysis of cerebrospinal fluid has replaced immunofluorescence analysis of a brain biopsy in the diagnosis for herpes encephalitis.

Virus Isolation

Virus isolation is the most definitive assay for the diagnosis of HSV infection. Virus can be obtained from vesicles but not crusted lesions. Specimens are collected by aspiration of the lesion fluid or by application of a cotton swab to the vesicles and direct inoculation of the sample into cell cultures.

HSV produces CPEs within 1 to 3 days in HeLa cells, HEp-2 cells, human embryonic fibroblasts, and rabbit kidney cells. Infected cells become enlarged and appear ballooned (see Figure 51–4). Some isolates induce fusion of neighboring cells, giving rise to multinucleated giant cells (syncytia). A new, sensitive approach to isolation and identification uses a cell line that expresses β-galactosidase in HSV-infected cells (enzyme-linked viral inducible system [ELVIS]). Addition of the appropriate substrate produces color and allows detection of the enzyme in the infected cells.

HSV type–specific DNA probes, specific DNA primers for PCR and antibodies are used to differentiate HSV-1 and HSV-2. The distinction between HSV-1 or HSV-2 and different strains of either virus can also be made by restriction endonuclease cleavage patterns of the viral DNA.

Serology

Serologic procedures are useful only for diagnosing a primary HSV infection and for epidemiologic studies. They are not useful for diagnosing recurrent disease, because a significant rise in antibody titers does not usually accompany recurrent disease.

TREATMENT, PREVENTION, AND CONTROL

HSV encodes several target enzymes for antiviral drugs (Box 54–5) (see Chapter 50). Most antiherpes drugs are nucleoside analogues and other inhibitors of the viral DNA polymerase, an enzyme essential for viral replication and the best antiviral drug target. Treatment prevents or shortens the course of primary or recurrent disease. None of the drug treatments can eliminate latent infection.

The prototype U.S. Food and Drug Administration (FDA)-approved anti-HSV drug is **acyclovir (ACV). Valacyclovir** (the valyl ester of ACV), **penciclovir,** and **famciclovir** (a derivative of penciclovir) are related to ACV in their mechanisms of action but have different pharmacologic properties. Vidarabine (adenosine arabinoside [Ara A]), idoxuridine (iododeoxyuridine), and trifluridine, also FDA-approved for treatment of HSV, are less effective. Although **Cidofovir** and **adefovir** are active against HSV, cidofovir is only approved for treatment of CMV.

BOX 54–5. FDA-Approved Antiviral Treatments for Herpesvirus Infections

Herpes Simplex 1 and 2	Epstein-Barr Virus
Acyclovir	None
Penciclovir	
Valacyclovir	***Cytomegalovirus***
Famciclovir	Ganciclovir*
Adenosine arabinoside	Valganciclovir*
Iododeoxyuridine	Foscarnet*
Trifluridine	Cidofovir*
Varicella-Zoster Virus	
Acyclovir	
Famciclovir	
Valacyclovir	
Varicella-zoster immune globulin	
Zoster immune plasma	
Live vaccine	

*FDA, U.S. Food and Drug Administration.
*Also inhibits herpes simplex and varicella-zoster viruses.

ACV is the most-prescribed anti-HSV drug. Phosphorylation of ACV and penciclovir by the viral **thymidine kinase** and cellular enzymes activates the drug as a substrate for the viral **DNA polymerase.** These drugs are then incorporated into and **prevent the elongation of the viral DNA** (see Figure 50–2). ACV, valaciclovir, penciclovir, and famciclovir (1) are relatively nontoxic, (2) are effective in treating serious presentations of HSV disease and first episodes of genital herpes, and (3) are also used for prophylactic treatment.

The most prevalent form of resistance to these drugs results from mutations that inactivate the thymidine kinase, thereby preventing conversion of the drug to its active form. Mutation of the viral DNA polymerase also produces resistance. Fortunately, resistant strains appear to be less virulent.

Ara A is less soluble, less potent, and more toxic than ACV. Trifluridine, penciclovir, and ACV have replaced iododeoxyuridine as topical agents for the treatment of herpetic keratitis. Tromantadine, an amantadine derivative, is approved for topical use in countries other than the United States. It works by inhibiting penetration and syncytia formation. Various nonprescription treatments may be effective for specific individuals.

HSV-1 is transmitted most often from an active mucocutaneous lesion, so avoidance of direct contact with lesions reduces the risk of infection. Unfortunately, the symptoms may be inapparent and thus the virus can be transmitted unknowingly. Physicians, nurses, dentists, and technicians must be especially careful when handling potentially infected tissue or fluids. The wearing of gloves can prevent the acquisition of infections of the fingers (herpetic whitlow). People with recurrent herpetic whitlow disease are very contagious and can spread the infection to patients. Washing with soap readily disinfects the virus.

Patients who have a history of genital HSV infection must be instructed to refrain from sexual intercourse while they have prodromal symptoms or lesions and to resume sexual intercourse only after lesions are completely reepithelialized, because virus may be transmitted from lesions that have crusted over. Condoms may be useful and are undoubtedly better than nothing but may not be fully protective.

A pregnant woman who has active genital HSV infection or who is asymptomatically shedding the virus in the vagina at term may transmit HSV to the neonate if the infant is delivered vaginally. Such transmission can be prevented by cesarean section.

No vaccine is currently available for HSV. However, killed, subunit, vaccinia hybrid, and DNA vaccines are being developed to prevent acquisition of the virus or to treat infected people. The glycoprotein D is being used in several subunit vaccines. Defective infectious single-cycle (DISC) vaccines are being developed that use live, defective mutant viruses lacking essential genes. On administration, the vaccine virus produces noninfectious virions.

Varicella-Zoster Virus

VZV causes **chickenpox (varicella)** and, upon recurrence, causes herpes **zoster, or shingles.** VZV shares many characteristics with HSV, including: (1) the ability to establish latent infection of neurons and recurrent disease, (2) the importance of cell-mediated immunity in controlling and preventing serious disease, and (3) the characteristic blisterlike lesions. Like HSV, VZV encodes a **thymidine kinase** and is susceptible to **antiviral drugs.** Unlike HSV, VZV spreads predominantly by the **respiratory route.** Viremia occurs after local replication of the virus in the respiratory tract, leading to the formation of skin lesions over the entire body.

STRUCTURE AND REPLICATION

VZV has the smallest genome of the human herpesviruses. VZV replicates in a similar manner but slower and in fewer types of cells than HSV. Human diploid fibroblasts in vitro, and activated T cells, epithelial and epidermal cells in vivo, support productive VZV replication. Like HSV, VZV establishes a latent infection of neurons, but unlike HSV, several viral RNAs and specific viral proteins can be detected in the cells.

PATHOGENESIS AND IMMUNITY

VZV is generally acquired by inhalation, and primary infection begins in the mucosa of the respiratory tract. Virus replication in the lung is a major source of contagion. The virus then progresses via the bloodstream and lymphatic system to the cells of the reticuloendothelial system (Box 54–6 and Figures 54–8 and 54–9). A secondary viremia occurs after 11 to 13 days and spreads the virus throughout the body and to the skin. The virus remains cell associated and is transmitted on cell-cell interaction, except for terminally differentiated epithelial cells in the lungs and keratinocytes of skin lesions, which can release infectious virus. These cells are the source of virus in vesicles and for contagion. The virus causes a dermal vesiculopustular rash that develops over time in successive crops. Fever and systemic symptoms occur with the rash.

The virus becomes latent in the dorsal root or cranial nerve ganglia after the primary infection. The virus can be reactivated in older adults or in patients with impaired cellular immunity. On reactivation, the virus replicates and is released along the entire neural pathway to infect the skin, causing a vesicular rash along the entire dermatome, known as herpes zoster, or shingles.

Antibody is important in limiting the viremic spread of VZV, and if present, can limit the spread of virus. Cell-mediated immunity is essential for limiting the progression of and resolving the disease. The virus causes more disseminated and more serious disease in the absence of cell-mediated immunity (e.g., in children with leukemia) and may recur on immunosuppression. Although

BOX 54–6. Disease Mechanisms of Varicella-Zoster Virus (VZV)

Initial replication is in the respiratory tract.
VZV infects epithelial cells, fibroblasts, T cells, and neurons.
VZV can form syncytia and spread directly from cell to cell.
Virus is spread by viremia to skin and causes lesions in successive crops.
VZV can escape antibody clearance, and cell-mediated immune response is essential to control infection. Disseminated, life-threatening disease can occur in immunocompromised people.
Virus establishes latent infection of neurons, usually dorsal root and cranial nerve ganglia.
Herpes zoster is a recurrent disease; it results from virus replication along the entire dermatome.
Herpes zoster may result from depression of cell-mediated immunity and other mechanisms of viral activation.

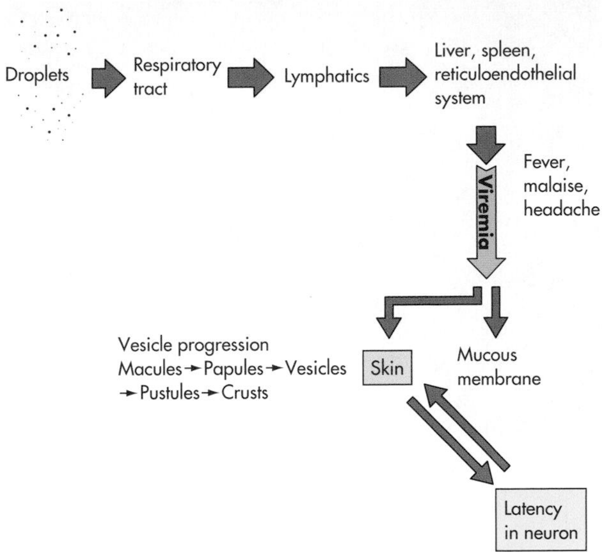

FIGURE 54–8. Mechanism of spread of varicella-zoster virus (VZV) within the body. VZV initially infects the respiratory tract and is spread by the reticuloendothelial system and by viremia to other parts of the body.

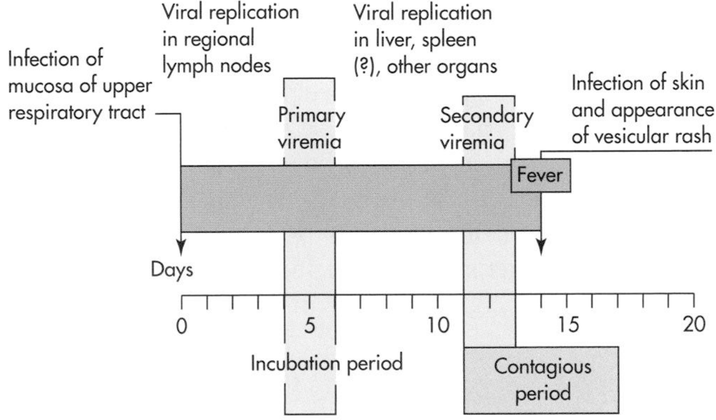

FIGURE 54–9. Time course of varicella (chickenpox). The course in young children, as presented in this figure, is generally shorter and less severe than that in adults.

important for protection, cell-mediated immune responses contribute to the symptomatology. An overzealous response in adults is responsible for causing more extensive cell damage and a more severe manifestation (especially in the lung) in primary infection than that seen in children. Waning of the immune response later in life is the major factor that allows VZV recurrence and herpes zoster.

EPIDEMIOLOGY

VZV is extremely communicable, with rates of infection exceeding 90% among susceptible household contacts (Box 54–7). The disease is spread principally by the respiratory route but may also be spread through contact with skin vesicles. Patients are contagious before and during symptoms. More than 90% of adults in developed countries have the VZV antibody. Herpes zoster results from the reactivation of a patient's latent virus. The disease develops in approximately 10% to 20% of the population infected with VZV, and the incidence rises with age. Herpes zoster lesions contain viable virus and therefore may be a source of varicella infection in a nonimmune person (child).

BOX 54–7. Epidemiology of Varicella-Zoster Virus

Disease/Viral Factors
Virus causes lifelong infection.
Recurrent disease is a source of contagion.

Transmission
Virus is transmitted mainly by respiratory droplets but also by direct contact.

Who Is at Risk?
Children (ages 5 to 9): Mild classic disease.
Teens and adults: At risk for more severe disease with potential pneumonia.
Immunocompromised people and newborns: At risk for life-threatening pneumonia, encephalitis, and progressive-disseminated varicella.
Elderly and immunocompromised people: At risk for recurrent disease (herpes zoster [shingles]).

Geography/Season
Virus is found worldwide.
There is no seasonal incidence.

Modes of Control
Antiviral drugs are available.
Immunity may wane in the elderly population.
Varicella-zoster immunoglobulin is available for immunocompromised people and staff exposed to virus, as well as newborns of mothers showing symptoms within 5 days of birth.
Live vaccine (Oka strain) for children.

CLINICAL SYNDROMES

Varicella (chickenpox) is one of the five **classic childhood exanthems** (along with rubella, roseola, fifth disease, and measles). The disease results from a primary infection with VZV; it is usually a mild disease of childhood and is normally symptomatic, although asymptomatic infection can occur (see Figure 54–9). Varicella characteristics include fever and a maculopapular rash that appear after an incubation period of approximately 14 days (Figure 54–10). Within hours, each maculopapular

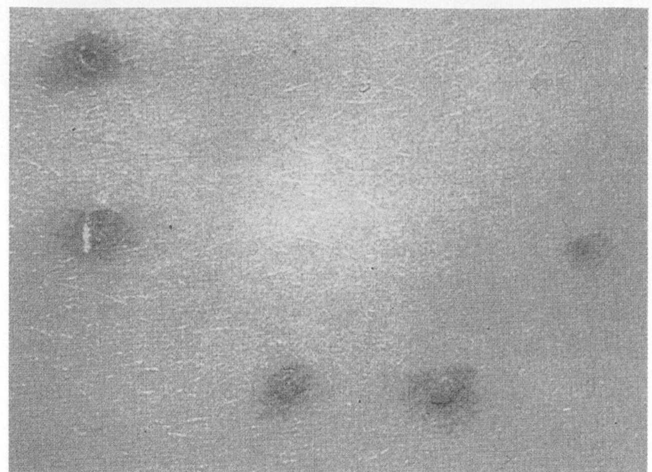

FIGURE 54–10. Characteristic rash of varicella in all stages of its evolution. (From Hart CA, Broadhead RL: *A color atlas of pediatric infectious diseases,* London, 1992, Wolfe.)

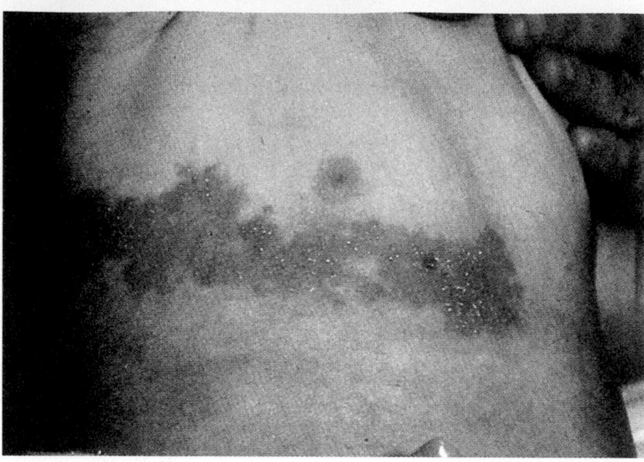

FIGURE 54–11. Herpes zoster ("shingles") in a thoracic dermatome.

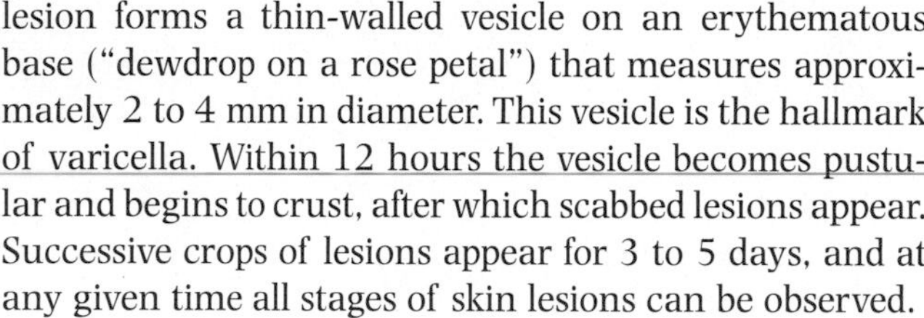

lesion forms a thin-walled vesicle on an erythematous base ("dewdrop on a rose petal") that measures approximately 2 to 4 mm in diameter. This vesicle is the hallmark of varicella. Within 12 hours the vesicle becomes pustular and begins to crust, after which scabbed lesions appear. Successive crops of lesions appear for 3 to 5 days, and at any given time all stages of skin lesions can be observed.

The rash spreads across the entire body but is more severe on the trunk than on the extremities. Its presence on the scalp distinguishes it from many other rashes. The lesions itch and cause scratching, which may lead to bacterial superinfection and scarring. Lesions on the mucous membrane typically occur in the mouth, conjunctivae, and vagina.

Primary infection is usually more severe in adults than in children. **Interstitial pneumonia** may occur in 20% to 30% of adult patients and may be fatal. The pneumonia results from inflammatory reactions at this primary site of infection.

As noted earlier, **herpes zoster** (*zoster* means "belt" or "girdle") is a recurrence of a latent varicella infection acquired earlier in the patient's life. Severe pain in the area innervated by the nerve usually precedes the appearance of the chickenpox-like lesions. The rash is usually limited to a dermatome and resembles varicella (Figure 54–11). A chronic pain syndrome called **postherpetic neuralgia,** which can persist for months to years, occurs in as many as 30% of patients older than 65 years in whom herpes zoster develops.

VZV infection in immunocompromised patients or neonates can result in serious, progressive, and potentially fatal disease. Defects of cell-mediated immunity in such patients increase the risk for dissemination of the virus to the lungs, brain, and liver, which may be fatal. The disease may occur in response to a primary exposure to varicella or because of recurrent disease.

LABORATORY DIAGNOSIS

Cytology

The CPEs in VZV-infected cells are similar to those seen in HSV-infected cells and include Cowdry type A intranuclear inclusions and syncytia. These cells may be seen in skin lesions, respiratory specimens, or organ biopsy specimens. Syncytia may also be seen in Tzanck smears of scrapings from a vesicle's base. A direct fluorescent antibody to membrane antigen test can also be used to examine skin lesion scrapings or biopsy specimens for membrane antigens. Antigen detection and PCR are sensitive means of diagnosing VZV infection.

Virus Isolation

Isolation of VZV is not routinely done because the virus is labile during transport to the laboratory and replicates poorly in vitro. Cultures of material from skin lesions that are crusted over (5 or more days after onset) are usually negative for the virus. Human diploid fibroblasts can support VZV replication and exhibit a CPE similar to that seen in HSV-infected cells, but after a longer incubation period.

Serology

Serologic tests that detect antibodies to VZV are used to screen people for immunity to VZV. However, antibody levels are normally low, so sensitive tests such as immunofluorescence and enzyme-linked immunosorbent assay (ELISA) must be performed to detect the antibody. A significant increase in antibody level can be detected in people experiencing herpes zoster.

TREATMENT, PREVENTION, AND CONTROL

Treatment may be appropriate for adults and immunocompromised patients with VZV infections and for people with shingles, but no treatment is usually necessary for children with varicella. **ACV, famciclovir,** and **valacyclovir** have been approved for the treatment of VZV infections. The VZV DNA polymerase is much less sensitive to ACV treatment than the HSV enzyme, requiring large doses of ACV or the improved pharmacodynamics of famciclovir and valacyclovir (see Box 54–5). There is no good treatment, but analgesics and other painkillers, topical anesthetics, or capsacin cream may provide some relief from the postherpetic neuralgia that follows zoster.

As with other respiratory viruses, it is difficult to limit the transmission of VZV. Because VZV infection in children is generally mild and induces lifelong immunity, exposure of children to VZV early in life is often encouraged. However, high-risk people (e.g., immunosuppressed children) should be protected from exposure to VZV.

Immunosuppressed patients susceptible to severe disease may be protected from serious disease through the administration of **varicella-zoster immunoglobulin (VZIg).** VZIg is prepared through the pooling of plasma from seropositive people. VZIg prophylaxis can prevent viremic spread leading to disease but is ineffective as a therapy for patients already suffering from active varicella or herpes zoster disease.

A **live attenuated vaccine** for VZV (Oka strain) has been licensed for use in the United States and elsewhere and is administered after 2 years of age, on the same schedule as the measles, mumps, and rubella vaccine. The vaccine induces the production of protective antibody and cell-mediated immunity. It is effective as a prophylactic treatment in people even after exposure to VZV. Most significantly, the vaccine promotes protection in immunodeficient children. Vaccination of older adults is also effective at boosting antiviral responses to limit the onset of zoster.

Epstein-Barr Virus

EBV has developed into the ultimate B-lymphocyte parasite, and the diseases it causes reflect this association. EBV was discovered by electron-microscopic observation of characteristic herpes virions in biopsy specimens of a B-cell neoplasm, African Burkitt's lymphoma (AfBL). Its association with infectious mononucleosis was discovered accidentally when serum collected from a laboratory technician convalescing from infectious mononucleosis was found to contain the antibody that recognized AfBL cells. This finding was later confirmed in a large serologic study performed on college students.

EBV causes **heterophile antibody-positive infectious mononucleosis** and has been causally associated with **AfBL (endemic Burkitt's lymphoma), Hodgkin's disease,** and **nasopharyngeal carcinoma.** EBV has also been associated with B-cell lymphomas in patients with acquired or congenital immunodeficiencies. **EBV stimulates the growth and immortalizes B cells** in tissue culture.

STRUCTURE AND REPLICATION

EBV is a member of the subfamily Gammaherpesvirinae, with a very limited host range and a **tissue tropism** defined by the limited cellular expression of its receptor. This receptor is also **the receptor for the C3d component of the complement system (also called CR2 or CD21).** It is expressed on B cells of humans and New World monkeys and on some epithelial cells of the oropharynx and nasopharynx. EBV also uses class II MHC molecules as a co-receptor.

EBV infection has the following three potential outcomes:

1. EBV can replicate in B cells or epithelial cells permissive for EBV replication.
2. EBV can cause latent infection of B cells in the presence of competent T cells.
3. EBV can stimulate and immortalize B cells.

EBV encodes more than 70 proteins, different groups of which are expressed for the different types of infections.

Permissive epithelial and B cells allow the transcription and translation of the ZEBRA (peptide encoded by the Z gene region) transcriptional activator protein, which activates the immediate early genes of the virus and the lytic cycle. After synthesis of the DNA polymerase and replication of DNA, the viral capsid and glycoproteins are synthesized. They include gp350/220 (related glycoproteins of 350,000 and 220,000 Da), which is the viral attachment protein, and gp85 (85,000 Da). The viral proteins produced during a productive infection are serologically defined and grouped as **early antigen (EA), viral capsid antigen (VCA),** and the glycoproteins of the **membrane antigen (MA)** (Table 54–3).

During nonpermissive infection of B cells, the cells contain a small number of circular, plasmidlike EBV genomes that replicate only during cell division. Select viral genes are expressed depending on the state of the B cell; they include **Epstein-Barr nuclear antigens (EBNAs)** 1, 2, 3A, 3B, and 3C; latent proteins **(LPs); latent membrane proteins (LMPs) 1 and 2;** and two small Epstein-Barr–encoded RNA (EBER) molecules, EBER-1 and EBER-2. The EBNAs and LPs are DNA-binding proteins that are essential for establishing and maintaining the infection (EBNA-1), immortalization (EBNA-2), and other purposes. The LMPs are membrane proteins

TABLE 54–3. Markers of Epstein-Barr Virus (EBV) Infection

Name	Abbreviation	Characteristics	Biologic Association	Clinical Association
EBV nuclear antigens	EBNAs	Nuclear	EBNAs are nonstructural antigens and are the first antigens to appear; EBNAs are seen in all infected and transformed cells and bind to cell DNA.	Anti-EBNA develops late in infection.
Early antigen	EA-R	Only cytoplasmic	EA-R appears before EA-D; its appearance is first sign that infected cell has entered lytic cycle.	Anti–EA-R is seen in Burkitt's lymphoma.
	EA-D	Diffuse in cytoplasm and nucleus	—	Anti–EA-D is seen in infectious mononucleosis.
Viral capsid antigen	VCA	Cytoplasmic	VCA is a late antigen; it is found in virus producer cells.	Anti-VCA IgM is transient; anti-VCA IgG is persistent.
Lymphocyte-defined membrane antigen (LYDMA)	LYDMA	—	LYDMA is not found on Burkitt's lymphoma cells; it is found on cells infected in vitro and on nonproducer cells.	LYDMA is not detectable by antibody.
Membrane antigen	MA	Cell surface	MAs are the envelope glycoproteins.	Same as VCA.
Heterophile antibody		Recognition of Paul-Bunnell antigen on sheep, horse, or bovine erythrocytes	EBV-induced B-cell proliferation promotes production of heterophile antibody.	Early symptom occurs in more than 50% of patients.

EA, Early antigen; EBNA = Epstein-Barr nuclear antigen; MA, membrane antigen; VCA, viral capsid antigen.

with oncogene-like activity. These proteins stimulate the growth of and immortalize the B cell. EBV establishes latency in memory B cells in which only the EBNA-1 and LMP-2 are expressed, maintaining the genome in the cells but with minimal potential for immune recognition of the infected cell.

PATHOGENESIS AND IMMUNITY

EBV has adapted to the human B cell and manipulates and uses the different phases of B-cell development to establish lifelong infection of the individual and still promote its transmission. The diseases of EBV result from either an overactive immune response (infectious mononucleosis) or the lack of effective immune control (lymphoma and hairy cell leukoplakia).

The productive infection of B cells and epithelial cells of the oropharynx, such as in the tonsils (Box 54–8 and Figure 54–12), promotes virus shedding into saliva to transmit the virus to other hosts and establishes a viremia to spread the virus to other B cells in lymphatic tissue and blood.

EBV proteins activate B-cell growth and also prevent apoptosis (programmed cell death). T cells usually control the B-cell proliferation. In the absence of T cells (e.g., in tissue culture), EBV can immortalize B cells and promote the development of B-lymphoblastoid cell lines. In vivo, B-cell activation and proliferation occurs and is indicated by the spurious production of an IgM antibody to the Paul-Bunnell antigen, termed the *heterophile antibody* (see later discussion of serology). Continued B-cell proliferation in conjunction with the effects of other cofactors may result in the development of lymphoma.

BOX 54–8. Disease Mechanisms of Epstein-Barr Virus

- Virus in saliva initiates infection of oral epithelia and spreads to B cells in lymphatic tissue.
- There is productive infection of epithelial and B cells.
- Virus promotes growth of B cells (immortalizes).
- T cells kill and limit B-cell outgrowth. T cells are *required for controlling infection*. Antibody role is limited.
- EBV establishes latency in memory B cells and is reactivated when the B cell is activated.
- T-cell response (lymphocytosis) contributes to symptoms of **infectious mononucleosis.**
- There is causative association with lymphoma in immunosuppressed people and African children living in malarial regions (African Burkitt's lymphoma) and with nasopharyngeal carcinoma in China.

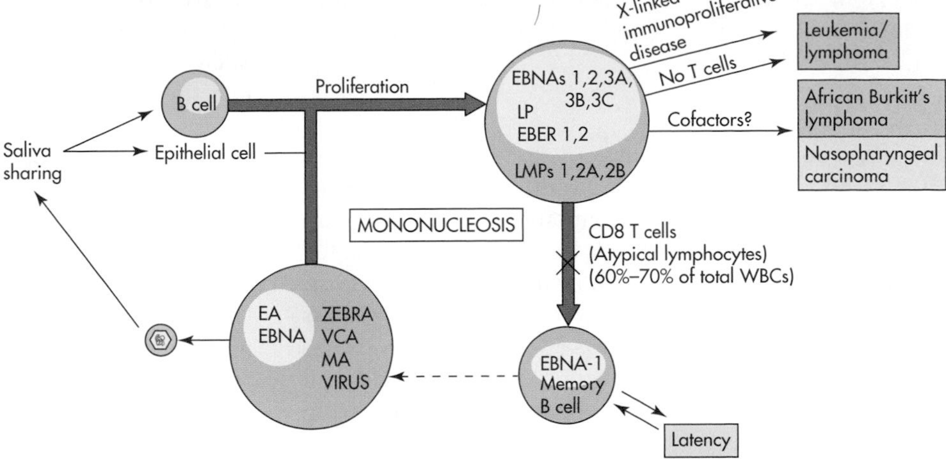

FIGURE 54–12. Progression of Epstein-Barr virus (EBV) infection. Infection may result in lytic, latent, or immortalizing infection, which can be distinguished on the basis of production of virus and expression of different viral proteins and antigens. T cells limit the outgrowth of the EBV-infected cells and maintain the latent infection. EA, Early antigen; EBER, Epstein-Barr–encoded RNA; EBNA, Epstein-Barr nuclear antigen; LMP, latent membrane protein; LP, latent protein; MA, membrane antigen; VCA, viral capsid antigen; ZEBRA, peptide encoded by the Z gene region.

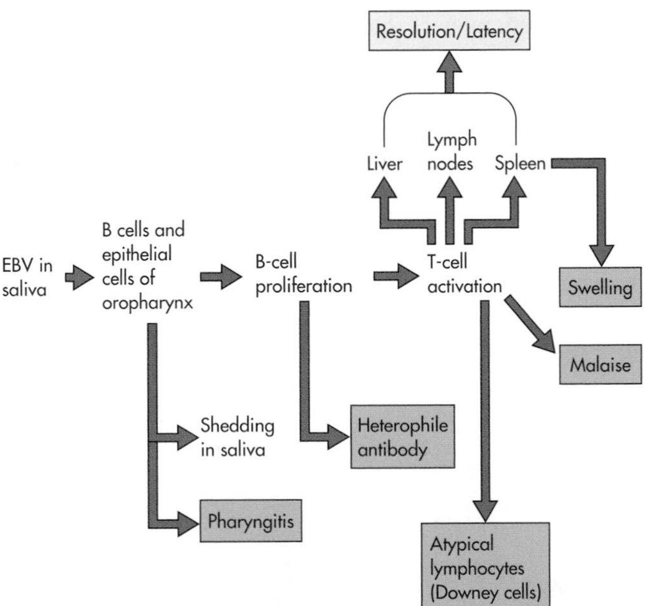

FIGURE 54–13. Pathogenesis of Epstein-Barr virus (EBV). EBV is acquired by close contact between persons through saliva and infects the B cells. The resolution of the EBV infection and many of the symptoms of infectious mononucleosis result from the activation of T cells in response to the infection.

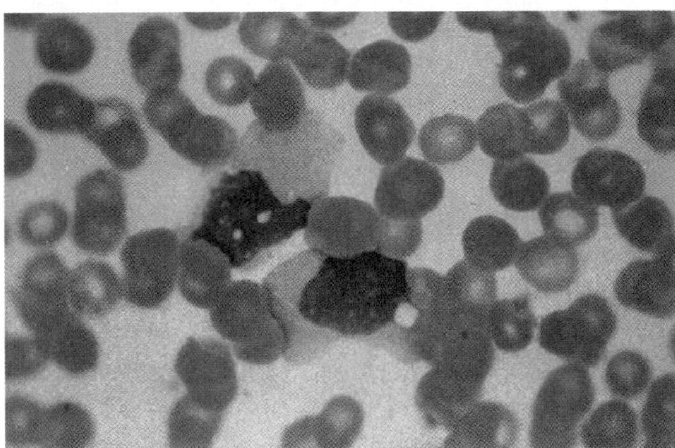

FIGURE 54–14. Atypical T-cell (Downey cell) characteristic of infectious mononucleosis. The cells have a more basophilic and vacuolated cytoplasm than normal lymphocytes, and the nucleus may be oval, kidney shaped, or lobulated. The cell margin may seem to be indented by neighboring red blood cells.

During productive infection, antibody is first developed against the components of the virion, VCA and MA, and later against the EA. After resolution of the infection (lysis of the productively infected cells), antibody against the nuclear antigens (EBNAs) is produced. T cells are essential for limiting the proliferation of EBV-infected B cells and controlling the disease (Figure 54–13). EBV counteracts some of the protective action of TH1 CD4 T-cell responses by producing an interleukin-10 analogue (BCRF-1) during productive infection that inhibits the protective TH1 CD4 T-cell responses and also stimulates B-cell growth.

Infectious mononucleosis results from a "civil war" between the EBV-infected B cells and the protective T cells. The T cells are surrounded by infected B cells and are activated by viral antigenic peptides presented on both the MHC I and II molecules. The classic **lymphocytosis** (increase in mononuclear cells), swelling of lymphoid organs (lymph nodes, spleen, and liver), and malaise associated with infectious mononucleosis results mainly from the activation and proliferation of T cells. The T cells appear as **atypical lymphocytes** (also called **Downey cells**) (Figure 54–14). They increase in number in the peripheral blood during the second week of infection, accounting for 10% to 80% of the total white blood cell count at this time (hence the "mononucleosis"). Children have a less active immune response to EBV infection and therefore have very mild disease.

The virus persists in at least one memory B cell per milliliter of blood for the person's lifetime. EBV may be reactivated when the memory B cell is activated (especially in the tonsils or oropharynx) and may be shed in saliva.

EPIDEMIOLOGY

EBV is transmitted in saliva (Box 54–9). More than 90% of EBV-infected people intermittently shed the virus for life, even when totally asymptomatic. Children can acquire the virus at an early age by sharing contaminated drinking glasses. *Children generally have subclinical disease.* Saliva sharing between adolescents and young adults often occurs during kissing; thus EBV mononucleosis has earned the nickname "the kissing disease." Disease in these people may go unnoticed or may manifest in varying degrees of severity. At least 70% of the population of the United States is infected by age 30.

The geographic distribution of some EBV-associated neoplasms indicates a possible association with cofactors. The immunosuppressive potential of malaria has been suggested as a cofactor in the progression of chronic or latent EBV infection to AfBL. The restriction of nasopharyngeal carcinoma to people living in certain regions of China indicates a possible genetic predisposition to the cancer or the presence of cofactors in the food or environment. More subtle mechanisms may facilitate the role of EBV in 30% to 50% of cases of Hodgkin's disease.

Transplant recipients, patients with the acquired immune deficiency syndrome (AIDS), and genetically immunodeficient people are at high risk for lymphoproliferative disorders initiated by EBV. These disorders may appear as polyclonal and monoclonal B-cell lymphomas. Such people are also at high risk for a productive EBV infection in the form of **hairy oral leukoplakia.**

BOX 54–9. Epidemiology of Epstein-Barr Virus

Disease/Viral Factors
Virus causes lifelong infection.
Recurrent disease is cause of contagion.
Virus may cause asymptomatic shedding.

Transmission
Transmission occurs via saliva, close oral contact ("kissing disease"), or sharing of items such as toothbrushes and cups.

Who Is at Risk?
Children: Asymptomatic disease or mild symptoms.
Teenagers and adults: At risk for infectious mononucleosis.
Immunocompromised people: At highest risk for life-threatening neoplastic disease.

Geography/Season
Infectious mononucleosis has worldwide distribution.
There is causative association with African Burkitt's lymphoma in malarial belt of Africa.
There is no seasonal incidence.

Modes of Control
There are no modes of control.

CLINICAL SYNDROMES

Heterophile Antibody-Positive Infectious Mononucleosis

Like infections caused by other herpesviruses, EBV infection in a child is much milder than infection in an adolescent or adult. In fact, infection in children is usually subclinical. The triad of classic symptoms for infectious mononucleosis is **lymphadenopathy** (swollen glands), **splenomegaly** (large spleen), and **exudative pharyngitis** accompanied by high fever, malaise, and often, hepatosplenomegaly (large liver and spleen). A rash may occur, especially after ampicillin treatment (for the sore throat). The major complaint of people with infectious mononucleosis is fatigue (Figure 54–15). The disease is rarely fatal in healthy people but can cause serious complications resulting from neurologic disorders, laryngeal obstruction, or rupture of the spleen. Neurologic complications include meningoencephalitis and the Guillain-Barré syndrome. Mononucleosis-like syndromes can also be caused by CMV, HHV6, *Toxoplasma gondii,* and human immunodeficiency virus (HIV).

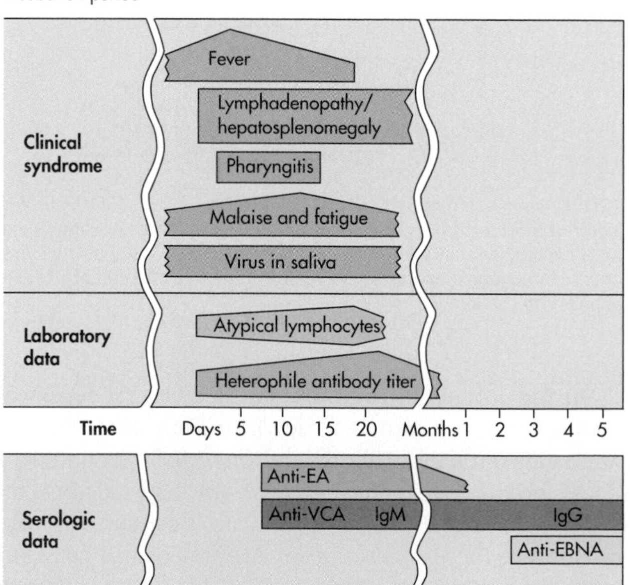

FIGURE 54–15. Clinical course of infectious mononucleosis and laboratory findings of those with the infection. Epstein-Barr virus (EBV) infection may be asymptomatic or may produce the symptoms of mononucleosis. The incubation period can last as long as 2 months. EA, Early antigen; EBNA, Epstein-Barr nuclear antigen; VCA, viral capsid antigen.

Chronic Disease

EBV can cause cyclic recurrent disease in some people. These patients experience chronic tiredness and may also have low-grade fever, headaches, and sore throat. This disorder is different from chronic fatigue syndrome, which has an unknown etiology.

Epstein-Barr Virus–Induced Lymphoproliferative Diseases

On infection with EBV, people lacking T-cell immunity are likely to suffer life-threatening polyclonal leukemia-like B-cell proliferative disease and lymphoma instead of infectious mononucleosis. People with congenital deficiencies of T-cell function are likely to suffer life-threatening X-linked lymphoproliferative disease. One such X-linked genetic defect in a T-cell gene (SLAM [signaling lymphocyte activation molecule]-associated protein) prevents the T cell from controlling B-cell growth during a normal immune response to antigen or to EBV. Transplant recipients undergoing immunosuppressive treatment are at high risk for **post-transplant lymphoproliferative** disease instead of infectious mononucleosis after exposure to the virus or on reactivation of latent virus. Similar diseases are seen in patients with AIDS.

African Burkitt's lymphoma (endemic lymphoma) is a poorly differentiated monoclonal B-cell lymphoma of the jaw and face that is endemic in children living in the malarial regions of Africa. The tumors contain EBV DNA sequences but express only the EBNA-1 viral antigen. Virions can occasionally be seen on electron micrographs of infected material. In addition to EBV DNA, the tumor cells contain chromosomal translocations that juxtapose the *C-myc* oncogene to a very active promoter, such as an immunoglobulin gene promoter [t(8;14), t(8;22), t(8;2)]. The tumor cells are also relatively invisible to immune control. It is not known how malaria acts to promote EBV involvement with AfBL. EBV is also associated with Burkitt's lymphomas in people living in other parts of the world but to a much smaller extent. Many **Hodgkin's lymphomas** can also be attributed to EBV.

As noted earlier, **nasopharyngeal carcinoma** is endemic in Asia, occurs in adults, and contains EBV DNA within the tumor cells. Unlike Burkitt's lymphoma, in which the tumor cells are derived from lymphocytes, the tumor cells of nasopharyngeal carcinoma are of epithelial origin.

Hairy Oral Leukoplakia

Hairy oral leukoplakia is an unusual manifestation of a productive EBV infection of epithelial cells characterized by lesions of the mouth. It is an opportunistic manifestation that occurs in patients with AIDS.

BOX 54–10. Diagnosis of Epstein-Barr Virus

1. Symptoms
   a. Mild headache, fatigue, fever
   b. Triad: Lymphadenopathy, splenomegaly, exudative pharyngitis
   c. Other: Hepatitis, ampicillin-induced rash
2. Complete blood cell count
   a. Hyperplasia
   b. Atypical lymphocytes (Downey cells) (T cells)
3. Heterophile antibody (transient)
4. EBV-antigen specific antibody

LABORATORY DIAGNOSIS

EBV-induced infectious mononucleosis is diagnosed on the basis of the **symptoms** (Box 54–10), the finding of atypical lymphocytes, and the presence of **lymphocytosis** (mononuclear cells constituting 60% to 70% of the white blood cell count with 30% atypical lymphocytes), **heterophile antibody,** and antibody to viral antigens. Virus isolation is not practical. PCR and DNA probe analysis for the viral genome and immunofluorescent identification of viral antigens are used to detect evidence of infection.

Atypical lymphocytes are probably the earliest detectable indication of an EBV infection. These cells appear with the onset of symptoms and disappear with resolution of the disease.

Heterophile antibody results from the nonspecific, mitogen-like activation of B cells by EBV and the production of a wide repertoire of antibodies. These antibodies include an IgM heterophile antibody that recognizes the Paul-Bunnell antigen on sheep, horse, and bovine erythrocytes but not that on guinea pig kidney cells. The heterophile antibody response can usually be detected by the end of the first week of illness and lasts for as long as several months. It is an excellent indication of EBV infection in adults but is not as reliable in children or infants. The horse cell (Monospot) test and ELISA are rapid and widely used for the detection of the heterophile antibody.

Serologic tests for antibody to viral antigens are a more dependable method than heterophile antibody to confirm the diagnosis of EBV mononucleosis (Figure 54–15; also see Table 54–4). EBV infection is indicated by the finding of any of the following: (1) IgM antibody to the VCA, (2) the presence of VCA antibody and the absence of EBNA antibody, or (3) elevation of antibodies to VCA and early antigen. The finding of both VCA and EBNA antibodies in serum indicates that the person had a previous infection. Generation of antibody to EBNA requires lysis of the infected cell and usually indicates T-cell control of active disease.

TABLE 54–4. Serologic Profile for Epstein-Barr Virus (EBV) Infections

Patient's Clinical Status	Heterophile Antibodies	EBV-Specific Antibodies				
		VCA-IgM	VCA-IgG	EA	EBNA	Comment
Susceptible	–	–	–	–	–	–
Acute primary infection	+	+	+	±	–	–
Chronic primary infection	–	–	+	+	–	–
Past infection	–	–	+	–	+	–
Reactivation infection	–	–	+	+	+	EA restricted or diffuse
Burkitt's lymphoma	–	–	+	+	+	EA restricted only
Nasopharyngeal carcinoma	–	–	+	+	+	EA diffuse only

Modified from Balows A et al, editors: *Laboratory diagnosis of infectious diseases: Principles and practices,* New York, 1988, Springer-Verlag.
EA, Early antigen; EBNA = Epstein-Barr nuclear antigen; Ig, immunoglobulin; VCA, viral capsid antigen.

TREATMENT, PREVENTION, AND CONTROL

No effective treatment or vaccine is available for EBV disease (see Box 54–5). The ubiquitous nature of the virus and the potential for asymptomatic shedding make control of infection difficult. However, infection elicits lifelong immunity. Therefore, the best means of preventing infectious mononucleosis is exposure to the virus early in life, because the disease is more benign in children.

Cytomegalovirus

CMV is a common human pathogen, infecting 0.5% to 2.5% of all newborns and approximately 40% of women visiting clinics for sexually transmitted diseases. It is the most common viral cause of **congenital defects.** Although usually causing mild or asymptomatic disease in children and adults, CMV is particularly important as an **opportunistic pathogen in immunocompromised patients.**

STRUCTURE AND REPLICATION

CMV is a member of the subfamily Betaherpesvirinae and is considered lymphotropic. It has the largest genome of the human herpesviruses. In contrast to the traditional definition of a virus, which states that a virion particle contains DNA or RNA, studies now indicate that CMV carries specific mRNAs into the cell in the virion particle to facilitate infection. Human CMV replicates only in human cells. Fibroblasts, epithelial cells, macrophages, and other cells are permissive for CMV replication. CMV establishes latent infection in mononuclear lymphocytes, the stromal cells of the bone marrow, and other cells.

BOX 54–11. Disease Mechanisms of Cytomegalovirus (CMV)

CMV is acquired from blood, tissue, and most body secretions.
CMV causes productive infection of epithelial and other cells.
CMV establishes latency in T cells, macrophages, and other cells.
Cell-mediated immunity is required for resolution and contributes to symptoms; role of antibody is limited.
Suppression of cell-mediated immunity allows recurrence and severe presentation.
CMV generally causes subclinical infection.

PATHOGENESIS AND IMMUNITY

The pathogenesis of CMV is similar to that of other herpesviruses in many respects (Box 54–11). CMV is an excellent parasite and readily establishes persistent and latent infections rather than an extensive lytic infection. CMV is highly cell-associated and is spread throughout the body within infected cells, especially lymphocytes and leukocytes. The virus is reactivated by immunosuppression (e.g., corticosteroids, infection with HIV) and possibly by allogeneic stimulation (i.e., the host response to transfused or transplanted cells).

Cell-mediated immunity is essential for resolving and controlling the outgrowth of CMV infection. However, CMV has several means for evading the immune response. CMV infection alters the function of lymphocytes and leukocytes. The virus prevents antigen presentation to both CD8 cytotoxic T cells and CD4 T cells by preventing the expression of MHC I molecules on the cell surface and by interfering with cytokine-induced expression of MHC II molecules on antigen-presenting cells (including the infected cells). A viral protein also blocks natural killer cell attack of CMV-infected cells. Like EBV, CMV also encodes an interleukin-10 analogue that would inhibit TH1 protective immune responses.

EPIDEMIOLOGY AND CLINICAL SYNDROMES

In most cases, CMV replicates and is shed without causing symptoms (Table 54–5). Activation and replication of CMV in the kidney and secretory glands promote its secretion in urine and bodily secretions. CMV can be isolated from urine, blood, throat washings, saliva, tears, breast milk, semen, stool, amniotic fluid, vaginal and cervical secretions, and tissues obtained for transplantation (Table 54–6 and Box 54–12). Virus can be transmitted to other individuals by means of blood transfusions and organ transplants. The congenital, oral, and sexual routes, blood transfusion, and tissue transplantation are the major means by which CMV is transmitted. CMV disease is an opportunistic disorder, rarely causing symptoms in the immunocompetent host but causing serious disease in an immunosuppressed or immunodeficient person, such as a patient with AIDS, or a neonate (Figure 54–16).

TABLE 54–5. Sources of Cytomegalovirus Infection

Age Group	Source
Neonate	Transplacental transmission, intrauterine infections, cervical secretions
Baby or child	Body secretions: breast milk, saliva, tears, urine
Adult	Sexual transmission (semen), blood transfusion, organ graft

Congenital Infection

CMV is the most prevalent viral cause of congenital disease. A significant percentage (0.5% to 2.5%) of all newborns in

TABLE 54–6. Cytomegalovirus Syndromes

Tissue	Children/Adults	Immunosuppressed Patients
Predominant presentation	**Asymptomatic**	**Disseminated disease, severe disease**
Eyes	—	Chorioretinitis
Lungs	—	Pneumonia, pneumonitis
Gastrointestinal tract	—	Esophagitis, colitis
Nervous system	Polyneuritis, myelitis	Meningitis and encephalitis, myelitis
Lymphoid system	Mononucleosis syndrome, post-transfusion syndrome	Leukopenia, lymphocytosis
Major organs	Carditis,* hepatitis*	Hepatitis
Neonates	**Deafness, intracerebral calcification, microcephaly, mental retardation**	—

*Complication of mononucleosis or postperfusion syndrome.

BOX 54–12. Epidemiology of Cytomegalovirus Infection

Disease/Viral Factors
Virus causes lifelong infection.
Recurrent disease is source of contagion.
Virus may cause asymptomatic shedding.

Transmission
Transmission occurs via blood, organ transplants, and all secretions (urine, saliva, semen, cervical secretions, breast milk, and tears).
Virus is transmitted orally and sexually, in blood transfusions, in tissue transplants, in utero, at birth, and by nursing.

Geography/Season
Virus is found worldwide.
There is no seasonal incidence.

Who Is at Risk?
Babies.
Babies of mothers who experience seroconversion during term: At high risk for congenital defects.
Sexually active people.
Blood and organ recipients.
Burn victims.
Immunocompromised people: Symptomatic and recurrent disease.

Modes of Control
Antiviral drugs are available for patients with acquired immune deficiency syndrome.
Screening potential blood and organ donors for cytomegalovirus reduces transmission of virus.

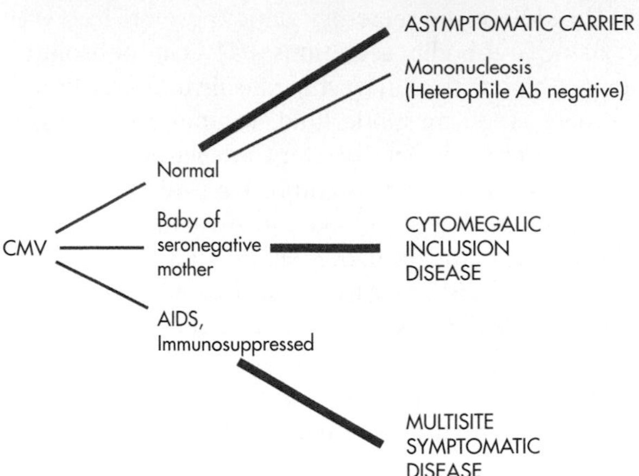

FIGURE 54–16. Outcomes of cytomegalovirus (CMV) infections. The outcome of CMV infection depends very heavily on the immune status of the patient.

the United States are infected with CMV prior to birth, and a large percentage of babies are infected within the first months of life. Approximately 10% of affected newborns (4000 per year) show clinical evidence of disease, such as small size, thrombocytopenia, microcephaly, intracerebral calcification, jaundice, hepatosplenomegaly, and rash **(cytomegalic inclusion disease).** Unilateral or bilateral hearing loss and mental retardation are common consequences of congenital CMV infection. The risk for serious birth defects is extremely high for infants born to mothers who underwent primary CMV infections during their pregnancies.

Fetuses are infected by virus in the mother's blood (primary infection) or by virus ascending from the cervix (after a recurrence). The symptoms of congenital infection are less severe or can be prevented by the immune response of a seropositive mother. Congenital CMV infection is best documented by isolation of the virus from the infant's urine during the first week of life.

Perinatal Infection

In the United States, as many as 20% of pregnant women harbor CMV in the cervix at term and are likely to experience reactivation of the virus during pregnancy. Approximately half the neonates born through an infected cervix acquire CMV infection and become excreters of the virus at 3 to 4 weeks of age. Neonates may also acquire CMV from maternal milk or colostrum. Perinatal infection causes no clinically evident disease in healthy full-term infants.

Another means by which neonates can acquire CMV is through blood transfusions. Of the seronegative babies who are exposed to blood from seropositive donors, 13.5% acquire CMV infection in the immediate postnatal period. Significant clinical infection may occur in premature infants who acquire CMV from transfused blood, usually resulting in pneumonia and hepatitis.

Infection in Children and Adults

Only 10% to 15% of adolescents are infected with CMV, but this number increases to 50% to 85% of adults in the United States by the age of 40. CMV is more prevalent among people in low socioeconomic brackets living in crowded conditions and in people living in developing countries. CMV is a **sexually transmitted disease.** The titer of the CMV in semen is the highest of that in any body secretion. Approximately 40% of women seen at a venereal disease clinic had recently acquired the virus.

Although most CMV infections acquired in young adulthood are asymptomatic, patients may show a **heterophile-negative mononucleosis syndrome.** The symptoms of CMV disease are similar to those of EBV infection but with less severe pharyngitis and lymphadenopathy (see Figure 54–16). Although the presence of CMV-infected cells promotes a T-cell outgrowth (atypical lymphocytosis) similar to that seen in EBV infection, heterophile antibody is not present. The absence of this antibody reflects the differences in the target cell and the action of the viruses on the target cell. CMV disease should be suspected in a patient who has heterophile-negative mononucleosis or in whom there are signs of hepatitis but results of tests for hepatitis A, B, and C are negative.

Transmission via Transfusion and Transplantation

Transmission of CMV by blood most often results in an asymptomatic infection; if symptoms are present, they typically resemble those of mononucleosis. Fever, splenomegaly, and atypical lymphocytosis usually begin 3 to 5 weeks after transfusion. Pneumonia and mild hepatitis may also occur. CMV may also be transmitted by organ transplantation (e.g., kidneys, bone marrow), and CMV infection is often reactivated in transplant recipients during periods of intense immunosuppression.

Infection in the Immunocompromised Host

CMV is a prominent opportunistic infectious agent. In immunocompromised people, it causes symptomatic primary or recurrent disease (see Table 54–6).

CMV disease of the lung **(pneumonia and pneumonitis)** is a common outcome in immunosuppressed patients and can be fatal if not treated. In addition, CMV often causes **retinitis** in patients who are severely immunodeficient (e.g., in as many as 10% to 15% of patients with AIDS). Interstitial pneumonia and encephalitis may also be caused by CMV but may be difficult to distinguish from infections caused by other opportunistic agents. CMV **colitis or esophagitis** may develop in as many as 10% of patients with AIDS. CMV esophagitis may mimic candidal esophagitis. A smaller percentage of immunocompromised patients may experience CMV infection of the gastrointestinal tract. Patients with CMV colitis usually have diarrhea, weight loss, anorexia, and fever.

CMV is also responsible for the **failure of many kidney transplants.** This may be the result of virus replication in the graft after reactivation in the transplanted kidney or infection from the host.

LABORATORY DIAGNOSIS

Histology

The histologic hallmark of CMV infection is the **cytomegalic cell,** which is an **enlarged cell** (25 to 35 mm in diameter) that contains a dense, **central, "owl's eye," basophilic intranuclear inclusion body** (Table 54–7; Figure 54–17). Such infected cells may be found in any tissue of the body and in urine and are thought to be epithelial in origin. The inclusions are readily seen with Papanicolaou or hematoxylin-eosin staining.

Immune and DNA Probe Techniques

A rapid, sensitive diagnosis can be obtained by detection of viral antigen using immunofluorescence or an ELISA or the viral genome using PCR and related techniques in cells of a biopsy, blood, bronchoalveolar lavage, or urine sample (see Figure 17–3).

Culture

CMV grows only in diploid fibroblast cell cultures and, normally, must be maintained for at least 4 to 6 weeks because the characteristic CPE develops very slowly in specimens with very low titers of the virus. Isolation of CMV is especially reliable in immunocompromised patients, who often have high titers of virus in their secretions. For example, in the semen of patients with AIDS, titers of viable virus may be greater than 10^6.

More rapid results are achieved by centrifuging a patient's sample onto cells grown on a coverslip within a shell vial. Specimens are examined after 1 to 2 days of incubation by indirect immunofluorescence for the presence of one or more of the immediate early viral antigens.

Serology

Seroconversion is usually an excellent marker for primary CMV infection. Titers of CMV-specific IgM antibody may be very high in patients with AIDS. However, CMV-specific IgM antibody may also develop during the reactivation of CMV and is therefore not a dependable indicator of primary infection.

TREATMENT, PREVENTION, AND CONTROL

Ganciclovir (dihydroxypropoxymethyl guanine), **valganciclovir** (valyl ester of ganciclovir), **cidofovir,** and **foscarnet** (phosphonoformic acid) have been approved by the FDA for the treatment of specific diseases resulting from CMV infections of immunosuppressed patients (see Box 54–5). Ganciclovir is structurally similar to ACV; it is phosphorylated and activated by a CMV-encoded protein kinase, inhibits the viral DNA polymerase, and causes DNA chain termination (see Chapter 50). Ganciclovir is more toxic than ACV. Ganciclovir can be used to treat severe CMV infections in immunocompromised patients. Valganciclovir is a prodrug of ganciclovir that can be taken orally, is converted to ganciclovir in the liver, and has better bioavailability than ganciclovir. Cidofovir is a phosphorylated cytidine nucleoside analogue that does

TABLE 54–7. Laboratory Tests for Diagnosing Cytomegalovirus Infection

Test	Finding
Cytology and histology*	"Owl's-eye" inclusion body Antigen detection In situ DNA probe hybridization Polymerase chain reaction (PCR)
Cell culture	Cytologic effect in human diploid fibroblasts Immunofluorescence detection of early antigens (most common) PCR
Serology:	Primary infection

*Samples taken for analysis include urine, saliva, blood, bronchoalveolar lavage specimens, and tissue biopsy specimens.

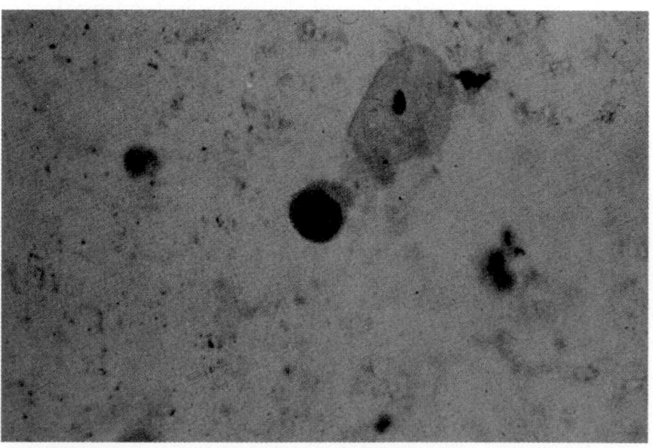

FIGURE 54–17. Cytomegalovirus-infected cell with basophilic nuclear inclusion body.

not require a viral enzyme for activation. Foscarnet is a simple molecule that inhibits the viral DNA polymerase by mimicking the pyrophosphate portion of nucleotide triphosphates.

CMV spreads mainly by the sexual, tissue transplantation, and transfusion routes, and spread by these means is preventable. Semen is a major vector for the sexual spread of CMV to both heterosexual and homosexual contacts. The use of condoms or abstinence would limit viral spread. Transmission of the virus can also be reduced through the screening of potential blood and organ donors for CMV seronegativity. Screening is especially important for donors of blood transfusions to be given to infants. Although congenital and perinatal transmission of CMV cannot effectively be prevented, a seropositive mother is least likely to produce a baby with symptomatic CMV disease. No vaccine for CMV is available.

Human Herpesviruses 6 and 7

The two variants of HHV6, HHV6A and HHV6B, and HHV7, are members of the genus *Roseolovirus* of the subfamily Betaherpesvirinae. HHV6 was first isolated from the blood of patients with AIDS and grown in T-cell cultures. It was identified as a herpesvirus because of its characteristic morphology within infected cells. Like CMV, HHV6 is lymphotropic and ubiquitous. At least 45% of people are seropositive for HHV6 by age 2 years, and almost 100% by adulthood. In 1988, HHV6 was serologically associated with a common disease of children, **exanthem subitum**, commonly known as **roseola.** HHV7 was isolated in a similar manner from the T cells of a patient with AIDS who was also infected with HHV6, and later it was also shown to cause exanthem subitum.

PATHOGENESIS AND IMMUNITY

HHV6 infection occurs very early in life, indicating that it must be shed and spread readily. It is present in the saliva of most adults and is spread by oral secretions.

HHV6, like CMV, infects lymphocytes, monocytes, and epithelial and endothelial cells. Replication of the virus in salivary glands is the source of the virus secreted in saliva. HHV6 establishes a latent infection in T cells and monocytes but may replicate on activation of the cells. Cells in which the virus is replicating appear large and refractile and have occasional intranuclear and intracytoplasmic inclusion bodies. T-cell leukemia cell lines also support replication of the virus.

Like the replication of CMV, the replication of HHV6 is controlled by cell-mediated immunity. The virus is likely to become activated in patients with AIDS or other lymphoproliferative and immunosuppressive disorders.

CLINICAL SYNDROMES (BOX 54–13)

Exanthem subitum, or roseola, is caused by either HHV6B or HHV7 and is one of the five classic childhood exanthems previously mentioned (Figure 54–18). It is characterized by the rapid onset of high fever of a few days' duration, which is followed by a generalized rash that lasts only 24 to 48 hours. The presence of infected T cells or the activation of delayed-type hypersensitivity T cells in the skin may be the cause of the rash. The disease is effectively controlled and resolved by cell-mediated immunity, but the virus establishes a lifelong latent infection of T cells.

HHV6 may also cause a mononucleosis syndrome and lymphadenopathy in adults and may be a cofactor in the pathogenesis of AIDS.

Other Human Herpesviruses

HUMAN HERPESVIRUS 8 (KAPOSI'S SARCOMA–ASSOCIATED HERPESVIRUS)

HHV8 DNA sequences were discovered in biopsy specimens of **Kaposi's sarcoma, primary effusion lymphoma** (a rare type of B-cell lymphoma), **and multicentric Castleman's disease** through the use of PCR analysis. Kaposi's sarcoma is one of the characteristic opportunistic diseases associated with AIDS. Genome sequence analysis showed that the virus was unique and a member of the subfamily Gammaherpesvirinae. Like EBV, the B cell is the primary target cell for HHV8, but the virus also infects a limited number of endothelial cells, monocytes, and epithelial and sensory nerve cells. Within the Kaposi's sarcoma tumors, endothelial spindle cells contain the virus.

HHV8 encodes several proteins with homology to human proteins that promote the growth and prevent apoptosis of the infected and surrounding cells. These proteins include an interleukin-6 homologue (growth and antiapoptosis), a Bcl-2 analogue (antiapoptosis), chemokines, and a chemokine receptor. These proteins can promote the growth and development of polyclonal Kaposi's sarcoma cells in AIDS patients and others. HHV8 DNA is present and is associated with peripheral blood lymphocytes, most likely B cells, in approximately 10% of immunocompetent people. HHV8 is limited to certain geographic areas (Italy, Greece, Africa) and to patients

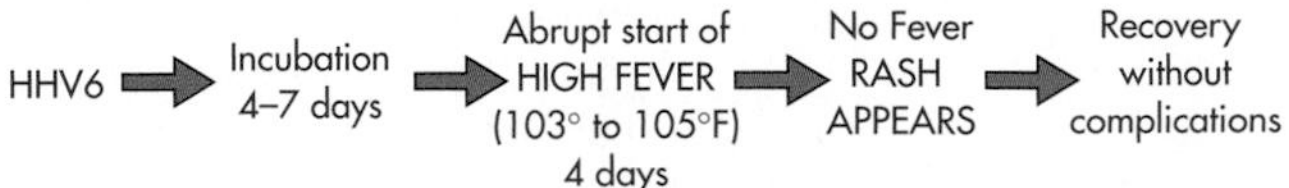

FIGURE 54–18. Time course of symptoms of exanthema subitum (roseola) caused by human herpesvirus 6 (HHV6). Compare these symptoms and this time course with those of fifth disease, which is caused by parvovirus B19 (see Chapter 56).

Box 54–13. Clinical Summaries

Primary oral herpes: A 5-year-old boy has an ulcerative rash with vesicles around the mouth. Vesicles and ulcers are also present within the mouth. Results of a Tzanck smear show multinucleated giant cells (syncytia) and Cowdry type A inclusion bodies. The lesions resolve after 18 days.

Recurrent oral herpes HSV: A 22-year-old medical student studying for examinations feels a twinge at the crimson border of his lip and 24 hours later has a single vesicular lesion at the site.

Recurrent genital HSV: A sexually active 32-year-old woman has a recurrence of ulcerative vaginal lesions with pain, itching, dysuria, and systemic symptoms 48 hours after being exposed to UVB light while skiing. The lesions resolve within 8 days. Results of a Papanicolaou smear shows multinucleated giant cells (syncytia) and Cowdry type A inclusion bodies.

Encephalitis HSV: A patient has focal neurologic symptoms and seizures. Magnetic resonance imaging results show destruction of a temporal lobe. Erythrocytes are present in the cerebrospinal fluid, and polymerase chain reaction is positive for viral DNA.

Varicella-Zoster Virus

Varicella (chickenpox): A 5-year-old boy develops a fever and maculopapular rash on his abdomen 14 days after meeting with his cousin, who also developed the rash. Successive crops of lesions appeared for 3 to 5 days, and the rash spread peripherally.

Zoster (shingles): A 65-year-old woman has a belt of vesicles along the thoracic dermatome and experiences severe pain localized to the region.

Epstein-Barr Virus

Infectious mononucleosis: A 23-year-old college student develops malaise, fatigue, fever, swollen glands, and pharyngitis. After empirical treatment with ampicillin for sore throat, a rash appears. Heterophile antibody and atypical lymphocytes were detected from blood.

Cytomegalovirus

Congenital CMV disease: A neonate exhibits microcephaly, hepatosplenomegaly, and rash. Intracerebral calcification is noted on the radiograph. The mother had symptoms similar to mononucleosis during the third trimester of her pregnancy.

Human Herpes Virus 6

Roseola (exanthem subitum): A 4-year-old child experiences a rapid onset of high fever that lasts for 3 days and then suddenly returns to normal. Two days later, a maculopapular rash appears on the trunk and spreads to other parts of the body.

with AIDS. The virus is most likely a sexually transmitted disease but may be spread by other means.

Herpesvirus simiae (B virus) (subfamily Alphaherpesvirinae; the simian counterpart of HSV), is indigenous to Asian monkeys. The virus is transmitted to humans by monkey bites or saliva, or even by tissues and cells widely used in virology laboratories. Once infected, a human may have pain, localized redness, and vesicles at the site where the virus entered. An encephalopathy develops and is often fatal; most people who survive have serious brain damage. Virus isolation or serologic tests can be used to establish the diagnosis of B-virus infections.

CASE STUDIES AND QUESTIONS

A 2-year-old child with fever for 2 days has not been eating and has been crying often. On examination the physician notes that the mucous membranes of the mouth are covered with numerous shallow, pale ulcerations. A few red papules and blisters are also observed around the border of the lips. The symptoms worsen over the next 5 days and then slowly resolve, with complete healing after 2 weeks.

1. The physician suspects that this is an HSV infection. How would the diagnosis be confirmed?
2. How could you determine whether this infection was caused by HSV-1 or HSV-2?
3. What immune responses were most helpful in resolving this infection, and when were they activated?
4. HSV escapes complete immune resolution by causing latent and recurrent infections. What was the site of latency in this child, and what might promote future recurrences?
5. What were the most probable means by which the child was infected with HSV?
6. Which antiviral drugs are available for the treatment of HSV infections? What are their targets? Were they indicated for this child? Why or why not?

A 17-year-old high school student has had low-grade fever and malaise for several days, followed by sore throat, swollen cervical lymph nodes, and increasing fatigue. The patient also notes some discomfort in the left upper quadrant of the abdomen. The sore throat, lymphadenopathy, and fever gradually resolve over the next 2 weeks, but the patient's full energy level does not return for another 6 weeks.

1. What laboratory tests would confirm the diagnosis of EBV-induced infectious mononucleosis and distinguish it from CMV infection?
2. To what characteristic diagnostic feature of the disease does *mononucleosis* refer?
3. What causes the swollen glands and fatigue?
4. Who is at greatest risk for a serious outcome of an EBV infection? What is the outcome? Why?

Bibliography

Belshe RB: *Textbook of human virology*, ed 2, St Louis, 1991, Mosby.

Cohen J, Powderly WG, editors: *Infectious diseases*, ed 2, St Louis, 2004, Mosby.

Flint SJ et al: *Principles of virology: Molecular biology, pathogenesis and control of animal viruses*, ed 2, Washington, 2003, American Society for Microbiology Press.

Garcia-Blanco MA, Cullen BR: Molecular basis of latency in pathogenic human viruses, *Science* 254:815-820, 1991.

Gorbach SL, Bartlett JG, Blacklow NR, editors: *Infectious diseases*, ed 2, Philadelphia, 1997, WB Saunders.

Knipe DM, Howley PM, editors: *Fields virology*, ed 4, New York, 2001, Lippincott-Williams and Wilkins.

Mandell GL, Bennet JE, Dolin R, editors: *Principles and practice of infectious diseases*, ed 6, Philadelphia, 2004, Churchill Livingstone.

McGeoch DJ: The genomes of the human herpesviruses: Contents, relationships and evolution, *Annu Rev Microbiol* 43:235-265, 1989.

Strauss JH, Strauss EG: *Viruses and human disease*, San Diego, 2002, Academic Press.

White DO, Fenner FJ: *Medical virology*, ed 4, New York, 1994, Academic.

Herpes Simplex Virus

Arbesfeld DM, Thomas I: Cutaneous herpes simplex infections, *Am Fam Physician* 43:1655-1664, 1991.

Dawkins BJ: Genital herpes simplex infections, *Prim Care* 17:95-113, 1990.

Landy HJ, Grossman JH III: Herpes simplex virus, *Obstet Gynecol Clin North Am* 16:495-515, 1989.

National Institute of Allergy and Infectious Diseases: Herpes simplex virus fact sheet: Available at www.niaid.nih.gov/factsheets/stdherp.htm

Rouse BT: Herpes simplex virus: Pathogenesis, immunobiology and control, *Curr Top Microbiol Immunol* 179:1-179, 1992.

Wald A: New therapies and prevention strategies for genital herpes, *Clin Infect Dis* 28(suppl 1):S4-S13, 1999.

Whitley RJ, Kimberlin DW, Roizman B: Herpes simplex virus: State of the art clinical article, *Clin Infect Dis* 26:541-555, 1998.

Varicella-Zoster Virus

Arvin AM, Moffat JF, Redman R: Varicella-zoster virus: Aspects of pathogenesis and the host response to natural infection and varicella vaccine, *Adv Virus Res* 46:263-309, 1996.

Croen KD, Strauss SE: Varicella zoster latency, *Annu Rev Microbiol* 45:265-282, 1991.

Ostrove JM: Molecular biology of varicella zoster virus, *Adv Virus Res* 38:45-98, 1990.

White CJ: Varicella-zoster virus vaccine, *Clin Infect Dis* 24:753-761; quiz 762-763, 1997.

Epstein-Barr Virus

Basgoz N, Preiksaitis JK: Post-transplant lymphoproliferative disorder, *Infect Dis Clin North Am* 9:901-923, 1995.

Cohen JI: The biology of Epstein-Barr virus: Lessons learned from the virus and the host, *Curr Opin Immunol* 11:365-370, 1999.

Englund JA: The many faces of Epstein-Barr virus, *Postgrad Med* 83:167-179, 1988.

Faulkner GC, Krajewski AS, Crawford DH: The ins and outs of EBV infection, *Trends Microbiol* 8:185-189, 2000.

Khanna R, Burrows SR, Moss DJ: Immune regulation in EBV-associated diseases, *Microbiol Rev* 59:387-405, 1995.

Sugden B: EBV's open sesame, *Trends Biochem Sci* 17:239-240, 1992.

Takada K: Epstein Barr virus and human cancer, *Curr Top Microbiol Immunol* 258, 2001.

Thorley-Lawson DA: Epstein-Barr virus and the B cell: That's all it takes, *Trends Microbiol* 4:204-208, 1996.

Thorley-Lawson DA, Babcock GJ: A model for persistent infection with Epstein-Barr virus: The stealth virus of human B cells, *Life Sci* 65:1433-1453, 1999.

Cytomegalovirus and Human Herpesviruses 6, 7, and 8

Ablashi DV et al: Human herpesvirus-6 (HHV6) (short review), *In Vivo* 5:193-200, 1991.

Bigoni B et al: Human herpesvirus 8 is present in the lymphoid system of healthy persons and can reactivate in the course of AIDS, *J Infect Dis* 173:542-549, 1996.

Gnann JW Jr, Pellett PE, Jaffe HW: Human herpesvirus 8 and Kaposi's sarcoma in persons infected with human immunodeficiency virus, *Clin Infect Dis* 30:S72-S76, 2000.

McDougall JK: Cytomegalovirus, *Curr Top Microbiol Immunol* 154:1-279, 1990.

Pellet PE, Black JB, Yamamoto Y: Human herpesvirus 6: The virus and the search for its role as a human pathogen, *Adv Virol* 41:1-52, 1992.

Plachter B, Sinzger C, Jahn G: Cell types involved in replication and distribution of human cytomegalovirus, *Adv Virus Res* 46:197-264, 1996.

Proceedings of a conference on pathogenesis of cytomegalovirus diseases, *Transplant Proc* 23(suppl 3):1-182, 1991.

Stoeckle MY: The spectrum of human herpesvirus 6 infection: From roseola infantum to adult disease, *Annu Rev Med* 51:423-430, 2000.

Wyatt LS, Frenkel N: Human herpesvirus 7 is a constitutive inhabitant of adult human saliva, *J Virol* 66:3206-3209, 1992.

Yamanishi K et al: Identification of human herpesvirus-6 as a causal agent for exanthema subitum, *Lancet* 1:1065-1067, 1988.

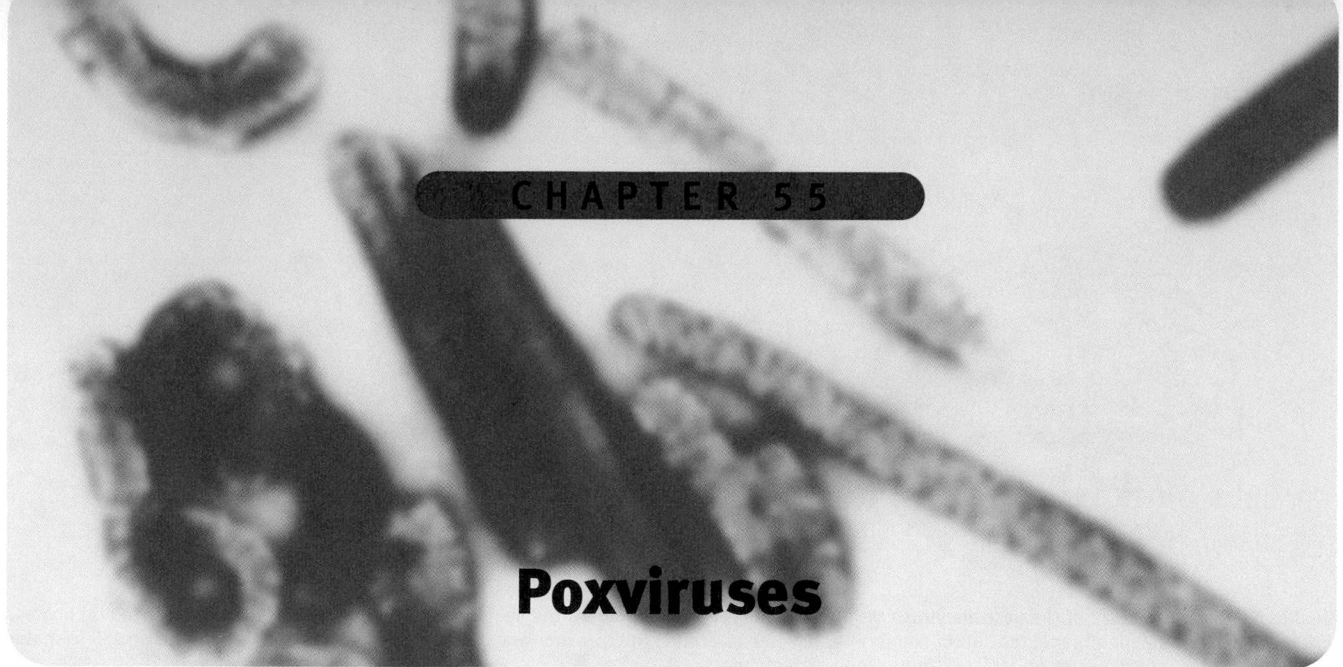

CHAPTER 55

Poxviruses

The poxviruses include the human viruses **variola (smallpox)** (genus *Orthopoxvirus*) and **molluscum contagiosum** (genus *Molluscipoxvirus*), as well as some viruses that naturally infect animals but can cause incidental infection in humans **(zoonosis)**. Many of these viruses share antigenic determinants with smallpox, allowing the use of an animal poxvirus for a human vaccine.

In eighteenth-century England, smallpox accounted for 7% to 12% of all deaths and the deaths of one third of children. However, the development of the first live vaccine in 1796 and the later worldwide distribution of this vaccine led to the eradication of smallpox by 1980. As a result, reference stocks of smallpox virus in two World Health Organization (WHO) laboratories were destroyed in 1996 after an international agreement to do so had been reached. Unfortunately, smallpox did not disappear. Stocks of the virus still exist in the United States and in Russia. While the world was successfully eliminating natural smallpox, the former U.S.S.R. (Union of Soviet Socialist Republics) was stockpiling immense amounts of weaponized smallpox virus for biowarfare. Smallpox is considered a category A agent by the U.S. Centers for Disease Control and Prevention (CDC), with anthrax, plague, botulism, tularemia, and viral hemorrhagic fevers, because of their great potential as bioterrorism-biowarfare agents capable of large-scale dissemination and serious disease. The potential for these stocks of smallpox to be acquired and used by a terrorist has been the impetus to renew interest in developing new smallpox vaccine programs and antiviral drugs.

On a positive note, the vaccinia and canary pox viruses have found a beneficial use as gene delivery vectors and for the development of hybrid vaccines. These hybrid viruses contain and express the genes of other infectious agents and infection results in immunization against both agents.

Structure and Replication

Poxviruses are the largest viruses, almost visible on light microscopy (Box 55–1). They measure 230 × 300 nm and are ovoid to brick shaped with a complex morphology. The poxvirus virion particle must carry many enzymes, including a deoxyribonucleic acid (DNA)-dependent ribonucleic acid (RNA) polymerase, to allow viral mRNA synthesis to occur in the cytoplasm. The viral genome consists of a large double-stranded, linear DNA that is fused at both ends. The structure and replication of vaccinia virus is representative of the other poxviruses (Figure 55–1). The genome of vaccinia virus consists of 86,000 base pairs (molecular weight, approximately 120×10^6 Da).

The replication of poxviruses is unique among the DNA-containing viruses, in that the entire multiplication cycle takes place within the host cell cytoplasm (Figure 55–2). As a result, *poxviruses must encode the enzymes required for messenger RNA (mRNA) and DNA synthesis, as well as activities that other DNA viruses normally obtain from the host cell.*

After binding to a cell surface receptor, the poxvirus outer envelope fuses with cellular membranes, either at the cell surface or within the cell. Early gene transcription is initiated on removal of the outer membrane. The virion core contains a specific transcriptional activator and all the enzymes necessary for transcription, including a multisubunit RNA polymerase, as well as enzymes for polyadenylate addition and capping mRNA. Among the early proteins produced is an uncoating protein (uncoatase) that removes the core membrane, thereby liberating viral DNA into the cell cytoplasm. Viral DNA then replicates in electron-dense cytoplasmic inclusions (Guarnieri's inclusion bodies), referred to as factories. Late viral mRNA is translated into structural and virion

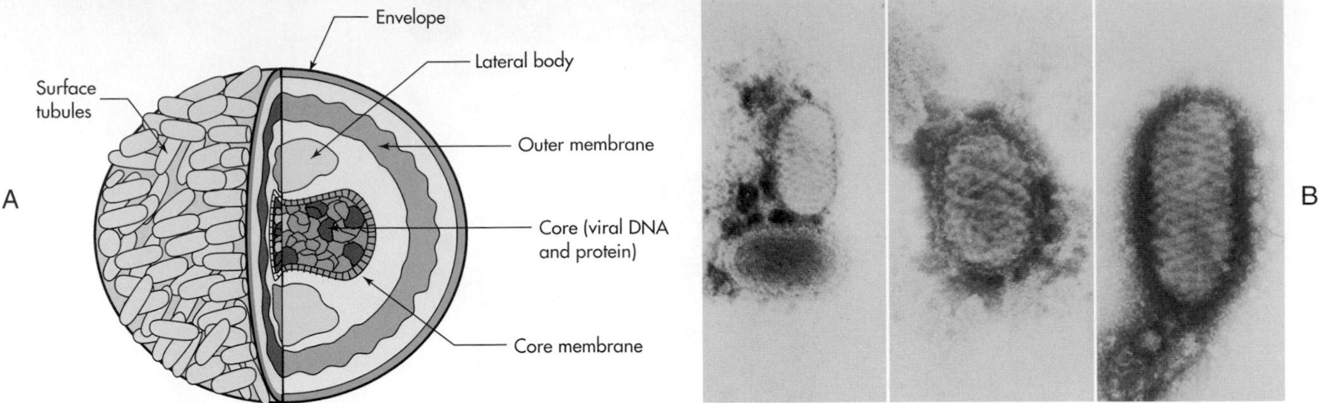

FIGURE 55–1. A, Structure of the vaccinia virus. Within the virion, the core assumes the shape of a dumbbell because of the large lateral bodies. Virions have a double membrane; the "outer membrane" assembles around the core in the cytoplasm, and the envelope is acquired on exit from the cell. **B,** Electron micrographs of orf virus. Note its complex structure.

BOX 55–1. Unique Properties of Poxviruses

- Poxviruses are the largest, most complex viruses.
- Poxviruses have complex, oval to brick-shaped morphology with internal structure.
- Poxviruses have a linear, double-stranded DNA genome with fused ends.
- Poxviruses are **DNA viruses that replicate in the cytoplasm.**
- Virus encodes and carries all proteins necessary for mRNA synthesis.
- Virus also encodes proteins for functions such as DNA synthesis, nucleotide scavenging, and immune escape mechanisms.
- Virus is assembled in inclusion bodies (Guarnieri's bodies), where it acquires its outer membranes.

proteins. In poxviruses, unlike other viruses, the membranes assemble around the core factories. Approximately 10,000 viral particles are produced per infected cell and are released on cell lysis.

The vaccinia and canarypox viruses are being used as expression vectors to produce live recombinant/hybrid vaccines for more virulent infectious agents (Figure 55–3). For this process, a plasmid is constructed that contains the foreign gene that encodes the immunizing molecule flanked by specific poxvirus gene sequences to promote recombination. This plasmid is inserted into a host cell, which is then infected with the poxvirus. The foreign gene is incorporated into the "rescuing" poxvirus genome because of the homologous viral sequences included on the plasmid. Immunization with the recombinant poxvirus results from expression of the foreign gene and its presentation to the immune response almost as if by infection with the other agent. A vaccinia hybrid

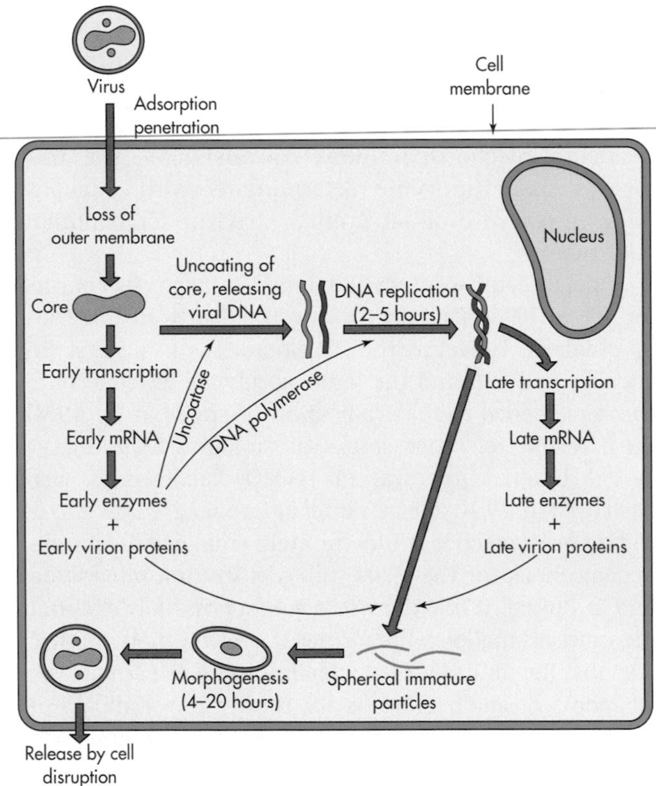

FIGURE 55–2. Replication of vaccinia virus. The core is released into the cytoplasm, where virion enzymes initiate transcription. A viral-encoded "uncoatase" enzyme then causes the release of DNA. Viral polymerase replicates the genome, and late transcription occurs. DNA and protein are assembled into cores with the core membrane. An outer membrane shrouds the core containing the lateral bodies and the enzymes required for infectivity. The virion buds through the plasma membrane or is released by cell lysis. mRNA, Messenger RNA.

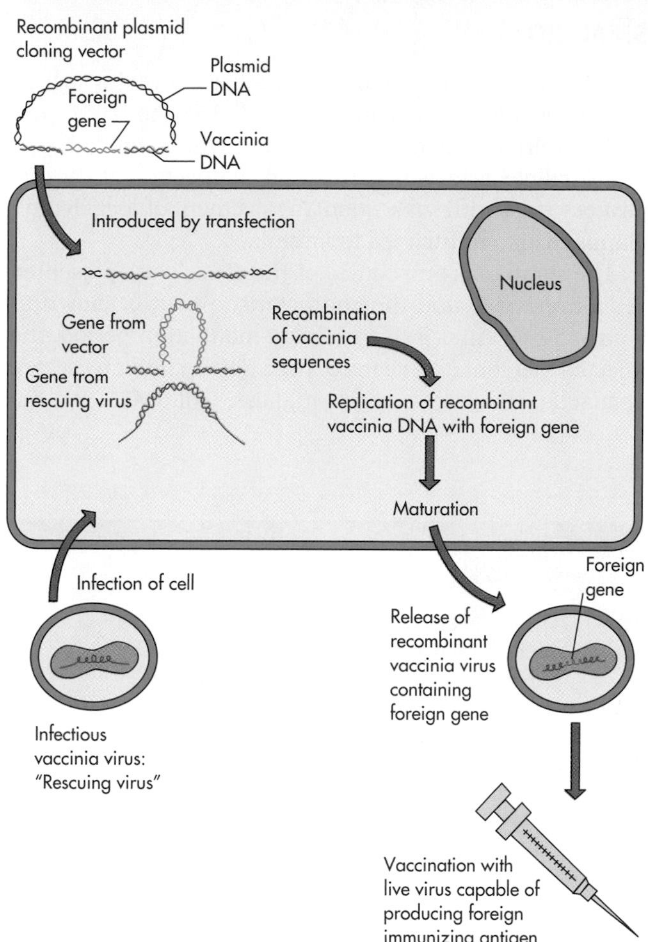

FIGURE 55–3. Vaccinia virus as an expression vector for the production of live recombinant vaccines. (Modified from Piccini A, Paoletti E: *Adv Virus Res* 34:43-64, 1988.)

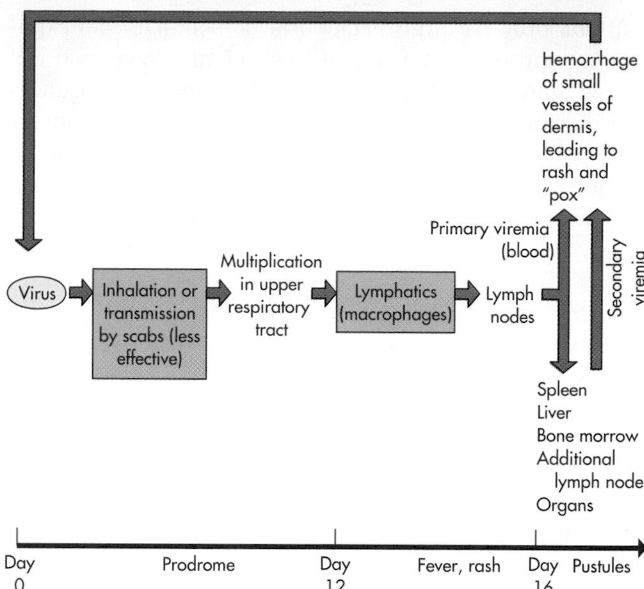

FIGURE 55–4. Spread of smallpox within the body. The virus enters and replicates in the respiratory tract without causing symptoms or contagion. The virus infects macrophages, which enter the lymphatic system and carry the virus to regional lymph nodes. The virus then replicates and initiates a viremia, causing the infection to spread to the spleen, bone marrow, lymph nodes, liver, and all organs, followed by the skin (rash). A secondary viremia causes the development of additional lesions throughout the host, followed by death or recovery with or without sequelae. Recovery from smallpox was associated with prolonged immunity and lifelong protection.

virus containing the G protein of rabies virus soaked onto a bait food and dropped into forests has been used successfully to immunize raccoons, foxes, and other mammals. Experimental vaccines for human immunodeficiency virus, hepatitis B, influenza, and other viruses have also been prepared using these techniques. The potential for producing other vaccines in this manner is unlimited.

Pathogenesis and Immunity

After being inhaled, smallpox virus replicates in the upper respiratory tract (Figure 55–4). Dissemination occurs via lymphatic and cell-associated viremic spread. Internal and dermal tissues are inoculated after a second, more intense viremia, causing the simultaneous eruption of the characteristic "pocks." Molluscum contagiosum and the other poxviruses, however, are acquired through direct contact with lesions and do not spread extensively.

The poxviruses encode many proteins that facilitate their replication and pathogenesis in the host. They include proteins that initially stimulate host cell growth and then lead to cell lysis and viral spread. Molluscum contagiosum causes a wartlike lesion rather than a lytic infection.

Cell-mediated immunity is essential for resolving a poxvirus infection. However, poxviruses encode activities that help the virus evade immune control. These include the cell-to-cell spread of the virus to avoid antibody and proteins that impede the interferon, complement, and inflammatory responses. The disease mechanisms of poxviruses are summarized in Box 55–2.

Epidemiology

Smallpox and molluscum contagiousum are strictly human viruses. In contrast, the natural hosts for the other poxviruses important to humans are vertebrates other than humans (e.g., cow, sheep, goats). The viruses infect humans only through accidental or occupational exposure (zoonosis). A recent outbreak of monkeypox in the United States is such an example. The infected individuals had purchased prairie dog pets that had been in contact with Gambian giant rats, which were the probable source of the virus.

Smallpox (variola) was very contagious and, as just noted, was spread primarily by the respiratory route. It was also spread less efficiently through close contact with dried virus on clothes or other materials. Despite the severity of the disease and its tendency to spread, several factors contributed to its elimination, as listed in Box 55–3.

Clinical Syndromes

The diseases associated with poxviruses are listed in Table 55–1.

BOX 55–2. Disease Mechanisms of Poxvirus

Smallpox is initiated by respiratory tract infection and is spread mainly by the lymphatic system and cell-associated viremia.
Molluscum contagiosum and **zoonoses** are transmitted by contact.
Virus may cause initial stimulation of cell growth and then cell lysis.
Virus encodes immune escape mechanisms.
Cell-mediated immunity and humoral immunity are important for resolution.
Most poxviruses share antigenic determinants allowing preparation of "safe" live vaccines from animal poxviruses.

SMALLPOX

The two variants of smallpox were variola major, which was associated with a mortality of 15% to 40%, and variola minor, which was associated with a mortality of 1%. Smallpox was usually initiated by infection of the respiratory tract with subsequent involvement of local lymph glands, which in turn led to viremia.

The symptoms and course of the disease are presented in Figure 55–4, and the characteristic rash is shown in Figure 55–5. After a 5- to 17-day incubation period, the infected person experienced high fever, fatigue, severe headache, backache, and malaise, followed by the

BOX 55–3. Properties of Natural Smallpox That Led to Its Eradication

Viral Characteristics
Exclusive human host range (no animal reservoirs or vectors)
Single serotype (immunization protected against all infections)

Disease Characteristics
Consistent disease presentation with visible pustules (identification of sources of contagion allowed quarantine and vaccination of contacts)

Vaccine
Immunization with animal poxviruses protects against smallpox
Stable, inexpensive, and easy-to-administer vaccine
Presence of scar indicating successful vaccination

Public Health Service
Successful worldwide WHO program combining vaccination and quarantine

TABLE 55–1. Diseases Associated with Poxviruses

Virus	Disease	Source	Location
Variola	Smallpox (now extinct)	Humans	Extinct
Vaccinia	Used for smallpox vaccination	Laboratory product	—
Orf	Localized lesion	Zoonosis—sheep, goats	Worldwide
Cowpox	Localized lesion	Zoonosis—rodents, cats, cows	Europe
Pseudocowpox	Milker's nodule	Zoonosis—dairy cows	Worldwide
Monkeypox	Generalized disease	Zoonosis—monkeys, squirrels	Africa
Bovine papular stomatitis virus	Localized lesion	Zoonosis—calves, beef cattle	Worldwide
Tanapox	Localized lesion	Rare zoonosis—monkeys	Africa
Yabapox	Localized lesion	Rare zoonosis—monkeys, baboons	Africa
Molluscum contagiosum	Many skin lesions	Humans	Worldwide

Modified from Balows A et al, editors: *Laboratory diagnosis of infectious diseases: Principles and practice*, vol 2, New York, 1988, Springer-Verlag.

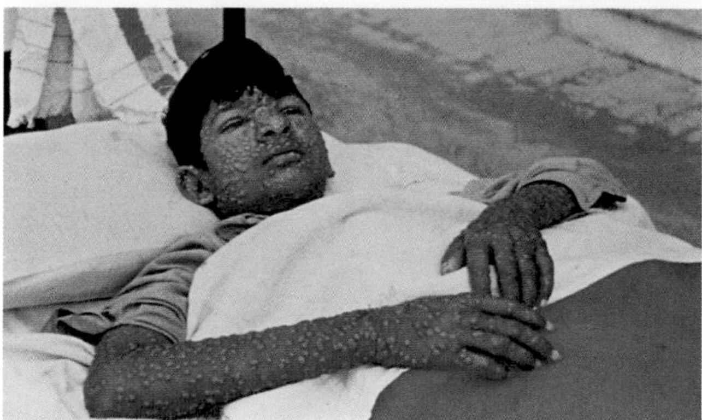

FIGURE 55–5. Child with smallpox. Note the characteristic rash.

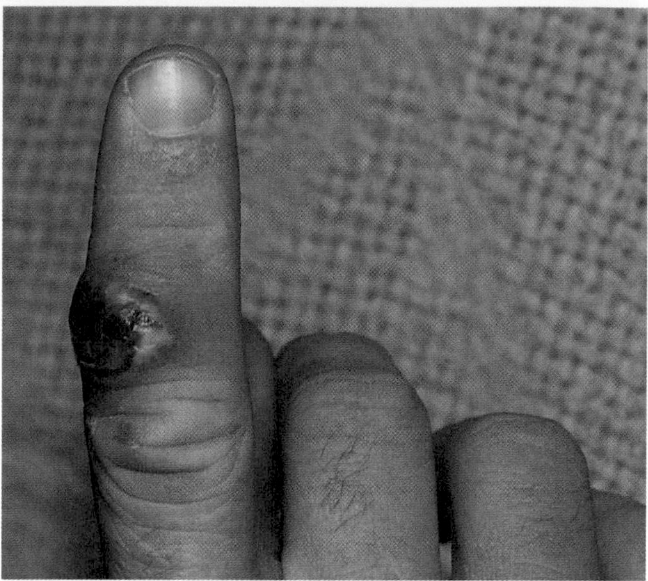

FIGURE 55–6. Orf lesion on the finger of a taxidermist. (Courtesy Joe Meyers, MD, Akron, Ohio.)

vesicular rash in the mouth and, soon after, on the body. Vomiting, diarrhea, and excessive bleeding would soon follow. The simultaneous outbreak of the vesicular rash distinguishes smallpox from the vesicles of varicella-zoster, which erupt in successive crops.

Smallpox was usually diagnosed clinically but was confirmed by growth of the virus in embryonated eggs or cell cultures. Characteristic lesions (pocks) appeared on the chorioallantoic membrane of embryonated eggs. New polymerase chain reaction and rapid DNA sequencing techniques are available at the CDC.

Smallpox was the first disease to be controlled by immunization, and its eradication is one of the greatest triumphs of medical epidemiology. Eradication resulted from a massive WHO campaign to vaccinate all susceptible people, especially those exposed to anyone with the disease, and thereby interrupt the chain of human-to-human transmission. The campaign began in 1967 and succeeded. The last case of naturally acquired infection was reported in 1977, and eradication of the disease was acknowledged in 1980.

Variolation, an early approach to immunization, involved the inoculation of susceptible people with the virulent smallpox pus. It was first performed in the Far East and later in England. Cotton Mather introduced the practice to America. Variolation was associated with a fatality rate of approximately 1%, a better risk than that associated with smallpox itself. In 1796, Jenner developed and then popularized a vaccine using the less virulent cowpox virus, which shares antigenic determinants with smallpox.

As the eradication program neared its goal, it became apparent that the rate of serious reactions to vaccination (see the following discussion of vaccinia) exceeded the risk of infection in the developed world. Therefore, routine smallpox vaccination began to be discontinued in the 1970s and was totally discontinued after 1980. Newer, safer vaccines are being stockpiled in response to concerns regarding the use of smallpox in biowarfare.

Renewed interest is being paid to antiviral drugs that are effective against smallpox and other poxviruses. Cidofovir, a nucleotide analogue capable of inhibiting the viral DNA polymerase, is effective and approved for treatment of poxvirus infections.

VACCINIA

Vaccinia, a form of cowpox, was used for the smallpox vaccine. The vaccination procedure consisted of scratching live virus into the patient's skin and then observing for the development of vesicles and pustules to confirm a "take." As the incidence of smallpox waned, however, it became apparent that there were more complications related to vaccination than cases of smallpox. Several of these complications were severe and even fatal. They included encephalitis and progressive infection (vaccinia necrosum), the latter occurring occasionally in immunocompromised patients who were inadvertently vaccinated.

ORF, COWPOX, AND MONKEYPOX

Human infection with the orf (poxvirus of sheep and goat) or cowpox (vaccinia) virus is usually an occupational hazard resulting from direct contact with the lesions on the animal. A single nodular lesion usually forms on the point of contact, such as the fingers, hand, or forearm, and is hemorrhagic (cowpox) or granulomatous (orf or pseudocowpox) (Figure 55–6). Vesicular

Box 55–4. Clinical Summaries

Molluscum contagiosum: A 5-year-old girl has a group of wartlike growths on her arm that exude white material on squeezing.

lesions frequently develop and then regress in 25 to 35 days, generally without scar formation. The lesions may be mistaken for anthrax. The virus can be grown in culture or seen directly with electron microscopy but is usually diagnosed from the symptoms and patient history.

The more than 100 cases of illnesses resembling smallpox have been attributed to the monkeypox virus. Except for the outbreak in Illinois, Indiana, and Wisconsin in 2003, they all have occurred in western and central Africa, especially Zaire. Monkeypox causes a milder version of smallpox disease, including the pocklike rash.

MOLLUSCUM CONTAGIOSUM (BOX 55–4)

The lesions of molluscum contagiosum differ significantly from pox lesions in being nodular to wartlike (Figure 55–7*A*). They begin as papules and then become pearl-like, umbilicated nodules that are 2 to 10 mm in diameter and have a central caseous plug that can be readily expressed (squeezed out). They are most common on the trunk, genitalia, and proximal extremities and usually occur in a cluster of five to 20 nodules. The incubation period for molluscum contagiosum is 2 to 8 weeks, and the disease is spread by direct contact (e.g., sexual contact, wrestling) or fomites (e.g., towels). The disease is more common in children than adults, but its incidence is increasing in sexually active individuals.

The diagnosis of molluscum contagiosum is confirmed histologically by the finding of characteristic large, eosinophilic cytoplasmic inclusions (molluscum bodies) in epithelial cells (Figure 55–7*B*). These bodies can be seen in biopsy specimens or in the expressed caseous core of a nodule. The molluscum contagiosum virus cannot be grown in tissue culture or animal models.

Lesions of molluscum contagiosum disappear in 2 to 12 months, presumably as a result of immune responses. The nodules can be removed by curettage (scraping) or the application of liquid nitrogen or iodine solutions.

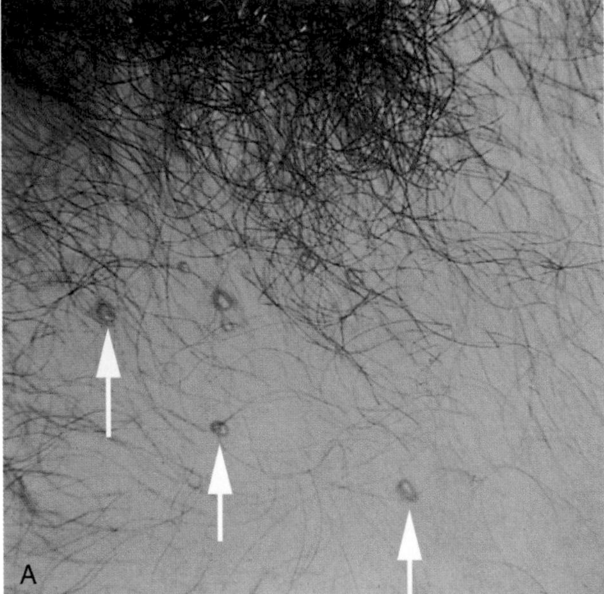

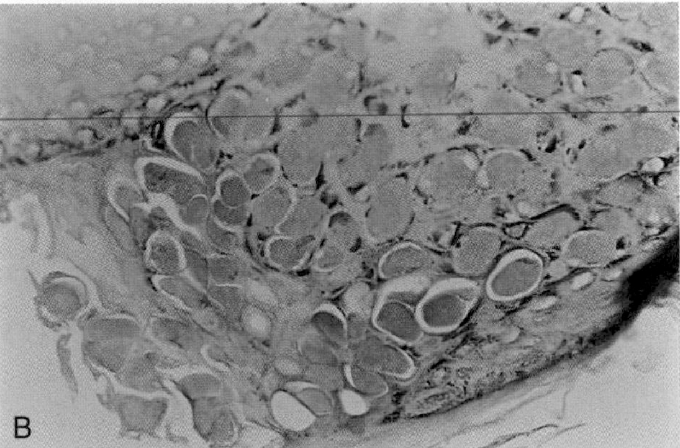

FIGURE 55–7. Molluscum contagiosum. **A,** Skin lesion. **B,** Microscopic view; epidermis is filled with molluscum bodies (Magnification 100X).

QUESTIONS

1. The structure of poxviruses is more complex than that of most other viruses. What problems does this complexity create for viral replication?
2. Poxviruses replicate in the cytoplasm. What problems does this feature create for viral replication?
3. How does the immune response to smallpox infection in an immunologically naïve person differ from that in a vaccinated person? When is antibody present in each case? What stage or stages of viral dissemination are blocked in each case?
4. What characteristics of smallpox facilitated its elimination?
5. Vaccinia virus is being used as a vector for the development of hybrid vaccines. Why is vaccinia virus well suited to this task? Which infectious agents would be appropriate for a vaccinia hybrid vaccine, and why?

Bibliography

Belshe RB, editor: *Textbook of human virology,* ed 2, St Louis, 1991, Mosby.

Cohen J, Powderly WG, editors: *Infectious diseases,* ed 2, St Louis, 2004, Mosby.

Fenner F: A successful eradication campaign: Global eradication of smallpox, *Rev Infect Dis* 4:916-930, 1982.

Flint SJ et al: *Principles of virology: Molecular biology, pathogenesis and control of animal viruses,* ed 2, Washington, 2003, American Society for Microbiology Press.

Gorbach SL, Bartlett JG, Blacklow NR, editors: *Infectious diseases,* ed 2, Philadelphia, 1997, WB Saunders.

Knipe DM, Howley PM, editors: *Fields virology,* ed 4, New York, 2001, Lippincott-Williams and Wilkins.

Mandell GL, Bennet JE, Dolin R, editors: *Principles and practice of infectious diseases,* ed 6, Philadelphia, 2004, Churchill Livingstone.

Moyer RW, Turner PC, editors: Poxviruses, *Curr Top Microbiol Immunol* 163:1-211, 1990.

Piccini A, Paoletti E: Vaccinia: Virus, vector, vaccine, *Adv Virus Res* 34:43-64, 1988.

Strauss JM, Strauss EG: *Viruses and human disease,* San Diego, 2002, Academic Press.

White DO, Fenner FJ: *Medical virology,* ed 4, New York, 1994, Academic.

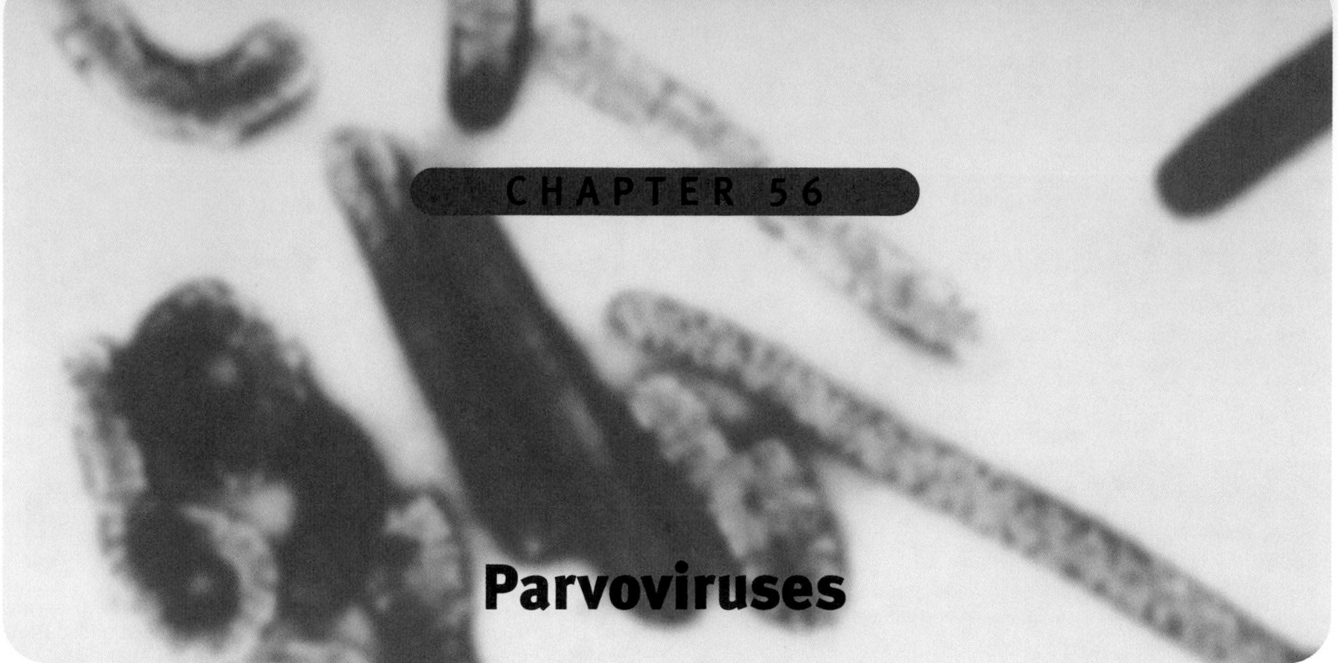

Parvoviruses

The Parvoviridae are the smallest of the deoxyribonucleic acid (DNA) viruses. Their small size and limited genetic repertoire make them more dependent than any other DNA virus on the host cell or require the presence of a helper virus to replicate. Only one member of the Parvoviridae, **B19,** a member of the genus *Parvovirus,* is known to cause human disease.

B19 normally causes **erythema infectiosum,** or **fifth disease,** a mild febrile exanthematous disease that occurs in children. It goes by the latter name because it was the fifth of the childhood exanthems (the first four being varicella, rubella, roseola, and measles). B19 is also responsible for episodes of **aplastic crisis in patients with chronic hemolytic anemia** and is associated with **acute polyarthritis** in adults. Intrauterine infection of a fetus may cause abortion.

Other parvoviruses, such as RA-1 (isolated from a person with rheumatoid arthritis) and fecal parvoviruses, have not been shown to cause human disease. Feline and canine parvoviruses do not cause human disease and are preventable with vaccination of the pet.

Adeno-associated viruses (AAVs) are members of the genus *Dependovirus* in the family Parvoviridae. They commonly infect humans but replicate only in association with a second "helper" virus, usually an adenovirus. Dependoviruses neither cause illness nor modify infection by their helper viruses. These properties and the propensity of AAVs to integrate into the host chromosome have made genetically modified AAVs candidates for use in **gene-replacement therapy.** A third genus of the family, *Densovirus,* infects only insects.

Structure and Replication

The parvoviruses are extremely small (18 to 26 nm in diameter) and have a nonenveloped, icosahedral capsid (Box 56–1 and Figure 56–1). The B19 virus genome contains one linear, single-stranded deoxyribonucleic acid (DNA) molecule with a molecular mass of 1.5 to 1.8×10^6 Da (5500 bases in length) (Box 56–2). Plus or minus DNA strands are packaged separately into virions. The genome encodes three structural and two major nonstructural proteins. Only one serotype of B19 is known to exist.

B19 virus replicates in mitotically active cells and prefers cells of the erythroid lineage, such as fresh human bone marrow cells, erythroid cells from fetal liver, and erythroid leukemia cells (Figure 56–2). After binding to the erythrocyte blood group P antigen (globoside) and its internalization, the virion is uncoated, and the single-stranded DNA genome is delivered to the nucleus. Factors available only during the S phase of the cell's growth cycle and cellular DNA polymerases are required to generate a complementary DNA strand.

The single-stranded DNA virion genome is converted to a double-stranded DNA version, which is required for transcription and replication. Inverted repeat sequences of DNA at both ends of the genome fold back and hybridize with the genome to create a primer for the cell's DNA polymerase. This creates the complementary strand and replicates the genome. The two major nonstructural proteins and the VP1 and VP2 structural capsid proteins are translated from larger ribonucleic acid strands. Viral proteins are synthesized in the cytoplasm and then return to the nucleus, where the virion is assembled. The VP2 protein is cleaved later to produce VP3. The nuclear and cytoplasmic membrane degenerates, and the virus is released on cell lysis.

Pathogenesis and Immunity

B19 targets and is cytolytic for erythroid precursor cells (Box 56–3). B19 disease is determined by the direct killing

BOX 56–1. Unique Properties of Parvoviruses

Smallest DNA virus
Naked icosahedral capsid
Single-stranded (+ or – sense) DNA genome
Requirement of growing cells (B19) or helper virus (dependovirus) for replication

BOX 56–2. Parvovirus Genome

Single-stranded linear DNA genome.
Approximately 5.5 kilobases in length
Plus and minus strands packaged into separate B19 virions
Ends of the genome have inverted repeats that hybridize to form hairpin loops and a primer for DNA synthesis

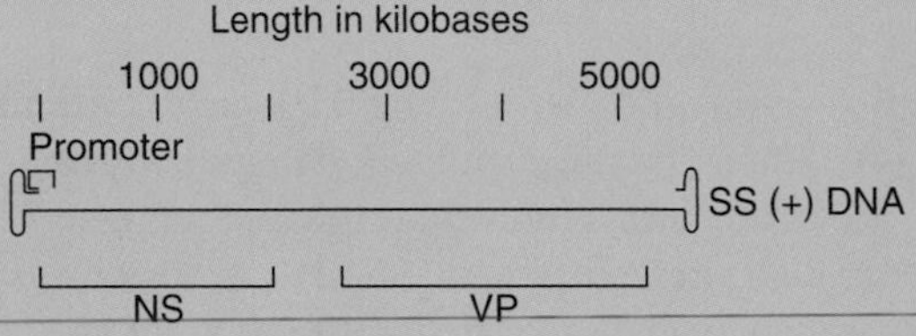

Separate coding regions for nonstructural (NS) and structural proteins (VP)

BOX 56–3. Disease Mechanisms of B19 Parvovirus

Virus spreads by **respiratory** and **oral** secretions.
Virus **infects mitotically active erythroid precursor** cells in bone marrow and establishes lytic infection.
Virus establishes large **viremia** and can **cross the placenta.**
Antibody is important for resolution and prophylaxis.
Virus causes **biphasic disease:**
- Initial phase is related to viremia:
  - Flulike symptoms and viral shedding.
- Later phase is related to immune response:
  - Circulating immune complexes of antibody and virions that do not fix complement.
- Result: Erythematous maculopapular rash, arthralgia, and arthritis.

Depletion of erythroid precursor cells and destabilization of erythrocytes initiate **aplastic crisis in people with chronic anemia.**

of these cells and the subsequent immune response to the infection (rash and arthralgia).

Studies performed in volunteers suggest that B19 virus first replicates in the nasopharynx or upper respiratory tract, then spreads by viremia to the bone marrow and elsewhere, where it replicates and kills erythroid precursor cells (Figure 56–3). The disease has a **biphasic course.**

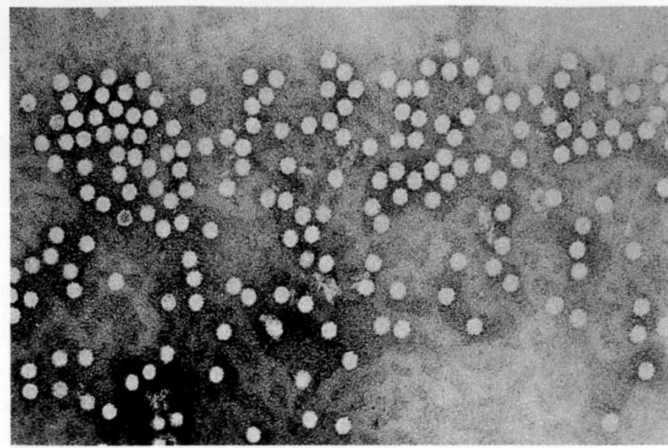

FIGURE 56–1. Electron micrograph of parvovirus. Parvoviruses are small (18 to 26 nm), nonenveloped viruses with single-stranded DNA. (Courtesy Centers for Disease Control and Prevention, Atlanta.)

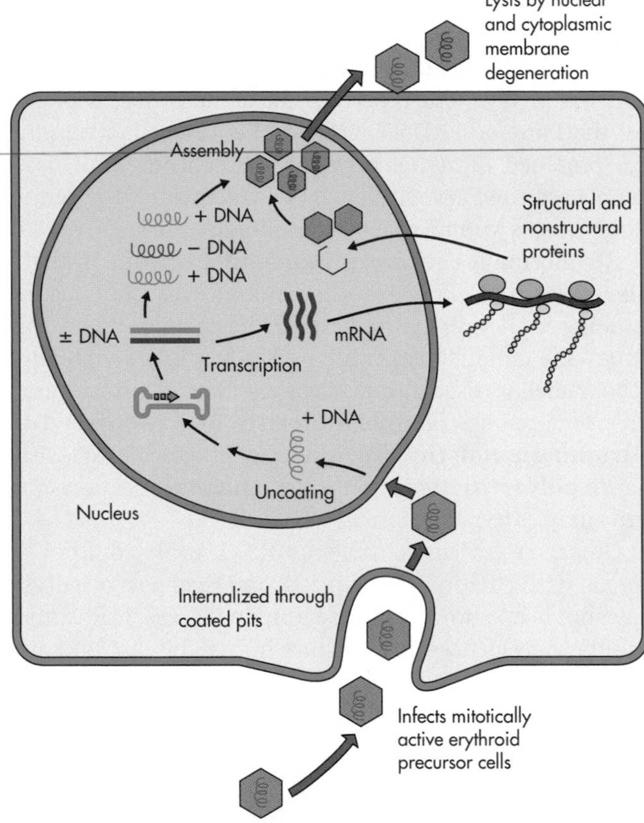

FIGURE 56–2. Postulated replication of parvovirus (B19) based on information from related viruses (minute virus of mice). The internalized parvovirus delivers its genome to the nucleus, where the single-stranded (plus or minus) DNA is converted to double-stranded DNA by host factors and DNA polymerases present only in growing cells. Transcription, replication, and assembly occur in the nucleus. Virus is released by cell lysis.

The *initial febrile stage is the infectious stage.* During this time, erythrocyte production is stopped for approximately 1 week as a result of the viral killing of erythroid precursor cells. A large viremia occurs within 8 days of infection and is accompanied by nonspecific flulike symptoms.

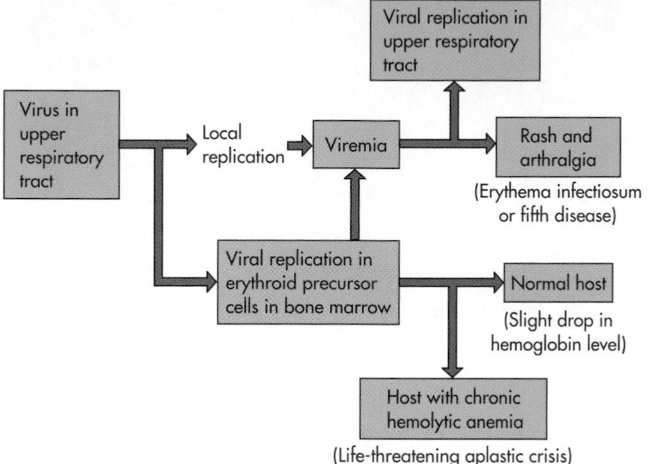

FIGURE 56–3. Mechanism of spread of parvovirus within the body.

Large numbers of virus are also released into oral and respiratory secretions. Antibody stops the viremia and is important for resolution of the disease but contributes to the symptoms.

The *second, symptomatic stage is immune mediated.* The rash and arthralgia seen in this stage coincide with the appearance of virus-specific antibody, the disappearance of detectable B19 virus, and the formation of immune complexes.

Hosts with chronic hemolytic anemia (e.g., sickle cell anemia) who are infected with B19 are at risk for a life-threatening reticulocytopenia, which is referred to as an **aplastic crisis.** The reticulocytopenia results from the combination of (1) B19 depletion of the red blood cell precursors and (2) shortened life span of the erythrocytes caused by the underlying anemia.

BOX 56–4. Epidemiology of B19 Parvovirus Infection

Disease/Viral Factors
Capsid virus is resistant to inactivation.
Contagious period precedes symptoms.
Virus crosses placenta and infects fetus.

Transmission
Transmitted via respiratory droplets.

Who Is at Risk?
Children, especially those in elementary school: Erythema infectiosum (fifth disease).
Parents of children with B19 infection are at risk.
Pregnant women: Fetal infection and disease.
People with chronic anemia: Aplastic crisis.

Geography/Season
Virus is found worldwide.
Fifth disease is more common in late winter and spring.

Modes of Control
There are no modes of control.

BOX 56–5. Clinical Consequences of Parvovirus (B19) Infection

Mild, flulike illness (fever, headache, chills, myalgia, malaise)
Erythema infectiosum (fifth disease)
Aplastic crisis in people with chronic anemia
Arthropathy (polyarthritis: symptoms in many joints)
Risk of fetal loss as a result of B19 virus crossing the placenta, causing anemia-related disease but not congenital anomalies

Epidemiology

Approximately 65% of the adult population have been infected with B19 by 40 years of age (Box 56–4). Erythema infectiosum is most common in children and adolescents ages 4 to 15 years, who are a source of contagion. Arthralgia and arthritis are likely to occur in adults. Respiratory droplets and oral secretions most probably transmit the virus. Disease usually occurs in late winter and spring. Parenteral transmission of the virus by blood-clotting factor concentrate has also been described.

Clinical Syndromes

B19 virus is the cause of erythema infectiosum (fifth disease) (Box 56–5). Infection starts with an unremarkable prodromal period of 7 to 10 days, during which the person is contagious. Infection of a normal host may cause either no noticeable symptoms or fever and nonspecific symptoms, such as sore throat, chills, malaise, and myalgia, as well as a slight decrease in hemoglobin levels (Figure 56–4). This period is followed by a distinctive rash on the cheeks, which appear as if they have been slapped. The rash then usually spreads, especially to exposed skin such as the arms and legs (Figure 56–5), and then subsides over 1 to 2 weeks. Relapse of the rash is common.

B19 infection in adults causes polyarthritis, with or without a rash, that can last for weeks, months, or longer. Arthritis of the hands, wrists, knees, and ankles predominates. The rash may precede the arthritis but often does not occur. B19 infection of immunocompromised people may result in chronic disease.

The most serious complication of parvovirus infection is the aplastic crisis that occurs in patients with chronic hemolytic anemia (e.g., sickle cell anemia). Infection in these people causes a transient reduction in erythropoiesis

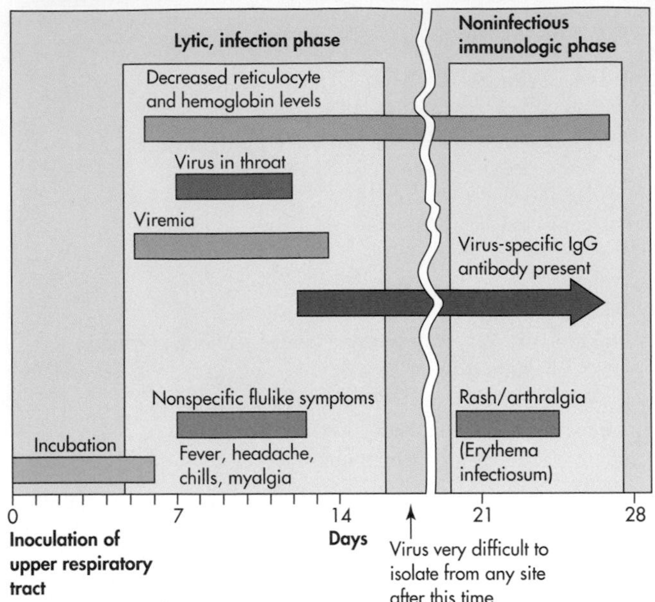

FIGURE 56–4. Time course of parvovirus (B19) infection. B19 causes biphasic disease: first, an initial, lytic infection phase characterized by febrile, flulike symptoms and then a noninfectious immunologic phase characterized by a rash and arthralgia.

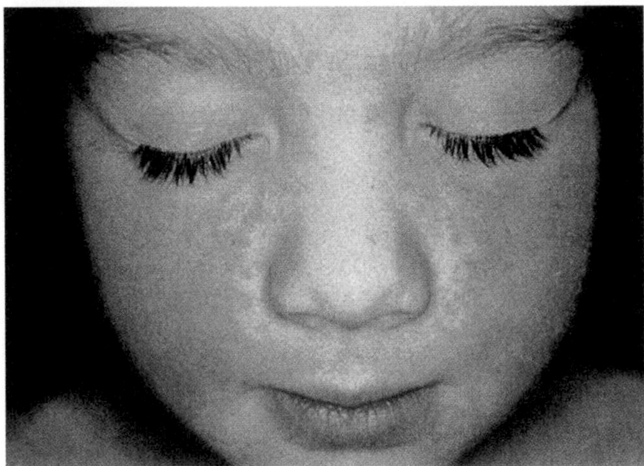

FIGURE 56–5. A "slapped-cheek" appearance is typical of the rash for erythema infectiosum. (From Hart CA, Broadhead RL: *A color atlas of pediatric infectious diseases,* London, 1992, Wolfe.)

in the bone marrow. The reduction results in a transient reticulocytopenia that lasts 7 to 10 days and a decrease in hemoglobin level. An aplastic crisis is accompanied by fever and nonspecific symptoms, such as malaise, myalgia, chills, and itching. A maculopapular rash with arthralgia and some joint swelling may also be present.

B19 infection of a seronegative mother increases the risk for fetal death. The virus can infect the fetus and kill erythrocyte precursors, causing anemia and congestive heart failure **(hydrops fetalis).** Infection of seropositive pregnant women often has no adverse effect on the fetus.

BOX 56–6. Clinical Summaries

A 10-year-old patient has a five-day history of a flulike illness (headache, fever, muscle pain, tired), then develops an intensely red rash over the cheeks and a fainter, "lacy" rash over the trunk and extremities. Also, the patient's mother just learned she is pregnant.

There is no evidence that B19 causes congenital abnormalities (see Box 56–5, Box 56–6).

Laboratory Diagnosis

The diagnosis of erythema infectiosum is usually based on the clinical presentation. For B19 disease to be definitively diagnosed, however, specific immunoglobulin M (IgM) or viral DNA must be detected (i.e., to distinguish the rash of B19 from that of rubella in a pregnant woman). Enzyme-linked immunosorbent assays for B19 IgM and IgG are available. The polymerase chain reaction test is a very sensitive method for detecting the B19 genome in clinical samples. Virus isolation is not performed.

Treatment, Prevention, and Control

No specific antiviral treatment or means of control is available. Vaccines are available for dog and cat parvoviruses.

CASE STUDY AND QUESTIONS

Mrs. Doe brought her daughter to the pediatrician with the complaint of a rash. The daughter's face appeared as if it had been slapped, but she had no fever or other notable symptoms. On questioning, Mrs. Doe reported that her daughter had had a mild cold within the previous 2 weeks and that she, herself, was currently having more joint pain than usual and was very tired.

1. What features of this history indicate a parvovirus B19 etiology?
2. Was the child infectious at presentation? If not, when was she contagious?
3. What caused the symptoms?
4. Were the symptoms of the mother and daughter related?
5. What underlying condition would put the daughter at increased risk for serious disease after B19 infection? The mother?
6. Why is quarantine a poor means of limiting the spread of B19 parvovirus?

Bibliography

Anderson LJ: Human parvoviruses, *J Infect Dis* 161:603-608, 1990.

Anderson MJ: Parvoviruses. In Belshe RB, editor: *Textbook of human virology*, ed 2, St Louis, 1991, Mosby.

Balows A, Hausler WJ Jr, Lennette EH, editors: *Laboratory diagnosis of infectious diseases: Principles and practice*, vol 2, New York, 1988, Springer-Verlag.

Berns KI: *The parvoviruses*, New York, 1984, Plenum.

Berns KI: Parvovirus replication, *Microbiol Rev* 54:316-329, 1990.

Brown KE, Young NS: Parvovirus B19 in human disease, *Annu Rev Med* 48:59-67, 1997.

Chorba T et al: The role of parvovirus B19 in aplastic crisis and erythema infectiosum (fifth disease), *J Infect Dis* 154:383-393, 1986.

Cohen J, Powderly WG, editors: *Infectious diseases*, ed 2, St Louis, 2004, Mosby.

Flint SJ et al: *Principles of virology: Molecular biology, pathogenesis and control of animal viruses*, ed 2, Washington, 2003, American Society for Microbiology Press.

Gorbach SL, Bartlett JG, Blacklow NR, editors: *Infectious diseases*, ed 2, Philadelphia, 1997, WB Saunders.

Knipe DM, Howley PM, editors: *Fields virology*, ed 4, New York, 2001, Lippincott-Williams and Wilkins.

Mandell GL, Bennet JE, Dolin R, editors: *Principles and practice of infectious diseases*, ed 6, Philadelphia, 2004, Churchill Livingstone.

Naides SJ et al: Rheumatologic manifestations of human parvovirus B19 infection in adults, *Arthritis Rheum* 33:1297-1309, 1990.

Törk TJ: Parvovirus B19 and human disease, *Adv Intern Med* 37:431-455, 1992.

Ware RE: Parvovirus infections. In Katz SL et al: *Krugman's Infectious diseases of children*, ed 10, St Louis, 1998, Mosby.

White DO, Fenner FJ: *Medical virology*, ed 4, New York, 1994, Academic.

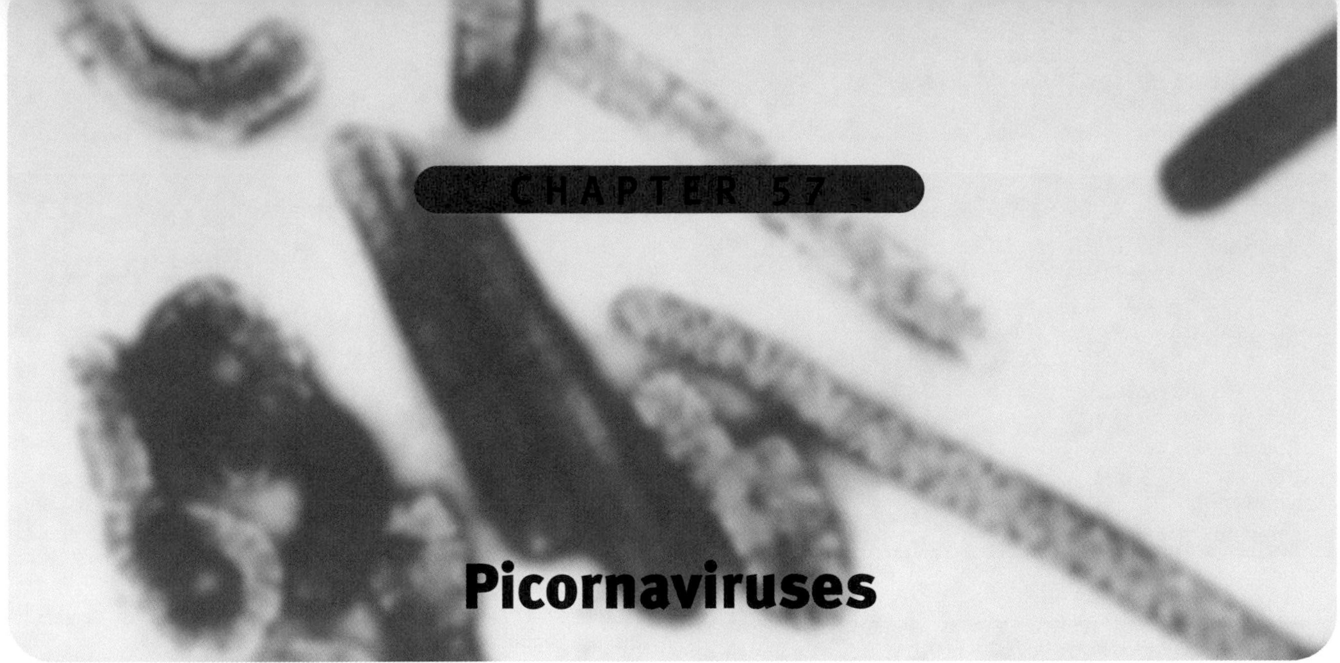

Picornaviruses

Picornaviridae is one of the largest families of viruses and includes some of the most important human and animal viruses (Box 57–1). As the name indicates, these viruses are **small *(pico)* RNA** (ribonucleic acid) viruses that have a **naked capsid** structure. The family has more than 230 members, which are divided into five genera: *Enterovirus, Rhinovirus, Heparnavirus, Cardiovirus,* and *Aphthovirus*. The enteroviruses are distinguished from the rhinoviruses by the stability of the capsid at pH 3, the optimum temperature for growth, the mode of transmission, and their diseases (Box 57–2).

At least 71 serotypes of human enteroviruses exist, which are members of the polioviruses, group A or B Coxsackie viruses, or echoviruses. Several different disease syndromes may be caused by a specific serotype of enterovirus. Likewise, several different serotypes may cause the same disease, depending on the target tissue affected. Hepatitis A virus was included in this group but has been reclassified as a hepatovirus in the *Heparnavirus* genus, and is discussed separately in Chapter 66.

The capsids of enteroviruses are *very resistant to harsh environmental conditions* (sewage systems) and the conditions in the gastrointestinal tract, a fact that facilitates their transmission by the fecal-oral route. Although they may initiate infection in the gastrointestinal tract, the enteroviruses rarely cause enteric disease. In fact, most infections are usually asymptomatic. The best-known and most-studied picornavirus is poliovirus, of which there are three serotypes.

Coxsackieviruses are named after the town of Coxsackie, N.Y., where they were first isolated. They are divided into two groups, A and B, on the basis of certain biologic and antigenic differences, and are further subdivided into numeric serotypes on the basis of additional antigenic differences.

The name **echovirus** is derived from **e**nteric **c**ytopathic **h**uman **o**rphan, because these agents were not initially thought to be associated with clinical disease. Thirty-two serotypes are currently recognized. Since 1967, newly isolated enteroviruses have been distinguished numerically.

The human rhinoviruses consist of at least 100 serotypes and are the major cause of the common cold. They are *sensitive to acidic pH and replicate poorly at temperatures above 33°C.* This sensitivity usually limits rhinoviruses to causing upper respiratory tract infections.

Structure

The plus-strand RNA of the picornaviruses is surrounded by an **icosahedral capsid** approximately 30 nm in diameter. The icosahedral capsid has 12 pentameric vertices, each of which is composed of five protomeric units of proteins. The protomers are made of four virion polypeptides (VP1 to VP4). VP2 and VP4 are generated by the cleavage of a precursor, VP0. VP4 in the virion solidifies the structure, but it is not generated until the genome is incorporated into the capsid. This protein is released on binding of the virus to the cellular receptor. The capsids are stable in the presence of heat and detergent and, except for the rhinoviruses, are also stable in acid. The capsid structure is so regular that paracrystals of virions often form in infected cells (Figures 57–1 and 57–2).

The **genome of the picornaviruses resembles a messenger RNA** (mRNA) (Figure 57–3). It is a single strand of plus-sense RNA of approximately 7200 to 8450 bases that has a poly A at the 3′-end and a small protein, VPg (22 to 24 amino acids), attached to the 5-′end. The poly A sequence enhances the infectivity of the RNA, and the VPg may be important in packaging the genome into the capsid and initiating viral RNA synthesis. *The naked picornavirus genome is sufficient to infect a cell.*

BOX 57–1. Picornaviridae

Enterovirus
- Poliovirus types 1, 2, and 3
- Coxsackie A virus types 1 to 22 and 24
- Coxsackie B virus types 1 to 6
- Echovirus (ECHO virus) types 1 to 9, 11 to 27, and 29 to 34
- Enterovirus 68 to 71

Rhinovirus types 1 to 100+
Cardiovirus
Aphthovirus
Heparnavirus
- Hepatitis A virus

BOX 57–2. Unique Properties of Human Picornaviruses

Virion is **naked, small** (25 to 30 nm) **icosahedral** capsid enclosing a single-stranded positive RNA genome.
Enteroviruses are resistant to pH 3 to pH 9, detergents, mild sewage treatment, and heat.
Rhinoviruses are labile at acidic pH; optimum growth temperature is 33°C.
Genome is an mRNA.
Naked genome is sufficient for infection.
Virus replicates in cytoplasm.
Viral RNA is translated into polyprotein, which is then cleaved into enzymatic and structural proteins.
Most viruses are **cytolytic.**

The genome encodes a polyprotein that is proteolytically cleaved to produce the enzymatic and structural proteins of the virus. In addition to the capsid proteins and VPg, the picornaviruses encode at least two proteases and an RNA-dependent RNA polymerase. Poliovirus also produces a protease that degrades the 200,000-Da cap-binding protein of eukaryotic ribosomes, thereby blocking the translation of most cellular mRNA.

Replication

The specificity of the picornavirus interaction for cellular receptors is the major determinant of the target tissue tropism and disease (see Figure 6–13). The VP1 proteins at the vertices of the virion contain a canyon structure to which the receptor binds. The site of binding is protected from antibody neutralization. Pleconaril and related antiviral compounds contain a 3-methylisoxazole group that binds to the floor of this canyon and alters its conformation to prevent the uncoating of the virus.

The picornaviruses can be categorized according to their cell surface receptor specificity. The receptors for polioviruses, some coxsackieviruses, and rhinoviruses are members of the immunoglobulin superfamily of proteins.

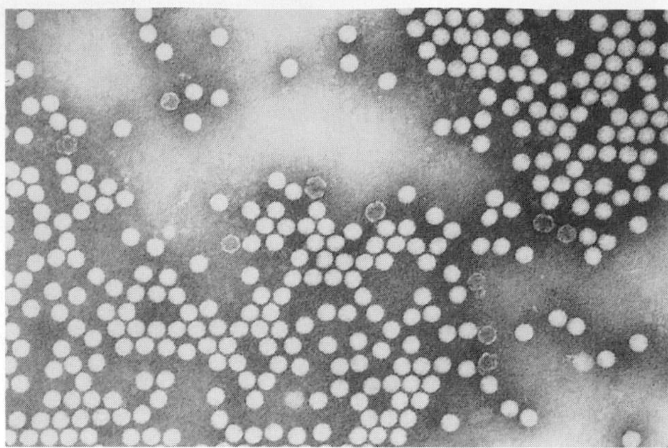

FIGURE 57–1. Electron micrograph of poliovirus. (Courtesy Centers for Disease Control and Prevention, Atlanta.)

At least 80% of the rhinoviruses and several serotypes of coxsackievirus bind to the intercellular adhesion molecule-1 (ICAM-1), which is expressed on epithelial cells, fibroblasts, and endothelial cells. Several coxsackieviruses, echoviruses, and other enteroviruses bind to decay accelerating factor (CD55). Poliovirus binds to a different molecule (PVR/CD155) that is similar to the receptor for herpes simplex virus. The poliovirus receptor is present on many different human cells, but not all of these cells will replicate the virus.

On binding to the receptor the VP4 is released and the virion weakened. The genome is then injected directly across the membrane through a channel created at one of the vertices of the virion. The genome binds directly to ribosomes despite the lack of a 5′-cap structure. The ribosomes recognize a unique internal RNA loop in the genome. A polyprotein containing all the viral protein sequences is synthesized within 10 to 15 minutes of infection. This polyprotein is cleaved by viral proteases encoded in it. The viral RNA-dependent RNA polymerase generates a negative-strand RNA template from which the new mRNA/genome can be synthesized. The amount of viral mRNA increases rapidly in the cell, with the number of viral RNA molecules reaching 400,000 per cell.

Most picornaviruses inhibit cellular RNA and protein synthesis during infection. For example, cleavage of the 200,000-Da cap-binding protein (EIF4-G) of the ribosome by a poliovirus protease prevents most cellular mRNA from binding to the ribosome. Inhibition of transcription factors decrease cellular mRNA synthesis, and permeability changes induced by picornaviruses reduce the ability of cellular mRNA to bind to the ribosome. In addition, viral mRNA can outcompete cellular mRNA for the factors required in protein synthesis. These activities contribute to the cytopathologic effect of the virus on the target cell.

As the viral genome is being replicated and translated, the structural proteins VP0, VP1, and VP3 are cleaved from the polyprotein by a viral-encoded protease and

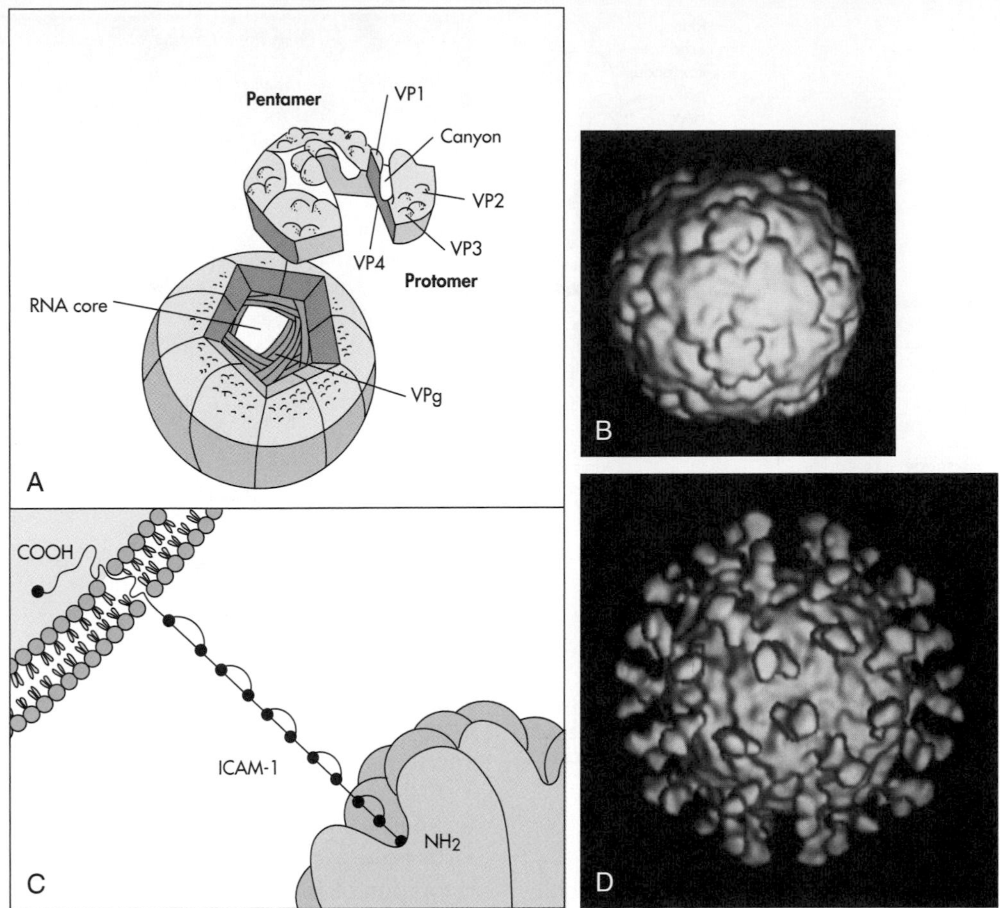

FIGURE 57–2. A, Structure of the human rhinovirus and its interaction with ICAM-1 on the target cell. **B,** Cryoelectron microscopy computer-generated reconstruction of the human rhinovirus 16. **C,** Binding of the ICAM-1 molecule within the canyon of the virion triggers the opening of capsid for release of the genome into the cell. **D,** Cryoelectron microscopy reconstruction of the interaction of a soluble form of ICAM-1 with human rhinovirus 16. *Note:* There is one ICAM-1 per capsomere. ICAM-1, Intercellular adhesion molecule-1. (**B** and **D** courtesy Tim Baker, Purdue University, West Lafayette, Ind.)

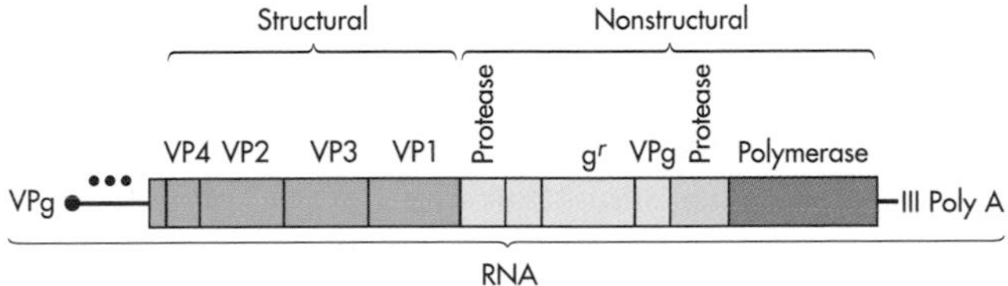

FIGURE 57–3. Structure of the picornavirus genome. The genome (7200 to 8400 bases) is translated as a polyprotein, which is cleaved by viral-encoded proteases into individual proteins. g, Guanidine resistance marker (a genetic locus involved in the initiation of RNA synthesis); Poly A, polyadenylate, •••, internal ribosomal entry site for initiation of protein synthesis.

assembled into subunits. Five **subunits** associate into **pentamers**, and 12 **pentamers** associate to form the **procapsid.** After insertion of the genome, VP0 is cleaved into VP2 and VP4 to complete the **capsid.** As many as 100,000 virions per cell may be produced and released on cell lysis.

Enteroviruses

PATHOGENESIS AND IMMUNITY

Contrary to their name, enteroviruses do not usually cause enteric disease but are transmitted by the fecal-oral route. The diseases produced by the enteroviruses are determined mainly by differences in tissue tropism and the cytolytic capacity of the virus (Figure 57–4; Box 57–3). The upper respiratory tract, the oropharynx, and the intestinal tract are the portals of entry for enteroviruses. The virions are impervious to stomach acid, proteases, and bile. Viral replication is initiated in the mucosa and lymphoid tissue of the tonsils and pharynx, and the virus later infects lymphoid cells of Peyer's patches underlying the intestinal mucosa. Primary viremia spreads the virus to receptor-bearing target tissues, including the reticuloendothelial cells of the lymph nodes, spleen, and liver, to initiate a second phase of viral replication, resulting in a secondary viremia and symptoms.

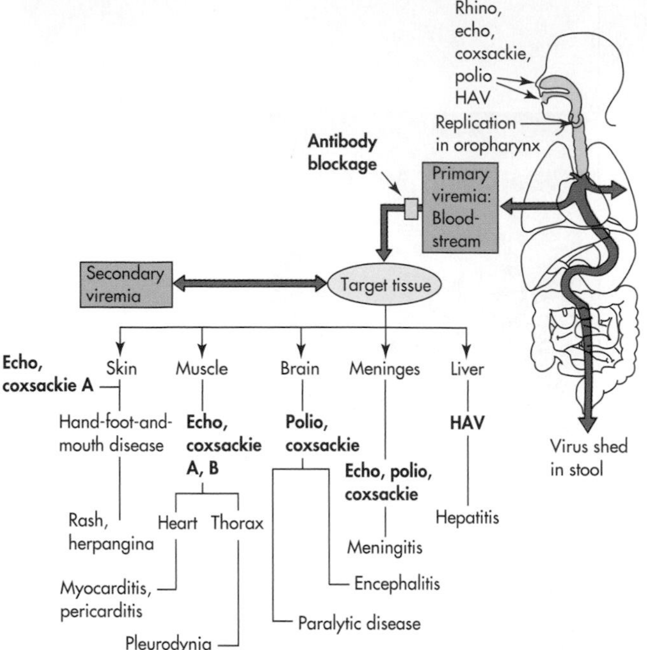

FIGURE 57–4. Pathogenesis of enterovirus infection. The target tissue infected by the enterovirus determines the predominant disease caused by the virus. Coxsackie, coxsackievirus; echo, echovirus; HAV, hepatitis A virus; polio, poliovirus; Rhino, rhinovirus.

BOX 57–3. Disease Mechanisms of Picornaviruses

Enteroviruses enter via the oropharynx, intestinal mucosa, or upper respiratory tract and infect the underlying lymphatic tissue; rhinoviruses are restricted to the upper respiratory tract.
In the absence of serum antibody, enterovirus spreads by viremia to cells of a receptor-bearing target tissue.
Different picornaviruses bind to different receptors, many of which are members of the immunoglobulin superfamily (i.e., ICAM-1).
The infected target tissue determines the subsequent disease.
Viral, rather than immune, pathologic effects are usually responsible for causing disease symptoms.
The secretory antibody response is transitory but can prevent the initiation of infection.
Serum antibody blocks viremic spread to target tissue, preventing symptoms.
Enterovirus is shed in feces for long periods.
Infection is often asymptomatic or causes mild, flulike or upper respiratory tract disease.

Most enteroviruses are cytolytic, replicating rapidly and causing direct damage to the target cell. The hepatitis A virus is the exception because it is not very cytolytic. The kinetics of the immune response to hepatitis A correlate with the appearance of symptoms, indicating immunopathogenesis.

In the case of poliovirus, the virus gains access to the brain by infecting skeletal muscle and traveling up the innervating nerves to the brain, like the rabies virus (see Chapter 61). The virus is cytolytic for the motor neurons of the anterior horn and brain stem. Which of these nerve cells are killed by the virus determine which tissue becomes paralyzed. The number of neurons killed will determine whether paralysis will occur, and whether and when other neurons can reinnervate the muscle and restore activity. The loss of neurons to polio and to old age may result in paralysis later in life, termed postpolio syndrome.

Viral shedding from the oropharynx can be detected for a short time before symptoms begin, whereas viral production and shedding from the intestine may last for 30 days or longer, even in the presence of a humoral immune response.

Antibody is the major protective immune response to the enteroviruses. Secretory antibody can prevent the initial establishment of infection in the oropharynx and gastrointestinal tract, and serum antibody prevents viremic spread to the target tissue and therefore disease. The time course for antibody development after infection with a live vaccine is presented in Figure 57–10.

Cell-mediated immunity is not usually involved in protection but may play a role in pathogenesis. Hepatitis A virus is the exception, in that T cells are important for the resolution of the disease and are a major determinate of the pathogenesis. T cells also appear to contribute to the pathogenesis of Coxsackie B virus–induced myocarditis in mice.

EPIDEMIOLOGY

The enteroviruses are exclusively human pathogens (Box 57–4). As the name implies, these viruses primarily spread via the **fecal-oral** route. **Asymptomatic shedding** can occur for up to a month, putting virus into the environment. Poor sanitation and crowded living conditions foster transmission of the viruses (Figure 57–5). Sewage contamination of water supplies can result in enterovirus epidemics. Outbreaks of enterovirus disease are seen in schools and daycare settings, and summer is the major season for such disease. The coxsackieviruses and echoviruses may also be spread in aerosol droplets and cause respiratory tract infections.

With the success of the polio vaccines, the wild-type poliovirus has been eliminated from the western hemisphere (Figure 57–6) but not from the world. Paralytic polio is still prevalent in Africa and other areas where the vaccine is not available and in communities where vaccination is contrary to religious beliefs or other teachings. A small but significant number of vaccine-related cases of polio result from the reversion of the live vaccine virus and its reestablishing neurovirulence. This development has

BOX 57–4. Epidemiology of Enterovirus Infections

Disease/Viral Factors

Nature of disease correlates with specific enterovirus and age of person.
Infection is often asymptomatic, with viral shedding.
Virion is resistant to environmental conditions (detergents, acid, drying, mild sewage treatment, and heat).

Transmission

Fecal-oral route: Poor hygiene, dirty diapers (especially in daycare settings).
Ingestion via contaminated food and water.
Contact with infected hands and fomites.
Inhalation of infectious aerosols.

Who Is at Risk?

Young children: at risk for polio (asymptomatic or mild disease).
Older children and adults: At risk for polio (asymptomatic to paralytic disease).
Newborns and neonates: At highest risk for serious coxsackievirus and enterovirus disease.

Geography/Season

Viruses have worldwide distribution; wild-type polio is virtually eradicated in developed countries because of vaccination program.
Disease is more common in summer.

Modes of Control

For polio, live oral polio vaccine (trivalent OPV) or inactivated trivalent polio vaccine (IPV) is administered.
For other enteroviruses, there is no vaccine; good hygiene limits spread.

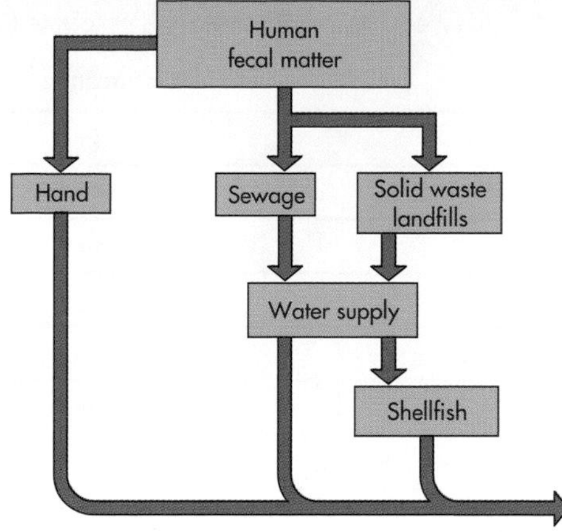

FIGURE 57–5. Transmission of enteroviruses. The capsid structure is resistant to mild sewage treatment, salt water, detergents, and temperature changes, allowing these viruses to be transmitted by fecal-oral routes, fomites, and on hands.

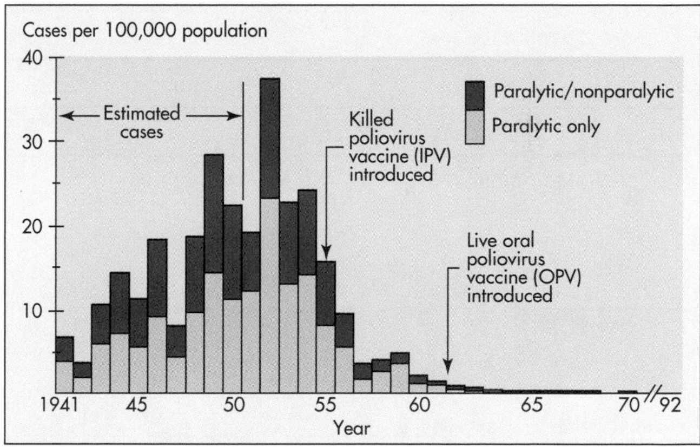

FIGURE 57–6. Incidence of polio in the United States. Killed (inactivated) poliovirus vaccine (IPV) was introduced in 1955, and live (oral) poliovirus vaccine (OPV) was introduced in 1961 and 1962. Wild-type polio has been eradicated in the United States. (Courtesy Centers for Disease Control and Prevention: *Immunization against disease: 1972,* Washington, 1973, U.S. Government Printing Office.)

prompted a change to promote the use of the inactivated polio vaccine. Polioviruses are spread most often during the summer and autumn.

Paralytic polio was once considered a middle-class disease because good hygiene would delay exposure of a person to the virus until late childhood, the adolescent years, or adulthood, when infection would produce the most severe symptoms. Infection during early childhood generally results in asymptomatic or very mild disease.

Like poliovirus infection, Coxsackie A virus disease is generally more severe in adults than in children. However, Coxsackie B virus and some of the echoviruses (especially echovirus 11) can be particularly harmful to infants.

CLINICAL SYNDROMES

The clinical syndromes produced by the enteroviruses are determined by several factors, including: (1) viral serotype, (2) infecting dose, (3) tissue tropism, (4) portal of entry, (5) patient's age, gender, and state of health, and (6) pregnancy (Table 57–1). The incubation period for enterovirus disease varies from 1 to 35 days, depending on the virus, the target tissue, and the person's age. Viruses that affect oral and respiratory sites have the shortest incubation periods.

Poliovirus Infections

Wild-type polio infections are becoming rarer because of the success of the polio vaccines (see Figure 57–6). As noted earlier, however, vaccine-associated cases of polio do occur, and some populations remain unvaccinated, putting them at risk for infection. Poliovirus may cause one of the following four outcomes in unvaccinated people, depending on the progression of the infection (Figure 57–7):

TABLE 57–1. Summary of Clinical Syndromes Associated with Major Enterovirus Groups

Syndrome	Occurrence	Polioviruses	Coxsackie A Viruses	Coxsackie B Viruses	Echoviruses
Paralytic disease	Sporadic	+	+	+	+
Encephalitis, meningitis	Outbreaks	+	+	+	+
Carditis	Sporadic		+	+	+
Neonatal disease	Outbreaks			+	+
Pleurodynia	Outbreaks			+	
Herpangina	Common		+		
Hand-foot-and-mouth disease	Common		+		
Rash disease	Common		+	+	+
Acute hemorrhagic conjunctivitis	Epidemics		+		
Respiratory tract infections	Common	+	+	+	+
Undifferentiated fever	Common	+	+	+	+
Diarrhea, gastrointestinal disease	Uncommon				+
Diabetes, pancreatitis	Uncommon			+	
Orchitis	Uncommon			+	
Disease in immunodeficient patients	—	+	+		+
Congenital anomalies	Uncommon		+	+	

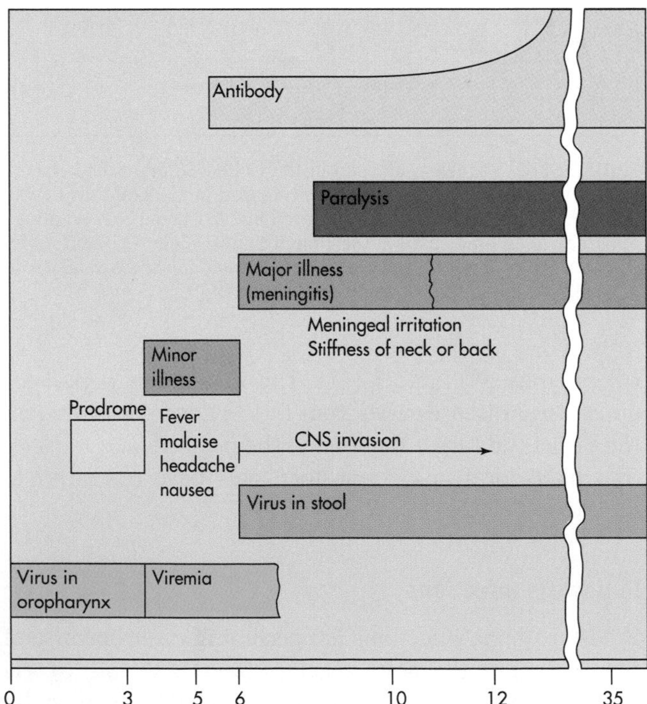

FIGURE 57–7. Progression of poliovirus infection. Infection may be asymptomatic or may progress to minor or major disease. CNS, Central nervous system.

1. **Asymptomatic illness** results if the viral infection is limited to the oropharynx and the gut. At least 90% of poliovirus infections are asymptomatic.
2. **Abortive poliomyelitis,** the **minor illness,** is a nonspecific febrile illness occurring in approximately 5% of infected people. Fever, headache, malaise, sore throat, and vomiting occur in such people within 3 to 4 days of exposure.
3. **Nonparalytic poliomyelitis** or **aseptic meningitis** occurs in 1% to 2% of patients with poliovirus infections. In this disease, the virus progresses into the central nervous system and the meninges, causing back pain and muscle spasms in addition to the symptoms of the minor illness.
4. **Paralytic polio, the major illness,** occurs in 0.1% to 2.0% of persons with poliovirus infections and is the most severe outcome. It appears 3 to 4 days after the minor illness has subsided, thereby producing a biphasic illness. In this disease, the virus spreads from the blood to the **anterior horn cells** of the spinal cord and the motor cortex of the brain. The severity of the paralysis is determined by the extent of the neuronal infection and which neurons are affected. Spinal paralysis may involve one or more limbs, whereas bulbar (cranial) paralysis may involve a combination of cranial nerves and even the medullary respiratory center.

Paralytic poliomyelitis is characterized by an asymmetrical flaccid paralysis with no sensory loss. Poliovirus type 1 is responsible for 85% of the cases of paralytic polio. Reversion of the attenuated vaccine virus types 2 and 3 to virulence can cause vaccine-associated disease.

The degree of paralysis varies in that it may involve only a few muscle groups (e.g., one leg) or there may be complete flaccid paralysis of all four extremities. The paralysis may then progress over the first few days and may result in complete recovery, residual paralysis, or death. Most recoveries occur within 6 months, but as long as 2 years may be required for complete remission.

Bulbar poliomyelitis can be more severe, may involve the muscles of the pharynx, vocal cords, and respiration, and may result in death in 75% of patients. Iron lungs, chambers that provided external respiratory compression, were used during the 1950s to assist the breathing of patients with such polio disease. Before vaccination programs, iron lungs filled the wards of children's hospitals.

Postpolio syndrome is a sequela of poliomyelitis that may occur much later in life (30 to 40 years later) in 20% to 80% of the original victims. Affected people suffer a deterioration of the originally affected muscles. Poliovirus is not present, but the syndrome is believed to result from a loss of neurons in the initially affected nerves.

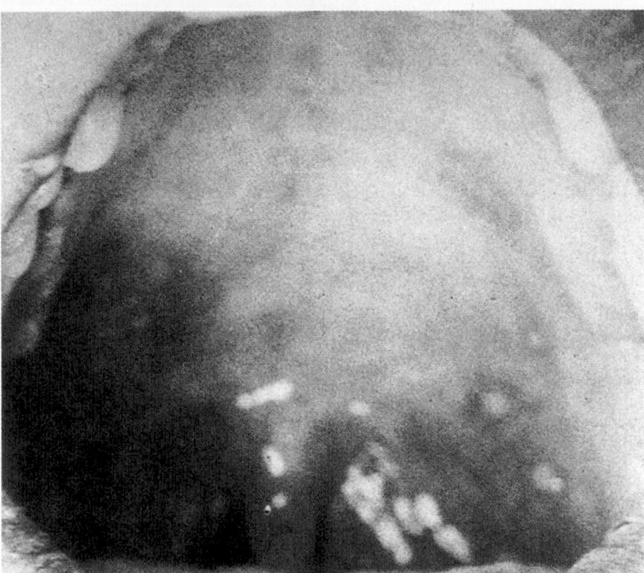

FIGURE 57–8. Herpangina. Characteristic discrete vesicles are seen on the anterior tonsillar pillars. (Courtesy Dr. GDW McKendrick. From Lambert HP et al: *Infectious diseases illustrated,* London, 1982, Gower.)

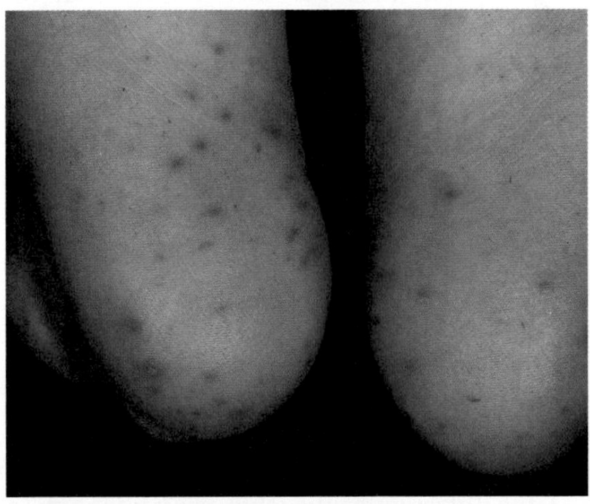

FIGURE 57–9. Hand-foot-and-mouth disease caused by Coxsackie A virus. Lesions initially appear in the oral cavity and then develop within 1 day on the palms and, as seen here, on soles. (From Habif TP: *Clinical dermatology: A color guide to diagnosis and therapy,* ed 3, St Louis, 1996, Mosby.)

Coxsackievirus and Echovirus Infections

Several clinical syndromes may be caused by either a coxsackievirus or an echovirus (e.g., aseptic meningitis), but certain illnesses are specifically associated with coxsackieviruses. Coxsackie A viruses are associated with diseases involving vesicular lesions (e.g., herpangina), whereas Coxsackie B viruses **(B for *body*)** are most frequently associated with myocarditis and pleurodynia. These viruses can also cause a polio-like paralytic disease. The most common result of infection is lack of symptoms or a mild upper respiratory tract or flulike disease.

Herpangina is caused by several types of coxsackie A virus and is not related to a herpesvirus infection. Fever, sore throat, pain on swallowing, anorexia, and vomiting characterize this disorder. The classic finding is vesicular ulcerated lesions around the soft palate and uvula (Figure 57–8). Less typically, the lesions affect the hard palate. The virus can be recovered from the lesions or from feces. The disease is self-limited and requires only symptomatic management.

Hand-foot-and-mouth disease is a vesicular exanthem usually caused by coxsackievirus A16. The name is descriptive because the main features of this infection consist of vesicular lesions on the hands, feet, mouth, and tongue (Figure 57–9). The patient is mildly febrile, and the illness subsides in a few days.

Pleurodynia (Bornholm disease), also known as the devil's grip, is an acute illness in which patients have a sudden onset of fever and unilateral low thoracic, pleuritic chest pain that may be excruciating. Abdominal pain and even vomiting may also occur, and muscles on the involved side may be extremely tender. Pleurodynia lasts an average of 4 days but may relapse after the condition has been asymptomatic for several days. Coxsackie B virus is the causative agent.

Myocardial and **pericardial infections** caused by Coxsackie B virus occur sporadically in older children and adults but are most threatening in newborns. Neonates with these infections have febrile illnesses and sudden and unexplained onset of heart failure. Cyanosis, tachycardia, cardiomegaly, and hepatomegaly occur. Electrocardiographic changes are found in patients with myocarditis. The mortality associated with the infection is high, and autopsy typically reveals the involvement of other organ systems, including the brain, liver, and pancreas. Acute benign pericarditis affects young adults but may be seen in older people. The symptoms resemble those of myocardial infarction with fever.

Viral (aseptic) meningitis is an acute febrile illness accompanied by headache and signs of meningeal irritation, including nuchal rigidity. Petechiae or a rash may occur in patients with enteroviral meningitis. Recovery is usually uneventful, unless the illness is associated with encephalitis (meningoencephalitis) or occurs in children younger than 1 year. Outbreaks of picornavirus meningitis (echovirus 11) occur each year during the summer and autumn.

Fever, rash, and **common cold-like symptoms** may occur in patients infected with echoviruses or coxsackieviruses. The rash is usually maculopapular but may occasionally be petechial or even vesicular. The petechial type of eruption must be differentiated from that of meningococcemia. The symptoms of enteroviral infection are less intense for the child than meningococcemia. Coxsackieviruses A21 and A24 and echoviruses 11 and 20 can cause rhinovirus-like, coldlike symptoms.

Other Enterovirus Diseases

Enterovirus 70 and a variant of coxsackievirus A24 have been associated with an extremely contagious ocular disease, **acute hemorrhagic conjunctivitis.** The infection causes subconjunctival hemorrhages and conjunctivitis. The disease has a 24-hour incubation period and resolves within 1 or 2 weeks. Some strains of Coxsackie B virus and echovirus can be transmitted transplacentally to the fetus. Infection of the fetus or an infant by this or another route may produce severe disseminated disease. Coxsackie B virus infections of the pancreas have been suspected of causing insulin-dependent diabetes as a result of the destruction of the islets of Langerhans.

LABORATORY DIAGNOSIS

Clinical Chemistry

Cerebrospinal fluid (CSF) from poliovirus or enterovirus aseptic meningitis reveals a predominantly lymphocytic pleocytosis (presence of 25 to 500 cells/mm^3). In contrast with bacterial meningitis, the CSF in viral meningitis lacks neutrophils, and the glucose level is usually normal or slightly low. The CSF protein level is normal to slightly elevated. The CSF is rarely positive for the virus.

Culture

Polioviruses may be isolated from the patient's pharynx during the first few days of illness, from the feces for as long as 30 days, but only rarely from the CSF. The virus grows well in monkey kidney tissue culture. Coxsackieviruses and echoviruses can usually be isolated from the throat and stool during infection and often from the CSF in patients with meningitis. Virus is rarely isolated in patients with myocarditis, however, because the symptoms occur several weeks after the initial infection. The Coxsackie B viruses can be grown on primary monkey or human embryo kidney cells. Many strains of Coxsackie A virus do not grow in tissue culture, however, and must still be grown in suckling mice.

Genome and Serology Studies

The specific type of enterovirus can be determined through the use of specific antibody and antigen assays (e.g., neutralization, immunofluorescence, enzyme-linked immunosorbent assay) or reverse transcriptase polymerase chain reaction (RT-PCR) detection of specific viral RNA. RT-PCR of clinical samples has become a rapid and routine method for confirming a diagnosis of echovirus 11 meningitis in an infant and other picornavirus diseases.

Serology is used to confirm an enterovirus infection through detection of specific immunoglobulin (Ig)M or the finding of a fourfold increase in the antibody titer between the time of the acute illness and the period of convalescence. This approach may not be practical for detection of echovirus and coxsackievirus because of their many serotypes, unless a specific virus is suspected.

TREATMENT, PREVENTION, AND CONTROL

A new antiviral drug, pleconaril, is available on a limited basis. The drug inhibits the penetration of picornaviruses into the cell. It must be administered early in the course of the infection.

The prevention of paralytic poliomyelitis is one of the triumphs of modern medicine. By 1979, infections with the wild-type poliovirus disappeared from the United States, with the number of cases of polio decreasing from 21,000 per year in the prevaccine era to 18 in unvaccinated patients in 1977. Like smallpox, polio has been targeted for elimination. Health care delivery to underdeveloped countries is more difficult, and for this reason, wild-type viral disease still exists in Africa, the Middle East, and Asia. Misinformation, misunderstanding, and political unrest in Africa and other parts of the world have also limited acceptance of polio vaccination. New worldwide vaccination programs have been developed to reach the goal.

TABLE 57–2. Advantages and Disadvantages of Polio Vaccines

Vaccine	Advantages	Disadvantages
Live (oral polio vaccine)	Effective Lifelong immunity Induction of secretory antibody response similar to that of natural infection Spread of attenuated virus circulating to contacts promotes indirect immunization (herd immunity) Inexpensive and easy to administer No need for repeated booster vaccine	Risk of vaccine-associated poliomyelitis in vaccine recipients or contacts Spread of vaccine to contacts without their consent Not safe for administration to immunodeficient patients
Inactivated polio vaccine	Effective Good stability during transport and in storage Safe administration in immunodeficient patients No risk of vaccine-related disease	Lack of induction of secretory antibody Booster vaccine needed for lifelong immunity Requires sterile syringes and needles Injection more painful than oral administration Higher community immunization levels needed than with live vaccine

The two types of poliovirus vaccine are (1) **inactivated polio vaccine (IPV)**, developed by Jonas Salk, and (2) **live attenuated oral polio vaccine (OPV),** developed by Albert Sabin. Both vaccines incorporate the three strains of polio, are stable, are relatively inexpensive, and induce a protective antibody response (Figure 57–10). The IPV was proven effective in 1955, but the oral vaccine took its place because it is inexpensive, easy to administer, and elicits lifelong immunity (Table 57–2).

The OPV was *attenuated* (i.e., rendered less virulent) by passage in human or monkey cell cultures. Attenuation yielded a virus that can replicate in the oropharynx and intestinal tract but cannot infect neuronal cells. A mixed blessing of the live vaccine strain is that it is shed in feces for weeks and may be spread to close contacts. The spread will immunize or reimmunize close contacts, thus promoting mass immunization. The major drawbacks of the live vaccine are that (1) the vaccine virus may infect an immunologically compromised individual and (2) there is a remote potential for the virus to revert to its virulent form and cause paralytic disease. The incidence of paralytic disease is estimated to be one per 4 million doses administered (versus one in 100 people infected with the wild-type poliovirus).

In the absence of wild-type poliovirus, new recommendations call for the use of the IPV for routine vaccination. Children should receive the IPV at 2, 4, and 15 months and then at 4 to 6 years of age. Alternatively, the first two doses of IPV can be followed by OPV.

There are no vaccines for coxsackieviruses or echoviruses. Transmission of these viruses can presumably be reduced by improvements in hygiene and living conditions.

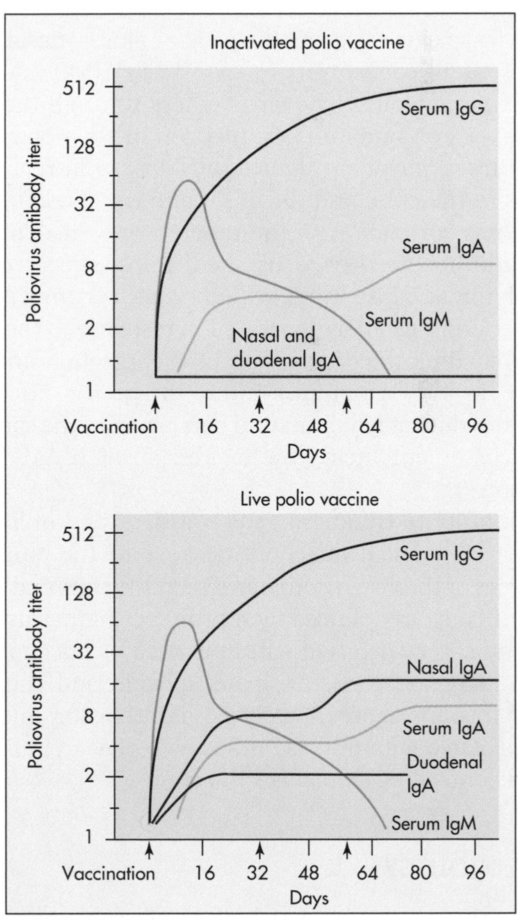

FIGURE 57–10. Serum and secretory antibody response to intramuscular inoculation of inactivated polio vaccine and to live attenuated oral polio vaccine. Note the presence of secretory IgA induced by the live polio vaccine. (Redrawn from Ogra P et al: *Rev Infect Dis* 2:352-369, 1980. Copyright 1980, University of Chicago Press.)

Rhinoviruses

Rhinoviruses are the most important cause of the **common cold** and upper respiratory tract infections. Such infections are self-limited, however, and do not cause serious disease. More than 100 serotypes of rhinovirus have been identified. At least 80% of the rhinoviruses have a common receptor that is also used by some of the coxsackieviruses. This receptor has been identified as ICAM-1, a member of the immunoglobulin superfamily, which is expressed on epithelial, fibroblast, and B-lymphoblastoid cells.

BOX 57–5. Epidemiology of Rhinovirus Infections

Disease/Viral Factors

Virion is resistant to drying and detergents.

Multiple serotypes preclude prior immunity

Replication occurs at optimum temperature of 33°C and cooler temperatures.

Transmission

Direct contact via infected hands and fomites.

Inhalation of infectious droplets.

Who Is at Risk?

People of all ages.

Geography/Season

Virus is found worldwide.

Disease is more common in early autumn and late spring.

Modes of Control

Washing hands and disinfecting contaminated objects help prevent spread.

PATHOGENESIS AND IMMUNITY

Unlike the enteroviruses, rhinoviruses are **unable to replicate in the gastrointestinal tract** (see Box 57–3). The rhinoviruses are **labile to acidic pH.** Also, they **grow best at 33°C,** a feature that may partly account for their predilection for the cooler environment of the nasal mucosa. Infection can be initiated by as little as one infectious viral particle. During the peak of illness, nasal secretions contain concentrations of 500 to 1000 infectious virions per milliliter. The virus enters through the nose, mouth, or eyes and initiates infection of the upper respiratory tract, including the throat. Most viral replication occurs in the nose, and the onset and the severity of the symptoms correlate with the time of viral shedding and the quantity (titer) of virus shed. Infected cells release bradykinin and histamine, which cause a "runny nose."

Interferon, which is generated in response to the infection, may limit the progression of the infection and contribute to the symptoms. Interestingly, the release of cytokines during inflammation can promote the spread of the virus by enhancing the expression of ICAM-1 viral receptors.

Immunity to rhinoviruses is transient and unlikely to prevent subsequent infection, because of the numerous serotypes of the virus. Both nasal secretory IgA and serum IgG antibody are induced by a primary rhinovirus infection and can be detected within a week of infection. The secretory IgA response dissipates quickly, and immunity begins to wane approximately 18 months after infection. Cell-mediated immunity is not likely to play an important role in controlling rhinovirus infections.

EPIDEMIOLOGY

Rhinoviruses cause at least half of all upper respiratory tract infections (Box 57–5). Other agents likely to cause the symptoms of the common cold are enteroviruses, coronaviruses, adenoviruses, and parainfluenza viruses. Rhinoviruses can be transmitted by two mechanisms, as aerosols and on fomites (e.g., by hands or on contaminated inanimate objects). Hands appear to be the major vector, and direct person-to-person contact is the predominant mode of spread. These nonenveloped viruses are extremely stable and can survive on such objects for many hours.

Rhinoviruses produce clinical illness in only half of the people infected. Asymptomatic people are also capable of spreading the virus, even though they may produce less of the virus.

Rhinovirus "colds" occur most often in early autumn and late spring in people living in temperate climates. This may reflect social patterns (e.g., return to school and daycare) rather than any change in the virus itself.

Rates of infection are highest in infants and children. Children younger than 2 years "share" their colds with their families. Secondary infections occur in approximately 50% of family members, especially other children.

Many different rhinovirus serotypes may be found in a given community during a specific cold season, but the predominant strains are usually the newly categorized serotypes. This pattern indicates the existence of a gradual antigenic drift (mutation), similar to that seen for the influenza virus.

CLINICAL SYNDROMES (BOX 57–6)

Common cold symptoms caused by rhinoviruses cannot readily be distinguished from those caused by other viral respiratory pathogens (e.g., enteroviruses, paramyxoviruses, coronaviruses). An upper respiratory tract infection usually begins with sneezing, which is soon followed by rhinorrhea (runny nose). The rhinorrhea increases and

BOX 57–6. Clinical Summaries

Polio: A 12-year-old girl from Kenya has headache, fever, nausea, and stiff neck. Symptoms improve and then recur several days later, with weakness and paralysis of her legs. She has no history of polio immunization.

Coxsackie A virus

Herpangina: Vesicular lesions on the tongue and roof of the mouth of a 7-year-old patient accompany fever, sore throat, and pain on swallowing.

Coxsackie B (*B for body*) virus

Pleurodynia: A 13-year-old boy has fever and severe chest pain with headache, fatigue, and aching muscles lasting for 4 days.

Coxsackie or echovirus

Aseptic meningitis: A 7-month-old infant with fever and rash appears listless, with a stiff neck. A sample of his cerebrospinal fluid contains lymphocytes but has normal glucose and no bacteria. Full recovery occurs within 1 week.

Common cold (Rhinovirus)

A 25-year-old person develops runny nose, mild cough, and malaise with a low-grade fever. A co-worker in the office has had similar symptoms for the past few days.

is then accompanied by symptoms of nasal obstruction. Mild sore throat also occurs, along with headache and malaise. The illness peaks in 3 to 4 days, but the cough and nasal symptoms may persist for 7 to 10 days or longer. Fever and rigors sometimes accompany rhinovirus infections.

LABORATORY DIAGNOSIS

The clinical syndrome of the common cold is usually so characteristic that laboratory diagnosis is unnecessary. Virus can be obtained from nasal washings. Rhinoviruses are grown in human diploid fibroblast cells (e.g., WI-38) at 33°C. Virus is identified by the typical cytopathologic effect and the demonstration of acid lability. Serotyping is rarely necessary but can be performed with the use of pools of specific neutralizing sera. The performance of serologic testing to document rhinovirus infection is not practical.

TREATMENT, PREVENTION, AND CONTROL

There are many over-the-counter remedies for the common cold. Nasal vasoconstrictors may provide relief, but their use may be followed by rebound congestion and a worsening of symptoms. Rigorous studies of vitamin C therapy have not shown it to be efficacious.

Pleconaril inhibits rhinovirus replication but has not proved therapeutically useful in controlling rhinovirus infections. Experimental antiviral drugs similar to pleconaril (e.g., arildone, rhodanine, disoxaril), and their analogues, contain a 3-methylisoxazole group that inserts into the base of the receptor-binding canyon and blocks uncoating of the virus. Enviroxime inhibits the viral RNA–dependent RNA polymerase. A polypeptide receptor analogue based on the ICAM-1 protein structure may have potential as an antiviral drug. The intranasal administration of interferon can block infection for a short time after a known exposure, but its long-term use (e.g., throughout the "cold season") could cause symptoms at least as bad as those of the rhinovirus infection.

Rhinovirus is not a good candidate for a vaccine program. The multiple serotypes, the apparent antigenic drift in rhinoviral antigens, the requirement for secretory IgA production, and the transience of the antibody response pose major problems for the development of vaccines. In addition, the benefit-to-risk ratio would be very low because rhinoviruses do not cause significant disease.

Hand washing and the disinfection of contaminated objects are the best means of preventing the spread of the virus. Facial tissues have been impregnated with antiviral chemicals to limit the spread of the virus.

CASE STUDY AND QUESTIONS

A 6-year-old girl was brought to the doctor's office at 4:30 PM because she had a sore throat, had been unusually tired, and was napping excessively. Her temperature was 39°C. She had a sore throat with enlarged tonsils and a faint rash on her back. At 10:30 PM, the patient's mother reported that the child had vomited three times, continued to nap excessively, and complained of a headache when awake.

The doctor examined the child at 11:30 PM and noted that she was lethargic and aroused only when her head was turned, complaining that her back hurt. Her CSF contained no red blood cells, but there were 28 white blood cells/mm^3, half polymorphonuclear neutrophils and half lymphocytes. The glucose and protein levels in the CSF were normal, and Gram stain of a specimen of CSF showed no bacteria.

1. What were the key signs and symptoms in this case?
2. What was the differential diagnosis?
3. What signs and symptoms suggested an enterovirus infection?
4. How would the diagnosis be confirmed?
5. What were the most likely sources and means of infection?
6. What were the target tissue and mechanism of pathogenesis?

Bibliography

Ansardi D et al: Poliovirus assembly and encapsidation of genomic RNA, *Adv Virus Res* 46:2-70, 1996.

Cohen J, Powderly WG, editors: *Infectious diseases*, ed 2, St Louis, 2004, Mosby.

Flint SJ et al: *Principles of virology: Molecular biology, pathogenesis and control of animal viruses*, ed 2, Washington, 2003, American Society for Microbiology Press.

Knipe DM, Howley PM, editors: *Fields virology*, ed 4, New York, 2001, Lippincott-Williams and Wilkins.

Levandowski RA: Rhinoviruses. In Belshe RB, editor: *Textbook of human virology*, ed 2, St Louis, 1991, Mosby.

McKinlay MA et al: Treatment of the picornavirus common cold by inhibitors of viral uncoating and attachment, *Ann Rev Microbiol* 46:635-654, 1992.

Moore M, Morens DM: Enteroviruses including polioviruses. In Belshe RB, editor: *Textbook of human virology*, ed 2, St Louis, 1991, Mosby.

Plotkin SA, Vidor E: Poliovirus vaccine—Inactive. In Plotkin SA, Orenstein WA: *Vaccines*, ed 4, Philadelphia, 2004, WB Saunders.

Racaniello VR: Picornaviruses, *Curr Top Microbiol Immunol* 161:1-192, 1990.

Ren R, Racaniello VR: Human poliovirus receptor gene expression and poliovirus tissue tropism in transgenic mice, *J Virol* 66:296-304, 1992.

Robbins FC: The history of Polio vaccine development. In Plotkin SA, Orenstein WA: *Vaccines*, ed 4, Philadelphia, 2004, WB Saunders.

Strauss JM, Strauss EG: *Viruses and human disease*, San Diego, 2002, Academic Press.

Sutter RW et al: Poliovirus vaccine—Live. In Plotkin SA, Orenstein WA: *Vaccines*, ed 4, Philadelphia, 2004, WB Saunders.

Tracy S, Chapman NM, Mahy BWJ: Coxsackie B viruses, *Curr Topics Microbiol Immunol*, Vol 223, Berlin, 1997, Springer-Verlag.

Wilfert CM et al: Enteroviruses and meningitis, *Pediatr Infect Dis* 2:333-341, 1983.

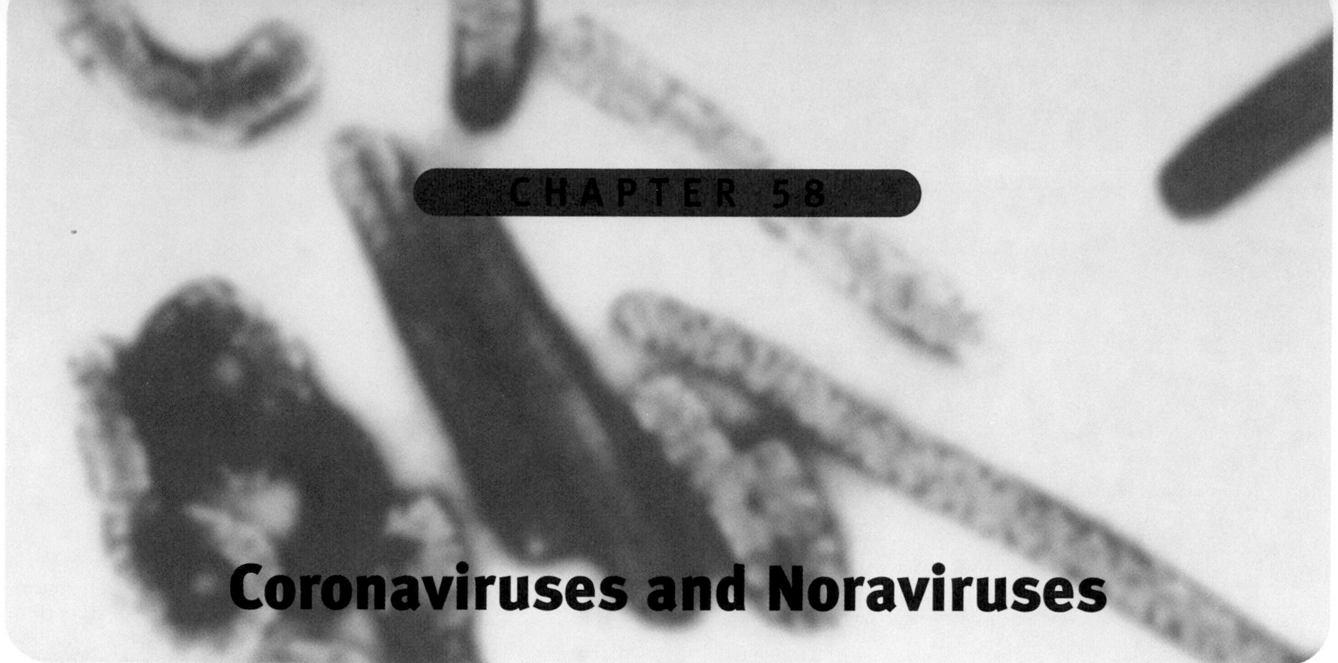

CHAPTER 58

Coronaviruses and Noraviruses

Coronaviruses

Coronaviruses are named for the solar corona-like appearance (the surface projections) of their virions when viewed with an electron microscope (Figure 58–1). Coronaviruses are the second most prevalent cause of the **common cold** (rhinovirus is the first). In 2002, an outbreak of **severe acute respiratory syndrome (SARS)** in Guangdong Province, South China spread to Hong Kong and then around the world. It was shown that the disease was caused by a coronavirus **(SARS-CoV).** Electron microscopy findings have also linked coronaviruses to gastroenteritis in children and adults.

STRUCTURE AND REPLICATION

Coronaviruses are **enveloped virions** with the longest **positive (+) RNA** genome. Virions measure 80 to 160 nm in diameter (Box 58–1). The glycoproteins on the surface of the envelope appear as club-shaped projections that are 20 nm long and 5 to 11 nm wide and appear as a halo (corona) around the virus. Unlike most enveloped viruses, the "corona" formed by the glycoproteins allows the virus to endure the conditions in the gastrointestinal tract and be spread by the fecal-oral route.

The large, plus-stranded RNA genome (27,000 to 30,000 bases) associates with the N protein to form a helical nucleocapsid. Protein synthesis occurs in two phases, similar to that of the togaviruses. On infection, the genome is translated to produce a polyprotein that is cleaved to produce an RNA-dependent RNA polymerase (L [225,000 Da]). The polymerase generates a negative-sense template RNA. The L protein then uses the template RNA to replicate new genomes and produce five to seven **individual messenger ribonucleic acids (mRNAs)** for the individual viral proteins. Generation of the individual mRNAs may also promote recombination events between viral genomes to promote genetic diversity.

Virions contain the glycoproteins E1 (20,000 to 30,000 Da) and E2 (160,000 to 200,000 Da) and a core nucleoprotein (N [47,000 to 55,000 Da]); some strains also contain a hemagglutinin-neuraminidase (E3 [120,000 to 140,000 Da]) (Table 58–1). The E2 glycoprotein is responsible for mediating viral attachment and membrane fusion and is the target of neutralizing antibodies. The E1 glycoprotein is a transmembrane matrix protein. The replication scheme for coronaviruses is shown in Figure 58–2.

PATHOGENESIS AND CLINICAL SYNDROMES

Coronaviruses inoculated into the respiratory tracts of human volunteers have been found to infect epithelial cells. Infection remains localized to the upper respiratory tract because the *optimum temperature for viral growth is 33° to 35°C* (Box 58–2). The virus is most likely spread by aerosols and in large droplets (e.g., sneezes). Most human coronaviruses cause an upper respiratory tract infection similar to the colds caused by rhinoviruses but with a longer incubation period (average, 3 days). The infection may exacerbate a preexisting chronic pulmonary disease, such as asthma and bronchitis, and on rare occasions may cause pneumonia.

Infections occur mainly in infants and children. Coronavirus disease appears either sporadically or in outbreaks in the winter and spring. Usually, one strain predominates in an outbreak. Findings from serologic studies show that coronaviruses cause approximately 10% to 15% of upper respiratory tract infections and pneumonias in humans. Antibodies to coronaviruses are uniformly present by adulthood, but reinfections are common despite the preexisting serum antibodies.

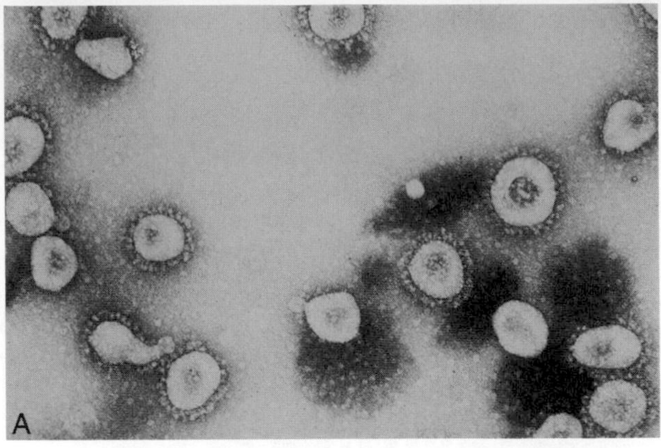

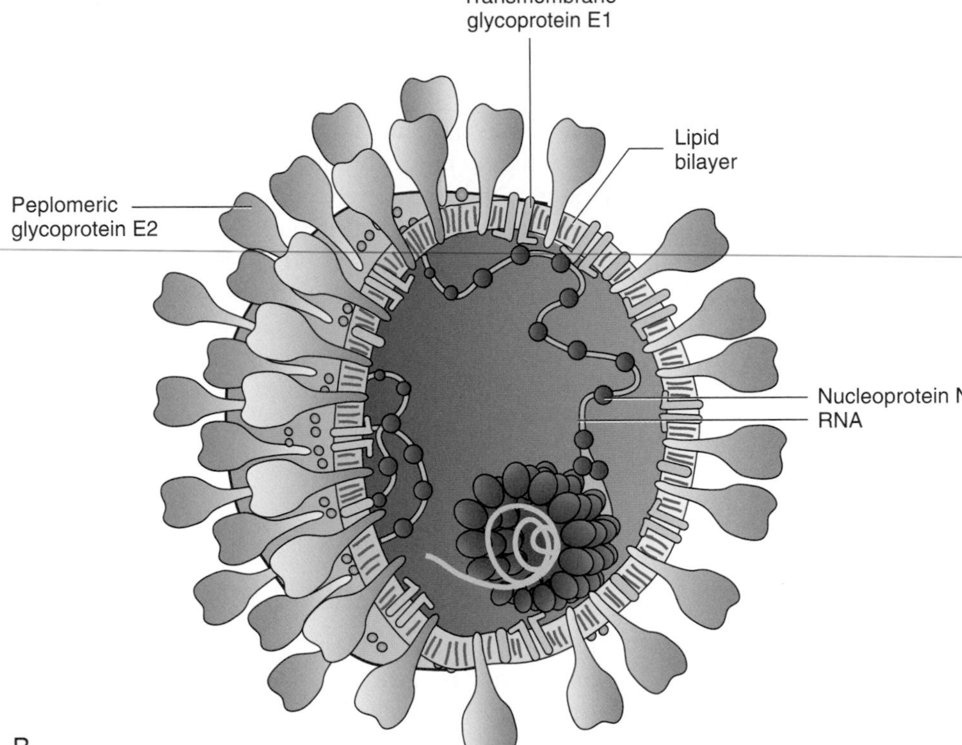

FIGURE 58–1. A, Electron micrograph of the human respiratory coronavirus. (magnification 90,000X.) **B,** Model of a coronavirus. The viral nucleocapsid is a long, flexible helix composed of the positive-strand genomic RNA and many molecules of the phosphorylated nucleocapsid protein N. The viral envelope consists of a lipid bilayer derived from the intracellular membranes of the host cell and two viral glycoproteins (E1 and E2). (**A** courtesy Centers for Disease Control and Prevention, Atlanta; **B** redrawn from Fields BF, Knipe DM, editors: *Virology,* New York, 1985, Raven.)

BOX 58–1. Unique Features of Coronaviruses

Virus has medium-sized virions with a solar corona-like appearance.
Single-stranded, positive-sense RNA genome is enclosed in an envelope containing the E2 viral attachment protein, E1 matrix protein, and N nucleocapsid protein.
Translation of genome occurs in two phases: (1) the early phase produces an RNA polymerase (L), and (2) the late phase, from a negative-sense RNA template, yields structural and nonstructural proteins.
Virus assembles at the rough endoplasmic reticulum.
Virus is difficult to isolate and grow in routine cell culture.

BOX 58–2. Disease Mechanisms of Human Coronaviruses

Virus infects epithelial cells of upper respiratory tract.
Virus replicates best at 33° to 35°C; therefore it prefers the upper respiratory tract.
Reinfection occurs in presence of serum antibodies.
The glycoprotein "corona" helps this enveloped virus survive the gastrointestinal tract.
Severe acute respiratory syndrome infection is exacerbated by inflammatory responses.

TABLE 58–1. Major Human Coronavirus Proteins

Proteins	Molecular Weight (kDa)	Location	Functions
E2 (peplomeric glycoprotein)	160-200	Envelope spikes (peplomer)	Binding to host cells; fusion activity
H1 (hemagglutinin protein)	60-66	Peplomer	Hemagglutination
N (nucleoprotein)	47-55	Core	Ribonucleoprotein
E1 (matrix glycoprotein)	20-30	Envelope	Transmembrane protein
L (polymerase)	225	Infected cell	Polymerase activity

Modified from Balows A et al, editors: *Laboratory diagnosis of infectious diseases: Principles and practice*, New York, 1988, Springer-Verlag.

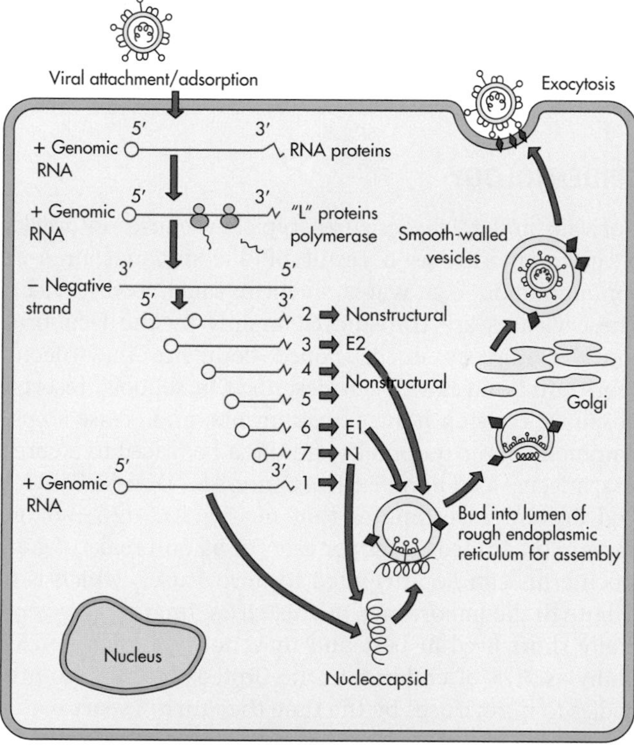

FIGURE 58–2. Replication of human coronaviruses. The E2 glycoprotein interacts with receptors on epithelial cells, the virus fuses or is endocytosed into the cell, and the genome is released into the cytoplasm. Protein synthesis is divided into early and late phases, similar to that in the togaviruses. The genome binds to ribosomes, and an RNA-dependent RNA polymerase is translated. This enzyme generates a full-length, negative-sense RNA template for the production of new virion genomes and six individual mRNAs for the other coronavirus proteins. The genome associates with rough endoplasmic reticulum membranes modified by virion proteins and buds into the lumen of the rough endoplasmic reticulum. Vesicles that contain virus migrate to the cell membrane, and virus is released by exocytosis. (Redrawn from Balows A et al, editors: *Laboratory diagnosis of infectious diseases: Principles and practice,* New York, 1988, Springer-Verlag.)

Coronavirus-like particles have also been seen in electron micrographs of stool specimens obtained from adults and children with diarrhea and gastroenteritis and infants with neonatal necrotizing enterocolitis.

SARS is a form of atypical pneumonia characterized by high fever (> 38°C), chills, rigors, headache, dizziness, malaise, and myalgia, cough or breathing difficulty, and a history of exposure to a person or place associated with SARS within the previous 10 days. Up to 20% of patients will also develop diarrhea. Mortality is at least 10% of people with indication of SARS infection. Although SARS-CoV is most likely transmitted in respiratory droplets, it is also present in sweat, urine, and feces.

As already mentioned, the outbreak of SARS started in November 2002 in South China's Guangdong Province, was brought to Hong Kong by a physician working within the original outbreak, and then was brought to Vietnam, Toronto, and other places by travelers. The virus was shown to be a coronavirus by its electron microscopic morphology and by reverse transcriptase polymerase chain reaction (RT-PCR). The virus apparently jumped to man from animals (masked-palm civets, raccoon dogs, and Chinese ferret badgers) raised for food. A World Health Organization WHO global alert prompted containment measures to limit the spread of the virus and controlled the outbreak to 8000 infected individuals. Travel restrictions and public concern resulted in a loss of hundreds of millions of dollars in travel and other business.

LABORATORY DIAGNOSIS

Laboratory tests are not routinely performed to diagnose coronavirus infections other than SARS. The method of choice for coronaviruses, including SARS-CoV, is detection of the viral RNA genome in respiratory and stool samples by RT-PCR. Virus isolation of the coronaviruses is difficult and for SARS-CoV, requires stringent biosafety level 3 (BSL-3) conditions. Testing of samples suspected of containing SARS-CoV must be performed with appropriate BSL-2 precautions attainable in many virology laboratories. Serology using enzyme-linked immunosorbent assay (ELISA) can be used to evaluate acute and convalescent sera. Electron microscopy has also been used to detect coronavirus-like particles in stool specimens.

TREATMENT, PREVENTION, AND CONTROL

Control of the respiratory transmission of the common cold form of coronavirus would be difficult and is probably unnecessary because of the mildness of the infection. Strict quarantine of individuals infected with SARS-CoV and screening of travelers for fever from a region with an outbreak of SARS is necessary to limit the spread of the virus. No vaccine or specific antiviral therapy is available.

Noroviruses

The noroviruses include the Norwalk-like viruses, caliciviruses, astroviruses, and other small, round gastroenteritis viruses. Norwalk virus was discovered on electron microscopic examination of stool samples from adults during an epidemic of acute gastroenteritis in Norwalk, Ohio. Many of the other viruses in this family also bear the names of the geographic locations where they were identified (Box 58–3).

STRUCTURE AND REPLICATION

Noroviruses resemble and are approximately the same size as the picornaviruses. Their **positive-sense RNA genome** (approximately 7500 bases) has a VPg protein and a 3′ terminal poly adenosine sequence similar to picornaviruses. The genome is contained in a 27-nm **naked capsid** consisting of 60,000-Da capsid proteins. Norwalk virions are round with a ragged outline, whereas other calicivirions have cup-shaped indentations and a six-point star shape. The virions of the astroviruses have a five- or six-point star shape on the surface but no indentations. Antibodies from seropositive people can also be used to distinguish these viruses.

Caliciviruses and astroviruses can be grown in cell culture, but the Norwalk viruses cannot. Expression of the structural protein genes of different Norwalk viruses in tissue culture cells produces Norwalk virus–like particles. These particles were used to show that Norwalk viruses bind to the carbohydrate of the A, B, or O blood group antigen on the cell surface. The noraviruses replicate similar to the picornaviruses, except that there is an early and late mRNA similar to the togaviruses and coronaviruses. The early mRNA encodes a polyprotein containing the RNA polymerase while the late mRNA for the capsid protein is transcribed from the replicative intermediate (-strand RNA) and the protein is expressed as a single protein.

BOX 58–3. Characteristics of Noroviruses

- Viruses are small capsid viruses distinguishable by **capsid** morphology.
- Viruses are resistant to environmental pressure: Detergents, drying, and acid.
- Viruses are transmitted by **fecal-oral** route in contaminated water and food.
- Viruses cause **outbreaks of gastroenteritis.**
- Disease resolves after 48 hours, without serious consequences.

PATHOGENESIS

The virus compromises the function of the intestinal brush border, preventing proper absorption of water and nutrients. Although no histologic changes occur in the gastric mucosa, gastric emptying may be delayed. Examination of jejunal biopsy specimens from human volunteers infected with noroviruses revealed the existence of blunted villi, cytoplasmic vacuolation, and infiltration with mononuclear cells. Shedding of the virus may continue for 2 weeks after symptoms have ceased.

EPIDEMIOLOGY

Norwalk and related viruses typically cause outbreaks of gastroenteritis as a result of a common source of contamination (e.g., water, shellfish, salad, food service). These viruses are transmitted mainly by the fecal-oral route. Outbreaks in developed countries may occur year-round and have been described in schools, resorts, hospitals, nursing homes, restaurants, and cruise ships. Common-source outbreaks can often be traced to a careless, infected food handler. The Centers for Disease Control and Prevention estimates that nearly 50% (23 million cases in the United States per year) of all outbreaks of gastroenteritis can be attributed to noroviruses, which is a tribute to the importance of this virus. Immunity is generally short lived at best and may not be protective. As many as 70% of children in the United States have antibodies to noroviruses by the time they turn 7 years old.

CLINICAL SYNDROMES (BOX 58–4)

Norwalk and related viruses cause symptoms similar to those caused by the rotaviruses. Infection causes an acute onset of **diarrhea with nausea and vomiting,** with abdominal cramps and nausea, especially in children (Figure 58–3). Bloody stools do not occur. Fever may occur in as many as a third of the patients. The incubation period is usually 24 to 48 hours, and the illness resolves within 12 to 60 hours without problems.

LABORATORY DIAGNOSIS

The use of RT-PCR for detection of the norovirus genome in stool or emesis samples has enhanced the speed and detection of the virus during outbreaks. Immunoelectron microscopy can be used to concentrate and identify the virus from stool. The addition of an antibody directed

BOX 58–4. Clinical Summaries

Coronaviruses

Common cold: A 25-year-old person develops runny nose, mild cough, and malaise with a low-grade fever. A co-worker in the office has had similar symptoms for the past few days.

SARS: A 45-year-old businessman returned from a 2-week trip to China. Five days after returning home to the United States, he developed a fever of 101.5°F (38.6°C) and cough. Now he observes that it is harder to catch his breath.

Norovirus

Norwalk virus: On the third day of a cruise (incubation period of 24 to 60 hours), a group of 45 passengers on a cruise ship experienced watery diarrhea, nausea, and vomiting for 12 to 60 hours, depending on the individual.

CASE STUDY AND QUESTIONS

Several adults complained of serious diarrhea, nausea, vomiting, and a mild fever 2 days after visiting Le Café Grease. The symptoms were too severe to result from food poisoning or a routine gastroenteritis but lasted only 24 hours.

1. What characteristics distinguished this disease from a rotavirus infection?
2. What was the most likely means of viral transmission?
3. What physical characteristics of the virus allowed it to be transmitted by these means?
4. What public health measures could be followed to prevent such outbreaks?

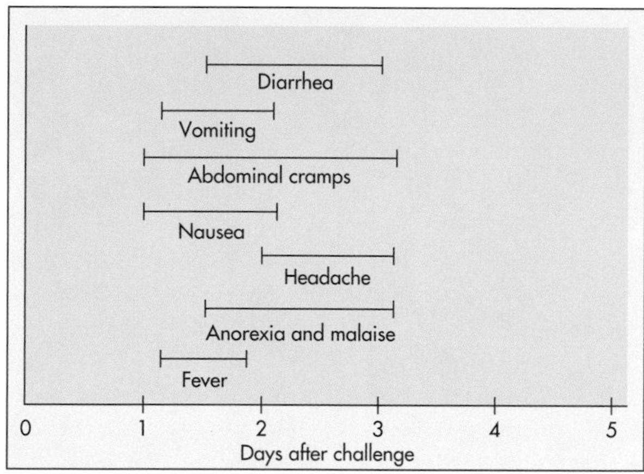

FIGURE 58–3. Response to ingestion of Norwalk virus. Symptoms vary in severity.

against the suspected agent causes the virus to aggregate, thereby facilitating recognition. Radioimmunoassay (RIA) and ELISA have been developed to detect the virus and viral antigen. Confirmation of the diagnosis by serology can be used to confirm a diagnosis. RIA or ELISA can detect antibody to the Norwalk agent. Antibodies to the other calicivirus-like agents are more difficult to detect.

TREATMENT, PREVENTION, AND CONTROL

No specific treatment for infection with the calicivirus or other small, round gastroenteritis viruses is available. Bismuth subsalicylate may reduce the severity of the gastrointestinal symptoms. Outbreaks may be minimized by handling food carefully and by maintaining the purity of the water supply. Norwalk virus is resistant to heat (60°C), pH 3, detergent, and even the chlorine levels of drinking water, which is more resistant than polioviruses or rotaviruses.

Bibliography

Balows A, Hausler WJ Jr, Lennette EH: *Laboratory diagnosis of infectious diseases: Principles and practice,* New York, 1988, Springer-Verlag.

Belshe RB, editor: *Textbook of human virology,* ed 2, St Louis, 1991, Mosby.

Bishop RF: Other small virus-like particles in humans. In Tyrrell DAJ, Kapikian AZ, editors: *Virus infections of the gastrointestinal tract,* New York, 1982, Marcel Dekker.

Blacklow NR, Greenberg HB: Viral gastroenteritis, *N Engl J Med* 325:252-264, 1991.

Christensen ML: Human viral gastroenteritis, *Clin Microbiol Rev* 2:51-89, 1989.

Cohen J, Powderly WG, editors: *Infectious diseases,* ed 2, St Louis, 2004, Mosby.

Flint SJ et al: *Principles of virology: Molecular biology, pathogenesis and control of animal viruses,* ed 2, Washington, 2003, American Society for Microbiology Press.

Knipe DM, Howley PM, editors: *Fields virology,* ed 4, New York, 2001, Lippincott-Williams and Wilkins.

Meulen V, Siddell S, Wege H, editors: *Biochemistry and biology of coronaviruses,* New York, 1981, Plenum.

Strauss JM, Strauss EG: *Viruses and human disease,* San Diego, 2002, Academic Press.

Tan M et al: Mutations within the P2 domain of norovirus capsid affect binding to human histo-blood group antigens: Evidence for a binding pocket, J Virol 77: 12562-12571.

Xi JN et al: Norwalk virus genome cloning and characterization, *Science* 250:1580-1583, 1990.

Websites

Kamps BS, Hoffmann C: SARS reference, 2003: www.sarsreference.com/sarsref/preface.htm

National Institute of Allergy and Infectious Diseases research on SARS: www.niaid.nih.gov/factsheets/sars.htm

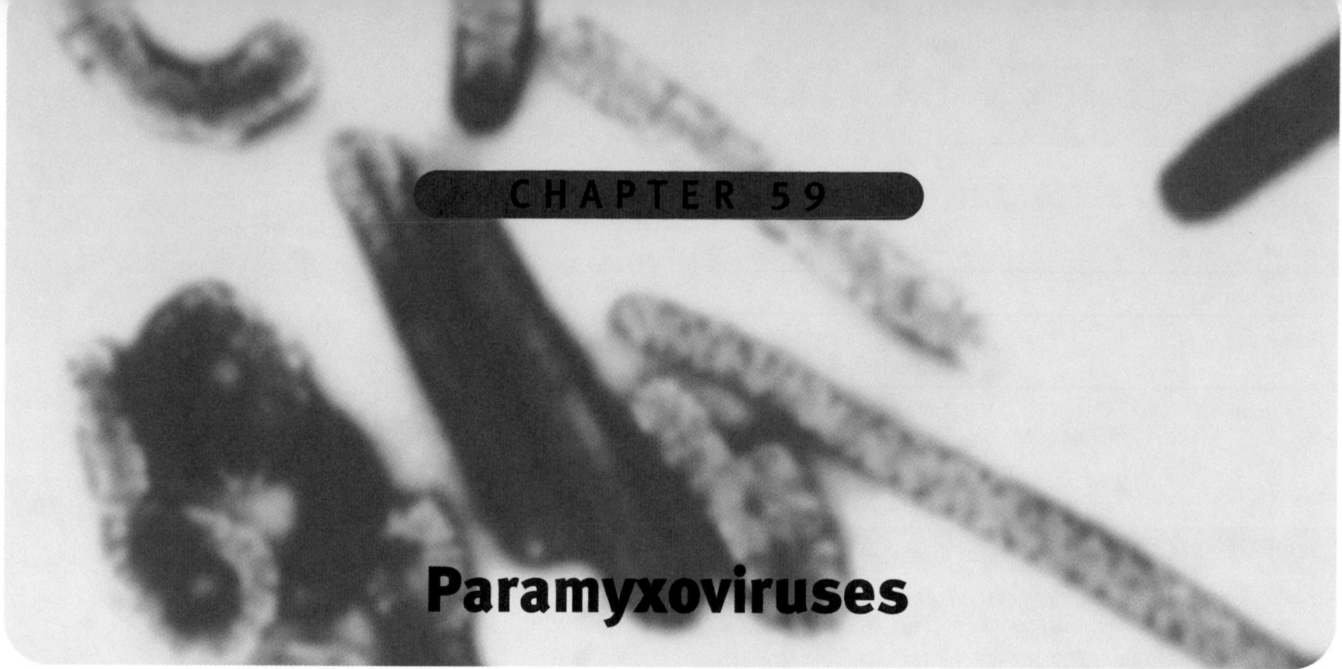

CHAPTER 59

Paramyxoviruses

The Paramyxoviridae include the following genera: *Morbillivirus, Paramyxovirus,* and *Pneumovirus* (Table 59–1). Human pathogens within the morbilliviruses include the **measles** virus; within the paramyxoviruses, the **parainfluenza** and **mumps** viruses; and within the pneumoviruses, the **respiratory syncytial virus (RSV)** and newly discovered, but relatively common, **metapneumovirus.** Their virions have similar morphologies and protein components, and they share the capacity to induce **cell-cell fusion** (syncytia formation and multinucleated giant cells). A new group of highly pathogenic paramyxoviruses, including two zoonosis-causing viruses, **Nipah virus** and **Hendra virus,** was identified in 1998 after an outbreak of severe encephalitis in Malaysia and Singapore.

These agents cause some well-known major diseases. Measles virus causes a potentially serious generalized infection characterized by a maculopapular rash **(rubeola).** Parainfluenza viruses cause upper and lower respiratory tract infections, primarily in children, including pharyngitis, croup, bronchitis, bronchiolitis, and pneumonia. Mumps virus causes a systemic infection whose most prominent clinical manifestation is parotitis. RSV causes mild upper respiratory tract infections in children and adults but can cause life-threatening pneumonia in infants.

Measles and mumps viruses have *only one serotype,* and protection is provided by an effective **live vaccine.** In the United States and other developed countries, successful vaccination programs using the live attenuated measles and mumps vaccines have made measles and mumps rare. In particular, these programs have led to the virtual elimination of the serious sequelae of measles.

Structure and Replication

Paramyxoviruses consist of **negative-sense, single-stranded ribonucleic acid (RNA)** (5 to 8 × 10^6 Da) in a helical nucleocapsid surrounded by a pleomorphic **envelope** of approximately 156 to 300 nm (Figure 59–1). They are similar in many respects to orthomyxoviruses but are larger and do not have the segmented genome of the influenza viruses (Box 59–1). Although significant homology exists among paramyxovirus genomes, the order of the protein-coding regions differs for each genus. The gene products of the measles virus are listed in Table 59–2.

The nucleocapsid consists of the negative-sense, single-stranded RNA associated with the nucleoprotein **(NP),** polymerase phosphoprotein **(P),** and large **(L)** protein. The L protein is the RNA polymerase, the P protein facilitates RNA synthesis, and the NP protein helps maintain genomic structure. The nucleocapsid associates with the matrix **(M)** protein lining the inside of the virion envelope. The envelope contains two glycoproteins, a fusion **(F)** protein, which promotes fusion of the viral and host cell membranes, and a viral attachment protein (hemagglutinin-neuraminidase **[HN],** hemagglutinin **[H],** or **G** protein) (see Box 59–1). The F protein must be activated by proteolytic cleavage, which produces F_1 and F_2 glycopeptides held together by a disulfide bond, to express membrane-fusing activity.

Replication of the paramyxoviruses is initiated by the binding of the HN, H, or G protein on the virion envelope to sialic acid on the cell surface glycolipids. The measles virus binds to a protein, CD46 (membrane cofactor protein, MCP). This receptor is present on most cell types,

TABLE 59–1. Paramyxoviridae

Genus	Human Pathogen
Morbillivirus	Measles virus
Paramyxovirus	Parainfluenza viruses 1 to 4 Mumps virus
Pneumovirus	Respiratory syncytial virus Metapneumovirus

BOX 59–1. Unique Features of the Paramyxoviridae

Large virion consists of a negative RNA genome in a helical nucleocapsid surrounded by an envelope containing a viral attachment protein (hemagglutinin-neuraminidase [HN], parainfluenza virus and mumps virus; hemagglutinin [H], measles virus; and glycoprotein [G], respiratory syncytial virus [RSV]) and a fusion glycoprotein (F).

The three genera can be distinguished by the activities of the viral attachment protein: HN of parainfluenza virus and mumps virus has hemagglutinin and neuraminidase, and H of measles virus has hemagglutinin activity, but G of RSV lacks these activities.

Virus replicates in the cytoplasm.

Virions penetrate the cell by fusion with and exit by budding from the plasma membrane.

Viruses induce cell-cell fusion, causing multinucleated giant cells.

Paramyxoviridae are transmitted in respiratory droplets and initiate infection in the respiratory tract.

Cell-mediated immunity causes many of the symptoms but is essential for control of the infection.

protects the cell from complement by regulating complement activation, and is also the receptor for human herpes virus 6 and some strains of adenovirus. The F protein promotes fusion of the envelope with the plasma membrane. Paramyxoviruses are also able to induce cell-cell fusion, thereby creating multinucleated giant cells (syncytia).

The replication of the genome occurs in a manner similar to that of other negative-strand RNA viruses (i.e., rhabdoviruses). The RNA polymerase is carried into the cell as part of the nucleocapsid. Transcription, protein synthesis, and replication of the genome all occur in the host cell's cytoplasm. The genome is transcribed into individual messenger RNAs (mRNAs) and a full-length positive-sense RNA template. New genomes associate with the L, N, and NP proteins to form nucleocapsids, which associate with the M proteins on viral glycoprotein–modified plasma membranes. The glycoproteins are synthesized and processed like cellular glycoproteins. Mature virions then bud from the host cell plasma membrane and exit the cell. Replication of the paramyxoviruses is represented by the RSV infectious cycle shown in Figure 59–2.

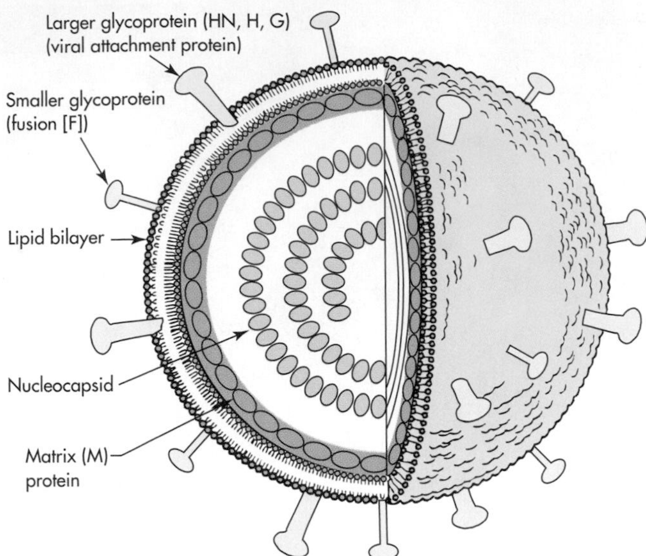

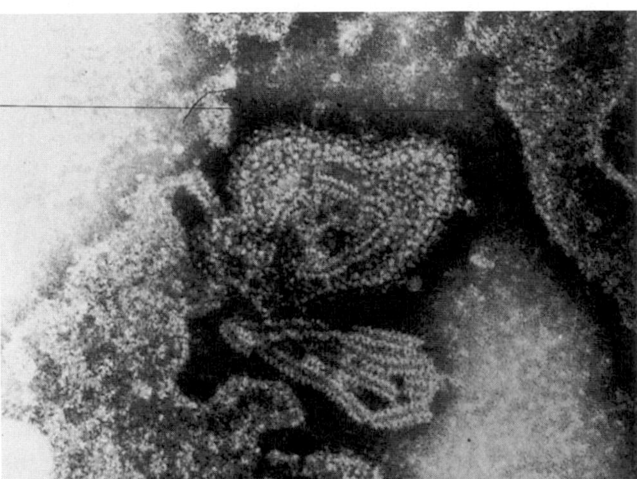

FIGURE 59–1. A, Model of paramyxovirus. The helical nucleocapsid–consisting of negative-sense, single-stranded RNA and the P protein, nucleoprotein (NP), and large (L) protein—associates with the matrix (M) protein at the envelope membrane surface. The nucleocapsid contains RNA transcriptase activity. The envelope contains the viral attachment glycoprotein (hemagglutinin-neuraminidase [HN], hemagglutinin [H], or G protein [G]) and the fusion (F) protein. **B,** Electron micrograph of a disrupted paramyxovirus showing the helical nucleocapsid. (**A** redrawn from Jawetz E, Melnick JL, Adelberg EA: *Review of medical microbiology,* ed 17, Norwalk, Conn, 1987, Appleton & Lange; **B** courtesy Centers for Disease Control and Prevention, Atlanta.)

Measles Virus

Measles is one of the five classic childhood exanthems, along with rubella, roseola, fifth disease, and chickenpox. Historically, measles was one of the most common and unpleasant viral infections with potential sequelae. Before 1960, more than 90% of the population younger than 20 years had experienced the rash, high fever, cough,

TABLE 59–2. Viral-Encoded Proteins of Measles Virus

Gene Products*	Virion Location	Function
Nucleoprotein (NP)	Major internal protein	Protection of viral RNA
Polymerase phosphoprotein (P)	Association with nucleoprotein	Possible part of transcription complex
Matrix (M)	Inside virion envelope	Assembly of virions
Fusion factor (F)	Transmembranous envelope glycoprotein	Factor active in fusion of cells, hemolysis, and viral entry
Hemagglutinin-neuraminidase (HN): hemagglutinin (H); glycoprotein (G)	Transmembranous envelope glycoprotein	Viral attachment proteins
Large protein (L)	Association with nucleoprotein	Polymerase

Modified from Fields BN, editor: *Virology,* New York, 1985, Raven.
*In order of transcription.

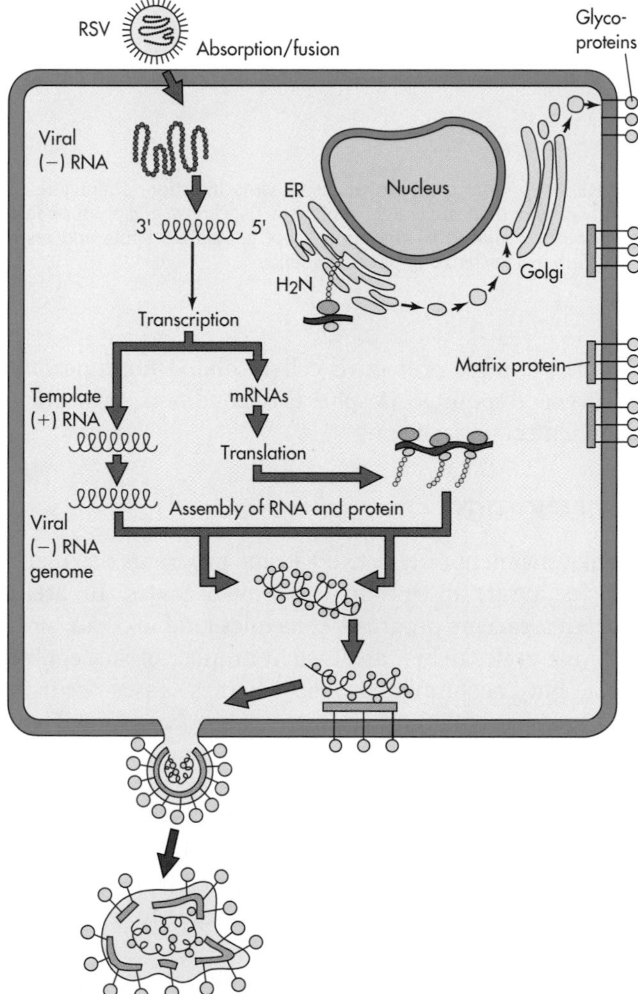

FIGURE 59–2. Replication of paramyxoviruses. The virus binds to glycolipids or proteins and fuses with the cell surface. Individual mRNAs for each protein and a full-length template are transcribed from the genome. Replication occurs in the cytoplasm. The nucleocapsid associates with matrix and glycoprotein-modified plasma membranes and leaves the cell by budding. (–), Negative sense; (+), positive sense; ER, endoplasmic reticulum; RSV, respiratory syncytial virus. (Redrawn from Balows A, Hausler WJ Jr, Lennette-EH: *Laboratory diagnosis of infectious diseases: Principles and practice,* New York, 1988, Springer-Verlag.)

conjunctivitis, and coryza of measles. Since the use of the live vaccine began in 1993, fewer than 1000 cases have been reported in the United States. Measles is still one of the most prominent causes of disease (30 to 40 million cases per year) and death (1 to 2 million per year) worldwide in unvaccinated populations.

PATHOGENESIS AND IMMUNITY

Measles is known for its propensity to cause cell fusion, leading to the formation of giant cells (Box 59–2). As a result, the virus can pass directly from cell to cell and escape antibody control. Inclusions occur most commonly in the cytoplasm and are composed of incomplete viral particles. Infection usually leads to cell lysis, but persistent infections without lysis can occur in certain cell types (e.g., human brain cells).

Measles is **highly contagious** and is transmitted from person to person by **respiratory droplets** (Figure 59–3). Local replication of virus in the respiratory tract precedes its spread to the lymphatic system and cell-associated viremia. The wide dissemination of the virus causes infection of the conjunctiva, respiratory tract, urinary tract, small blood vessels, lymphatic system, and the central nervous system. During the incubation period, measles causes a decrease in eosinophils and lymphocytes, including B and T cells, and a depression of their response to activation (mitogens). *The characteristic **maculopapular** measles rash is caused by immune T cells targeted to measles-infected endothelial cells lining small blood vessels.* Recovery follows the rash in most patients, who then have **lifelong immunity** to the virus. The time course of measles infection is shown in Figure 59–4.

Measles can cause encephalitis in three ways: (1) direct infection of neurons, (2) a postinfectious encephalitis, which is believed to be immune mediated, and (3) subacute sclerosing panencephalitis (SSPE) caused by a defective variant of measles generated during the acute disease.

BOX 59–2. Disease Mechanisms of Measles Virus

Virus infects epithelial cells of respiratory tract.
Virus spreads systemically in lymphocytes and by **viremia.**
Virus replicates in cells of conjunctivae, respiratory tract, urinary tract, lymphatic system, blood vessels, and central nervous system.
Rash is caused by T-cell response to virus-infected epithelial cells lining capillaries.
Cell-mediated immunity is essential to control infection; antibody is not sufficient because of measles' ability to spread cell to cell.
Sequelae in central nervous system may result from immunopathogenesis (postinfectious measles encephalitis) or development of defective mutants (subacute sclerosing panencephalitis).

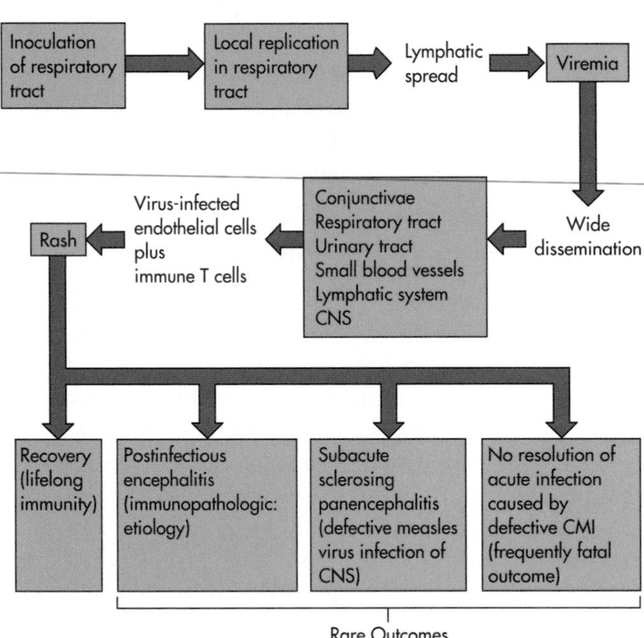

FIGURE 59–3. Mechanisms of spread of the measles virus within the body and the pathogenesis of measles. CMI, Cell-mediated immunity; CNS, central nervous system.

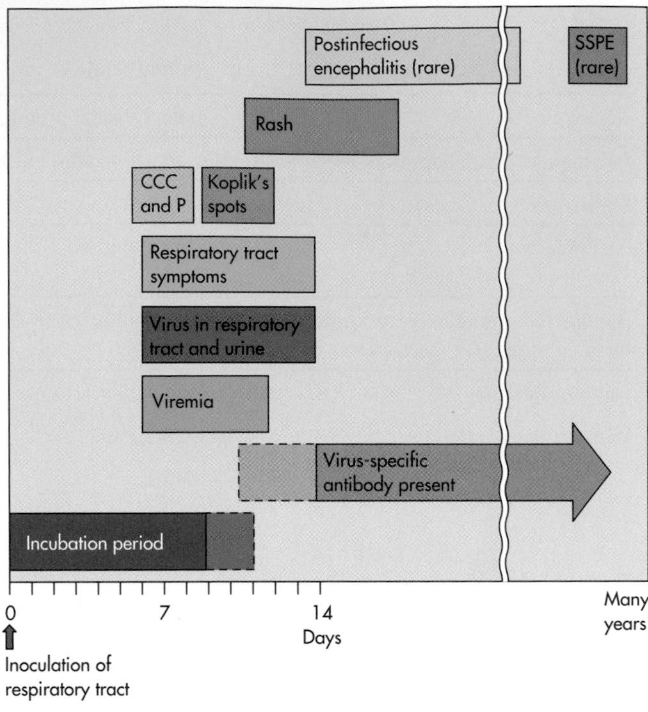

FIGURE 59–4. Time course of measles virus infection. Characteristic prodrome symptoms are cough, conjunctivitis, coryza, and photophobia (CCC and P), followed by the appearance of Koplik's spots and rash. SSPE, Subacute sclerosing panencephalitis.

The SSPE virus acts as a slow virus and causes cytopathologic effect in neurons and symptoms many years after acute disease.

Cell-mediated immunity is responsible for most of the symptoms and is essential for the control of measles infection. T-cell–deficient children who are infected with measles have an atypical presentation consisting of **giant cell pneumonia without a rash.** During measles infection, and for weeks after, the virus depresses the immune response by directly infecting monocytes, T and B cells and by promoting a switch to T cell production of TH2-associated cytokines, especially interleukin 4 (IL4), IL5, IL10, and IL13. These cytokines reduce the host's ability to mount protective cell–mediated immune and DTH-type responses. Despite this condition, protection from reinfection is lifelong.

EPIDEMIOLOGY

The development of effective vaccine programs has made measles a rare disease in the United States. In areas without a vaccine program, epidemics tend to occur in 1- to 3-year cycles, when a sufficient number of susceptible people have accumulated. Many of these cases occur in preschool-age children who have not been vaccinated and who live in large urban areas. The incidence of infection peaks in the winter and spring. Measles is still common in people living in developing countries and is the most significant cause of death in children 1 to 5 years of age in several countries. Immunocompromised and malnourished people with measles may not be able to resolve the infection, resulting in death.

Measles, which can be spread in respiratory secretions before and after the onset of characteristic symptoms, is one of the most contagious infections known (Box 59–3). In a household, approximately 85% of exposed susceptible people become infected, and 95% of these people develop clinical disease.

The measles virus has only one serotype and infects only humans, and infection usually manifests as symptoms. These properties facilitated the development of an effective vaccine program. Once vaccination was introduced, the yearly incidence of measles dropped dramatically in the United States, from 300 to 1.3 per 100,000 (U.S. statistics for 1981 to 1988). This change represented a 99.5% reduction in the incidence of the infection from that in the prevaccination period from 1955 to 1962.

Poor compliance with vaccination programs and the prevaccinated population (<2 years old) provide susceptible individuals to measles. The virus may surface from within the community or can be imported by immigration from areas of the world lacking an effective vaccine program. An outbreak of measles in a daycare center (10 infants, too young to have been vaccinated, and two adults) was traced to an infant from the Philippines.

BOX 59–3. Epidemiology of Measles

Disease/Viral Factors

Virus has large enveloped virion that is easily inactivated by dryness and acid.
Contagion period precedes symptoms.
Host range is limited to humans.
Only one serotype exists.
Immunity is lifelong.

Transmission

Inhalation of large-droplet aerosols.

Who Is at Risk?

Unvaccinated people.
Immunocompromised people, who have more serious outcomes.

Geography/Season

Virus is found worldwide.
Virus is endemic from autumn to spring, possibly because of crowding indoors.

Modes of Control

Live attenuated vaccine (Schwartz or Moraten variants of Edmonston B strain) can be administered.
Immune serum globulin can be administered after exposure.

CLINICAL SYNDROMES

Measles is a serious febrile illness (Table 59–3). The incubation period lasts 7 to 13 days, and the prodrome starts with **high fever** and CCC and P—**cough, coryza, conjunctivitis,** and **photophobia.** The disease is most infectious during this time.

After 2 days of illness, the typical mucous membrane lesions, known as **Koplik's spots** (Figure 59–5), appear. They are seen most commonly on the buccal mucosa across from the molars, but they may appear on other mucous membranes as well, including the conjunctivae and the vagina. The lesions, which last 24 to 48 hours, are usually small (1 to 2 mm) and are best described as grains of salt surrounded by a red halo. Their appearance in the mouth establishes with certainty the diagnosis of measles.

Within 12 to 24 hours of the appearance of Koplik's spots, the **exanthem** of measles starts below the ears and

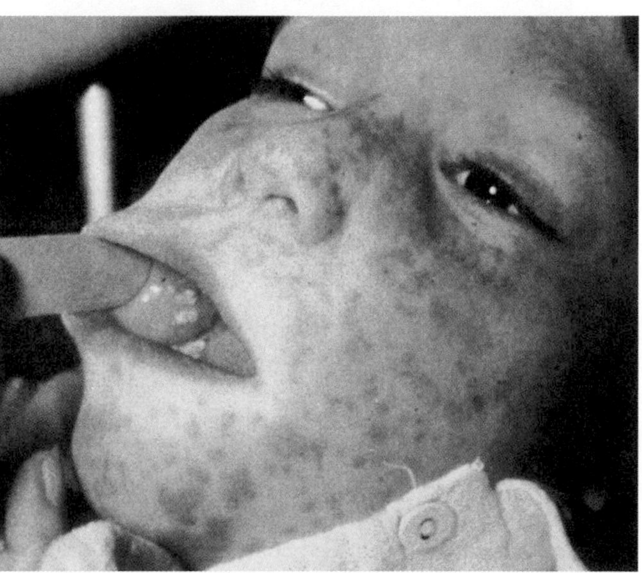

FIGURE 59–5. Koplik's spots in the mouth and exanthem. Koplik's spots usually precede the measles rash and may be seen for the first day or two after the rash appears. (Courtesy Dr. J.I. Pugh, St. Albans; from Emond RTD, Rowland HAK: *A color atlas of infectious diseases,* ed 3, London, 1995, Mosby.)

TABLE 59–3. Clinical Consequences of Measles Virus Infection

Disorder	Symptoms
Measles	Characteristic maculopapular rash, cough, conjunctivitis, coryza, photophobia, Koplik's spots *Complications:* Otitis media, croup, bronchopneumonia, and encephalitis
Atypical measles	More intense rash (most prominent in distal areas); possible vesicles, petechiae, purpura, or urticaria
Subacute sclerosing panencephalitis	Central nervous system manifestations (e.g., personality, behavior, and memory changes; myoclonic jerks; spasticity; and blindness

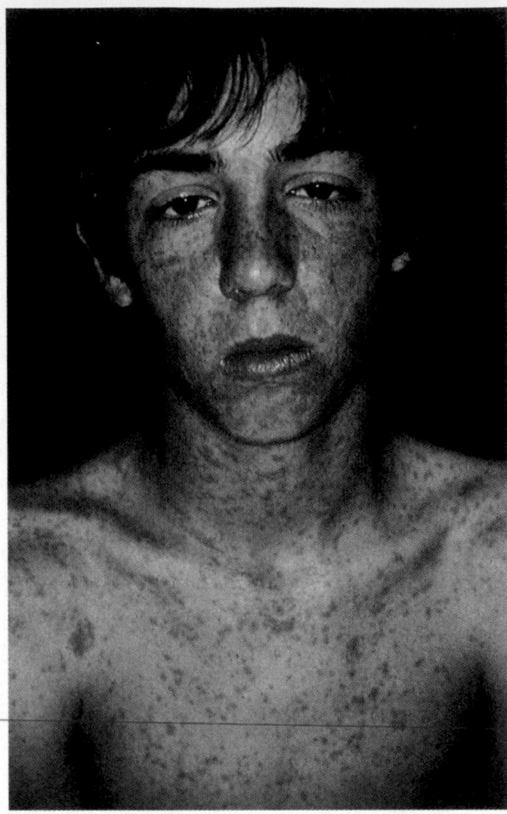

FIGURE 59–6. Measles rash. (From Habif TP: *Clinical dermatology: Color guide to diagnosis and therapy,* St Louis, 1985, Mosby.)

spreads over the body. The **rash is maculopapular** and usually very extensive, and often the lesions become confluent. The rash, which takes 1 or 2 days to cover the body, fades in the same order in which it appeared over the body. The fever is highest and the patient is sickest on the day the rash appears (Figure 59–6).

Pneumonia, which can also be a serious complication, accounts for 60% of the deaths caused by measles. The mortality associated with pneumonia, like the incidence of the other complications associated with measles, is higher in the malnourished and for the extremes of age. **Bacterial superinfection** is common in patients with pneumonia caused by the measles virus.

One of the most feared complications of measles is **encephalitis,** which may occur in as many as 0.5% of those infected and may be fatal in 15% of cases. Encephalitis can rarely occur during acute disease, but usually begins 7 to 10 days after the onset of illness. This **postinfectious encephalitis** is caused by immunopathologic reactions, is associated with demyelination of neurons, and occurs more often in older children and adults.

Atypical measles occurred in people who received the older inactivated measles vaccine and were subsequently exposed to the wild-type measles virus. It may also rarely occur in those vaccinated with the attenuated virus vaccine. Prior sensitization with insufficient protection enhances the immunopathologic response to the challenge by wild measles virus. The illness begins abruptly and is a more intense presentation of measles.

Subacute sclerosing panencephalitis is an extremely serious, very late neurologic sequela of measles that afflicts approximately seven of every 1 million patients. The incidence of SSPE has decreased markedly as the result of the measles vaccination programs.

This disease occurs when a defective measles virus persists in the brain and acts as a slow virus. The virus can replicate and spread directly from cell to cell but is not released. SSPE is most prevalent in children who were initially infected when younger than 2 years and occurs approximately 7 years after clinical measles. The patient demonstrates changes in personality, behavior, and memory, followed by myoclonic jerks, blindness, and spasticity. Unusually high levels of measles antibodies are found in the blood and cerebrospinal fluid of patients with SSPE.

The immunocompromised and malnourished child is at highest risk for severe outcome of measles. **Giant cell pneumonia without rash** occurs in children lacking T-cell immunity. Severe bacterial superinfection and pneumonia occur in malnourished children, with up to 25% mortality.

LABORATORY DIAGNOSIS

The clinical manifestations of measles are usually so characteristic that it is rarely necessary to perform laboratory tests to establish the diagnosis. The measles virus is difficult to isolate and grow, although it can be grown in primary human or monkey cell cultures. Respiratory tract secretions, urine, blood, and brain tissue are the recommended specimens. It is best to collect respiratory and blood specimens during the prodromal stage and up until 1 to 2 days after the appearance of the rash.

Measles antigen can be detected with immunofluorescence in pharyngeal cells or urinary sediment or the measles genome by reverse transcriptase polymerase chain reaction (RT-PCR) in any of the aforementioned specimens. Characteristic cytopathologic effects, including multinucleated giant cells with cytoplasmic inclusion bodies, can be seen in Giemsa-stained cells taken from the upper respiratory tract and urinary sediment.

Antibody, especially immunoglobulin (Ig)M, can be detected when the rash is present. Measles infection can be confirmed by the finding of seroconversion or a fourfold increase in the titer of measles-specific antibodies between sera obtained during the acute stage and the convalescent stage.

BOX 59–4. Measles-Mumps-Rubella (MMR) Vaccine

Composition: Live attenuated viruses
Measles: Schwartz or Moraten substrains of Edmonston B strain
Mumps: Jeryl Lynn strain
Rubella: RA/27-3 strain
Vaccination schedule: At age 15–24 months and at age 4–6 years or before junior high school (12 years of age)
Efficiency: 95% lifelong immunization with a single dose

*Data from update on adult immunization, *MMWR Morb Mortal Wkly Rep* 40(RR-12), 1991.

BOX 59–5. Disease Mechanisms of Parainfluenza Viruses

There are four serotypes of viruses.
Infection is **limited to respiratory tract;** upper respiratory tract disease is most common, but significant disease can occur with lower respiratory tract infection.
Parainfluenza viruses do *not* cause viremia or become systemic
Diseases include **coldlike** symptoms, **bronchitis** (inflammation of bronchial tubes), and **croup** (laryngotracheobronchitis).
Infection induces protective immunity of short duration.

TREATMENT, PREVENTION, AND CONTROL

A live attenuated measles vaccine, in use since 1963, has been responsible for a significant reduction in the incidence of measles in the United States. The current Schwartz or Moraten attenuated strains of the original Edmonston B vaccine are being used in the United States. Live attenuated vaccine is given to all children at 2 years of age, in combination with mumps and rubella **(MMR vaccine)** and the varicella vaccines (Box 59–4). Although immunization is successful in more than 95% of vaccinees, revaccination is required in much of the United States for children before grade school or junior high school. As noted earlier, a killed measles vaccine, which was introduced in 1963, was not protective, and its use was subsequently discontinued because recipients were at risk for the more serious atypical measles presentation on infection. Although measles is a good candidate for eradication, because it is strictly a human virus and there is only one serotype, this is prevented by difficulties in distributing the vaccine to regions that lack proper refrigeration facilities (e.g., Africa) and distribution networks.

Hospitals in areas experiencing endemic measles may wish to vaccinate or check the immune status of their employees to decrease the risk of nosocomial transmission. Exposed susceptible people who are immunocompromised should be given immune globulin to lessen the risk and severity of clinical illness. This product is most effective if given within 6 days of exposure. No specific antiviral treatment is available for measles.

Parainfluenza Viruses

Parainfluenza viruses, which were discovered in the late 1950s, are respiratory viruses that usually cause **mild coldlike symptoms** but can also cause **serious respiratory tract disease.** Four serologic types within the parainfluenza genus are human pathogens. Types 1, 2, and 3 are second only to RSV as important causes of severe lower respiratory tract infection in infants and young children. They are especially associated with **laryngotracheobronchitis (croup).** Type 4 causes only mild upper respiratory tract infection in children and adults.

PATHOGENESIS AND IMMUNITY

Parainfluenza viruses infect epithelial cells of the upper respiratory tract (Box 59–5). The virus replicates more rapidly than measles and mumps viruses and can cause giant cell formation and cell lysis. Unlike measles and mumps viruses, the parainfluenza viruses rarely cause viremia. The viruses generally stay in the upper respiratory tract, causing only coldlike symptoms. In approximately 25% of cases the virus spreads to the lower respiratory tract, and in 2% to 3%, disease may take the severe form of laryngotracheobronchitis.

The cell-mediated immune response both causes cell damage and confers protection. IgA responses are protective but short-lived. Parainfluenza viruses manipulate cell-mediated immunity to limit development of memory. Multiple serotypes and the short duration of immunity after natural infection make reinfection common, but the reinfection disease is milder, suggesting at least partial immunity.

EPIDEMIOLOGY

Parainfluenza viruses are ubiquitous, and infection is common (Box 59–6). The virus is transmitted by person-to-person contact and respiratory droplets. Primary infections usually occur in infants and children younger than 5 years. Reinfections occur throughout life, indicating short-lived immunity. Infections with parainfluenza viruses 1 and 2, the major causes of croup, tend to occur in the autumn, whereas parainfluenza virus 3 infections occur throughout the year. All of these viruses spread readily within hospitals and can cause outbreaks in nurseries and pediatric wards.

CLINICAL SYNDROMES

Parainfluenza viruses 1, 2, and 3 may cause respiratory tract syndromes ranging from a **mild coldlike upper respiratory tract infection** (coryza, pharyngitis, mild bronchitis, wheezing, and fever) to **bronchiolitis** and **pneumonia.** Older children and adults generally experience milder infections than those seen in young children, although pneumonia may occur in the elderly.

A parainfluenza virus infection in infants may be more severe than infections in adults, causing bronchiolitis, pneumonia, and, most notably, croup (laryngotracheobronchitis). **Croup** results in subglottal swelling, which may close the airway. Hoarseness, a "seal bark" cough, tachypnea, tachycardia, and suprasternal retraction develop in infected patients after a 2- to 6-day incubation period. Most children recover within 48 hours. The principal differential diagnosis is epiglottitis caused by *Haemophilus influenzae.*

LABORATORY DIAGNOSIS

Parainfluenza virus is isolated from nasal washings and respiratory secretions and grows well in primary monkey kidney cells. Like other paramyxoviruses, the virions are labile during transit to the laboratory. The presence of virus-infected cells in aspirates or in cell culture is indicated by the finding of syncytia and is identified with immunofluorescence. Like the hemagglutinin of the influenzaviruses, the hemagglutinin of the parainfluenza viruses promotes hemadsorption and hemagglutination. The serotype of the virus can be determined through the use of specific antibody to block hemadsorption or hemagglutination (hemagglutination inhibition). Rapid RT-PCR techniques are becoming the method of choice to detect and identify parainfluenza viruses from respiratory secretions.

BOX 59–6. Epidemiology of Parainfluenza Virus Infections

Disease/Viral Factors
Virus has large enveloped virion that is easily inactivated by dryness and acid.
Contagion period precedes symptoms and may occur in absence of symptoms.
Host range is limited to humans.
Reinfection can occur later in life.

Transmission
Inhalation of large-droplet aerosols.

Who Is at Risk?
Children: At risk for mild disease or croup.
Adults: At risk for reinfection with milder symptoms.

Geography/Season
Virus is ubiquitous and worldwide.
Incidence is seasonal.

Modes of Control
There are no modes of control.

TREATMENT, PREVENTION, AND CONTROL

Treatment of croup consists of the administration of nebulized cold or hot steam and careful monitoring of the upper airway. On rare occasions, intubation may become necessary. No specific antiviral agents are available.

Vaccination with killed vaccines is ineffective, possibly because they fail to induce local secretory antibody and appropriate cellular immunity. No live attenuated vaccine is available.

Mumps Virus

Mumps virus is the cause of acute, benign viral **parotitis** (painful swelling of the salivary glands). Mumps is rarely seen in countries that promote use of the live vaccine, which is administered with the measles and rubella live vaccines.

Mumps virus was isolated in embryonated eggs in 1945 and in cell culture in 1955. The virus is most closely related to parainfluenza virus 2, but there is no cross-immunity with the parainfluenza viruses.

PATHOGENESIS AND IMMUNITY

The mumps virus, of which only one serotype is known, causes a lytic infection of cells (Box 59–7). The virus initiates infection in the epithelial cells of the upper respiratory tract and infects the parotid gland either by way of Stensen's duct or by means of a viremia. The virus is spread by the viremia throughout the body to the testes, ovary, pancreas, thyroid, and other organs. Infection of the central nervous system, especially the meninges, with symptoms (meningoencephalitis) occurs in as many as

BOX 59–7. Disease Mechanisms of Mumps Virus

Virus infects epithelial cells of respiratory tract.
Virus spreads systemically by viremia.
Infection of parotid gland, testes, and central nervous system occurs.
Principal symptom is swelling of parotid glands caused by inflammation.
Cell-mediated immunity is essential for control of infection and is responsible for causing some of the symptoms. Antibody is not sufficient because of virus' ability to spread cell to cell.

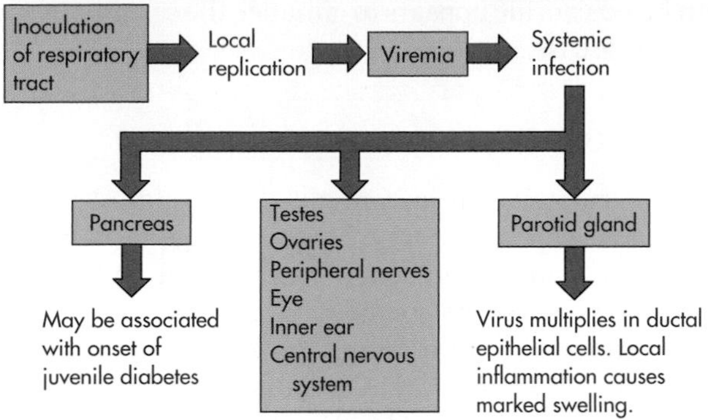

FIGURE 59–7. Mechanism of spread of mumps virus within the body.

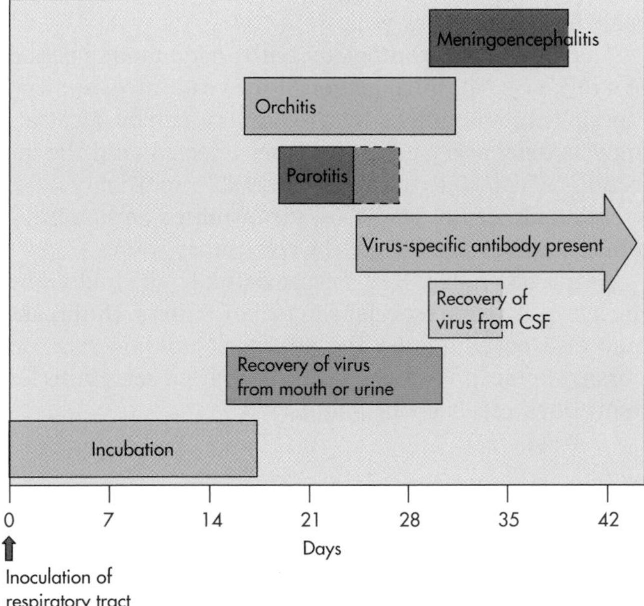

FIGURE 59–8. Time course of mumps virus infection.

50% of those infected (Figure 59–7). Inflammatory responses are mainly responsible for the symptoms. The time course of human infection is shown in Figure 59–8. Immunity is lifelong.

EPIDEMIOLOGY

Mumps, like measles, is a very communicable disease with only one serotype, and it infects only humans (Box 59–8). In the absence of vaccination programs, infection occurs in 90% of people by the age of 15. The virus spreads by direct person-to-person contact and respiratory droplets. The virus is released in respiratory secretions from patients who are asymptomatic and during the 7-day period before clinical illness, so it is virtually impossible to control the spread of the virus. Living or working in close quarters promotes the spread of the virus, and the incidence of the infection is greatest in the winter and spring.

BOX 59–8. Epidemiology of Mumps Virus

Disease/Viral Factors

Virus has large enveloped virion that is easily inactivated by dryness and acid.
Contagion period precedes symptoms.
Virus may cause asymptomatic shedding.
Host range is limited to humans.
Only one serotype exists.
Immunity is lifelong.

Transmission

Inhalation of large-droplet aerosols.

Who Is at Risk?

Unvaccinated people.
Immunocompromised people, who have more serious outcomes.

Geography/Season

Virus is found worldwide.
Virus is endemic in late winter and early spring.

Modes of Control

Live attenuated vaccine (Jeryl Lynn strain) is part of MMR vaccine.

CLINICAL SYNDROMES

Mumps infections are often asymptomatic. Clinical illness manifests as a parotitis that is almost always bilateral and accompanied by fever. Onset is sudden. Oral examination reveals redness and swelling of the ostium of Stensen's (parotid) duct. The swelling of other glands (epididymo-orchitis, oophoritis, mastitis, pancreatitis, and thyroiditis) and meningoencephalitis may occur a few days after the onset of the viral infection but can occur in the absence of parotitis. The swelling that results from mumps orchitis may cause sterility. Mumps virus involves the central nervous system in approximately 50% of patients; and 10% of those affected may exhibit clinical evidence of such an infection.

LABORATORY DIAGNOSIS

Virus can be recovered from saliva, urine, the pharynx, secretions from Stensen's duct, and cerebrospinal fluid. Virus is present in saliva for approximately 5 days after the onset of symptoms and in urine for as long as 2 weeks. Mumps virus grows well in monkey kidney cells, causing the formation of multinucleated giant cells. The hemadsorption of guinea pig erythrocytes also occurs on virus-infected cells, due to the viral hemagglutinin.

A clinical diagnosis can be confirmed by serologic testing. A fourfold increase in the virus-specific antibody level or the detection of mumps-specific IgM antibody indicates active infection. Enzyme-linked immunosorbent assay, immunofluorescence tests, and hemagglutination inhibition can be used to detect the mumps virus, antigen, or antibody.

TREATMENT, PREVENTION, AND CONTROL

Vaccines provide the only effective means for preventing the spread of mumps infection. Since the introduction of the live attenuated vaccine (Jeryl Lynn vaccine) in the United States in 1967 and its administration as part of the MMR vaccine, the yearly incidence of the infection has declined from 76 to 2 per 100,000. Antiviral agents are not available.

Respiratory Syncytial Virus

RSV, first isolated from a chimpanzee in 1956, is a member of the *Pneumovirus* genus. Unlike the other paramyxoviruses, RSV lacks hemagglutinin and neuraminidase activities. It is the most common cause of **fatal acute respiratory tract infection** in infants and young children. It infects virtually everyone by 2 years of age, and reinfections occur throughout life, even among elderly persons.

PATHOGENESIS AND IMMUNITY

RSV produces an infection that is localized to the respiratory tract (Box 59–9). As the name suggests, RSV induces syncytia. The pathologic effect of RSV is mainly caused by direct viral invasion of the respiratory epithelium, which is followed by immunologically mediated cell injury. Necrosis of the bronchi and bronchioles leads to the formation of "plugs" of mucus, fibrin, and necrotic material within smaller airways. The narrow airways of young infants are readily obstructed by such plugs. Natural immunity does not prevent reinfection, and vaccination with killed vaccine appears to enhance the severity of subsequent disease.

BOX 59–9. Disease Mechanisms of Respiratory Syncytial Virus

- Virus causes localized infection of respiratory tract.
- Virus does not cause viremia or systemic spread.
- Pneumonia results from cytopathologic spread of virus (including syncytia).
- Bronchiolitis is most likely mediated by host's immune response.
- Narrow airways of young infants are readily obstructed by virus-induced pathologic effects.
- Maternal antibody does not protect infant from infection.
- Natural infection does not prevent reinfection.
- Improper vaccination increases severity of disease.

EPIDEMIOLOGY

RSV is very prevalent in young children; almost all children have been infected by 2 years of age (Box 59–10) with global annual infection rates of 64 million and mortality of 160,000. As many as 25% to 33% of these cases involve the lower respiratory tract, and 1% are severe enough to necessitate hospitalization (occurring in as many as 95,000 children in the United States each year).

RSV infections almost always occur in the winter. Unlike influenza, which may occasionally skip a year, RSV epidemics occur every year.

The virus is very contagious, with an incubation period of 4 to 5 days. The introduction of the virus into a nursery, especially into an intensive care nursery, can be devastating. Virtually every infant becomes infected, and the infection is associated with considerable morbidity and, occasionally, death. The virus is transmitted on hands, by fomites, and to some degree by respiratory routes.

As already noted, RSV infects virtually all children by the age of 4 years, especially in urban centers. Outbreaks may also occur among the elderly population (e.g., in nursing homes). Virus is shed in respiratory secretions for many days, especially by infants.

BOX 59–10. Epidemiology of Respiratory Syncytial Virus

Disease/Viral Factors

- Virus has large enveloped virion that is easily inactivated by dryness and acid.
- Contagion period precedes symptoms and may occur in absence of symptoms.
- Host range is limited to humans.

Transmission

- Inhalation of large-droplet aerosols.

Who Is at Risk?

- Infants: Lower respiratory tract infection (bronchiolitis and pneumonia).
- Children: Spectrum of disease—mild to pneumonia.
- Adults: Reinfection with milder symptoms.

Geography/Season

- Virus is ubiquitous and found worldwide.
- Incidence is seasonal.

Modes of Control

- Immune globulin is available for infants at high risk.
- Aerosol ribavirin is available for infants with serious disease.

BOX 59–11. Clinical Summaries

Measles: An 18-year-old woman had been home for 10 days after a trip to Haiti when she developed a fever, cough, runny nose, mild redness of her eyes, and now has a red, slightly raised rash over her face, trunk, and extremities. There are several 1-mm white lesions inside her mouth. She was never immunized for measles because of an "egg allergy."

Mumps: A 30-year-old man returning from a trip to Russia began with a 1- to 2-day period of headache and decreased appetite, followed by swelling over both sides of his jaw. The swelling extends from the bottom of the jaw to in front of the ear. Five days after the jaw swelling appeared, the patient began complaining of nausea and lower abdominal and testicular pain.

Croup: A grumpy 2-year-old toddler with little appetite has a sore throat, fever, hoarse voice, and coughs with the sound of a barking seal. A high-pitched noise (stridor) is heard on inhalation. Flaring of the nostrils indicates difficulty breathing.

TABLE 59–4. Clinical Consequences of Respiratory Syncytial Virus Infection

Disorder	Age Group Affected
Bronchiolitis, pneumonia, or both	Fever, cough, dyspnea, and cyanosis in children younger than 1 year
Febrile rhinitis and pharyngitis	Children
Common cold	Older children and adults

CLINICAL SYNDROMES (BOX 59–11)

RSV can cause any respiratory tract illness, from a **common cold** to **pneumonia** (Table 59–4). Upper respiratory tract infection with prominent rhinorrhea (runny nose) is most common in older children and adults. A more severe lower respiratory tract illness, **bronchiolitis,** may occur in infants. Because of inflammation at the level of the bronchiole, there is air trapping and decreased ventilation. Clinically, the patient usually has low-grade fever, tachypnea, tachycardia, and expiratory wheezes over the lungs. Bronchiolitis is usually self-limited, but it can be a frightening disease to observe in an infant. It may be fatal in premature infants, persons with underlying lung disease, and immunocompromised people.

LABORATORY DIAGNOSIS

RSV is difficult to isolate in cell culture. The presence of the viral genome in infected cells and nasal washings can be detected by RT-PCR techniques, and commercially available immunofluorescence and enzyme immunoassay tests are available for detection of the viral antigen. The finding of seroconversion or a fourfold or greater increase in the antibody titer can confirm the diagnosis for epidemiologic purposes.

TREATMENT, PREVENTION, AND CONTROL

In otherwise healthy infants, treatment is supportive, consisting of the administration of oxygen, intravenous fluids, and nebulized cold steam. **Ribavirin,** a guanosine analogue, is approved for the treatment of patients predisposed to a more severe course (e.g., premature or immunocompromised infants). It is administered by inhalation (nebulization).

Passive immunization with anti-RSV immunoglobulin is available for premature infants. Infected children must be isolated. Control measures are required for hospital staff caring for infected children, to avoid transmitting the virus to uninfected patients. These measures include hand washing and wearing gowns, goggles, and masks.

No vaccine is currently available for RSV prophylaxis. A previously available vaccine containing inactivated RSV caused recipients to have more severe RSV disease when subsequently exposed to the live virus. This development is thought to be the result of a heightened immunologic response at the time of exposure to the wild virus.

Human Metapneumovirus

Human metapneumovirus is a recently recognized member of the pneumovirus family. Use of RT-PCR methods was and remains the means of detection and distinction of the pneumoviruses from other respiratory disease viruses. Its identity was unknown until recently because it is difficult to grow in cell culture. The virus is ubiquitous and almost all 5-year-old children have experienced a virus infection and are seropositive.

Infections by human metapneumovirus, like its close cousin, RSV, may be asymptomatic, cause common cold–like disease or serious bronchiolitis and pneumonia. Seronegative children, elderly persons and immunocompromised people are at risk to disease. Human metapneumovirus probably causes 15% of common colds in children, especially those of which are complicated by otitis media. Signs of disease usually include cough, sore throat, runny nose, and high fever. Approximately 10% of patients with metapneumovirus will experience wheezing, dyspnea, pneumonia, bronchitis, or bronchiolitis. As with other common cold agents, laboratory identification of the virus is not performed routinely but can be performed by RT-PCR. Supportive care is the only therapy available for these infections.

Nipah and Hendra Viruses

A new paramyxovirus, Nipah virus, was isolated from patients after an outbreak of severe encephalitis in Malaysia and Singapore in 1998. Nipah virus is more closely related to the Hendra virus, discovered in 1994 in Australia, than to other paramyxoviruses. Both viruses have broad host ranges, including pigs, man, dogs, horses, cats, and other mammals. For Nipah virus, the reservoir is a fruit bat (flying fox). The virus can be obtained from fruit contaminated by infected bats or amplified in pigs and then spread to humans. The human is an accidental host for these viruses, but the outcome of human infection is severe. Disease signs include flulike symptoms, seizures, and coma. Of the 269 cases occurring in 1999, 108 were fatal. Another epidemic in Bangladesh in 2004 had a higher mortality rate.

CASE STUDIES AND QUESTIONS

An 18-year-old college freshman complained of a cough, runny nose, and conjunctivitis. The physician in the campus health center noticed small white lesions inside the patient's mouth. The next day, a confluent red rash covered his face and neck.

1. What clinical characteristics of this case were diagnostic for measles?
2. Are any laboratory tests readily available to confirm the diagnosis? If so, what are they?
3. Is there a possible treatment for this patient?
4. When was this patient contagious?
5. Why is this disease not common in the United States?
6. Provide several possible reasons for this person's susceptibility to measles at 18 years of age.

A 13-month-old child had a runny nose, mild cough, and low-grade fever for several days. The cough got worse and sounded like "barking." The child made a wheezing sound when agitated. The child appeared well except for the cough. A lateral radiograph of the neck showed a subglottic narrowing.

1. What is the specific and common name for these symptoms?
2. What other agents would cause a similar clinical presentation (differential diagnosis)?
3. Are there readily available laboratory tests to confirm this diagnosis? If so, what are they?
4. Was there a possible treatment for this child?
5. When was this child contagious, and how was the virus transmitted?

Bibliography

Balows A et al: *Laboratory diagnosis of infectious diseases: Principles and practice,* New York, 1988, Springer-Verlag.

Belshe RB, editor: *Textbook of human viruses,* ed 2, St Louis, 1991, Mosby.

Centers for Disease Control: Public-sector vaccination efforts in response to the resurgence of measles among preschool-aged children: United States, 1989-1991, *MMWR Morb Mortal Wkly Rep* 41:522-525, 1992.

Cohen J, Powderly WG, editors: *Infectious diseases,* ed 2, St Louis, 2004, Mosby.

Flint SJ et al: *Principles of virology: Molecular biology, pathogenesis and control of animal viruses,* ed 2, Washington, 2003, American Society for Microbiology Press.

Galinski MS: Paramyxoviridae: Transcription and replication, *Adv Virus Res* 40:129-163, 1991.

Hart CA, Broadhead RL: *Color atlas of pediatric infectious diseases,* St Louis, 1992, Mosby.

Hinman AR: Potential candidates for eradication, *Rev Infect Dis* 4:933-939, 1982.

Katz SL et al: *Krugman's infectious diseases of children,* ed 10, St Louis, 1998, Mosby.

Knipe DM, Howley PM, editors: *Fields virology,* ed 4, New York, 2001, Lippincott-Williams and Wilkins.

Meulen V, Billeter MA: Measles virus, *Curr Top Microbiol Immunol* 191:1-196, 1995.

Strauss JM, Strauss EG: *Viruses and human disease,* San Diego, 2002, Academic Press.

White DO, Fenner F: *Medical virology,* ed 4, San Diego, 1994, Academic.

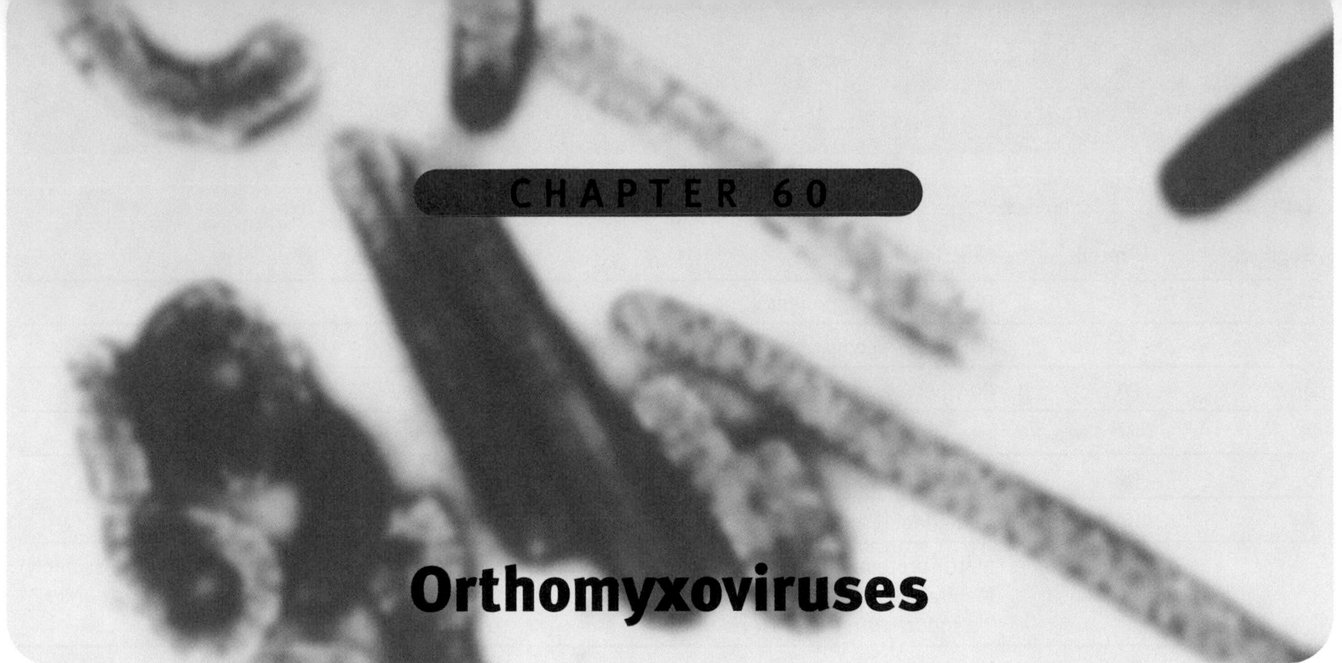

Orthomyxoviruses

Influenza A, B, and C viruses are the only members of the Orthomyxoviridae family, and only influenza A and B viruses cause significant human disease. The orthomyxoviruses are **enveloped and have a segmented negative-sense RNA genome.** The segmented genome of these viruses facilitates the development of new strains through the mutation and reassortment of the gene segments among different human and animal strains of virus. This genetic instability is responsible for the annual **epidemics (mutation: drift)** and **periodic pandemics (reassortment: shift)** of influenza infection worldwide.

Influenza is one of the most prevalent and significant viral infections. There are even descriptions of influenza **epidemics (local dissemination)** that occurred in ancient times. Probably the most famous influenza **pandemic (worldwide)** is the Spanish influenza that swept the world in 1918 to 1919, killing 20 million to 40 million people. In fact, more people died of influenza during this time than in the battles of World War I. Pandemics caused by novel influenza viruses occurred in 1918, 1947, 1957, 1968, and 1977, but, fortunately, none have occurred since. New virus strains have been detected since the last pandemic, including a limited outbreak in Hong Kong in 1997 ("chicken flu"). Fortunately, prophylaxis, in the form of vaccines and antiviral drugs, is now available for people at risk for serious outcomes.

Influenza viruses are respiratory viruses that cause respiratory symptoms and the classic flulike symptoms of fever, malaise, headache, and myalgias (body aches). The term *flu,* however, has been mistakenly used to refer to many other respiratory and viral infections (e.g., "intestinal flu").

Structure and Replication

Influenza virions are pleomorphic, appearing spherical or tubular (Box 60–1 and Figure 60–1) and ranging in diameter from 80 to 120 nm. The envelope contains two glycoproteins, **hemagglutinin (HA)** and **neuraminidase (NA),** and is internally lined by the **matrix (M_1)** and **membrane (M_2)** proteins. The genome of the influenza A and B viruses consists of **eight different helical nucleocapsid segments,** each of which contains a negative-sense RNA associated with the **nucleoprotein (NP)** and the **transcriptase (RNA polymerase components: PB1, PB2, PA)** (Table 60–1). Influenza C has only seven genomic segments.

The genomic segments in the influenza A virus range from 890 to 2340 bases. All the proteins are encoded on separate segments, with the exception of the nonstructural proteins (NS_1 and NS_2) and the M_1 and M_2 proteins, which are transcribed from one segment each.

The **HA** forms a spike-shaped trimer; each unit is activated by a protease and is cleaved into two subunits held together by a disulfide bond (see Figure 6–8). The HA has several functions: It is the viral attachment protein, binding to sialic acid on epithelial cell surface receptors; it promotes fusion of the envelope to the cell membrane; it hemagglutinates (binds and aggregates) human, chicken, and guinea pig red blood cells; and it elicits the protective neutralizing antibody response. Mutation-derived changes in HA are responsible for the minor ("drift") and major ("shift") changes in antigenicity. *Shifts occur only with influenza A virus, and the different HAs are designated H1, H2, and so on.*

The **NA** glycoprotein forms a tetramer and has enzyme activity. The NA cleaves the sialic acid on glycoproteins, including the cell receptor. Cleavage of the sialic acid on

TABLE 60–1. Products of Influenza Gene Segments

Segment*	Protein	Function
1	PB2	Polymerase component
2	PB1	Polymerase component
3	PA	Polymerase component
4	HA	Hemagglutinin, viral attachment protein, fusion protein, target of neutralizing antibody
5	NP	Nucleocapsid
6	NA	Neuraminidase (cleaves sialic acid and promotes virus release)
7†	M_1 M_2	Matrix protein: Viral structural protein (interacts with nucleocapsid and envelope, promotes assembly) Membrane protein (forms membrane channel and target for amantadine, facilitates uncoating and HA production)
8†	NS_1 NS_2	Nonstructural protein (inhibits cellular messenger RNA translation) Nonstructural protein (important but unknown function)

*Listed in decreasing order of size.
†Encodes two messenger RNAs.

BOX 60–1. Unique Features of the Influenza A and B Viruses

Enveloped virion has a genome of **eight unique negative-sense RNA nucleocapsid segments.**
Hemagglutinin glycoprotein is the viral attachment protein and fusion protein, and it elicits neutralizing, protective antibody responses.
Influenza transcribes and replicates its genome in the target cell nucleus but assembles and buds from the plasma membrane.
The antiviral drugs **amantadine** and **rimantadine** inhibit an uncoating step and target the M_2 (membrane) protein for influenza A *only.*
The antiviral drugs **zanamivir** and **oseltamivir** inhibit the NA protein of influenza A and B.
The segmented genome promotes **genetic diversity** caused by **mutation** and **reassortment** of segments on infection with two different strains.
Influenza A infects humans, mammals, and birds (zoonosis).

virion proteins prevents clumping and facilitates the release of virus from infected cells sufficiently such that NA is a target for two antiviral drugs, **zanamivir (Relenza)** and **oseltamivir (Tamiflu).** The NA of influenza A virus also undergoes antigenic changes, and major differences acquire the designations N1, N2, and so on.

The **M_1**, **M_2**, and **NP** proteins are typespecific and are therefore used to differentiate influenza A from B or C viruses. The M_1 proteins line the inside of the virion and promote assembly. The M_2 protein forms a proton channel in membranes and promotes uncoating and viral release. The M_2 of influenza A is a target for the antiviral drugs amantadine and rimantadine.

Viral replication begins with the binding of HA to specific sialic acid structures on cell surface glycoproteins (Figure 60–2). The virus is then internalized into a coated vesicle and transferred to an endosome. Acidification of the endosome causes the HA to bend over and expose hydrophobic fusion-promoting regions of the protein. The viral envelope then fuses with the endosome membrane. The proton channel formed by the M_2 protein promotes acidification of the envelope contents to break the interaction between the M_1 protein and the NP, to allow uncoating and delivery of the nucleocapsid into the cytoplasm. The nucleocapsid travels to the nucleus, where it is transcribed into messenger ribonucleic acid (mRNA).

The influenza transcriptase (PA, PB1, PB2) uses host cell mRNA as a primer for viral mRNA synthesis. In so doing, it steals the methylated cap region of the RNA, the sequence required for efficient binding to ribosomes. All the genomic segments are transcribed into 5′-capped, 3′-polyadenylated (poly A) mRNA for individual proteins, except the segments for the M and NS proteins, which are each differentially spliced (using cellular enzymes) to produce two different mRNAs. The mRNAs are translated into protein in the cytoplasm. The HA and NA glycoproteins are processed by the endoplasmic reticulum and Golgi apparatus. The M_2 protein inserts into cellular membranes. Its proton channel prevents acidification of Golgi and other vesicles, thus preventing acid-induced folding and inactivation of the HA within the cell. The HA and NA are then transported to the cell surface.

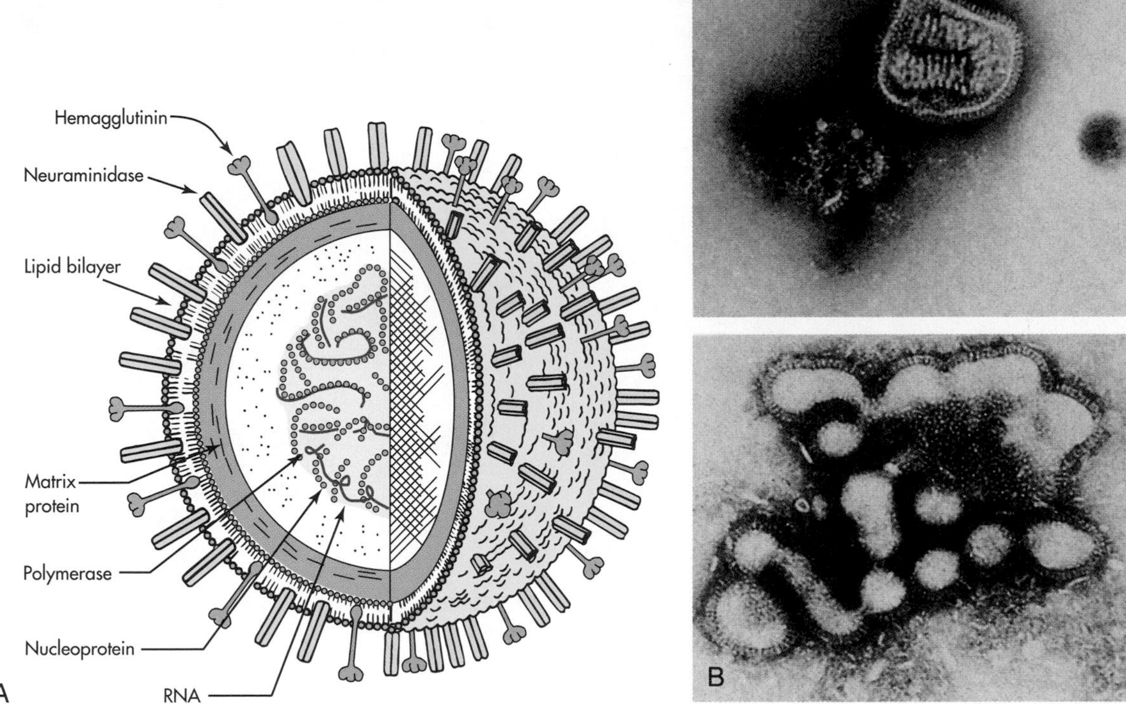

FIGURE 60–1. A, Model of influenza A virus. **B,** Electron micrographs of influenza A virus. (**A** from Kaplan MM, Webster RG: The epidemiology of influenza, *Sci Am* 237:88-106, 1977; **B** from Balows A et al, editors: *Laboratory diagnosis of infectious diseases: Principles and practice,* vol 2, Heidelberg, Germany, 1988, Springer-Verlag.)

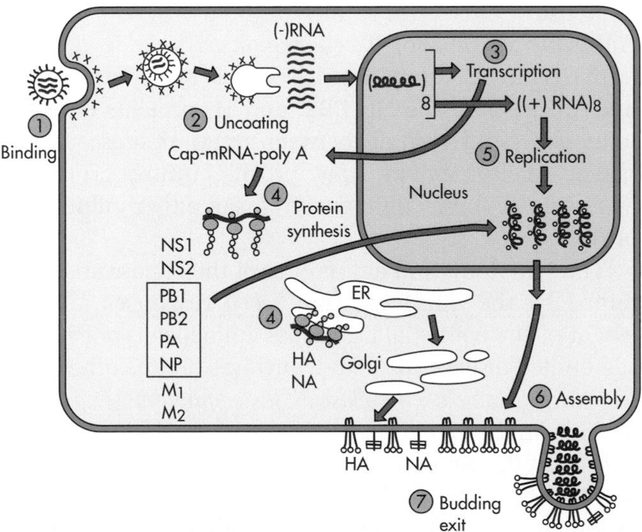

FIGURE 60–2. Replication of influenza A virus. After binding (*1*) to sialic acid–containing receptors, influenza is endocytosed and fuses (*2*) with the vesicle membrane. Unlike for most other RNA viruses, transcription (*3*) and replication (*5*) of the genome occur in the nucleus. Viral proteins are synthesized (*4*), helical nucleocapsid segments form and associate (*6*) with the M_1 protein–lined membranes containing M_2 and the HA and NA glycoproteins. The virus buds (*7*) from the plasma membrane with 11 nucleocapsid segments. (–), Negative sense; (+), positive sense; ER, endoplasmic reticulum.

Positive-sense RNA templates for each segment are produced, and the negative-sense RNA genome is replicated in the nucleus. The genomic segments are then transported to the cytoplasm and associate with polymerase and NP proteins to form nucleocapsids, which interact with the M_1 protein lining plasma membrane sections containing M_2, HA, and NA. The genomic segments are enveloped in a random manner, with 11 segments per virion. This process produces a small number of virions with a complete set of the 8 genomic segments and numerous defective particles. The particles are antigenic and can also cause interference, which may limit the progression of the infection. The virus buds selectively from the apical surface of the cell as a result of the preferential insertion of the HA in this membrane. Virus is released approximately 8 hours after infection.

Pathogenesis and Immunity

Influenza initially establishes a local upper respiratory tract infection (Box 60–2). To do so, the virus first targets and kills mucus-secreting, ciliated, and other epithelial cells, causing the loss of this primary defense system. NA

BOX 60–2. Disease Mechanisms of Influenza A and B Viruses

Virus can establish infection of upper and lower respiratory tract.
Systemic symptoms are caused by the interferon and lymphokine response to the virus. Local symptoms result from epithelial cell damage, including ciliated and mucus-secreting cells.
Interferon and cell-mediated immune responses (NK [natural killer] and T cell) are important for immune resolution and immunopathogenesis.
Infected people are predisposed to bacterial superinfection because of the loss of natural barriers and exposure of binding sites on epithelial cells.
Antibody is important for future protection against infection and is specific for defined epitopes on HA and NA proteins.
The HA and NA of influenza A virus can undergo **major (reassortment: shift)** and **minor (mutation: drift)** antigenic changes to ensure the presence of immunologically naïve, susceptible people.
Influenza B virus undergoes only minor antigenic changes.

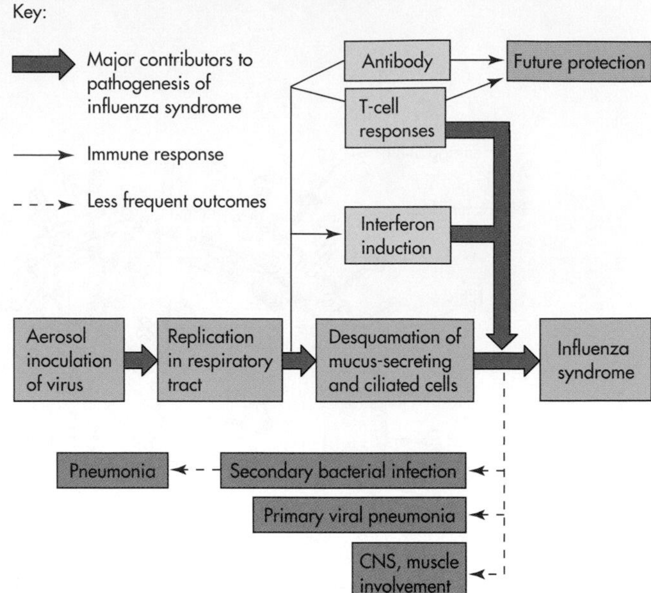

FIGURE 60–3. Pathogenesis of influenza A virus. The symptoms of influenza are caused by viral pathologic and immunopathologic effects, but the infection may promote secondary bacterial infection. CNS, Central nervous system.

facilitates the development of the infection by cleaving sialic acid residues of the mucus, thereby providing access to tissue. Preferential release of the virus at the apical surface of epithelial cells and into the lung promotes cell-to-cell spread and transmission to other hosts. If the virus spreads to the lower respiratory tract, the infection can cause severe desquamation (shedding) of bronchial or alveolar epithelium down to a single-cell basal layer or to the basement membrane.

In addition to compromising the natural defenses of the respiratory tract, influenza infection promotes bacterial adhesion to the epithelial cells. Pneumonia may result from a viral pathogenesis or from a secondary bacterial infection. Influenza may also cause a transient or low-level viremia but rarely involves tissues other than the lung.

Histologically, influenza infection leads to an inflammatory cell response of the mucosal membrane, which consists primarily of monocytes and lymphocytes and few neutrophils. Submucosal edema is present. Lung tissue may reveal hyaline membrane disease, alveolar emphysema, and necrosis of the alveolar walls (Figure 60–3).

Interferon and cytokine responses peak at almost the same time as virus in nasal washes and are concomittant with the febrile phase of disease. T-cell responses are important for effecting recovery and immunopathogenesis. However, influenza infection depresses macrophage and T-cell function, hindering immune resolution. Interestingly, recovery often precedes detection of antibody in serum or secretions.

Protection against reinfection is primarily associated with the development of antibodies to HA, but antibodies to NA are also protective. The antibody response is specific for each strain of influenza, but the cell-mediated immune response is more general and is capable of reacting to influenza strains of the same type (influenza A or B virus). Antigenic targets for T-cell responses include peptides from HA but also from the nucleocapsid proteins (NP, PB2) and M_1 protein. The NP, PB2, and M_1 proteins differ for influenza A and B but not between strains of these viruses; hence T-cell memory may provide future protection against infection by different strains of either influenza A or B.

The symptoms and time course of the disease are determined by the interferon and T-cell responses and the extent of the epithelial tissue loss. Influenza is normally a self-limited disease that rarely involves organs other than the lung. *Many of the classic "flu" symptoms (e.g., fever, malaise, headache, and myalgia) are associated with interferon induction.* Repair of the compromised tissue is initiated within 3 to 5 days of the start of symptoms but may take as long as a month or more, especially for elderly people. The time course of influenza virus infection is illustrated in Figure 60–4.

Epidemiology

Strains of influenza A virus are classified by the following four characteristics:

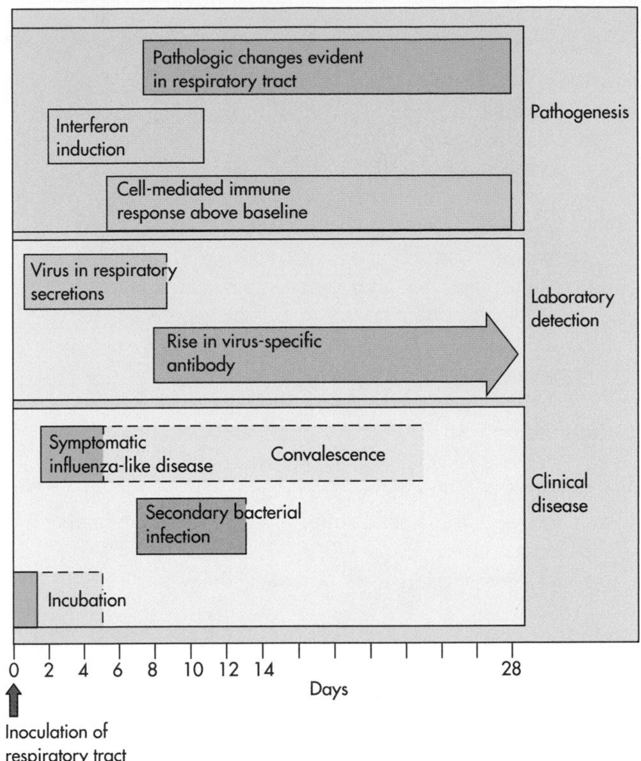

FIGURE 60–4. Time course of influenza A virus infection. The classic "flu syndrome" occurs early. Later, pneumonia may result from bacterial pathogenesis, viral pathogenesis, or immunopathogenesis.

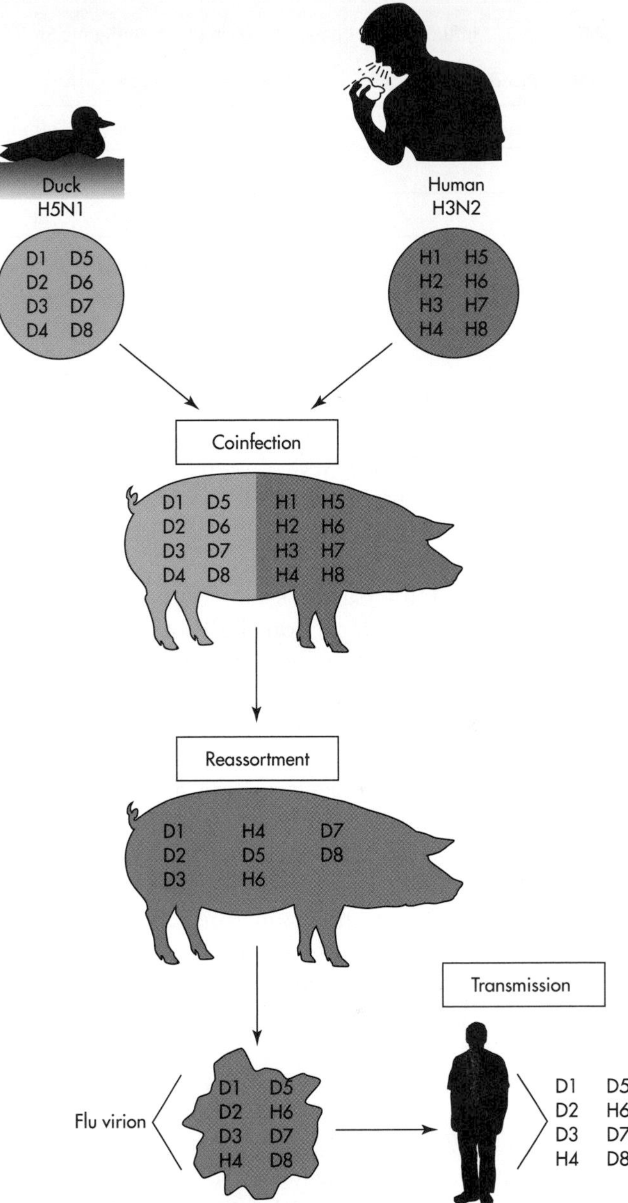

FIGURE 60–5. Example of reassortment of genomic fragments of influenza A virus. Diagram of the origin of a new human virus with a shift from H3N2 to H5N1. Pigs were infected with a duck influenza virus, and another set of pigs with the human influenza virus. At some time, a pig underwent mixed infection with both viruses. The resulting virus created by reassortment of the viral gene segments could be transmitted to and infect humans.

1. Type (A, B, and C)
2. Place of original isolation
3. Date of original isolation
4. Antigen (HA and NA)

For example, a current strain of influenza virus might be designated A/Bangkok/1/79 (H3N2), meaning that it is an influenza A virus that was first isolated in Bangkok in January 1979 and contains HA (H3) and NA (N2) antigens.

Strains of influenza B are designated by (1) type, (2) geography, and (3) date of isolation (e.g., B/Singapore/3/64), but without specific mention of HA or NA antigens because influenza B does not undergo antigenic shift nor pandemics like influenza A does.

New influenza A strains are generated through mutation and reassortment. The genetic diversity of influenza A is fostered by its segmented genomic structure and ability to infect and replicate in humans and many animal species **(zoonose),** including birds and pigs. Hybrid viruses are created by coinfection of a cell with different strains of influenza A virus, allowing the genomic segments to randomly associate into new virions. An exchange of the HA glycoproteins may generate a new virus that can infect an immunologically naïve human population. For example, an H5N1 duck virus and an H3N2 human virus infected pigs, reassortants were isolated from the pig, and the resulting virus was able to infect humans (Figure 60–5).

This type of reassortment is postulated to be the source of pathogenic human strains. Because of its high population density and proximity of humans, pigs, chickens, and ducks, China is thought to be a breeding ground for new reassortant viruses and the source of many of the pandemic strains of influenza. In 1997, an avian influenza

TABLE 60–2. Influenza Pandemics Resulting from Antigenic Shift

Year of Pandemic	Influenza A Subtype
1918	$H_{SW}N1$; probable swine flu strain
1947	H1N1
1957	H2N2; Asian flu strain
1968	H3N2; Hong Kong flu strain
1977	H1N1

virus (H5N1) strain was isolated from at least 18 humans and caused six deaths. A similar outbreak occurred in 2003. Although relatively few humans were infected, the H5N1 virus was unusual because it was not a reassortant, it was very virulent, and passed directly from bird to man. Avian influenza is transmitted in bird feces and not by human-to-human transmission. Outbreaks of avian influenza require the destruction of all potentially infected birds, such as for the 1.6 million chickens in Hong Kong, to destroy the potential source of the virus. There is concern that a reassortant with a human influenza virus might generate a pandemic.

Minor antigenic changes resulting from mutation of the HA and NA genes are called **antigenic drift.** This process occurs every 2 to 3 years, causing local outbreaks of influenza A and B infection. Major antigenic changes **(antigenic shift)** result from the reassortment of genomes among different strains, including animal strains. *This process occurs only with the influenza A virus.* Such changes are often associated with the occurrence of pandemics.

Antigenic shifts occur infrequently but can be devastating (Table 60–2). For example, the prevalent influenza A virus in 1947 was the H1N1 subtype. In 1957, there was a shift in both antigens, resulting in an H2N2 subtype. H3N2 appeared in 1968, and H1N1 reappeared in 1977. The reappearance of H1N1 put the population younger than age 30 at risk to disease. Prior exposure and an anamnestic antibody response protected the members of the population older than 30 years. *In contrast to influenza A, influenza B is predominantly a human virus and does not undergo antigenic shift.*

The changing antigenic nature of influenza ensures a large proportion of immunologically naïve, susceptible people (especially children) in the population (Box 60–3). An influenza outbreak can be readily detected from the increased absenteeism in schools and work and the number of emergency department visits. During the winter, influenza outbreaks occur annually in temperate climates. Fortunately, influenza virus is present in a community for only a short time (4 to 6 weeks).

Influenza infection is spread readily via small airborne droplets expelled during talking, breathing, and coughing.

BOX 60–3. Epidemiology of Influenza A and B Viruses

Disease/Viral Factors

Virus has large enveloped virion that is easily inactivated by dryness, acid, and detergents.

Segmented genome facilitates major genetic changes, especially on HA and NA proteins.

Influenza A infects many vertebrate species, including other mammals and birds.

Coinfection with animal and human strains of influenza can generate very different virus strains by genetic reassortment.

Transmission of virus often precedes symptoms.

Transmission

Virus is spread by inhalation of small aerosol droplets expelled during talking, breathing, and coughing.

Virus likes cool, less humid atmosphere (e.g., winter heating season).

Virus is extensively spread by school children.

Who Is at Risk?

Seronegative people.

Adults: Classic flu syndrome.

Children: Asymptomatic to severe respiratory tract infections.

High-risk groups: Elderly and immunocompromised people, and people with underlying cardiac or respiratory problems (including asthma sufferers and smokers).

Geography/Season

There is worldwide occurrence: Epidemics are local; pandemics are worldwide.

Disease is more common in winter.

Modes of Control

Amantadine, rimantadine, zanamivir, and oseltamivir have been approved for prophylaxis or early treatment.

Killed and live vaccines contain predicted yearly strains of influenza A and B viruses.

The virus can also survive on countertops for as long as a day.

The most susceptible population is children, and school-age children are most likely to spread the infection. Contagion precedes symptoms and lasts for a long time, especially in children. Children, immunosuppressed people (including pregnant women), elderly people, and people with heart and lung ailments (including smokers) are at highest risk for more serious disease, pneumonia, or other complications of infection. More than 90% of the mortalities occur in patients who are older than 65 years.

Extensive surveillance of influenza A and B outbreaks is conducted to identify the new strains that should be incorporated into new vaccines. The prevalence of a particular strain of influenza A or B virus changes each year

BOX 60–4. Clinical Summaries

Influenza A: A 70-year-old woman has rapid onset of fever with headache, myalgia, sore throat, and nonproductive cough. The disease progresses to pneumonia with bacterial involvement. There is no history of recent immunization with influenza A vaccine. Her husband is treated with amantadine or a neuraminidase inhibitor.

and reflects the particular immunologic naïveté of the population at that time. Surveillance also extends into the animal populations because of the possible presence of recombinant animal influenza A strains that can cause human pandemics.

Clinical Syndromes (Box 60–4)

Depending on the degree of immunity to the infecting strain of virus and other factors, infection may range from asymptomatic to severe. Patients with underlying cardiorespiratory disease, people with immune deficiency (even that associated with pregnancy), and smokers are more prone to have a severe case.

After an incubation period of 1 to 4 days, the "flu syndrome" begins with a brief prodrome of malaise and headache lasting a few hours. The prodrome is followed by the abrupt onset of fever, chills, severe myalgias, loss of appetite, and, usually, a nonproductive cough. The fever persists for 3 to 8 days, and unless a complication occurs, recovery is complete within 7 to 10 days. Influenza in young children resembles other severe respiratory tract infections, causing bronchiolitis, croup, otitis media, vomiting, and abdominal pain in children younger than 3 years, and, rarely, febrile convulsions (Table 60–3). Complications of influenza include bacterial pneumonia, myositis, and Reye's syndrome. The central nervous system can also be involved. Influenza B disease is similar to influenza A disease.

Influenza may directly cause pneumonia, but it more commonly promotes a secondary bacterial superinfection that leads to bronchitis or pneumonia. The tissue damage caused by progressive influenza virus infection of alveoli can be extensive, leading to hypoxia and bilateral pneumonia. Secondary bacterial infection usually involves *Streptococcus pneumoniae, Haemophilus influenzae,* or *Staphylococcus aureus.* In these infections, sputum usually is produced and becomes purulent.

Although the infection generally is limited to the lung, some strains of influenza can spread to other sites in certain people. For example, myositis (inflammation of muscle) may occur in children. Encephalopathy, although rare, may accompany an acute influenza illness and may be fatal. Postinfluenza encephalitis occurs 2 to 3 weeks after recovery from influenza. It is associated with evidence of inflammation and is rarely fatal.

TABLE 60–3. Diseases Associated with Influenza Virus Infection

Disorder	Symptoms
Acute influenza infection in adults	Rapid onset of fever, malaise, myalgia, sore throat, and nonproductive cough
Acute influenza infection in children	Acute disease similar to that in adults but with higher fever, gastrointestinal tract symptoms (abdominal pain, vomiting), otitis media, myositis, and more frequent croup
Complications of influenza virus infection	Primary viral pneumonia Secondary bacterial pneumonia Myositis and cardiac involvement Neurologic syndromes: Guillain-Barré syndrome Encephalopathy Encephalitis Reye's syndrome

Reye's syndrome is an acute encephalitis that affects children and occurs after a variety of acute febrile viral infections, including varicella and influenza B and A diseases. Children given salicylates (aspirin) are at increased risk for this syndrome. In addition to encephalopathy, hepatic dysfunction is present. The mortality rate may be as high as 40%.

Laboratory Diagnosis

The diagnosis of influenza is usually based on the characteristic symptoms, the season, and the presence of the virus in the community. Laboratory methods that distinguish influenza from other respiratory viruses and identify its type and strain confirm the diagnosis (Table 60–4).

Influenza viruses are obtained from respiratory secretions. The virus is generally isolated in primary monkey kidney cell cultures or the Madin-Darby canine kidney cell line. Nonspecific cytopathologic effects are often difficult to distinguish but may be noted within as few as 2 days (average, 4 days). Before the cytopathologic effects develop, the addition of guinea pig erythrocytes may reveal **hemadsorption** (the adherence of these erythrocytes to HA-expressing infected cells) (see Figure 51–5). The addition of influenza virus–containing media to erythrocytes promotes the formation of a gel-like aggregate due to **hemagglutination.** Hemagglutination and hemadsorption are not specific to influenza viruses,

TABLE 60–4. Laboratory Diagnosis of Influenza Virus Infection

Test	Detects
Cell culture in primary monkey kidney or Madin-Darby canine kidney cells	Presence of virus; limited cytopathologic effects
Hemadsorption to infected cells	Presence of HA protein on cell surface
Hemagglutination	Presence of virus in secretions
Hemagglutination inhibition	Type and strain of influenza virus or specificity of antibody
Antibody inhibition of hemadsorption	Identification of influenza type and strain
Immunofluorescence, ELISA	Influenza virus antigens in respiratory secretions or tissue culture
Serology: Hemagglutination inhibition, hemadsorption inhibition, ELISA, immunofluorescence, complement fixation	Seroepidemiology
Genomics: RT-PCR	Identification of influenza type and strain

ELISA, Enzyme-linked immunosorbent assay.

however; parainfluenza and other viruses also exhibit these properties.

More rapid techniques detect and identify the influenza genome or antigens of the virus. Rapid antigen assays (less than 30 min) can detect and distinguish influenza A and B. Reverse transcriptase polymerase chain reaction, using generic influenza primers, can be used to detect and distinguish influenza A and B, and more specific primers can be used to distinguish the different strains, such as H1N1. Enzyme immunoassay or immunofluorescence can be used to detect viral antigen in exfoliated cells, respiratory secretions, or cell culture and are more sensitive assays. Immunofluorescence, or inhibition of hemadsorption or hemagglutination (hemagglutination inhibition [HI]) with specific antibody (see Chapter 51), can also detect and distinguish different influenza strains. Laboratory studies are primarily used for epidemiologic purposes.

Treatment, Prevention, and Control

Hundreds of millions of dollars are spent on acetaminophen, antihistamines, and similar drugs to relieve the symptoms of influenza. The antiviral drug **amantadine** and its analogue **rimantadine** inhibit an uncoating step of the influenza A virus but do not affect the influenza B and C viruses. The target for their action is the M_2 protein. **Zanamivir** and **oseltamivir** inhibit both influenza A and B as enzyme inhibitors of the neuraminidase. Without the neuraminidase, the hemagglutinin of the virus binds to sialic acid on other viral particles to form clumps, thereby preventing virus release. Zanamivir is inhaled, whereas oseltamivir is taken orally as a pill. These drugs are effective for prophylaxis and for treatment during the first 24 to 48 hours after the onset of influenza A illness. Treatment cannot prevent the later host-induced immunopathogenic stages of the disease.

The airborne spread of influenza is almost impossible to limit. However, the best way to control the virus is through immunization. Natural immunization, which results from prior exposure, is protective for long periods. A killed-virus vaccine representing the "strains of the year" and antiviral drug prophylaxis can also prevent infection.

Killed (formalin-inactivated) influenza vaccine is available every year. Killed whole-virus vaccines are prepared from virus grown in embryonated eggs and then chemically inactivated. Detergent-treated virion preparations and HA- and NA-containing detergent extracts of virus are also available. Ideally the vaccine incorporates antigens of the A and B influenza strains that will be prevalent in the community during the upcoming winter. For instance, the trivalent influenza vaccine used in 1992 and 1993 consisted of inactivated A/Texas/91–like (H1N1), A/Beijing/89–like (H3N2), and B/Panama/90–like virus strains. Vaccination is routinely recommended for persons older than 50, healthcare workers, pregnant women who will be in their second or third trimester during flu season, people with chronic pulmonary heart disease, and others. Persons with allergies to eggs should not get the vaccine.

A live vaccine is also available for administration as a nasal spray. The trivalent vaccine consists of reassortants for the HA and NA gene segments of different influenza strains with a master donor virus that is cold adapted to optimum growth at 25°C. This vaccine will elicit a more natural protection, including cell-mediated, antibody and mucosal-secretory immunoglobulin (Ig)A antibody. Currently, the vaccine is recommended for people ages 5 to 50.

CASE STUDY AND QUESTIONS

In late December, a 22-year-old man suddenly experienced headache, myalgia, malaise, dry cough, and fever. He basically felt lousy. After a couple of days, he had a sore throat, his cough had worsened, he started to feel nauseated, and he began vomiting. Several of his family members had experienced similar symptoms during the previous 2 weeks.

1. In addition to influenza, what other agents could cause similar symptoms (differential diagnosis)?
2. How would the diagnosis of influenza be confirmed?
3. Amantadine is effective against influenza. What is its mechanism of action? Will it be effective for this patient? For uninfected family members or contacts?
4. When was the patient contagious, and how was the virus transmitted?
5. What family members were at greatest risk for serious disease, and why?
6. Why is influenza so difficult to control even when there is a national vaccination program?

Bibliography

Cohen J, Powderly WG, editors: *Infectious diseases,* ed 2, St Louis, 2004, Mosby.

Cox NJ, Subbarao K: Global epidemiology of influenza: Past and present, *Annu Rev Med* 51:407-421, 2000.

Flint SJ et al: *Principles of virology: Molecular biology, pathogenesis and control of animal viruses,* ed 2, Washington, 2003, American Society for Microbiology Press.

Hay AJ et al: Influenza viruses. In Belshe RB, editor: *Textbook of human virology,* ed 2, St Louis, 1991, Mosby.

Helenius A: Unpacking the incoming influenza virus, *Cell* 69:577-578, 1992.

Knipe DM, Howley PM, editors: *Fields virology,* ed 4, New York, 2001, Lippincott-Williams and Wilkins.

Laver WG, Bischofberger N, Webster RG: Disarming flu viruses, *Sci Am* 280:78-87, 1999.

Laver WG, Bischofberger N, Webster RG: The origin and control of pandemic influenza, *Perspect Biol Med* 43:173-192, 2000.

Strauss JM, Strauss EG: *Viruses and human disease,* San Diego, 2002, Academic Press.

Stuart-Harris C: The epidemiology and prevention of influenza, *Am Sci* 69:166-172, 1981.

Webster RG: Predictions for future human influenza pandemics, *J Infect Dis* 176(suppl 1):S14-S19, 1997.

Webster RG et al: Evolution and ecology of influenza viruses, *Microbiol Rev* 56:152-179, 1992.

Website

National Institute of Allery and Infectious Disease: Influenza fact sheet: Available at www.niaid.nih.gov/publications/flu.htm

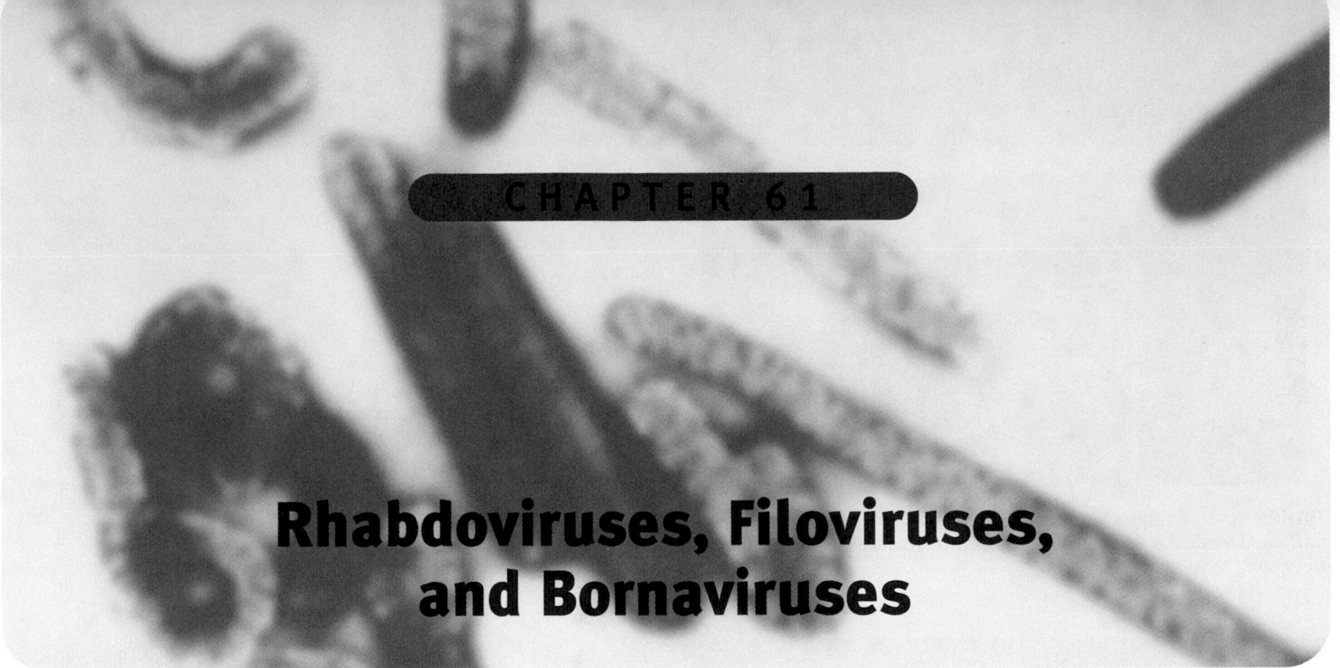

Rhabdoviruses, Filoviruses, and Bornaviruses

The members of the family Rhabdoviridae (from the Greek word *rhabdos,* meaning "rod") include pathogens for a variety of mammals, fish, birds, and plants. The family contains *Vesiculovirus* (vesicular stomatitis viruses [VSVs]); *Lyssavirus* (rabies and rabieslike viruses), an unnamed genus constituting the plant rhabdovirus group; and other ungrouped rhabdoviruses of mammals, birds, fish, and arthropods.

Rabies virus is the most significant pathogen of the rhabdoviruses. Until Louis Pasteur developed the killed-rabies vaccine, a bite from a "mad" dog always led to the characteristic symptoms of **hydrophobia** and certain death.

Physiology, Structure, and Replication

Rhabdoviruses are simple viruses encoding only five proteins and appearing as **bullet-shaped, enveloped virions** with a diameter of 50 to 95 nm and length of 130 to 380 nm (Box 61–1, Figure 61–1). Spikes composed of a trimer of the glycoprotein (G) cover the surface of the virus. The viral attachment protein, G protein, generates neutralizing antibodies. The G protein of the vesicular stomatitis virus is a simple glycoprotein with *N*-linked glycan. This G protein has been used as the prototype for studying eukaryotic glycoprotein processing.

Within the envelope the **helical nucleocapsid** is coiled symmetrically into a cylindrical structure, giving it the appearance of striations (see Figure 61–1). The nucleocapsid is composed of one molecule of **single-stranded, negative-sense RNA** (ribonucleic acid) of approximately 12,000 bases and the nucleoprotein (N), large (L) and nonstructural (NS) proteins. The matrix (M) protein lies between the envelope and the nucleocapsid. The N protein is the major structural protein of the virus. It protects the RNA from ribonuclease digestion and maintains the RNA in a configuration acceptable for transcription. The L and NS proteins constitute the RNA-dependent RNA polymerase.

The replicative cycle of VSV is the prototype for the rhabdoviruses and other negative-strand RNA viruses (see Figure 6–14). The viral G protein attaches to the host cell and is internalized by endocytosis. The viral envelope then fuses with the membrane of the endosome on acidification of the vesicle. This uncoating releases the nucleocapsid to be released into the cytoplasm, where replication takes place.

The RNA-dependent RNA polymerase associated with the nucleocapsid transcribes the viral genomic RNA, producing five individual messenger RNAs (mRNAs). These mRNAs are then translated into the five viral proteins. The viral genomic RNA is also transcribed into a full-length positive-sense RNA template that is used to generate new genomes. The G protein is synthesized by membrane-bound ribosomes, processed by the Golgi apparatus, and delivered to the cell surface in membrane vesicles. The M protein associates with the G protein–modified membranes.

Assembly of the virion occurs in two phases: (1) assembly of the nucleocapsid in the cytoplasm and (2) envelopment and release at the cell plasma membrane. The genome associates with the N protein and then with the polymerase proteins L and NS to form the nucleocapsid. Association of the nucleocapsid with the M protein at the plasma membrane induces coiling into its condensed form. The virus then buds through the plasma membrane and is released when the entire nucleocapsid is enveloped. Cell death and lysis occur after infection with most rhabdoviruses, with the important exception of rabies virus, which produces little discernible cell damage.

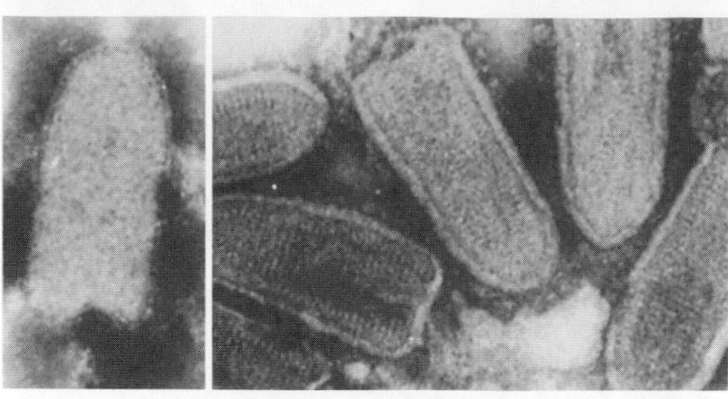

FIGURE 61–1. Rhabdoviridae seen by electron microscopy: rabies virus (*left*) and vesicular stomatitis virus (*right*). (From Fields BN: *Virology,* New York, 1985, Raven.)

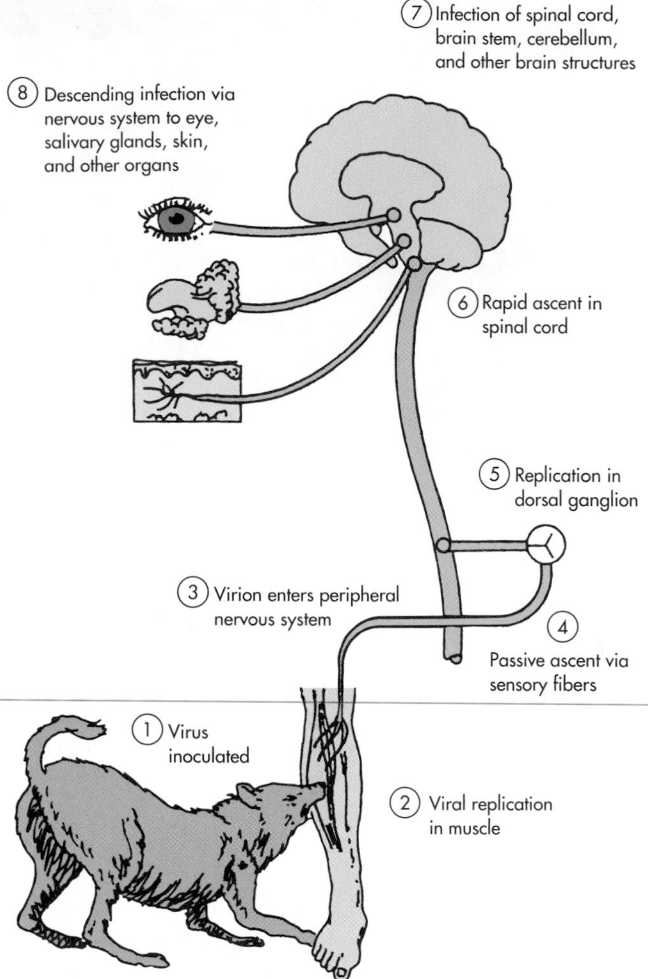

FIGURE 61–2. Pathogenesis of rabies virus infection. Numbered steps describe the sequence of events. (Redrawn from Belshe RB, editor: *Textbook of human virology,* ed 2, St Louis, 1991, Mosby.)

BOX 61–1. Unique Features of Rhabdoviruses

Bullet-shaped, enveloped, negative, single-stranded RNA viruses that encode five proteins.
Prototype for replication of negative-stranded enveloped viruses.
Replication in the cytoplasm.

BOX 61–2. Disease Mechanisms of Rabies Virus

Rabies is usually transmitted in saliva and is acquired from the bite of a rabid animal.
Rabies virus is **not very cytolytic** and seems to remain cell associated.
Virus replicates in the muscle at the site of the bite, with minimal or no symptoms (*incubation phase*).
The length of the incubation phase is determined by the infectious dose and the proximity of the infection site to the central nervous system (CNS) and brain.
After weeks to months, the virus infects the peripheral nerves and travels up the CNS to the brain (*prodrome phase*).
Infection of the brain causes classic symptoms, coma, and death (*neurologic phase*).
During the neurologic phase the virus spreads to the glands, skin, and other body parts, including the salivary glands, from where it is transmitted.
Rabies infection does not elicit an antibody response until the late stages of the disease, when the virus has spread from the CNS to other sites.
Antibody can block the progression of the virus and disease.
The long incubation period allows **active immunization as a postexposure treatment.**

Pathogenesis and Immunity

Only the pathogenesis of rabies virus infection is discussed here (Box 61–2). Rabies infection usually results from the bite of a rabid animal. Rabies infection of the animal causes secretion of the virus in the animal's saliva and promotes aggressive behavior ("mad" dog), which in turn promotes transmission of the virus. The virus can also be transmitted through the inhalation of aerosolized virus (as may be found in bat caves), in transplanted infected tissue (e.g., cornea), and by inoculation through intact mucosal membranes.

Virus may directly infect nerve endings by binding to nicotinic acetylcholine or ganglioside receptors of neurons or muscle at the site of inoculation. The virus remains at the site for days to months (Figure 61–2) before progressing to the central nervous system (CNS). Rabies virus travels by retrograde axoplasmic transport to the dorsal root ganglia and to the spinal cord. Once the virus gains access to the spinal cord, the brain becomes rapidly infected. The affected areas are the hippocampus, brain stem, ganglionic cells of the pontine nuclei, and Purkinje cells of the cerebellum. The virus then disseminates from the CNS via afferent neurons to highly innervated sites, such as the skin of the head and neck, **salivary glands,** retina, cornea, nasal mucosa, adrenal medulla, renal parenchyma, and pancreatic acinar cells. After the virus invades the brain and spinal cord, an encephalitis develops, and neurons degenerate. Despite the extensive CNS involvement and impairment of CNS function, little histopathologic change can be observed in the affected tissue other than the presence of Negri bodies (see section on Laboratory Diagnosis).

With rare exception (three known cases), rabies is fatal once clinical disease is apparent. The length of the incubation period is determined by (1) the concentration of the virus in the inoculum, (2) the proximity of the wound to the brain, (3) the severity of the wound, (4) the host's age, and (5) the host's immune status.

In contrast to other viral encephalitis syndromes, rabies rarely causes inflammatory lesions. Neutralizing antibodies are not apparent until after the clinical disease is well established. Little antigen is released, and the infection probably remains hidden from the immune response. Cell-mediated immunity appears to play little or no role in protection against rabies virus infection.

Antibody can block the spread of virus to the CNS and to the brain if administered or generated during the incubation period. *The incubation period is usually long enough to allow generation of a therapeutic protective antibody response after active immunization with the killed rabies vaccine.*

BOX 61–3. Epidemiology of Rabies Virus

Disease/Viral Factors

Virus-induced aggressive behavior in animals promotes virus spread.

Disease has long, asymptomatic incubation period.

Transmission

Zoonosis:

Reservoir: Wild animals.

Vector: Wild animals and unvaccinated dogs and cats.

Source of virus:

Major: Saliva in bite of rabid animal.

Minor: Aerosols in bat caves containing rabid bats.

Who Is at Risk?

Veterinarians and animal handlers.

Person bitten by a rabid animal.

Inhabitants of countries with no pet vaccination program.

Geography/Season

Virus is found worldwide, except in some island nations.

There is no seasonal incidence.

Modes of Control

Vaccination program is available for pets.

Vaccination is available for at-risk personnel.

Vaccination programs have been implemented to control rabies in forest mammals.

Epidemiology

Rabies is the **classic zoonotic infection,** spread from animals to humans (Box 61–3). It is endemic in a variety of animals worldwide, except in Australia. Rabies is maintained and spread in two ways: In urban rabies, dogs are the primary transmitter, and in sylvatic (forest) rabies, many species of wildlife can serve as the transmitter. In the United States, rabies is more prevalent in cats because they are not vaccinated. Virus-containing aerosols, bites, and scratches from infected bats also spread the disease. The principal reservoir for rabies in most of the world, however, is the dog. In Latin America and Asia, this feature is a problem because of the existence of many stray, unvaccinated dogs and the absence of rabies-control programs. These two factors are responsible for thousands of rabies cases in dogs each year in these countries.

Because of the excellent vaccination program in the United States, sylvatic rabies accounts for most of the cases of animal rabies in this country. Statistics for animal rabies are collected by the U.S. Centers for Disease Control and Prevention, which in 1999 recorded more than 8000 documented cases of rabies in raccoons, skunks, bats, and farm animals, in addition to dogs and cats (Figure 61–3). Badgers and foxes are also major carriers of rabies in Western Europe. In South America, vampire bats transmit rabies to cattle, resulting in losses of millions of dollars each year.

The distribution of human rabies approximates the distribution of animal cases in each country. It is estimated that rabies accounts for between 40,000 and as high as 70,000 deaths annually worldwide, and at least 25,000 deaths in India, where the virus is transmitted by dogs in 96% of cases. In Latin America, cases of human rabies primarily result from contact with rabid dogs in urban areas. In Indonesia, an outbreak of more than 200 human cases of rabies in 1999 promoted the killing of more than 40,000 dogs on the islands. The incidence of human rabies in the United States is approximately one case per year, because of effective dog vaccination programs and limited human contact with skunks, raccoons, and bats. Since 1990, human cases of rabies in the United States have been caused primarily by bat variants of the virus. The World Health Organization estimates that 10 million people per year receive treatment after exposure to animals suspected of being rabid.

Clinical Syndromes (Box 61–4)

Rabies is virtually always fatal unless treated by vaccination. After a long but highly variable incubation period, the prodrome phase of rabies ensues (Table 61–1). The

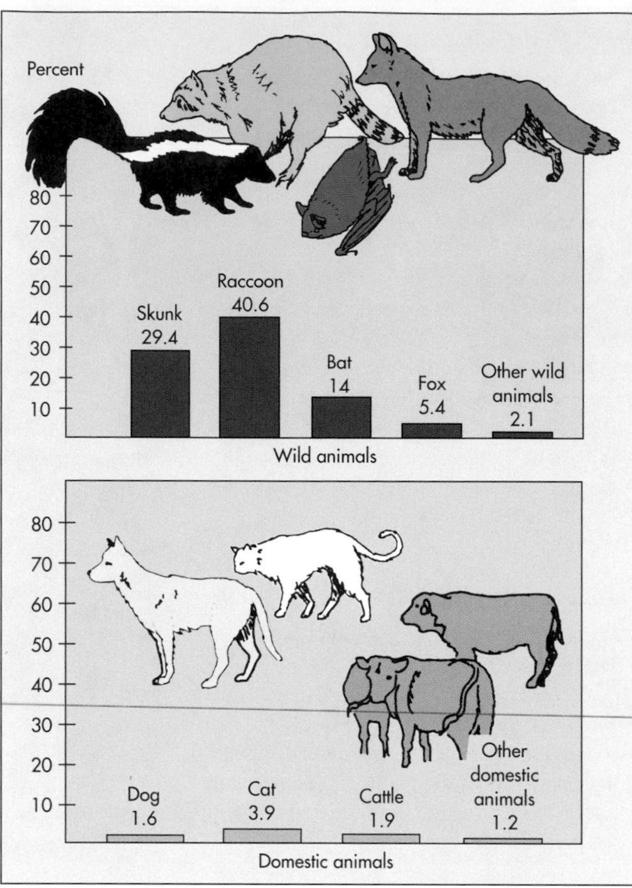

FIGURE 61–3. Distribution of animal rabies in the United States, 1999. The percentages relate to the total number of cases of animal rabies. (Data from Krebs JW et al: *JAVMA* 217:1799-1811, 2000.)

patient has symptoms such as fever, malaise, headache, pain or paresthesia (itching) at the site of the bite, gastrointestinal symptoms, fatigue, and anorexia. The prodrome usually lasts 2 to 10 days, after which the neurologic symptoms specific to rabies appear. **Hydrophobia** (fear of water), the most characteristic symptom of rabies, occurs in 20% to 50% of patients. It is triggered by the pain associated with the patient's attempts to swallow water. Focal and generalized seizures, disorientation, and hallucinations are also common during the neurologic phase. From 15% to 60% of patients exhibit paralysis as the only manifestation of rabies. The paralysis may lead to respiratory failure.

The patient becomes comatose after the neurologic phase, which lasts from 2 to 10 days. This phase almost universally leads to death due to neurologic and pulmonary complications.

Box 61–4. Clinical Summaries

Rabies: A 3-year-old girl was found to have a bat flying in her bedroom. The bat apparently was there all night. There was no evidence of any bite wound or contact, and the bat was caught and released. Three weeks later the child developed a change in behavior, in which she was irritable and agitated. She quickly became confused and uncontrollable, thrashing about and unable to handle her secretions. She eventually became comatose and died from respiratory arrest.

TABLE 61–1. Progression of Rabies Disease

Disease Phase	Symptoms	Time (days)	Viral Status	Immunologic Status
Incubation phase	Asymptomatic	60–365 after bite	Low titer, virus in muscle	—
Prodrome phase	Fever, nausea, vomiting, loss of appetite, headache, lethargy, pain at site of bite	2–10	Low titer, virus in CNS and brain	—
Neurologic phase	Hydrophobia, pharyngeal spasms, hyperactivity, anxiety, depression CNS symptoms: loss of coordination, paralysis, confusion, delirium	2–7	High titer, virus in brain and other sites	Detectable antibody in serum and CNS
Coma	Coma: cardiac arrest, hypotension, hypoventilation, secondary infections	0–14	High titer, virus in brain and other sites	—
Death	—	—	—	—

CNS, Central nervous system.

Laboratory Diagnosis

The occurrence of neurologic symptoms in a person who has been bitten by an animal generally establishes the diagnosis of rabies. Unfortunately, **evidence of infection, including symptoms and the detection of antibody, does not occur until it is too late for intervention.** Laboratory tests are usually performed to confirm the diagnosis and to determine whether a suspected individual or animal is rabid (postmortem).

The diagnosis of rabies is made through detection of viral antigen in the CNS or skin, isolation of the virus, detection of the genome, and serologic findings. The hallmark diagnostic finding has been the detection of intracytoplasmic inclusions consisting of aggregates of viral nucleocapsids **(Negri bodies)** in affected neurons (see Figure 51–3). Although their finding is diagnostic of rabies, Negri bodies are seen in only 70% to 90% of brain tissue from infected humans.

Antigen detection using direct immunofluorescence or genome detection using reverse transcriptase polymerase chain reaction (RT-PCR) are relatively quick and sensitive assays that are the preferred methods for diagnosing rabies. Samples of saliva, serum, spinal fluid, skin biopsy material from the nape of the neck, brain biopsy or autopsy material, and impression smears of corneal epithelial cells are the specimens that are examined.

Rabies can also be grown in cell culture or in intracerebrally inoculated infant mice. Inoculated cell cultures or brain tissues are subsequently examined with direct immunofluorescence.

Rabies antibody titers in serum and cerebrospinal fluid are usually measured by enzyme-linked immunosorbant assay (ELISA) or a rapid fluorescent focus inhibition test. Antibody usually is not detectable until late in the disease, however.

Treatment and Prophylaxis

Clinical rabies is almost always fatal unless treated. Once the symptoms have appeared, little other than supportive care can be given.

Postexposure prophylaxis is the only hope for preventing overt clinical illness in the affected person. Although human cases of rabies are rare, appoximately 20,000 people receive rabies prophylaxis each year in the United States alone. Prophylaxis should be initiated for anyone exposed by bite or by contamination of an open wound or mucous membrane to the saliva or brain tissue of an animal suspected to be infected with the virus, unless the animal is tested and shown not to be rabid.

The first protective measure is local treatment of the wound. The wound should be washed immediately with soap and water or another substance that inactivates the virus. The World Health Organization Expert Committee on Rabies also recommends the instillation of antirabies serum around the wound.

Subsequently, immunization with vaccine in combination with administration of one dose of human rabies immunoglobulin (HRIG) or equine antirabies serum is recommended. Passive immunization with HRIG provides antibody until the patient produces antibody in response to the vaccine. A series of five immunizations is then administered over the course of a month. The slow course of rabies disease allows active immunity to be generated in time to afford protection.

The rabies vaccine is a killed-virus vaccine prepared through the chemical inactivation of rabies-infected tissue culture human diploid cells (HDCV) or fetal rhesus lung cells. These vaccines cause fewer negative reactions than the older vaccines (Semple and Fermi), which were prepared in the brains of adult or suckling animals. The HDCV is administered intramuscularly on the day of exposure and then on days 3, 7, 14, and 28 or intradermally with a lower dose of vaccine to multiple sites on days 0, 3, 7, 28, and 90.

Preexposure vaccination should be performed on animal workers, laboratory workers who handle potentially infected tissue, and people traveling to areas where rabies is endemic. HDCV administered intramuscularly or intradermally in three doses is recommended and provides 2 years of protection.

Ultimately, the prevention of human rabies hinges on the effective control of rabies in domestic and wild animals. Its control in domestic animals depends on the removal of stray and unwanted animals and the vaccination of all dogs and cats. A variety of attenuated oral vaccines have also been used successfully to immunize foxes. A live recombinant vaccinia virus vaccine expressing the rabies virus G protein is in use in the United States. This vaccine, which is injected into bait and parachuted into the forest, successfully immunizes raccoons, foxes, and other animals.

Filoviruses

The **Marburg** and **Ebola** viruses (Figure 61–4) were classified as members of the family Rhabdoviridae but are now classified as **filoviruses.** They are **filamentous, enveloped, negative-strand RNA viruses.** These agents cause **severe or fatal hemorrhagic fevers** and are **endemic in Africa.** Awareness of the Ebola virus increased after an outbreak of the disease in Zaire in 1995, in Gabon in 1996, and also after the release of the movie "Outbreak," based on the book by Robin Cook, and the book *The Hot Zone* by Richard Preston.

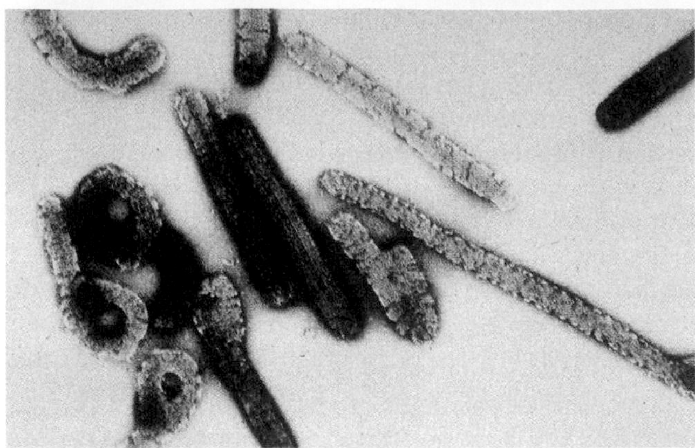

Figure 61–4. Electron micrograph of the Ebola virus. (Courtesy Centers for Disease Control and Prevention, Atlanta.)

STRUCTURE AND REPLICATION

Filoviruses have a single-stranded RNA genome (4.5×10^6 Da) that encodes seven proteins. The virions form enveloped filaments with a diameter of 80 nm but may also assume other shapes. They vary in length from 800 nm to as long as 1400 nm. The nucleocapsid is helical and enclosed in an envelope containing one glycoprotein. The virus replicates in the cytoplasm like the rhabdoviruses.

PATHOGENESIS

The filoviruses replicate efficiently, producing large amounts of virus and causing extensive tissue necrosis in parenchymal cells of the liver, spleen, lymph nodes, and lungs. The breakdown of endothelial cells leading to vascular injury can be attributed to the Ebola glycoprotein. Strains with mutations in this protein lack the hemorrhagic component of disease. The widespread hemorrhage that occurs in affected patients causes edema and hypovolemic shock.

EPIDEMIOLOGY

Marburg virus infection was first detected among laboratory workers in Marburg, Germany, who had been exposed to tissues from apparently healthy African green monkeys. Rare cases of Marburg virus infection have been seen in Zimbabwe and Kenya.

Ebola virus was named for the river in the Democratic Republic of Congo (formerly Zaire) where it was discovered. Outbreaks of Ebola virus disease have occurred in the Democratic Republic of Congo and Sudan. During an outbreak, the Ebola virus is so lethal that it eliminates the susceptible population before it can be spread extensively. However, in rural areas of central Africa as much as 18% of the population have antibody to this virus, indicating that subclinical infections do occur.

These viruses may be endemic in wild monkeys but can be spread from monkeys to humans and between humans. Contact with the animal reservoir or direct contact with infected blood or secretions can spread the disease. These viruses have been transmitted by accidental injection and through the use of contaminated syringes. Health care workers tending the sick and monkey handlers may be at risk.

CLINICAL SYNDROMES

Marburg and Ebola viruses are the most severe causes of viral hemorrhagic fevers. The illness usually begins with flulike symptoms such as headache and myalgia. Nausea, vomiting, and diarrhea occur within a few days; a rash also may develop. Subsequently, hemorrhage from multiple sites, especially the gastrointestinal tract, and death occur in as many as 90% of patients with clinically evident disease. The 1995 outbreak in Kikwit, Congo, killed 245 people.

LABORATORY DIAGNOSIS

All specimens from patients with a suspected filovirus infection must be handled with extreme care to prevent accidental infection. Handling of these viruses requires **level 4 isolation** procedures that are not routinely available. Marburg virus may grow rapidly in tissue culture (Vero cells), but animal (e.g., guinea pig) inoculation may be necessary to recover Ebola virus.

Infected cells have large eosinophilic cytoplasmic inclusion bodies. Viral antigens can be detected in tissue by direct immunofluorescence analysis, and fluids by enzyme-linked immunosorbent assay (ELISA). RT-PCR amplification of the viral genome in secretions can be used to confirm the diagnosis and minimize handling of samples.

Immunoglobulin (Ig)G and IgM antibody to filovirus antigens can be detected by immunofluorescence, ELISA, or radioimmunoassay.

TREATMENT, PREVENTION, AND CONTROL

Antibody-containing serum and interferon therapies have been tried in patients with filovirus infections. Infected patients should be quarantined, and contaminated animals should be sacrificed. Handling of the viruses or contaminated materials requires very stringent (level 4) isolation procedures.

Borna Disease Virus

Borna disease virus (BDV) is the only member of a new family of enveloped, negative strand RNA viruses. BDV was first associated with infection of horses in Germany. The virus has received considerable recent interest because of its association with specific neuropsychiatric diseases, such as schizophrenia.

STRUCTURE AND REPLICATION

The 8910 nucleotide long genome of BDV encodes five detectable proteins, including a polymerase (L), nucleoprotein (N), phosphoprotein (P), matrix protein (M) and envelope glycoprotein (G). Unlike most negative-strand viruses, BDV replicates in the nucleus. Although this is similar to the orthomyxoviruses, BDV differs in that its genome is unsegmented. Also unusual for an RNA virus, one of the positive-strand RNAs that is transcribed from the genome is processed to remove introns to produce three mRNAS for three different proteins.

PATHOGENESIS

BDV is highly neurotropic and capable of spreading throughout the CNS. BDV also infects parenchymal cells of different organs and peripheral blood mononuclear cells. The virus is not very cytolytic and establishes a persistent infection in the infected individual. T cell immune responses are important for controlling BDV infections but also contribute to tissue damage leading to disease.

DISEASE

Although there is limited understanding of the BDV disease in humans, infection of animals can result in subtle losses of learning and memory and in fatal immune-mediated meningoencephalitis. Many of the outcomes of BDV infection of laboratory animals resemble human neuropsychiatric diseases, including depression, biopolar disorder, schizophrenia, and autism. The presence of antibodies to the virus and/or infected peripheral blood mononuclear cells in higher than background numbers of patients with schizophrenia, autism, and other neuropsychiatric diseases suggest that BDV either causes or exacerbates these mental illnesses.

EPIDEMIOLOGY

BDV is a zoonose capable of infecting many different mammalian species including horses, sheep, and humans. Most outbreaks of the virus have occurred in central Europe, but the virus has also been detected in North America and Asia. Neither the reservoir nor the mode of transmission of BDV is known. Higher levels of infection of humans are present where outbreaks in horses have been observed.

LABORATORY DIAGNOSIS

Infection can be detected by direct analysis of the viral genome and mRNA in peripheral blood mononuclear cells using RT-PCR. Serologic analysis of antibody to the viral proteins continues to be used to identify an association of BDV with human diseases.

TREATMENT

Like many other RNA viruses, BDV is sensitive to ribavirin treatment. Ribavirin treatment may be a reasonable treatment approach for some psychoneurologic disorders if BDV was demonstrated as a cofactor.

CASE STUDY AND QUESTIONS

An 11-year-old boy was brought to a hospital in California after falling; his bruises were treated and he was released. The following day he refused to drink water with his medicine, and he became more anxious. That night he began to act up and hallucinate. He also was salivating and had difficulty breathing. Two days later, he had a fever of 40.8°C (105.4°F) and experienced two episodes of cardiac arrest. Although rabies was suspected, no remarkable data were obtained from a computed tomographic image of the brain or cerebrospinal fluid analysis. A skin biopsy from the nape of the neck was negative for viral antigen on day 3 but was positive for rabies on day 7. The patient's condition continued to deteriorate, and he died 11 days later. When the parents were questioned, it was learned that the boy had been bitten on the finger by a dog 6 months earlier while on a trip to India.

1. What clinical features of this case suggested rabies?
2. Why does rabies have such a long incubation period?
3. What treatment should have been given immediately after the dog bite? What treatment should be given as soon as the diagnosis was suspected?
4. How do the clinical aspects of rabies differ from those of other neurologic viral diseases?

Bibliography

Anderson LJ et al: Human rabies in the United States, 1960-1979: Epidemiology, diagnosis, and prevention, *Ann Intern Med* 100:728-735; 1984.

Baer GM et al: Rhabdoviruses. In Fields BN, Knipe DM, editors: *Virology*, New York, 1990, Raven.

Cohen J, Powderly WG, editors: *Infectious diseases*, ed 2, St Louis, 2004, Mosby.

Fishbein DB: Rabies, *Infect Dis Clin North Am* 5:53-71, 1991.

Flint SJ et al: *Principles of virology: Molecular biology, pathogenesis and control of animal viruses*, ed 2, Washington, 2003, American Society for Microbiology Press.

Knipe DM, Howley PM, editors: *Fields virology*, ed 4, New York, 2001, Lippincott-Williams and Wilkins.

Krebs JW et al: Rabies surveillance in the United States during 1999. *JAVMA* 217:1799-1811, 2000. (Available online at www.cdc.gov/ncidod/dvrd/rabies/Professional/Surveillance99/index.htm)

Immunization Practices Advisory Committee: Rabies prevention: Supplementary statement on the preexposure use of human diploid cell rabies vaccine by the intradermal route, *MMWR Morb Mortal Wkly Rep* 35:767-768, 1986.

Plotkin SA: Rabies: State of the art clinical article. *Clin Infect Dis* 30:4-12,2000.

Rabies vaccine, absorbed: A new rabies vaccine for use in humans, *MMWR Morb Mortal Wkly Rep* 37: No. 14; 217, 223, 1988.

Robinson PA: Rabies virus. In Belshe RB, editor: *Textbook of human virology*, ed 2, St Louis, 1991, Mosby.

Steele JH: Rabies in the Americas and remarks on the global aspects, *Rev Infect Dis* 10(suppl 4):S585-S597, 1988.

Strauss JM, Strauss EG: *Viruses and human disease*, San Diego, 2002, Academic Press.

Warrell DA, Warrell MJ: Human rabies and its prevention: An overview, *Rev Infect Dis* 10(suppl 4):S726-S731, 1988.

Winkler WG, Bogel K: Control of rabies in wildlife, *Sci Am* 266:86-92, 1992.

Wunner WH et al: The molecular biology of rabies viruses, *Rev Infect Dis* 10(suppl 4):S771-S784, 1988.

Filoviruses

Klenk HD: *Marburg and Ebola viruses, Current topics in microbiology and immunology*, vol 235, Berlin, New York, 1999, Springer-Verlag.

Preston R: *The hot zone*, New York, 1994, Random House.

Sodhi A: Ebola virus disease, *Postgrad Med* 99:75-76, 1996.

Borna Viruses

Hatalski CG, Lewis AJ, Lipkin WI: Borna disease, *Emerging Infectious Diseases*, 3(2), 1997. (Available online at www.cdc.gov/ncidod/EID/vol3no2/hatalski.htm#ref1)

Jordan I, Lipkin WI: Borna disease virus, *Rev Med Virol* 11:37-57, 2001.

Website

Rabies virus fact sheet: Available online at www.cdc.gov/ncidod/dvrd/rabies/Professional/professi.htm

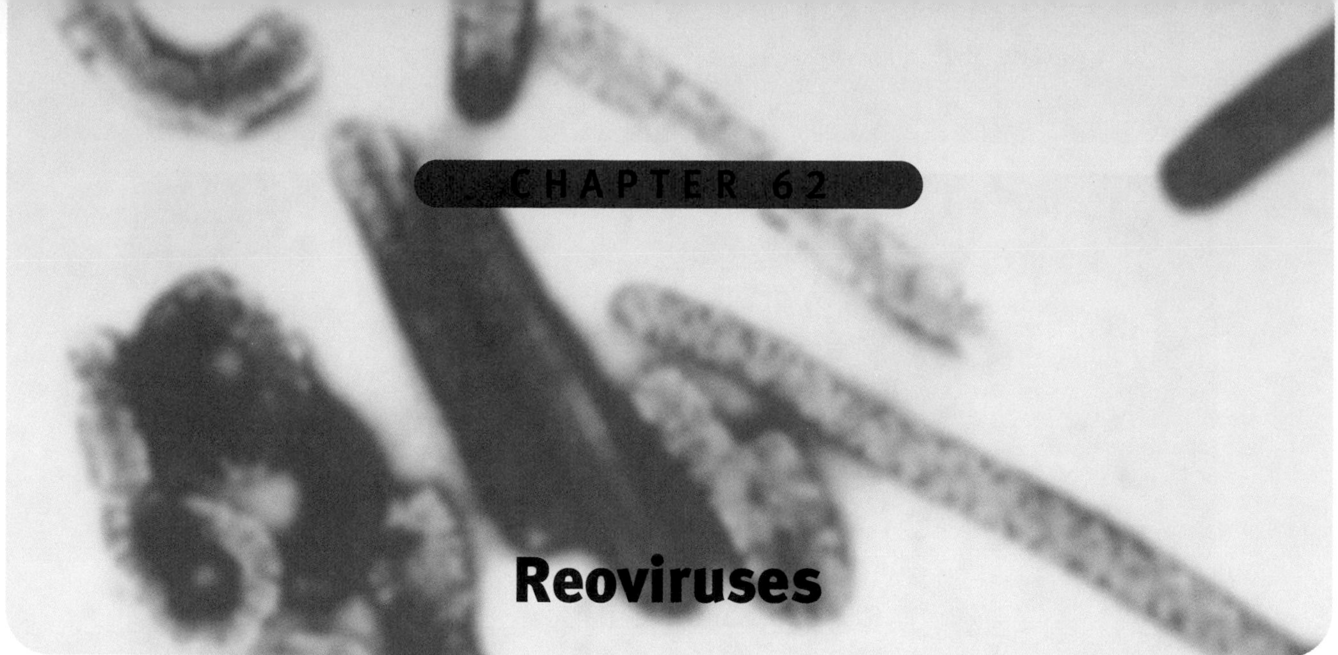

Reoviruses

The **Reoviridae** consist of the orthoreoviruses, rotaviruses, orbiviruses, and coltiviruses (Table 62–1). The name reovirus was proposed in 1959 by Albert Sabin for a group of respiratory and enteric viruses that were not associated with any known disease **(respiratory, enteric, orphan).** The Reoviridae are nonenveloped viruses with **double-layered protein capsids** containing **10 to 12 segments of the double-stranded ribonucleic acid (RNA) genomes.** These viruses are stable over wide pH and temperature ranges and in airborne aerosols. The orbiviruses and coltiviruses are spread by arthropods and are arboviruses.

The **orthoreoviruses,** also referred to as mammalian reoviruses or, simply, reoviruses, were first isolated in the 1950s from the stools of children. They are the prototype of this virus family, and the molecular basis of their pathogenesis has been studied extensively. In general, these viruses cause asymptomatic infections in humans.

Rotaviruses cause **human infantile gastroenteritis,** a very common disease. In fact, rotaviruses account for approximately 50% of all cases of diarrhea in children requiring hospitalization because of dehydration (70,000 cases per year in the United States). Rotaviruses are even more of a problem in underdeveloped countries, where they may be responsible for at least 1 million deaths each year from uncontrolled viral diarrhea in undernourished children.

Structure

Rotaviruses and reoviruses share many structural, replicative, and pathogenic features. Reoviruses and rotaviruses have an icosahedral morphology with a double-layered capsid (60 to 80 nm in diameter) (Box 62–1; Figure 62–1) and a double-stranded segmented genome **("double:double").** The name rotavirus is derived from the Latin word *rota,* meaning "wheel," which refers to the virion's appearance in negative-stained electron micrographs (Figure 62–2). Proteolytic cleavage of the outer capsid (as occurs in the gastrointestinal tract) activates the virus for infection and produces an **intermediate/infectious subviral particle (ISVP).**

The outer capsid is composed of structural proteins (Figure 62–3), which surround a nucleocapsid core that includes enzymes for RNA synthesis and 10 (reo) or 11 (rota) different double-stranded RNA genomic segments. Like the influenza virus capsid, the reovirus and rotavirus capsids are randomly filled with more than 10 or 11 genome segments to generate virions with a complete set of different segments. In addition, **reassortment of gene segments** can occur and thus create hybrid viruses.

Interestingly, rotaviruses resemble enveloped viruses in that they (1) have glycoproteins that act as the viral attachment proteins, (2) acquire but then lose an envelope during assembly, and (3) appear to have a fusion protein activity that promotes direct penetration of the target cell membrane.

The genomic segments of rotaviruses and reoviruses encode structural and nonstructural proteins. The genomic segments of reovirus, the proteins they encode, and their functions are summarized in Table 62–2; those of rotavirus are summarized in Table 62–3. Core proteins include enzymatic activities required for the transcription of messenger RNA (mRNA). They include a 5′-methyl guanosine mRNA capping enzyme and an RNA polymerase. The σ1 protein (reo) and VP4 (rota) are located at the vertices of the capsid and extend from the surface like spike proteins. They have several functions, including hemagglutination and viral attachment, and they elicit neutralizing antibodies. VP4 is activated by protease cleavage, exposing a structure similar to that of the fusion proteins of paramyxoviruses. Its cleavage is necessary for

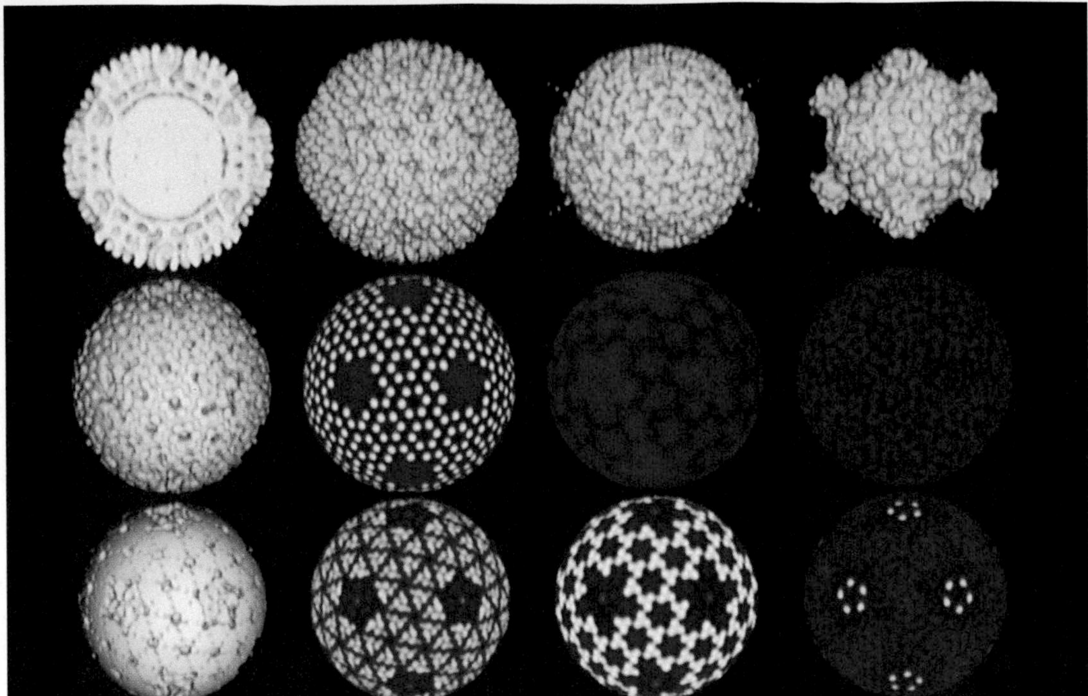

FIGURE 62–1. Computer reconstruction of cryoelectron micrographs of human reovirus type 1 (Lang). *Top, left to right,* Cross section of virion, intermediate/infectious subviral particle (ISVP), and core particle. The ISVP and core particles are generated by proteolysis of the virion and play important roles in the replication cycle. *Center and bottom,* Computer-generated images of the virions at different radii after the outer layers of features have been shaved off. The colors help one visualize the symmetry and molecular interactions within the capsid. (Courtesy Tim Baker, Purdue University.)

TABLE 62–1. Reoviridae Responsible for Human Disease

Virus	Disease
Orthoreovirus*	Mild upper respiratory tract illness, gastrointestinal tract illness, biliary atresia
Orbivirus/coltivirus	Febrile illness with headache and myalgia (zoonosis)
Rotavirus	Gastrointestinal tract illness, respiratory tract illness (?)

*Reovirus is the common name for the family Reoviridae and for the specific genus *Orthoreovirus.*

BOX 62–1. Unique Features of Reoviridae

Double-layered capsid virion (60 to 80 nm) has icosahedral symmetry containing 10 to 12 unique **double-stranded genomic segments** (depending on the virus) (*double:double virus).*

Virion is **resistant** to environmental and gastrointestinal conditions (e.g., detergents, acidic pH, drying).

Rotavirus and orthoreovirus virions are activated by mild proteolysis to intermediate/infectious subviral particles, increasing their infectivity.

Inner capsid contains a complete transcription system, including RNA-dependent RNA polymerase and enzymes for 5′ capping and polyadenylate addition.

Viral replication occurs in the cytoplasm. Double-stranded RNA remains in the inner core.

Inner capsid aggregates around (+) RNA and transcribes (–) RNA in the cytoplasm.

Rotavirus-filled inner capsid buds into the endoplasmic reticulum, acquiring its outer capsid and a membrane, which is then lost.

Virus is released by cell lysis.

productive entry of the virus into cells. The viral attachment proteins, σ3 of reoviruses and VP7 of rotaviruses, elicit neutralizing antibody.

Replication

The replication of reoviruses and rotaviruses starts with ingestion of the virus (Figure 62–4). The virion outer capsid protects the inner nucleocapsid and core from the environment, especially the acidic environment of the gastrointestinal tract. The complete virion is then partially digested in the gastrointestinal tract and presumably activated by protease cleavage and loss of the external capsid proteins (σ3/VP7) and cleavage of the σ1/VP4 protein to produce the ISVP. The σ1/VP4 protein at the

TABLE 62–2. Functions of Reovirus Gene Products

Genomic Segments (Molecular Weight, Da)	Protein	Function (If Known)
Large segments (2.8×10^6)		
1	λ3 (inner capsid)	Polymerase
2	λ2 (outer capsid)	Capping enzyme
3	λ1 (inner capsid)	Transcriptase component
Medium segments (1.4×10^6)		
1	μ2 (inner capsid)	—
2	μ1C (outer capsid)	Cleaved from μ1, complexes with σ3, promotes entry
3	μNS	Promotes viral assembly*
Small segments (0.7×10^6)		
1	σ1 (outer capsid)	Viral attachment protein, hemagglutinin, determines tissue tropism†
2	σ2 (inner capsid)	Facilitates viral RNA synthesis
3	σNS	Facilitates viral RNA synthesis
4	σ3 (outer capsid)	Major component of outer capsid with μ1C

Modified from Field BN et al, editors: *Virology,* ed 3, New York, 1996, Lippincott-Raven.
*Proteins are not found in the virion.
†Neutralizing antibodies.

TABLE 62–3. Functions of Rotavirus Gene Products

Gene Segment	Protein (Location)	Function
1	VP1 (inner capsid)	Polymerase
2	VP2 (inner capsid)	Transcriptase component
3	VP3 (inner capsid)	mRNA capping
4	VP4 (outer capsid spike protein at vertices of virion)	Activation by protease to VP5 and VP8 in ISVP, hemagglutinin, viral attachment protein
5	NSP1 (NS53)	RNA binding
6	VP6 (inner capsid)	Major structural protein of inner capsid, binding to NS28 at ER to promote assembly of outer capsid
7	NSP3 (NS34)	RNA binding
8	NSP2 (NS35)	RNA binding
9	VP7 (outer capsid)	Type-specific antigen, major outer capsid component that is glycosylated in ER and facilitates attachment and entry
10	NSP4 (NS28)	Glycosylated protein in ER that promotes inner capsid binding to ER, transient envelopment, and addition of outer capsid; acts as enterotoxin to mobilize calcium
11	NSP5 (NS26)	RNA binding

ER, Endoplasmic reticulum; ISVP, intermediate/infectious subviral particle.
Modified from Field BN et al, editors: *Virology,* ed 3, New York, 1996, Lippincott-Raven.

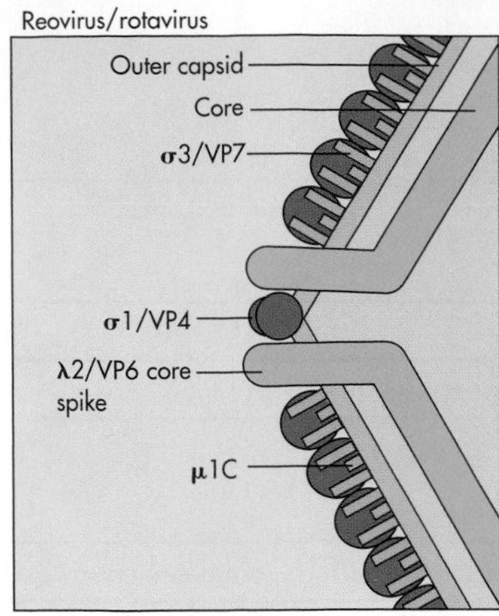

FIGURE 62–2. Structure of reovirus/rotavirus core and outer proteins. σ1/VP4, Viral attachment protein; σ3/VP7, major capsid component; λ2/VP6, major inner capsid protein; μ1C, minor outer capsid protein. (Redrawn from Sharpe AH, Fields BN: *N Engl J Med* 312:486-497, 1985.)

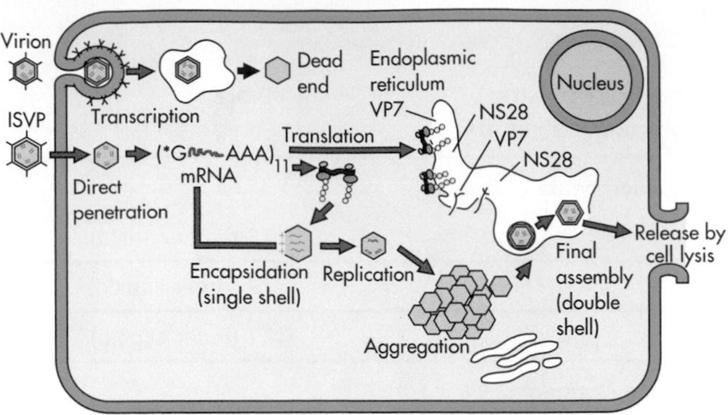

FIGURE 62–4. Replication of rotavirus. Rotavirus virions are activated by protease (e.g., in the gastrointestinal tract) to an intermediate/infectious subviral particle (ISVP). The ISVP binds, penetrates the cell, and loses its outer capsid. The inner capsid contains the enzymes for mRNA transcription using the (±) strand as a template. Some mRNA segments are transcribed early; others are transcribed later. Enzymes in the virion cores attach 5′-methyl capped guanosine (***G**) and 3′ poly A (**AAA**) to mRNA. VP7 and NS28 are synthesized as glycoproteins and expressed in the endoplasmic reticulum. (+) RNA is mRNA and is also enclosed into inner capsids as a template to replicate the ± segmented genome. The capsids aggregate and "dock" onto the NS28 protein in the endoplasmic reticulum, acquiring VP7 and its outer capsid and an envelope. The virus loses the envelope and leaves the cell on cell lysis.

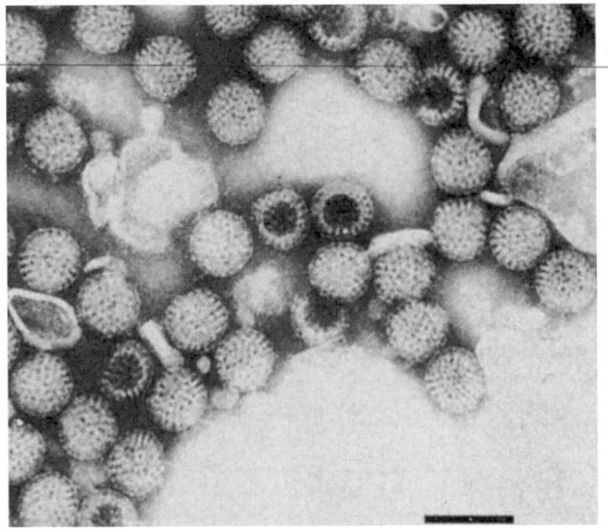

FIGURE 62–3. Electon micrograph of rotavirus. *Bar* = 100 nm. (From Fields BN et al, editors: *Virology,* New York, Raven, 1985.)

vertices of the ISVP binds to sialic acid–containing glycoproteins on epithelial and other cells, which include the β-adrenergic receptor for reovirus and integrin molecules for rotavirus. The ISVP of rotavirus appears to penetrate through the target cell membrane directly. Whole virions of reovirus and rotavirus can be taken up by receptor-mediated endocytosis; however, this is a dead-end pathway for rotavirus.

The ISVP releases the core into the cytoplasm, and the enzymes in the core initiate mRNA production. The **double-stranded RNA always remains in the core.** Transcription of the genome occurs in two phases, early and late, before replication of the genome. In a manner similar to a negative-sense RNA virus, each of the negative-sense (−) RNA strands is used as a template by virion core enzymes, which synthesize individual mRNAs. Virus-encoded enzymes within the core add a 5′-methyl guanosine cap and a 3′-polyadenylate tail. The mRNA then leaves the core and is translated. Later, virion proteins and positive-sense (+) RNA segments associate together into corelike structures that aggregate into large cytoplasmic inclusions. The (+) RNA segments are copied to produce (−) RNAs in the new cores, replicating the double-stranded genome. The new cores either generate more (+) RNA or are assembled into virions.

The assembly processes for reovirus and rotavirus differ. In the assembly of reovirus the outer capsid proteins associate with the core, and the virion leaves the cell upon cell lysis. Assembly of rotavirus resembles that of an enveloped virus, in that the rotavirus cores associate with the NS28 viral protein on the outside of the endoplasmic reticulum (ER) and, on budding into the ER, acquire its VP7 outer capsid protein. The membrane is lost in the ER, and the virus leaves the cell during cell lysis. Reovirus inhibits cellular macromolecular synthesis within 8 hours of infection.

Orthoreoviruses (Mammalian Reoviruses)

The orthoreoviruses are ubiquitous. The virions are very stable and have been detected in sewage and river water. The mammalian reoviruses occur in three serotypes, referred to as reovirus types 1, 2, and 3; these serotypes are based on neutralization and hemagglutination-inhibition tests. All three serotypes share a common complement-fixing antigen.

PATHOGENESIS AND IMMUNITY

Orthoreoviruses do not cause significant disease in humans. However, studies of reovirus disease in mice have advanced our understanding of the pathogenesis of viral infections in humans. Depending on the reovirus strain, the virus can be neurotropic or viscerotropic in mice. The functions and virulence properties of the reovirus proteins were identified through comparison of the activities of interstrain hybrid viruses that differ in only one genomic segment (encoding one protein). With this approach, the new activity is attributable to the genomic segment from the other virus strain.

After ingestion and proteolytic production of the ISVP, the orthoreoviruses bind to M cells in the small intestine, which then transfer the virus to the lymphoid tissue of Peyer's patches lining the intestines. The viruses then replicate and initiate a viremia. Although the virus is cytolytic in vitro, it causes few if any symptoms before entering the circulation and producing infection at a distant site. In the mouse model, the outer capsid protein responsible for causing hemagglutinin activity (δ1) also facilitates viral spread to the mesenteric lymph nodes and determines whether the virus is neurotropic.

Mice, and presumably humans, mount protective humoral and cellular immune responses to outer capsid proteins. Although orthoreoviruses are normally lytic, they can also establish persistent infection in cell culture.

EPIDEMIOLOGY

As already mentioned, the orthoreoviruses have been found worldwide. Seroprevalence studies suggest that most people are probably infected during childhood, because approximately 75% of adults have the antibody. Most animals, including chimpanzees and monkeys, are infected with reoviruses that are serologically related to human reovirus. It is not known whether animals are a reservoir for human infections.

CLINICAL SYNDROMES

Orthoreoviruses infect people of all ages, but linking specific diseases to these agents has been difficult. Most infections are thought to be asymptomatic or are so mild that they go undetected. Thus far, these viruses have been linked to common cold–like, mild upper respiratory tract illness (low-grade fever, rhinorrhea, pharyngitis), gastrointestinal tract disease, and biliary atresia.

LABORATORY DIAGNOSIS

Human orthoreovirus infection can be detected through assay of the viral antigen or RNA in clinical material, virus isolation, or serologic assays for virus-specific antibody. Throat, nasopharyngeal, and stool specimens from patients with suspected upper respiratory tract or diarrheal disease are used as samples. Human orthoreoviruses can be isolated using mouse L-cell fibroblasts, primary monkey kidney cells, and HeLa cells. Serologic assays can be performed for epidemiologic purposes.

TREATMENT, PREVENTION, AND CONTROL

Orthoreovirus disease is mild and self-limited. For this reason, treatment has not been necessary, and prevention and control measures have not been investigated.

Rotaviruses

Rotaviruses are common agents of infantile diarrhea worldwide. The rotaviruses are a large group of gastroenteritis-causing viruses found in many different mammals and birds.

Rotavirus virions are relatively stable at room temperature and to treatment with detergents, at pH extremes of 3.5 to 10, and even with repeated freezing and thawing. Proteolytic enzymes such as trypsin enhance infectivity.

Human and animal rotaviruses are divided into serotypes, groups, and subgroups. Serotypes are distinguished primarily by the VP7 outer capsid protein and, to a lesser extent, by the VP4 minor outer capsid protein. Groups are determined primarily on the basis of the antigenicity of VP6 and the electrophoretic mobility of the genomic segments. Seven groups (A to G) of human and animal rotaviruses have been identified on the basis of the VP6 inner capsid protein. Human disease is caused by group A rotavirus and, occasionally, group B and C rotaviruses.

PATHOGENESIS AND IMMUNITY

The rotavirus can survive the acidic environment in a buffered stomach or in a stomach after a meal (Box 62–2). Viral replication occurs after adsorption to columnar epithelial cells covering the villi of the small intestine. Approximately 8 hours after infection, cytoplasmic inclusions are seen that contain newly synthesized proteins and RNA. As many as 10^{10} viral particles per gram of stool may be released during disease. Studies of the small intestine, either of experimentally infected animals or in biopsy specimens from infants, show shortening and blunting of the microvilli and mononuclear cell infiltration into the lamina propria.

BOX 62–2. Disease Mechanisms of Rotavirus

Virus is spread by the **fecal-oral route** and possibly the respiratory route.
Cytolytic and toxinlike action on the intestinal epithelium causes loss of electrolytes and prevents readsorption of water.
Disease can be significant in infants younger than 24 months, but it is asymptomatic in adults.
Large amounts of virus are released during the diarrheal phase.

Like cholera, rotavirus infection prevents the absorption of water, causing a net secretion of water and loss of ions, which together result in a watery diarrhea. The NSP4 protein of rotavirus acts in a toxinlike manner to promote calcium ion influx into enterocytes, release of neuronal activators, and a neuronal alteration in water absorption. The loss of fluids and electrolytes can lead to severe dehydration and even death if therapy does not include electrolyte replacement.

Immunity to infection requires the presence of antibody, primarily immunoglobulin (Ig)A, in the lumen of the gut. Actively or passively acquired antibody (including antibody in colostrum and mothers' milk) can lessen the severity of disease but does not consistently prevent reinfection. In the absence of antibody, the inoculation of even small amounts of virus causes infection and diarrhea. Infection in infants and small children is generally symptomatic, whereas that in adults is usually asymptomatic.

BOX 62–3. Epidemiology of Rotavirus

Disease/Viral Factors
Capsid virus is resistant to environmental and gastrointestinal conditions.
Large amounts of virus are released in fecal matter.
Asymptomatic infection can result in release of virus.

Transmission
Virus is transmitted in fecal matter, especially in daycare settings.
Respiratory transmission may be possible.

Who Is at Risk?
Rotavirus type A
- Infants younger than 24 months of age: At risk for infantile gastroenteritis with potential dehydration.
- Older children and adults: At risk for mild diarrhea.
- Undernourished people in underdeveloped countries: At risk for diarrhea, dehydration, and death.

Rotavirus type B (adult diarrhea rotavirus, ADRV)
- Infants, older children, and adults in China: At risk for severe gastroenteritis.

Geography/Season
Virus is found worldwide.
Disease is more common in autumn, winter, and spring.

Modes of Control
Hand washing and isolation of known cases are modes of control.
Experimental live vaccines use human, bovine, or monkey reassorted rotavirus.

EPIDEMIOLOGY

Rotaviruses are ubiquitous worldwide, with 95% of children infected by 3 to 5 years of age (Box 62–3). It is assumed that rotaviruses are passed from person to person by the **fecal-oral route.** Maximal shedding of the virus occurs 2 to 5 days after the start of diarrhea but can occur without symptoms. The virus survives well on fomites (e.g., furniture and toys) and on hands, because it can withstand drying. Although domestic animals are known to harbor serologically related rotaviruses, they are not believed to be a common source of human infection. Outbreaks occur in preschools and daycare centers and among hospitalized infants.

Rotaviruses are **one of the most common causes of serious diarrhea in young children** worldwide, affecting more than 18 million infants and children and accounting for close to one million deaths due to dehydration per year. In North America, outbreaks occur annually during the autumn, winter, and spring. More severe disease occurs in severely malnourished children. Rotavirus diarrhea is a very contagious, severe, life-threatening disease for infants in developing countries, and it occurs year-round. Several outbreaks of type B Rotavirus have occurred in China because of contaminated water supplies that affected millions of people.

BOX 62–4. Clinical Summary

Rotavirus: A one-year-old infant has watery diarrhea, vomiting, and fever for 4 days. Enzyme-linked immunosorbent assay analysis of stool confirm rotavirus. The baby is very dehydrated.

CLINICAL SYNDROMES (BOX 62–4)

Rotavirus is a major cause of gastroenteritis. The incubation period for rotavirus diarrheal illness is estimated to be 48 hours. The major clinical findings in hospitalized patients are **vomiting, diarrhea, fever,** and **dehydration.** Neither fecal leukocytes nor blood occurs in stool for this form of diarrhea. Rotavirus gastroenteritis is a self-limited disease, and recovery is generally complete and without sequelae. However, the infection may prove fatal in infants who live in developing countries and who are malnourished and dehydrated before the infection.

LABORATORY DIAGNOSIS

The clinical findings in patients with rotavirus infection resemble those of other viral diarrheas (e.g., Norwalk virus). Most patients have large quantities of virus in stool, making the direct detection of viral antigen the method of choice for diagnosis. Enzyme immunoassay and latex agglutination are quick, easy, and relatively inexpensive ways to detect rotavirus in stool. Viral particles in specimens can also be readily detected on electron microscopy.

The cell culture of rotavirus is difficult and not reliable for diagnostic purposes. Serologic studies are primarily used for research and epidemiologic purposes. Because so many people have rotavirus-specific antibody, a fourfold rise in antibody titer is necessary for the diagnosis of recent infection or active disease.

TREATMENT, PREVENTION, AND CONTROL

Rotaviruses are acquired very early in life. Their ubiquitous nature makes it difficult to limit the spread of the virus and infection. Hospitalized patients with disease must be isolated, however, to limit spread of the infection to other susceptible patients.

No specific antiviral therapy is available for a rotavirus infection. The morbidity and mortality associated with rotavirus diarrhea result from dehydration and electrolyte imbalance. The purpose of supportive therapy is to replace fluids so that the blood volume and electrolyte and acid-base imbalances are corrected.

Development of a safe rotavirus vaccine is a high priority for protecting children, especially those in underdeveloped countries, from potentially fatal disease. Experimental vaccines have been prepared from animal rotaviruses, such as the rhesus monkey rotavirus and the Nebraska calf diarrhea virus. These vaccines share antigenic determinants with human rotaviruses, do not cause disease in humans, and afford protection against infection. The two vaccines in human trials include a live attenuated vaccine based on single isolate of human virus and a mixture of five antigens from different strains of virus prepared as a live attenuated bovine-human reassortant virus. A recent U.S. Food and Drug Administration (FDA) approved vaccine based on a human-rhesus monkey reassortant elicited protection but was recalled in 1999 because of the incidence of intussusception. The vaccines may not protect against all serotypes of rotavirus.

Coltiviruses and Orbiviruses

The coltiviruses and orbiviruses infect vertebrates and invertebrates. The coltiviruses cause Colorado tick fever and related human disease. The orbiviruses mainly cause disease in animals, including blue tongue disease of sheep, African horse sickness, and epizootic hemorrhagic disease of deer.

Colorado tick fever, an acute disease characterized by fever, headache, and severe myalgia, was originally described in the nineteenth century and is now believed to be one of the most common tick-borne viral diseases in the United States. Although hundreds of infections occur annually, the exact number is not known because Colorado tick fever is not a reportable disease.

The structure and physiology of the coltiviruses and orbiviruses are similar to those of the other Reoviridae, with the following major exceptions:

1. The outer capsid of the orbiviruses has no discernible capsomeric structure, even though the inner capsid is icosahedral.
2. The virus causes viremia, infects erythrocyte precursors, and remains in the mature red blood cells protected from the immune response.
3. The orbivirus life cycle includes vertebrates and invertebrates (insects).

Colorado tick fever viruses have 12 double-stranded RNA genomic segments, and orbiviruses have 10.

PATHOGENESIS

Colorado tick fever virus infects erythroid precursor cells without severely damaging them. The virus remains within the cells, even after they mature into red blood cells; this factor protects the virus from clearance. The resulting viremia can persist for weeks or months, even after symptomatic recovery. Both of these factors promote transmission of the virus to the tick vector.

Serious hemorrhagic disease can result from the infection of vascular endothelial and vascular smooth muscle cells and pericytes, thereby weakening capillary structure. The weakness leads to leakage and hemorrhage and, potentially, hypotension and shock. Neuronal infection can lead to meningitis and encephalitis.

EPIDEMIOLOGY

Colorado tick fever occurs in western and northwestern areas of the United States and western Canada, where the wood tick *Dermacentor andersoni* is distributed (elevations of 4000 to 10,000 feet) (Figure 62–5). Ticks acquire the virus by feeding on a viremic host and subsequently

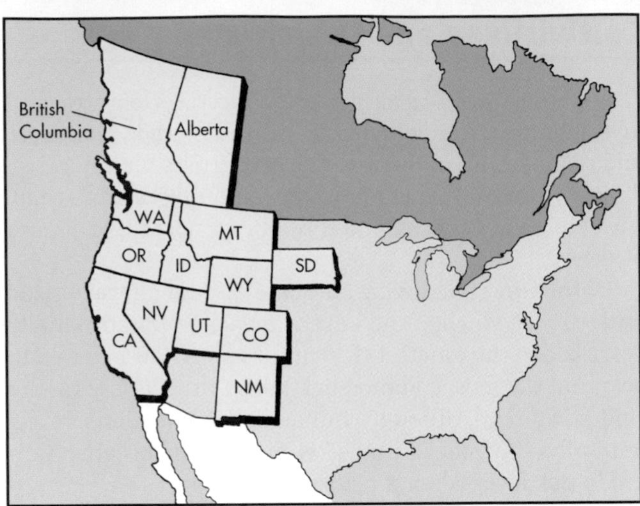

FIGURE 62–5. Geographic distribution of Colorado tick fever.

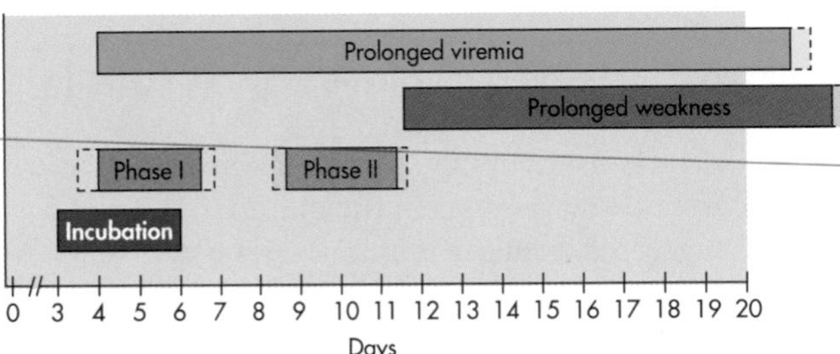

FIGURE 62–6. Time course of Colorado tick fever.

transmit the virus in saliva when feeding on a new host. Natural hosts of this virus constitute many mammals, including squirrels, chipmunks, rabbits, and deer. Human disease is observed during the spring, summer, and autumn, seasons when humans are more likely to invade the habitat of the tick.

CLINICAL SYNDROMES

Colorado tick fever virus generally causes mild or subclinical infection. The symptoms of the acute disease resemble those of dengue fever. After a 3- to 6-day incubation period, symptomatic infections start with the sudden onset of fever, chills, headache, photophobia, myalgia, arthralgia, and lethargy (Figure 62–6). Characteristics of the infection include a biphasic fever and conjunctivitis, and possibly lymphadenopathy, hepatosplenomegaly, and a maculopapular or petechial rash. A leukopenia involving both neutrophils and lymphocytes is an important hallmark of the disease. Children occasionally have a more severe hemorrhagic disease. Colorado tick fever must be differentiated from Rocky Mountain spotted fever, a tick-borne rickettsial infection characterized by a rash, because the latter disease may require antibiotic treatment.

LABORATORY DIAGNOSIS

A diagnosis of Colorado tick fever can be established through the direct detection of viral antigens, virus isolation, or serologic tests. The best, most rapid method is detection of viral antigen on the surfaces of erythrocytes in a blood smear through the use of immunofluorescence. Laboratory tests may be available through state Public Health departments or the Centers for Disease Control and Prevention.

The titers of antibody in acute and convalescent specimens must be compared for a serologically based diagnosis to be rendered, because subclinical infections can occur and antibody may persist for a lifetime. Specific IgM is present for approximately 45 days after the onset of illness, and its detection is also presumptive evidence of an acute or a very recent infection. Immunofluorescence is the best technique, but complement fixation, neutralization, and enzyme immunoassay are also used to detect Colorado tick fever antibody.

TREATMENT, PREVENTION, AND CONTROL

No specific treatment is available for Colorado tick fever. The disease is generally self-limited, indicating that supportive care is sufficient. The viremia is long lasting, implying that infected patients should not donate blood soon after recovery. Prevention consists of (1) avoiding tick-infested areas, (2) using protective clothing and tick repellents, and (3) removing ticks before they bite. Unlike tick-borne rickettsial disease, in which prolonged feeding is required for the bacteria to be transmitted, the coltivirus from the tick's saliva can enter the bloodstream rapidly. A formalinized Colorado tick fever vaccine has been developed and evaluated, but because of the mildness of the disease, its distribution to the general public is not warranted.

CASE STUDY AND QUESTIONS

In January a 6-month-old boy was seen in the emergency department after 2 days of persistent watery diarrhea and vomiting accompanied by a low-grade fever and mild cough. The infant appeared dehydrated and required hospitalization. The patient attended a daycare center.

1. In addition to rotavirus, what other viral agents must be considered in the differential diagnosis of this infant's disease? What agents would need consideration if the patient were a teenager or an adult?
2. How would the diagnosis of rotavirus have been confirmed?
3. How was the virus transmitted? How long was the patient contagious?
4. Who was at risk for serious disease?

Bibliography

Balows A et al, editors: *Laboratory diagnosis of infectious diseases: Principles and practice,* New York, 1988, Springer-Verlag.

Bellamy AR, Both GW: Molecular biology of rotaviruses, *Adv Virol* 38:1-44, 1990.

Belshe RB, editor: *Textbook of human virology,* ed 2, St Louis, 1991, Mosby.

Blacklow NR, Greenberg HB: Viral gastroenteritis, *N Engl J Med* 325:252-264, 1991.

Christensen ML: Human viral gastroenteritis, *Clin Microbiol Rev* 2:51–89, 1989.

Cohen J, Powderly WG, editors: *Infectious diseases,* ed 2, St Louis, 2004, Mosby.

Feigin RD, et al, editors: *Textbook of pediatric infectious disease,* ed 5, Philadelphia, 2004, WB Saunders.

Flint SJ et al: *Principles of virology: Molecular biology, pathogenesis and control of animal viruses,* ed 2, Washington, 2003, American Society for Microbiology Press.

Joklik WK, editor: *The Reoviridae,* New York, 1983, Plenum.

Knipe DM, Howley PM, editors: *Fields virology,* ed 4, New York, 2001, Lippincott-Williams and Wilkins.

Nibert ML et al: Mechanisms of viral pathogenesis: Distinct forms of reovirus and their roles during replication in cells and host, *J Clin Invest* 88:727-734, 1991.

Ramig RF: Rotaviruses, *Curr Top Microbiol Immunol* 185:1-380, 1994.

Sharpe AH, Fields BN: Pathogenesis of viral infections: Basic concepts derived from the reovirus model, *N Engl J Med* 312:486-497, 1985.

Strauss JM, Strauss EG: *Viruses and human disease,* San Diego, 2002, Academic Press.

Tyler KL, Oldstone MBA, editors: Reoviruses, *Curr Top Microbiol Immunol,* vol 233, Berlin, New York, 1998, Springer.

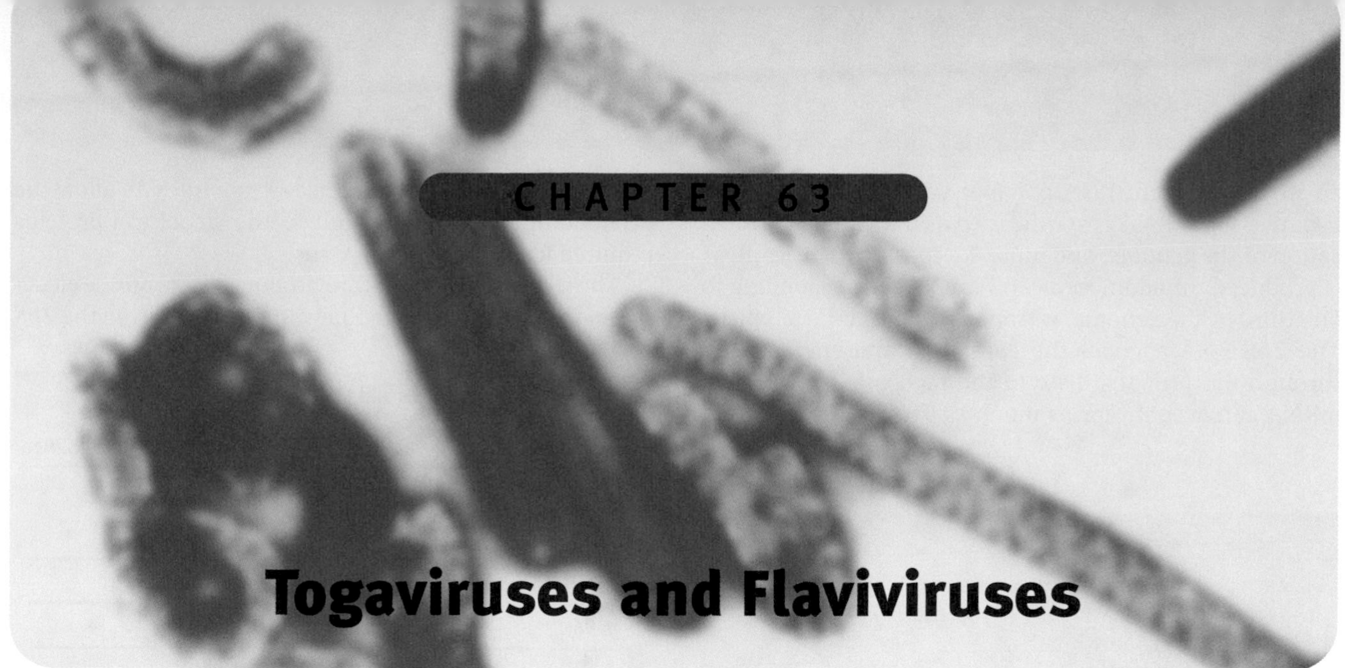

Togaviruses and Flaviviruses

The members of the Togaviridae and Flaviviridae families are enveloped, positive, single-stranded ribonucleic acid (RNA) viruses (Box 63–1). Alphavirus and Flavivirus are discussed together because of similarities in the diseases that they cause, as well as in epidemiology. Most are transmitted by arthropods and are therefore **arboviruses (*ar*thropod-*bo*rne viruses).** They differ in size, morphology, gene sequence, and replication.

The togaviruses can be classified into the following major genera (Table 63–1): Alphavirus, Rubivirus, and Arterivirus. No known arteriviruses cause disease in humans, so this genus is not discussed further. **Rubella** virus is the only member of the Rubivirus group; it is discussed separately, however, because its disease manifestation *(German measles)* and its means of spread differ from those of the alphaviruses. The Flaviviridae include the flaviviruses, pestiviruses, and hepaciviruses (hepatitis C and G viruses). Hepatitis C and G are discussed in Chapter 62.

Alphaviruses and Flaviviruses

The alphaviruses and flaviviruses were classified as arboviruses because they are usually spread by arthropod vectors. These viruses have a very **broad host range,** including vertebrates (e.g., mammals, birds, amphibians, reptiles) and invertebrates (e.g., mosquitoes, ticks). Diseases spread by animals or with an animal reservoir are called **zoonoses.** Examples of pathogenic alphaviruses and flaviviruses are listed in Table 63–2.

STRUCTURE AND REPLICATION OF ALPHAVIRUSES

The alphaviruses are similar to the picornaviruses in having an **icosahedral capsid** and a positive-sense, single-strand RNA genome that resembles messenger RNA (mRNA). They differ from picornaviruses by being slightly larger (45 to 75 nm in diameter) and are surrounded by an **envelope** (Latin *toga,* "cloak"). In addition, the togavirus genome encodes **early** and **late proteins.**

Alphaviruses have two or three glycoproteins that associate to form a single spike. The COOH-terminus of the glycoproteins is anchored in the capsid, forcing the envelope to wrap tightly ("shrink-wrap") and take on the shape of the capsid (Figure 63–1). The capsid proteins of all the alphaviruses are similar in structure and are antigenically cross-reactive. The envelope glycoproteins express unique antigenic determinants that distinguish the different viruses and also express antigenic determinants that are shared by a group, or "complex," of viruses.

The alphaviruses attach to specific receptors expressed on many different cell types from many different species (Figure 63–2). The host range for these viruses includes vertebrates, such as humans, monkeys, horses, birds, reptiles, and amphibians, and invertebrates, such as mosquitoes and ticks. However, the individual viruses have different tissue tropisms, accounting somewhat for the different disease presentations.

The virus enters the cell by means of receptor-mediated endocytosis (see Figure 63–2). The viral envelope then fuses with the membrane of the endosome on acidification of the vesicle to deliver the capsid and genome into the cytoplasm.

Once released into the cytoplasm the alphavirus genomes bind to ribosomes as mRNA. The alphavirus genome is translated in early and late phases. The initial two thirds of the alphavirus RNA is translated into a polyprotein, which is subsequently cleaved by proteases into four nonstructural early proteins (NSPs 1 through 4). Each of these proteins contains a protease activity and an RNA-dependent RNA polymerase. A full-length, 42S, negative-sense RNA is synthesized as a template for replication of the genome, and more 42S positive-sense mRNA is produced. In addition, a 26S mRNA, corresponding to one third of the genome, is transcribed from the template. The 26S RNA encodes the capsid (C) and envelope (E1 through E3) proteins. Late in the replication cycle, viral mRNA can account for as much as 90% of the mRNA in the infected cell. The abundance of late mRNAs allow the production of a large amount of the structural proteins required for packaging the virus.

The structural proteins are produced by protease cleavage of the late polyprotein that was produced from the 26S

BOX 63–1. Unique Features of Togaviruses and Flaviviruses

Viruses have enveloped, single-stranded, positive-sense RNA.
Togavirus replication includes early (nonstructural) and late (structural) protein synthesis.
Togaviruses replicate in the cytoplasm and bud at the plasma membranes.
Flaviviruses replicate in the cytoplasm and bud at internal membranes.

TABLE 63–1. Togaviruses and Flaviviruses

Virus Group	Human Pathogens
Togaviruses	
Alphavirus	Arboviruses
Rubivirus	Rubella virus
Pestivirus	None
Arterivirus	None
Flaviviruses	Arboviruses
Hepaciviridae	Hepatitis C virus

TABLE 63–2. Arboviruses

Disease	Vector	Host	Distribution	Disease
Alphaviruses				
Sindbis*	*Aedes* and other mosquitoes	Birds	Africa, Australia, India	Subclinical
Semliki Forest*	*Aedes* and other mosquitoes	Birds	East and West Africa	Subclinical
Venezuelan equine encephalitis	*Aedes*, *Culex*	Rodents, horses	North, South, and Central America	Mild systemic; severe encephalitis
Eastern equine encephalitis	*Aedes*, *Culiseta*	Birds	North and South America, Caribbean	Mild systemic; encephalitis
Western equine encephalitis	*Culex*, *Culiseta*	Birds	North and South America	Mild systemic; encephalitis
Chikungunya	*Aedes*	Humans, monkeys	Africa, Asia	Fever, arthralgia, arthritis
Flaviviruses				
Dengue*	*Aedes*	Humans, monkeys	Worldwide, especially tropics	Mild systemic; break-bone fever, dengue hemorrhagic fever, and dengue shock syndrome
Yellow fever*	*Aedes*	Humans, monkeys	Africa, South America	Hepatitis, hemorrhagic fever
Japanese encephalitis	*Culex*	Pigs, birds	Asia	Encephalitis
West Nile encephalitis	*Culex*	Birds	Africa, Europe, central Asia, North America	Fever, encephalitis, hepatitis
St. Louis encephalitis	*Culex*	Birds	North America	Encephalitis
Russian spring-summer encephalitis	*Ixodes* and *Dermacentor* ticks	Birds	Russia	Encephalitis
Powassan encephalitis	*Ixodes* ticks	Small mammals	North America	Encephalitis

*Prototypical viruses.

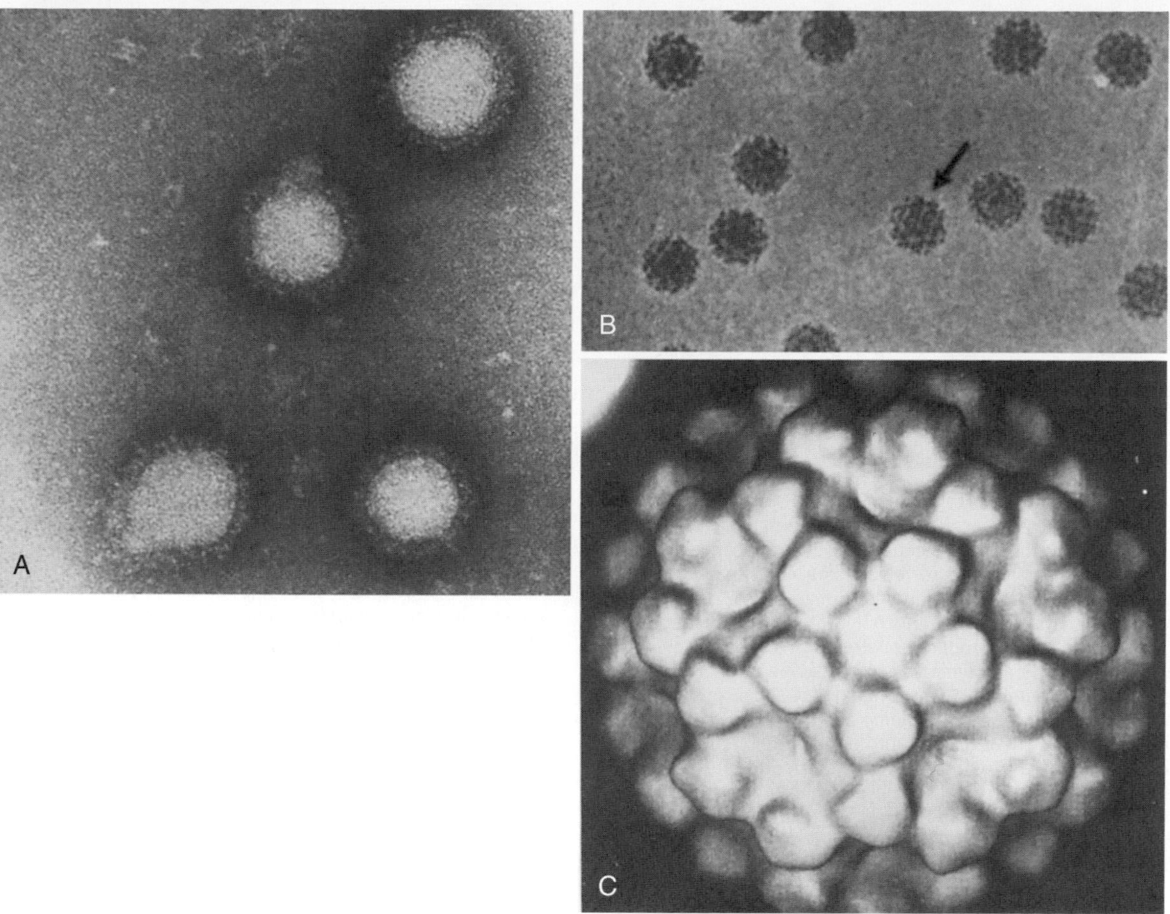

FIGURE 63–1. Alphavirus morphology. **A,** The outline of the envelope and the glycoprotein spikes of the Sindbis virus are visualized by negative staining. **B,** More detail on the morphology of the virion is obtained from cryoelectron microscopy. **C,** Surface representation of the Sindbis virus obtained by image processing of the cryoelectron micrographs indicates that the envelope is held tightly and conforms to the shape and symmetry of the capsid. (From Fuller SD: *Cell* 48:923-934, 1987.)

mRNA. The C protein is translated first and is cleaved from the polyprotein (see Figure 63–2). A signal sequence is then made that associates the nascent polypeptide with the endoplasmic reticulum. Thereafter, envelope glycoproteins are translated, glycosylated, and cleaved from the remaining portion of the polyprotein to produce the E1, E2, and E3 glycoprotein spikes. The E3 is released from most alphavirus glycoprotein spikes. The glycoproteins are processed by the normal cellular machinery in the endoplasmic reticulum and Golgi apparatus and are also acetylated and acylated with long-chain fatty acids (see Figure 63–2). Alphavirus glycoproteins are then transferred efficiently to the plasma membrane.

The C proteins associate with the genomic RNA soon after their synthesis and form an icosahedral capsid. Once this step is completed the capsid associates with portions of the membrane expressing the viral glycoproteins. The alphavirus capsid has binding sites for the C-terminus of the glycoprotein spike, which pulls the envelope tightly around itself in a manner like shrink-wrapping (see Figures 63–1 and 63–2). Alphaviruses are released on budding from the plasma membrane.

STRUCTURE AND REPLICATION OF FLAVIVIRUSES

The flaviviruses also have a positive-strand RNA genome and an envelope. However, the virions of the flavivirus are slightly smaller than those of an alphavirus (37 to 50 nm in diameter), the RNA does not have a polyadenylate sequence, and the virus lacks a visible capsid structure in the virion. Most of the flaviviruses are serologically related, and antibodies to one virus may neutralize another virus.

The attachment and penetration of the flaviviruses occur in the same way as described for the alphaviruses, but the flaviviruses can also attach to the Fc receptors on macrophages, monocytes, and other cells when the virus is coated with antibody. The antibody actually enhances the infectivity of these viruses by providing new receptors

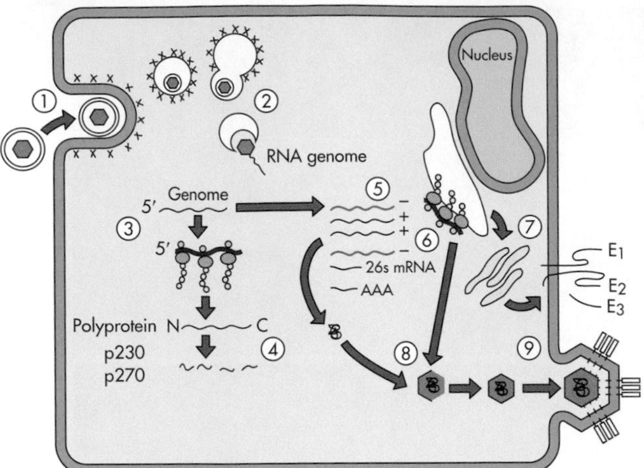

FIGURE 63–2. Replication of a togavirus. Semliki Forest virus. *1,* Semliki Forest virus binds to cell receptors and is internalized in a coated vesicle. *2,* On acidification of the endosome, the viral envelope fuses with the endosomal membrane to release the nucleocapsid into the cytoplasm. *3,* Ribosomes bind to the positive-sense RNA genome, and the p230 or p270 (full-length) early polyproteins are made. *4,* The polyproteins are cleaved to produce nonstructural proteins 1 to 4 (NSP1 to NSP4), which include a polymerase to transcribe the genome into a negative-sense RNA template. *5,* The template is used to produce a full-length 42S positive-sense mRNA genome and a late 26S mRNA for the structural proteins. *6,* The C (capsid) protein is translated first, exposing a protease cleavage site and then a signal peptide for association with the endoplasmic reticulum. *7,* The E glycoproteins are then synthesized, glycosylated, processed in the Golgi apparatus, and transferred to the plasma membrane. *8,* The capsid proteins assemble on the 42S genomic RNA and then associate with regions of cytoplasmic and plasma membranes containing the E1, E2, and E3 spike proteins. *9,* Budding from the plasma membrane releases the virus.

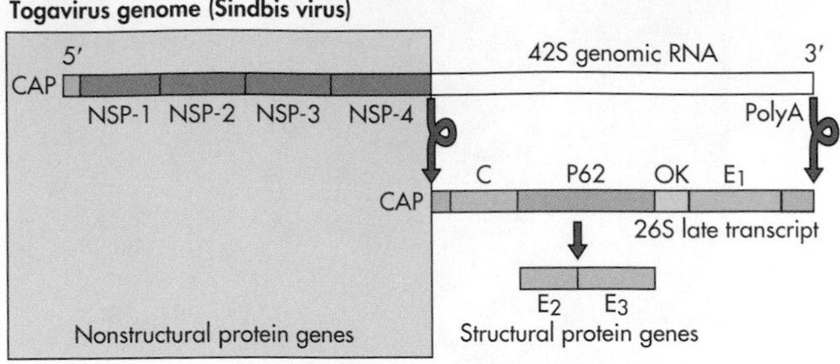

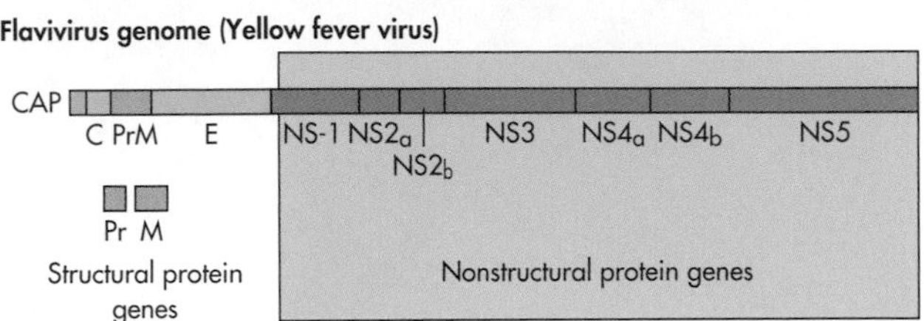

FIGURE 63–3. Comparison of the togavirus (alphavirus) and flavivirus genomes. *Alphavirus:* The enzymatic activities are translated from the 5′-end of the input genome, promoting their early rapid translation. The structural proteins are translated later from a smaller mRNA transcribed from the genomic template. *Flavivirus:* The genes for the structural proteins of the flaviviruses are at the 5′-end of the genome/mRNA, and only one species of polyprotein is made, which represents the entire genome. Poly A, polyadenylate. (Redrawn from Hahn CS et al: *Annu Rev Microbiol* 44:649-688, Copyright 1990 by Annual Reviews, www.AnnualReviews.org.)

for the virus and by promoting viral uptake into these target cells.

The major differences between alphaviruses and flaviviruses are in the organization of their genomes and their mechanisms of protein synthesis. The entire flavivirus genome is translated into a single polyprotein, in a manner more similar to the process for picornaviruses than for alphaviruses (Figure 63–3). As a result, there is no temporal distinction in the translation of the different viral proteins. The polyprotein produced from the yellow fever genome contains four nonstructural proteins, including a protease and an RNA-dependent RNA polymerase, plus the capsid and envelope structural proteins.

Unlike in the alphavirus genome, the structural genes are at the 5′-end of the flavivirus genome. As a result, the portions of the polyprotein containing the structural (not the catalytic) proteins are synthesized first and with the greatest efficiency. This arrangement may allow the production of more structural proteins, but it decreases the efficiency of nonstructural protein synthesis and the initiation of viral replication. This feature of flaviviruses may contribute to the lag before detection of their replication.

Another distinction of the flaviviruses is that they acquire their envelope by budding into intracellular vesicles rather than at the cell surface. The virus is then released by exocytosis or cell lysis mechanisms. This route is less efficient, and the virus may remain cell-associated.

PATHOGENESIS AND IMMUNITY

Because the arboviruses are acquired from the bite of an arthropod such as a mosquito, a knowledge of the course of infection in both the vertebrate host and the invertebrate vector is important for an understanding of the diseases. These viruses can cause lytic or persistent infections of both vertebrate and invertebrate hosts (Box 63–2). Infections of invertebrates are usually persistent, with continued virus production.

The death of an infected cell results from a combination of virus-induced insults. The large amount of viral RNA produced on the replication and transcription of the genome blocks cellular mRNA from binding to ribosomes. Increased permeability of the target cell membrane and changes in ion concentrations can alter enzyme activities and favor the translation of viral mRNA over cellular mRNA. The displacement of cellular mRNA from the protein synthesis machinery prevents rebuilding and maintenance of the cell and is a major cause of the death of the virus-infected cell. Some alphaviruses, such as western equine encephalitis (WEE) virus, make a nucleotide triphosphatase that degrades

BOX 63–2. Disease Mechanisms of Togaviruses and Flaviviruses

Viruses are cytolytic, except for rubella.
Viruses establish systemic infection and viremia.
Viruses are good inducers of interferon, which can account for the flulike symptoms of infection.
Viruses, except rubella and hepatitis C, are arboviruses.
Flaviviruses can infect cells of the monocyte-macrophage lineage. Non-neutralizing antibody can enhance flavivirus infection via Fc receptors on the macrophage.

	Flulike Syndrome	Encephalitis	Hepatitis	Hemorrhage	Shock
Dengue	+		+	+	+
Yellow fever	+		+	+	+
St. Louis encephalitis	+	+			
West Nile encephalitis	+	+			
Venezuelan encephalitis	+	+			
Western equine encephalitis	+	+			
Eastern equine encephalitis	+	+			
Japanese encephalitis	+	+			

deoxyribonucleotides, depleting even the substrate pool for deoxyribonucleic acid (DNA) production.

Female mosquitoes acquire the alphaviruses and flaviviruses by taking a blood meal from a **viremic vertebrate host.** *A sufficient viremia must be maintained in the vertebrate host to allow acquisition of the virus by the mosquito.* The virus then infects the epithelial cells of the midgut of the mosquito, spreads through the basal lamina of the midgut to the circulation, and infects the salivary glands. The virus sets up a persistent infection and replicates to high titers in these cells. The salivary glands can then release virus into the saliva. Not all arthropod species support this type of infection, however. For example, the normal vector for the WEE virus is the *Culex tarsalis* mosquito, but certain strains of virus are limited to the midgut of this mosquito, cannot infect its salivary glands, and therefore cannot be transmitted to humans.

On biting a host, the female mosquito regurgitates virus-containing saliva into the victim's bloodstream. The virus then circulates freely in the host's plasma and comes into contact with susceptible target cells, such as the endothelial cells of the capillaries, monocytes, and macrophages.

The nature of alphavirus and flavivirus disease is determined primarily by (1) the specific tissue tropisms of the individual virus type, (2) the concentration of infecting virus, and (3) individual responses to the infection. These viruses are associated with **mild systemic disease, encephalitis, arthrogenic disease,** or **hemorrhagic disease.**

The initial viremia produces systemic symptoms, such as fever, chills, headaches, backaches, and other flulike symptoms, within 3 to 7 days of infection. Some of these symptoms can be attributed to the effects of the interferon produced in response to the viremia and infection of host cells. The viremia is considered a mild systemic disease, and most viral infections do not progress beyond this point.

After replication in cells of the monocyte-macrophage system, a secondary viremia may result. This viremia can produce sufficient virus to infect target organs such as the brain, liver, skin, and vasculature, depending on the tissue tropism of the virus (Figure 63–4). The virus gains access to the brain by infecting the endothelial cells lining the small vessels of the brain or the choroid plexus.

The primary target cells of the flaviviruses are of the monocyte-macrophage lineage. Although these cells are found throughout the body and may have different characteristics, they express Fc receptors for antibody and release cytokines on challenge. Flavivirus infection is enhanced 200- to 1000-fold by non-neutralizing antiviral antibody that promotes binding of the virus to the Fc receptors and its uptake into the cell.

IMMUNE RESPONSE

Both humoral immunity and cellular immunity are elicited and are important to the control of primary infection and the prevention of future infections with the alphaviruses and flaviviruses.

Replication of the alphaviruses and flaviviruses produces a double-stranded RNA replicative intermediate that is a good inducer of interferon-α and interferon-β. The interferon is released into the bloodstream and

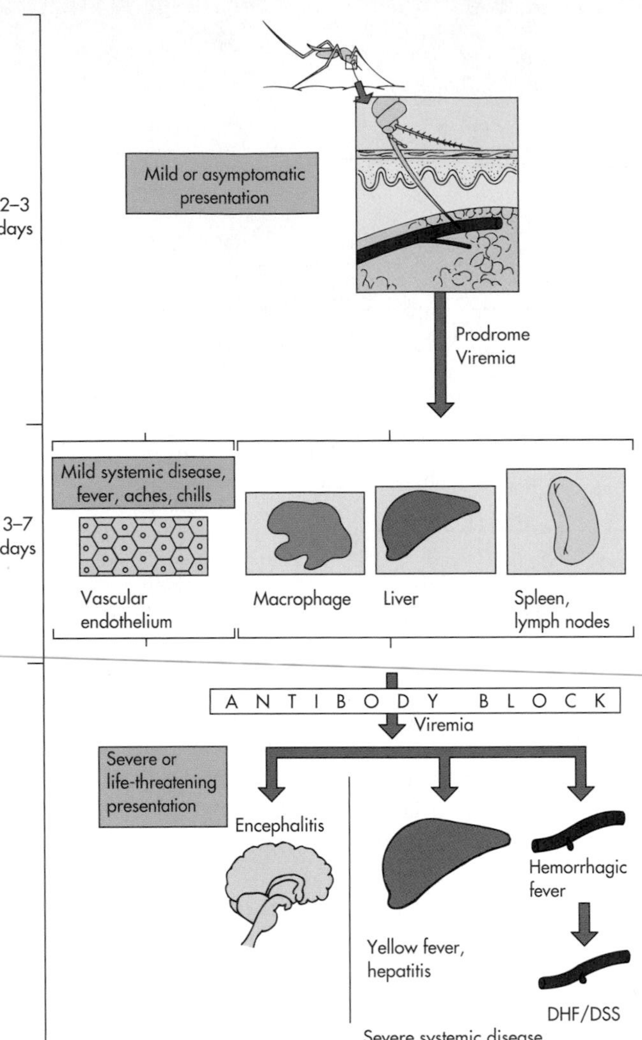

FIGURE 63–4. Disease syndromes of the alphaviruses and flaviviruses. Primary viremia may be associated with mild systemic disease. Most infections are limited to this. If sufficient virus is produced during the secondary viremia to escape immune protection and to reach critical target tissues, severe systemic disease or encephalitis may result. For dengue virus, rechallenge with another strain can result in severe dengue hemorrhagic fever (DHF), which can cause dengue shock syndrome (DSS) because of the loss of fluids from the vasculature.

limits replication of the virus; it also stimulates the immune response but, in doing so, causes the rapid onset of the flulike symptoms characteristic of mild systemic disease.

Circulating immunoglobulin (Ig)M is produced within 6 days of infection, followed by the production of IgG. The antibody blocks the viremic spread of the virus and the subsequent infection of other tissues. Immunity to one flavivirus can provide some protection against infection with other flaviviruses, through recognition of the type-common antigens expressed on all viruses in the family. Cell-mediated immunity is also important in controlling the primary infection.

Immunity to these viruses is a double-edged sword. A non-neutralizing antibody can enhance the uptake of flaviviruses into macrophages and other cells that express Fc receptors. Such an antibody can be generated to a related strain of virus in which the neutralizing epitope is not expressed or is different. Inflammation resulting from the cell-mediated immune response can destroy tissues and significantly contribute to the pathogenesis of encephalitis. Hypersensitivity reactions, such as delayed-type hypersensitivity, the formation of immune complexes with virions and viral antigens, and the activation of complement, can also occur. They can weaken the vasculature and cause it to rupture, leading to hemorrhagic symptoms. Immune responses to a related strain of dengue virus that do not prevent infection can promote immunopathogenesis, leading to dengue hemorrhagic fever or dengue shock syndrome.

EPIDEMIOLOGY

Alphaviruses and most flaviviruses are prototypical arboviruses (Box 63–3). To be an arbovirus, the virus must be able to (1) infect both vertebrates and invertebrates, (2) initiate a sufficient viremia in a vertebrate host for a sufficient time to allow acquisition of the virus by the invertebrate vector, and (3) initiate a persistent productive infection of the salivary gland of the invertebrate to provide virus for the infection of other host animals. **Humans are usually "dead-end" hosts,** in that they cannot spread the virus back to the vector because they do not maintain a persistent viremia. *If the virus is not in the blood, the mosquito cannot acquire it.* A full cycle of infection occurs when the virus is transmitted by the arthropod vector and amplified in a susceptible, immunologically naïve host **(reservoir)** that allows the reinfection of other arthropods (Figure 63–5). The vectors, natural hosts, and geographic distribution of representative alphaviruses and flaviviruses are listed in Table 63–2.

These viruses are usually restricted to a specific arthropod vector, its vertebrate host, and their ecologic niche. The most common vector is the mosquito, but ticks and sandflies spread some arboviruses. Even in a tropical region overrun with mosquitoes, the spread of these viruses is still restricted to a specific genus of mosquitoes. Not all arthropods can act as good vectors for each virus. For example, *Culex quinquefasciatus* is resistant to infection by the WEE virus (alphavirus) but is an excellent vector for St. Louis encephalitis virus (flavivirus).

Birds and small mammals are the usual reservoir hosts for the alphaviruses and flaviviruses, but reptiles and amphibians can also act as hosts. A large population of viremic animals can develop in these species to continue the infection cycle of the virus.

A 1999 epidemic of West Nile encephalitis virus (WNV) in New York was marked by the unusual deaths of

BOX 63–3. Epidemiology of Togavirus and Flavivirus Infection

Disease/Viral Factors

Enveloped virus must stay wet and can be inactivated by drying, soap, and detergents.

Virus can infect mammals, birds, reptiles, and insects.

Asymptomatic or nonspecific (flulike fever or chills), encephalitis, hemorrhagic fever, or arthritis.

Transmission

Specific arthropods characteristic of each virus (zoonosis: arbovirus).

Who Is at Risk?

People who enter ecologic niche of arthropod: arboviruses.

Geography/Season

Endemic regions for each arbovirus are determined by habitat of mosquito or other vector.

Aedes mosquito, which carries dengue and yellow fever, is found in urban areas and in pools of water.

Culex mosquito, which carries St. Louis encephalitis and West Nile encephalitis viruses, is found in forest and urban areas.

Disease is more common in summer.

Modes of Control

Mosquito breeding sites and mosquitoes should be eliminated.

Live attenuated vaccines are available for yellow fever virus and Japanese encephalitis virus.

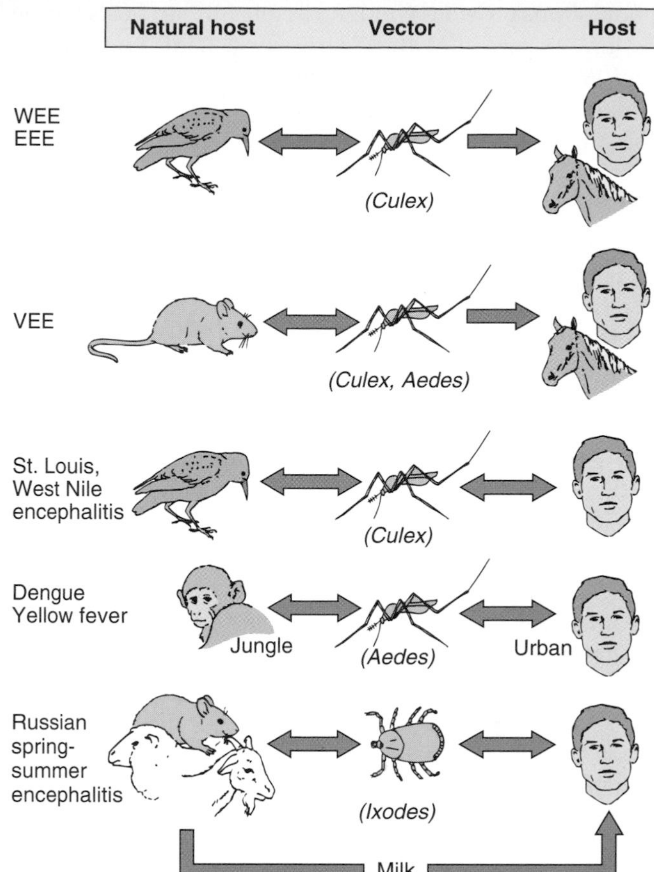

FIGURE 63–5. Patterns of alphavirus and flavivirus transmission. Birds and small mammals are the hosts that maintain and amplify an arbovirus, which is spread by the insect vector upon a blood meal. A double arrow indicates a cycle of replication in both host (including man) and vector. "Dead-end" infections with no transmission of the virus back to the vector are indicated by the single arrow. EEE, Eastern equine encephalitis; VEE, Venezuelan equine encephalitis; WEE, western equine encephalitits.

captive birds at the Bronx Zoo, as well as of crows, blue jays, and other wild birds. Representative birds and *Culex pipiens* mosquitoes in the region were demonstrated to be positive for the viral genome through the use of reverse transcriptase polymerase chain reaction (RT-PCR) testing. Each year since 1999, WNV has moved westward across the United States. WNV establishes a sufficient viremia in humans to be a risk factor for transmission through blood transfusions. Documentation of two such cases has led to screening blood donors for WNV and rejecting donors who have fever and headache during the week of blood donation.

Arbovirus diseases occur during the summer months and rainy seasons, when the arthropods breed and the arboviruses are cycled among a host reservoir (birds), an arthropod (e.g., mosquitoes), and human hosts. This cycle maintains and increases the amount of virus in the environment. In the winter the vector is not present to maintain the virus. The virus may either (1) persist in arthropod larvae or eggs or in reptiles or amphibians that remain in the locale or (2) migrate with the birds and then return during the summer.

When humans travel into the ecologic niche of the mosquito vector, they risk being infected by the virus. Pools of standing water, drainage ditches, and trash dumps in cities can also provide breeding grounds for mosquitoes such as *Aedes aegypti,* the vector for yellow fever, dengue, and chikungunya. An increase in the population of these mosquitoes therefore puts the human population at risk for infection. Health departments in many areas monitor birds and mosquitoes caught in traps for arboviruses and initiate control measures such as insecticide spraying when necessary.

Urban outbreaks of arbovirus infections occur when the reservoirs for the virus are humans or urban animals. Humans can be reservoir hosts for yellow fever, dengue, and chikungunya viruses (see Figure 63–5). These viruses are maintained by *Aedes* mosquitoes in a **sylvatic** or **jungle cycle,** in which monkeys are the natural host, and also in an **urban cycle,** in which humans are the host. *A. aegypti,* a vector for each of these viruses, is a household mosquito. It breeds in pools of water, open sewers, and other accumulations of water in cities. The occurrence of numerous inapparent infections in high-density populations provides enough viremic human hosts for the continued spread of these viruses. St. Louis encephalitis and West Nile encephalitis viruses are maintained in an urban environment because their vectors, *Culex* mosquitoes, breed in stagnant water, including puddles and sewage, and the reservoir group includes common city birds (e.g., crows).

CLINICAL SYNDROMES

More humans are infected with alphaviruses and flaviviruses than show significant, characteristic symptoms. The incidence of arbovirus disease is sporadic. Alphaviruses infections are usually asymptomatic or cause low-grade disease such as **flulike symptoms** (chills, fever, rash, aches) that correlate with systemic infection during the initial viremia. Eastern equine encephalitis (EEE), WEE, and Venezuelan equine encephalitis (VEE) virus infections can progress to **encephalitis** in humans. The equine encephalitis viruses are usually more of a problem to livestock than to humans. An affected human may experience fever, headache, and decreased consciousness 3 to 10 days after infection. Unlike herpes simplex virus encephalitis, the disease generally resolves without sequelae, but there is the possibility of paralysis, mental disability, seizures, and death. The name **chikungunya** (Swahili for "that which bends up") refers to the crippling arthritis associated with serious disease caused by infection with these viruses. Although predominant in South America and western Africa, this disease may spread to the United States because of the return of the *A. aegypti* mosquito, its vector.

Most flavivirus infections are relatively benign, but serious **aseptic meningitis** and **encephalitic** or **hemorrhagic disease** can occur. The encephalitis viruses include St. Louis, **West Nile,** Japanese, Murray Valley, and Russian spring-summer viruses. Symptoms and outcomes are similar to those of the togavirus encephalitides. Hundreds to thousands of cases of St. Louis encephalitis virus disease are noted in the United States annually. Approximately 20% of individuals infected with WNV will develop West Nile Fever characterized by fever, headache, tiredness, and body aches, occasionally with a skin rash on the trunk of the body and swollen lymph glands usually lasting only a few days. Encephalitis, meningitis, or meningoencephalitis occurs in approximately 1% of WNV-infected individuals.

The hemorrhagic viruses are dengue and yellow fever viruses. **Dengue virus** is a major worldwide problem, with up to 100 million cases of dengue fever and 300,000 cases of **dengue hemorrhagic fever (DHF)** occurring per year. Although not endemic in the United States, the virus and its vector are present in central and northern South America. The incidence of the more serious DHF has quadrupled since 1985. Dengue fever is also known as **break-bone fever;** the symptoms and signs consist of high fever, headache, rash, and back and bone pain that last 6 to 7 days. On rechallenge with another of the four related strains, dengue can also cause DHF and **dengue shock syndrome (DSS).** Non-neutralizing antibody promotes uptake of the virus into macrophages, which causes memory T cells to become activated, release inflammatory cytokines, and initiate hypersensitivity reactions. These reactions result in weakening and rupture of the vasculature, internal bleeding, and loss of plasma, leading to shock symptoms and internal bleeding. In 1981 in Cuba, dengue-2 virus infected a population previously exposed to dengue-1 virus between 1977 and 1980, leading to an epidemic of more than 100,000 cases of DHF/DSS and 168 deaths.

Yellow fever infections are characterized by severe systemic disease, with degeneration of the liver, kidney, and heart, as well as hemorrhage. Liver involvement causes the jaundice from which the disease gets its name, but massive gastrointestinal hemorrhages ("black vomit") may also occur. The mortality rate associated with yellow fever during epidemics is as high as 50%.

LABORATORY DIAGNOSIS

The alphaviruses and flaviviruses can be grown in both vertebrate and mosquito cell lines, but most are difficult to isolate. Infection can be detected through the use of cytopathologic studies, immunofluorescence, and the hemadsorption of avian erythrocytes. Detection and characterization can be performed by RT-PCR testing of genomic RNA or viral mRNA in blood or other samples. After isolation, the viral RNA can also be distinguished by the finding of RNA "fingerprints" of the genomic RNA. Monoclonal antibodies to the individual viruses have become a useful tool for distinguishing the individual species and strains of viruses.

A variety of serologic methods can be used to diagnose infections, including hemagglutination inhibition, enzyme-linked immunosorbent assays, and latex agglutination. The presence of specific IgM or a fourfold increase in titer between acute and convalescent sera is used to indicate a recent infection. The serologic cross-reactivity among viruses limits distinction of the actual viral species in many cases.

TREATMENT, PREVENTION, AND CONTROL

No treatments exist for arbovirus diseases other than supportive care. *The easiest means of preventing the spread of any arbovirus is elimination of its vector and breeding grounds.* After 1900, when Walter Reed and his colleagues discovered that yellow fever was spread by *A. aegypti,* the number of cases was reduced from 1400 to none within 2 years purely through control of the mosquito population. Many

Public Health departments monitor the bird and mosquito populations in a region for arboviruses and periodically spray to reduce the mosquito population. Avoidance of the breeding grounds of a mosquito vector is also a good preventive measure.

A live vaccine against yellow fever virus and killed vaccines against EEE, WEE, Japanese, and Russian spring-summer encephalitis viruses are available. These vaccines are meant for people working with the virus or at risk for contact. A live vaccine against VEE virus is available but only for use in domestic animals. A vaccine against dengue virus has not been developed because of the potential risk for immune enhancement of the disease on subsequent challenge.

The yellow fever vaccine is prepared from the 17D strain isolated from a patient in 1927 and grown for long periods in monkeys, mosquitoes, embryonic tissue culture, and embryonated eggs. The vaccine is administered intradermally and elicits lifelong immunity to yellow fever and, possibly, other cross-reacting flaviviruses.

Rubella Virus

Rubella virus has the same structural properties and mode of replication as the other togaviruses. However, unlike the other togaviruses, rubella is a **respiratory virus** and **does not cause readily detectable cytopathologic effects.**

Rubella is one of the five **classic childhood exanthems,** along with measles, roseola, fifth disease, and chickenpox. Rubella, meaning "little red" in Latin, was first distinguished from measles and other exanthems by German physicians; thus the common name for the disease, **German measles.** In 1941, an astute Australian ophthalmologist, Norman McAlister Gregg, recognized that maternal rubella infection was the cause of congenital cataracts. Maternal rubella infection has since been correlated with several other **severe congenital defects.** This finding prompted the development of a unique program to vaccinate children to prevent infection of pregnant women and neonates.

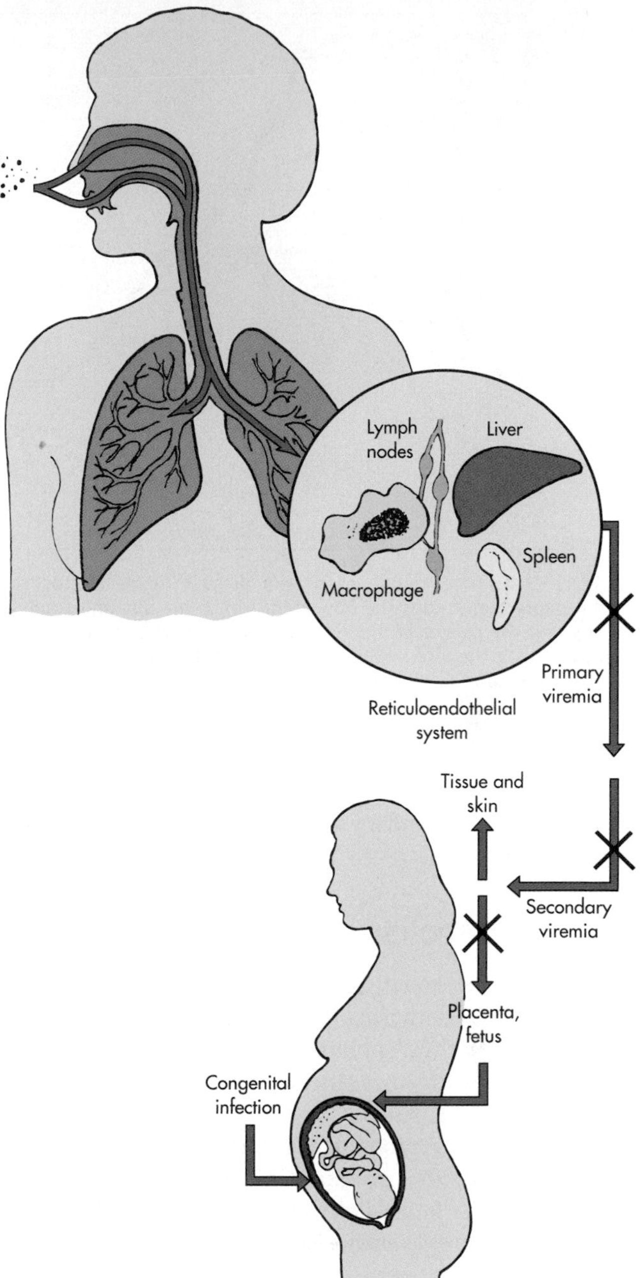

FIGURE 63–6. Spread of rubella virus within the host. Rubella enters and infects the nasopharynx and lung and then spreads to the lymph nodes and monocyte-macrophage system. The resulting viremia spreads the virus to other tissues and the skin. Circulating antibody can block the transfer of virus at the indicated points (*X*). In an immunologically deficient pregnant woman, the virus can infect the placenta and spread to the fetus.

PATHOGENESIS AND IMMUNITY

Rubella virus is not cytolytic but does have limited cytopathologic effects in certain cell lines, such as Vero and RK13. The replication of rubella prevents (in a process known as **heterologous interference**) the replication of superinfecting picornaviruses. This property allowed the first isolations of rubella virus in 1962.

Rubella infects the upper respiratory tract and then spreads to local lymph nodes, which coincides with a period of lymphadenopathy (Figure 63–6). This stage is followed by establishment of viremia, which spreads the virus throughout the body. Infection of other tissues and the characteristic mild rash result. The prodromal period lasts approximately 2 weeks (Figure 63–7). The person can shed virus in respiratory droplets during the

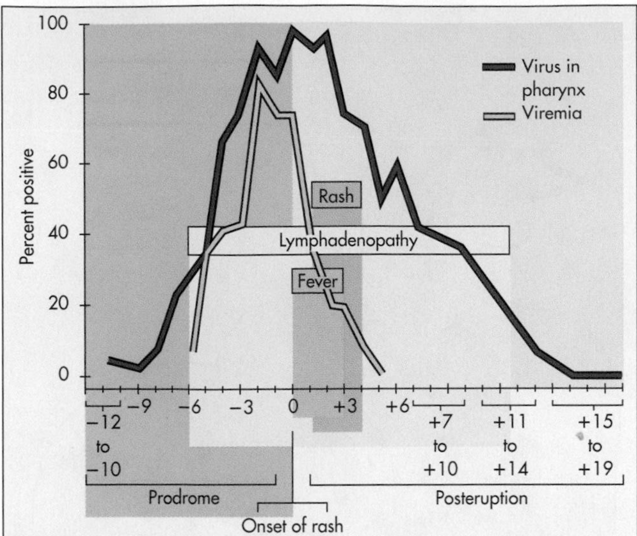

FIGURE 63–7. Time course of rubella disease. Rubella production in the pharynx precedes the appearance of symptoms and continues throughout the course of the disease. The onset of lymphadenopathy coincides with the viremia. Fever and rash occur later. The person is infectious as long as the virus is produced in the pharynx. (Redrawn from Plotkin SA: Rubella vaccine. In Plotkin SA, Mortimer EA, editors: *Vaccines,* Philadelphia, 1988, WB Saunders.)

prodromal period and for as long as 2 weeks after the onset of the rash.

IMMUNE RESPONSE

Antibody is generated after the viremia, and its appearance correlates with the appearance of the rash. The antibody limits viremic spread, but cell-mediated immunity plays an important role in resolving the infection. Only one serotype of rubella exists, and natural infection produces lifelong protective immunity. Most important, serum antibody in a pregnant woman prevents spread of the virus to the fetus. *Immune complexes most likely cause the rash and arthralgia associated with rubella infection.*

CONGENITAL INFECTION

Rubella infection in a pregnant woman can result in serious congenital abnormalities in the child. If the mother does not have antibody, the virus can replicate in the placenta and spread to the fetal blood supply and throughout the fetus. Rubella can replicate in most tissues of the fetus. The virus may not be cytolytic, but the normal growth, mitosis, and chromosomal structure of the cells of the fetus can be altered by the infection. The alterations can lead to improper development of the fetus, small size of the infected baby, and the **teratogenic effects** associated with congenital rubella infection. The nature of the disorder is determined by (1) the tissue affected and (2) the stage of development disrupted.

BOX 63–4. Epidemiology of Rubella Virus

Disease/Viral Factors
Rubella infects only humans.
Virus causes asymptomatic disease.
There is one serotype.

Transmission
Respiratory route.

Who Is at Risk?
Children: Mild exanthematous disease.
Adults: More severe disease with arthritis or arthralgia.
Neonates younger than 20 weeks: Congenital defects.

Modes of Control
Live attenuated vaccine is administered as part of measles, mumps, and rubella (MMR) vaccine.

The virus may persist in tissues, such as the lens of the eye, for 3 to 4 years and may be shed up to a year after birth. The presence of the virus during the development of the baby's immune response may even have a tolerative effect on the system, preventing effective clearance of the virus after birth. Immune complexes that produce further clinical abnormalities may also form in the neonate or infant.

EPIDEMIOLOGY

Humans are the only host for rubella (Box 63–4). The virus is spread in respiratory secretions and is generally acquired during childhood. Spread of virus, before or in the absence of symptoms, and crowded conditions, such as those in daycare centers, promote contagion.

Approximately 20% of women of childbearing age escape infection during childhood and are susceptible to infection unless vaccinated. Programs in many states in the United States test expectant mothers for antibodies to rubella.

Before the development and use of the rubella vaccine, cases of rubella in school children would be reported every spring, and major epidemics of rubella occurred at regular 6- to 9-year intervals. The severity of the 1964 to 1965 epidemic in the United States is indicated in Table 63–3. Congenital rubella occurred in as many as 1% of all the children born in cities such as Philadelphia during this epidemic. Since the development of the vaccine, however, the incidence of rubella and congenital rubella is now less than 1 and 0.1 per 100,000 pregnancies, respectively.

CLINICAL SYNDROMES

Rubella disease is normally benign in children. After a 14- to 21-day incubation period, the symptoms in children

TABLE 63–3. Estimated Morbidity Associated with the 1964-1965 U.S. Rubella Epidemic

Clinical Events	Number Affected
Rubella cases	12,500,000
Arthritis-arthralgia	159,375
Encephalitis	2,084
Deaths	
Excess neonatal deaths	2,100
Other deaths	60
Total deaths	2160
Excess fetal wastage	6250
Congenital rubella syndrome	
Deaf children	8055
Deaf/blind children	3580
Mentally retarded children	1790
Other congenital rubella syndrome symptoms	6575
Total congenital rubella syndrome	20,000
Therapeutic abortions	5000

From National Communicable Disease Center: *Rubella surveillance*, U.S. Department of Health, Education and Welfare, No 1, June 1969.

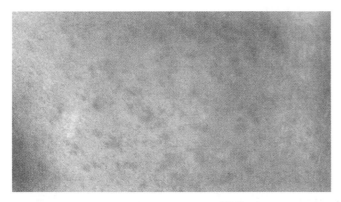

FIGURE 63–8. Close-up of the rubella rash. Small erythematous macules are visible. (From Hart CA, Broadwell RL: *A color atlas of pediatric infectious disease,* London, 1992, Wolfe.)

consist of a 3-day **maculopapular** or **macular rash** and swollen glands (Figure 63–8). Infection in adults, however, can be more severe and include problems such as bone and joint pain (arthralgia and arthritis) and (rarely) thrombocytopenia or postinfectious encephalopathy. Immunopathologic effects resulting from cell-mediated immunity and hypersensitivity reactions are a major cause of the more severe forms of rubella in adults.

Congenital disease is the most serious outcome of rubella infection. The fetus is at major risk until the 20th week of pregnancy. Maternal immunity to the virus resulting from prior exposure or vaccination prevents spread of the virus to the fetus. The most common manifestations of congenital rubella infection are cataracts, mental retardation, and deafness (Boxes 63–5 and 63–6; see Table 63–3). The mortality in utero and within the first year after birth is high for affected babies.

BOX 63–5. Prominent Clinical Findings in Congenital Rubella Syndrome

Cataracts and other ocular defects
Heart defects
Deafness
Intrauterine growth retardation
Failure to thrive
Mortality within the first year
Microcephaly
Mental retardation

BOX 63–6. Clinical Summaries

West Nile Encephalitis: During August, a 70-year-old man from a swampy area of Louisiana develops fever, headache, muscle weakness, nausea, and vomiting. He has difficulty answering questions. He progresses into a coma. Magnetic resonance imaging results show no specific localization of lesions (unlike in herpes simplex virus encephalitis). His disease progresses to respiratory failure and death. His 25-year-old niece, living next door, complains of sudden onset of fever (39°C [102.2°F]), headache, and myalgias, with nausea and vomiting lasting 4 days.
http://www.postgradmed.com/issues/2003/07_03/gelfand.htm

Yellow fever: A 42-year-old man had fever (103°F), headache, vomiting, and backache, which started 3 days after returning from a trip to Central America. He appeared normal for a short time, but then his gums started to bleed and he had bloody urine, vomited blood, and developed petechiae, jaundice, and a slower and weakened pulse. He started to improve 10 days after the onset of disease.

Rubella: A 6-year-old girl from Romania develops a faint rash on her face and is accompanied by mild fever and lymphadenopathy. Over the next 3 days the rash progresses to other parts of the body. She has no history of rubella immunization.

LABORATORY DIAGNOSIS

Isolation of the rubella virus is difficult and rarely attempted. The presence of the virus can be detected by RT-PCR detection of viral RNA. The diagnosis is usually confirmed by the presence of anti–rubella-specific IgM. A fourfold increase in specific IgG antibody titer between

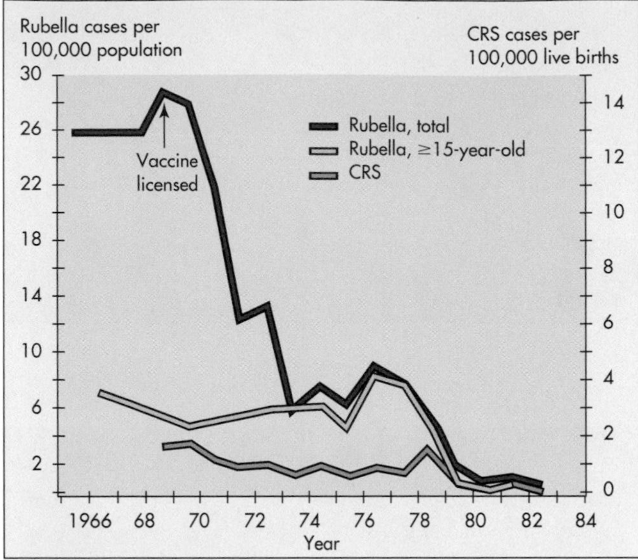

FIGURE 63–9. Effect of rubella virus vaccination on the incidence of rubella and congenital rubella syndrome (CRS). (Redrawn from Williams MN, Preblud SR: Current trends: Rubella and congenital rubella—United States, 1983, *MMWR Morbid Mortal Wkly Rep* 33:237-247, 1984.)

acute and convalescent sera is also used to indicate a recent infection. Antibodies to rubella are assayed early in pregnancy to determine the immune status of the woman; this test is required in many states.

When isolation of the virus is necessary, the virus is usually obtained from urine and is detected as interference with replication of echovirus 11 in primary African green monkey kidney cell cultures.

TREATMENT, PREVENTION, AND CONTROL

No treatment has been found for rubella. The best means of preventing rubella is vaccination with the live cold-adapted RA27/3 vaccine strain of virus (Figure 63–9). The live rubella vaccine is usually administered with the measles and mumps vaccines **(MMR vaccine)** at 24 months of age. The triple vaccine is included routinely in well-baby care. Vaccination promotes both humoral and cellular immunity.

The primary reason for the rubella vaccination program is to prevent congenital infection by decreasing the number of susceptible people in the population, especially children. As a result, there are fewer seronegative mothers and smaller chance that they will be exposed to the virus from contact with the children. Because only one serotype for rubella exists and humans are the only reservoir, vaccination of a large proportion of the population can significantly reduce the likelihood of exposure to the virus.

CASE STUDIES AND QUESTIONS

A 27-year-old businessman experienced a high fever, serious retroorbital headache, and severe joint and back pain 5 days after he and his family returned from a trip to Malaysia. The symptoms lasted for 4 days, and then a rash appeared on his palms and soles that lasted for 2 days.

At the same time the man's 5-year-old son experienced mild flulike symptoms and then collapsed after 2 to 5 days. The boy's hands were cold and clammy, his face was flushed, and his body was warm. There were petechiae on his forehead and ecchymoses elsewhere. He bruised very easily. He was breathing rapidly and had a weak rapid pulse. He then rapidly recovered after 24 hours.

1. What features of these cases pointed to the diagnosis of dengue virus infection?
2. Of what significance was the trip to Malaysia?
3. What was the source of infection in the father and son?
4. What were the significance of and the pathogenic basis for the petechiae and ecchymoses in the child?

Two weeks after returning from a trip to Mexico, a 25-year-old man had arthralgia (joint aches) and a mild rash that started on his face and spread to his body. He recalled that he had felt as if he had the flu a few days before the onset of the rash. The rash disappeared in 4 days.

1. What features of this case pointed to the diagnosis of rubella infection?
2. Why is it significant that the symptoms started after a trip outside the United States?
3. What precaution could the man have taken to prevent this infection?
4. How was this infection transmitted?
5. Who was at risk for a serious outcome of this infection?
6. If this disease is normally mild in children, why is their immunization so important?

Bibliography

Belshe RB, editor: *Textbook of human virology,* ed 2, St Louis, 1991, Mosby.

Chambers TJ, Monath TP, editors: *The flaviviruses,* vol 60, *Pathogenesis and immunity; Advances in virus research,* vol 61, *Detection, diagnosis and vaccine development,* San Diego, CA, 2003, Elsevier-Academic Press.

Cohen J, Powderly WG, editors: *Infectious diseases,* ed 2, St Louis, 2004, Mosby.

Flint SJ et al: *Principles of virology: Molecular biology, pathogenesis and control of animal viruses,* ed 2, Washington, 2003, American Society for Microbiology Press.

Hahn CS et al: Flavivirus genome organization, expression, and replication, *Annu Rev Microbiol* 44:663-188, 1990.

Johnson RT: *Viral infections of the nervous system,* Philadelphia, 1998, Lippincott-Raven.

Knipe DM, Howley PM, editors: *Fields virology*, ed 4, New York, 2001, Lippincott-Williams and Wilkins.

Koblet H: The "merry-go-round": Alphaviruses between vertebrate and invertebrate cells, *Adv Virus Res* 38:343-403, 1990.

Mackenzie JS, Barrett ADT, Deubel V: Japanese Encephalitis and West Nile Viruses, *Curr Top Microbiol Immunol* 267, 2002.

Monath TP: Yellow fever vaccine. In: Plotkin SA, Orenstein WA: *Vaccines*, ed 4, Philadelphia, 2004, WB Saunders.

Plotkin SA, Reef S: Rubella vaccine. In: Plotkin SA, Orenstein WA: *Vaccines*, ed 4, Philadelphia, 2004, WB Saunders.

Stollar V: Approaches to the study of vector specificity for arboviruses: Model systems using cultured mosquito cells. In Maramorosch K et al, editors: *Advances in virus research*, vol 33, New York, 1987, Academic Press.

Strauss JH, Strauss EG: *Viruses and human disease*, San Diego, 2002, Academic Press.

Tsai TF: Arboviral infections in the United States, *Infect Dis Clin North Am* 5:73-102, 1991.

West Nile virus: National Institte of Allergy and Infectious Diseases fact sheet: Available online at www.niaid.nih.gov/factsheets/westnile.htm/

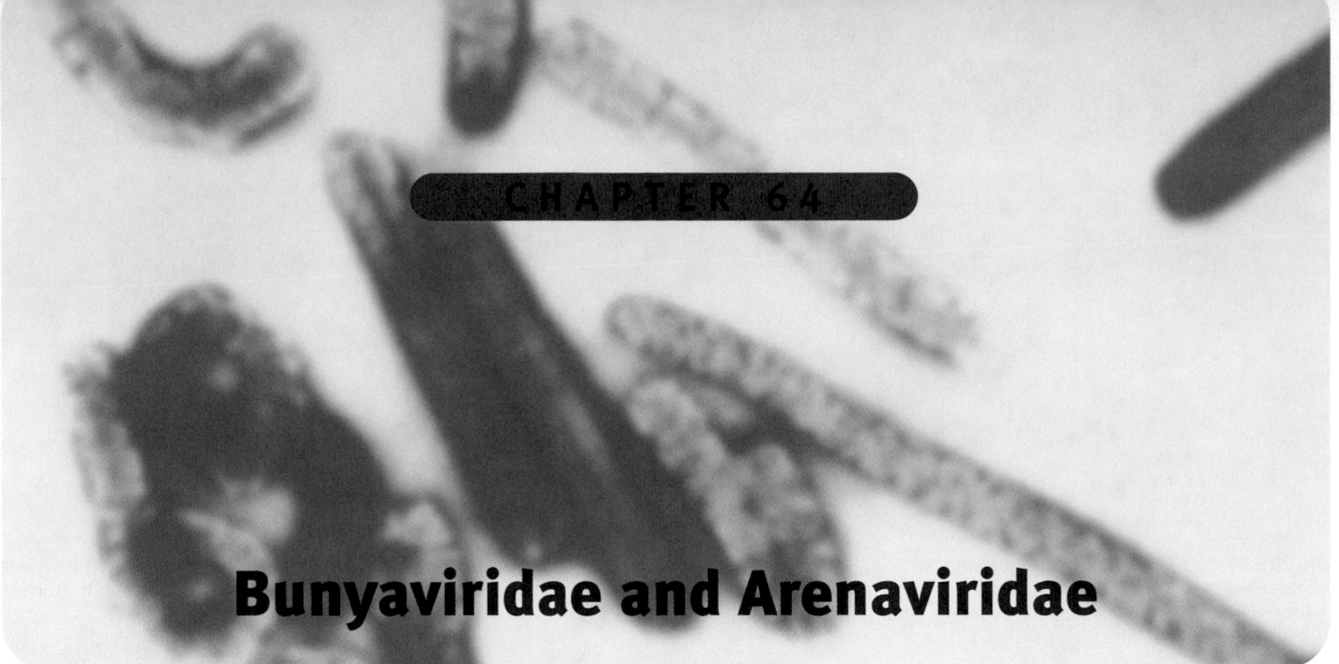

Bunyaviridae and Arenaviridae

The Bunyaviridae and Arenaviridae share several similarities. The viruses of these families are negative-strand ribonucleic acid (RNA) enveloped viruses with similar modes of replication. They are zoonoses, and most of the Bunyaviridae but not the Arenaviridae are arboviruses. Many of the viruses from these families cause encephalitis or hemorrhagic disease.

Bunyaviridae

The Bunyaviridae constitute a "supergroup" of at least **200 enveloped, segmented, negative-strand RNA viruses.** The supergroup is further broken down into the following five genera on the basis of structural and biochemical features: *Bunyavirus, Phlebovirus, Uukuvirus Nairovirus,* and *Hantavirus* (Table 64–1). Most of the Bunyaviridae are **arboviruses** (*ar*thropod-*bo*rne) that are spread by mosquitoes, ticks, or flies and are endemic to the environment of the vector. The **hantaviruses** are the exception; they are carried by **rodents.**

STRUCTURE

The bunyaviruses are roughly spherical particles 90 to 120 nm in diameter (Box 64–1). The envelope of the virus contains two glycoproteins (G1 and G2) and encloses three unique negative-strand RNAs, the large **(L)**, medium **(M)**, and small **(S)** RNAs that are associated with protein to form nucleocapsids (Table 64–2). The genome segments for the La Crosse and related California encephalitis viruses are circular. The nucleocapsids include the RNA-dependent RNA polymerase (L protein) and two nonstructural proteins (NS_s, NS_m) (Figure 64–1). Unlike other negative-strand RNA viruses, the Bunyaviridae **do not have a matrix protein.** The five genera of Bunyaviridae are distinguished by differences in (1) the number and sizes of the virion proteins, (2) the lengths of the L, M, and S strands of the genome, and (3) their transcription.

REPLICATION

The Bunyaviridae replicate in the same way as other enveloped, negative-strand viruses. For most bunyaviridae, the G1 glycoprotein interacts with β integrins on the cell surface and the virus is internalized by endocytosis. After fusion of the envelope with endosomal membranes on acidification of the vesicle, the nucleocapsid is released into the cytoplasm and messenger RNA (mRNA) and protein synthesis begin. Like influenza, the bunyaviruses steal the 5′-capped portion of mRNAs to prime the synthesis of viral mRNAs; but unlike influenza, this occurs in the cytoplasm.

The M strand encodes the NS_m nonstructural protein and the G1 (viral attachment) and G2 proteins, and the L strand encodes the L protein (polymerase) (see Table 64–2). The S strand of RNA encodes two nonstructural proteins, N and NS_s. For the phlebo and tospovirus groups, the S strand is ambisense, such that one protein is translated from the (+) strand and the other from the (−) RNA template.

Replication of the genome by the L protein also provides new templates for transcription, thereby increasing the rate of mRNA synthesis. The glycoproteins are then synthesized and glycosylated in the endoplasmic reticulum, after which they are transferred to the Golgi apparatus but not translocated to the plasma membrane. Virions are assembled by budding into the Golgi apparatus and are released by cell lysis or exocytosis.

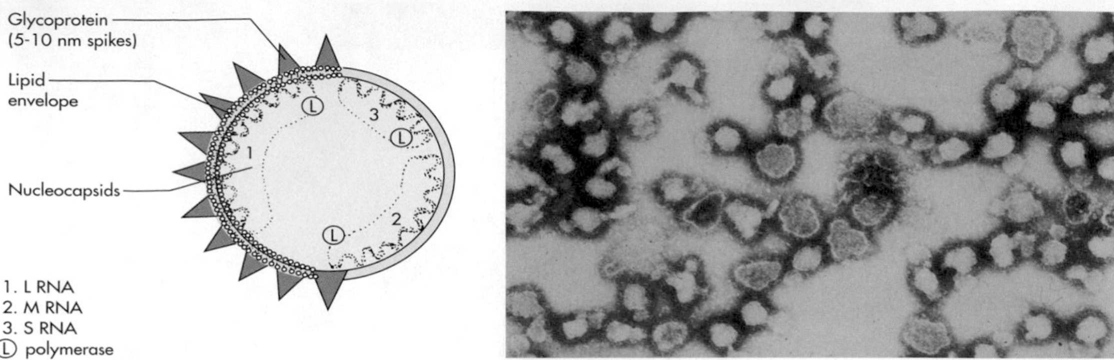

FIGURE 64–1. A, Model of the bunyavirus particle. **B,** Electron micrograph of La Crosse variant of bunyavirus. Note the spike proteins at the surface of the virion envelope. (**A** redrawn from Fraenkel-Conrat H, Wagner RR, editors: *Comprehensive virology,* vol 14, New York, 1979, Plenum; **B** courtesy Centers for Disease Control and Prevention, Atlanta.)

TABLE 64–1. Notable Bunyaviridae Genera*

Genus	Members	Insect Vector	Pathologic Conditions	Vertebrate Hosts
Bunyavirus	Bunyamwera virus, California encephalitis virus, La Crosse virus, Oropouche virus; 150 members	Mosquito	Febrile illness, encephalitis, febrile rash	Rodents, small mammals, primates, marsupials, birds
Phlebovirus	Rift Valley fever virus, sandfly fever virus; 36 members	Fly	Sandfly fever, hemorrhagic fever, encephalitis, conjunctivitis, myositis	Sheep, cattle, domestic animals
Nairovirus	Crimean-Congo hemorrhagic fever virus; 6 members	Tick	Hemorrhagic fever	Hares, cattle, goats, seabirds
Uukuvirus	Uukuniemi virus; 7 members	Tick	—	Birds
Hantavirus	Hantaan virus	None	Hemorrhagic fever with renal syndrome, adult respiratory distress syndrome	Rodents
	Sin Nombre	None	Hantavirus pulmonary syndrome, shock, pulmonary edema	Deer mouse

*An additional 35 viruses possess several common properties with Bunyaviridae but are as yet unclassified.

TABLE 64–2. Genome and Proteins of California Encephalitis Virus

Genome*	Proteins
L	RNA polymerase, 170 kDa
M	Spike glycoprotein, 75 kDa Spike glycoprotein, 65 kDa Nonstructural protein, 15-17 kDa
S	Nucleocapsid protein, 25 kDa Nucleocapsid protein, 10 kDa

*Negative-strand RNA.

BOX 64–1. Unique Features of Bunyaviruses

There are at least 200 related viruses in five genera that share a common morphology and basic components.
Virion is enveloped with three (L, M, S) negative RNA nucleocapsids but no matrix proteins.
Virus replicates in the cytoplasm.
Virus can infect humans and arthropods.
Virus in arthropod can be transmitted to its eggs.

BOX 64–2. Disease Mechanisms for Bunyaviruses

Virus is acquired from an arthropod bite (e.g., mosquito)
Initial viremia may cause flulike symptoms.
Establishment of secondary viremia may allow virus access to specific target tissues, including the central nervous system, organs, and vascular endothelium.
Antibody is important in controlling viremia; interferon and cell-mediated immunity may prevent the outgrowth of infection.

PATHOGENESIS

Most of the Bunyaviridae are arboviruses and possess many of the same pathogenic mechanisms as the togaviruses and flaviviruses (Box 64–2). For example, the viruses are spread by an arthropod vector and are injected into the blood to initiate a viremia. Progression past this stage to secondary viremia and further dissemination of the virus can deliver the virus to target sites typically involved in that particular viral disease, such as the central nervous system, liver, kidney, and vascular endothelium.

Many Bunyaviridae cause neuronal and glial damage and cerebral edema, leading to encephalitis. In certain viremic infections (e.g., Rift Valley fever), hepatic necrosis may occur. In others (e.g., Crimean-Congo hemorrhagic fever and Hantaan hemorrhagic disease), the primary lesion involves the leakage of plasma and erythrocytes through the vascular endothelium. In the latter infection, these changes are most prominent in the kidney and are accompanied by hemorrhagic necrosis of the kidney.

Unlike the other bunyaviruses, rodents are the reservoir and vector for hantaviruses, and humans acquire the virus by breathing aerosols contaminated with infected urine. The virus initiates infection and remains in the lung, where it causes hemorrhagic tissue destruction and lethal pulmonary disease.

BOX 64–3. Epidemiology of Bunyavirus Infections

Disease/Viral Factors

Virus is able to replicate in mammalian and arthropod cells.
Virus is able to pass into ovary and infect arthropod eggs, allowing virus to survive during winter.

Transmission

Via arthropods through break in skin. California encephalitis group: *Aedes* mosquito.
Aedes mosquitoes are daytime feeders and live in forest.
Aedes mosquitoes lay eggs in small pools of water trapped in places such as trees and tires.

Who Is at risk?

People in habitat of arthropod vector.
California encephalitis group: Campers, forest rangers, woodsmen.

Geography/Season

Disease incidence correlates with distribution of vector.
Disease is more common in summer.

Modes of Control

Elimination of vector or vector's habitat.
Avoidance of vector's habitat.

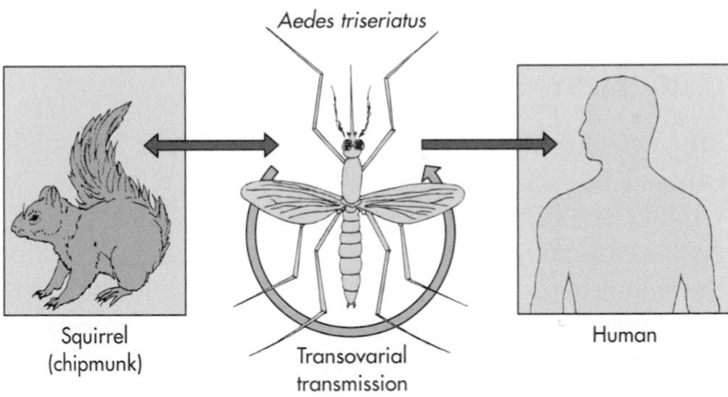

FIGURE 64–2. Transmission of La Crosse (California) encephalitis virus.

Epidemiology

Most bunyaviruses are transmitted by infected mosquitoes, ticks, or *Phlebotomus* flies to rodents, birds, and larger animals (Box 64–3). The animals then become the **reservoirs** for the virus, thereby continuing the cycle of infection. Humans are infected when they enter the environment of the insect vector (Figure 64–2). Transmission occurs during the summer, but unlike many other arboviruses, many of the Bunyaviridae can survive a winter in the ova of the mosquito and remain in a locale.

Many of the members of this virus family are found in South America, southeastern Europe, southeast Asia, and Africa and bear the exotic names of their ecologic niches. Viruses of the **California encephalitis virus group** (e.g., La Crosse virus) are spread by mosquitoes found in the forests of North America (Figure 64–3). Up to 150 cases of encephalitis occur during the summer each year in the United States, but most infections are asymptomatic. These viruses are spread mainly by *Aedes triseriatus* and by *Culiseta,* which breeds in the water in tree holes and in discarded tires.

The hantaviruses do not have an arthropod vector but are maintained in a rodent species specific for each virus. Humans are infected by close contact with rodents or through the inhalation of aerosolized rodent urine. In May 1993, an outbreak of **hantavirus pulmonary syndrome** occurred in the Four Corners area of New Mexico.

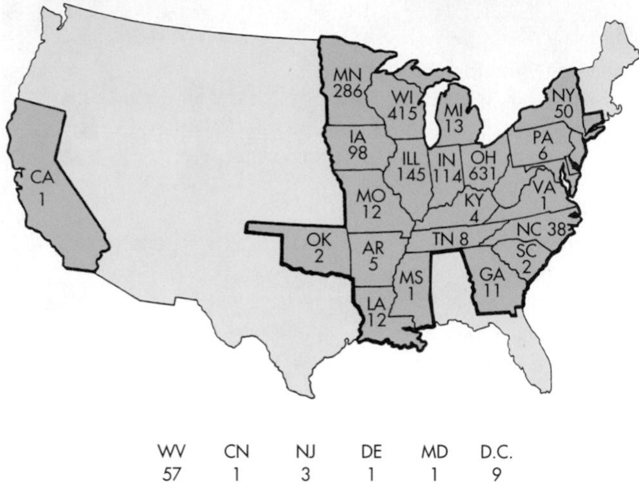

FIGURE 64–3. Distribution of California encephalitis, 1964 to 1989. (Redrawn from Tsai TF: *Infect Dis Clin North Am* 5:73-102, 1991.)

The outbreak is attributed to increased contact with the deer mouse vector during a season of unusually high rainfall, greater availability of food, and rise in the rodent population. Viruses of the Sin Nombre subfamily were isolated from the victims and rodents. Since this incident, viruses from this subfamily have been associated with outbreaks of respiratory tract disease in the Eastern and Western United States and Central and South America.

CLINICAL SYNDROMES

Bunyaviridae, which are mosquito-borne viruses, usually cause a nonspecific febrile, flulike illness related to the viremia (see Table 64–1) that is indistinguishable from illnesses caused by other viruses. The incubation period for these illnesses is approximately 48 hours, and the fevers last approximately 3 days. Most patients with infections, even those infected by agents known to cause severe disease (e.g., Rift Valley fever virus, La Crosse virus), have mild illness.

Encephalitis illnesses (e.g., La Crosse virus) are sudden in onset after an incubation period of approximately 1 week, and symptoms at this time consist of fever, headache, lethargy, and vomiting. Seizures occur in 50% of patients with encephalitis, usually early in the illness. Signs of meningitis may also be present. The illness lasts an average of 7 days. Death occurs in less than 1% of patients, but seizure disorders may occur as sequelae in as much as 20%.

Hemorrhagic fevers such as Rift Valley fever are characterized by petechial hemorrhages, ecchymosis, epistaxis, hematemesis, melena, and bleeding of the gums. Death occurs in as many as half of patients with hemorrhagic phenomena. The **hantavirus pulmonary syndrome** is a terrible disease consisting of a prodrome of fever and muscle aches, followed rapidly by interstitial pulmonary edema, respiratory failure, and death within days.

Laboratory Diagnosis

Detection of viral RNA by reverse transcriptase polymerase chain reaction (RT-PCR) has become the accepted method for detecting and identifying bunyaviruses. The Sin Nombre and Convict Creek hantaviruses were identified through the use of the RT-PCR test. Viral RNA from patient tissue was converted to complementary DNA with the use of the reverse transcriptase of a retrovirus, and then DNA primers representing conserved sequences of hantaviruses were used to promote synthesis of the characteristic hantavirus sequences.

Serologic tests are generally performed to confirm a diagnosis of bunyavirus infection. Virus neutralization assays can be used to identify the virus. Assays specific for immunoglobulin (Ig)M are useful in the documentation of acute infection. Seroconversion or a fourfold increase in the titer of the IgG antibody is used to document recent infection, but cross-reactions within viral genera are common. Enzyme-linked immunosorbent assay (ELISA) may detect antigen in clinical specimens from patients with an intense viremia (e.g., Rift Valley fever, hemorrhagic fever with renal syndrome, Crimean-Congo hemorrhagic fever). ELISAs that can detect viral antigen in mosquitoes have been developed.

TREATMENT, PREVENTION, AND CONTROL

No specific therapy for infections of the Bunyaviridae is available. Human disease is prevented by interruption of the contact between humans and the vector, whether arthropod or mammal. Arthropod vectors are controlled by (1) eliminating the growth conditions for the vector, (2) spraying with insecticide, (3) installing netting or screening at windows and doors, (4) wearing protective clothing, and (5) controlling the tick infestation of animals. Rodent control minimizes the transmission of many viruses, especially hantaviruses. Rift Valley fever vaccines have been developed for use in humans and animals (sheep and cattle).

Arenaviruses

The arenaviruses include **lymphocytic choriomeningitis (LCM)** and **hemorrhagic fever viruses,** such as the **Lassa, Junin,** and **Machupo** viruses. These viruses cause persistent infections in specific rodents and can be transmitted to humans as **zoonoses.**

STRUCTURE AND REPLICATION

Arenaviruses are seen in electron micrographs as **pleomorphic, enveloped viruses** (diameter, 120 nm) that have a **sandy appearance** (the name comes from the Greek word *arenosa,* meaning "sandy") because of the

ribosomes in the virion (Box 64–4). Although functional, the ribosomes do not seem to serve a purpose. Virions contain a beaded nucleocapsid with **two single-stranded RNA circles** (S, 3400 nucleotides; L, 7200 nucleotides) and a transcriptase. The L strand is a negative-sense RNA and encodes the polymerase. The S strand encodes the nucleoprotein (N protein) and the glycoproteins but is **ambisense.** Whereas the mRNA for the N protein is transcribed directly from the ambisense S strand, the mRNA for the glycoprotein is transcribed from a full-length template of the genome. As a result, the glycoproteins are produced as late proteins after genome replication. Arenaviruses replicate in the cytoplasm and acquire their envelope by budding from the host cell plasma membrane.

Arenaviruses readily cause persistent infections. This may result from inefficient transcription of the glycoprotein genes and thus poor virion assembly.

PATHOGENESIS

Arenaviruses are able to infect macrophages and possibly cause the release of mediators of cell and vascular damage. T-cell-induced immunopathologic effects significantly exacerbate tissue destruction. Persistent infection of rodents results from neonatal infection and the induction of immune tolerance. The incubation period for arenavirus infections averages 10 to 14 days.

EPIDEMIOLOGY

Most arenaviruses, except for the virus that causes LCM, are found in the tropics of Africa and South America. The arenaviruses, like the hantaviruses, infect specific rodents and are endemic to the rodents' habitats. Chronic asymptomatic infection is common in these animals and leads to a chronic viremia and long-term viral shedding in saliva, urine, and feces. Humans may become infected through the inhalation of aerosols, the consumption of contaminated food, or contact with fomites. Bites are not a usual mechanism of spread.

The virus that causes LCM infects hamsters and house mice *(Mus musculus)*. It was found in 20% of mice in Washington, DC. LCM disease in the United States is associated with contact with pet hamsters and with the animals in rodent-breeding facilities. Lassa fever virus infects *Mastomys natalensis*, an African rodent. The Lassa fever virus is spread from human to human through contact with infected secretions or body fluids, but the viruses that cause LCM or other hemorrhagic fevers are rarely, if ever, spread in this way.

During 1999 and 2000, three cases of fatal hemorrhagic disease in California were found to be caused by the Whitewater Arroyo arenavirus. This virus is normally found in the white-throated wood rat, so its occurrence in humans constitutes a newly emergent disease. The disease association was made by a special RT-PCR assay.

BOX 64–4. Characteristics of Arenaviruses

Virus has **enveloped** virion with two **circular, negative RNA** genome segments (L, S). Virion appears **sandy because of ribosomes.**
S genome segment is ambisense.
Arenavirus infections are zoonoses, establishing persistent infections in rodents.
Pathogenesis of arenavirus infections is largely attributed to T-cell immunopathogenesis.

CLINICAL SYNDROMES (Box 64–5)

Lymphocytic Choriomeningitis

The name of this virus, lymphocytic choriomeningitis, suggests that meningitis is a typical clinical event, but actually, LCM causes a febrile illness with flulike myalgia more often than meningeal illness. Only approximately 10% of infected persons exhibit clinical evidence of a central nervous system infection. The meningeal illness, if it occurs, will start 10 days after the initial phase of illness, with full recovery. Perivascular mononuclear infiltrates may be seen in neurons of all sections of the brain and in the meninges of an affected patient.

Lassa and Other Hemorrhagic Fevers

Lassa fever, which is endemic to West Africa, is the best known of the hemorrhagic fevers caused by an arenavirus. Other agents, however, such as the Junin and Machupo viruses, cause similar syndromes in the inhabitants of different geographic areas (Argentina and Bolivia, respectively).

Clinical illness is characterized by fever, coagulopathy, petechiae, and occasional visceral hemorrhage, as well as liver and spleen necrosis, but not vasculitis. Hemorrhage and shock also occur, as does occasional cardiac and liver damage. In contrast to LCM, hemorrhagic fevers cause no lesions in the central nervous system. Pharyngitis, diarrhea, and vomiting may be prevalent, especially in patients with Lassa fever. Death occurs in as many as 50% of those with Lassa fever and in a smaller percentage of

Box 64–5. Clinical Summaries

Lassa fever: Approximately 10 days after returning from a trip to visit family in Nigeria, a 47-year-old man developed flulike symptoms with a higher than expected fever and malaise. The disease got progressively worse and after 3 days, the patient developed abdominal pain, nausea, vomiting, diarrhea, pharyngitis, bleeding gums, and began vomiting blood. He developed shock and then died.

those infected with the other arenaviruses that cause hemorrhagic fevers. The diagnosis is suggested by recent travel to endemic areas.

LABORATORY DIAGNOSIS

An arenavirus infection is usually diagnosed on the basis of serologic and genomic (RT-PCR) findings. These viruses are too dangerous for routine isolation. Throat specimens can yield arenaviruses; urine is a source for the Lassa fever virus but not for the LCM virus. The risk of infection is substantial for laboratory workers handling body fluids. Therefore, if the diagnosis is suspected, laboratory personnel should be so warned and the specimens processed only in facilities that specialize in the isolation of contagious pathogens **(level 3 for LCM and level 4 for Lassa fever and other arenaviruses).**

TREATMENT, PREVENTION, AND CONTROL

The antiviral drug **ribavirin** has limited activity against arenaviruses and can be used to treat Lassa fever. However, supportive therapy is usually all that is available for patients with arenavirus infections.

These rodent-borne infections can be prevented by limiting contact with the vector. For example, improved hygiene to limit contact with mice reduced the incidence of LCM in Washington, DC. In the geographic areas where hemorrhagic fever occurs, trapping rodents and carefully storing food may decrease exposure to the virus.

The incidence of laboratory-acquired cases can be reduced if samples submitted for arenavirus isolation are processed in at least level 3 or 4 biosafety facilities and not in the usual clinical virology laboratory.

CASE STUDIES AND QUESTIONS

A 58-year-old woman complained of flulike symptoms, severe headache, stiff neck, and photophobia. She was lethargic and had a mild fever. The cerebrospinal fluid specimen contained 900 white blood cells per ml, mostly lymphocytes, and lymphocytic choriomeningitis virus. She recovered after a week. Her home was infested with gray mice (Mus musculus).

1. What were the significant symptoms of this disease?
2. How was the virus transmitted?
3. What type of immune response is most important in controlling this infection?

A 15-year-old summer camp counselor in Ohio suddenly complained of a headache, nausea, and vomiting; she had a fever and experienced a stiff neck. She was admitted to the hospital, where a spinal tap and examination of cerebrospinal fluid revealed inflammatory cells. She became lethargic over the next day but became alert again after 4 to 5 days.

1. The physician suspected La Crosse encephalitis virus as the agent. What clues pointed to La Crosse virus?
2. What other agents would also be considered in the differential diagnosis?
3. How was the patient infected?
4. How would the transmission of this agent be prevented?
5. How could the local Public Health department determine the prevalence of La Crosse virus in the environment of the summer camp? What samples would they obtain, and how would they test them?

Bibliography

Bishop DHL, Shope RE: Bunyaviridae. In Fraenkel-Conrat H, Wagner RR, editors: *Comprehensive virology*, vol 14, New York, 1979, Plenum.

Cohen J, Powderly WG, editors: *Infectious diseases*, ed 2, St Louis, 2004, Mosby.

Flint SJ et al: *Principles of virology: Molecular biology, pathogenesis and control of animal viruses*, ed 2, Washington, 2003, American Society for Microbiology Press.

Knipe DM, Howley PM, editors: *Fields virology*, ed 4, New York, 2001, Lippincott-Williams and Wilkins.

Kolakofsky D: Bunyaviridae, *Curr Top Microbiol Immunol* 169:1-256, 1991.

McKee KT, LeDuc JW, Peters CJ: Hantaviruses. In Belshe RB, editor: *Textbook of human virology*, ed 2, St Louis, 1991, Mosby.

Oldstone MBA: Arenaviruses I and II, *Curr Top Microbiol Immunol* vol. 262-263, 2002.

Peters CJ, LeDuc JW: Bunyaviruses, phleboviruses and related viruses. In Belshe RB, editor: *Textbook of human virology*, ed 2, St Louis, 1991, Mosby.

Peters CJ, Simpson GL, Levy H: Spectrum of hantavirus infection: Hemorrhagic fever with renal syndrome and hantavirus pulmonary syndrome, *Annu Rev Med* 50:531-545, 1999.

Schmaljohn CS, Nichol ST: Hantaviruses, *Curr Top Microbiol Immunol* 256, 2001.

Strauss JH, and Strauss EG, *Viruses and human disease*, San Diego, 2002, Academic Press.

Tsai TF: Arboviral infections in the United States, *Infect Dis Clin North Am* 5:73-102, 1991.

Wrobel S: Serendipity, science and a new hantavirus, *FASEB J* 9:1247-1254, 1995.

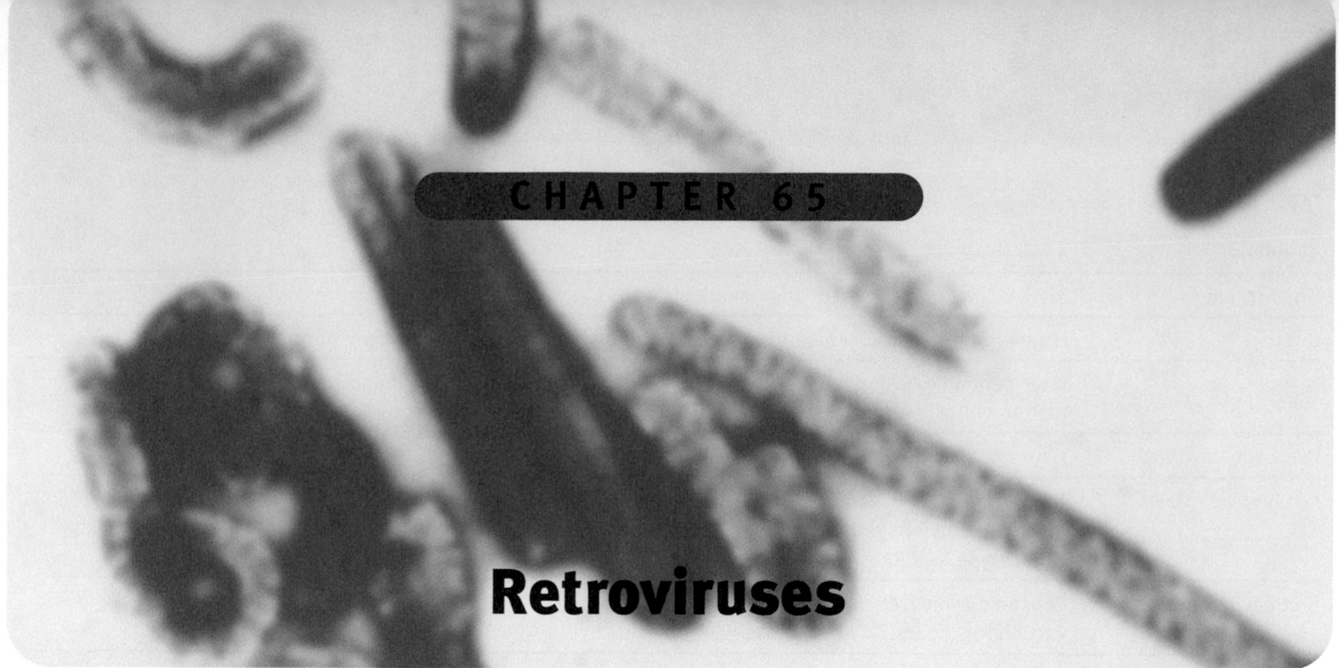

Retroviruses

The retroviruses are probably the most studied group of viruses in molecular biology. These viruses are **enveloped, positive-strand ribonucleic acid (RNA)** viruses with a unique morphology and means of replication. In 1970, Baltimore and Temin showed that the retroviruses encode an **RNA-dependent deoxyribonucleic acid (DNA) polymerase (reverse transcriptase [RT])** and replicate through a DNA intermediate. The DNA copy of the viral genome is then integrated into the host chromosome to become a cellular gene. This discovery, which earned the Nobel Prize, contradicted what had been the central dogma of molecular biology—that genetic information passed from DNA to RNA and then to protein.

The first retrovirus to be isolated was the Rous sarcoma virus, shown by Peyton Rous to produce solid tumors (sarcomas) in chickens. Like most retroviruses, the Rous sarcoma virus proved to have a very limited host and species range. Cancer-causing retroviruses have since been isolated from other animal species and are classified as RNA tumor viruses or **oncornaviruses.** Many of these viruses alter cellular growth by expressing analogues of cellular growth–controlling genes **(oncogenes).** Not until 1981, however, when Robert Gallo and his associates isolated human T-lymphotropic virus (HTLV-1) from a person with adult human T-cell lymphotropic, was a human retrovirus isolated and associated with human disease.

In the late 1970s and early 1980s, an unusual number of young homosexual men, Haitians, heroin addicts, and hemophiliacs in the United States (the initial "4H club" of risk groups) were noted to be dying of normally benign opportunistic infections. Their symptoms defined a new disease, the **acquired immune deficiency syndrome (AIDS).** However, as is now known, AIDS proved not to be limited to these groups but can occur in anyone exposed to the virus. Now approximately 40 million men, women, and children around the world are living with the virus that causes AIDS. Montagnier and associates in Paris, and Gallo and colleagues in the United States, reported the isolation of the human immunodeficiency virus (HIV-1) from patients with lymphadenopathy and AIDS. A variant of HIV-1, designated **HIV-2,** was isolated later and is prevalent in West Africa. HIV appears to have evolved since the 1930s from a simian virus and then rapidly spread through Africa and the world by an increasingly mobile population. Although a devastating disease that cannot be completely cured, the development of antiviral drug cocktails (HAART, highly active antiretroviral therapy) has allowed many HIV patients to resume a normal life.

Our understanding of the retroviruses has paralleled progress in molecular biology. In turn, the retroviruses have provided a major tool for molecular biology, the reverse transcriptase enzyme, and through the study of viral oncogenes have also provided a means of advancing our understanding of cell growth, differentiation, and oncogenesis.

The three subfamilies of human retroviruses are the **Oncovirinae,** or oncovirus (HTLV-1, HTLV-2, HTLV-5); the **Lentivirinae** (HIV-1, HIV-2); and the **Spumavirinae** (Table 65–1). Although a spumavirus was the first human retrovirus to be isolated, no such virus has been associated with human disease. **Endogenous retroviruses,** the ultimate parasite, have integrated, are transmitted vertically, and may take up as much as 1% of the human chromosome. Although they may not produce virions, their gene sequences have been detected in many animal species and in humans.

Classification

The retroviruses are classified by the diseases they cause, tissue tropism and host range, virion morphology, and

TABLE 65–1. Classification of Retroviruses

Subfamily	Characteristics	Examples
Oncovirinae	Are associated with cancer and neurologic disorders	—
B	Have eccentric nucleocapsid core in mature virion	Mouse mammary tumor virus
C	Have centrally located nucleocapsid core in mature virion	Human T-lymphotropic virus* (HTLV-1, HTLV-2, HTLV-5), Rous sarcoma virus (chickens)
D	Have nucleocapsid core with cylindrical form	Mason-Pfizer monkey virus
Lentivirinae	Have slow onset of disease: cause neurologic disorders and immunosuppression; are viruses with D-type, cylindrical nucleocapsid core	Human immunodeficiency virus* (HIV-1, HIV-2), visna virus (sheep), caprine arthritis/encephalitis virus (goats)
Spumavirinae	Cause no clinical disease but characteristic vacuolated "foamy" cytopathology	Human foamy virus*
Endogenous viruses	Have retrovirus sequences that are integrated into human genome	Human placental virus

*Also classified as complex retroviruses because of the requirement for accessory proteins for replication.

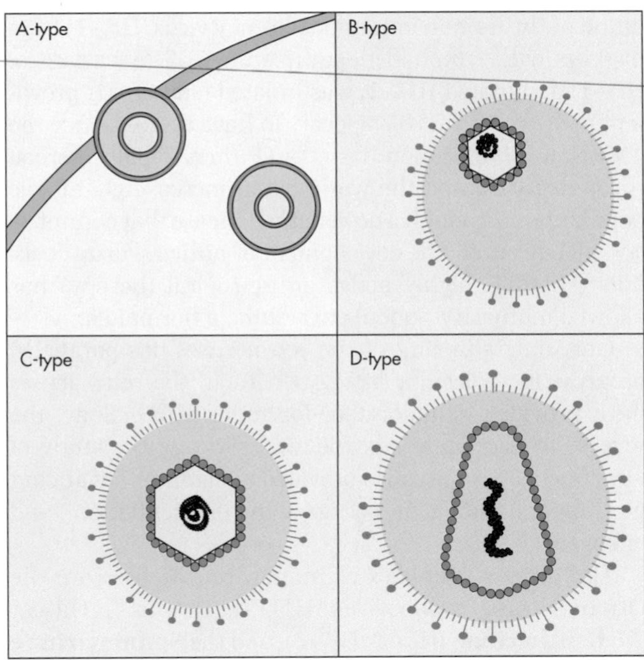

FIGURE 65–1. Morphologic distinction of retrovirions. The morphology and position of the nucleocapsid core are used to classify the viruses. A-type particles are immature intracytoplasmic forms that bud through the plasma membrane into mature B-type, C-type, and D-type particles.

BOX 65–1. Unique Characteristics of Retroviruses

Virus has an **enveloped** spherical virion that is 80 to 120 nm in diameter and encloses a capsid containing **two** copies of the **positive-strand RNA** genome (approximately 9 kilobases for HIV and HTLV).
RNA-dependent DNA polymerase **(reverse transcriptase)** and integrase enzymes are carried in the virion.
Virus receptor is the initial determinant of tissue tropism.
Replication proceeds through a DNA intermediate, termed the *provirus*.
The provirus **integrates** randomly into the host chromosome and becomes a cellular gene.
Transcription of the genome is regulated by the interaction of host transcription factors with promoter and enhancer elements in the long-terminal repeat (LTR) portion of the genome.
Simple retroviruses encode *gag, pol,* and *env* genes. **Complex viruses** also encode accessory genes (e.g., *tat, rev, nef, vif, vpu* for HIV).
Virus assembles and buds from the plasma membrane.
Final morphogenesis of HIV *requires* protease cleavage of gag and gag-pol polypeptides after envelopment.

HIV, Human immunodeficiency virus; HTLV, human T-lymphotropic virus.

genetic complexity (see Table 65–1). The **oncoviruses** include the only retroviruses that can *immortalize or transform target cells.* These viruses are also categorized by the morphology of their core and capsid as type A, B, C, or D, as seen in electron micrographs (Figure 65–1; see Table 65–1). The **lentiviruses** *are slow viruses associated with neurologic and immunosuppressive diseases.* The spumaviruses, represented by a foamy virus, cause a distinct cytopathologic effect but, as already noted, do not seem to cause clinical disease.

Structure

The retroviruses are roughly spherical, enveloped RNA viruses with a diameter of 80 to 120 nm (Figure 65–2 and Box 65–1). The envelope contains viral glycoproteins and is acquired by budding from the plasma membrane. The **envelope surrounds a capsid that contains two identical copies of the positive-strand RNA genome** inside an electron-dense core. The virion also contains 10 to 50 copies of the **reverse transcriptase and**

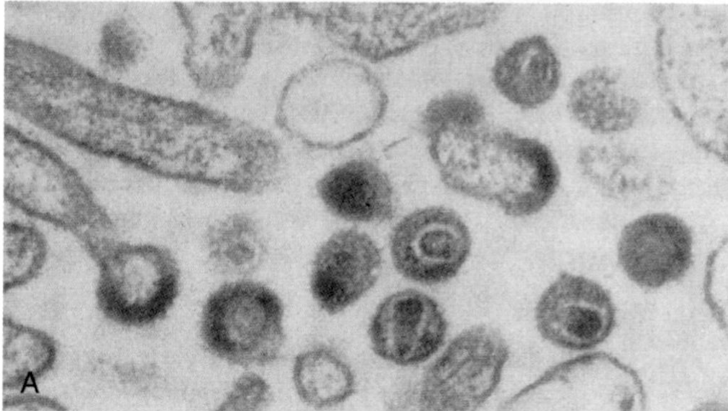

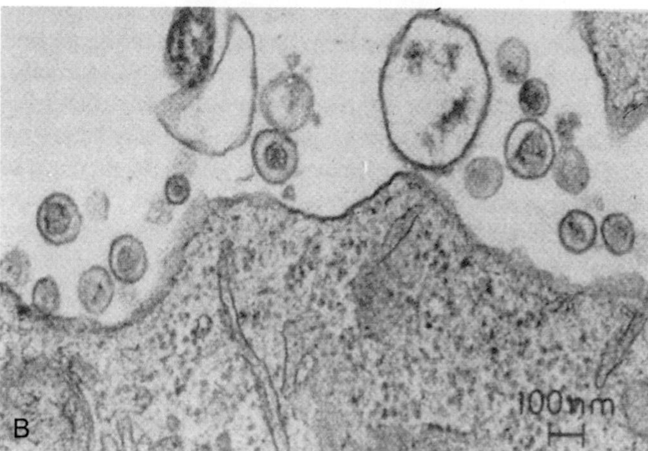

FIGURE 65–2. Electron micrographs of two retroviruses. **A,** Human immunodeficiency virus. Note the cone-shaped nucleocapsid in several of the virions. **B,** Human T-leukemia virus. Note the C-type morphology characterized by a central symmetrical nucleocapsid. (From Belshe RB, editor: *Textbook of human virology,* ed 2, St Louis, 1991, Mosby.)

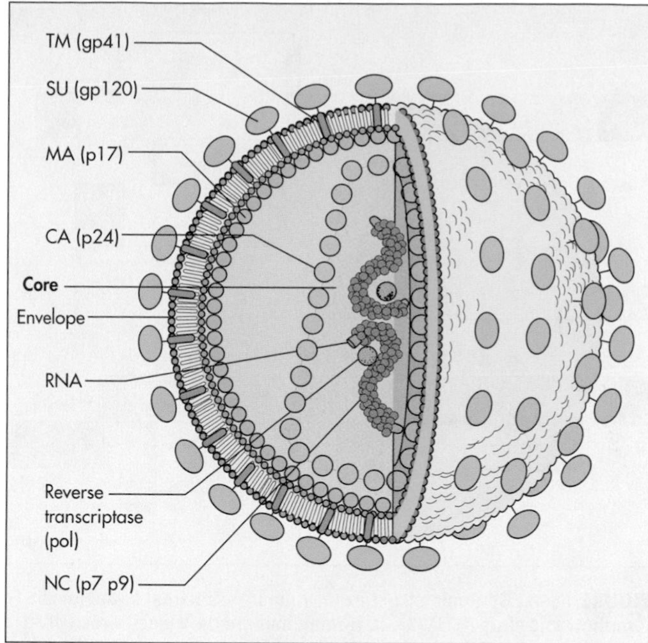

FIGURE 65–3. Cross section of human immunodeficiency virus. The enveloped virion contains two identical RNA strands, RNA polymerase, integrase, and two transfer RNAs (tRNAs) base-paired to the genome within the protein core. This is surrounded by proteins and a lipid bilayer. The envelope spikes are the glycoprotein (gp) 120 attachment protein and gp41 fusion protein. (Redrawn from Gallo RC, Montagnier L: *Sci Am* 259:41-51, 1988.)

integrase enzymes and **two cellular transfer RNA** (tRNAs). These tRNAs are base-paired to each copy of the genome to be used as a primer for the reverse transcriptase. The morphology of the core differs for different viruses and is used as a means of classifying the retroviruses (see Figure 65–1). The HIV virion core resembles a truncated cone (Figure 65–3).

The retrovirus genome has a 5′-cap and is polyadenylated at the 3′-end (Figure 65–4 and Table 65–2). Although the genome resembles a messenger RNA (mRNA), it is not infectious because it does not encode a polymerase that can directly generate more mRNA. The genome of the **simple retroviruses** *consists of three major genes that encode polyproteins* for the following enzymatic and structural proteins of the virus: **gag** (group-specific antigen, *capsid, matrix and nucleic acid binding proteins*), **pol** *(polymerase, protease,* and *integrase),* and **env** (envelope, *glycoproteins*). At each end of the genome are **long-terminal repeat (LTR)** sequences. The LTR sequences contain promoters, enhancers, and other gene sequences used for binding different cellular transcription factors. Oncogenic viruses may also contain a growth-regulating **oncogene.** The **complex retroviruses,** HTLV, and the lentiviruses (including HIV) also *encode several regulatory proteins* that require more complex transcriptional processing (splicing) than the simple retroviruses.

The viral glycoproteins are produced by proteolytic cleavage of the polyprotein encoded by the *env* gene. The size of the glycoproteins differs for each group of viruses. For example, the (glycoprotein) gp62 of HTLV-1 is cleaved into gp46 and p21, and the *gp160 of HIV is cleaved into gp41 and gp120.* These glycoproteins form lollipop-like trimer spikes that are visible on the surface of the virion. The larger of the glycoproteins binds to cell surface receptors, initially determines the tissue tropism of the virus, and is recognized by neutralizing antibody. The smaller subunit (gp41 in HIV) forms the lollipop stick and promotes cell-cell fusion. The gp120 of HIV is extensively glycosylated, and *its antigenicity and receptor specificity can drift during the course of a chronic HIV infection.* These factors impede immune clearance of the virus.

Replication

Replication of the human retroviruses (HIV and HTLV) starts with binding of the viral glycoprotein spikes (trimer

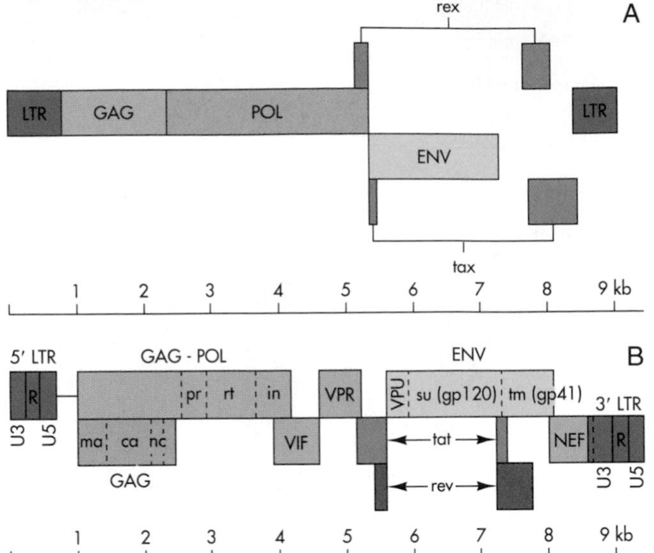

FIGURE 65–4. Genomic structure of human retroviruses. **A,** Human T-lymphotropic virus (HTLV-1). **B,** Human immunodeficiency virus (HIV-1). The genes are defined in Table 65–2 and Figure 65–7. Unlike the other genes of these viruses, production of the messenger RNA for tax and rex (HTLV-1) and tat and rev (HIV) requires excision of two intron units. HIV-2 has a similar genome map. The vpu for HIV-2 is termed *vpx.* LTR, Long-terminal repeat. Protein nomenclature for HIV: ca, capsid protein; in, integrase; ma, matrix protein; nc, nucleocapsid protein; pr, protease; rt, reverse transcriptasesu, surface glycoprotein component; tm, transmembrane glycoprotein component. (Redrawn from Belshe RB, editor: *Textbook of human virology,* ed 2, St Louis, 1991, Mosby.)

of gp120 and gp41 molecules) to the **CD4 protein, the primary receptor** (Figure 65–5). For newly transmitted HIV, the gp120 binds to the CD4 protein on cells of the macrophage lineage (e.g., macrophage, dendritic cells, microglial cells) and activated T cells, as well as a second receptor, a 7-transmembrane G-protein–coupled chemokine receptor **(CCR5 on macrophages and activated T cells).** Variants of HIV bind to CD4 and a different chemokine receptor **[CXCR4]** on naïve and other helper T cells **(T-tropic)** (Figure 65–6). Chemokines are small peptides involved in promoting inflammatory responses and chemotaxis. A small percentage of people are resistant to infection because they are genetically deficient in these co-receptors. Binding to the chemokine receptor brings the viral envelope and cell plasma membrane close together and allows the gp41 to interact with and promote the fusion of the two membranes. The fusion step is the target for an antiviral drug that interferes with the action of gp41.

Once released into the cytoplasm, the early phase of replication begins. The reverse transcriptase, encoded by the *pol* gene, uses the tRNA in the virion as a primer and synthesizes a **complementary**, negative-strand DNA **[cDNA]**. The reverse transcriptase also acts as a ribonuclease H, degrades the RNA genome, and then synthesizes the positive strand of DNA (Figure 65–7). The reverse

TABLE 65–2. Retrovirus Genes and Their Function

Gene	Virus	Function
gag	All	Group-specific antigen: core and capsid proteins
int	All	Integrase
pol	All	Polymerase: reverse transcriptase, protease, integrase
pro	All	Protease
env	All	Envelope: glycoproteins
tax	HTLV	Transactivation of viral and cellular genes
tat	HIV-1	Transactivation of viral and cellular genes
rex	HTLV	Regulation of RNA splicing and promotion of export to cytoplasm
rev	HIV-1	Regulation of RNA splicing and promotion of export to cytoplasm
nef	HIV-1	Alteration of cell activation signals; progression to AIDS (essential)
vif	HIV-1	Virus infectivity, promotion of assembly, blocks a cellular antiviral protein
vpu	HIV-1	Facilitates virion assembly and release, decrease of cell surface CD4
vpr (vpx*)	HIV-1	Transport of complementary DNA to nucleus, arresting of cell growth
LTR	All	Promoter, enhancer elements

HIV, Human immunodeficiency virus; HTLV, human T-lymphotropic virus; LTR, long-terminal repeat (sequence).
*In HIV-2.

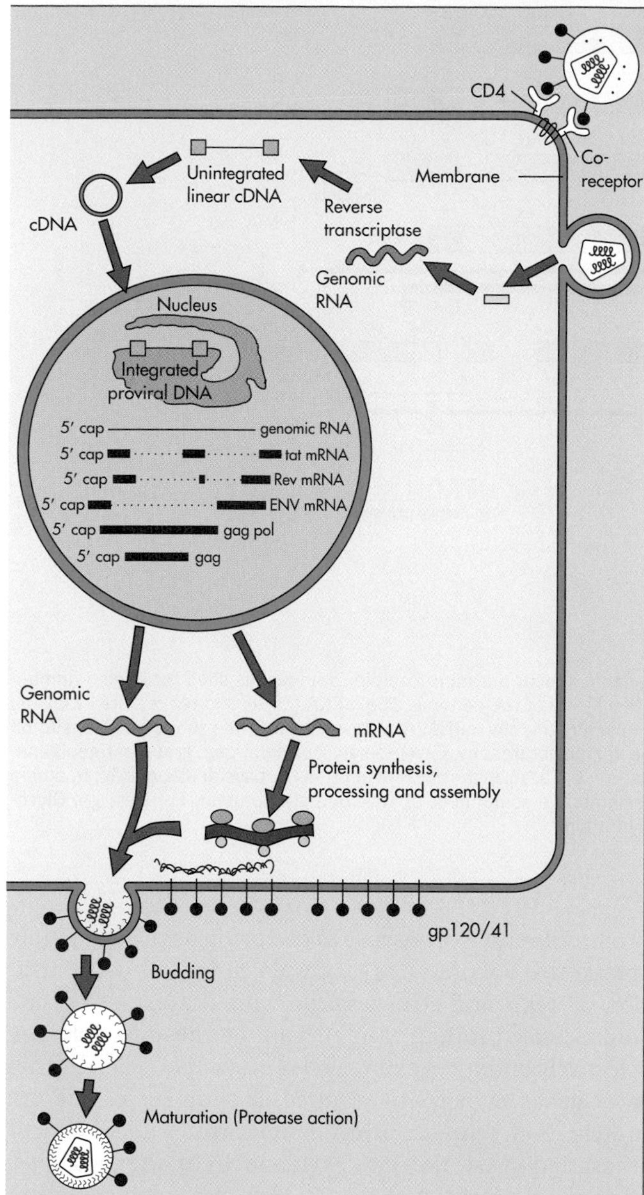

FIGURE 65–5. The life cycle of human immunodeficiency virus (HIV). HIV binds to CD4 and chemokine co-receptors and enters by fusion. The genome is reverse transcribed into DNA in the cytoplasm and integrated into the nuclear DNA. Transcription and translation of the genome occur in a fashion similar to that of human T-lymphotropic virus (HTLV-1) (see Figure 65–7). The virus assembles at the plasma membrane and matures after budding from the cell. cDNA, complementary DNA. (Redrawn from Fauci AS: *Science* 239:617-622, 1988.)

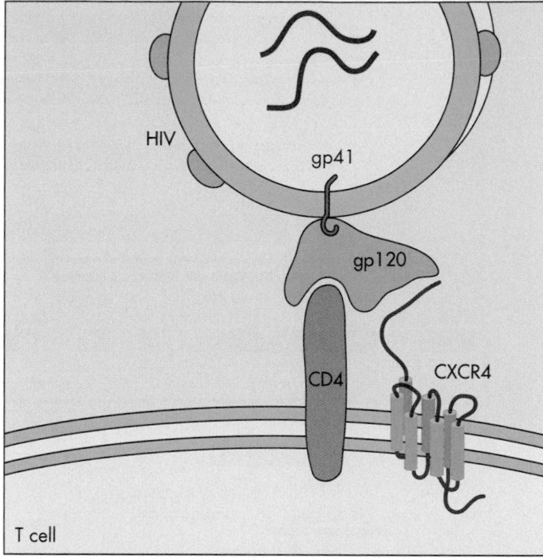

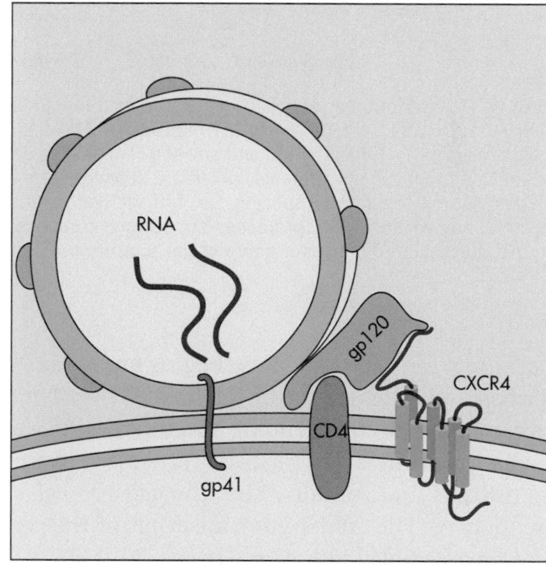

FIGURE 65–6. Target cell binding of human immunodeficiency virus. (Redrawn from Balter M: *Science* 274:1988, 1996.)

transcriptase is the major target for antiviral drugs. During the synthesis of the virion DNA **(provirus)**, sequences from each end of the genome (U3 and U5) are duplicated, thus attaching the LTRs to both ends. This process creates sequences necessary for integration and *creates enhancer and promoter sequences within the LTR for the regulation of transcription.* The DNA copy of the genome is larger than the original RNA.

Reverse transcriptase is very error prone. For example, the error rate for the reverse transcriptase from HIV is one error per 2000 bases, or approximately five errors per genome (HIV, 9000 base pairs), the equivalent of at least one typo on every page of this text, but different for every book. This genetic instability of HIV is responsible for promoting the generation of new strains of virus during a person's disease, a property that may alter the pathogenicity of the virus and promote immune escape.

The double-stranded cDNA is then delivered to the nucleus and spliced into the host chromosome with the aid of a virus-encoded, virion-carried enzyme, **integrase.** Integration requires cell growth, but the cDNA of HIV and other lentiviruses can remain in the nucleus and cytoplasm in a nonintegrated circular DNA form until the cell is activated.

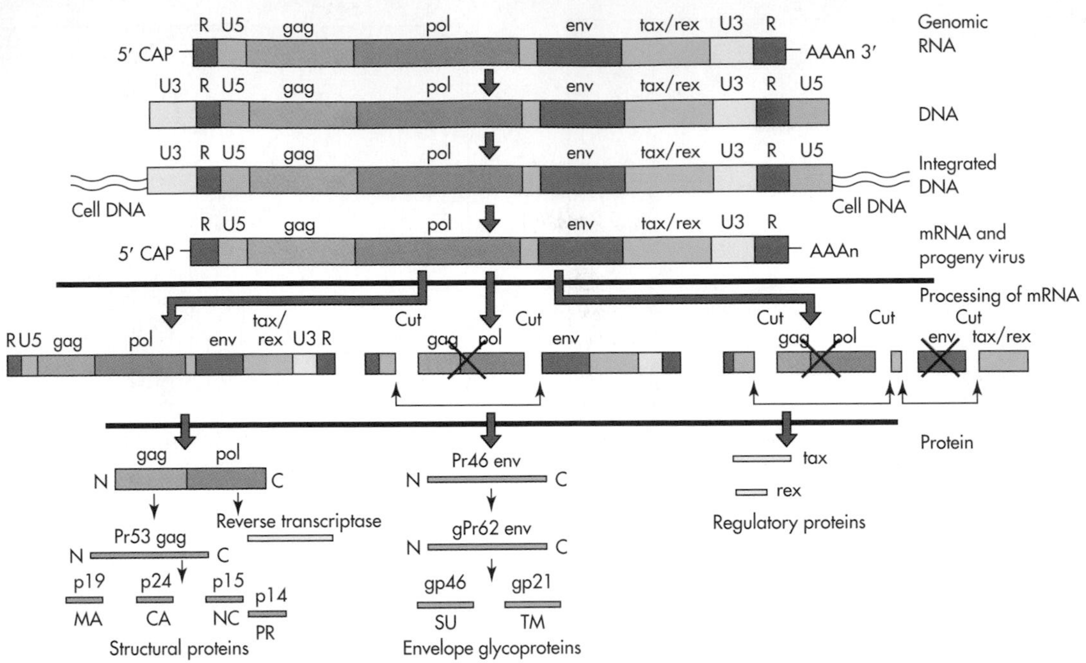

FIGURE 65–7. Transcription and translation of human T-leukemia virus (HTLV-1). (A similar but more complex approach is used for human immunodeficiency virus [HIV].). All HTLV-1 and HIV messenger RNA (mRNA) include the 5′-end of the genome. The mRNA for tax and rex requires excision of two sequences (*red X*), the gag-pol and env sequences. The other mRNAs, including the env mRNA, require excision of one sequence. Translation of these mRNAs produces polyproteins, which are subsequently cleaved. Gene nomenclature: env, Envelope glycoprotein; gag, group antigen gene; pol, polymerase; rex, regulator of splicing; tax, transactivator. Protein nomenclature: C, Carboxyl terminus of peptide CA, capsid; MA, matrix; N, amino terminus; NC, nucleocapsid; PR, protease; SU, surface component; TM, transmembrane component of envelope glycoprotein. Prefixes: gp, Glycoprotein; gPr, glycosylated precursor polyprotein; p, protein; PR, precursor polyprotein.

Once integrated, the late phase begins and viral DNA is transcribed as a cellular gene by the host RNA polymerase II. Transcription of the genome produces a full-length RNA, which for simple retroviruses is processed to produce several mRNAs that contain either the *gag*, *gag-pol*, or *env* gene sequences. The full-length transcripts of the genome can also be assembled into new virions.

Because the virus acts as a cellular gene, its replication depends on the extent of methylation of the viral DNA and on the cell's growth rate, but mostly on the ability of the cell to recognize the enhancers and promoter sequences encoded in the LTR region. Stimulation of the cell in response to other infections, through the action of cytokines, or mitogens, produces transcription factors that bind to the LTR and can activate transcription of the virus. If the virus encodes viral oncogenes, they can promote cell growth, stimulate transcription and hence viral replication. *The ability of a cell to transcribe the retroviral genome is the second major determinant of tissue tropism and host range for a retrovirus.*

HTLV and HIV are complex retroviruses. HTLV-1 encodes two proteins, **tax** and **rex,** that regulate viral replication. Unlike the other viral mRNAs, the mRNA for tax and rex requires more than one splicing step. The *rex* gene encodes two proteins that bind to a structure on the viral mRNA and thereby prevents further splicing and promotes mRNA transport to the cytoplasm. The doubly spliced tax/rex mRNA is expressed early (low concentration of rex), and structural proteins are expressed late (high concentration of rex). Late in the infection, rex selectively enhances expression of the singly spliced structural genes, which are required in abundance. The tax protein is a **transcriptional activator** and enhances transcription of the viral genome from the promoter gene sequence in the 5′ LTR. Tax also activates other genes, including interleukin-2 (IL-2), IL-3, granulocyte-macrophage colony-stimulating factor, and the receptor for IL-2. Activation of these genes promotes the growth of the infected T cell.

HIV replication is regulated by as many as six **"accessory" gene products** (see Table 65–2). The **tat,** like tax, is a transactivator of the transcription of viral and cellular genes. The **rev** acts like the rex protein to regulate and promote transport of viral mRNA into the cytoplasm. The **nef** protein reduces cell surface expression of CD4 and major histocompatibility class I molecules, alters T-cell signaling pathways, regulates the cytotoxicity of the virus, and is required to maintain high viral loads. The nef protein appears to be essential for causing the infection to progress to AIDS. The **vif** protein promotes assembly and maturation and binds to an antiviral cellular protein to prevent it from hypermutating the cDNA and helps the virus replicate in myeloid and other cells. The **vpu** reduces cell surface CD4 expression and enhances virion release. The **vpr** (vpx in HIV-2) is important for transport of the cDNA into the nucleus and for virus replication in non-growing cells, like macrophages. VPR also arrests the cell in the G2 phase of the growth cycle, which is likely to be optimal for HIV replication. The cell also controls HIV replication, and activation of the T cell by a mitogen or antigen also promotes virus replication.

The proteins translated from the gag, gag-pol, and env mRNAs are synthesized as polyproteins and are subsequently cleaved to functional proteins (see Figure 65–7). The viral glycoproteins are synthesized, glycosylated, and processed by the endoplasmic reticulum and Golgi apparatus. These glycoproteins are then cleaved into membrane-spanning and extracellular subunits of the viral attachment protein, which associate to form trimers and migrate to the plasma membrane.

The gag and the gag-pol polyproteins are acylated and then bind to the plasma membrane containing the envelope glycoprotein. The association of two copies of the genome and cellular transfer RNA molecules promotes budding of the virion. After envelopment and release from the cell, the viral protease cleaves the gag and gag-pol polyproteins to release the reverse transcriptase and form the virion core, thus ensuring the inclusion of these components into the virion. The protease step is required for the production of infectious virions and is a target for antiviral drugs.

The envelopment and release of retroviruses occur at the cell surface. Replication and budding of the retrovirus does not necessarily kill the cell. HIV can also spread from cell to cell through the production of multinucleated giant cells, or syncytia. Syncytia are fragile, and their formation enhances the cytolytic activity of the virus.

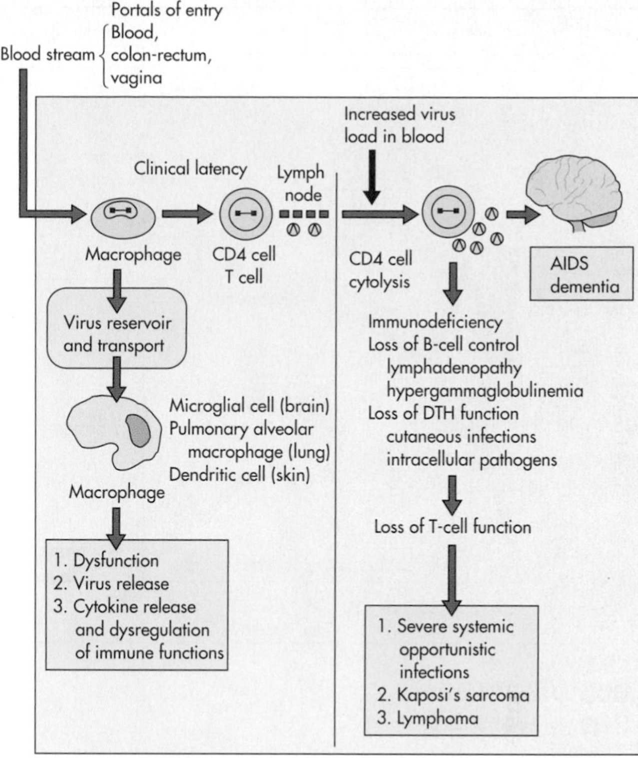

FIGURE 65–8. Pathogenesis of human immunodeficiency virus (HIV). HIV causes lytic and latent infection of CD4 T cells and persistent infection of cells of the monocyte macrophage family and disrupts neurons. The outcomes of these actions are immunodeficiency and acquired immune deficiency syndrome (AIDS) dementia. DTH, Delayed-type hypersensitivity. (Redrawn from Fauci AS: *Science* 239:617–622, 1988.)

BOX 65–2. Disease Mechanisms of HIV

Human immunodeficiency virus primarily infects CD4 T cells and cells of the macrophage lineage (e.g., monocytes, macrophages, alveolar macrophages of the lung, dendritic cells of the skin, and microglial cells of the brain).
Virus causes lytic infection of CD4 T cells and persistent low-level productive infection of macrophage lineage cells.
Virus causes syncytia formation, with cells expressing large amounts of CD4 antigen (T cells) with subsequent lysis of the cells.
Virus alters T-cell and macrophage cell function.

Human Immunodeficiency Virus

PATHOGENESIS AND IMMUNITY

The major determinant in the pathogenesis and disease caused by HIV is the **virus tropism for CD4-expressing T cells and macrophages** (Box 65–2 and Figure 65–8). HIV-induced immunosuppression (AIDS) results from a reduction in the number of CD4 T cells, which decimates the helper and delayed-type hypersensitivity (DTH) functions of the immune response.

During vaginal or anal intercourse, HIV-1 infects and sticks to Langerhans and dendritic cells in the epithelium, and these can then travel to lymph nodes. HIV binds and can remain on the surface of dendritic cells through a lectin molecule, DC-SIGN, and use the dendritic cell to deliver the virus and promote infection of CD4 T cells. Anal sex may be of greater risk than other routes of infection. Special T cells bearing a greater number of co-receptors for the virus are separated by only a single layer of cells from the colon. On injection of virus into blood, the virus is likely to infect dendritic, other monocyte-macrophage lineage cells, and CCR5 expressing T cells. Macrophage-lineage cells can be infected by CCR5 and CXCR4 binding variants of HIV. Macrophages are persistently infected with HIV and are probably the major reservoirs and means of distribution of HIV. Mutation in the *env* gene for the gp120 shifts the tropism of the virus from

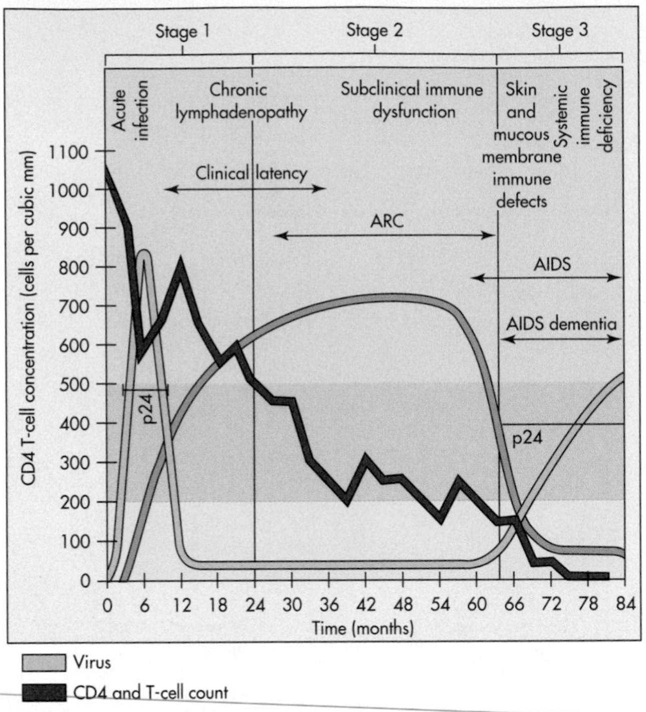

FIGURE 65–9. Time course and stages of human immunodeficiency virus (HIV) disease. A long clinical latency period follows the initial mononucleosis-like symptoms. The progressive decrease in the number of CD4 T cells, even during the latency period, allows opportunistic infections to occur. The stages in HIV disease are defined by the CD4 T-cell levels and occurrence of opportunistic diseases. ARC, acquired immune deficiency syndrome (AIDS)-related complex. (Redrawn from Redfield RR, Buske DS: *Sci Am* 259:90–98, 1988, updated 1996.)

macrophages to CD4 T cells. Continuous replication of the virus occurs in the lymph nodes, with subsequent release of the virus and infected T cells into the blood. Reductions in the numbers of CD4 T cells may result from HIV-induced cytolysis, cytotoxic T-cell immune cytolysis, or chronic activation in response to the large HIV antigen challenge leading to a rapid terminal differentiation and death of T cells. The development of the symptoms of AIDS correlates with increased release of virus into the blood and a decrease in total T cell numbers (CD3 bearing cells) (Figure 65–9).

HIV induces several cytopathologic effects that may kill the infected T cell (Table 65–3). These include an accumulation of nonintegrated circular DNA copies of the genome, increased permeability of the plasma membrane, syncytia formation, and induction of apoptosis (programmed cell death). The relative ability of HIV to kill the target cell correlates with the amount of CD4 expressed by the cell. Macrophages may be spared the cytolytic action of HIV because they express less CD4 than T cells. The accessory proteins of HIV are important for replication and virulence. As noted earlier, the nef protein appears to be essential for promoting the progression of HIV infection

TABLE 65–3. Means of HIV Escape from the Immune System

Characteristic	Function
Infection of lymphocytes and macrophages	Inactivation of key element of immune defense
Inactivation of CD4 helper cells	Loss of activator of the immune system and delayed-type hypersensitivity
Antigenic drift of gp120	Evasion of antibody detection
Heavy glycosylation of gp120	Evasion of antibody detection

to AIDS. Individuals infected with natural mutants of nef, and primates infected with mutants of the simian immunodeficiency virus, which lacks nef, have lived beyond their expected lifetimes (nonprogressors).

The immune response to HIV restricts viral infection but contributes to pathogenesis. Neutralizing antibodies are generated against gp120 and participate in antibody-dependent cellular cytotoxicity responses. Antibody-coated virus is infectious, however, and is taken up by macrophages. CD8 T cells are critical for controlling HIV disease progression. CD8 T cells can kill infected cells by direct cytotoxic action and by producing suppressive factors that restrict viral replication, including chemokines that also block the binding of virus to its coreceptor. However, CD8 T cells require activation by CD4 T cells, CD8 T-cell numbers decrease with CD4 T-cell number, and their reduction correlates with disease progression to AIDS.

HIV has several ways of escaping immune control. Most significant is the virus's ability to undergo mutation and, hence, alter its antigenicity and escape antibody clearance. By targeting the CD4 T cell that controls other T cells, B cells, and macrophages through cytokine production, HIV compromises the entire immune system. Persistent infection of macrophages and CD4 T cells maintains the virus in an immune-privileged cell and cells in immune-privileged tissues (e.g., central nervous system and genital organs) (see Table 65–3).

The course of HIV disease parallels the reduction in CD4 T-cell numbers and the amount of virus in the blood (see Figure 65–9). Initially, (acute phase) there is a large burst of virus production (10^7 particles per ml of plasma) and viremia. T cell proliferation and responses to the infected lymphoid and myeloid cells promotes a mononucleosis-like syndrome. Virus levels in the blood decrease during a clinically latent period, but viral replication continues in the lymph nodes. Virus also remains latent in macrophage and resting T cells. Late in the disease, virus levels in the blood increase, CD4 levels are significantly decreased, the

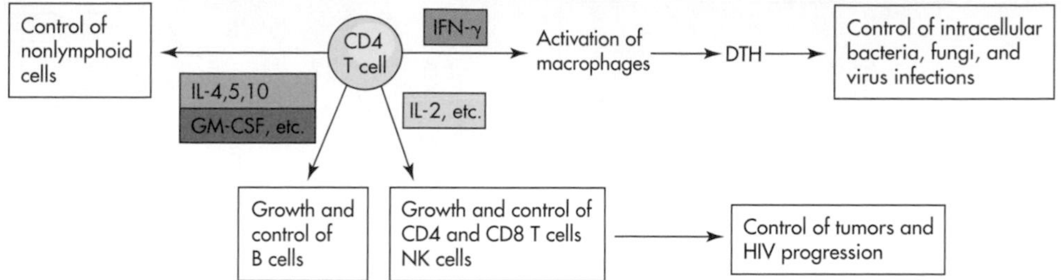

FIGURE 65–10. CD4 T cells have a critical role in the regulation of the human immune response by mediating the release of soluble factors and the delayed-type hypersensitivity (DTH) response toward intracellular pathogens. Human immunodeficiency virus–induced loss of the CD4 T cells results in loss of the functions shown, especially the DTH responses and the lymphokine control of immune responses.

structure of the lymph nodes is destroyed, and the patient becomes immunodepressed.

The central role of the CD4 helper T cells in the initiation of an immune response and DTH is indicated by the extent of the loss of immune response caused by HIV infection (Figure 65–10). Activated CD4 T cells initiate immune responses by the release of cytokines required for the activation of macrophages, other T cells, B cells, and natural killer cells. When CD4 T cells are unavailable or not functional (CD4 numbers less than 200 per microliter), antigen-specific immune responses (especially cellular immune responses) are incapacitated, and humoral responses are uncontrolled. The loss of the CD4 T cells responsible for activating DTH allows the outgrowth of many of the opportunistic intracellular infections characteristic of AIDS (e.g., fungi and intracellular bacteria).

In addition to immunodepression, HIV can also cause neurologic abnormalities. The microglial cell and macrophage are the predominant cell types of a brain infected with HIV, but neurons and glial cells may also be infected. Infected monocytes and microglial cells may release neurotoxic substances or chemotactic factors that promote inflammatory responses in the brain. Direct cytopathologic effects of the virus on neurons are also possible.

EPIDEMIOLOGY

AIDS was first noted in homosexual men in the United States but has spread in epidemic proportions throughout the population (Box 65–3). In 2003, it was estimated that 5 million new HIV infections occur per year, with 3 million deaths per year due to AIDS (according to Joint United Nations Programme on HIV/AIDS [UNAIDS] and World Health Organization [WHO] data) (Figures 65–11 and 65–12).

HIV is thought to be derived from simian immunodeficiency virus, and, in fact, HIV-2 is similar to simian immunodeficiency virus. The initial human infection occurred in Africa in the 1930s but went unnoticed in rural areas. The migration of infected people to the cities after the 1960s brought the virus into population centers, and cultural acceptance of prostitution promoted its transmission throughout the population.

BOX 65–3. Epidemiology of HIV Infections

Disease Viral Factors

Enveloped virus is easily inactivated and must be transmitted in body fluids.

Disease has a long prodromal period.

Virus can be shed before development of identifiable symptoms.

Transmission

Virus is present in blood, semen, and vaginal secretions.

See Table 65–4 for modes of transmission.

Who Is at Risk?

Intravenous drug abusers; sexually active people with many partners (homosexual and heterosexual); prostitutes; newborns of HIV–positive mothers.

Blood and organ transplant recipients and hemophiliacs: Before 1985 (prescreening programs).

Geography Season

There is an expanding epidemic worldwide.

There is no seasonal incidence.

Modes of Control

Antiviral drugs limit progression of disease.

Vaccines for prevention and treatment are in trials.

Safe, monogamous sex helps limit spread.

Sterile injection needles should be used.

Large-scale screening programs for blood for transfusions, organs for transplants, and clotting factors used by hemophiliacs.

Clades and Geographic Distribution

HIV-1 infections are spreading worldwide, with the largest number of AIDS cases in sub-Saharan Africa but with a growing number of cases in Asia, the United States, and

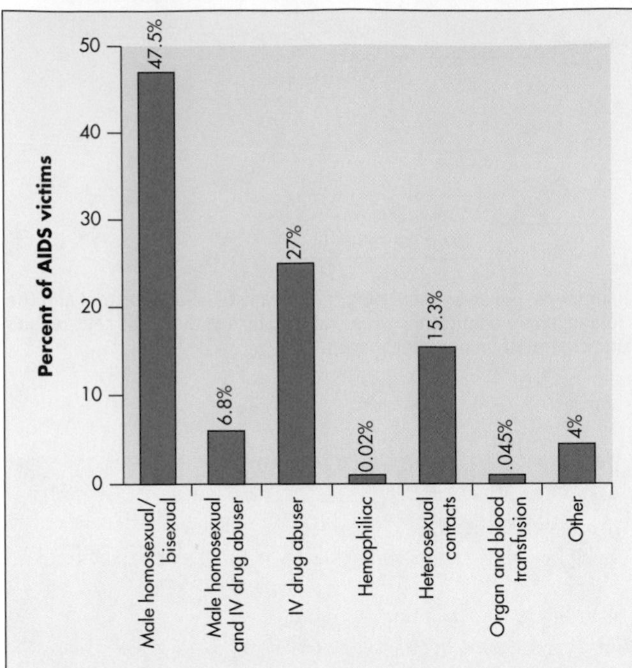

FIGURE 65–11. Acquired immune deficiency syndrome (AIDS) statistics for the United States as of December 2003. The percentages of AIDS cases are presented by exposure category for men, women, and children younger than 13 years. In the United States, unlike Africa and many other parts of the world, male homosexuals are the largest exposure category. However, intravenous (IV) drug abusers and heterosexual partners are becoming more prevalent. (From the Centers for Disease Control and Prevention: *HIV/AIDS surveillance report,* available at www.cdc.gov/hiv/stats/hasrlink.htm)

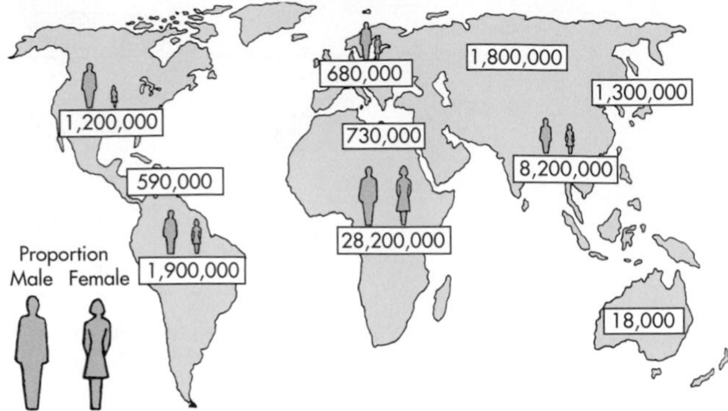

FIGURE 65–12. Upper estimates of cumulative global distribution of human immunodeficiency virus (HIV) infections as of the end of 2003. The estimated cumulative global total of HIV-infected adults in 2003 was approximately 46 million. Infection rates vary widely in different regions of the world. The highest rates are in sub-Saharan Africa. (Modified from AIDS Epidemic Update, Dec 2003 www.unaids.org)

the rest of the world (see Figure 65–12). HIV-2 is more prevalent in Africa (especially West Africa) than in the United States and other parts of the world. Heterosexual transmission is the major means of spread of HIV-1 and HIV-2 in Africa, with men and women equally affected by these viruses. HIV-2 produces a disease similar to but less severe than AIDS. There are at least nine subtypes, or **clades,** of HIV-1, designated A through H, M, and O, and for HIV-2, A-E, based on the sequence of their *env* and *gag* genes. The gp120 and capsid proteins of viruses in different clades differ, and these are the major antigens for antibody and T cells. The different clades have different worldwide geographic distributions.

TABLE 65–4. Transmission of HIV Infection

Routes	Specific Transmission
Known Routes of Transmission	
Inoculation in blood	Transfusion of blood and blood products
	Needle sharing among intravenous drug abusers
	Needlestick, open wound, and mucous membrane exposure in health care workers
	Tattoo needles
Sexual transmission	Anal and vaginal intercourse
Perinatal transmission	Intrauterine transmission
	Peripartum transmission
	Breast milk
Routes Not Involved in Transmission	
Close personal contact	Household members
	Health care workers not exposed to blood

Transmission

The presence of **HIV in the blood, semen, and vaginal secretions** of infected people and **the long asymptomatic period of infection** are factors that have promoted the spread of the disease through sexual contact and exposure to contaminated blood and blood products (Table 65–4). The virus can also be transmitted perinatally to newborns. HIV is ***not,*** however, transmitted by casual contact, touching, hugging, kissing, coughing, sneezing, insect bites, water, food, utensils, toilets, swimming pools, or public baths.

Populations at Highest Risk

Sexually active people (homosexual and heterosexual), intravenous drug abusers and their sexual partners, and the newborns of HIV-positive mothers are at highest risk for HIV infections, with black and Hispanic persons disproportionally represented in the HIV-positive population.

As already noted, AIDS was initially described in young, promiscuous homosexual men and is still prevalent in the gay community. Anal intercourse is an efficient means of viral transmission. However, heterosexual transmission by vaginal intercourse and intravenous drug abuse have become the major routes by which HIV is being spread in the population. The prevalence of HIV in drug abusers stems from sharing contaminated syringe needles, a common practice in "shooting galleries." In New York alone, more than 80% of intravenous drug abusers are positive for the HIV antibody, and these people are now the major source of heterosexual and congenital transmission of the virus.

Before 1985, people receiving blood transfusions or organ transplants and hemophiliacs receiving clotting factors from pooled blood were at high risk for HIV infection. HIV was spread in many countries by health care workers using shared or improperly sterilized syringe needles or instruments. Proper screening of the blood supply and transplant tissue in the United States and elsewhere has practically eliminated the danger of HIV being transmitted in blood transfusions (see Figure 65–12). Hemophiliacs who receive pooled clotting factors are protected further by the proper handling of the factor (prolonged heating) to kill the virus.

Health care workers are at risk for HIV infection from accidental needlesticks or cuts or through the exposure of broken skin and mucosal membranes to contaminated blood. Fortunately, studies of needlestick victims have shown that seroconversion occurs in fewer than 1% of those exposed to HIV-positive blood. Tattoo needles and contaminated inks are other potential means by which HIV can be transmitted.

BOX 65–4. Potential Antiviral Therapies for HIV Infection

Nucleoside Analogue Reverse Transcriptase Inhibitors
Azidothymidine (AZT) (Zidovudine/retrovir)
Dideoxycytidine (ddC) (Zalcitabine)
Dideoxyinosine (ddI) (Didanosine)
d4T (Stavudine)
3TC (Lamivudine)
Tenofovir disoproxil fumarate (adenosine class) (Viread)
ABC (Abacavir)

Non-nucleoside Reverse Transcriptase Inhibitors
Nevirapine (Viramune)
Delavirdine (Rescriptor)
Efavirenz (Sustiva)

Protease Inhibitors
Saquinavir (Invirase/Fortovase)
Ritonavir (Norvir)
Indinavir (Crixivan)
Lopinavir (Kaletra)
Nelfinavir (Viracept)
Amprenavir (Agenerase)
Fosamprevavir (Lexavir)
Atazanavir (Reyataz)

Fusion Inhibitor
T-20 (enfuvirtide/Fuzeon)

Highly Active Antiretroviral Therapy (HAART) (Combination)
Abacavir/zidovudine/lamivudine (Trizivir)
Indinavir/AZT/3TC
Ritonavir/AZT/3TC
Nelfinavir/AZT/3TC
Nevirapine/AZT/ddI
Nevirapine/indinavir/3T

CLINICAL SYNDROMES

AIDS is one of the most devastating epidemics ever recorded. Most HIV-infected people will become symptomatic, and the overwhelming majority of them will ultimately succumb to the disease without treatment. HIV disease progresses from an asymptomatic infection to profound immunosuppression, referred to as full-blown AIDS (see Figure 65–9). The diseases related to AIDS mainly consist of opportunistic infections, cancers, and the direct effects of HIV on the central nervous system (Table 65–5). Although rare, there are cases of long-term survivors. Some of these result from infection with HIV strains that lack a functional nef protein. Resistance to the virus correlates with a lack of expression of the chemokine co-receptor for the virus.

The initial symptoms following HIV infection (acute phase, 2 to 4 weeks after infection) may resemble those of influenza or infectious mononucleosis, with an "aseptic" meningitis or a rash occurring up to 3 months after infection (Box 65–5). As in mononucleosis, the symptoms stem from immune responses triggered by a widespread infection of lymphoid cells. These symptoms subside spontaneously after 2 to 3 weeks and are followed by a period of asymptomatic infection or a persistent generalized lymphadenopathy that may last for several years. During this period, the virus is replicating in the lymph nodes.

BOX 65–5. Clinical Summary

A 32-year-old ex-heroin addict had a mononucleosis-like illness for 2 weeks, occasional night sweats and fever for 3 years and then presented with thrush, cytomegalovirus retinitis, and pneumocystis pneumonia. His CD4 T-cell count is less than 200 per μl. He was started on highly active antiretroviral therapy treatment.

Deterioration of the immune response is indicated by increased susceptibility to opportunistic pathogens, especially those controlled by CD4 T cells, activated macrophages, CD8 T-cells, and DTH responses (e.g.,

TABLE 65–5. Indicator Diseases of AIDS*

Infection	Disease
Opportunistic infections	
Protozoal	Toxoplasmosis of the brain Cryptosporidiosis with diarrhea Isosporiasis with diarrhea
Fungal	Candidiasis of the esophagus, trachea, and lungs *Pneumocystis jiroveci* (previously called *Pneumocystis carinii*) pneumonia Cryptococcosis (extrapulmonary) Histoplasmosis (disseminated) Coccidioidomycosis (disseminated)
Viral	Cytomegalovirus disease Herpes simplex virus infection (persistent or disseminated) Progressive multifocal leukoencephalopathy Hairy leukoplakia caused by Epstein-Barr virus
Bacterial	*Mycobacterium avium-intracellulare* complex (disseminated) Any "atypical" mycobacterial disease Extrapulmonary tuberculosis *Salmonella* septicemia (recurrent) Pyogenic bacterial infections (multiple or recurrent)
Opportunistic neoplasias	Kaposi's sarcoma Primary lymphoma of the brain Other non-Hodgkin's lymphomas
Others	HIV wasting syndrome HIV encephalopathy Lymphoid interstitial pneumonia

Modified from Belshe RB, editor: *Textbook of human virology*, ed 2, St Louis, 1991, Mosby.
HIV, human immunodeficiency virus.
*Manifestations of HIV infection–defining acquired immune deficiency syndrome according to criteria of Centers for Disease Control and Prevention.

yeasts, herpesviruses, or intracellular bacteria). The onset of symptoms correlates with a reduction in the number of CD4 T cells to less than 450/μl and increased levels of virus (as determined by polymerase chain reaction [PCR]-related techniques) and protein p24 in the blood. Full-blown AIDS occurs when the CD4 T-cell counts are less than 200/μl and involves the onset of more significant diseases, including HIV wasting syndrome (weight loss and diarrhea for more than 1 month) and the occurrence of indicator diseases such as **Kaposi's sarcoma** or specific opportunistic diseases, especially **pneumocystis pneumonia, *Mycobacterium avium-intracellulare* complex** infection, and **severe cytomegalovirus disease** (see Table 65–5).

AIDS may be manifested in several different ways, including lymphadenopathy and fever, opportunistic infections, malignancies, and AIDS-related dementia.

Lymphadenopathy and Fever

Lymphadenopathy and fever can occur, and this combination of clinical findings has been called the **AIDS-related complex (ARC).** It is a process that develops insidiously and may be accompanied by weight loss and malaise. These findings may persist indefinitely or may progress. Symptoms may also include opportunistic infections, diarrhea, night sweats, and fatigue. The wasting disease is termed *slim disease* in Africa.

Opportunistic Infections

Normally benign infections caused by agents such as *Candida albicans* and other fungi, DNA viruses capable of recurrent disease, parasites, and intracellularly growing bacteria cause significant disease after the HIV depletion of CD4 T cells (See Table 65–5). ***Pneumocystis jiroveci*** (previously called *Pneumocystis carinii*) **induced pneumocystis (PCP) pneumonia** is a major sign of AIDS. Oral candidiasis (thrush), cerebral toxoplasmosis, and cryptococcal meningitis also often occur, as do prolonged and severe infections caused by the herpesviruses (e.g., herpes simplex virus; varicella-zoster virus; Epstein-Barr virus [EBV, hairy leukoplakia of the mouth, EBV–associated lymphomas]; cytomegalovirus [especially retinitis, pneumonia, and bowel disease]; and papovaviruses [JC virus causing progressive multifocal leukoencephalopathy]). Tuberculosis and other mycobacterial diseases and diarrhea caused by common pathogens (*Salmonella*, *Shigella*, and *Campylobacter* species) and uncommon agents (cryptosporidia, mycobacteria, *Amoeba* species) are also common problems.

Malignancies

The most notable malignancy to develop in patients with AIDS is the human herpesvirus 8–associated Kaposi's sarcoma, a rare and otherwise benign skin cancer that disseminates to involve visceral organs in immunodeficient patients. Non-Hodgkin's lymphoma and EBV-related lymphomas are also prevalent.

Dementia Related to AIDS

AIDS-related dementia may result from opportunistic infection or HIV infection of the microglial cells and neurons of the brain. Patients with this condition may undergo a slow deterioration of their intellectual abilities and other signs of a neurologic disorder, similar to the signs of the early stages of Alzheimer's disease. Neurologic deterioration could also result from infection with one of the many opportunistic infections.

TABLE 65–6. Laboratory Analysis for HIV

Test	Purpose
Serology	
Enzyme-linked immunosorbent assay	Initial screening
Latex agglutination	Initial screening
Rapid oral antibody test	Initial screening
Western blot analysis	Confirmation test
Immunofluorescence	Confirmation test
Virion RNA RT-PCR	Detection of virus in blood
Real-time RT-PCR	Quantitation of virus in blood
Branched-chain DNA	Quantitation of virus in blood
p24 antigen	Early marker of infection
Isolation of virus	Test not readily available
CD4 : CD8 T-cell ratio	Correlate of human immunodeficiency virus disease

RT-PCR, Teverse transcriptase polymerase chain reaction.

LABORATORY DIAGNOSIS

Tests for HIV infection are performed for one of three reasons: (1) to identify those with the infection, so that antiviral drug therapy can be initiated, (2) to identify carriers who may transmit infection to others (specifically blood or organ donors, pregnant women, and sex partners), or (3) to follow the course of disease and confirm the diagnosis of AIDS (Table 65–6). The chronic nature of the disease allows the use of serologic tests to document HIV infection as supplemented by genomic detection and quantitation using PCR-related techniques. Unfortunately, serologic tests cannot identify recently infected people. HIV is very difficult to grow in tissue culture, and virus isolation is not performed. Recent infection or late stage disease are indicated by the presence of the p24 viral antigen, the reverse transcriptase enzyme, or large quantities of viral RNA in blood samples (see Figure 65–9). Viral RNA (in virions) in blood can be detected by the reverse transcriptase polymerase chain reaction (RT-PCR), real-time PCR, and related methods. Blood levels of viral RNA are also useful as a monitor for the success of antiviral drug therapy.

Genomics

Newer methods for detection and quantitation of HIV genomes in blood have become a mainstay for following the course of an HIV infection and the efficacy of antiviral therapy. After converting viral RNA into DNA with a reverse transcriptase (laboratory provided), the cDNA of the genome can be detected by PCR and quantitated by real-time PCR, branched-chain DNA amplification, and other methods (see Chapter 17). Determination of the viral load (amount of genome in blood) allows monitoring of the course of disease and efficacy of therapy.

Serology

Enzyme-linked immunosorbent assays (ELISAs) or agglutination procedures are used for routine screening. The ELISA test, however, can yield false-positive results and will not detect a recent infection. More specific procedures, such as the Western blot analysis, are subsequently used to confirm seropositive results. The Western blot assay (see Chapter 51 and Figure 51–7), on the other hand, determines the presence of antibody to the viral antigens (p24 or p31) and glycoproteins (gp41 and gp120/160). HIV antibody may develop slowly, taking 4 to 8 weeks in most patients; however, it may take 6 months or more in as much as 5% of those infected (see Figure 65–9).

Immunologic Studies

The status of an HIV infection can be implied from an analysis of the T-cell subsets. The absolute number of CD4 lymphocytes and the ratio of helper to inducer lymphocytes (CD4:CD8 ratio) are abnormally low in HIV-infected people. The particular concentration of CD4 lymphocytes identifies the stage of AIDS.

TREATMENT, PREVENTION, AND CONTROL

An extensive effort to develop antiviral drugs and vaccines effective against HIV has been initiated worldwide. The principal (as of summer 2004) anti-HIV therapies are listed in Box 65–4. The anti-HIV drugs approved by the U.S. Food and Drug Administration can be classified as **fusion-penetration, nucleoside analogue reverse transcriptase inhibitors, non-nucleoside reverse transcriptase inhibitors, or protease inhibitors.** Inhibition of the initial viral envelope-cell membrane fusion event with a peptide (T-20: enfuviritide) that blocks the action of the gp41 molecule prevents infection of the cell. Inhibition of the reverse transcriptase prevents the initiation of virus replication by blocking cDNA synthesis. Azidothymidine (AZT), dideoxyinosine (ddI), and dideoxycytidine (ddC) and the other nucleotide analogues are phosphorylated by cellular enzymes and are incorporated into cDNA by the reverse transcriptase to cause DNA chain termination. Non-nucleoside reverse transcriptase inhibitors (nevirapine) inhibit the enzyme by other mechanisms. Protease inhibitors block the morphogenesis of the virion by inhibiting the cleavage of the gag and gag-pol polyproteins. The resulting virion is inactive. Other anti-HIV drugs being developed include different nucleotide analogues and other inhibitors of reverse transcriptase, receptor antagonists (CD4 and gp120 analogues), inhibitors of tat function (Ro 24-7429), glycoprotein glycosylation inhibitors, interferon and interferon inducers, and antisense DNA to essential genome sequences.

In the current guidelines, AZT is recommended for the treatment of asymptomatic or mildly symptomatic people with CD4 counts of less than 500/µl and for the treatment of infected pregnant women to reduce the likelihood of transmission of the virus to the fetus. The significant toxic side effects associated with high-dose AZT therapy can be minimized by administering AZT early in the disease and in smaller, repeated doses. Unfortunately, the high mutation rate of HIV promotes the development of resistance to these drugs. A cocktail of several antiviral drugs (e.g., AZT, 3TC, protease inhibitor) termed **highly active antiretroviral treatment,** each with different mechanisms of action, has less potential to breed resistance and has become a recommended therapy. Multidrug therapy can reduce blood levels of virus to nearly zero and reduce morbidity and mortality in many patients with advanced AIDS. Although HAART is a difficult and expensive drug regimen, many patients return to nearly normal health on this therapy.

Education

The principal way in which HIV infection can be controlled is by educating the population about the methods of transmission and the measures that may curtail viral spread. For instance, monogamous relationships, the practice of safe sex, and the use of condoms reduce the possibility of exposure. Because contaminated needles are a major source of HIV infection in intravenous drug abusers, people must be taught that needles must not be shared. The reuse of contaminated needles in clinics was the source of outbreaks of AIDS in the former Soviet bloc and other countries. In some places, efforts have been launched to provide sterile equipment to intravenous drug abusers. A successful anti-HIV education campaign in Uganda has been cited as more effective than antiviral drugs for saving lives.

Blood, Blood Product, and Organ Screening

Potential blood and organ donors are screened before they donate blood, tissue, and blood products. People testing positive for HIV must not donate blood. People who anticipate a future need for blood, such as those awaiting elective surgery, should consider donating blood beforehand. To limit the worldwide epidemic, blood screening must be initiated in developing nations as well.

Infection Control

The infection-control procedures for HIV infection are the same as those for hepatitis B virus. They include the use of universal blood and body fluid precautions, which are based on the assumption that all patients are infectious for HIV and other blood-borne pathogens. The precautions include wearing protective clothing (e.g., gloves, mask, gown) and using other barriers to prevent exposure to blood products. Syringes and surgical instruments should never be reused unless carefully disinfected. Contaminated surfaces should be disinfected with 10% household bleach, 70% ethanol or isopropanol, 2% glutaraldehyde, 4% formaldehyde, or 6% hydrogen peroxide. Washing laundry in hot water with detergent should be sufficient to inactivate HIV.

Vaccine Development

No vaccine against HIV is available despite several trials. A successful vaccine would prevent acquisition of the virus by adults and transmission of the virus to infants of HIV-positive mothers; it would also block the progression of the disease.

Most HIV vaccines being investigated use gp120 or its precursor, gp160, as the immunogen to develop neutralizing antibody. The gene for this protein has been cloned, expressed in different eukaryotic cell systems (e.g., yeast, baculovirus), and developed as a subunit vaccine. The *env* gene has also been incorporated into the vaccinia, canarypox, and other carrier viruses to create hybrid vaccines.

Specific epitopes and T-cell antigens from the *gag* gene product are also being investigated as possible peptide vaccines. Creating DNA vaccines consisting of eukaryotic expression vectors (plasmids) containing the gene for gp160 or other HIV genes is the newest approach to immunization. The hybrid and DNA vaccines have the potential to elicit both humoral and cellular protective immune responses.

The development of a vaccine against HIV is, however, fraught with several problems unique to the virus. For instance, initial protection would require the production of secretory antibody to prevent sexual transmission and acquisition of the virus. Both antibody and cell-mediated immunity are necessary to protect against and resolve an HIV infection. Although a live attenuated vaccine would be ideal (e.g., deletion of the *nef* gene), these viruses still have some virulence in tests on primates. Protective antibody is difficult to establish because the antigenicity of the gp120 is different for virus in different HIV clades and changes readily through mutation during the infection of the individual. A further problem is that the virus can be spread through syncytia and remains latent, thereby hiding from antibody. HIV also infects and inactivates the cells required to initiate an immune response. Testing of the vaccine would be a problem because HIV is a human disease and long-term follow-up is required to monitor the efficacy of the vaccine.

Human T-Leukemia Virus and Other Oncogenic Retroviruses

The Oncovirinae were originally called the *RNA tumor viruses* and have been associated with the development of leukemias, sarcomas, and lymphomas in many animals. These viruses are not cytolytic. The members of this family are distinguished by the mechanism of cell transformation and thus the length of the latency period between infection and the development of disease (Table 65–7).

TABLE 65–7. Mechanisms of Retrovirus Oncogenesis

Disease	Speed	Effect
Acute leukemia or sarcoma	Fast: Oncogene	Direct effect Provision of growth-enhancing proteins
Leukemia	Slow: Transactivation	Indirect effect Transactivation protein (tax) or long-terminal repeat promoter sequences that enhance expression of cellular growth genes

The **sarcoma and acute leukemia viruses** have incorporated modified versions of cellular genes (protooncogenes) encoding growth-controlling factors into their genome **(v-onc)**. These include genes that encode growth hormones, growth hormone receptors, protein kinases, guanosine triphosphate–binding proteins, and nuclear DNA-binding proteins. These viruses can cause transformation of cells relatively rapidly and are highly oncogenic. *No human virus of this type has been identified.*

At least 35 different viral oncogenes have been identified (Table 65–8). Transformation results from the overproduction or altered activity of the growth-stimulating oncogene product. Increased cell growth then promotes transcription, which also promotes viral replication. Incorporation of the oncogene into many of these viruses causes the coding sequences for the *gag, pol,* or *env* genes to be replaced, such that most of these viruses are defective and require helper viruses for replication. Many of these viruses remain endogenous and are transmitted vertically through the germ line of the animal.

The **leukemia viruses,** including HTLV-1, are competent in terms of replication but cannot transform cells in vitro. They cause cancer after a **long latency period** of at least 30 years. The leukemia viruses promote cell growth in more indirect ways than the oncogene-encoding viruses. Specifically, a transcriptional regulator, tax, is produced and is capable of activating promoters in the LTR region and specific cellular genes (including growth-controlling and cytokine genes such as IL-2 and granulocyte-macrophage colony-stimulating factor) to promote the outgrowth of that cell. Alternatively, by integrating near cellular growth–controlling genes, the enhancer and promoter gene sequences encoded in the viral LTR region can promote the expression of growth-stimulating proteins. Uncontrolled cell growth may be sufficient to transform the cell neoplastically or may promote other genetic aberrations over a long period. These viruses are also associated with non-neoplastic neurologic disorders and other diseases. For example, HTLV-1 causes **adult acute T-cell lymphocytic leukemia (ATLL)** and **HTLV-1–**associated myelopathy (tropical spastic paraparesis), a nononcogenic neurologic disease.

The human oncoviruses include HTLV-1, HTLV-2, and HTLV-5, but only HTLV-1 has been definitively associated with disease (i.e., ATLL). HTLV-2 was isolated from atypical forms of hairy cell leukemia, and HTLV-5 was isolated from a malignant cutaneous lymphoma. HTLV-1 and HTLV-2 share as much as 50% homology.

PATHOGENESIS AND IMMUNITY

HTLV-1 is cell associated and is spread in cells after blood transfusion, sexual intercourse, or breastfeeding. The

TABLE 65–8. Representative Examples of Oncogenes

Function	Oncogene	Virus
Tyrosine kinase	*Src*	Rous sarcoma virus
	Abl	Abelson murine leukemia virus
	Fes	ST feline sarcoma virus
Growth factor receptors	*erb*-B (EGF receptor)	Avian erythroblastosis virus
	erb-A (thyroid hormone receptor)	Avian erythroblastosis virus
Guanosine triphosphate–binding proteins	Ha-*ras*	Harvey murine sarcoma virus
	Ki-*ras*	Kirsten murine sarcoma virus
Nuclear proteins	*Myc*	Avian myelocytomatosis virus
	Myb	Avian myeloblastosis virus
	Fos	Murine osteosarcoma virus FBJ
	Jun	Avian sarcoma virus 17

Based on data from Jawetz E et al: *Medical microbiology*, ed 18, Los Altos, Calif, 1989, Appleton & Lange.

virus enters the bloodstream and infects the CD4 helper and DTH T cells. These T cells have a tendency to reside in the skin, thus contributing to the symptoms of ATLL. Neurons also express a receptor for HTLV-1.

HTLV is competent for replication, with the *gag, pol,* and *env* genes transcribed, translated, and processed as described earlier. In addition to its action on viral genes, the tax protein transactivates the cellular genes for the T-cell growth factor, IL-2 and its receptor (IL-2R), which activates growth in the infected cell. The virus may remain latent or may replicate slowly for many years but may also induce the clonal outgrowth of particular T-cell clones. There is a long latency period (approximately 30 years) before the onset of leukemia.

Although the virus can induce a polyclonal outgrowth of T cells, the HTLV-1–induced adult T-cell leukemia is usually monoclonal. Chromosomal aberrations and rearrangements in the T-cell antigen receptor β gene may accumulate in the HTLV growth-stimulated cells, and it may be this that causes the transition to leukemia.

Antibodies are elicited to the gp46 and other proteins of HTLV-1. HTLV-1 infection also causes immunosuppression.

EPIDEMIOLOGY

HTLV-1 is transmitted and acquired by the same routes as HIV. It is endemic in southern Japan, the Caribbean, Central Africa, and among African Americans in the southeastern United States. In the endemic regions of Japan, the children acquire HTLV-1 in breast milk from their mothers, whereas the adults are infected sexually. The number of seropositive people in some regions of Japan may be as high as 35% (Okinawa), with twice the mortality rate from leukemia compared to other regions. Intravenous drug abuse and blood transfusion are becoming the most prominent means of transmitting the virus in the United States. In the United States, the high-risk groups for HTLV-1 infection are the same as those for HIV infection, and the seroprevalence of HTLV-1 is approaching that of HIV.

CLINICAL SYNDROMES

HTLV infection is usually asymptomatic but can progress to ATLL in approximately one in 20 persons over a 30- to 50-year period. ATLL caused by HTLV-1 is a neoplasia of the CD4 helper T cells that can be acute or chronic. The malignant cells have been termed "flower cells" because they are pleomorphic and contain lobulated nuclei. In addition to an elevated white blood cell count, this form of ATLL is characterized by skin lesions similar to those seen in another leukemia, Sézary's syndrome. ATLL is usually fatal within a year of diagnosis, regardless of treatment.

LABORATORY DIAGNOSIS

HTLV-1 infection is detected using ELISA to find virus-specific antigens in blood, using RT-PCR for viral RNA, or using ELISA to detect specific antiviral antibodies.

TREATMENT, PREVENTION, AND CONTROL

A combination of AZT and interferon-α has been effective in some patients with ATLL. However, no particular treatment has been approved for the management of HTLV-1 infection.

The measures used to limit the spread of HTLV-1 are the same as those used to limit the transmission of HIV. Sexual precautions, screening of the blood supply, and increased awareness of the potential risks and diseases all are ways to prevent transmission of the virus. Routine screening for HTLV-1, HIV, hepatitis B virus, and hepatitis C virus are performed to protect the blood supply. Maternal infection of children is very difficult to control, however.

Endogenous Retroviruses

Different retroviruses have integrated into and become a part of the chromosomes of humans and animals. In fact, retrovirus sequences may make up at least 1% of the human genome. Complete and partial provirus sequences with gene sequences similar to those of HTLV, mouse mammary tumor virus, and other retroviruses can be detected in humans. These endogenous viruses generally lack the ability to replicate because of deletions or the insertion of termination codons or because they are poorly transcribed. One such retrovirus can be detected in placental tissue and is activated by pregnancy. This virus may facilitate placental function.

CASE STUDY AND QUESTIONS

A 28-year-old man had several complaints. He had a bad case of thrush (oral candidiasis) and low-grade fever, had serious bouts of diarrhea, had lost 20 pounds in the past year without dieting, and, most seriously, complained of difficulty breathing. His lungs showed a bilateral infiltrate on radiographic examination, characteristic of P. carinii *pneumonia. A stool sample was positive for* Giardia *organisms. He was a heroin addict and admitted to sharing needles at a "shooting gallery."*

1. What laboratory tests should have been done to support and confirm a diagnosis of HIV infection and AIDS?
2. How did this man acquire the HIV infection? What are other high-risk behaviors for HIV infection?
3. What was the immunologic basis for the increased susceptibility of this patient to opportunistic infections?
4. What precautions should have been taken in handling samples from this patient?
5. Several forms of HIV vaccines are being developed. What are possible components of an HIV vaccine? Who would be appropriate recipients of an HIV vaccine?

Bibliography

AIDS: Ten years later, *FASEB J* 5:2338-2455, 1991.

Anderson RM: Understanding the AIDS pandemic, *Sci Am* 266: 58-66, 1992.

Antiretroviral therapy for HIV infection in 1996: Consensus statement, *JAMA* 276:146-154, 1996.

Arts EJ, Wainberg MA: Human immunodeficiency virus type 1 reverse transcriptase and early events in reverse transcription, *Adv Virus Res* 46:99-166, 1996.

Caldwell JC, Caldwell P: The African AIDS epidemic, *Sci Am* 274:62-68, 1996.

Carpenter CC et al: Antiretroviral therapy in adults: Updated recommendations of the International AIDS Society—USA Panel, *JAMA* 283:381-390, 2000.

Centers for Disease Control and Prevention: Updated U.S. Public Health Service guidelines for the management of exposures to HBV, HCV, and HIV and recommendations for postexposure prophylaxis, *MMWR* 50 (RR11):1-42, 2001.

Cohen J, Powderly WG, editors: *Infectious diseases*, ed 2, St Louis, 2004, Mosby.

Fauci AS: The human immunodeficiency virus: Infectivity and mechanisms of pathogenesis, *Science* 239:617-622, 1988.

Flint SJ et al: *Principles of virology: Molecular biology, pathogenesis and control of animal viruses*, ed 2, Washington, 2003, American Society for Microbiology Press.

Hehlmann R: Human retroviruses. In Belshe RB, editor: *Textbook of human virology*, ed 2, St Louis, 1991, Mosby.

Hehlmann R, Erfle V: Introduction to retroviruses: Human retroviruses. In Belshe RB, editor: *Textbook of human virology*, ed 2, St Louis, 1991, Mosby.

Knipe DM, Howley PM, editors: *Virology*, ed 4, New York, 2001, Lippincott-Williams and Wilkins.

Kräusslich HG: Morphogenesis and maturation of retroviruses, *Curr Top Microbiol Immunol* 214:1-344, 1996.

Löwer R: The pathogenic potential of endogenous retroviruses: Facts and fantasies, *Trends Microbiol* 7:350-356, 1999.

Ng VL, McGrath MS: Human T-cell leukemia virus involvement in adult T-cell leukemia, *Cancer Bull* 40:276-280, 1988.

Oldstone MBA, Vitkovic L: HIV and dementia, *Curr Top Microbiol Immunol* 202:1-279, 1995.

Pantaleo G, Fauci AS: Immunopathology of HIV infection, *Annu Rev Microbiol* 50:825-854, 1996.

Strauss JM, Strauss EG: *Viruses and human disease*, San Diego, 2002, Academic Press.

The new face of AIDS, *Science* 272:1879-1890, 1996.

The science of AIDS 1989: Readings from Scientific American, New York, 1989, Scientific American Books.

Williams AO: *AIDS: An African perspective*, Boca Raton, Fla, 1992, CRC.

World Health Organization UNAIDS: HIV/AIDS information and data: Available online at http://www.unaids.org/

HIV/AIDS Web Sites

AIDS Education Global Information System: general information available at www.aegis.com

HIV InSite: http://hivinsite.ucsf.edu

National Institute of Allergy and Infectious Diseases: http://www.niaid.nih.gov/spotlight/daids

NIAID fact sheet: http://www.niaid.nih.gov/publications/aids.htm

Treatment options: Available at www.hivatis.org

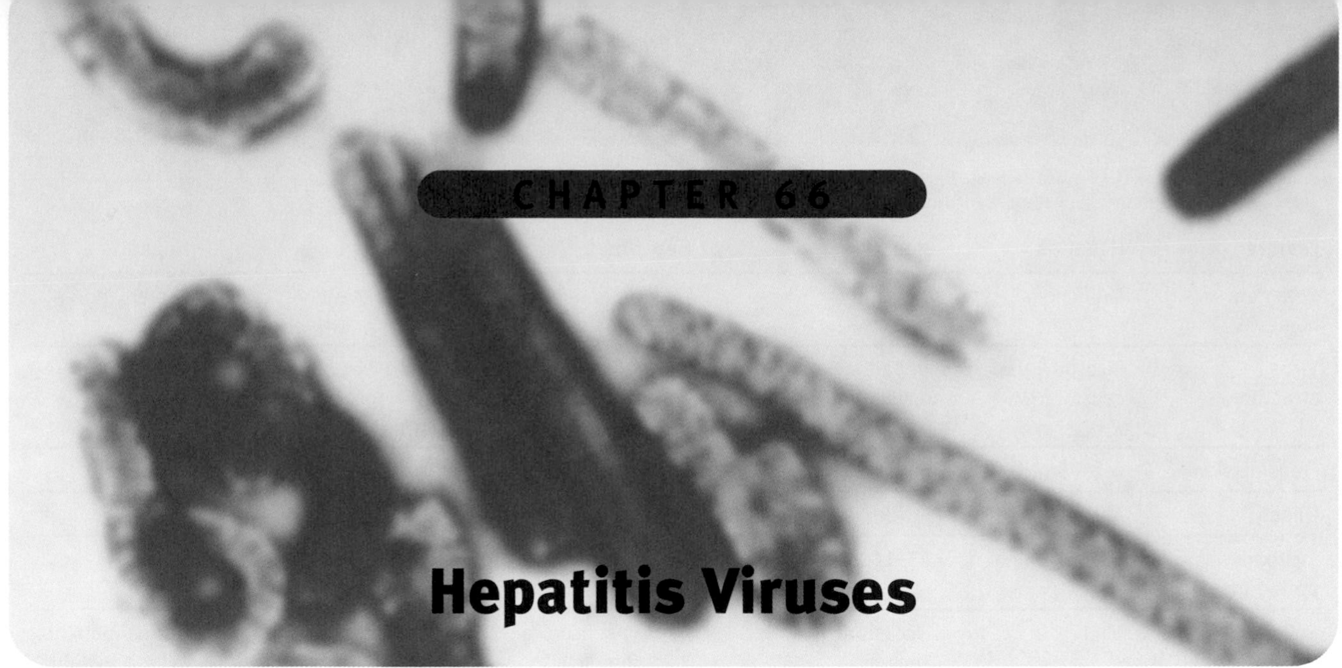

Hepatitis Viruses

The hepatitis alphabet of viruses includes at least six viruses, A through E, and G (Table 66–1). Although the target organ for each of these viruses is the liver and the basic hepatitis symptoms are similar, they differ greatly in their structure, mode of replication, mode of transmission, and in the time course and sequelae of the disease they cause. **Hepatitis A virus (HAV)** and **hepatitis B virus (HBV)** are the classical hepatitis viruses, and **hepatitis C, G, E,** and **hepatitis D virus (HDV),** the delta agent, are called **non-A non-B hepatitis (NANBH) viruses.** Additional non-A, non-B agents also exist.

Each of the hepatitis viruses infects and damages the liver, causing the classic **icteric symptoms of jaundice and the release of liver enzymes.** The specific virus causing the disease can be distinguished by the course, nature, and serology of the disease. These viruses are readily spread because infected people are contagious before, or even without, showing symptoms.

Hepatitis A, which is sometimes known as infectious hepatitis, (1) is caused by a picornavirus, a ribonucleic acid (RNA) virus; (2) is spread by the fecal-oral route; (3) has an incubation period of approximately 1 month, after which icteric symptoms start abruptly; (4) does not cause chronic liver disease; and (5) rarely causes fatal disease.

Hepatitis B, previously known as serum hepatitis, (1) is caused by a hepadnavirus with a deoxyribonucleic acid (DNA) genome; (2) is spread parenterally by blood or needles, by sexual contact, and perinatally; (3) has a median incubation period of approximately 3 months, after which icteric symptoms start insidiously; (4) is followed by chronic hepatitis in 5% to 10% of patients; and (5) is causally associated with primary hepatocellular carcinoma (PHC). More than one third of the world's population has been infected with HBV, resulting in 1 to 2 million deaths per year. The incidence of HBV is decreasing, however, especially in infants, because of the development and use of the HBV subunit vaccine.

Hepatitis C virus (HCV) is also widely prevalent, with more than 170 million carriers of the disease. HCV is spread by the same routes as HBV but usually causes chronic disease. HCV is a flavivirus with an RNA genome. **Hepatitis G virus** is also a flavivirus and causes chronic infections. **Hepatitis E virus (HEV)** is an enteric virus in the Noravirus family, and its disease resembles HAV.

Hepatitis D, or delta hepatitis, is unique in that it requires actively replicating HBV as a "helper virus" and occurs only in patients who have active HBV infection. HBV provides an envelope for HDV RNA and its antigens. Delta agent exacerbates the symptoms caused by HBV.

Hepatitis A Virus

HAV causes infectious hepatitis and is spread by the fecal-oral route. HAV infections often result from consumption of contaminated water, shellfish, or other food. HAV is a **picornavirus** and was formerly called enterovirus 72, but it has been placed into a new genus, *Heparnavirus,* on the basis of its unique genome.

STRUCTURE

HAV has a 27-nm, **naked icosahedral capsid** surrounding a **positive-sense, single-stranded RNA** genome consisting of approximately 7470 nucleotides (Figure 66–1). The HAV genome has a VPg protein attached to the 5′ end and polyadenosine attached to the 3′ end. The capsid is even more stable than other picornaviruses to acid and other treatments (Box 66–1). There is only one serotype of HAV.

TABLE 66–1. Comparative Features of Hepatitis Viruses

Feature	Hepatitis A	Hepatitis B	Hepatitis C	Hepatitis D	Hepatitis E
Common name	"Infectious"	"Serum"	"Non-A, non-B–post-transfusion"	"Delta agent"	"Enteric non-A, non-B"
Virus structure	Picornavirus; capsid, RNA	Hepadnavirus; envelope, DNA	Flavivirus; envelope, RNA	Viroidlike; envelope, circular RNA	Norovirus; capsid, RNA
Transmission	Fecal-oral	Parenteral, sexual	Parenteral, sexual	Parenteral, sexual	Fecal-oral
Onset	Abrupt	Insidious	Insidious	Abrupt	Abrupt
Incubation period (days)	15–50	45–160	14–180	15–64	15–50
Severity	Mild	Occasionally severe	Usually subclinical; 70% chronicity	*Coinfection* with HBV occasionally severe; *superinfection* with HBV often severe	Normal patients, mild; pregnant women, severe
Mortality	<0.5%	1%–2%	~4%	High to very high	Normal patients, 1%–2%; pregnant women, 20%
Chronicity/carrier state	No	Yes	Yes	Yes	No
Other disease associations	None	Primary hepatocellular carcinoma, cirrhosis	Primary hepatocellular carcinoma, cirrhosis	Cirrhosis, fulminant hepatitis	None
Laboratory diagnosis	Symptoms and anti-HAV IgM	Symptoms and serum levels of HBsAg, HBeAg, and anti-HBc IgM	Symptoms and anti-HCV ELISA	Anti-HDV ELISA	—

ELISA, Enzyme-linked immunosorbent assay; HAV, hepatitis A virus; HCV, hepatitis C virus; HDV, hepatitis D virus; IgM, immunoglobulin M.

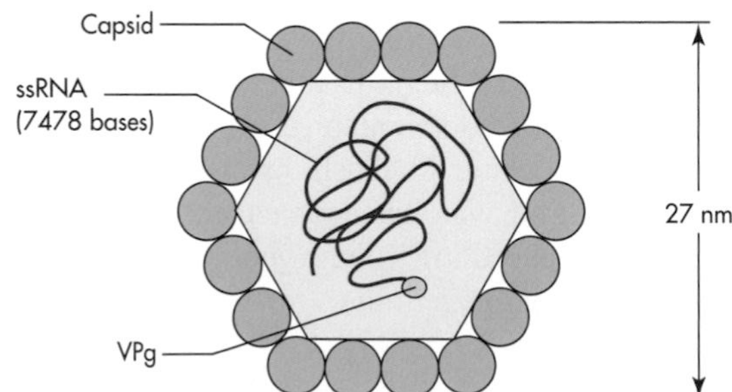

FIGURE 66–1. The picornavirus structure of hepatitis A virus. The icosahedral capsid is made up of four viral polypeptides (VP1 to VP4). Inside the capsid is a single-stranded, positive-sense RNA (ssRNA) that has a genomic viral protein (VPg) on the 5′ end.

BOX 66–1. Characteristics of Hepatitis A Virus

Stable to:
- Acid at pH 1
- Solvents (ether, chloroform)
- Detergents
- Salt water, groundwater (months)
- Drying (stable)
- Temperature
  - 4°C: weeks
  - 56°C for 30 minutes: Stable
  - 61°C for 20 minutes: Partial inactivation

Inactivated by:
- Chlorine treatment of drinking water
- Formalin (0.35%, 37°C, 72 hours)
- Peracetic acid (2%, 4 hours)
- β-Propiolactone (0.25%, 1 hour)
- Ultraviolet radiation (2 $\mu W/cm^2/min$)

REPLICATION

HAV replicates like other picornaviruses (see Chapter 57). It interacts specifically with a receptor expressed on liver cells and a few other cell types. Unlike other picornaviruses, however, HAV is not cytolytic and is released by exocytosis. Laboratory isolates of HAV have been adapted to growth in primary and continuous monkey kidney cell lines, but clinical isolates are difficult to grow in cell culture.

PATHOGENESIS

HAV is ingested and probably enters the bloodstream through the oropharynx or the epithelial lining of the intestines to reach its target, the parenchymal cells of the liver (Figure 66–2). The virus replicates in hepatocytes and Kupffer's cells. Virus is produced in these cells and is released into the bile and from there into the stool. Virus is shed in large quantity into the stool approximately 10 days before symptoms of jaundice appear or antibody can be detected.

HAV replicates slowly in the liver without producing apparent cytopathic effects. Although interferon limits viral replication, natural killer cells and cytotoxic T cells are required to eliminate infected cells. Antibody, complement, and antibody-dependent cellular cytotoxicity also facilitate clearance of the virus and induction of immunopathology. Icterus, resulting from damage to the liver, occurs when cell-mediated immune responses and antibody to the virus can be detected. Antibody protection against reinfection is lifelong.

The liver pathology caused by HAV infection is indistinguishable histologically from that caused by HBV. It is most likely caused by immunopathology and not virus-induced cytopathology. However, unlike HBV, HAV cannot initiate a chronic infection and is not associated with hepatic cancer.

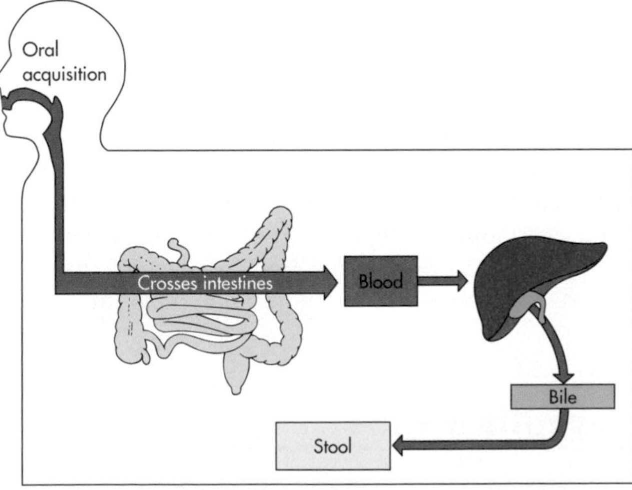

FIGURE 66–2. Spread of hepatitis A virus within the body.

EPIDEMIOLOGY

Approximately 40% of acute cases of hepatitis are caused by HAV (Box 66–2). The virus spreads readily in a community because most infected people are contagious 10 to 14 days before symptoms occur and 90% of infected children and 25% to 50% of infected adults have **inapparent but productive** infections.

The virus is released into stool in high concentrations and is spread via the **fecal-oral** route. Virus is spread in contaminated water, in food, and by dirty hands. HAV is resistant to detergents, acid (pH of 1), and temperatures as high as 60°C, and it can survive for many months in fresh water and salt water. Raw or improperly treated sewage can taint the water supply and contaminate shellfish. Shellfish, especially clams, oysters, and mussels, are important sources of the virus because they are efficient filter feeders and can therefore concentrate the viral particles, even from dilute solutions. This is exemplified by an epidemic of HAV that occurred in Shanghai, China, in

BOX 66–2. Epidemiology of Hepatitis A Virus and Hepatitis E Virus

Disease/Viral Factors
Capsid viruses are strongly resistant to inactivation.
Contagious period extends from before to after symptoms.
Virus may cause asymptomatic shedding.

Transmission
Virus can be transmitted via fecal-oral route.
Ingestion of contaminated food and water can cause infection.
HAV in shellfish is from sewage-contaminated water.
Virus can be transmitted by food handlers, daycare workers, and children.

Who Is at Risk?
People in overcrowded, unsanitary areas.
Children: Mild disease, possibly asymptomatic; daycare centers are a major source of spread of HAV.
Adults: Abrupt-onset hepatitis.
Pregnant women: High mortality associated with HEV.

Geography/Season
Virus is found worldwide.
There is no seasonal incidence.

Means of Control
Good hygiene.
HAV: Passive antibody protection for contacts.

Killed vaccine
Live vaccine in China

HAV, Hepatitis A virus; HEV, hepatitis E virus.

1988, when 300,000 people were infected with the virus as the result of eating clams obtained from a polluted river.

HAV outbreaks usually originate from a common source (e.g., water supply, restaurant, daycare center). Asymptomatic shedding and a long (15 to 40 days) incubation period make it difficult to identify the source. Daycare settings are a major source for spread of the virus among classmates and their parents. A further problem is posed by the fact that because the children and personnel in daycare centers may be transient, the number of contacts at risk for HAV infection from a single daycare center can be great.

A relatively high incidence of HAV infection is directly related to poor hygienic conditions and overcrowding. Most people infected with HAV in developing countries are children who have mild illness and then lifelong immune protection against reinfection. In the populations of more highly developed countries, infection occurs later in life. The seropositivity rate of adults ranges from a low of 13% of the adult population in Sweden to highs of 88% in Taiwan and 97% in Yugoslavia, with a 41% to 44% rate in the United States.

CLINICAL SYNDROMES

The symptoms caused by HAV are very similar to those caused by HBV and stem from immune-mediated damage to the liver. As already noted, disease in children is generally milder than that in adults and is usually asymptomatic. The **symptoms occur abruptly** 15 to 50 days after exposure and intensify for 4 to 6 days before the icteric (jaundice) phase (Figure 66–3). Initial symptoms include fever, fatigue, nausea, loss of appetite, and abdominal pain. Jaundice is observed in 70% to 80% of adults but in only 10% of children (<6 years of age). Symptoms generally wane during the jaundice period. Viral shedding in the stool precedes the onset of symptoms by approximately 14 days but stops before the cessation of symptoms. Complete recovery occurs 99% of the time.

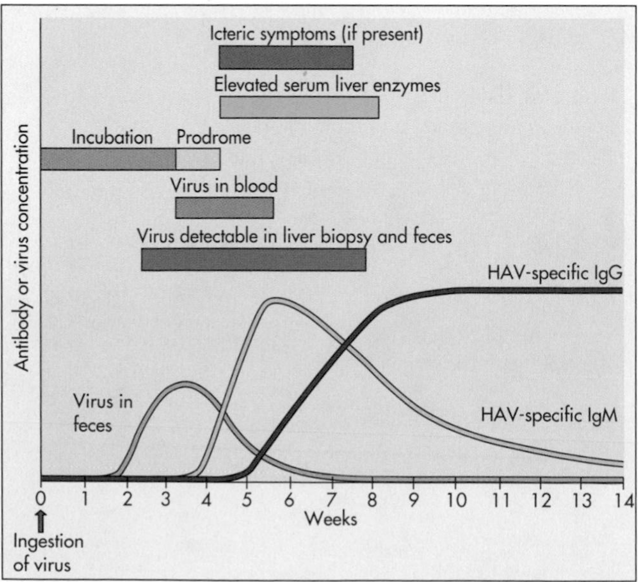

FIGURE 66–3. Time course of hepatitis A virus (HAV) infection.

Fulminant hepatitis in HAV infection occurs in one to three persons per 1000 and is associated with an 80% mortality rate. Unlike HBV, immune complex–related symptoms (e.g., arthritis, rash) rarely occur in people with HAV disease.

LABORATORY DIAGNOSIS

The diagnosis of HAV infection is generally made on the basis of the time course of the clinical symptoms, the identification of a known infected source, and, most reliably, the results yielded by specific serologic tests. The best way to demonstrate an acute HAV infection is by finding anti-HAV immunoglobulin M (IgM), as measured by an enzyme-linked immunosorbent assay (ELISA) or radioimmunoassay. Virus isolation is not performed because efficient tissue culture systems for growing the virus are not available.

TREATMENT, PREVENTION, AND CONTROL

The spread of HAV is reduced by interrupting the fecal-oral spread of the virus. This is accomplished by avoiding potentially contaminated water or food, especially uncooked shellfish. Proper hand washing, especially in daycare centers, mental hospitals, and other care facilities, is vitally important. Chlorine treatment of drinking water is generally sufficient to kill the virus.

Prophylaxis with immune serum globulin given before or early in the incubation period (i.e., less than 2 weeks after exposure) is 80% to 90% effective in preventing clinical illness.

A **killed HAV vaccine** has been approved by the U.S. Food and Drug Administration (FDA) and is available for all children, and for adults at high risk for infection, especially travelers to endemic regions. The vaccine is administered to infants at 2 years of age and can be administered with the HBV vaccine to adults. A live HAV vaccine has been developed in China. There is only one serotype of HAV, and HAV infects only humans, factors that help ensure the success of an immunization program.

Hepatitis B Virus

HBV is the major member of the **hepadnaviruses.** Other members of this family (Box 66–3) include woodchuck,

BOX 66–3. Unique Features of Hepadnaviruses

Virus has **enveloped** virion containing **partially double-stranded, circular DNA** genome.
Replication is through a circular **RNA intermediate.**
Virus encodes and carries a **reverse transcriptase.**
Virus encodes several proteins (HBsAg [L, M, S]; HBe/HBc) that share genetic sequences but with different in-frame start codons.
HBV has a strict tissue tropism to the liver.
HBV-infected cells produce and release large amounts of HBsAg particles lacking DNA.
The HBV genome can integrate into the host chromosome.

HBsAg, Hepatitis B surface antigen; HBV, hepatitis B virus.

ground squirrel, and duck hepatitis viruses. These viruses have limited tissue tropisms and host ranges. HBV infects the liver and, to a lesser extent, the kidneys and pancreas of only humans and chimpanzees. Advances in molecular biology have made it possible to study HBV despite the limited host range of the virus and the lack of a cell culture system in which to grow it.

STRUCTURE

HBV is a small, enveloped DNA virus with several unusual properties (Figure 66–4). Specifically, the **genome is a small, circular, partly double-stranded DNA** of only 3200 bases. Although a DNA virus, it encodes a **reverse transcriptase** and replicates through an **RNA intermediate.**

The virion, also called the **Dane particle,** is 42 nm in diameter. The virions are unusually stable for an enveloped virus. They resist treatment with ether, low pH, freezing, and moderate heating. These characteristics assist transmission from one person to another and hamper disinfection.

The HBV **virion includes a protein kinase and a polymerase** with reverse transcriptase and ribonuclease H activity, and a P protein attached to the genome, all of which is surrounded by the **hepatitis B core antigen (HBcAg)** and an envelope containing the glycoprotein **hepatitis B surface antigen (HBsAg).** A **hepatitis B e antigen (HBeAg)** protein is a minor component of the virion. The HBeAg and HBcAg proteins share most of their protein sequence. However, the HBeAg is processed differently by the cell, is primarily secreted into serum, does not self-assemble (like a capsid antigen), and expresses different antigenic determinants.

HBsAg-containing particles are released into the serum of infected people and outnumber the actual virions. These particles can be spherical (but smaller than the Dane particle) or filamentous (see Figure 66–4). They are immunogenic and were processed into the first commercial vaccine against HBV.

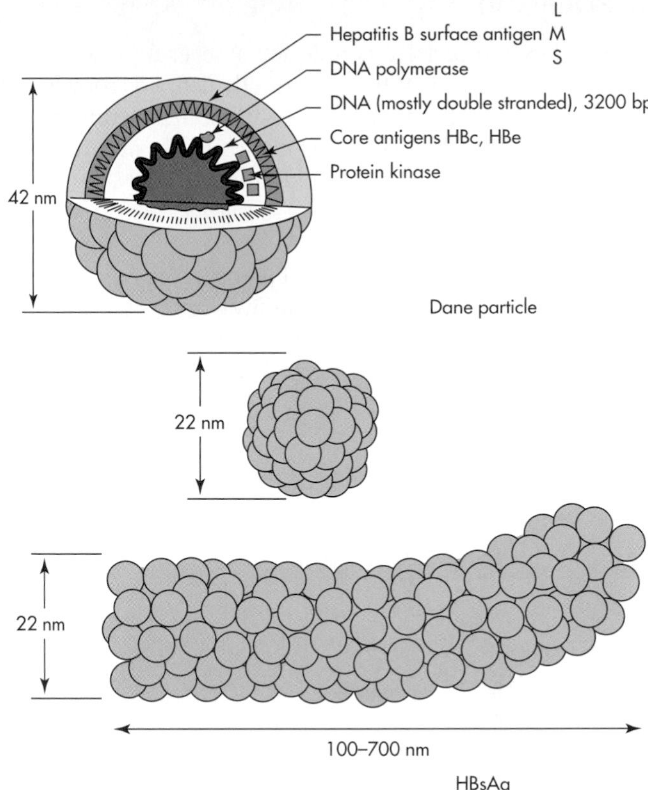

FIGURE 66–4. Hepatitis B virus (Dane particle) and hepatitis B surface antigen (HBsAg) particles. The spherical HBsAg consists mainly of the S form of HBsAg with some M. The fiber HBsAg has S, M, and L forms. Bp, Base pair; L, gp42; M, gp36; S, gp27.

HBsAg, originally termed the Australia antigen, includes three glycoproteins (L, M, and S) encoded by the same gene and read in the same frame but translated into protein from different AUG start codons. The S (gp27; 24 to 27 kDa) glycoprotein is completely contained in the M (gp36; 33 to 36 kDa) glycoprotein, which is contained in the L (gp42; 39 to 42 kDa) glycoprotein; all share the same C-terminal amino acid sequences. All three forms of HBsAg are found in the virion. The S glycoprotein is the major component of HBsAg particles; it self-associates into 22-nm spherical particles that are released from the cells. The filamentous particles of HBsAg found in serum contain mostly S but also small amounts of the M and L glycoproteins and other proteins and lipids. The L glycoprotein is an essential component for virion assembly and promotes filament formation and limits the secretion of these structures from the cell. The glycoproteins of HBsAg contain the group-specific (termed *a*) and type-specific determinants of HBV (termed *d* or *y* and *w* or *r*). Combinations of these antigens (e.g., ady, adw) result in eight subtypes of HBV that are useful epidemiologic markers.

REPLICATION

The replication of HBV is unique for several reasons (see Box 66–1). First, HBV has a distinctly defined tropism for the liver. Its small genome also necessitates economy, as illustrated by the pattern of its transcription and translation. In addition, *HBV replicates through an RNA intermediate and produces and releases antigenic decoy particles (HBsAg)* (Figure 66–5).

The attachment of HBV to hepatocytes is mediated by the HBsAg glycoproteins. Several liver cell receptors have been suggested, including the transferrin receptor, the asialoglycoprotein receptor, and human liver endonexin. The mechanism of entry is not known, but HBsAg binds to polymerized human serum albumin and other serum proteins, and this interaction may facilitate binding and uptake of the virus by the liver.

On penetration into the cell, the partial DNA strand of the genome is completed by being formed into a complete double-stranded DNA circle, and the genome is delivered to the nucleus. Transcription of the genome is controlled by cellular transcription elements found in hepatocytes. The DNA is transcribed into three major classes (2100, 2400, and 3500 bases) and two minor classes (900 bases) of overlapping messenger RNAs (mRNAs) (Figure 66–6). The 3500-base mRNA is larger than the genome. It

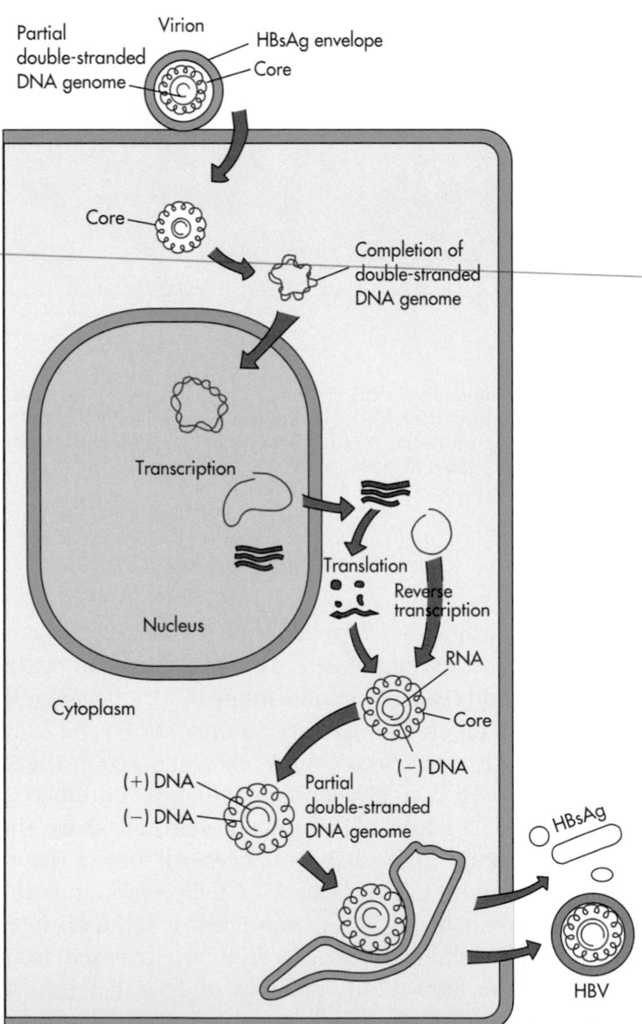

FIGURE 66–5. Replication of hepatitis B virus. After entry into the hepatocyte and uncoating of the nucleocapsid core, the partially double-stranded DNA genome is completed by enzymes in the core and then delivered to the nucleus. Transcription of the genome produces four messenger RNAs (mRNAs), including an mRNA larger than the genome (3500 bases). The mRNA then moves to the cytoplasm and is translated into protein. Core proteins assemble around the 3500-base mRNA, and negative-sense DNA is synthesized by a reverse transcriptase activity in the core. The RNA is then degraded as a positive-sense (+) DNA is synthesized. The core is enveloped before completion of the positive-sense DNA and then released by exocytosis.

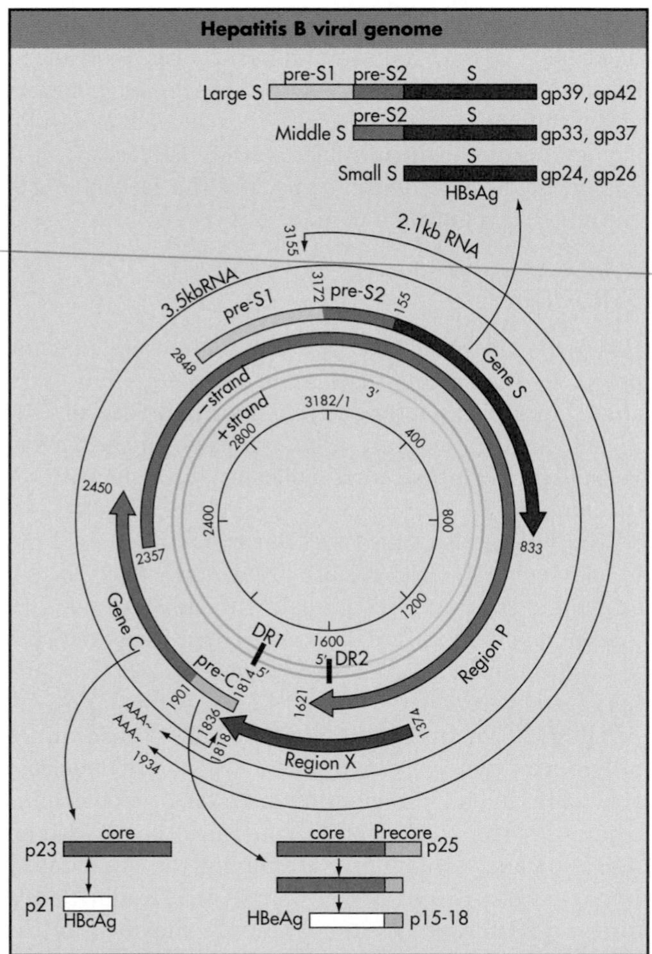

FIGURE 66–6. DNA, RNA, mRNA, and proteins of hepatitis B virus (HBV). The inner green circles represent the DNA genome with the nucleotide number at the center. DR1 and DR2 are direct repeat sequences of DNA and are important for replication and integration of the genome. The 3500-base transcript (outer black thin-line circle) is larger than the genome and is the template for replication of the genome. Bold arcs represent mRNA for viral proteins. Note that several proteins are translated from the same mRNA but from different AUG codons and that different mRNAs overlap. AAA, 3′ PolyA at end of mRN; C, C mRNA (HBcAg); E, E mRNA (HBeAg); l, large glycoprotein; m, medium glycoprotein; P, polymerase-protein primer for replication; s, small glycoprotein; S, S mRNA (HBsAg); X, X mRNA. (Modified from Armstrong D, Cohen J: *Infectious diseases,* St Louis, 1999, Mosby.)

encodes the HBc and HBe antigens, the polymerase, and a protein primer for DNA replication and acts as the template for replication of the genome. The HBe and HBc are related proteins that are translated from different in-phase start codons of closely related mRNA. This causes differences in their processing and structure, with shedding of the HBe and incorporation of HBc into the virion. Similarly, the 2100-base mRNA encodes the small and medium glycoproteins from different in-phase start codons. The 2400-base mRNA, which encodes the large glycoprotein, overlaps the 2100-base mRNA. The 900-base mRNA encodes the X protein, which promotes viral replication as a transactivator of transcription and as a protein kinase.

Replication of the genome begins with production of the larger-than-genome, 3500-base mRNA. This is packaged into the core nucleocapsid that contains the RNA-dependent DNA polymerase. This polymerase has **reverse transcriptase** and ribonuclease H activity but lacks the integrase activity of the retrovirus enzyme. The 3500-base RNA acts as a template, and negative-strand DNA is synthesized using a protein primer, which remains covalently attached to the 5′ end. After this, the RNA is degraded by the ribonuclease H activity as the positive-strand DNA is synthesized from the negative-sense DNA template. However, this process is interrupted by envelopment of the nucleocapsid at HBsAg-containing membranes of the endoplasmic reticulum, thereby capturing genomes containing RNA-DNA circles with different lengths of RNA. Continued degradation of the remainder of the RNA in the virion yields a partly double-stranded DNA genome. The virion is then released from the hepatocyte by exocytosis without killing the cell, and not by cell lysis.

The entire genome can also be integrated into the host cell chromatin. HBsAg, but not other proteins, can often be detected in the cytoplasm of cells containing integrated HBV DNA. The significance of the integrated DNA in the replication of the virus is not known, but integrated viral DNA has been found in hepatocellular carcinomas.

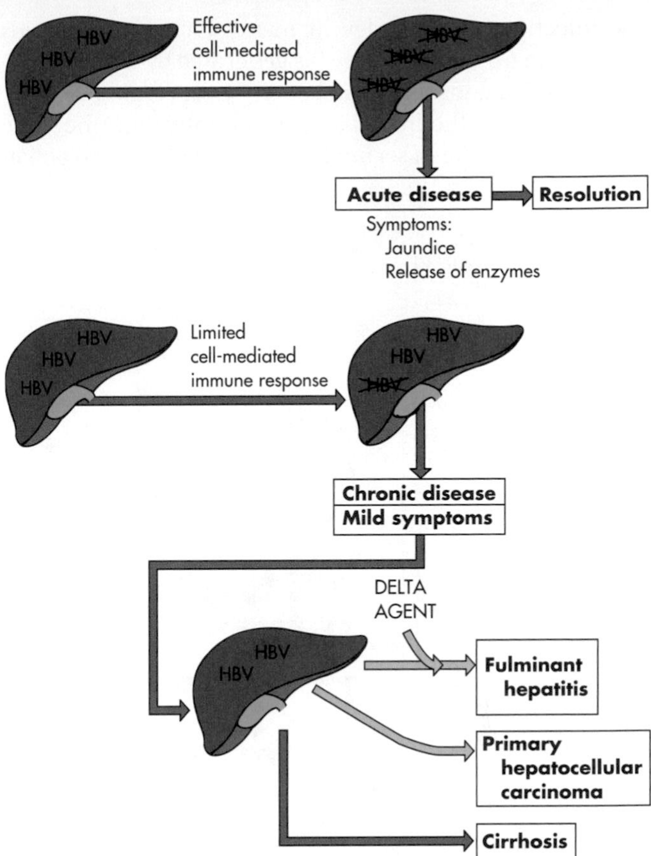

FIGURE 66–7. Major determinants of acute and chronic hepatitis B virus (HBV) infection. HBV infects the liver but does not cause direct cytopathology. Cell-mediated immune lysis of infected cells produces the symptoms and resolves the infection. Insufficient immunity can lead to chronic disease. Chronic HBV disease predisposes a person to more serious outcomes. Purple arrows indicate symptoms; green arrows indicate a possible outcome.

PATHOGENESIS AND IMMUNITY

HBV can cause acute or chronic, symptomatic or asymptomatic disease. Which of these occurs seems to be determined by the person's immune response to the infection (Figure 66–7). *Detection of both the HBsAg and the HBeAg components of the virion in the blood indicates the existence of an ongoing active infection.* HBsAg particles continue to be released into the blood even after virion release has ended and until the infection is resolved.

The major source of infectious virus is blood, but HBV can be found in semen, saliva, milk, vaginal and menstrual secretions, and amniotic fluid. The most efficient way to acquire HBV is through injection of the virus into the bloodstream (Figure 66–8). Common but less efficient routes of infection are sexual contact and birth.

The virus starts to replicate in the liver within 3 days of its acquisition, but as already noted, symptoms may not be observed for 45 days or longer, depending on the infectious dose, the route of infection, and the person. The virus replicates in hepatocytes with minimal cytopathic effect. Infection proceeds for a relatively long time without causing liver damage (i.e., elevation of liver enzyme levels) or symptoms. During this time, copies of the HBV genome integrate into the hepatocyte chromatin and remain latent. Intracellular buildup of filamentous forms of HBsAg can produce the ground-glass hepatocyte cytopathology characteristic of HBV infection.

Cell-mediated immunity and inflammation are responsible for causing the symptoms and effecting resolution of the HBV infection by eliminating the infected hepatocyte. Epitopes from the HBc antigen are prominent T-cell antigens. An insufficient T-cell response to the infection generally results in the occurrence of mild symptoms, an inability to resolve the infection, and the development of chronic hepatitis (see Figure 66–7). Antibody (as generated by vaccination) can protect against initial infection by preventing delivery of the virus to the liver. Later in the infection, the large amount of HBsAg in serum binds to and blocks the action of neutralizing antibody, which limits the antibody's capacity to resolve an infection. Immune complexes formed between HBsAg and anti-HBs contribute to the development of hypersensitivity reactions (type III), leading to problems such as vasculitis, arthralgia, rash, and renal damage.

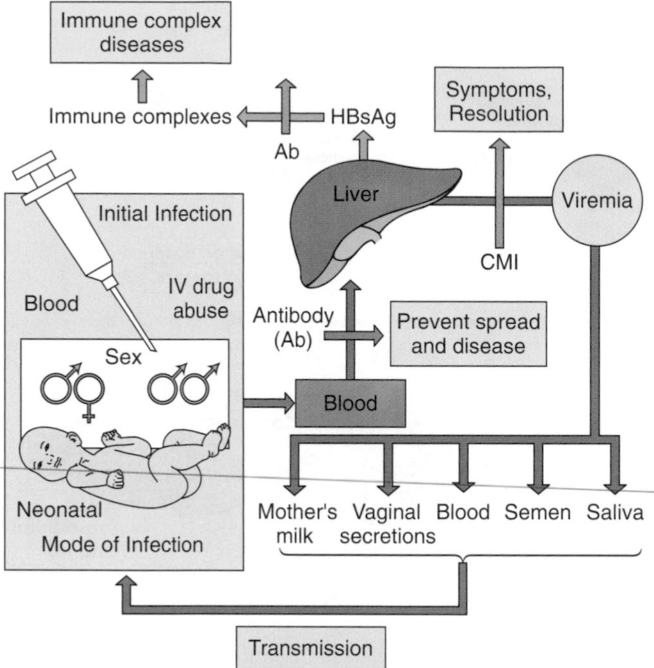

FIGURE 66–8. Spread of hepatitis B virus (HBV) in the body. Initial infection with HBV occurs through injection, heterosexual and homosexual sex, and birth. The virus then spreads to the liver, replicates, induces a viremia, and is transmitted in various body secretions in addition to blood to start the cycle again. Symptoms are caused by cell-mediated immunity (CMI) and immune complexes between antibody and hepatitis B surface antigen (HBsAg). IV, Intravenous.

Infants and young children have an immature cell-mediated immune response and are less able to resolve the infection, but they suffer less tissue damage and milder symptoms. As many as 90% of infants infected perinatally become chronic carriers. Viral replication persists in these people for long periods.

During the acute phase of infection, the liver parenchyma shows degenerative changes consisting of cellular swelling and necrosis, especially in hepatocytes surrounding the central vein of a hepatic lobule. The inflammatory cell infiltrate is mainly composed of lymphocytes. Resolution of the infection allows the parenchyma to regenerate. Fulminant infections, activation of chronic infections, or coinfection with the delta agent can lead to permanent liver damage and cirrhosis.

EPIDEMIOLOGY

In the United States, more than 300,000 persons are infected with HBV each year, resulting in 4000 deaths. However, even more people are infected in developing nations, with as much as 15% of the **population infected during birth or childhood.** High rates of seropositivity are observed in Italy, Greece, Africa, and southeast Asia (Figure 66–9). In some areas of the world (southern Africa and southeastern Asia), the seroconversion rate is as high as 50%. PHC, a long-term sequela of the infection, is also endemic in these regions.

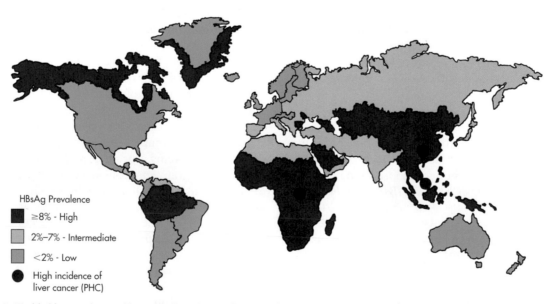

FIGURE 66–9. Worldwide prevalence of hepatitis B carriers and primary hepatocellular carcinoma. (Courtesy Centers for Disease Control and Prevention, Atlanta.)

BOX 66–4. High-Risk Groups for Hepatitis B Virus Infection

People from endemic regions (i.e., China, parts of Africa, Alaska, Pacific Islands)
Babies of mothers with chronic hepatitis B virus
Intravenous drug abusers
People with multiple sex partners: Homosexual and heterosexual
Hemophiliacs and other patients requiring blood and blood product treatments
Health care personnel who have contact with blood
Residents and staff members of institutions for the mentally retarded
Hemodialysis patients and blood and organ recipients

The many asymptomatic chronic carriers with virus in blood and other body secretions foster the spread of the virus. In the United States, 0.1% to 0.5% of the general population are chronic carriers, but this is very low in comparison with many areas of the world. Carrier status may be lifelong.

The virus is spread by sexual, parenteral, and perinatal routes. Transmission occurs through contaminated blood and blood components by transfusion, needle sharing, acupuncture, ear piercing, or tattooing and through very close personal contact involving the exchange of semen, saliva, and vaginal secretions (e.g., sex, childbirth) (see Figure 66–8). Medical personnel are at risk in accidents involving needlesticks or sharp instruments. People at particular risk are listed in Box 66–4. Sexual promiscuity and drug abuse are major risk factors for HBV infection. HBV can be transmitted to babies through contact with the mother's blood at birth and in the mother's milk. Babies born to chronic HBV-positive mothers are at highest risk for infection. Serologic screening of donor units in blood banks has greatly reduced the risk of acquisition of the virus from contaminated blood or blood products. Safer sex habits adopted to prevent HIV transmission and the administration of the HBV vaccine have also been responsible for decreasing the transmission of HBV.

One of the major concerns about HBV is its association with PHC. This type of carcinoma probably accounts for 250,000 to 1 million deaths per year worldwide; in the United States, approximately 5000 deaths per year are attributed to PHC.

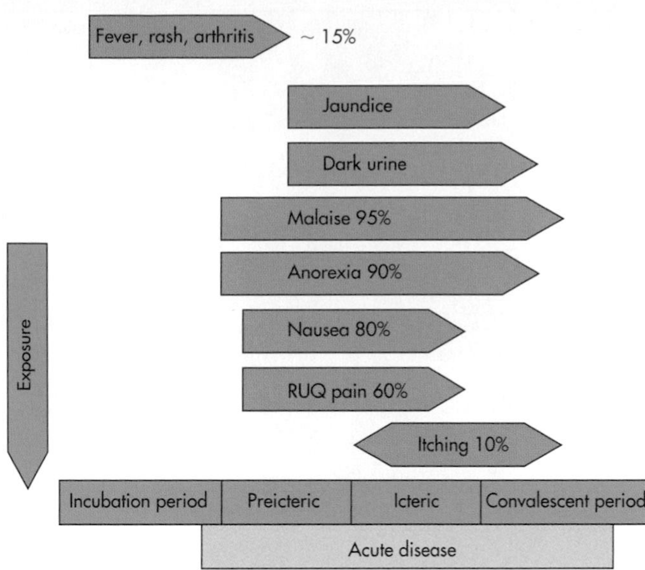

FIGURE 66–10. Symptoms of typical acute viral hepatitis B infection are correlated with the four clinical periods of this disease. RUQ, Right upper quadrant. (Redrawn from Hoofnagle JH: *Lab Med* 14:705-716, 1983.)

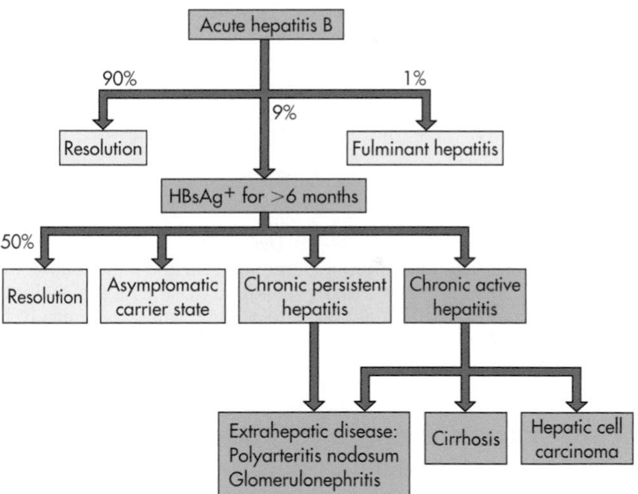

FIGURE 66–11. Clinical outcomes of acute hepatitis B infection. (Redrawn from White DO, Fenner F: *Medical virology*, ed 3, New York, 1986, Academic Press.)

CLINICAL SYNDROMES

Acute Infection

As already noted, the clinical presentation of HBV in children is less severe than that in adults, and infection may even be asymptomatic. Clinically apparent illness occurs in as many as 25% of those infected with HBV (Figures 66–10 to 66–12).

HBV infection is characterized by a **long incubation period and an insidious onset.** Symptoms during the prodromal period may include fever, malaise, and anorexia, followed by nausea, vomiting, abdominal discomfort, and chills. The classic icteric symptoms of liver damage (e.g., jaundice, dark urine, pale stools) follow soon thereafter. Recovery is indicated by a decline in the fever and renewed appetite.

Fulminant hepatitis occurs in approximately 1% of icteric patients and may be fatal. It is marked by more severe symptoms and indications of severe liver damage, such as ascites and bleeding.

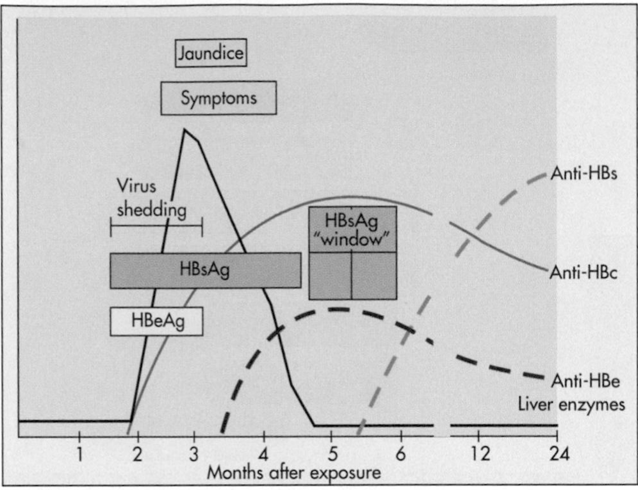

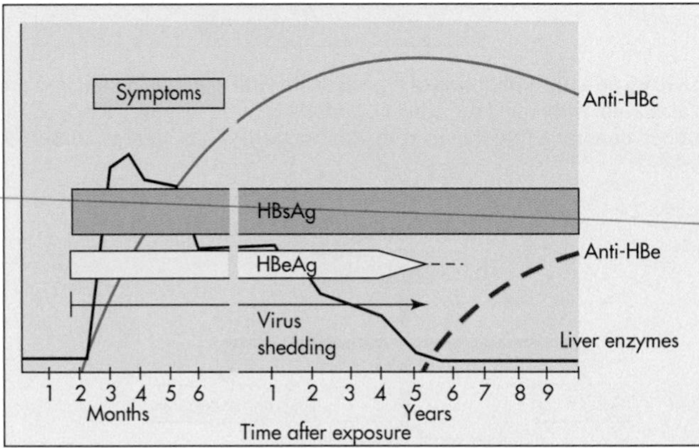

FIGURE 66–12. A, The serologic events associated with the typical course of acute hepatitis B disease. **B,** Development of the chronic hepatitis B virus carrier state. Routine serodiagnosis is difficult during the hepatitis B surface antigen (HBsAg) window, when HBs and anti-HBs are undetectable. Anti-HBs-antibody to HBsAg; anti-HBc-antibody to HBcAg; anti-HBe-antibody to HBeAg. (Redrawn from Hoofnagle JH: *Annu Rev Med* 32:1-11, 1981.)

HBV infection can promote hypersensitivity reactions that are caused by immune complexes of HBsAg and antibody. These may produce rash, polyarthritis, fever, acute necrotizing vasculitis, and glomerulonephritis.

Chronic Infection

Chronic hepatitis occurs in 5% to 10% of people with HBV infections, usually after mild or inapparent initial disease. Approximately one third of these people have chronic active hepatitis with continued destruction of the liver leading to scarring of the liver, cirrhosis, liver failure, or PHC. The other two thirds have chronic passive hepatitis and are less likely to have problems. Chronic hepatitis may be detected accidentally by finding elevated liver enzyme levels on a routine blood chemistry profile. Chronically infected people are the major source for spread of the virus and are at risk for fulminant disease if they become coinfected with HDV.

Primary Hepatocellular Carcinoma

The World Health Organization estimates that 80% of all cases of PHC can be attributed to chronic HBV infections. The HBV genome is integrated into these PHC cells, and the cells express HBV antigens. PHC is usually fatal and is one of the three most common causes of cancer mortality in the world. In Taiwan, at least 15% of the population are carriers of HBV, and nearly half die of PHC or cirrhosis. PHC may become the first vaccine-preventable human cancer.

HBV may induce PHC by promoting continued liver repair and cell growth in response to tissue damage or by integrating into the host chromosome and stimulating cell growth directly. Such integration could stimulate genetic rearrangements or juxtapose viral promoters next to cellular growth–controlling genes. Alternatively, a protein encoded by the HBV X gene may transactivate (turn on) the transcription of cellular proteins and stimulate cell growth. The presence of the HBV genome may allow a subsequent mutation to promote carcinogenesis. The latency period between HBV infection and PHC may be as short as 9 years or as long as 35 years.

LABORATORY DIAGNOSIS

The initial diagnosis of hepatitis can be made on the basis of the clinical symptoms and the presence of liver enzymes in the blood (see Figure 66–12). However, the serology of HBV infection describes the course and the nature of the disease (Table 66–2). Acute and chronic HBV infections can be distinguished by the presence of HBsAg and HBeAg in the serum and the pattern of antibodies to the individual HBV antigens.

HBsAg and HBeAg are secreted into the blood during viral replication. The detection of HBeAg is the best correlate to the presence of infectious virus. A chronic infection can be distinguished by the continued finding of HBeAg, HBsAg, or both, and a lack of detectable antibody to these antigens.

During the symptomatic phase of infection, detection of antibodies to HBeAg and HBsAg is obscured because the antibody is complexed with antigen in the serum. The best way to diagnose a recent acute infection, especially during the period when neither HBsAg nor anti-HBs can be detected (the window), is to measure IgM anti-HBc.

TREATMENT, PREVENTION, AND CONTROL

Although no treatment is available for acute infection, **Hepatitis B immune globulin** may be administered within a week of exposure and to newborn infants of HBsAg-positive mothers to prevent and ameliorate disease. Chronic HBV infection can be treated with drugs targeted at the polymerase, such as **lamivudine**

TABLE 66–2. Interpretation of Serologic Markers of Hepatitis B Virus Infection

	Disease State					Healthy State	
Serologic Reactivity	**Early (Presymptomatic)**	**Early Acute**	**Acute**	**Chronic**	**Late Acute**	**Resolved**	**Vaccinated**
Anti-HBc	–	–	–*	+	+/–	+	–
Anti-HBe	–	–	–	–	+/–	+/–†	–
Anti-HBs	–	–	–	–	–	+	+
HBeAg	–	+	+	+	–	–	–
HBsAg	+	+	+	+	+	–	–
Infectious virus	+	+	+	+	+	–	–

HBeAg, Hepatitis B e antigen; HbsAg, hepatitis B surface antigen.
*Anti-HBc IgM should be present.
†Anti-HBe may be negative after chronic disease.

(2′3′dideoxy-3′-thiacytidine), which is also an HIV (human immunodeficiency virus) reverse transcriptase inhibitor, or the nucleoside analogues, **adefovir dipivoxil and famciclovir.** These FDA-approved treatments are taken for 1 year. **Interferon-α** (INF-α) can also be effective and is taken for at least 4 months.

Transmission of HBV in blood or blood products has been greatly reduced by screening donated blood for the presence of HBsAg and anti-HBc. Additional efforts to prevent transmission of HBV consist of avoiding sex with a carrier of HBV and avoiding the lifestyles that facilitate spread of the virus. Household contacts and sexual partners of HBV carriers are at increased risk, as are patients undergoing hemodialysis, recipients of pooled plasma products, health care workers exposed to blood, and babies born of HBV-carrier mothers.

Vaccination is recommended for infants, children, and especially people in high-risk groups (see Box 66–4). Vaccination is useful even after exposure for newborns of HBsAg-positive mothers and people accidentally exposed either percutaneously or permucosally to blood or secretions from an HBsAg-positive person. Immunization of mothers should decrease the incidence of transmission to babies and older children, thus also reducing the number of chronic HBV carriers. Prevention of chronic HBV will reduce the incidence of PHC.

The HBV vaccines are subunit vaccines. The initial HBV vaccine was derived from the 22-nm HBsAg particles in human plasma obtained from chronically infected people. The current vaccine was genetically engineered and is produced by the insertion of a plasmid containing the S gene for HBsAg into a yeast, *Saccharomyces cerevisiae.* The protein self-assembles into particles, which enhances its immunogenicity.

The vaccine must be given in a series of three injections, with the second and third given 1 and 6 months after the first. More than 95% of individuals receiving the full three-dose course will develop protective antibody. The single serotype and limited host range (humans) help ensure the success of an immunization program.

Universal blood and body fluid precautions are used to limit exposure to HBV. It is assumed that all patients are infected. Gloves are required for handling blood and body fluids; wearing protective clothing and eyeglasses may also be necessary. Special care should be taken with needles and sharp instruments. HBV-contaminated materials can be disinfected with 10% bleach solutions, but unlike most enveloped viruses, HBV is not inactivated by detergents.

Hepatitis C and G Viruses

Hepatitis C virus was identified in 1989 after isolation of a viral RNA from a chimpanzee infected with blood from a person with NANBH. The viral RNA obtained from blood was converted to DNA with reverse transcriptase, its proteins were expressed, and antibodies from people with NANBH were then used to detect the viral proteins. These studies led to the development of ELISA and genomic and other tests for detection of the virus, which still cannot be grown in tissue culture.

HCV is the predominant cause of NANBH virus infections and was the major cause of post-transfusion hepatitis before routine screening of the blood supply for HCV. There are more than 170 million carriers of HCV in the world and more than 4 million in the United States. HCV is transmitted by means similar to HBV but has an even greater potential for establishing persistent, chronic hepatitis. The chronic hepatitis often leads to cirrhosis and potentially to hepatocellular carcinoma. The significance of the HCV epidemic has become more apparent with the development of laboratory screening procedures.

STRUCTURE AND REPLICATION

HCV is the only member of the *Hepacivirus* genus of the **Flaviviridae** family. It is 30 to 60 nm in diameter, with a **positive-sense RNA genome,** and is **enveloped.** The genome of HCV (9100 nucleotides) encodes 10 proteins, including two glycoproteins (E1, E2) that undergo variation during infection because of hypervariable regions within their genes. There are six major groups of variants (clades), which differ in their worldwide distribution.

HCV infects only humans and chimpanzees. Molecular biologic tricks have allowed expression and study of HCV replication. It coats itself with low-density lipoprotein, or very low-density lipoprotein, and then uses their receptor for uptake into hepatocytes. HCV binding to CD81 (tetraspanin) surface receptors, which are expressed on lymphocytes and other cells, allows these cells to harbor the virus outside the liver. The virus replicates like other flaviviruses. The virion buds into and remains in the endoplasmic reticulum, becoming cell associated. HCV proteins inhibit apoptosis and INF-α action by binding to the tumor necrosis factor receptor and to protein kinase R. These actions prevent the death of the host cell and promote persistent infection.

BOX 66–5. Epidemiology of Hepatitis B, C, and D Viruses

Disease/Viral Factors

Enveloped virus is labile to drying. HBV is less sensitive to detergents than other enveloped viruses.

Virus is shed during asymptomatic periods.

HBV (10%) and HCV (70%) cause chronic infection with potential shedding.

Transmission

In blood, semen, and vaginal secretions (HBV: saliva and mother's milk).

Via transfusion, needlestick injury, shared drug paraphernalia, sexual intercourse, and breast-feeding.

Who Is at Risk?

Children: Mild asymptomatic disease with establishment of chronic infection.

Adults: Insidious onset of hepatitis.

HBV-infected people coinfected or superinfected with HDV: Abrupt, more severe symptoms with possible fulminant disease.

Adults with chronic HBV or HCV: At high risk for cirrhosis and primary hepatocellular carcinoma.

Geography/Season

Viruses are found worldwide.

There is no seasonal incidence.

Modes of Control

Avoidance of high-risk behavior.

HBV: Viruslike particle (HBsAg) **vaccine.**

HBV and HCV screening of blood supply.

HBV, Hepatitis B virus; HCV, hepatitis C virus; HDV, hepatitis D virus.

PATHOGENESIS

The ability of HCV to remain cell associated and prevent host cell death promotes persistent infection but results in liver disease later in life. Cell-mediated immunopathology is responsible mainly for producing the tissue damage. The extent of lymphocytic infiltration, inflammation, portal and periportal fibrosis, and lobular necrosis in liver biopsies can be used to grade the severity of disease. It has been suggested that the continual liver repair and induction of cell growth occurring during chronic HCV infection, especially in cirrhotic livers, are predisposing factors in the development of PHC. Antibody to HCV is not protective, and findings yielded by experimental infection of chimpanzees indicate that immunity to HCV may not be lifelong.

EPIDEMIOLOGY

HCV is **transmitted primarily in infected blood** and sexually. Intravenous drug abusers, transfusion and organ recipients, and hemophiliacs receiving factors VIII or IX are at highest risk for infection (Box 66–5). Almost all (>90%) HIV-infected people who are or were intravenous drug users are infected with HCV. HCV is especially prevalent in southern Italy, Spain, central Europe, Japan, and parts of the Middle East (e.g., almost 20% of Egyptian blood donors are HCV positive). The **high incidence of chronic asymptomatic infections** promotes the spread of the virus in the population. Screening procedures have led to a reduction in the levels of transmission by blood transfusion and organ donation, but transmission by other routes is prevalent.

CLINICAL SYNDROMES

HCV causes three types of disease (Figure 66–13): (1) acute hepatitis with resolution of the infection and recovery in 15% of cases, (2) chronic persistent infection with possible progression to disease much later in life for 70% of infected persons, (3) and severe rapid progression to cirrhosis in 15% of patients. A viremia can be detected within 1 to 3 weeks of a transfusion of HCV-contaminated blood. The viremia lasts 4 to 6 months in people with an acute infection and longer than 10 years in those with a persistent infection. In its acute form, HCV infection is similar to acute HAV and HBV infection, but the inflammatory response is less intense and the symptoms are usually milder. More commonly (>70%), the initial disease is asymptomatic but establishes chronic persistent disease. The predominant symptom is a chronic fatigue. The chronic, persistent disease often progresses to chronic active hepatitis within 10 to 15 years and to cirrhosis

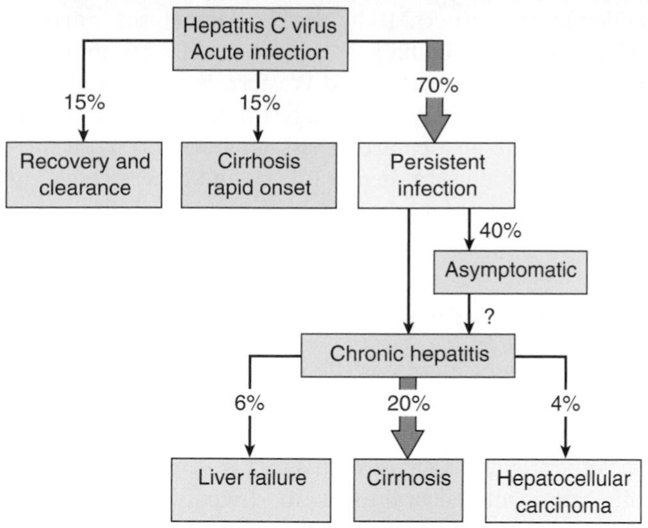

FIGURE 66–13. Outcomes of hepatitis C virus infection.

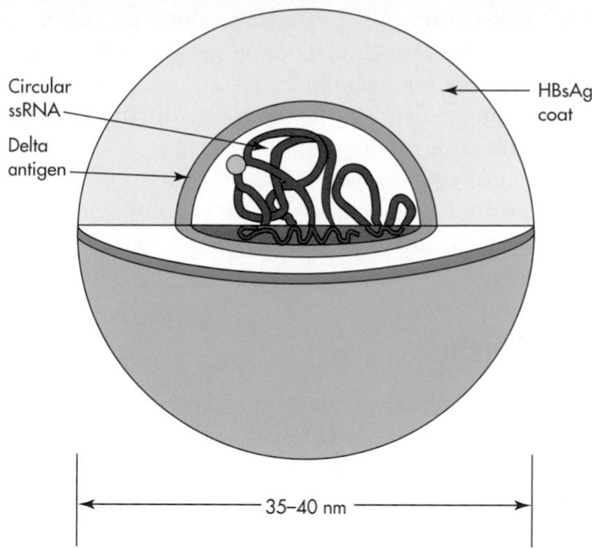

FIGURE 66–14. The delta hepatitis virion.

(20% of chronic cases) and liver failure (20% of cirrhotic cases) after 20 years. HCV-induced liver damage may be exacerbated by alcohol, certain medications, and other hepatitis viruses to promote cirrhosis. HCV promotes the development of hepatocellular carcinoma after 30 years in up to 5% of chronically infected patients.

LABORATORY DIAGNOSIS

The diagnosis and detection of HCV infection are based on ELISA recognition of anti-HCV antibody or detection of the RNA genome. Seroconversion occurs within 7 to 31 weeks of infection. ELISA is used for screening the blood supply from normal donors. As for HIV, results can be confirmed by Western immunoblot procedures. Antibody is not always detectable in viremic people, in immunocompromised patients, or in those receiving hemodialysis. Reverse transcriptase polymerase chain reaction (RT-PCR), branched-chain DNA, and other genetic techniques can detect HCV RNA in seronegative people and have become key tools in the diagnosis of HCV infection.

TREATMENT, PREVENTION, AND CONTROL

Recombinant INF-α or pegylated interferon (treated with polyethylene glycol to enhance its biologic lifetime), alone or with ribavarin, are the only known treatments for HCV. The combination therapy may yield up to 50% recovery rates.

Hepatitis G Virus

Hepatitis G virus resembles HCV in many ways. HGV is a flavivirus, is transmitted in blood, and has a predilection for chronic hepatitis disease. It is identified by detection of the genome by RT-PCR or other RNA detection methods.

Hepatitis D Virus

Approximately 15 million people in the world are infected with HDV (delta agent), and the virus is responsible for causing 40% of the **fulminant hepatitis** infections. HDV is unique in that it uses HBV and target cell proteins to replicate and produce its one protein. It is a viral parasite, proving that "even fleas have fleas." **HBsAg is essential for packaging the virus.** The delta agent resembles plant virus satellite agents and viroids in its size, genomic structure, and requirement for a helper virus for replication (Figure 66–14).

STRUCTURE AND REPLICATION

The **HDV RNA genome is very small** (approximately 1700 nucleotides), and unlike other viruses, the single-stranded RNA is circular and forms a rod shape as a result of its extensive base pairing. The virion is approximately the same size as the HBV virion (35 to 37 nm in diameter). The genome is surrounded by the delta antigen core, which in turn is surrounded by an HBsAg-containing envelope. The **delta antigen** exists as a small (24 kDa) or large (27 kDa) form; the small form is predominant.

The delta agent binds to and is internalized by hepatocytes in the same manner as HBV because it has HBsAg in its envelope. The transcription and replication processes of the HDV genome are unusual. The host cell's RNA polymerase II makes an RNA copy to replicate the genome. The genome then forms an RNA structure called a **ribozyme,** which cleaves the RNA circle to produce an mRNA for the small delta antigen. The gene for the delta antigen is mutated by a cellular enzyme (double-stranded RNA–activated adenosine deaminase) during infection, thereby allowing production of the large delta antigen. Production of this antigen limits replication of the virus but also promotes association of the genome with HBsAg to form a virion, and the virus is then released from the cell.

PATHOGENESIS

Similar to HBV, the delta agent is spread in blood, semen, and vaginal secretions. However, it can replicate and cause disease only in people with active HBV infections. Because the two agents are transmitted by the same routes, a person can be **coinfected** with HBV and the delta agent. A person with chronic HBV can also be **superinfected** with the delta agent. More rapid, severe progression occurs in HBV carriers superinfected with HDV than in people coinfected with HBV and the delta agent, because during coinfection HBV must first establish its infection before HDV can replicate (Figure 66–15), whereas superinfection of an HBV-infected person allows the delta agent to replicate immediately.

Replication of the delta agent results in cytotoxicity and liver damage. Persistent delta agent infection is often established in HBV carriers. Although antibodies are elicited against the delta agent, protection probably stems from the immune response to HBsAg because it is the external antigen and viral attachment protein for HDV. Unlike HBV disease, damage to the liver occurs as a result of the direct cytopathic effect of the delta agent combined with the underlying immunopathology of the HBV disease.

EPIDEMIOLOGY

The delta agent infects children and adults with underlying HBV infection (see Box 66–5), and people who are persistently infected with both HBV and HDV are a source for the virus. The agent has a worldwide distribution infecting approximately 5% of the 3×10^8 HBV carriers and is endemic in southern Italy, the Amazon Basin, parts of Africa, and the Middle East. Epidemics of HDV infection occur in North America and Western Europe, usually in illicit drug users. HDV is spread by the same routes as HBV, and the same groups are at risk for infection, with parenteral drug abusers, hemophiliacs and others receiving blood products at highest risk. Screening of the blood supply has reduced the risk for recipients of blood products.

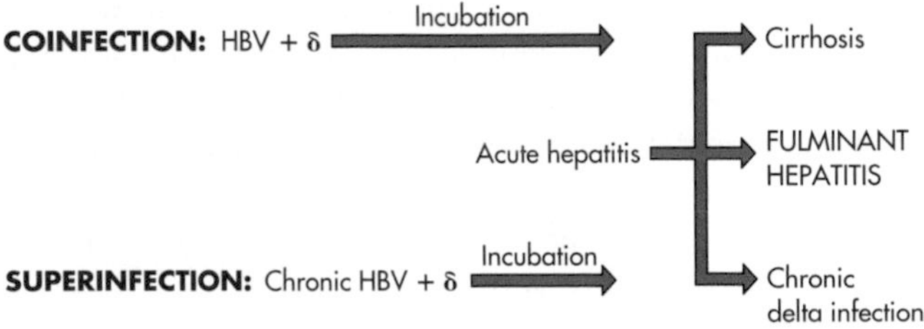

FIGURE 66–15. Consequences of delta virus infection. Delta virus (δ) requires the presence of hepatitis B virus (HBV) infection. Superinfection of a person already infected with HBV (carrier) causes more rapid, severe progression than coinfection *(shorter arrow)*.

CLINICAL SYNDROMES (BOX 66–6)

The delta agent increases the severity of HBV infections. Fulminant hepatitis is more likely to develop in people infected with the delta agent than in those infected with the other hepatitis viruses. This very severe form of hepatitis causes altered brain function (hepatic encephalopathy), extensive jaundice, and massive hepatic necrosis, which is fatal in 80% of cases. Chronic infection with the delta agent can occur in people with chronic HBV.

LABORATORY DIAGNOSIS

The only way to determine the presence of the agent is by detecting the RNA genome, the delta antigen, or anti-HDV antibodies. ELISA and radioimmunoassay procedures are available for detection.. The delta antigen can be detected in the blood during the acute phase of disease in a detergent-treated serum sample. RT-PCR techniques can be used to detect the virion genome in blood.

TREATMENT, PREVENTION, AND CONTROL

There is no known specific treatment for HDV hepatitis. Because the delta agent depends on HBV for replication and is spread by the same routes, prevention of infection with HBV prevents HDV infection. Immunization with HBV vaccine protects against subsequent deltavirus infec-

BOX 66–6. Clinical Summaries

Hepatitis A: A 37-year-old man develops fever, chills, headache, and fatigue 4 weeks after eating at a greasy spoon diner. Within 2 days he develops anorexia, vomiting, and right upper quadrant abdominal pain, followed by jaundice and with dark-colored urine and stools persisting for 12 days. Then symptoms decrease.

Hepatitis B: A 27-year-old intravenous (IV) drug user develops symptoms of hepatitis 2 months after using a dirty needle.

Hepatitis B and D: A different IV drug user develops symptoms of hepatitis, altered mental capacity, and massive hepatic necrosis and then dies.

Hepatitis C: Elevated liver enzymes were detected in an individual during a physical examination. HCV in the blood was detected by ELISA. Ten years later, cirrhosis and liver failure developed, requiring a liver transplant.

tion. If a person has already acquired HBV, delta agent infection may be prevented by halting illicit intravenous drug use and avoiding HDV-contaminated blood products.

Hepatitis E Virus

HEV (E-NANBH) (the E stands for enteric or epidemic) is predominantly spread by the fecal-oral route, especially in contaminated water (see Box 66–2). HEV is a separate genus within the Noroviruses, based on its size (27 to 34 nm) and structure. Although HEV is found throughout the world, it is most problematic in developing countries. Epidemics have been reported in India, Pakistan, Nepal, Burma, North Africa, and Mexico.

The symptoms and course of HEV disease are similar to those of HAV disease; it causes only acute disease. However, the symptoms for HEV may occur later than those of HAV disease. The mortality rate associated with HEV disease is 1% to 2%, approximately 10 times that associated with HAV disease. HEV infection is especially serious in pregnant women (mortality rate of approximately 20%).

CASE STUDIES AND QUESTIONS

A 55-year-old man ***(patient A)*** *was admitted to the hospital with fatigue, nausea, and abdominal discomfort. He had a slight fever, his urine was dark yellow, and his abdomen was distended and tender. He had returned from a trip to Thailand within the previous month.*

A 28-year-old woman ***(patient B)*** *was admitted to the hospital complaining of vomiting, abdominal discomfort, nausea, anorexia, dark urine, and jaundice. She admitted that she was a former heroin addict and that she had shared needles. In addition, she was 3 months pregnant.*

A 65-year-old man ***(patient C)*** *was admitted with jaundice, nausea, and vomiting 6 months after undergoing coronary artery bypass grafting.*

1. What clinical or epidemiologic clues would have assisted in the diagnosis of hepatitis A, B, and C?
2. What laboratory tests would have been helpful in distinguishing the different hepatitis infections?
3. What was the most likely means of viral acquisition in each case?
4. What personal and public health precautions should have been taken to prevent the transmission of virus in each case?
5. Which of the patients was susceptible to chronic disease?
6. What laboratory tests distinguish acute from chronic HBV disease?
7. How can HBV disease be prevented? Treated?

Bibliography

Blum HE, Gerok W, Vyas GN: The molecular biology of hepatitis B virus, *Trends Genet* 5:154-158, 1989.

Bradley DW, Krawczynski K, Kane MA: Hepatitis E. In Belshe RB, editor: *Textbook of human virology*, ed 2, St Louis, 1991, Mosby.

Catalina G, Navarro V: Hepatitis C: A challenge for the generalist. *Hosp Prac* 35:97-108, 2000.

Cohen J, Powderly WG, editors: *Infectious diseases*, ed 2, St Louis, 2004, Mosby.

Fallows DA, Goff AP: Hepadnaviruses: Current models of RNA encapsidation and reverse transcription, *Adv Virus Res* 46: 167-196, 1996.

Flint SJ et al: *Principles of virology: Molecular biology, pathogenesis and control of animal viruses*, ed 2, Washington, 2003, American Society for Microbiology Press.

Frosner G: Hepatitis A virus. In Belshe RB, editor: *Textbook of human virology*, ed 2, St Louis, 1991, Mosby.

Ganem D, Prince AM: Hepatitis B virus infection—natural history and clinical consequences. *NEJM* 350:1118-1119.

Hadler SC, Fields HA: Hepatitis delta virus. In Belshe RB, editor: *Textbook of human virology*, ed 2, St Louis, 1991, Mosby.

Hagedorn CH, Rice CM: The hepatitis C viruses, *Curr Top Microbiol Immunol* 242:1-380, 2000.

Hepatitis fact sheet: National Institute of Allergy and Infectious Diseases: Available online at www.niaid.nih.gov/publications/hepatitis.htm.

Hoofnagle JH: Type A and type B hepatitis, *Lab Med* 14:705-716, 1983.

Knipe DM, Howley PM, editors: *Fields virology*, ed 4, New York, 2001, Lippincott-Williams and Wilkins.

Lennette EH, Halonen P, Murphy FA, editors: *Laboratory diagnosis of infectious diseases: Principles and practice*, New York, 1988, Springer-Verlag.

Lutwick LI: Hepatitis B virus. In Belshe RB, editor: *Textbook of human virology*, ed 2, St Louis, 1991, Mosby.

Mason WS, Seeger C, editors: Hepadnaviruses: Molecular biology and pathogenesis, *Curr Top Microbiol Immunol* 162:1-206, 1991.

Plageman PGW: Hepatitis C virus, *Arch Virol* 120:165-180, 1991.

Reyes GR, Baroudy BM: Molecular biology of NANBH agents: Hepatitis C and hepatitis E viruses, *Adv Virus Res* 40:57-102, 1991.

Robinson W, Koike K, Will H, editors: *Hepadnavirus*, New York, 1987, Liss.

Strauss JH, Strauss EG: *Viruses and human disease*, San Diego, 2002, Academic Press.

Tam AW et al: Hepatitis E virus: Molecular cloning and sequencing of the full-length viral genome, *Virology* 185:120-131, 1991.

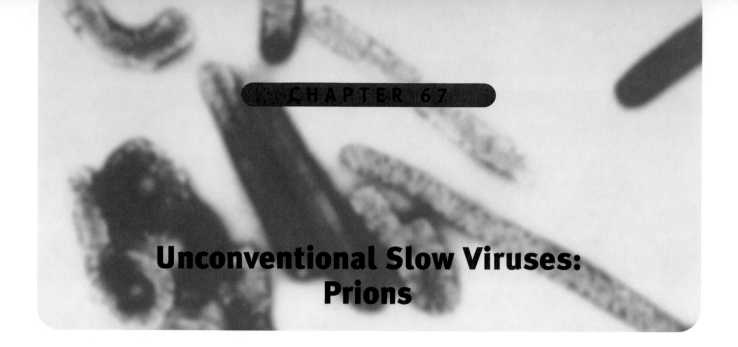

Unconventional Slow Viruses: Prions

The unconventional slow viruses cause spongiform encephalopathies, which are slow neurodegenerative diseases. These disorders include the human diseases kuru, Creutzfeldt-Jakob disease (CJD), Gerstmann-Sträussler-Scheinker (GSS) syndrome, and fatal familial insomnia (FFI) and the animal diseases scrapie, bovine spongiform encephalopathy (BSE) (mad cow disease), chronic wasting disease (in mule, deer, and elk), and transmissible mink encephalopathy (Box 67–1). In the late 1990s, there were outbreaks of BSE and a rapid progressing form of CJD affecting younger people (40 years) in the United Kingdom. CJD, FFI, and GSS syndrome are also genetic human disorders.

Slow virus agents are filterable and can transmit disease but otherwise do not conform to the standard definition of a virus (Table 67–1). Unlike conventional viruses, these agents have no virion structure or genome, elicit no immune response, and are extremely resistant to inactivation by heat, disinfectants, and radiation. The slow virus agent is a mutant or conformationally distinct form of a host protein known as a **prion (a small proteinaceous infectious particle),** which can transmit the disease.

After long incubation periods, these agents cause damage to the central nervous system that leads to a subacute spongiform encephalopathy. The long incubation period, which can last 30 years in humans, has made study of these agents difficult. Carlton Gajdusek won the Nobel Prize for showing that kuru has an infectious etiology and also for developing a method for analyzing the agent. Stanley Prusiner won the Nobel Prize in 1997 for developing a hamster infection model for the scrapie agent that allowed him and his co-workers to purify, characterize, and then clone the genes for the scrapie and other prion agents and for showing that the prion protein (PrP) is sufficient to cause disease.

Structure and Physiology

The slow virus agents were originally suspected to be viruses because they can pass through filters that block the passage of particles more than 100 nm in diameter and still transmit disease. Unlike viruses, the agents are resistant to a wide range of chemical and physical treatments, such as formaldehyde, ultraviolet radiation, and heat up to 80°C.

The prototype of these agents is scrapie, which has been adapted so that it can infect hamsters. Scrapie-infected hamsters have scrapie-associated fibrils in their brains. These fibrils are infectious and contain the prion. The prion, which lacks detectable nucleic acids, consists of aggregates of a protease-resistant, hydrophobic glycoprotein, which is termed $\mathbf{PrP^{Sc}}$ (scrapie-like prion protein) (27,000 to 30,000 Da). Humans and other animals encode a protein $\mathbf{PrP^{C}}$ (cellular prion protein) of unknown function that is held in the cell membrane by a linkage between its terminal serine and a special lipid, glycophosphatidyl inositol (GPI-linked protein). The PrP^{C} is closely related or can be identical to PrP^{Sc} in its protein sequence but differs in tertiary structure due to differences in the folding of the proteins (Table 67–2). PrP^{Sc} is protease resistant, aggregates into amyloid rods (fibrils), is found in cytoplasmic vesicles in the cell, and is secreted. The normal PrP^{C}, on the other hand, is protease sensitive and appears on the cell surface.

Many theories have been proposed to explain how an aberrant protein could cause disease. PrP^{Sc} binds to the normal PrP^{C} on the cell surface, causing it to refold and acquire the structure of PrP^{Sc}. The PrP^{Sc} is released from the cell and aggregates as amyloid-like plaques in the brain. The cell then replenishes the PrP^{C}, and the cycle continues. The human version of the PrP^{C} is encoded on

BOX 67–1. Slow Virus Diseases

Human
Kuru
Creutzfeldt-Jakob disease (CJD)
Gerstmann-Sträussler-Scheinker (GSS syndrome)
Fatal familial insomnia (FFI)

Animal
Scrapie (sheep and goats)
Transmissible mink encephalopathy
Bovine spongiform encephalopathy (BSE; mad cow disease)
Chronic wasting disease (mule, deer, and elk)

BOX 67–2. Pathogenic Characteristics of Slow Viruses

No cytopathologic effect in vitro
Long doubling time of at least 5.2 days
Long incubation period
Cause vacuolation of neurons (spongiform), amyloid-like plaques, gliosis
Symptoms that include loss of muscle control, shivering, tremors, dementia
Lack of antigenicity
Lack of inflammation
Lack of immune response
Lack of interferon production

TABLE 67–1. Comparison of Classic Viruses and Prions

	Virus	Prion
Filterable, infectious agents	Yes	Yes
Presence of nucleic acid	Yes	No
Defined morphology (electron microscopy)	Yes	No
Presence of protein	Yes	Yes
Disinfection by:		
Formaldehyde	Yes	No
Proteases	Some	No
Heat (80°C)	Most	No
Ionizing and ultraviolet radiation	Yes	No
Disease		
Cytopathologic effect	Yes	No
Incubation period	Depends on virus	Long
Immune response	Yes	No
Interferon production	Yes	No
Inflammatory response	Yes	No

TABLE 67–2. Comparison of Scrapie Prion Protein (PrP^{Sc}) and (Normal) Cellular Prion Protein (PrP^{C})

	PrP^{Sc}	PrP^{C}
Structure	Globular	Extended
Protease resistance	Yes	No
Presence in scrapie fibrils	Yes	No
Location in or on cells	Cytoplasmic vesicles and extracellular milieu	Plasma membrane
Turnover	Days	Hours

chromosome 20. The fact that these plaques consist of host protein may explain the lack of an immune response to these agents in patients with the spongiform encephalopathies.

Different strains of PrP^{Sc} occur because of mutations in the PrP^{C} or to self-perpetuating alternative folding patterns of the protein. Conformational, rather than genetic, mutation is another property that distinguishes prions from viruses. When the PrP^{Sc} aggregates, the PrP^{Sc} acts as a template to transmit its conformation onto each new PrP^{Sc}, analogous to a genetic template (DNA or RNA) transmitting its sequence onto a new viral genome. The different conformational strains can have different properties and varying disease aspects (e.g., incubation period).

Pathogenesis

Spongiform encephalopathy describes the appearance of the vacuolated neurons as well as their loss of function and the lack of an immune response or inflammation (Box 67–2). Vacuolation of the neurons, the formation of amyloid-containing plaques and fibrils, a proliferation and hypertrophy of astrocytes, and the fusion of neurons and adjacent glial cells are observed (Figure 67–1). The PrP^{Sc} is taken up by neurons and phagocytic cells but is difficult to degrade, a feature that may contribute to the vacuolation of the brain tissue. In addition, prions reach high concentrations in the brain, further contributing to the tissue damage. Prions can also be isolated from tissue other than the brain, but only the brain shows any disease. No inflammation or immune response to the agent is generated, distinguishing this disease from classic viral encephalitis. A protein marker (14-3-3 brain protein) can be detected in the cerebrospinal fluid of symptomatic persons.

The incubation period for CJD and kuru may be as long as 30 years, but once the symptoms become evident, the patient dies within a year.

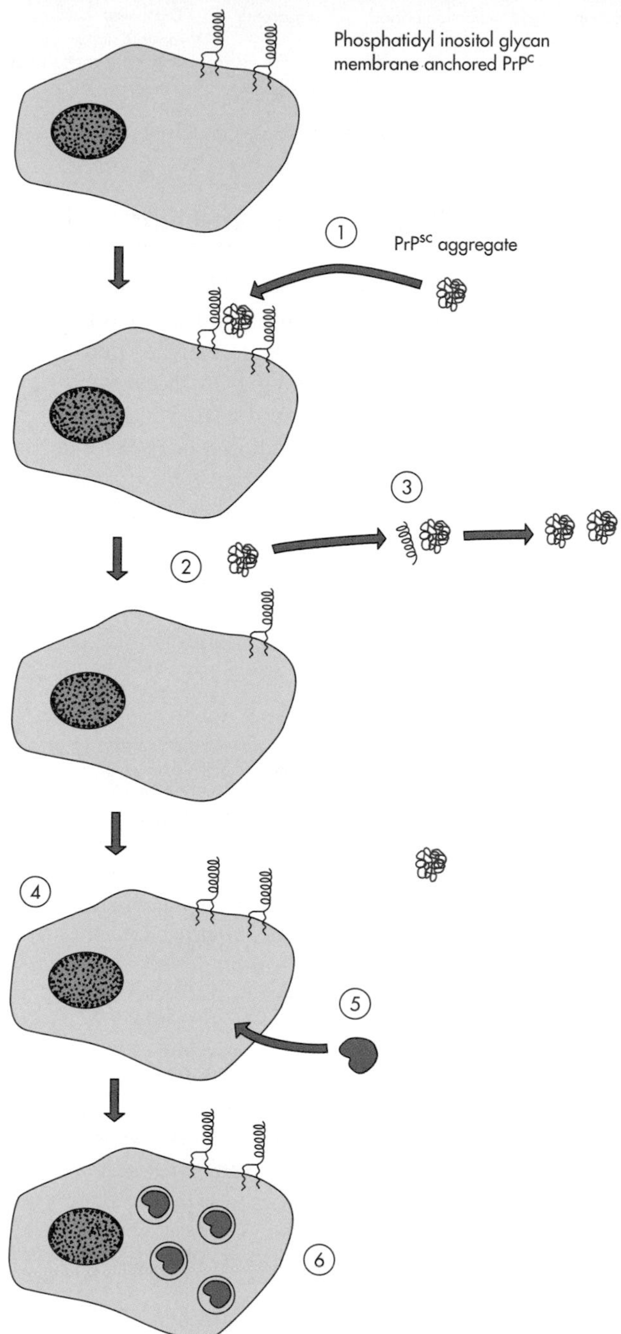

FIGURE 67–1. Model for proliferation of prions. PrP^{C} is a normal cellular protein that is anchored in the cell membrane by phosphatidyl inositol glycan. PrP^{Sc} is a hydrophobic globular protein that aggregates with itself and with PrP^{c} on the cell surface (1). PrP^{c} acquires the conformation of PrP^{Sc}, is released from the cell (2), and is converted to PrP^{Sc} (3). The cell synthesizes new PrP^{C} (4), and the cycle is repeated. A form of PrP^{Sc} is internalized by neurons (5) and accumulates (6), giving the cell a spongiform appearance. Other models have been proposed.

BOX 67–3. Epidemiology of Disease Caused by Slow Viruses

Disease/Viral Factors

Agents are impervious to standard viral disinfection procedures.

Diseases have very long incubation periods, as long as 30 years.

Transmission

Transmission is via **infected tissue,** or syndrome **may be inherited.**

Infection occurs through cuts in skin, transplantation of contaminated tissues (e.g., cornea), use of contaminated medical devices (e.g., brain electrodes), and by ingestion of infected tissue.

Who Is at Risk?

Women and children of the Fore tribe in New Guinea were at risk for kuru.

Surgeons, transplant and brain surgery patients, and others are at risk for CJD and GSS syndrome.

Geography/Season

GSS syndrome and CJD have sporadic occurrence worldwide.

There is no seasonal incidence.

Modes of Control

No treatments are available.

Cessation of ritual cannibalism has led to the disappearance of kuru.

Elimination of animal products from livestock feed to prevent vCJD transmission.

For GSS syndrome and CJD, neurosurgical tools and electrodes should be disinfected in 5% hypochlorite solution or 1.0 M sodium hydroxide or autoclaved at 15 psi for 1 hour.

CJD, Creutzfeldt-Jakob disease; GSS, Gerstman-Straüssler-Scheinker.

Epidemiology

CJD is transmitted predominantly by (1) injection, (2) transplantation of contaminated tissue (e.g., corneas), (3) contact with contaminated medical devices (e.g., brain electrodes), and (4) food (Box 67–3). CJD usually affects persons older than 50 years. CJD, FFI, and GSS syndrome are also inheritable, and families with genetic histories of these diseases have been identified. The diseases are rare but occur worldwide.

Kuru was limited to a very small area of the New Guinea highlands. The name of the disease means “shivering” or “trembling,” and the disease was related to the cannibalistic practices of the Fore tribe of New Guinea. Before Gajdusek intervened, it was the custom of these people to eat the bodies of their deceased kinsmen. When Gajdusek began his study, he noted that women and children in particular were the most susceptible to the disease, and he deduced that the reasons were that the women and children prepared the food and they were given the less

BOX 67–4. Clinical Summaries

CJD: A 63-year-old man complained of poor memory and difficulty with vision and muscle coordination. Over the course of the next year, he developed senile dementia and irregular jerking movements, progressively lost muscle function, and then died.

VCJD: A 25-year-old is seen by a psychiatrist for anxiety and depression. After 2 months, he has problems with balance and muscle control and has difficulty remembering. He develops myoclonus and dies within 12 months of onset.

desirable viscera and brains to eat. Their risk for infection was higher because they handled the contaminated tissue, making it possible for the agent to be introduced through the conjunctiva or cuts in the skin. In addition, they ingested the neural tissue, which contains the highest concentrations of the kuru agent. Cessation of this cannibalistic custom has stopped the spread of kuru.

An epidemic of BSE (mad cow disease) in 1980 in the United Kingdom and the unusual incidence of a more rapidly progressing CJD in younger people (younger than 45 years) in 1996 prompted concern that contaminated beef was the source of this new variant of CJD (vCJD). Infection of the cattle is most likely caused by the use of contaminated animal by-products (e.g., sheep entrails, brains) as a protein supplement in the cattle feed. Ingestion of contaminated beef is likely to be the cause of 153 cases of vCJD, more than 98% of which have occurred in the United Kingdom.

Clinical Syndromes (see Box 67–4)

As already noted, the slow virus agents cause a progressive, degenerative neurologic disease with a long incubation period but with rapid progression to death after the onset of symptoms (Figure 67–2). The spongiform encephalopathies are characterized by a loss of muscle control, shivering, myoclonic jerks and tremors, loss of coordination, rapidly progressive dementia, and death.

Laboratory Diagnosis

There are no methods for directly detecting prions in tissue through the use of electron microscopy, antigen detection, or nucleic acid probes. Also, no serologic tests can detect viral antibody. The initial diagnosis must be made on clinical grounds. Confirmation of the diagnosis can be made by detection of a proteinase K–resistant form of PrP in a Western blot using antibody to PrP in a tonsil biopsy. At autopsy, the characteristic amyloid plaques, spongiform vacuoles, and immunohistologically detected PrP can be observed.

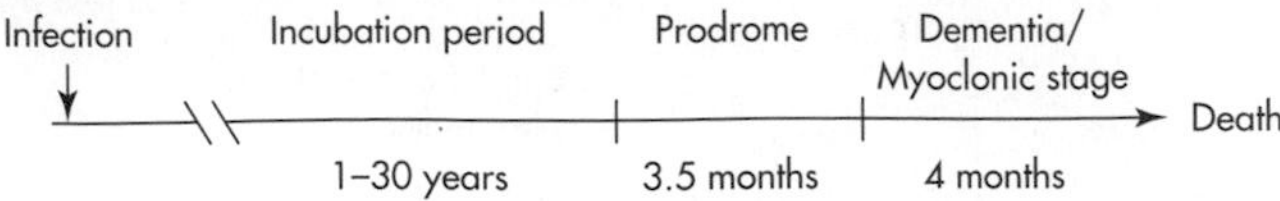

FIGURE 67–2. Progression of transmissible Creutzfeldt-Jakob disease.

Treatment, Prevention, and Control

No treatment exists for kuru or CJD. The causative agents are also impervious to the disinfection procedures used for other viruses, including formaldehyde, detergents, and ionizing radiation. Autoclaving at 15 psi for 1 hour instead of 20 minutes or treatment with 5% hypochlorite solution or 1.0 M sodium hydroxide can be used for decontamination. Because these agents can be transmitted on instruments and brain electrodes, such items should be carefully disinfected before being reused.

The outbreak of BSE and vCJD in the United Kingdom promoted legislation to ban animal products in livestock feed and encouraged more careful monitoring of cattle.

CASE STUDY AND QUESTIONS

A 70-year-old woman complained of severe headaches and appeared dull and apathetic with a constant tremor in the right hand. One month later, she experienced memory loss and moments of confusion. The patient's condition continued to deteriorate, and an abnormal electroencephalograph tracing showing periodic biphasic and triphasic slow-wave complexes was obtained at 2 months after onset of symptoms. By 3 months, the patient was in a comalike state. She also had occasional spontaneous clonic twitching of the arms and legs and a startle myoclonic jerking response to a loud noise. The patient died of pneumonia 4 months after the onset of symptoms. No gross abnormalities were noted at autopsy. Astrocytic gliosis of the cerebral cortex with fibrils and intracellular vacuolation throughout the cerebral cortex were seen on microscopic examination. There was no swelling and no inflammation.

1. What viral neurologic diseases would have been considered in the differential diagnosis formulated on the basis of the symptoms described? What other diseases?
2. What key features of the postmortem findings were characteristic of the diseases caused by unconventional slow virus agents (e.g., spongiform encephalopathies, prions)?
3. What key features distinguish the unconventional slow virus diseases from more conventional neurologic viral diseases?
4. What precautions should the pathologist have taken for protection against infection during the postmortem examination?

Bibliography

Belay ED: Transmissible spongiform encephalopathies in humans, *Annu Rev Microbiol* 53:283-314, 1999.

Brown P et al: Diagnosis of Creutzfeld-Jakob disease by Western blot identification, *N Engl J Med* 314:547-551, 1986.

Cohen J, Powderly WG, editors: *Infectious diseases*, ed 2, St Louis, 2004, Mosby.

Flint SJ et al: *Principles of virology: Molecular biology, pathogenesis and control of animal viruses*, ed 2, Washington, 2003, American Society for Microbiology Press.

Hsich G et al: The 14-3-3 brain protein in cerebrospinal fluid as a marker for transmissible spongiform encephalopathies, *N Engl J Med* 335:924-930, 1996.

Knipe DM, Howley PM, editors: *Fields virology*, ed 4, New York, 2001, Lippincott-Williams and Wilkins.

Manson JC: Understanding transmission of the prion diseases, *Trends Microbiol* 7:465-467, 1999.

Prusiner SB: Molecular biology and genetics of neurodegenerative diseases caused by prions, *Adv Virus Res* 41:241-280, 1992.

Prusiner SB: Prions, prions, prions, *Curr Top Microbiol Immunol* 207:1-162, 1996.

Websites

Freudenrich CC: How mad cow disease works. http://science.howstuffworks.com/mad-cow-disease6.htm

www.priondata.org

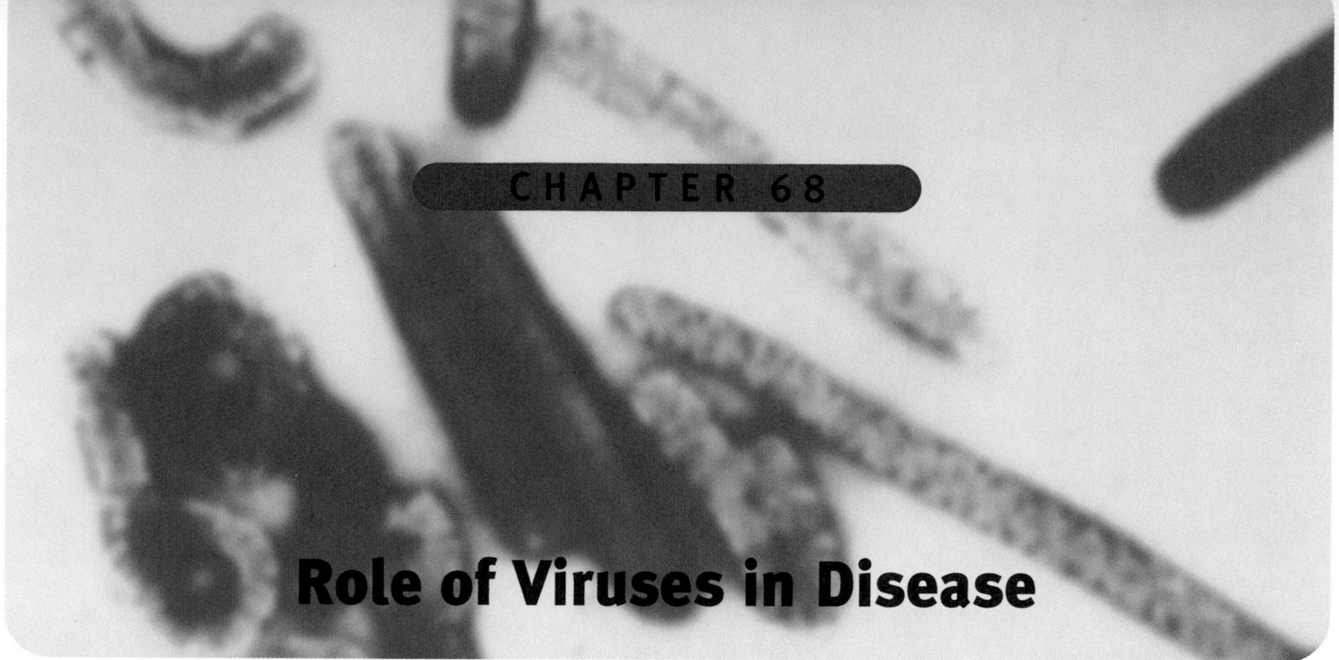

Role of Viruses in Disease

Most viral infections cause mild or no symptoms and do not require extensive treatment. The common cold, influenza, flulike syndromes, and gastroenteritis are common viral diseases. Other viral infections that target essential tissues and organs are very cytolytic, or induce immunopathologic effects, and can cause serious and even life-threatening disease. In general, the symptoms and severity of a viral infection are determined by (1) the patient's ability to prevent or rapidly resolve the infection before the virus can reach important organs or cause significant damage; (2) the target tissue and virulence of the virus; and (3) the ability of the body to repair the damage.

Previous chapters stressed the viral characteristics that promote disease. In this chapter, viral diseases are discussed with respect to their symptoms, the organ system they target, and the host factors that influence their presentation.

Viral Diseases

The major sites of viral disease are the respiratory tract; the gastrointestinal tract; the epithelial, mucosal, and endothelial linings of the skin, mouth, and genitalia; the lymphoid tissue; the liver and other organs; and the central nervous system (CNS) (Figure 68–1). The examples given in this chapter represent more common causes of disease.

ORAL AND RESPIRATORY TRACT INFECTIONS

The oropharynx and respiratory tract are the **most common sites** of viral infection and disease (Table 68–1). The viruses are spread in respiratory droplets and aerosols, food and water, and saliva; by close contact; and on hands. Similar respiratory symptoms can be caused by several different viruses. For example, bronchiolitis may be caused by respiratory syncytial or parainfluenza virus. Alternatively, one virus may cause different symptoms in different people. For example, influenza virus can cause a mild upper respiratory tract infection in one person and life-threatening pneumonia in another.

Many viral infections start in the oropharynx or respiratory tract, infect the lung, and spread without causing significant symptoms. Varicella-zoster virus (VZV) and the measles virus initiate infection in the lung and can cause pneumonia but generally cause systemic infections resulting in an exanthem (rash). Other viruses that establish primary infection of the oropharynx or respiratory tract and then progress to other sites are rubella, mumps, enteroviruses, and several human herpesviruses—herpes simplex virus (HSV), Epstein-Barr virus (EBV), cytomegalovirus (CMV), and human herpesvirus 6 (HHV-6).

The symptoms and severity of a respiratory viral disease depend on the nature of the virus, the site of infection (upper or lower respiratory tract), and the immune status and the age of the person. Conditions such as cystic fibrosis and smoking, which compromise the ciliated and mucoepithelial barriers to infection, increase the risk of serious disease.

Pharyngitis and oral disease are common viral presentations. Most enteroviruses infect the oropharynx and then progress by way of a viremia to other target tissues. For example, symptoms such as acute-onset pharyngitis, fever, and oral vesicular lesions are characteristic of Coxsackie A virus infections (herpangina, hand-foot-and-mouth disease) and some Coxsackie B virus and echovirus infections. Adenovirus and the early stages of EBV disease are characterized by sore throat and tonsillitis with an exudative membrane, and then EBV infects B lymphocytes to cause infectious mononucleosis. HSV causes local

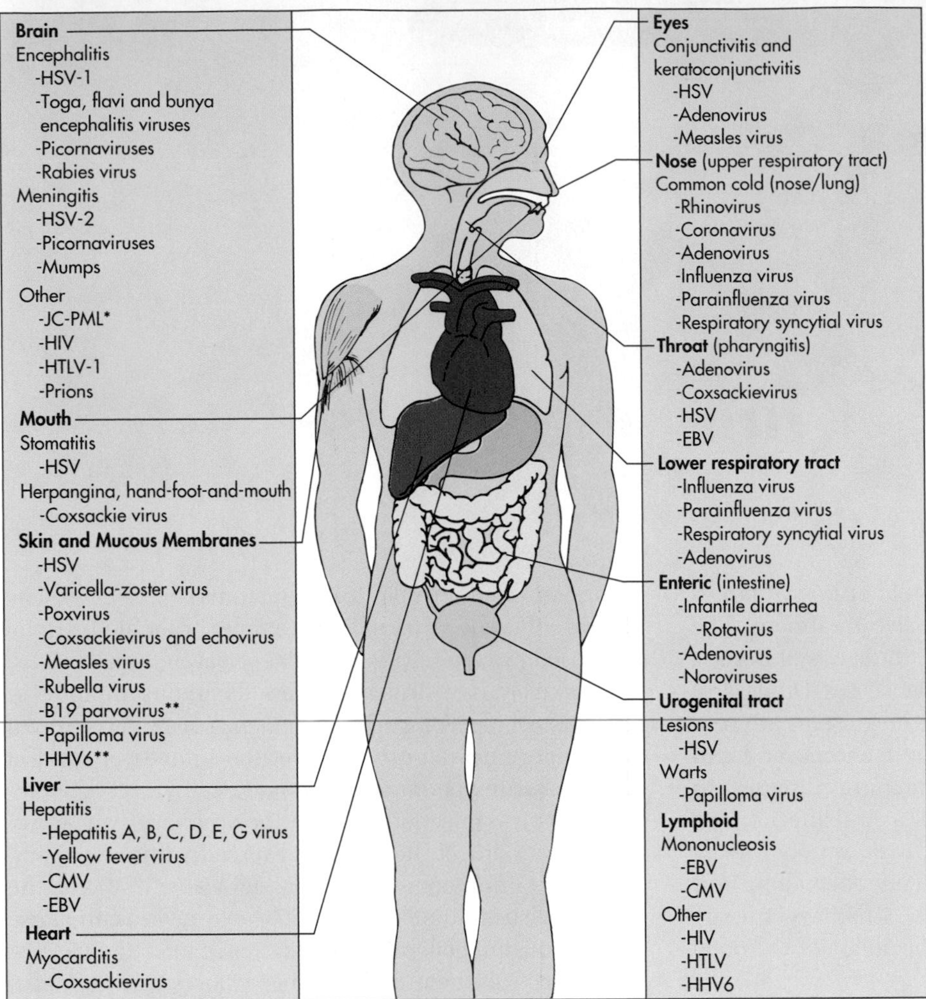

FIGURE 68–1. Major target tissues of viral disease. (*) indicates progressive multifocal leukoencephalopathy. Infection by viruses indicated by (**) results in an immune-mediated rash.

primary infections of the oral mucosa and face (gingivostomatitis) and then establishes a latent neuronal infection that can recur in the form of herpes labialis (cold sores, fever blisters). HSV is also a common cause of pharyngitis. Vesicular lesions on the buccal mucosa (Koplik's spots) are an early diagnostic feature of measles infection.

Although upper respiratory tract viral infections, including the common cold and pharyngitis, are generally benign, they still account for at least 50% of absenteeism from schools and the workplace. Rhinoviruses and coronaviruses are the predominant causes of upper respiratory tract infections. A runny nose (rhinitis) followed by congestion, cough, sneezing, conjunctivitis, headache, and sore throat are typical symptoms of the common cold. Other causes of the common cold and pharyngitis are specific serotypes of echoviruses and Coxsackie viruses, adenoviruses, influenza viruses, parainfluenza viruses, and respiratory syncytial virus.

Tonsillitis, laryngitis, and **croup** (laryngotracheobronchitis) may accompany certain respiratory tract viral infections. HSV and Coxsackie A viruses may also involve the tonsils, but with vesicular lesions. Laryngitis (adults) and croup (children) are caused by inflammatory responses to the viral infection that cause the trachea to narrow below the vocal cords (subglottic area). This narrowing causes loss of voice; a hoarse, barking cough; and the risk, especially in young children, for a blocked airway and choking. Children infected with parainfluenza viruses are especially at risk for croup.

Lower respiratory tract viral infections can also result in more serious disease. Symptoms of such infections include bronchiolitis (inflammation of the bronchioles), pneumonia, and related diseases. The parainfluenza and respiratory syncytial viruses are major problems for infants and children but cause only asymptomatic infections or common cold symptoms in adults. Parainfluenza 3 virus and especially respiratory syncytial virus infections are major causes of life-threatening pneumonia or bronchiolitis in infants younger than 6 months. Infection with these viruses does not provide lifelong immunity.

TABLE 68–1. Oral and Respiratory Diseases

Disease	Etiologic Agent
Common cold (including pharyngitis)	Rhinovirus* Coronavirus* Influenza viruses Parainfluenza viruses Respiratory syncytial virus Metapneumovirus Adenovirus Enteroviruses
Pharyngitis	Herpes simplex virus Epstein-Barr virus Adenovirus* Coxsackie A virus* (herpangina, hand-foot-and-mouth disease) and other enteroviruses
Croup, tonsillitis, laryngitis, and bronchitis (children younger than 2 years)	Parainfluenza virus 1* Parainfluenza virus 2 Influenza virus Adenovirus Epstein-Barr virus
Bronchiolitis	Respiratory syncytial virus* (infants) Metapneumovirus Parainfluenza virus 3* (infants and children) Parainfluenza viruses 1 and 2
Pneumonia	Respiratory syncytial virus* (infants) Metapneumovirus Parainfluenza virus* (infants) Influenza virus* Adenovirus Varicella-zoster virus (primary infection of adults or immunocompromised hosts) Cytomegalovirus (infection of immunocompromised host) Measles

*Most common causal agents.

Influenza virus is probably the best known and most feared of the common respiratory viruses, with the annual introduction of new strains of virus ensuring the presence of immunologically naive victims. Children are universally susceptible to new strains of virus, whereas older people may have been immunized during a prior outbreak of the annual strain. Despite such immunization, the elderly are especially susceptible to new strains of virus because they may not be able either to mount a sufficient primary immune response to the new strain of influenza virus or to repair the tissue damage caused by the disease. Other possible viral agents of pneumonia are adenovirus, paramyxoviruses, and primary VZV infections of adults.

BOX 68–1. Gastrointestinal Viruses

Infants
Rotavirus A*
Adenovirus 40, 41
Coxsackie A24 virus

Infants, Children, and Adults
Norwalk virus
Calicivirus
Astrovirus
Rotavirus B (outbreaks in China)
Reovirus

*Most common cause.

FLULIKE AND SYSTEMIC SYMPTOMS

Many viral infections cause classic **flulike symptoms** (e.g., fever, malaise, anorexia, headache, body aches), side effects caused by host responses to the infection. During the viremic phase, many viruses induce the release of interferon and cytokines. In addition to the respiratory viruses, flulike symptoms may accompany infections by arboencephalitis viruses, HSV type 2 (HSV-2), and other viruses.

Arthritis and other inflammatory diseases may result from immune hypersensitivity responses induced by the infection or immune complexes containing viral antigen. For example, B19 parvovirus infection of adults, rubella, and infection with several other togaviruses elicit arthritis. Immune complex disease that is associated with chronic hepatitis B virus (HBV) can result in various presentations, including arthritis and nephritis.

GASTROINTESTINAL TRACT INFECTIONS

Infections of the gastrointestinal tract can result in gastroenteritis, vomiting, diarrhea, or no symptoms (Box 68–1). Norwalk virus, caliciviruses, astroviruses, adenoviruses, reoviruses, and rotaviruses infect the small intestine but not the colon, damaging the epithelial lining and the absorptive villi. This damage leads to the malabsorption of water and an electrolyte imbalance. The resultant diarrhea in older children and adults is generally self-limited and can be treated with rehydration and restoration of the electrolyte balance. These viruses, especially rotavirus, are major problems for adults and children in regions where there is drought and starvation.

Viral gastroenteritis has a more significant effect on infants and may necessitate hospitalization. The extent of tissue damage and consequent loss of fluids and electrolytes is a more significant problem for infants. Rotavirus and adenovirus serotypes 40 and 41 are the major causes of infantile gastroenteritis.

Fecal-oral spread of the enteric viruses is promoted by poor hygiene and is especially prevalent in daycare centers. Norwalk virus and calicivirus outbreaks affecting older children and adults are generally linked to a common contaminated food or water source. Vomiting usually accompanies diarrhea in patients infected with the Norwalk virus and rotavirus. Although enteroviruses (picornaviruses) are spread by the fecal-oral route, they usually cause only mild or no gastrointestinal symptoms. Instead, these viruses establish a viremia, spread to other target organs, and then cause clinical disease.

EXANTHEMS AND HEMORRHAGIC FEVERS

Virus-induced skin disease (Table 68–2) can result from infection through the mucosa or small cuts or abrasions in the skin (HSV), as a secondary infection after establishment of a viremia (VZV and smallpox), or as a result of the inflammatory response mounted against viral antigens (parvovirus B19). The major classifications of viral rashes are maculopapular, vesicular, nodular, and hemorrhagic. **Macules** are flat, colored spots. **Papules** are slightly raised areas of the skin that may result from immune or inflammatory responses rather than the direct effects of the virus. **Nodules** are larger, raised areas of the skin. **Vesicular lesions** are blisters and are likely to contain virus. Papillomaviruses cause warts, and molluscum contagiosum causes wartlike growths (nodules) by stimulating the growth of skin cells.

The classic childhood exanthems are roseola infantum (exanthem subitum [HHV-6]), fifth disease (erythema infectiosum [parvovirus B19]), and, in unvaccinated children, varicella, measles, and rubella. The rash follows a viremia and is accompanied by fever. Rashes are also caused by enterovirus infections, dengue, and other infections caused by flaviviruses or alphaviruses. They also are occasionally seen in patients with infectious mononucleosis.

The yellow fever virus, dengue virus, Ebola virus, Lassa fever, Sin Nombre virus, and other hemorrhagic fever viruses establish a viremia and infect the endothelial cell lining of the vasculature, possibly compromising the structure of the blood vessel. Viral or immune cytolysis can then lead to greater permeability or rupture of the vessel, producing a hemorrhagic rash with petechiae (pinpoint hemorrhages under the skin) and ecchymoses (massive bruises) and hence internal bleeding, the loss of electrolytes, and shock.

TABLE 68–2. Viral Exanthems

Condition	Etiologic Agent
Rash	
Rubeola	Measles virus
German measles	Rubella virus
Roseola infantum	Human herpesvirus 6
Erythema infectiosum	Human parvovirus B19
Boston exanthem	Echovirus 16
Infectious mononucleosis	Epstein-Barr virus, cytomegalovirus
Vesicles	
Oral or genital herpes	Herpes simplex virus*
Chickenpox/shingles	Varicella-zoster virus*
Hand-foot-and-mouth disease, herpangina	Coxsackie A virus*
Papillomas	
Warts	Papillomavirus*
Molluscum	Molluscum contagiosum

*Most common cause.

INFECTIONS OF THE EYE

Infections of the eye result from direct contact with a virus or from viremic spread (Box 68–2). Conjunctivitis (pinkeye) is a normal feature of many childhood infections and is a characteristic of infections caused by specific adenovirus serotypes (3, 4a, and 7), the measles virus, and the rubella virus. Keratoconjunctivitis caused by adenovirus (8, 19a, and 37), HSV, or VZV involves the cornea and can cause severe damage. Enterovirus 70 and Coxsackie A24 virus can cause an acute hemorrhagic conjunctivitis. Cataracts are classic features of babies born with congenital rubella syndrome. Chorioretinitis is associated with CMV infection in newborns (congenital) as well as in immunosuppressed people (e.g., those with acquired immune deficiency syndrome [AIDS]).

INFECTIONS OF THE ORGANS AND TISSUES

Infection of the major organs may cause significant disease or may result in further spread or secretion of the virus (see Box 68–2). The symptoms may arise from tissue damage or inflammatory responses.

The liver is a prominent target for many viruses that reach the liver by means of a viremia or the mononuclear phagocyte (reticuloendothelial) system. The liver acts as a source for a secondary viremia but can also be damaged by the infection. The classic symptoms of hepatitis result from infections with hepatitis A, B, C, G, D, and E viruses

BOX 68–2. Infections of the Organs and Tissues

Liver
Hepatitis A,* B,* C,* G, D, and E viruses
Yellow fever virus
Epstein-Barr virus
Hepatitis in the neonate or immunocompromised person:
- Cytomegalovirus
- Herpes simplex virus
- Varicella-zoster virus
- Rubella virus (congenital rubella syndrome)

Heart
Coxsackie B virus

Kidney
Cytomegalovirus

Muscle
Coxsackie B virus (pleurodynia)

Glands
Cytomegalovirus
Mumps virus

Eye
Herpes simplex virus
Adenovirus*
Measles virus
Rubella virus
Enterovirus 70
Coxsackie A24 virus

*Most common cause.

and yellow fever virus and are often associated with EBV infectious mononucleosis and CMV infections. The liver is also a major target in disseminated HSV infection of neonates and infants.

The heart and other muscles are also susceptible to viral infection and damage. Coxsackie virus can cause myocarditis or pericarditis in newborns, children, and adults. Coxsackie B virus can infect muscle and cause pleurodynia (Bornholm's disease). Other viruses (e.g., influenza virus, CMV) can also infect the heart.

Infection of the secretory glands, accessory sexual organs, and mammary glands results in contagious spread of CMV. An inflammatory response to the infection, as occurs in **mumps** (parotitis, orchitis), may be the cause of the symptoms. CMV infection of the kidney and reactivation are problems for immunosuppressed people and a predominant reason for kidney transplant failure.

BOX 68–3. Central Nervous System Infections

Meningitis
Enteroviruses
- Echoviruses
- Coxsackie virus*
- Poliovirus

Herpes simplex virus 2
Adenovirus
Mumps virus
Lymphocytic choriomeningitis virus
Arboencephalitis viruses

Paralysis
Poliovirus
Enteroviruses 70 and 71
Coxsackie A7 virus

Encephalitis
Herpes simplex virus 1*
Varicella-zoster virus
Arboencephalitis viruses*
Rabies virus
Coxsackie A and B viruses
Polioviruses

Postinfectious Encephalitis (Immune Mediated)
Measles virus
Mumps virus
Rubella virus
Varicella-zoster virus
Influenza viruses

Other
JC virus (progressive multifocal leukoencephalopathy [in immunosuppressed people])
Measles variant (subacute sclerosing panencephalitis)
Prion (encephalopathy)
Human immunodeficiency virus (AIDS dementia)
Human T-cell lymphotrophic virus 1 (tropical spastic paraparesis)

*Most common cause.

INFECTIONS OF THE CENTRAL NERVOUS SYSTEM

Viral infections of the brain and CNS may cause the most serious viral diseases because of the importance of the CNS and its very limited capacity to repair damage (Box 68–3). Tissue damage is usually caused by a combination of viral pathogenesis and immunopathogenesis. Most neurotropic viral infections do not result in disease, however, because the virus does not reach the brain or does not cause sufficient tissue damage to produce symptoms.

Virus may spread to the CNS in blood (arboviruses) or in macrophages (human immunodeficiency virus [HIV]);

it may spread from a peripheral infection of the neurons (olfactory), or it may first infect skin (HSV) or muscle (polio, rabies) and then progress to the innervating neurons. The virus may have a predilection for certain sites in the brain. For example, the temporal lobe is targeted in HSV encephalitis, Ammon's horn in rabies, and the anterior horn of the spinal cord and motor neurons.

Viral infections of the CNS are usually distinguished from bacterial infections by the finding of mononuclear cells, low numbers of polymorphonuclear leukocytes, and normal or slightly reduced levels of glucose in the cerebrospinal fluid. Immunoassay detection of specific antigen, polymerase chain reaction detection of viral genomes or messenger RNA, or isolation of the virus from a cerebrospinal fluid or biopsy specimen confirms the diagnosis and identifies the viral agent. The season of the year also facilitates the diagnosis, in that enteroviral and arboviral diseases generally occur during the summer, whereas HSV encephalitis and other viral syndromes may be observed year-round.

Aseptic meningitis is caused by an inflammation and swelling of the meninges enveloping the brain and spinal cord in response to infection with enteroviruses (especially echoviruses and Coxsackie viruses), HSV-2, the mumps virus, or the lymphocytic choriomeningitis virus. The disease is usually self-limited and, unlike bacterial meningitis, resolves without sequelae unless the virus gains access to and infects neurons or the brain **(meningoencephalitis).** The viruses gain access to the meninges by means of a viremia.

Encephalitis and **myelitis** result from a combination of viral pathogenesis and immunopathogenesis in brain tissue and neurons and either are fatal or cause significant damage and permanent neurologic sequelae. HSV, VZV, rabies virus, California encephalitis viruses, West Nile and St. Louis encephalitis viruses, and measles virus are potential causes of encephalitis. Poliovirus and several other enteroviruses cause paralytic disease (myelitis).

HSV and VZV are ubiquitous and usually cause asymptomatic latent infections of the CNS but can also cause encephalitis. Most arboencephalitis virus infections result in flu-like symptoms rather than encephalitis. Postmeasles encephalitis and subacute sclerosing panencephalitis were rare sequelae of measles in the prevaccine era.

Other virus-induced neurologic syndromes are HIV dementia, human T-leukemia virus type 1 (HTLV-1) tropical spastic paraparesis, JC papovavirus–induced, progressive multifocal leukoencephalopathy in immunosuppressed people, and the prion-associated spongiform encephalopathies (kuru, Jakob-Creutzfeldt disease, Gerstmann-Sträussler-Scheinker disease). Progressive multifocal leukoencephalopathy and the spongiform encephalopathies have long incubation periods (conventional and unconventional slow viruses).

HEMATOLOGIC DISEASES

Lymphocytes and macrophages are not very permissive for viral replication but are targets for several viruses that establish persistent infections. Transient viral replication of EBV, HIV, or CMV elicits a large T-cell response, resulting in **mononucleosis-like syndromes.** In addition, CMV, measles virus, and HIV infections of T cells are immunosuppressive. HIV reduces the numbers of CD4 helper and delayed-type hypersensitivity T cells, further compromising the immune system. HTLV-1 infection causes little disease on infection but may lead to **adult T-cell leukemia** or tropical spastic paraparesis much later in life (Box 68–4).

Macrophages and cells of the macrophage lineage can be infected by many viruses. Macrophages act as vehicles for spreading the virus throughout the body because viruses replicate inefficiently in them and the cells are generally not lysed by the infection. This process promotes persistent and chronic infections. The macrophage is the primary target cell for the dengue virus. Non-neutralizing antibody can promote uptake of dengue virus and HIV into the cell through Fc receptors. Macrophages and cells of the macrophage lineage infected with HIV provide a reservoir for the virus and access to the brain. AIDS dementia is thought to result from the actions of HIV-infected macrophages and microglial cells in the brain.

SEXUALLY TRANSMITTED VIRAL DISEASES

Sexual transmission is a major route for the spread of papillomavirus, HSV, CMV, HIV, HTLV-1, HBV, hepatitis C virus (HCV), and hepatitis D virus (HDV) (Box 68–5). Such viruses establish chronic and latent-recurrent infections,

BOX 68–4. Viruses Transmitted in Blood

Hepatitis B, C, G, D
Human immunodeficiency virus
Human T-cell lymphotrophic virus 1
Cytomegalovirus
Epstein-Barr virus
West Nile encephalitis virus

BOX 68–5. Sexually Transmitted Viruses

Human papillomavirus 6, 11, 42
Human papillomavirus 16 and 18 (associated with human cervical carcinoma)
Herpes simplex virus (predominantly HSV-2)
Cytomegalovirus
Hepatitis B, C, and D viruses
Human immunodeficiency virus
Human T-cell lymphotrophic virus 1

with asymptomatic shedding into the semen and vaginal secretions. These viral properties foster dissemination via a route of transmission that is used relatively infrequently and might be avoided during symptomatic disease. The viruses can also be transmitted neonatally or perinatally to infants. Papillomaviruses and HSV establish local primary infections with recurrent disease at the same site. Lesions and asymptomatic shedding are sources for sexual transmission and for perinatal transmission to the newborn. CMV and HIV enter the bloodstream and infect lymphoid cells, whereas the hepatitis viruses are delivered to the liver. CMV, HIV, and the hepatitis viruses are present in blood, semen, and vaginal secretions, which can transmit the virus to sexual partners and neonates.

VIRUSES SPREAD BY TRANSFUSION AND TRANSPLANTATION

HBV, HCV, HDV, HIV, HTLV-1, and CMV are transmitted by blood and organ transplants. These viruses are also present in semen and therefore are sexually transmitted. The chronic nature of the infection, the persistent asymptomatic release of the virus, or the infection of macrophages and lymphocytes promotes transmission by these routes. West Nile encephalitis virus establishes a sufficient viremia for a long enough period that transmission by transfusion has occurred. Screening of the blood supply for HBV, HCV, HIV, and HTLV has controlled transmission of these viruses in blood transfusions (Box 68–6). Large-scale procedures for screening the other viruses have not been developed, so the risk remains for the spread of CMV by these routes.

VIRUSES SPREAD BY ARTHROPODS AND ANIMALS

Many of the toga, flavi, bunya, and the Colorado Tick fever reovirus establish sufficient viremia in birds or animals to allow their acquisition by mosquitos or ticks and subsequent transmission to humans. Arena, rhabdo, and hanta viruses are transmitted to humans in saliva, urine, feces or through the bite of an infected animal (Table 68–3).

SYNDROMES OF POSSIBLE VIRAL ETIOLOGY

Several diseases either produce symptoms or have epidemiologic or other characteristics that resemble those of viral infections or may be the sequelae of viral infections (e.g., inflammatory responses to a persistent viral infec-

BOX 68–6. Screening of the Blood Supply

Human immunodeficiency syndrome
Hepatitis B
Hepatitis C
Human T-cell lymphotropic virus type I and II
West Nile encephalitis virus*
Syphilis

*Trial initiated in 2003 on 6 million units with 818 positive units excluded from usage.

TABLE 68–3. Arboviruses and Zoonoses

Virus	Family	Reservoir/Vector
Eastern equine encephalitis	Toga	Birds/Aedes mosquito
Western equine encephalitis	Toga	Birds/Culex mosquito
West Nile encephalitis	Flavi	Birds/Culex mosquito
St. Louis encephalitis	Flavi	Birds/Culex mosquito
California encephalitis	Bunya	Small mammals/Aedes mosquito
La Crosse encephalitis	Bunya	Small mammals/Aedes mosquito
Yellow fever	Flavi	Birds/Aedes
Dengue	Flavi	Mosquito
Colorado tick fever	Reo	Tick
Lymphocytic choriomeningitis	Arena	Small mammals
Lassa fever	Arena	Rats
Sin Nombre virus	Hanta	Deer mice
Ebola	Filo	unknown
Rabies	Rhabdo	Bats, foxes, raccoons, etc.

tion). They include **multiple sclerosis, Kawasaki disease, arthritis, diabetes,** and **chronic fatigue syndrome.**

Chronic and Potentially Oncogenic Infections

Chronic infections occur when the immune system has difficulty resolving the infection. The DNA viruses (except parvovirus and poxvirus) and the retroviruses cause latent infections with the potential for recurrence. CMV and other herpesviruses; hepatitis B, C, G, and D viruses; and retroviruses cause chronic productive infections.

HBV, HCV, EBV, HHV-8, papillomavirus, and HTLV-1 are associated with **human cancers.** EBV, papillomavirus, and HTLV-1 can immortalize cells; after immortalization, cofactors, chromosomal aberrations, or both enable a clone of virus-containing cells to grow into a cancer. EBV normally causes infectious mononucleosis but is also associated with African Burkitt's lymphoma, Hodgkin's lymphoma, and nasopharyngeal carcinoma; HTLV-1 is associated with human adult T-cell leukemia. Many papillomaviruses induce a simple hyperplasia characterized by the development of a wart; however, several other strains of papillomaviruses have been associated with human cancers (e.g., type 16 and 18 associated with cervical carcinoma). Direct viral action or the chronic cell damage and repair in livers infected by HBV or HCV can result in a tumorigenic event leading to hepatocellular carcinoma. HSV-2 has been associated with human cervical carcinoma, most likely as a cofactor. Immunosuppression in patients who have AIDS, patients undergoing cancer chemotherapy, or transplant recipients also promotes the production of lymphoma by EBV. HHV-8 infection produces many cytokines to stimulate cell growth, and especially in persons with AIDS, this growth can progress to Kaposi's sarcoma.

Development of a worldwide vaccine program for HBV not only would reduce the spread of viral hepatitis but also would prevent the occurrence of primary hepatocellular carcinoma. The development of a vaccine for EBV and papillomavirus should also reduce the incidence of their associated cancers.

Infections in Immunocompromised Patients

Patients with **deficient cell-mediated immunity** are generally more susceptible to infection with enveloped viruses (especially the herpesviruses, measles virus, and even the vaccinia virus used for smallpox vaccinations) and to recurrences of infections with latent viruses (herpesviruses and papovaviruses). Severe T-cell deficiencies also affect the antiviral antibody response. Cell-mediated immunodeficiencies can be congenital or acquired. They may result from genetic defects (e.g., Duncan's disease, DiGeorge's syndrome, Wiskott-Aldrich syndrome), leukemia or lymphoma, infections (e.g., AIDS), or immunosuppressive therapy.

Viruses cause atypical and more severe presentations in immunosuppressed people. For example, infections with herpesviruses (e.g., HSV, CMV, VZV), which are normally benign and localized, can progress locally or can disseminate and cause visceral and neurologic infections that can be life threatening. A measles infection can cause a giant cell (syncytial) pneumonia rather than the characteristic rash.

People with immunoglobulin A deficiency or hypogammaglobulinemia (antibody deficiency) have more problems with respiratory and gastrointestinal viruses. Hypogammaglobulinemic people are more likely to suffer significant disease after infection by viruses that progress by viremia, including the live polio vaccine, echovirus, and VZV.

Congenital, Neonatal, and Perinatal Infections

The development and growth of the fetus are so ordered and rapid that a viral infection can damage or prevent the appropriate formation of important tissues, leading to miscarriage or congenital abnormalities. Infection can occur in utero (prenatal; e.g., rubella, parvovirus B19, CMV, HIV), during transit through the birth canal (neonatal; e.g., HSV, HBV, CMV), or soon after birth (postnatal; e.g., HIV, CMV, HBV, HSV, Coxsackie B virus, echovirus).

Neonates depend on the mother's immunity to protect them from viral infections. They receive maternal antibodies through the placenta and then in the mother's milk. This type of passive immunity can remain effective for 6 months to a year after birth. Maternal antibodies can (1) protect against spread of virus to the fetus during a viremia (e.g., rubella, B19), (2) protect against many enteric and respiratory tract viral infections, and (3) reduce the severity of other viral diseases after birth. Nevertheless, because the cell-mediated immune system is not mature at birth, newborns are susceptible to viruses that spread by cell-to-cell contact (e.g., HSV, VZV, CMV, HIV).

Rubella virus and CMV are examples of **teratogenic viruses** that can cause congenital infection and severe congenital abnormalities. HIV infection that is acquired in utero or from mother's milk initiates a chronic infection leading to lymphadenopathy, failure to thrive, or encephalopathy within 2 years of birth. HSV can be acquired during passage through an infected birth canal and can result in life-threatening disseminated disease. Nosocomial infection of newborns can result in a similar outcome. If parvovirus B19 is acquired in utero, it can cause spontaneous abortion.

Infection Control

Infection control is essential in hospital and health care settings. The spread of respiratory viruses is the most difficult to prevent. Viral spread can be controlled in the following ways:

1. Limiting personnel contact with sources of infection (e.g., wearing gloves, mask, goggles; using quarantine).
2. Improving hygiene, sanitation, and disinfection.
3. Ensuring that all personnel are immunized against common diseases.
4. Educating all personnel regarding points 1, 2, and 3 and in the ways to decrease high-risk behaviors.

Methods for disinfection differ for each virus and depend on its structure. Most viruses are inactivated by 70% ethanol, 15% chlorine bleach, 2% glutaraldehyde, 4% formaldehyde, or autoclaving (as described in "Guidelines for prevention of transmission of human immunodeficiency virus and hepatitis B virus to health-care and public-safety workers," issued in 1989 by the U.S. Centers for Disease Control and Prevention [CDC]). Most enveloped viruses do not require such rigorous treatment and are inactivated by soap and detergents. Other means of disinfection are also available.

Special "universal" precautions are required for the handling of human blood; that is, all blood should be assumed to be contaminated with HIV or HBV and should be handled with caution. In addition to these procedures, special care must be taken with syringe needles and surgical tools contaminated with blood to prevent needlesticks and cuts. Specific guidelines are available from the CDC.

Control of an outbreak usually requires identification of the source or reservoir of the virus, followed by cleanup, quarantine, immunization, or a combination of these measures. The first step in controlling an outbreak of gastroenteritis or hepatitis A is identification of the food, water, or possibly the daycare center that is the source of the outbreak.

Education programs can promote compliance with immunization programs and help people change lifestyles associated with viral transmission. Such programs have had a significant impact in reducing the prevalence of vaccine-preventable diseases such as smallpox, polio, measles, mumps, and rubella. It is hoped that educational programs will also promote changes in lifestyles and habits to restrict the spread of the blood-borne and sexually transmitted HBV and HIV.

QUESTIONS

1. What disinfection procedures are sufficient for inactivating the following viruses: HAV, HBV, HSV, and rhinovirus?
2. What precautions should health care workers take to protect themselves from infection with the following viruses: HBV, influenza A virus, HSV (whitlow), and HIV?
3. What predisposing conditions would exacerbate an infection with influenza A virus? VZV? Rotavirus?
4. Describe and compare the nature and mechanism of exanthem development for measles, VZV, HSV (primary and recurrence), and yellow fever.
5. A kidney transplant recipient undergoing immunosuppressive therapy has a lymphoma that regresses in response to a reduction in immunosuppressive therapy. The lymphoma cells are found to contain EBV. How might EBV be involved in this lymphoma? Why does the lymphoma regress in response to the reduction in the immunosuppressive therapy? For what other viral infections would this person be at increased risk during the immunosuppressive therapy?

Bibliography

Belshe RB, editor: *Textbook of human virology,* ed 2, St Louis, 1991, Mosby.

Cohen J, Powderly WG, editors: *Infectious diseases,* ed 2, St Louis, 2004, Mosby.

Ellner PD, Neu HC: *Understanding infectious disease,* St Louis, 1992, Mosby.

Emond RTD, Rowland HAK, Welsby P: *Colour atlas of infectious diseases,* ed 4, London, 2003, Mosby Ltd.

Gershon AA, Hotez PJ, Katz SL: *Krugman's infectious diseases of children,* ed 11, St Louis, 2004, Mosby.

Gorbach SL, Bartlett JG, Blacklow NR: *Infectious diseases,* ed 2, Philadelphia, 1997, WB Saunders.

Guidelines for prevention of transmission of human immunodeficiency virus and hepatitis B virus to health-care and public-safety workers, *MMWR Morb Mortal Wkly Rep* 38(suppl 6):1-37, 1989.

Hart CA, Broadhead RL: *Color atlas of pediatric infectious diseases,* St Louis, 1992, Mosby.

Haukenes G, Haaheim LR, Pattison JR: *A practical guide to clinical virology,* New York, 1989, John Wiley & Sons.

Knipe DM, Howley PM, editors: *Fields virology,* ed 4, New York, 2001, Lippincott-Williams and Wilkins.

Mandell GL, Bennet JE, Dolin R, editors: *Principles and practice of infectious diseases,* ed 6, Philadelphia, 2005, Churchill Livingstone.

Mims CA, White DO: *Viral pathogenesis and immunology,* Cambridge, Mass, 1984, Blackwell.
Shulman ST et al: *The biologic and clinical basis of infectious diseases,* ed 5, Philadelphia, 1997, WB Saunders.
White DO, Fenner FJ: *Medical virology,* ed 4, Orlando, Fla, 1994, Academic.

Website

All the virology on the Worldwide Web and specific viruses. Available at http://www.virology.net/

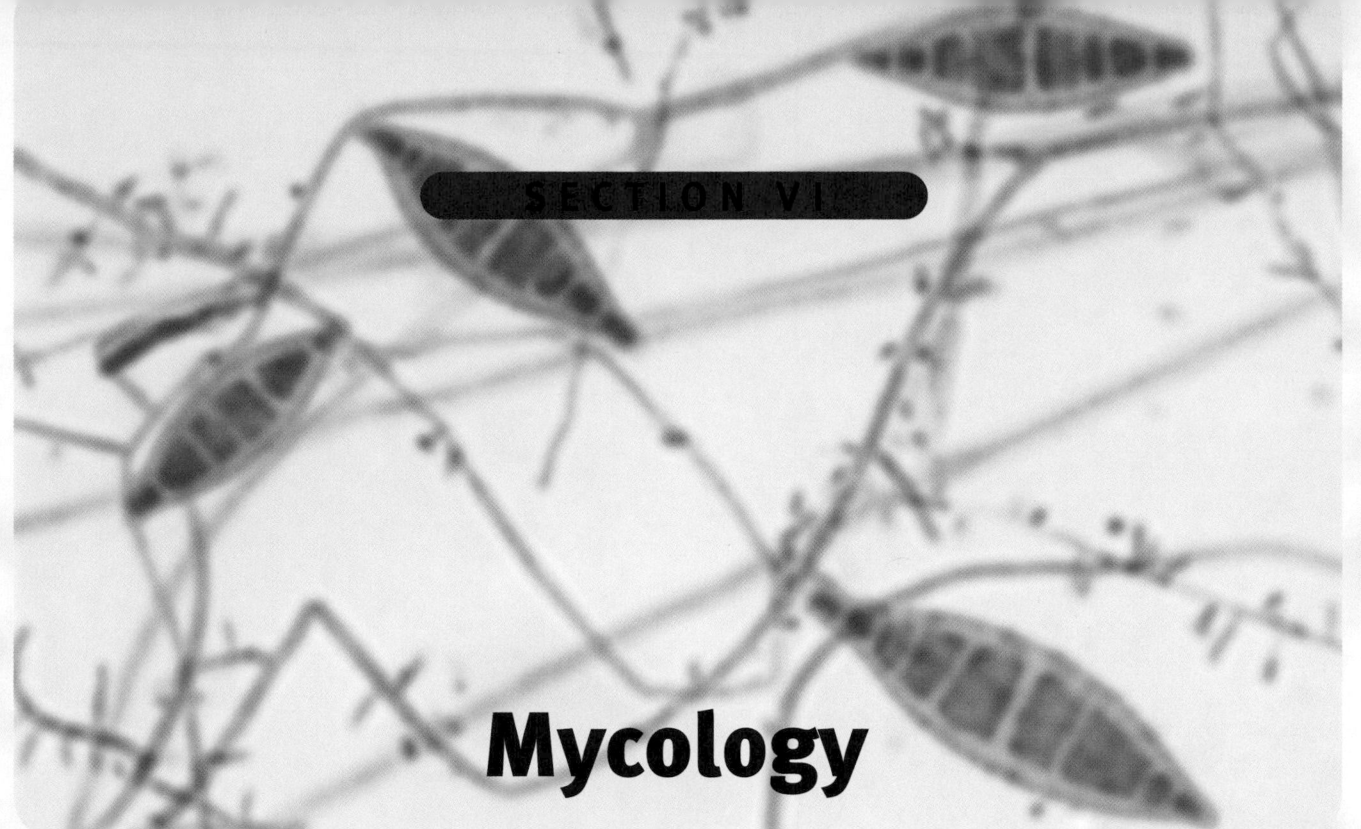

SECTION VI

Mycology

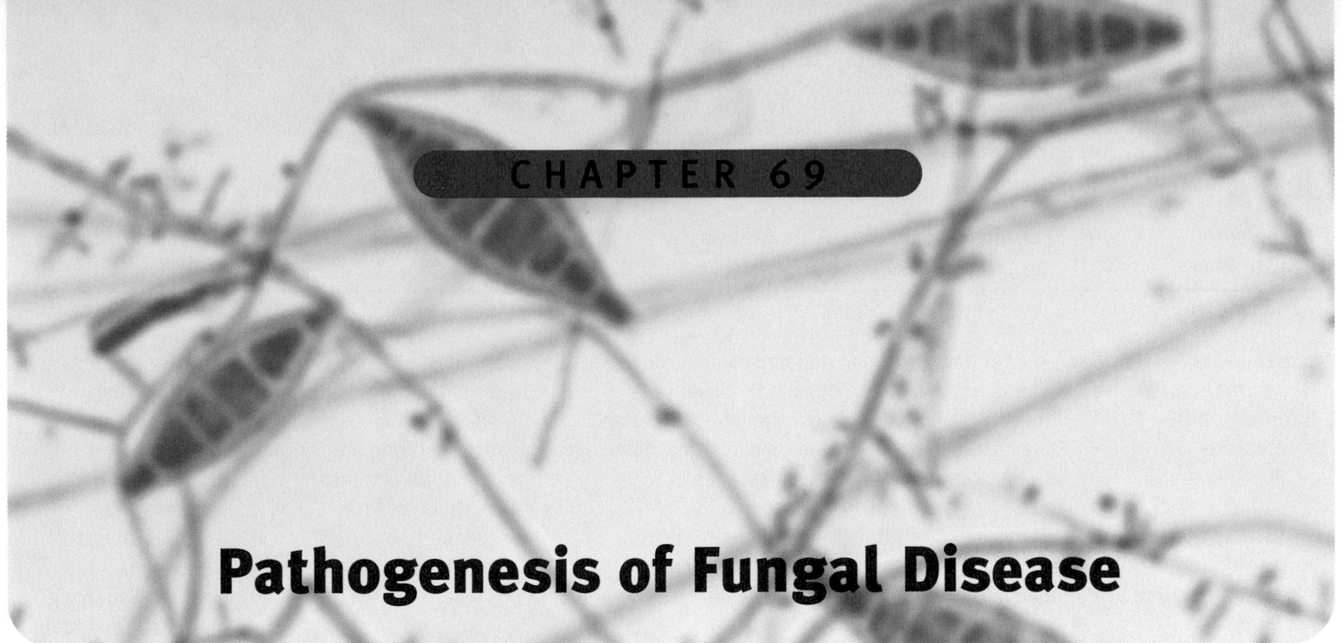

Pathogenesis of Fungal Disease

Although a great deal is known regarding the molecular and genetic basis for bacterial and viral pathogenesis, our understanding of the pathogenesis of fungal infections is limited. Relatively few fungi are sufficiently virulent to be considered **primary pathogens** (Table 69–1). Primary pathogens are capable of initiating infection in a normal, apparently immunocompetent host. They are able to colonize the host, find a suitable microenvironmental niche with sufficient nutritional substrates to avoid or subvert the normal host defense mechanisms, and then multiply within the microenvironmental niche. Among the acknowledged primary fungal pathogens are four ascomycetous fungi, the endemic dimorphic pathogens *Blastomyces dermatitidis, Coccidioides immitis* (and *Coccidioides posadasii*), *Histoplasma capsulatum*, and *Paracoccidioides brasiliensis*. Each of these organisms possesses putative virulence factors that allow them to actively breach host defenses that ordinarily restrict the invasive growth of other microbes (see Table 69–1). When large numbers of conidia of any of these four fungi are inhaled by humans, even if these persons are healthy and immunocompetent, infection and colonization, tissue invasion, and systemic spread of the pathogen commonly occur. As with most primary microbial pathogens, these fungi may also serve as **opportunistic pathogens,** given that the more severe forms of each mycosis are seen most often in individuals who are compromised in their innate and/or acquired immune defenses.

Generally, healthy immunocompetent persons have a high innate resistance to fungal infection, despite the fact that they are constantly exposed to the infectious forms of various fungi present as part of the normal commensal flora (endogenous) or in the environment (exogenous). The opportunistic fungal pathogens, such as *Candida* spp., *Cryptococcus neoformans,* and *Aspergillus* spp., generally only cause infection when there are disruptions in the protective barriers of the skin and mucous membranes or when defects in the host immune system allow them to penetrate, colonize, and reproduce in the host. However, even with these opportunists, there are factors associated with the organism rather than the host that contribute to the ability of the fungus to cause disease (see Table 69–1).

Primary Fungal Pathogens

Each of the primary systemic fungal pathogens are agents of respiratory infections and none are obligate parasites. Each has a **saprobic phase** that is characterized by filamentous septate hyphae typically found in soil or decaying vegetation and that produces the airborne infectious cells. Likewise, the **parasitic phase** of each fungus is adapted to grow at 37°C and to reproduce asexually in the alternative environmental niche of the host respiratory mucosa (see Figure 74–1). This ability to exist in alternate morphogenic forms (dimorphism) is one of several special characteristics (virulence factors) that allow these fungi to cope with the hostile environmental conditions of the host (see Table 69–1).

Blastomyces dermatitidis

Like the other endemic dimorphic fungal pathogens, *B. dermatitidis* often causes a self-limited respiratory infection (see Chapter 74). However, blastomycosis is distinguished from the other endemic mycoses by the high incidence of clinical disease compared with the mild or asymptomatic form among individuals infected in epidemics. The pathogenic potential of *B. dermatitidis* is underscored by the clinical severity of most sporadic cases of blastomycosis.

TABLE 69–1. Characteristics of Primary and Opportunistic Fungal Pathogens

Organism/ Growth Phase	Habitat/Infection	Pathogenesis	Putative Virulence Factors	Clinical Forms of Mycosis
Primary Pathogens				
Blastomyces dermatitidis Saprobic phase • Septate mycelium and conidia Parasitic phase • Large broad-based budding yeast	Saprobic habitat • Soil and organic debris • Endemic area Southeastern USA and Ohio-Mississippi River Valley Mode of infection • Inhalation of conidia	Inhaled conidia convert to yeast; localized yeast invasion of host invokes inflammatory reaction; yeast escapes recognition by macrophages and disseminates via bloodstream	• Growth at 37°C • Thermal dimorphism • Modulation of yeast-host immune system interactions • Generation of Th2 response • Shedding of WI-1	• Primary pulmonary blastomycosis • Chronic pulmonary blastomycosis • Disseminated blastomycosis — Cutaneous — Bone, genitourinary tract, and brain
Coccidioides immitis (posadasii) Saprobic phase • Septate hyphae and arthroconidia Parasitic phase • Spherules with endospores	Saprobic habitat • Desert soil • Southwestern USA, Mexico, regions of Central and South America Mode of infection • Inhalation of arthroconidia • Percutaneous inoculation (rare)	Inhaled arthroconidia reach alveoli; convert to spherule that gives rise to endospores; endospores phagocytosed but survive; large (60–100 μm) spherules escape phagocytosis; alkaline environment allows survival within phagosome	• Growth at 37°C • Thermal dimorphism • Resistance of conidia to phagocytic killing • Stimulation of ineffective Th2 response • Urease production • Extracellular proteinase production • Molecular mimicry	• Initial pulmonary infection • Chronic pulmonary coccidioidomycosis • Disseminated coccidioidomycosis — Meningitis — Bone and joints — Genitourinary tract — Cutaneous — Ophthalmic
Histoplasma capsulatum Saprobic phase • Septate hyphae, microconidia and tuberculate macroconidia Parasitic phase • Small intracellular budding yeast	Saprobic habitat • Soil enriched with bird/bat guano • Eastern half of USA, most of Latin America, parts of Asia, Europe, Middle East; var *duboisii* occurs in Africa Mode of infection • Inhalation of conidia	Inhaled conidia convert to yeast; yeast ingested by macrophages; survive and proliferate within phagosome; some yeast forms remain dormant within macrophage others proliferate and kill macrophages releasing daughter cells	• Growth at 37°C • Thermal dimorphism • Survival in macrophages • Modulate pH of phagosome • Iron and calcium uptake • Alteration of cell wall composition	• Clinically asymptomatic pulmonary and "cryptic dissemination" • Acute pulmonary histoplasmosis • Mediastinitis and pericarditis • Chronic pulmonary histoplasmosis — Mucocutaneous — Disseminated
Paracoccidioides brasiliensis Saprobic phase • Septate hyphae, conidia Parasitic phase • Yeast with multiple buds	Saprobic habitat • Soil and vegetation • Central and South America Mode of infection • Inhalation of conidia	Inhaled conidia convert to large multipolar budding yeast; ingested but not cleared by macrophages; may be dormant for up to 40 years; disseminate to oral and nasopharyngeal mucosa	• Growth at 37°C • Thermal dimorphism • Intracellular survival • Hormonal influences • Alteration of cell wall • Ineffective Th2 response to gp43	• Diverse clinical manifestations • Chronic single organ involvement • Chronic multifocal involvement (lungs, mouth, nose) • Juvenile progressive disease: lymph nodes, skin and visceral involvement

TABLE 69–1. Characteristics of Primary and Opportunistic Fungal Pathogens—cont'd

Organism/ Growth Phase	Habitat/Infection	Pathogenesis	Putative Virulence Factors	Clinical Forms of Mycosis
Opportunistic Pathogens				
Candida species Saprobic and Parasitic phases are the same: budding yeast, hyphae, pseudo-hyphae	Saprobic habitat • Gastrointestinal mucosa, vaginal mucosa, skin, nails Mode of infection • Gastrointestinal translocation • Intravascular catheters	Mucosal overgrowth with subsequent invasion; usually impaired mucosal barrier; hematogenous dissemination. Transfer from hands of health care worker to catheter hub; catheter colonization and hematogenous dissemination	• Growth at 37°C • Bud-hyphae transition • Adherence • Cell surface hydrophobicity • Cell wall mannans • Proteases and phospholipases • Phenotypic switching	• Simple mucosal colonization • Mucocutaneous candidiasis • Oral/vaginal thrush • Hematogenous dissemination • Hepatosplenic candidiasis • Endophthalmitis
Cryptococcus neoformans Saprobic and Parasitic phases are the same: encapsulated budding yeast	Saprobic habitat • Soil enriched with bird (pigeon) guano Mode of infection • Inhalation of aerosolized yeast • Percutaneous inoculation	Inhaled yeast cells ingested by macrophages; survive intracellularly; capsule inhibits phagocytosis; capsule and melanin protect from oxidative injury; hematogenous and lymphatic dissemination to brain	• Growth at 37°C • Polysaccharide capsule • Melanin • Alpha mating type	• Primary cryptococcal pneumonia • Meningitis • Hematogenous dissemination • Genitourinary (prostatic) cryptococcosis • Primary cutaneous cryptococcosis
Aspergillus species Saprobic phase • Septate mycelium, conidial heads and conidia Parasitic phase • Septate mycelium, conidia and conidial heads usually only seen in cavitary lesions	Saprobic habitat • Soil, plants, water, pepper, air Mode of infection • Inhalation of conidia • Transfer to wounds via contaminated tape/bandages	Inhaled conidia bind to fibrinogen and laminin in alveolus; conidia germinate and hyphal forms secrete proteases and invade epithelium; vascular invasion results in thrombosis and infarction of tissue; hematogenous dissemination	• Growth at 37°C • Binding to fibrinogen and laminin • Secretion of elastase and proteases • Catalase • Gliotoxin (?)	• Allergic bronchopulmonary aspergillosis • Sinusitis • Aspergilloma • Invasive aspergillosis — Lung — Brain — Skin — Gastrointestinal — Heart

Adapted from Cole GT: Fungal pathogenesis. In Anaissie EJ, McGinnis MR, Pfaller MA, editors: *Clinical mycology,* New York, 2003, Churchill Livingstone.

Important factors for the in vivo survival of *B. dermatitidis,* and any of the endemic dimorphic pathogens for that matter, are the ability of the inhaled pathogen to reach the alveoli, to undergo transformation to an alternate phase (yeast or spherule) capable of replicating at 37°C, and to colonize the respiratory mucosa. After inhalation of conidia or hyphal fragments of *B. dermatitidis,* the elements of the saprobic phase of the fungus presumably contact and adhere to the epithelial layer of the alveolus and then transform into the parasite yeast phase in a process known as **thermal dimorphism.** This conversion from conidia (2 to 10 μm diameter) to the larger yeast form (8 to 30 μm diameter) provides an important survival advantage to the fungus. Whereas the conidia are small enough to be readily ingested and killed by human neutrophils, the yeast cells are able to resist the phagocytic attack of neutrophils and mononuclear cells during the early stages of the inflammatory response. Rather than adapting to the intracellular microenvironment of phagolysosomes as does *H. capsulatum, B. dermatitidis* yeast cells shed their immunodominant antigen from the cell surface and subsequently modify their cell wall composition, allowing them to escape recognition by macrophages. Thus they are able to colonize tissue and disseminate through the bloodstream.

MODULATION OF YEAST AND HOST IMMUNE SYSTEM INTERACTIONS

The main immunoreactive moiety present on the surface of the yeast cells but not on the conidia of *B. dermatitidis* is a 120-kDa cell wall glycoprotein, WI-1. This glycoprotein appears to play a key role in the pathogenesis of *B. dermatitidis* in that it promotes adhesion of the yeast cell to macrophages and elicits a potent response of both the humoral and cellular immune systems. WI-1 is expressed by all virulent isolates of *B. dermatitidis* examined thus far.

It appears that avirulent mutant strains of *B. dermatitidis* with high levels of expression of WI-1 on their cell surface are recognized by macrophages, phagocytosed, and rapidly eliminated from the host. In contrast, virulent strains of this fungus shed copious amounts of WI-1 during growth and through this process are able to avoid recognition by macrophages. Thus presentation of WI-1, whether it remains associated with the cell surface or is shed into the milieu apart from the cell, is a key aspect of the pathogenicity of this fungus.

It also appears that the carbohydrate composition of the yeast cell wall plays a role in the presentation and shedding of WI-1 and thus in pathogenicity. One of the major components of the yeast cell wall is α-(1,3)-glucan. There is an inverse relationship between the amount of α-(1,3)-glucan present in the cell wall of *B. dermatitidis* and the amount of detectable WI-1 at the cell surface. Virulent strains of *B. dermatitidis* produce yeast cells that have thickened walls containing large amounts of α-(1,3)-glucan and, when mature, have little detectable WI-1 on their cell surface. Conversely, avirulent strains exhibit thin walls that lack α-(1,3)-glucan but have abundant WI-1 on their surface. It is speculated that the incorporation of α-(1,3)-glucan into the cell wall masks the WI-1 surface glycoprotein and plays a role in releasing a modified antigen (85-kDa component) into the microenvironment of the infection site. By masking the WI-1 antigen, the yeast is able to escape recognition by macrophages and disseminate hematogenously. Shedding the 85-kDa component of WI-1 may also facilitate immune evasion by binding or consuming antibody opsonins and complement away from the yeast cell surface. Likewise, the released WI-1 component may also saturate macrophage receptors and decrease the efficiency of binding and phagocytosis of yeast cells.

PRESENTATION OF SURFACE ANTIGEN MODULATES THE T-HELPER PATHWAY OF IMMUNE RESPONSE

Different subsets of CD4 T helper (Th) cells exist that secrete different patterns of cytokines in response to an antigenic stimulus. After an initial encounter with an antigen, Th cells may become polarized, secreting predominantly interleukin 2 (IL-2) and interferon γ (IFN-γ) (Th1 pattern) or predominantly IL-4, IL-5, and IL-10 (Th2 pattern). IFN-γ and IL-2 activate macrophages and cytotoxic T and natural killer (NK) cells, respectively, for clearance of intracellular organisms; whereas Th2 cytokines favor B cell growth and differentiation, isotype switching to immunoglobulin E (IgE), and eosinophil differentiation and activation, responses that may lead to protection against some pathogens but that have also been implicated in allergy and hypersensitivity reactions.

T cell–mediated immune response to *B. dermatitidis* is essential for immunoprotection against this pathogen. Mice immunized with WI-1 develop a robust Th2 response to the antigen. It is notable that, in a mouse infection model of blastomycosis, infected mice that developed features of a Th2 response died with a chronic, progressive infection, whereas those infected animals that developed a Th1 response restricted the spread of the pathogen and were able to respond to antifungal therapy and recover from the disease. Thus a robust Th2 response may not be helpful in clearing *B. dermatitidis* infection and may even retard its clearance. By releasing large amounts of the 85-kDa fragment of WI-1, the yeast cells of *B. dermatitidis* may be able to outmaneuver both arms of the immune response by evasion of the cellular response and stimulation of a dominant but ineffective humoral response.

Coccidioides immitis

C. immitis and *C. posadasii* are primary pathogens capable of causing a wide range of disease states (see Chapter 74). These fungi are endemic to the desert southwest of the United States and, although they both demonstrate different morphologies in their saprobic and parasite phases, they are distinguished from the other endemic dimorphic fungi by the unique features of the parasitic phase (see Figure 74–1). Among the various putative virulence factors that may contribute to the pathogenicity of this organism are the resistance of the infective conidia to phagocytic killing, the ability to stimulate an ineffective Th2 immune response (similar to *B. dermatitidis*), the production of urease and extracellular proteinases, and the capacity for molecular mimicry (see Table 69–1).

RESISTANCE OF CONIDIA TO PHAGOCYTIC KILLING

The saprobic phase of *C. immitis* (and *C. posadasii*) consists of septate filamentous hyphae that, when mature, produce barrel-shaped arthroconidia that are separated from one another by empty disjunctor cells (see Figures

7–2*B*, 74–1*C*, and 74–7). The arthroconidia are very hydrophobic and easily aerosolized. These conidia are small enough (3-5 × 2-4 μm) that when inhaled can be carried deep into the respiratory tract, frequently to the level of the alveoli. The outer wall of the conidia is composed primarily of protein (50%), including small cysteine-rich polypeptides known as hydrophobins due to their distinct hydropathic profiles. The remainder of the wall composition includes lipids (25%), carbohydrates (12%), and an unidentified pigment. It is thought that this hydrophobic outer layer has antiphagocytic properties since its removal resulted in increased phagocytosis of *C. immitis* arthroconidia by human polymorphonuclear neutrophils (PMNs) compared with their phagocytosis of intact arthroconidia. Importantly, neither the intact conidia nor the conidia with the outer wall layer removed were effectively killed after ingestion by PMNs. It appears that the infectious arthroconidia of *C. immitis* have both active and passive barriers against attack by the host's innate defenses in the lungs.

STIMULATION OF AN INEFFECTIVE TH2 IMMUNE RESPONSE BY *C. IMMITIS*

It is known that individuals with coccidioidal infections all produce antibody to a predominant glycoprotein (SOWgp) of an outer wall layer of the parasitic cells (spherules). Both arms of the T helper immune pathway, Th1 and Th2, are stimulated by SOWgp. Activation of the Th1 pathway is known to be associated with spontaneous resolution of coccidioidal infection in mice. Furthermore, it has been shown that mice that are susceptible to infection with *C. immitis* show a Th2 response to infection, whereas resistant strains show more of a Th1 response. Thus similar to that described for *B. dermatitidis*, Th2 responses to SOWgp may not contribute to clearance of *C. immitis* and may even be detrimental in control of the infection. The more severe forms of coccidioidomycosis are accompanied by depressed cell-mediated immunity and high serum levels of *C. immitis*–specific complement fixing antibody, consistent with a predominantly Th2 response. Although not much is known of the cytokine profile of humans during coccidioidal infections, it is reasonable to speculate that immunodominant antigens of *C. immitis* that elicit a profound increase in IL-10 and IL-4 may direct the immune response to a Th2 pathway. Such immunomodulation may contribute to increased severity of the mycotic infection.

UREASE PRODUCTION

The environmental niche for the saprobic form of *C. immitis* is alkaline desert soil. Both saprobic and parasitic phases of this organism have been shown to release ammonia and ammonium ions when grown in vitro, resulting in an alkalinization of the culture medium. The endospores of *C. immitis* release much more ammonia/ammonium ions than do spherules when grown in any acidic (pH 5.0) conditions. Newly released endospores have been shown to be surrounded by an alkaline halo produced by the ammonia/ammonium ions.

The endospores of *C. immitis* are readily phagocytosed by alveolar macrophages but, once ingested, are able to survive intracellularly. It has been shown that viable intracellular endospores are surrounded by an alkaline halo at their cell surface, suggesting that the production of ammonia/ammonium ions may contribute to the survival of the pathogen within the phagosome of the activated macrophage.

The ability of *C. immitis* to generate an alkaline microenvironment and to respond to acidification by increasing the amount of ammonia/ammonium ions released from its parasitic cells are features that may contribute to the pathogenesis of this fungus. Although the details of ammonia generation and how cell-surface alkalinity affects phagocyte function are poorly understood, it has been proposed that the major source of ammonia produced by *C. immitis* is due to urease activity. Urease is a metalloenzyme that is localized in the cytoplasmic fraction of microbial cells and that catalyzes the hydrolysis of urea to yield ammonia and carbamate. The carbamate subsequently hydrolyzes to yield another molecule of ammonia. The maximum amount of urease protein detected in *C. immitis* is in endosporulating spherules, which correlates with the developmental stage where the highest amounts of ammonia/ammonium ion have been recorded. Taken together, this information suggests that urease activity contributes to the pathogenicity of *C. immitis*.

EXTRACELLULAR PROTEINASES

Fungal pathogens produce an array of acid, neutral, and alkaline proteinases that are active over a wide pH range and exhibit a broad substrate specificity. It has been suggested that certain extracellular enzymes secreted by fungi may play key roles in invasive growth that may ultimately lead to the death of the infected host. Secreted proteinases may permit the ingress of skin and mucosal barriers, partial neutralization of active host defenses, transmigration of endothelial layers, and subsequent hematogenous dissemination leading to the establishment of infection in various anatomic sites.

C. immitis, as a primary fungal pathogen, is able to breach the respiratory mucosal barrier, enter the bloodstream and/or the lymphatic system, and disseminate to other organs of the body. Both the saprobic (conidial cell) and parasite forms of the fungus express several proteinases during cell growth. The conidial cell produces a 36-kDa extracellular proteinase capable of breaking down human collagen, elastin, and hemoglobin, as well as IgG and IgA. Cleavage of secretory immunoglobulins by opportunistic fungal pathogens has been correlated with the ability of these organisms to colonize the host mucosa. A 66-kDa alkaline proteinase capable of digesting structural proteins found in lung tissue is thought to be secreted during the entire course of disease caused by *C. immitis*. All patients with coccidioidomycosis produce antibodies directed against this enzyme, and it is thought that this alkaline proteinase may play an important role in host tissue colonization and invasion by spherules and endospores of *C. immitis*.

MOLECULAR MIMICRY

The production of molecules by a pathogenic microbe that are structurally, antigenically and functionally similar to host molecules is termed *molecular mimicry*. In some instances, infection may result in the generation of antibodies by the host that cross-react with host tissues and produce an autoimmune-type pathology. Fungi have been shown to produce molecules that are functionally, but not necessarily structurally, similar to host molecules ("functional mimicry"). Fungal molecules have been identified that function similarly to integrins, complement receptors, and sex hormones.

An estrogen-binding protein has been isolated from cytosolic fractions of *C. immitis*. It is known that physiologic concentrations of progesterone and 17-β-estradiol stimulate the rate of *C. immitis* growth and endospore release. This information coincides with the recognition of pregnancy, especially during the third trimester, as a major risk factor for disseminated coccidioidomycosis.

Histoplasma capsulatum

It is well known that most people infected with *H. capsulatum* recover without complications and without specific antifungal therapy (see Chapter 74). Nevertheless, reactivation of pulmonary and extrapulmonary histoplasmosis in immunocompromised patients who originally experienced cryptic dissemination of the fungus is documented throughout the literature. Inhalation of conidia from the environment coupled with failure to evacuate the fungus by mucociliary mechanisms provides the opportunity for the inhaled conidia to transform into yeasts that are ingested by mononuclear phagocytes. *H. capsulatum* is found almost exclusively within host cells where it may actively replicate or remain dormant.

H. CAPSULATUM RESIDES IN HOST MACROPHAGES

Conversion of inhaled conidia of *H. capsulatum* to yeast cells is critical for survival of the pathogen within the host and occurs within hours of infection. Although theoretically a single conidium may be sufficient to establish an infection, it is usually assumed that a very large conidial inoculum is necessary to establish disseminated disease in a healthy, immunocompetent person. The phagocytes that are mobilized to the site of infection are effective in killing ingested conidia but are less so against the yeast form.

It is known that the organism facilitates uptake by the host phagocytes by producing substances that contribute to the chemotaxis of alveolar macrophages; however, the details of how the pathogen resists the destructive efforts of the macrophages remain unclear. It is suggested that certain phosphoinositol-containing sphingolipids in the yeast cell wall may interfere with the oxidative response of the macrophage to the fungal pathogen. The fact that the macrophages are the primary host cells in which the yeast phase of *H. capsulatum* resides is thought to be an important strategy for survival and dissemination of the pathogen. There are several factors that are thought to be important in the ability of the fungus to persist within the phagolysosome of the macrophage and add significantly to the pathogenicity of organism: pH modulation, iron and calcium uptake, and alteration of the yeast cell wall.

MODULATION OF THE pH OF THE PHAGOLYSOSOME

The yeast cells of *H. capsulatum* are rapidly ingested by alveolar macrophages. After ingestion, the pH of the phagolysosome containing one or more yeast cells is elevated (6.0 to 6.5) above that which is optimal for many of the lysosomal enzymes. This pH modulation not only interferes with enzyme activity but also influences antigen processing within the cell and contributes to the survival of the pathogen in vivo. Although it is tempting to implicate *H. capsulatum* urease in this process, it is not considered to be a major factor since the pH is only elevated in the phagosome containing the yeast cell. If the fungal urease was involved, the ammonia/ammonium ions produced would be expected to diffuse out of the phagosome and raise the pH in the rest of the host cell as well.

IRON AND CALCIUM UPTAKE

Iron is an important cofactor of several different metalloenzymes and heme-containing proteins. Microorganisms obtain iron from the environment by producing siderophores that chelate ferric iron and form soluble iron complexes. *H. capsulatum* traps iron by virtue of a hydroxamic siderophore, although the role of this siderophore in survival of the fungus within the macrophage is unknown. The ability of the fungus to modulate the intraphagolysosomal pH between 6.0 and 6.5 is key in the uptake of iron by yeast cells. A pH greater than 6.5 renders iron inaccessible to *H. capsulatum*.

As with iron, yeast cells within the phagolysosome must have an efficient mechanism for binding and transporting Ca^{2+}. Yeast cells, but not mycelial cells, release large amounts of a calcium-binding protein, CBP1, into the surrounding microenvironment. CBP1 has been suggested to be important in calcium acquisition during intracellular parasitism. The yeast phase-specific expression of CBP1 may provide *H. capsulatum* with another important adaptive mechanism for its survival within the phagolysosome of the macrophage.

ALTERATION OF YEAST CELL WALL COMPOSITION

Similar to *B. dermatitidis*, most *H. capsulatum* strains have α-(1,3)-glucan in their cell wall. Spontaneous mutants of *H. capsulatum* that have lost the α-(1,3)-glucan component have been shown to infect and persist within macrophages without apparent harm to the host cell. In contrast, normal wild-type yeasts with α-(1,3)-glucan can infect and survive within macrophages but also can proliferate within the phagolysosome and ultimately kill the phagocyte releasing yeast cells that go on to infect new macrophages. Thus, it appears that distinctive microenvironments found within host cells can influence the selection of variants that have the potential for long-term persistence within the host, as well as those that produce a more rapidly proliferative process.

Paracoccidioides brasiliensis

Infection due to *P. brasiliensis* is initiated by the inhalation of conidia into the lungs, after which the fungus may disseminate hematogenously or lymphatically to virtually all parts of the body (Chapter 74). A unique feature of paracoccidioidomycosis compared with the other endemic mycoses is that primary pulmonary infections that subsequently disseminate most often manifest as mucosal lesions of the mouth, nose, and occasionally the gastrointestinal tract.

The yeast cell wall of *P. brasiliensis* is rich in alkali-soluble glucans such as α-(1,3)-glucan. As with several other of the endemic dimorphic fungal pathogens, it is thought that the presence of α-(1,3)-glucan in the outermost layer of the yeast cell wall is essential for the survival of the fungus in vivo. It appears that macrophages are key elements of the innate response to infection by *P. brasiliensis*. Macrophages are able to contain *P. brasiliensis* infection but usually do not eliminate the yeast cells. Despite an early clinical resolution of infection, residual lesions containing viable yeast cells may reactivate up to 40 years later, causing relapse and serious sequelae. Characteristics of *P. brasiliensis* that are considered important in the pathogenesis of infection include response to hormonal factors, expression of α-(1,3)-glucan, and immune responses to an immunodominant antigen, gp43.

HORMONAL INFLUENCES ON INFECTION

Although skin test reactivity to paracoccidioidin is comparable among both males and females living in areas endemic for paracoccidioidomycosis, the male/female ratio of symptomatic disease is 78 : 1. Subclinical infection appears to occur at the same rate in both genders; however, progression to clinically overt disseminated disease is much more frequent in males. This observation has led to the hypothesis that hormonal factors play a very important role in the pathogenesis of paracoccidioidomycosis.

In contrast to *C. immitis*, in which estrogen stimulates fungal growth and endosporulation, the transition from conidia to the yeast form of *P. brasiliensis* is inhibited by estrogen. This results in rapid clearance of the infection in females whereas the infection is allowed to progress in males. An alternative explanation is that male sex hormones have an immunoinhibitory effect that facilitates the establishment of infection. This remains an area of active investigation. Regardless, it appears that the early events of host-fungal interaction after natural infection are hormonally modulated and therefore are significantly different in males and females. These differences could account for the markedly higher susceptibility of males to paracoccidioidomycosis.

ROLE OF CELL WALL GLUCANS IN THE PATHOGENESIS OF *P. BRASILIENSIS*

The cell wall of *P. brasiliensis* contains four main polysaccharides: galactomannan, α-(1,3)-glucan, β-(1,3)-glucan, and chitin. The α-(1,3)-glucan component is only expressed in the yeast form of the organism, and its expression correlates with virulence. Mutant strains of *P. brasiliensis* that lack this glucan are avirulent and are much more susceptible to digestion by neutrophils.

The β-(1,3)-glucan fraction of the cell wall acts as an important immunomodulator and when exposed on the fungal cell wall elicits an intense inflammatory response. β-glucans are unmasked when levels of α-(1,3)-glucan are reduced, leading to the hypothesis that the ratio of α-(1,3)-glucan to β-(1,3)-glucan in the cell wall of *P. brasiliensis* may be more important in pathogenesis than the individual polysaccharide components. It is important to realize that the relationship between the α-/β-glucan ratio in the *P. brasiliensis* cell wall and the type of immune response is similar to that seen in both histoplasmosis and blastomycosis. In each case, a high α-(1,3)-glucan content of the yeast cell is related to increased virulence and absent or decreased levels of this component to reduced virulence. Alteration in the cell wall composition of the yeast cells of all three of these dimorphic pathogens is also related to their ability to become sequestered within cells and tissues and to persist as viable elements for years after infection.

RESPONSES TO AN IMMUNODOMINANT ANTIGEN, gp43

The yeast phase of *P. brasiliensis* secretes an immunodominant 43-kDa glycoprotein (gp43) that is both an important serodiagnostic antigen and a putative virulence factor. The gp43 antigen is a receptor for laminin-1 and may be responsible for adhesion of the yeast cell to the host basement membrane. This antigen also binds to macrophages and elicits both a strong humoral response and a delayed-type hypersensitivity response in humans.

The immunologic defense against infection with *P. brasiliensis* depends on cellular rather than humoral immunity. An impaired delayed-type hypersensitivity response correlates with increased severity of disease. Mice immunized with gp43 develop both a Th1- and Th2-type immune response, whereas gp43 and a second antigen gp70 are major contributors to a humoral response in humans. It is possible that patient immune reactivity to gp43 and gp70 is dominated by a Th2 pathway with inadequate T-cell response. If patient cell-mediated immunity to *P. brasiliensis* is actually compromised by such T-cell hyporesponsiveness, this could be a mechanism, as seen in histoplasmosis and coccidioidomycosis, underlying the immunopathogenesis of paracoccidioidomycosis.

Opportunistic Pathogens

The state of the host is of primary importance in determining the pathogenicity of opportunistic fungal pathogens such as *Candida* spp., *C. neoformans,* and *Aspergillus* spp. In most instances, these organisms may exist as benign colonizers or as environmental saprobes and only cause serious infection when there is a breakdown of host defenses. There are factors associated with these organisms, however, that may be considered "virulence factors" in that they contribute to the disease process and in some instances may explain the differences in pathogenicity of the various organisms.

CANDIDA SPECIES

Candida spp. are the most common of the opportunistic fungal pathogens (see Chapter 75). It is now well established that *Candida* spp. colonize the gastrointestinal mucosa and reach the bloodstream through gastrointestinal translocation or via contaminated vascular catheters, interact with host defenses, and exit the intravascular compartment to invade deep tissues of target organs such as the liver, spleen, kidneys, heart, and brain. Characteristics of the organism that are thought to contribute to pathogenicity include the ability to adhere to tissues, the ability to exhibit yeast-hyphal dimorphism, cell surface hydrophobicity, proteinase secretion, and phenotypic switching (see Table 69–1).

The ability of *Candida* spp. to adhere to a variety of tissues and inanimate surfaces is considered important in the early stages of infection. The adherence capability of the various species of *Candida* is directly related to their virulence ranking in various experimental models. Adherence is achieved by a combination of specific (ligand-receptor interaction) and nonspecific (electrostatic, van der Waals forces) mechanisms.

The ability to undergo the yeast-to-hypha transformation has long been considered to have some importance in pathogenicity. Most species of *Candida* are capable of such transformation, which has been shown to be regulated by both pH and temperature. The yeast-hyphal transformation is one way for *Candida* spp. to respond to changes in the microenvironment. The hyphae of *C. albicans* exhibit **thigmotropism** (a sense of touch), which allows them to grow along grooves and through pores and may aid in infiltration of epithelial surfaces.

The composition of the cell surface of *Candida* spp. may affect both the hydrophobicity of the cell and the immune response to the cell. The type and the degree of glycosylation of the mannoproteins on the cell surface may affect the hydrophobicity of the cell and therefore adhesion to epithelial cells. The germ tubes of *C. albicans* are hydrophobic whereas the buds or blastoconidia are hydrophilic. The various glycoproteins of *C. albicans* also suppress the immune response to the organism by mechanisms that are not well understood.

As discussed with the primary pathogens, the ability of *Candida* spp. to secrete various enzymes may also influence the pathogenicity of the organism. Several species of *Candida* secrete aspartyl proteinases that hydrolyze host proteins involved in defenses against infection, thus allowing the yeasts to breach connective tissue barriers. Likewise, phospholipases are produced by most species of *Candida* causing infection in humans. These enzymes damage host cells and are considered important in tissue invasion.

The ability of *Candida* spp. to rapidly switch from one morphotype to another has been termed *phenotypic switching.* Although originally applied to changes in gross colony morphology, it is now known that the different switch phenotypes observed on solid culture media represent differences in bud and hypha formation, expression of cell wall glycoproteins, proteolytic enzyme secretion, susceptibility to oxidative damage by neutrophils, and antifungal susceptibility and resistance. Phenotypic switching contributes to the virulence of *Candida* spp. by allowing the organism to rapidly adapt to changes in its microenvironment, thereby facilitating its ability to survive, invade tissues, and escape from host defenses.

CRYPTOCOCCUS NEOFORMANS

C. neoformans is an encapsulated yeast that causes human infection throughout the world. Although this organism can infect apparently normal hosts, it causes disease much more frequently, and with greater severity, in immunocompromised hosts. In considering the pathogenesis of cryptococcosis, it is useful consider both host defenses and putative virulence factors.

There are three main lines of defense against infection by *C. neoformans:* alveolar macrophages, inflammatory phagocytic cells, and T and B cell responses. Development of cryptococcosis largely depends on the competence of the host's cellular defenses and the number and virulence of the inhaled yeast cells.

The first line of defense is the alveolar macrophages. These cells are capable of ingesting the yeast cells but are limited in their ability to kill them. Macrophages that contain ingested yeast cells produce various cytokines for the recruitment of neutrophils, monocytes, NK cells, and cells from the bloodstream into the lung. They also act as antigen-presenting cells and induce the differentiation and proliferation of T and B lymphocytes that are specific for *C. neoformans.* The recruited cells are effective in killing *C. neoformans* by intracellular and extracellular mechanisms (both oxidative and non-oxidative).

The antibody response to this organism is nonprotective but serves to opsonize the yeast cells, thus enhancing cell-mediated cytotoxicity. Likewise, the complement system enhances the efficacy of the antibody response and provides opsonins and chemotactic factors for phagocytosis and recruitment of inflammatory cells.

An effective host response to *C. neoformans* is a complex interaction of cellular and humoral immune factors. When these factors are impaired the infection disseminates, usually by migration of macrophages containing viable yeast cells, from the lung to the lymphatics and the bloodstream to the brain.

The main factors that are inherent in *C. neoformans* and that allow the yeast to evade the host defenses and establish infection include the ability to grow at 37°C, to produce a thick polysaccharide capsule, to synthesize melanin, and to be an alpha-mating phenotype (MATalpha) (see Table 69–1).

The capsule of *C. neoformans* protects the cell from phagocytosis and from cytokines induced by the phagocytic process and suppresses both cellular and humoral immunity. The capsule can physically block the opsonic effect of complement and anticryptococcal antibodies and the negative change that it confers produces an electrostatic repulsion between the yeast cells and the host effector cells. Furthermore, the capsular material interferes with antigen presentation and limits the production of nitric oxide (toxic for cryptococcal cells) by the host cells.

Melanin is produced by the fungus by virtue of a membrane-bound phenol-oxidase enzyme and is deposited within the cell wall. It is thought that melanin enhances the integrity of the cell wall and increases the net negative charge of the cell, further protecting it from phagocytosis. Melanization is thought to be responsible for the neurotropism of *C. neoformans* and may protect the cell from oxidative stress, temperature extremes, iron reduction, and microbicidal peptides.

The alpha-mating phenotype is associated with the presence of the gene ***STE12alpha,*** which has been proven to modulate the expression of several other genes whose functions are important for the production of the capsule and melanin.

ASPERGILLUS SPECIES

Aspergillosis is the most common invasive mould infection worldwide. Aspergilli are ubiquitous saprobes in nature and can be found in soil, potted plants, decaying vegetation, pepper, and construction sites. *Aspergillus* spp. can cause disease in humans by airway colonization with subsequent allergic reactions, through colonization of preexisting cavities (aspergilloma), or by tissue invasion.

The primary route of infection in aspergillosis is by inhalation of aerosolized conidia (2.5 to 3 μm) that settle in the lungs, nasopharynx, or sinuses. In the lungs, alveolar macrophages and neutrophils play a major role in the host defense against *Aspergillus* spp. The macrophages ingest and kill the conidia, whereas the neutrophils adhere to and kill the hyphae that arise upon germination of the conidia. Those hyphal forms that are not killed may invade the pulmonary tissue and vasculature, leading to thrombosis and local tissue necrosis, as well as to hematogenous dissemination to other target organs (brain).

Aspergilli secrete various metabolic products, such as gliotoxins, and a variety of enzymes including elastase, phospholipase, various proteases, and catalase, which may play a role in virulence. Gliotoxin inhibits macrophage phagocytosis and T-cell activation and proliferation; however, it is not known whether clinically significant amounts of gliotoxin are produced in human disease.

A. fumigatus conidia bind to human fibrinogen, as well as to laminin in the alveolar basement membrane. It is thought that this could be an important first step that allows the fungus to establish residence in host tissues. Thus, binding to fibrinogen and laminin could facilitate adherence of conidia whereas secretion of elastase and acid proteases could assist with host cell invasion by the hyphae.

Invasive aspergillosis is highly associated with neutropenia and impaired neutrophil function. Aspergillus conidia are resistant to killing by neutrophils whereas germinating conidia and hyphae are readily killed. In chronic granulomatous disease, neutrophils are unable to generate the respiratory burst to kill catalase-producing microorganisms. Aspergilli produce catalase, an enzyme that breaks down hydrogen peroxide. The strong association of aspergillosis with chronic granulomatous disease underscores the importance of neutrophil function in the host defense against aspergillosis and provides indirect evidence for catalase as a virulence factor. The increased risk of aspergillosis in individuals receiving high doses of corticosteroids is generally thought to be due to impairment of macrophage and perhaps T-cell function. In addition, corticosteroids have been shown to enhance the growth of *Aspergillus* spp. in culture. It is not known whether *Aspergillus* spp. have specific steroid-binding proteins analogous to those that have been found on other fungi.

QUESTIONS

1. What distinguishes a primary pathogen from an opportunistic pathogen?
2. What are the common themes that are seen in the pathogenesis of the primary fungal pathogens?
3. What is the most important line of defense against the endemic dimorphic fungi?
4. What putative virulence factor is common to both the primary and opportunistic fungal pathogens discussed in this chapter?

Bibliography

Cole GT: Fungal pathogenesis. In Anaissie EJ, McGinnis MR, Pfaller MA, editors: *Clinical mycology*, New York, 2003, Churchill Livingstone.

Dignani MC et al: *Candida*. In Anaissie EJ, McGinnis MR, Pfaller, MA, editors: *Clinical mycology*, New York, 2003, Churchill Livingstone.

Hogan LH et al: Virulence factors of medically important fungi. *Clin Microbiol Rev* 9:469-488, 1996.

Viviani MA et al: Cryptococcus. In Anaissie EJ, McGinnis MR, Pfaller MA, editors: *Clinical mycology*, New York, 2003, Churchill Livingstone.

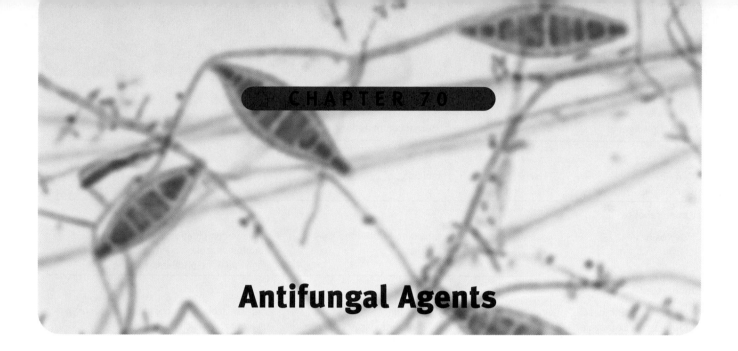

Antifungal Agents

Antifungal therapy has undergone a tremendous transformation in recent years. Once the sole domain of the agents amphotericin B and 5-fluorocytosine (flucytosine, 5-FC), which were toxic and difficult to use, the treatment of mycotic disease has now been advanced by the availability of several new, systemically active agents and new formulations of other older agents that provide comparable, if not superior, efficacy with significantly less toxicity.

In this chapter we will review the antifungal agents, both systemic and topical (Table 70–1). We will discuss their spectrum, potency, mode of action, and clinical indications for their use as therapeutic agents. Furthermore, we will discuss the mechanisms of resistance to the various classes of antifungal agents and the in vitro methods for determining the susceptibility and resistance of fungi to the available agents.

The terminology appropriate for this discussion is summarized in Box 70–1 and Figure 70–1.

Systemically Active Antifungal Agents

POLYENES

Amphotericin B and its lipid formulations are polyene macrolide antifungal agents used in the treatment of serious life-threatening mycoses (see Table 70–1). Another polyene, nystatin, is a topical agent. A lipid formulation of nystatin has been developed for systemic use but remains investigational.

The basic structure of polyenes consists of a large lactone ring, with a rigid lipophilic chain containing three to seven double bonds, and a flexible hydrophilic portion bearing several hydroxyl groups (Figure 70–2). Amphotericin B contains seven conjugated double bonds and may be inactivated by heat, light, and extremes of pH. It is poorly soluble in water and is not absorbed by the oral or intramuscular route of administration. The conventional formulation of amphotericin B for intravenous administration is amphotericin B deoxycholate. The lipid formulations of amphotericin B were developed in an effort to circumvent the nephrotoxic nature of conventional amphotericin B and, in many instances, have replaced the deoxycholate form.

Amphotericin B and its lipid formulations exert their antifungal action by at least two mechanisms. The primary mechanism involves the binding of amphotericin B to ergosterol, the principal membrane sterol of fungi. This binding produces ion channels that destroy the osmotic integrity of the fungal cell membrane and lead to leakage of intracellular constituents and cell death (Figure 70–3). Amphotericin B also binds to cholesterol, the main membrane sterol of mammalian cells, but it does so less avidly than to ergosterol. The binding of amphotericin B to cholesterol accounts for most of the toxicity observed when amphotericin B is administered to humans. An additional mechanism of action of amphotericin B involves direct membrane damage caused by the generation of a cascade of oxidative reactions triggered by the oxidation of amphotericin B itself. This process may be a major contributor to the rapid fungicidal activity of amphotericin B via the generation of toxic free radicals.

The spectrum of activity of amphotericin B is broad and includes most strains of *Candida, Cryptococcus neoformans, Aspergillus* spp., the zygomycetes, and the endemic dimorphic pathogens *(Blastomyces dermatitidis, Coccidioides immitis, Histoplasma capsulatum, Paracoccidioides brasiliensis,* and *Penicillium marneffei)* (Table 70–2). *Aspergillus terreus, Fusarium* spp., *Pseudallescheria boydii, Scedosporium prolificans, Trichosporon* spp., and certain dematiaceous fungi may be resistant to amphotericin B. Likewise, reduced susceptibility to amphotericin B has

TABLE 70–1. Systemic and Topical Antifungal Agents in Use and in Development

Antifungal Agents	Route	Mechanism of Action	Comments
Allylamines			
Naftifine Terbinafine	Topical Oral, topical	Inhibition of squalene epoxidase	Terbinafine has very broad spectrum and acts synergistically with other antifungals
Antimetabolite			
Flucytosine	Oral	Inhibition of DNA and RNA synthesis	Used in combination with amphotericin B and fluconazole; toxicity and secondary resistance are problems
Imidazoles			
Ketoconazole, Bifonazole, Clotrimazole, Econazole, Miconazole, Oxiconazole, Sulconazole, Terconazole, Tioconazole	Oral, topical	Inhibits lanosterol 14 α-demethylase cytochrome P-450–dependent enzymes	Ketoconazole has modest broad spectrum activity and toxicity problems
Triazoles			
Fluconazole	Oral, IV	Same as imidazoles but more specific binding to target	Limited spectrum (yeasts); good central nervous system penetration; good in vivo activity; primary and secondary resistance seen with *Candida krusei* and *Candida glabrata*, respectively
Itraconazole	Oral, IV	Same as imidazoles but more specific binding to target enzyme	Broad-spectrum activity; erratic absorption; toxicity and drug interactions are problems
Voriconazole	Oral, IV	Same as imidazoles but more specific binding to target enzyme	Broad spectrum including yeasts and moulds; active vs. *Candida krusei;* many drug interactions
Posaconazole	Oral	Same as imidazoles but more specific binding to target enzyme	Investigational; broad spectrum including activity vs. zygomycetes
Ravuconazole	Oral, IV	Same as imidazoles but more specific binding to target enzyme	Investigational; broad spectrum including yeasts and moulds
Echinocandins			
Caspofungin Anidulafungin Micafungin	IV	Inhibition of fungal cell wall glucan synthesis	Caspofungin is approved for treatment of invasive candidiasis and aspergillosis; others are investigational; fungicidal activity against *Candida*
Polyenes			
Amphotericin B	IV, topical	Binds to ergosterol causing direct oxidative membrane damage	Established agent; broad spectrum; toxic
Lipid formulations (amphotericin B lipid complex or colloidal dispersion, liposomal amphotericin B)	IV	Same as amphotericin B	Broad spectrum; less toxic; expensive
Nystatin	Oral suspension, topical	Same as amphotericin B	Liposomal formulation (IV) under investigation

TABLE 70–1. Systemic and Topical Antifungal Agents in Use and in Development—cont'd

Antifungal Agents	Route	Mechanism of Action	Comments
Chitin synthesis inhibitor			
Nikkomycin Z	IV	Inhibition of fungal cell wall chitin synthesis	Investigational agent; possibly useful in combination with other antifungals
Sordarin and azasordarin derivatives			
		Inhibition of elongation factor 2 Inhibition of protein synthesis	Investigational agent; broad-spectrum activity including *Pneumocystis jiroveci (carinii)*
Other			
Amorolfine	Topical	Miscellaneous, varied	
Butenafine HC	Topical		
Ciclopirox olamine	Topical		
Griseofulvin	Oral		
Haloprogin	Topical		
Tolnaftate	Topical		
Undecylenate	Topical		

IV, Intravenous.

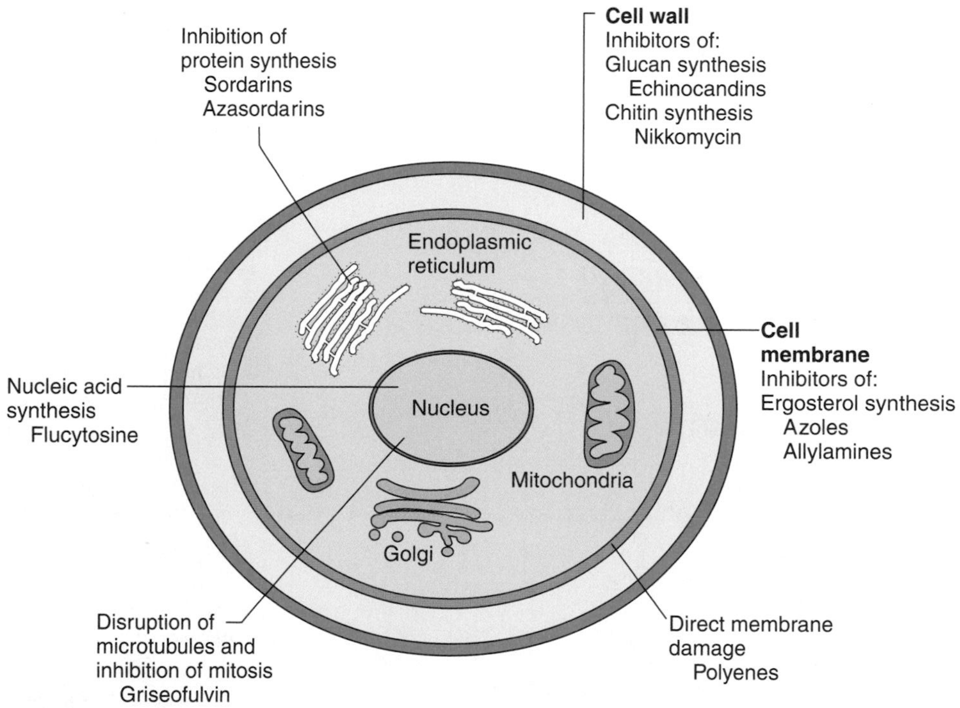

FIGURE 70–1. Sites of action of antifungal agents.

been noted among some strains of *Candida guilliermondii, Candida glabrata, Candida krusei, Candida lusitaniae,* and *Candida rugosa.* Resistance to amphotericin B has been associated with alterations in membrane sterols, usually a reduction in ergosterol.

Amphotericin B is widely distributed in various tissues and organs, including liver, spleen, kidney, bone marrow, and lung. Although negligible concentrations of amphotericin B can be found in the cerebrospinal fluid, it is generally effective in treating fungal infections of the central nervous system. Amphotericin B is considered to be fungicidal against most fungi.

The primary clinical indications for amphotericin B include invasive candidiasis, cryptococcosis, aspergillosis, zygomycosis, blastomycosis, coccidioidomycosis, histoplasmosis, paracoccidioidomycosis, penicilliosis marneffei, and sporotrichosis. The lipid formulations of amphotericin B offer an improved efficacy-to-toxicity

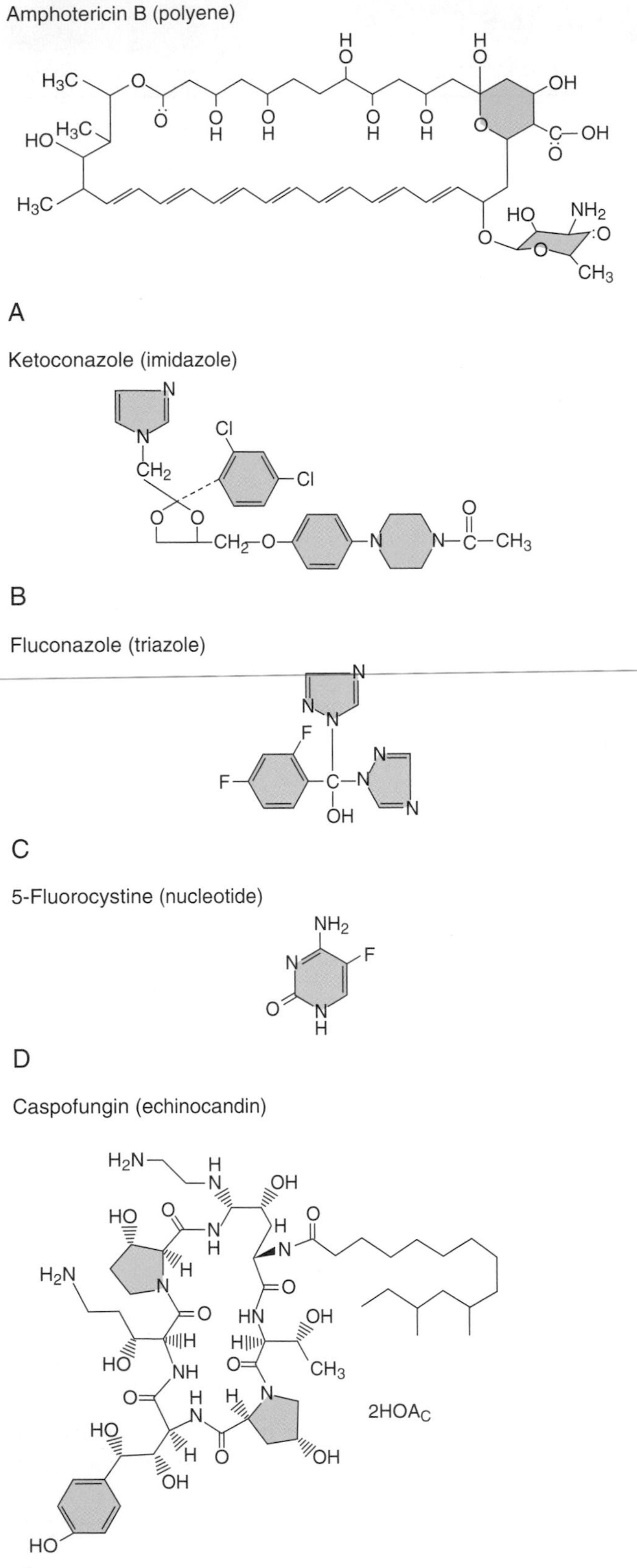

Amphotericin B (polyene)
A
Ketoconazole (imidazole)
B
Fluconazole (triazole)
C
5-Fluorocystine (nucleotide)
D
Caspofungin (echinocandin)
2HOAc
E

FIGURE 70–2. Chemical structures of antifungal agents representing five different classes.

Pore
Amphotericin B
Phospholipid
Heptaene segment
Ergosterol

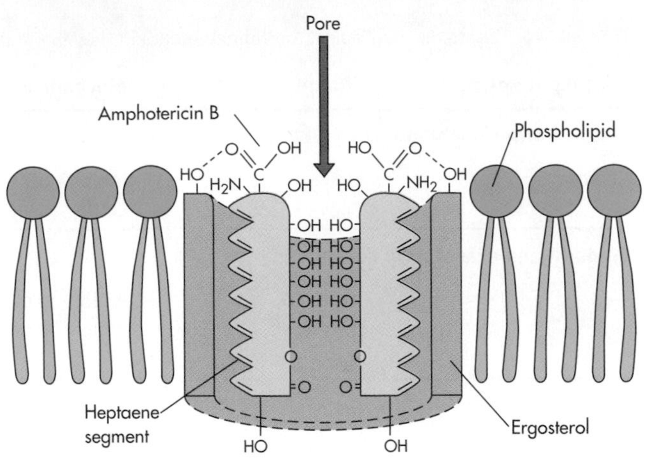

FIGURE 70–3. Mechanisms of action of amphotericin B.

BOX 70–1. Terminology

Antifungal spectrum: Range of activity of an antifungal agent against fungi. A *broad-spectrum* antifungal agent inhibits a wide variety of fungi, including both yeast-like fungi and moulds, whereas a *narrow-spectrum* agent is active only against a limited number of fungi.

Fungistatic activity: Level of antifungal activity that *inhibits* the growth of an organism. This is determined in vitro by testing a standardized concentration of organisms against a series of antifungal dilutions. The lowest concentration of the drug that inhibits the growth of the organism is referred to as the *minimum inhibitory concentration* (MIC).

Fungicidal activity: Ability of an antifungal agent to *kill* an organism in vitro or in vivo. The lowest concentration of the drug that kills 99.9% of the test population is called the *minimum fungicidal concentration* (MFC).

Antifungal combinations: Combinations of antifungal agents that may be used (1) to enhance efficacy in the treatment of a refractory fungal infection, (2) to broaden the spectrum of empiric antifungal therapy, (3) to prevent the emergence of resistant organisms, and (4) to achieve a synergistic killing effect.

Antifungal synergism: Combinations of antifungal agents that have enhanced antifungal activity when used together compared with the activity of each agent alone.

Antifungal antagonism: Combination of antifungal agents in which the activity of one of the agents interferes with the activity of the other agent.

Efflux pumps: Families of drug transporters that serve to actively pump antifungal agents out of the fungal cells, thus decreasing the amount of intracellular drug available to bind to its target.

TABLE 70–2. Spectrum and Relative Activity of Systemically Active Antifungal Agents

Organism	AMB	FC	KTZ	ITZ	FCZ	VCZ	CAS
Candida spp.							
C. albicans	++++	++++	+++	++++	++++	++++	++++
C. glabrata	+++	++++	++	++	++	+++	++++
C. parapsilosis	++++	++++	+++	++++	++++	++++	+++
C. tropicalis	+++	++++	+++	+++	++++	++++	++++
C. krusei	++	+	+	++	0	++++	++++
Cryptococcus neoformans	++++	+++	+	++	+++	++++	0
Aspergillus spp.	++++	0	0	++++	0	++++	+++
Fusarium spp.	+++	0	0	+	0	+++	0
Zygomycetes	++++	0	0	0	0	0	+
Blastomyces dermatitidis	++++	0	++	++++	+	++++	++
Coccidioides immitis	++++	0	++	++++	++++	++++	++
Histoplasma capsulatum	++++	0	++	++++	++	++++	++
Penicillium marneffei	++++	0	++	++++	++	++++	
Sporothrix schenckii	++++	0	++	++++	++		
Dematiaceous moulds	+++	+	++	+++	+	+++	0

AMB, Amphotericin B; CAS, caspofungin; FC, flucytosine; FCZ, fluconazole; ITZ, itraconazole; KTZ, ketoconazole; VCZ, voriconazole; 0, inactive or not recommended; +, occasional activity; ++, moderate activity with resistance noted; +++, reliable activity with occasional resistance; ++++, very active, resistance rare or not described.

profile and are primarily recommended for the treatment of documented fungal infections failing to respond to conventional amphotericin B or in persons with impaired renal function.

The main adverse effects of amphotericin B include nephrotoxicity and infusion-related side effects, such as fever, chills, myalgias, hypotension, and bronchospasm. The major advantage of the lipid formulations of amphotericin B are the significantly reduced side effects, especially nephrotoxicity. The lipid formulations are not superior to conventional amphotericin B in terms of efficacy and are much more expensive.

AZOLES

The azole class of antifungal agents can be divided in terms of structure into the imidazoles (two nitrogen molecules in the azole ring) and the triazoles (three nitrogens in the azole ring) (see Figure 70–2). Among the imidazoles, only ketoconazole has systemic activity. The triazoles all have systemic activity and include fluconazole, itraconazole, and voriconazole (see Table 70–1). Posaconazole and ravuconazole are also triazoles and are currently undergoing evaluation in clinical trials (see Table 70–1).

Both imidazoles and triazoles act by inhibiting the fungal cytochrome P-450–dependent enzyme lanosterol 14-α-demethylase (Figure 70–4). This enzyme is involved in the conversion of lanosterol to ergosterol, and its inhibition disrupts membrane synthesis in the fungal cell. Depending on the organism and specific azole, inhibition of ergosterol synthesis results in inhibition of fungal cell growth (fungistatic) or in cell death (fungicidal). In general, the azoles exhibit fungistatic activity against yeast-like fungi such as *Candida* spp. and *C. neoformans;* however, itraconazole, voriconazole, posaconazole, and ravuconazole appear to be fungicidal against *Aspergillus* spp.

Ketoconazole is an orally absorbed, lipophilic member of the imidazole class of antifungal agents. Its spectrum of activity includes the endemic dimorphic pathogens, *Candida* spp., *C. neoformans,* and *Malassezia* spp., although it is generally less active than the triazole antifungal agents (see Table 70–2). It is variably active against *P. boydii* and has little or no activity against the zygomycetes, *Aspergillus* spp., *S. prolificans,* or *Fusarium* spp.

The absorption of ketoconazole by the oral route of administration is erratic and requires an acid gastric pH. Its lipophilicity ensures penetration and concentration into fatty tissues and purulent exudates; however, because it is highly (>99%) protein bound it penetrates poorly into the central nervous system.

Ketoconazole may cause serious adverse effects including gastric and hepatic toxicity, nausea, vomiting and rash. At high doses, significant endocrinologic side effects

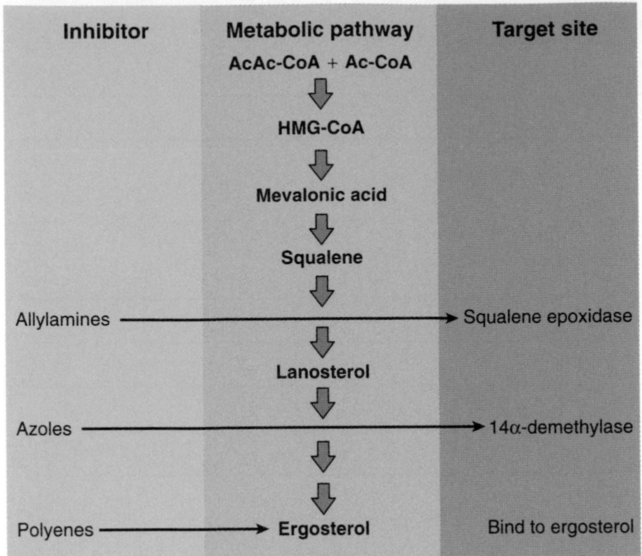

FIGURE 70–4. Metabolic pathway for the synthesis of ergosterol showing sites of inhibition by allylamine, azole, and polyene antifungal agents.

have been observed secondary to suppression of testosterone and cortisol levels.

Because of the availability of more potent and less toxic agents, the clinical indications for use of ketoconazole are quite limited. It is at best a second-line agent for the treatment of non-life threatening, non-meningeal forms of histoplasmosis, blastomycosis, coccidioidomycosis, and paracoccidioidomycosis in immunocompetent individuals. Similarly, it may be used in the treatment of mucocutaneous candidiasis and lymphocutaneous sporotrichosis.

Fluconazole is a first-generation triazole with excellent oral bioavailability and low toxicity. Fluconazole is used extensively and is active against most species of *Candida*, *C. neoformans*, dermatophytes, *Trichosporon* spp., *Histoplasma capsulatum*, *Coccidioides immitis*, and *Paracoccidioides brasiliensis* (see Table 70–2). Among *Candida* spp., decreased susceptibility is seen with *C. krusei* and *C. glabrata*. Whereas *C. krusei* must be considered to be intrinsically resistant to fluconazole, infections with *C. glabrata* may be treated successfully with high does (e.g. 800 mg/day) of fluconazole. Resistance may develop when fluconazole is used to treat histoplasmosis and it has only limited activity against *Blastomyces dermatitidis*. Fluconazole is not active against the opportunistic moulds including *Aspergillus* spp., *Fusarium* spp., and the zygomycetes.

Fluconazole is a water-soluble agent and may be administered orally or intravenously. Protein binding is low and it is distributed to all organs and tissues including the central nervous system. Severe side effects such as exfoliative dermatitis or liver failure are uncommon.

Because of its low toxicity, ease of administration, and fungistatic activity against most yeast-like fungi, fluconazole has an important role in the treatment of candidiasis, cryptococcosis, and coccidioidomycosis. It is used as primary therapy for candidemia and mucosal candidiasis and as prophylaxis in selected high-risk populations. It is used in maintenance therapy of cryptococcal meningitis in patients with AIDS and is the agent of choice in the treatment of meningitis caused by *Coccidioides immitis*. Fluconazole is a second-line agent in the treatment of histoplasmosis, blastomycosis and sporotrichosis.

Itraconazole is a lipophilic triazole that may be administered orally in capsule or in solution and also intravenously. Itraconazole has a broad spectrum of antifungal activity including *Candida* spp., *C. neoformans*, *Aspergillus* spp., dermatophytes, dematiaceous moulds, *P. boydii*, *Sporothrix schenckii*, and the endemic dimorphic pathogens (see Table 70–2). Itraconazole has activity against some, but not all, fluconazole-resistant strains of *C. glabrata* and *C. krusei*. Itraconazole-resistant strains of *Aspergillus fumigatus* have been reported; however, they are rare. The zygomycetes, *Fusarium*, and *S. prolificans* are resistant to itraconazole.

As with ketoconazole, the oral absorption of itraconazole is erratic and requires an acidic gastric pH. Absorption is enhanced with the oral solution when given in the fasting state. Itraconazole is highly protein bound and exhibits fungistatic activity against yeast-like fungi and fungicidal activity against *Aspergillus* spp.

The efficacy of itraconazole in the treatment of hematogenous candidiasis has not been adequately assessed, although it is useful in the treatment of cutaneous and mucosal forms of candidiasis. Itraconazole is often used in the treatment of dermatophytic infections and is the treatment of choice for lymphocutaneous sporotrichosis and non–life-threatening, non-meningeal forms of histoplasmosis, blastomycosis, and paracoccidioidomycosis. It may be useful in non-meningeal coccidioidomycosis, for maintenance treatment of cryptococcal meningitis and for some forms of phaeohyphomycosis (see Table 70–2). Itraconazole is considered a second-line agent for the treatment of invasive aspergillosis; however, it is not useful in the treatment of infections caused by *Fusarium* spp., the zygomycetes, or *S. prolificans*.

In contrast to fluconazole, drug interactions are common with itraconazole. Severe hepatotoxicity is rare and other side effects such as gastrointestinal intolerance, hypokalemia, edema, rash, and elevated transaminases occur infrequently.

Voriconazole is a new broad-spectrum triazole with activity against *Candida* spp., *C. neoformans*, *Trichosporon* spp., *Aspergillus* spp., *Fusarium* spp., dematiaceous fungi, and the endemic dimorphic pathogens (see Table 70–2). Among the *Candida* species, voriconazole is active against *C. krusei* and most but not all strains of *Candida albicans* and *C. glabrata* with reduced susceptibility to fluconazole. Although voriconazole has no activity against the zygomycetes, it is active against fungi that are resistant to amphotericin B including *Aspergillus terreus* and *P. boydii.*

Voriconazole is available in both oral and intravenous formulations. It has excellent penetration into the central nervous system and other tissues. Voriconazole exhibits fungistatic activity against yeast-like fungi and is fungicidal against *Aspergillus* spp.

Voriconazole has a primary indication for the treatment of invasive aspergillosis and of massive candidiasis. It is also approved for treatment of infections caused by *P. boydii* and *Fusarium* spp. in patients intolerant of or with infections refractory to other antifungal agents. Voriconazole has proven efficacy in the treatment of various forms of candidiasis and has been used successfully in the treatment of a variety of infections due to emerging or refractory pathogens, including brain abscesses caused by *Aspergillus* spp. and *P. boydii.*

Although approximately one third of patients experience transient visual disturbances, voriconazole is generally well tolerated. Other adverse effects include liver enzyme abnormalities, skin reactions, and hallucinations or confusion. Interactions with other drugs that are metabolized by the hepatic P-450 enzyme system are common.

ECHINOCANDINS

The echinocandins are a novel, highly selective class of semisynthetic lipopeptides (see Figure 70–2) that inhibit the synthesis of β-(1,3)-glucans, important constituents of the fungal cell wall (see Table 70–1 and Figure 70–1). Since mammalian cells do not contain β-(1,3)-glucans, this class of agents is selective in its toxicity for fungi in which the glucans play an important role in maintaining the osmotic integrity of the fungal cell. Glucans are also important in cell division and cell growth. Inhibition of the glucan synthesis enzyme complex results in fungicidal activity against *Candida* spp. and fungistatic activity against *Aspergillus* spp. At the present time, there are three echinocandins in various stages of development (see Table 70–1): caspofungin is licensed for use in patients with candidiasis and aspergillosis, and both anidulafungin and micafungin are under clinical investigation.

The spectrum of activity of the echinocandins is limited to those fungi where β-(1,3)-glucans compose the dominant cell wall glucan component. As such, they are active against *Candida* and *Aspergillus* spp. and have variable activity against the dematiaceous fungi and the endemic dimorphic pathogens (see Table 70–2). They are inactive against *C. neoformans, Trichosporon* spp., *Fusarium* spp., other hyaline moulds, and the zygomycetes. The echinocandins have excellent activity against fluconazole-resistant strains of *Candida* spp. Primary resistance to this class of agents appears to be rare among clinical isolates of *Candida* spp. and *Aspergillus* spp.

The echinocandins must be administered intravenously and are highly (>95%) protein bound. They are distributed to all major organs, although concentrations in cerebrospinal fluid are low. All of the echinocandins are very well tolerated and have few drug-drug interactions.

Among the three echinocandins, only caspofungin is licensed for the treatment of patients at the present time. Caspofungin is approved for the treatment of invasive candidiasis, including candidemia, and for the treatment of patients with invasive aspergillosis refractory to or intolerant of other approved antifungal therapies.

ANTIMETABOLITES

Flucytosine (5-fluorocytosine, 5FC) is the only available antifungal agent that functions as an antimetabolite. It is a fluorinated pyrimidine analogue that exerts antifungal activity by interfering with the synthesis of DNA, RNA, and proteins in the fungal cell (see Figure 70–1). Flucytosine enters the fungal cell via cytosine permease and is deaminated to 5-fluorouracil (5-FU) in the cytoplasm. The 5-FU is converted to 5-fluorouridylic acid, which then competes with uracil in the synthesis of RNA with resultant RNA miscoding and inhibition of DNA and protein synthesis.

The antifungal spectrum of flucytosine is limited to *Candida* spp., *C. neoformans, Saccharomyces cerevisiae* and selected dematiaceous moulds (see Table 70–2). Although primary resistance to flucytosine is rare among isolates of *Candida* spp., resistance can develop among *Candida* and *C. neoformans* during flucytosine monotherapy. Flucytosine is not active against *Aspergillus* spp., the zygomycetes, or other hyaline moulds.

Flucytosine is water soluble and has excellent bioavailability when administered orally. High concentrations of flucytosine can be achieved in serum, cerebrospinal fluid, and other body fluids. Major toxicities are observed when flucytosine serum concentrations exceed 100 μg/ml and include bone marrow suppression, hepatotoxicity, and gastrointestinal intolerance. Monitoring of serum concentrations of flucytosine is important in avoiding toxicity.

Flucytosine is not used as monotherapy because of the propensity for secondary resistance. Combinations of flucytosine with either amphotericin B or fluconazole have been shown to be efficacious in treating both cryptococcosis and candidiasis.

ALLYLAMINES

The allylamine class of antifungal agents includes terbinafine, which has systemic activity, and naftifine, which is a topical agent (see Table 70–1). These agents inhibit the enzyme squalene epoxidase, which results in a decrease in ergosterol and an increase in squalene within the fungal cell membrane (see Figures 70–1 and 70–4).

Terbinafine is a lipophilic antifungal agent with a broad spectrum of activity that includes dermatophytes, *Candida* spp., *Malassezia furfur, C. neoformans, Trichosporon* spp., *Aspergillus* spp., *S. schenckii*, and *Penicillium marneffei* (see Table 70–2). It is available in oral and topical formulations and achieves high concentrations in fatty tissues, skin, hair, and nails.

Terbinafine is efficacious in the treatment of virtually all forms of dermatomycoses, including onychomycosis, and exhibits few side effects. It has shown clinical effectiveness in the treatment of sporotrichosis, aspergillosis, and chromoblastomycosis and has shown promise for the treatment of infections caused by fluconazole-resistant *Candida* spp. when used in combination with fluconazole.

GRISEOFULVIN

Griseofulvin is an oral agent used in the treatment of infections caused by the dermatophytes. It is thought to inhibit fungal growth by interaction with microtubules within the fungal cell resulting in inhibition of mitosis (see Table 70–1 and Figure 70–1).

Griseofulvin is considered a second-line agent in the treatment of dermatomycoses. Newer agents such as itraconazole and terbinafine are more rapid acting and provide greater efficacy. Griseofulvin is also associated with a number of mild side effects including nausea, diarrhea, headache, hepatotoxicity, rash, and neurologic side effects.

Topical Antifungal Agents

A wide variety of topical antifungal preparations are available for the treatment of superficial cutaneous and mucosal fungal infections (see Table 70–1). Topical preparations are available for most classes of antifungal agents including polyenes (e.g., amphotericin B, nystatin, pimaracin), allylamines (e.g., naftifine and terbinafine), and numerous imidazoles and miscellaneous agents (see Table 70–1). Creams, lotions, ointments, powders, and sprays are available for use in the treatment of cutaneous infections and onychomycosis, whereas mucosal infections are best treated with suspensions, tablets, troches, or suppositories.

Whether one uses topical or systemic therapy for the treatment of cutaneous or mucosal fungal infections usually depends on the status of the host and the type and extent of infection. Whereas most cutaneous dermatophytic infections and oral or vaginal candidiasis will respond to topical therapy, the refractory nature of infections such as onychomycosis or tinea capitis ("ringworm" of the scalp) usually calls for long-term systemic therapy.

Investigational Antifungal Agents

At the present time there are several antifungal agents that are in various stage of clinical evaluation. These "investigational" agents include some with established modes of action, as well as some novel classes of antifungal agents, such as a liposomal formulation of nystatin, novel triazole agents (e.g., posaconazole and ravuconazole), echinocandins (e.g., anidulafungin and micafungin), an inhibitor of chitin synthesis (e.g., nikkomycin Z) and sordarin and azasordarin derivatives (see Table 70–1). The mechanisms of action and spectra of activity of liposomal nystatin, the novel triazoles, and the echinocandins are essentially the same as that of the currently available members of each class (see Tables 70–1 and 70–2). To a varying degree, the newer agents in each class offer the potential for more favorable pharmacokinetic and pharmacodynamic proprieties, decreased toxicities or drug-drug interactions, or possible improved activity against certain pathogens that are refractory to presently available agents. In contrast, completely new agents such as the sordarins and azasordarins interact with a novel target, elongation factor 2, which is essential for fungal protein synthesis. Inhibition of chitin synthesis in the fungal cell wall by nikkomycin Z provides another novel approach that may be useful in concert with other inhibitors of cell wall or cell membrane synthesis. The development of agents with novel mechanisms of action is both necessary and promising for future advances in the area of antifungal therapy.

Combinations of Antifungal Agents in the Treatment of Mycoses

The high mortality of opportunistic fungal infections has spurred the development of new antifungal agents, including some with novel mechanisms of action (see Table 70–1). In addition to aggressive use of new antifungal agents such as voriconazole and caspofungin as monotherapy, the use of azole-, echinocandin-, and polyene-based combinations for treatment of the more difficult to treat mycoses, such as opportunistic mould infections, is the focus of intense interest and discussion. The rationale behind combination therapy is that, by using combinations of antifungal agents, one can achieve a better clinical outcome than with monotherapy. The push toward the use of combination antifungal therapy is especially strong for those infections, such as invasive aspergillosis, for which the associated mortality is unacceptably high.

In considering combination therapy, one seeks to achieve **synergy** and avoid **antagonism.** Synergy is achieved when the outcome obtained with the combination of agents is significantly better than that obtained with either drug alone. Conversely, antagonism is when the combination is less active or efficacious than either drug alone. In the case of antifungal therapy, there are several mechanisms that one may consider in developing an effective combination treatment strategy:

1. Inhibition of different stages of the same biochemical pathway. This is a classical approach for achieving synergy with anti-infective agents. An example of this approach to antifungal therapy would be the combination of terbinafine with an azole, where both agents attack the sterol pathway at different points (see Figure 70–4) resulting in inhibition of ergosterol synthesis and disruption of the fungal cell membrane.
2. Increased penetration of one agent into the cell by virtue of the permeabilizing action of another agent on the fungal cell wall or cell membrane. The combination of amphotericin B (cell membrane disruption) and flucytosine (inhibition of nucleic acid synthesis intracellularly) is a classic example of this interaction.
3. Inhibition of the transport of one agent out of the cell by another agent. Many fungi use energy-dependent efflux pumps to actively pump antifungal agents out of the cell, thereby avoiding the toxic effects of the antifungal agent. Inhibition of these pumps by agents such as reserpine has been shown to enhance the activity of the azole antifungal agents against *Candida* spp.
4. Simultaneous inhibition of different fungal cell targets. Inhibition of fungal cell wall synthesis by an agent such as caspofungin coupled with disruption of cell membrane function by amphotericin B or azoles is an example of this type of combination.

Although the potential value of combination antifungal therapy is appealing, there are several possible downsides to this strategy that must be considered. Antagonism among antifungal agents when used in combination is also a distinct possibility and may occur via several different mechanisms: (1) The action of one agent results in a decrease in the target of another agent. The action of azole antifungal agents depletes the cell membrane of ergosterol, which is the primary target for amphotericin B. (2) The action of one antifungal agent results in the modification of the target of another agent. The inhibition of ergosterol synthesis by azole antifungal agents results in the accumulation of methylated sterols to which amphotericin B binds less well. (3) Blocking of the target site of one agent by another can occur. Lipophilic agents, such as itraconazole, may adsorb to the fungal cell surface and inhibit the binding of amphotericin B to membrane sterols.

Despite these possible positive and negative scenarios, the data supporting the achievement of synergy when various combinations are used clinically are limited. Likewise, antagonism may be demonstrated in the laboratory but significant antagonism has not been observed clinically with antifungal combinations. By considering all of the laboratory and clinical data for antifungal combination therapy, one arrives at a very limited number of instances in which combination therapy has been shown to be beneficial in the treatment of invasive mycoses (Table 70–3).

The strongest data exist for the treatment of cryptococcosis in which the combination of amphotericin B and

TABLE 70–3. Summary of Potentially Useful Antifungal Combinations for Treatment of Common Mycoses

Infection	Antifungal Combination	Comments
Candidiasis	AmB + FCZ	Good clinical success in humans with candidemia
	AmB + FC	Clinical success in humans with peritonitis
Cryptococcosis	AmB + FC	Good clinical success in humans with cryptococcal meningitis
	AmB + FCZ	Clinical success in humans with cryptococcal meningitis
	FC + FCZ	Clinical success in humans with cryptococcal meningitis
Aspergillosis	AmB + FC	In vivo benefit (animal model); no human data
	AmB + azoles	No benefit in animals
	AmB + echinocandins	In vivo benefit (animal model); no human data
	Triazoles + echinocandins	In vivo benefit (animal model); no human data

AmB, Amphotericin B; FC, flucytosine; FCZ, fluconazole.

flucytosine has been shown to be beneficial in the treatment of cryptococcal meningitis. The data are less strong for the combination of flucytosine with fluconazole or amphotericin B with triazoles; however, these combinations appear to be beneficial in treating cryptococcosis as well.

Candidiasis is generally treated adequately with a single antifungal agent such as amphotericin B, caspofungin, or fluconazole; however, combination therapy can be useful in selected situations. The combination of amphotericin B and fluconazole has proven benefits in treating candidemia. Likewise, the combination of terbinafine plus an azole is promising in the treatment of refractory oropharyngeal candidiasis. Flucytosine in combination with either amphotericin B or triazoles has positive effects on survival and tissue burden of infection in animal models of candidiasis. Currently, combination therapy of candidiasis should be reserved for specific individual settings such as meningitis, endocarditis, hepatosplenic infection, and candidiasis that is recurrent or refractory to single-agent therapy.

Although the clinical setting of invasive aspergillosis is where combination therapy is most attractive, the data to support its use are lacking. At the present time, there are no clinical trials published that evaluate the use of combination therapy in the treatment of invasive aspergillosis. Studies in vitro and in animals have produced variable results. Combinations of echinocandins with azoles or amphotericin B have yielded positive results. Likewise, amphotericin B plus rifampin appears synergistic. Studies with flucytosine or rifampin plus amphotericin B or azoles have been inconsistent. Despite the desperate need for better treatment options for invasive aspergillosis, there is little evidence that combination therapy will improve the clinical outcome. Combination therapy should be used with caution until more clinical data are available.

Mechanisms of Resistance to Antifungal Agents

Given the prominent role of *Candida* spp. as etiologic agents of invasive mycoses, it is not surprising that most of our understanding of the mechanisms of resistance to antifungal agents comes from studies of *C. albicans* and other species of *Candida*. Much less is known of resistance mechanisms in *Aspergillus* spp. and *C. neoformans*, and almost no information on antifungal resistance mechanisms is available for other opportunistic fungal pathogens.

In contrast to mechanisms of resistance to antibacterial agents, there is no evidence that fungi are capable of destroying or modifying antifungal agents as a means of achieving resistance. Likewise, antifungal resistance genes are not transmissible from cell-to-cell in the manner that occurs with many bacterial resistance genes. It is apparent, however, that multidrug efflux pumps, target alterations, and reduced access to drug targets are important mechanisms of resistance to antifungal agents, just as they are for antibacterial resistance (Table 70–4). In contrast to the rapid emergence and spread of high-level multidrug resistance that occurs in bacteria, antifungal resistance usually develops slowly and involves the emergence of intrinsically resistant species or a gradual, stepwise alteration of cellular structures or functions that results in resistance to an agent to which there has been prior exposure.

POLYENES

Resistance to polyenes, and amphotericin B in particular, remains uncommon despite extensive use over more than 30 years. Decreased susceptibility to amphotericin B has been reported in isolates of *C. lusitaniae*, *C. glabrata*, *C. krusei*, and *C. guilliermondii*. Although primary resistance may be seen, most resistance to amphotericin B among *Candida* spp. is secondary to amphotericin B exposure during therapy. *Aspergillus* spp. are generally susceptible to amphotericin B; however, *A. terreus* is unique in that it appears to be resistant both in vitro and in vivo. Although secondary resistance to amphotericin B has been reported in *C. neoformans*, it is quite rare.

The mechanisms of amphotericin B resistance appears to be a result of qualitative and quantitative alterations in the fungal cell. Amphotericin B–resistant mutants of *Candida* spp. and *C. neoformans* have been shown to have a reduced ergosterol content, replacement of polyene-binding sterols (e.g., ergosterol) by ones that bind polyenes less well (e.g., fecosterol), or masking of ergosterol in the cell membranes so that binding with polyenes is hindered because of steric or thermodynamic factors. The molecular mechanism of amphotericin B resistance has not been determined; however, sterol analysis of resistant strains of *Candida* spp. and *C. neoformans* suggest that they are defective in *ERG2* or *ERG3*, genes encoding for the C-8 sterol isomerase and C-5 sterol desaturase enzymes, respectively.

AZOLES

The ubiquitous use of azoles, especially fluconazole, for the treatment and prevention of fungal infections has given rise to reports of emerging resistance to this class of antifungal agents. Fortunately, primary resistance to fluconazole is rare among most species of *Candida* causing bloodstream infection. Among the five most common species of *Candida* isolated from the blood of infected patients (i.e., *C. albicans*, *C. glabrata*, *parapsilosis*, *tropicalis*, and *C. krusei*), only *C. krusei* is considered intrinsically

TABLE 70–4. Mechanisms Involved in the Development of Resistance to Antifungal Agents in Pathogenic Fungi

Fungus	Amphotericin B	Flucytosine	Itraconazole	Fluconazole	Caspofungin
Aspergillus fumigatus			• Altered target enzyme, 14α-demethylase • Decreased azole accumulation		
Candida albicans	• Decrease in ergosterol • Replacement of polyene-binding sterols • Masking of ergosterol	• Loss of permease activity • Loss of cytosine deaminase activity • Loss of uracil phosphoribosyl-transferase activity		• Overexpression or mutation of 14α-demethylase • Overexpression of efflux pumps, *CDR* and *MDR* genes	• Mutation in *FKS*1 gene
Candida glabrata	• Alteration or decrease in ergosterol content	• Loss of permease activity		• Overexpression of efflux pumps (*CgCDR* genes)	
Candida krusei	• Alteration or decrease in ergosterol content			• Active efflux • Reduced affinity for target enzyme, 14α-demethylase	• Mutation in *FKS*1 gene
Candida lusitaniae	• Alteration or decrease in ergosterol content • Production of modified sterols				

resistant to fluconazole. Among the remaining species, approximately 10% of *C. glabrata* exhibit primary resistance to fluconazole and less than 2% of *C. albicans, C. parapsilosis,* and *C. tropicalis* are resistant to this agent. The new triazoles (voriconazole, posaconazole, and ravuconazole) are more potent than fluconazole against *Candida* spp., including activity against *C. krusei* and some fluconazole-resistant strains of other *Candida* spp.; however, there is a strong positive correlation between the activity of fluconazole and that of the other triazoles, suggesting some degree of cross-resistance within the class.

Primary resistance to fluconazole is also rare among clinical isolates of *C. neoformans.* Secondary resistance has been described in isolates obtained from individuals with AIDS and relapsing cryptococcal meningitis.

Only a small number of isolates of *Aspergillus* spp. have been shown to demonstrate resistance to itraconazole. In contrast to *Candida,* cross-resistance between itraconazole and the new triazoles is not complete among isolates of *Aspergillus* spp.: cross-resistance between itraconazole and posaconazole, but not voriconazole, has been reported.

Azole resistance in *Candida* spp. can be caused by the following mechanisms: a modification in the quantity or quality of the target enzymes, reduced access of the drug to the target, or some combination of these mechanisms. Thus, point mutations in the gene (*ERG*11) encoding the target enzyme, lanosterol 14 α-demethylase, leads to an altered target with decreased affinity for azoles. Overexpression of *ERG*11 results in overproduction of the target enzyme, creating the need for higher concentrations of the drug within the cell to inactivate all of the target enzyme molecules. Upregulation of genes encoding for multidrug efflux pumps results in active efflux of the azole antifungal agents out of the cell. Upregulation of genes encoding the **major facilitator type efflux pump** (MDR) leads to fluconazole resistance, and upregulation of genes encoding the **ATP-binding cassette transporters** (CDR) leads to resistance to multiple azoles. These mechanisms may act individually, sequentially, or simultaneously, resulting in strains of *Candida* that exhibit progressively higher levels of azole resistance.

The mechanisms of azole resistance in *Aspergillus* spp. are poorly characterized given the paucity of strains with documented resistance. It appears that both increased drug efflux and alterations in the 14 α-demethylase target enzyme serve as mechanisms for resistance to itraconazole among isolates of *Aspergillus* spp.

Similarly, secondary resistance to fluconazole among isolates of *C. neoformans* has been associated with overexpression of MDR efflux pumps and alteration of the target enzyme. *C. neoformans* has also been shown to have a CDR-type efflux pump.

ECHINOCANDINS

Caspofungin, anidulafungin, and micafungin all demonstrate potent fungicidal activity against *Candida* spp., including azole-resistant strains. Clinical isolates of *Candida* spp. with reduced susceptibility to the echinocandins are very rare. Efforts to produce caspofungin-resistant mutants of *C. albicans* in the laboratory have shown that the frequency with which these mutants arise is very low (1 in 10^8 cells), suggesting a low potential for the emergence of resistance in the clinical setting. Clinical isolates of *Aspergillus* spp. with reduced susceptibility to echinocandins are nonexistent at the present time, and efforts to produce resistance in the laboratory setting have been unsuccessful.

The mechanism of resistance to caspofungin that has been characterized in laboratory-derived mutants of *C. albicans* is one of an altered glucan synthesis enzyme complex that shows a decreased sensitivity to inhibition by caspofungin. These strains have point mutations in the *FKS*1 gene that encodes for an integral membrane protein (*FKS*1), which is the catalytic subunit of the glucan synthesis enzyme complex. The *FKS*1 mutation results in strains that are resistant to all of the echinocandins but retain susceptibility to polyene and azole antifungal agents. Although the *FKS*1 gene is essential in *Aspergillus* species as well, similar mutations have not been demonstrated thus far.

FLUCYTOSINE

Primary resistance to flucytosine is uncommon among clinical isolates of *Candida* spp. and *C. neoformans*. Secondary resistance, however, is well documented to occur among both *Candida* spp. and *C. neoformans* during monotherapy with this agent.

Flucytosine resistance may develop because of decreased uptake of the drug (loss of permease activity) or by loss of enzymatic activity necessary to convert flucytosine to 5-FU (cytosine deaminase) and 5-fluorouridylic acid (FUMP pyrophosphorylase). Uracil phosphoribosyltransferase, another enzyme in the pyrimidine salvage pathway, is also important in the formation of 5-fluorouracilmonophosphate (FUMP), and loss of its activity is sufficient to confer resistance to flucytosine.

ALLYLAMINES

Although clinical failures can occur during treatment of fungal infections with terbinafine and naftifine, they have not been shown to be due to resistance to these agents. It has been shown that the CDR1 multidrug efflux pump can use terbinafine as a substrate, suggesting that efflux-mediated resistance to allylamines is a possibility.

CLINICAL FACTORS CONTRIBUTING TO RESISTANCE

Antifungal therapy may fail clinically despite the fact that the drug used is active against the infecting fungus. The complex interaction of the host, the drug, and the fungal pathogen may be influenced by a wide variety of factors including the immune status of the host, the site and severity of the infection, presence of foreign body (e.g., catheter, vascular graft), the activity of the drug at the site of infection, the dose and duration of therapy, and patient compliance with the antifungal regimen. It must be recognized that the presence of neutrophils, use of immunomodulating drugs, concomitant infections (e.g., HIV), surgical procedures, and the age and nutritional status of the host all may be more important in determining the outcome of the infection than the ability of the antifungal agent to inhibit or kill the infecting organism.

ANTIFUNGAL SUSCEPTIBILITY TESTING

In vitro susceptibility testing of antifungal agents is designed to determine the relative activity of one or more agents against the infecting pathogen in hopes of selecting the best option for treatment of the infection. Thus antifungal susceptibility tests are performed for the same reasons that tests with antibacterial agents are performed. Antifungal susceptibility tests will do the following: (1) provide a reliable estimate of the relative activity of two or more antifungal agents against the tested organism; (2) correlate with in vivo antifungal activity and predict the likely outcome of therapy; (3) provide a means with which to monitor the development of resistance among a normally susceptible population of organisms; and (4) predict the therapeutic potential of newly developed investigational agents.

Standardized methods for performing antifungal susceptibility testing are reproducible, accurate, and available for use in clinical laboratories. Antifungal susceptibility testing is now increasingly and appropriately used as a routine adjunct to the treatment of fungal infections. Guidelines for the use of antifungal testing as a complement to other laboratory studies have been developed. Selective application of antifungal susceptibility testing, coupled with broader identification of fungi to the species level, is especially useful in difficult to manage fungal infections. One must keep in mind, however, that the in vitro susceptibility of an infecting organism to the antimicrobial agent is only one of several factors that may influence the likelihood that therapy for an infection will be successful. (See previous section.)

QUESTIONS

1. What is the mechanism of action of the echinocandin antifungal agents? Why is this an advantage for this class of agents?
2. Describe the mechanisms of resistance to the azoles that are known for *Candida albicans.*
3. Why is combination therapy with antifungal agents attractive? Give an example of a mechanism that would likely produce synergy.

Biblography

Espinel-Ingroff A, Pfaller MA: Susceptibility test methods: Yeasts and filamentous fungi. In Murray PR et al, editors: *Manual of clinical microbiology,* ed 8, Washington, 2003, American Society for Microbiology.

Ghannoum MA, Rice LB: Antifungal agents: Mode of action, mechanisms of resistance, and correlation of these mechanisms with bacterial resistance, *Clin Microbiol Rev* 12:501-517, 1999.

Johnson MD et al: Combination antifungal therapy, *Antimicrob Agents Chemother* 48:693-715, 2004.

Revankar SG, Graybill JR: Antifungal therapy. In Anaissie EJ, McGinnis MR, Pfaller MA, editors: *Clinical mycology,* New York, 2003, Churchill Livingstone.

Rex JH, Pfaller MA: Has antifungal susceptibility come of age? *Clin Infect Dis* 35:982-989, 2002.

White TC: Mechanisms of resistance to antifungal agents. In Murray PR et al, editors: *Manual of clinical microbiology,* ed 8, Washington, 2003, American Society for Microbiology.

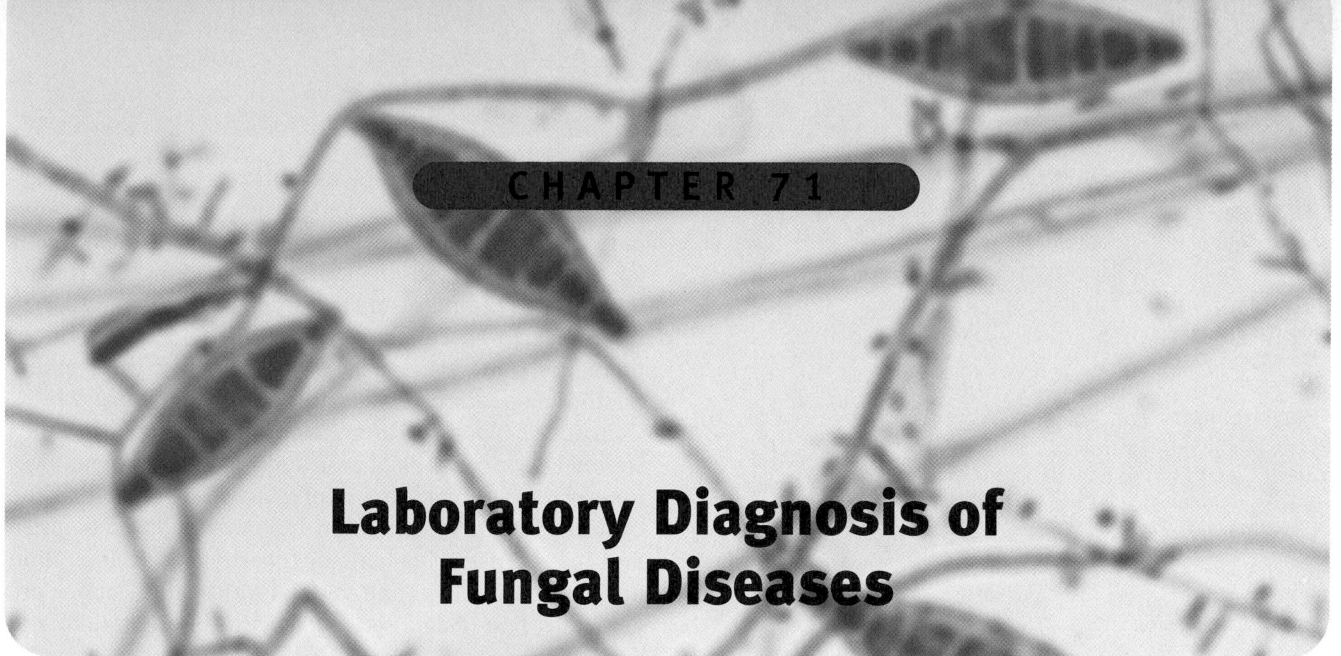

CHAPTER 71

Laboratory Diagnosis of Fungal Diseases

The spectrum of mycotic disease ranges from superficial cutaneous and mucosal infections that may be locally irritating to highly invasive processes associated with classic systemic and opportunistic pathogens. Serious infections are being reported with an ever increasing array of pathogens, including the well-known pathogenic fungi such as *Candida, Cryptococcus neoformans, Histoplasma capsulatum*, and *Aspergillus*, as well as lesser known hyaline and dematiaceous moulds (see Tables 7–1 and 7–2). Modern medical mycology has become the study of mycoses caused by a variety of taxonomically diverse fungi.

Opportunistic mycoses pose a significant diagnostic challenge to clinicians and mycologists alike due to the complexity of the patient population at risk and the increasing array of fungi that can infect these individuals. Successful diagnosis and treatment of mycotic infections in the compromised patient is highly dependent on a team approach involving clinicians, medical mycologists, and pathologists.

This chapter provides a general description of the principles of specimen collection and processing necessary for the diagnosis of most fungal infections. An overview of direct microscopy, culture, and immunologic and molecular diagnostic testing is also provided. Specific details of these and other procedures used in the diagnosis of fungal infections can be found in several reference texts listed in the bibliography.

Clinical Recognition of Fungal Infections

Prompt diagnosis of invasive mycoses requires a high index of suspicion and an appreciation of specific risk factors that may predispose a patient to such infections. Clinical suspicion, thorough history and physical examination including a search for cutaneous and mucosal lesions, inspection of all implanted devices (catheters, etc.), a careful ophthalmologic examination, diagnostic imaging studies, and finally, procurement of appropriate specimens for laboratory diagnosis are all essential steps that must be taken to optimize the diagnosis and treatment of fungal infections. Unfortunately, although specific fungi may be associated with "classic" case scenarios such as onychomycosis and lower extremity skin lesions due to *Fusarium* spp. in a patient with neutropenia or sinus infection due to *Rhizopus* spp. in a diabetic with ketoacidosis, clinical signs and symptoms are not specific for fungal infections and are often not helpful in distinguishing between bacterial and fungal infections in a patient at risk for both types of infection. Increasingly, it is also important to know not only that the patient is infected with a fungus but what the fungus is in order to provide the best treatment and clinical support. Thus, diagnosis of fungal infections depends on three basic laboratory approaches: microbiologic, immunologic, and histopathologic (Box 71–1). These approaches can be supplemented by molecular and biochemical methods of organism detection and identification. Use of the newer methods for detection of fungal antigens and nucleic acids offer great promise for rapid diagnosis of fungal infections.

Conventional Laboratory Diagnosis

SPECIMEN COLLECTION AND PROCESSING

As with all types of infectious processes, the laboratory diagnosis of fungal infection is directly dependent on the proper collection of appropriate clinical material and

BOX 71–1. Laboratory Methods for Diagnosing Fungal Disease

Conventional Microbiologic Methods
Direct microscopy (Gram, Giemsa, and Calcofluor stains)
Culture
Identification
Susceptibility testing

Histopathologic
Routine stains (H&E)
Special stains (GMS, PAS, mucicarmine)
Direct immunofluorescence
In situ hybridization

Immunologic
Antibody
Antigen

Molecular
Direct detection (nucleic acid amplification)
Identification
Strain typing

Biochemical
Metabolites
Cell wall components
Enzymes

H&E, hematoxylin and eosin; GMS, Gomori methenamine silver; PAS, periodic acid-Schiff.

prompt delivery of the specimens to the clinical laboratory. Selection of specimens for culture and microscopic examination is based not only on information obtained from clinical examination and radiographic studies, but also on consideration of the most likely fungal pathogen that may cause a specific type of infection (Table 71–1). Specimens should be collected aseptically or after proper cleaning and decontamination of the site to be sampled. An adequate amount of clinical material must be submitted promptly for culture and microscopy. Unfortunately, many specimens submitted to the laboratory are of poor quality and insufficient amount and are not appropriate to make a diagnosis. Specimens should be submitted, whenever possible, in a sterile leak-proof container and should be accompanied by a relevant clinical history. The laboratory depends on clinical information in making decisions as to the best way to process the specimen to ensure recovery of the etiologic agent. The clinical history is also useful in interpreting the results of culture and other laboratory testing, especially when dealing with specimens from nonsterile sites such as sputum and skin. Furthermore, clinical information alerts the laboratory personnel that they may be dealing with a potentially dangerous pathogen such as *Coccidioides immitis* or *Histoplasma capsulatum*.

Transportation of specimens to the laboratory should be prompt; however, delayed processing of specimens for fungal culture may not be as detrimental as with specimens for bacteriologic, virologic or parasitologic examination. In general, if processing is delayed, the specimens for fungal culture can be stored at 4°C for a short time without loss of organism viability.

Similar to specimens for bacteriologic examination, there are some specimens that are better than others for the diagnosis of fungal infections (see Table 71–1). Cultures of blood and other normally sterile body fluids should be done if clinical indications suggest a hematogenous process or involvement of a closed space such as the central nervous system. Skin lesions should be biopsied and material sent for both histopathologic examination and for culture. Oral and vaginal mucosal infections are generally best diagnosed by clinical presentation and direct microscopic examination of secretions or mucosal scrapings because cultures often yield growth that represents normal flora or even contaminants. Similarly, diagnosis of gastrointestinal fungal infections are best made by biopsy and histopathologic examination rather than by culture. Twenty-four-hour collections of sputum or urine are not appropriate for mycologic examination because they typically become overgrown with both bacterial and fungal contaminants.

STAINS AND DIRECT MICROSCOPIC EXAMINATION

Direct microscopic examination of tissue sections and clinical specimens is generally considered to be among the most rapid and cost-effective means of diagnosing fungal infections. Detection of yeasts or hyphal structures microscopically in tissue may be accomplished in less than an hour, whereas culture results may not be available for days or even weeks. In certain instances, the fungus may not only be detected but identified by microscopy due to the fact that it possesses a distinctive morphology. Specifically, detection of characteristic cysts, yeast cells, or spherules can provide an etiologic diagnosis of infections due *Pneumocystis jiroveci (carinii)*, *H. capsulatum*, *Blastomyces dermatitidis*, or *C. immitis*, respectively. Although the morphologic appearance of *Candida*, a zygomycete, or *Trichosporon* in tissue may lead to the diagnosis of the type of infection (i.e., candidiasis, zygomycosis, trichosporonosis), the actual species of fungus causing the infection would remain unknown pending culture. Microscopic detection of fungi in tissue serves to guide the laboratory in selecting the most appropriate means to culture the specimen and also is helpful in determining the significance of culture results. The latter is especially true when the organism isolated in culture is a known component of the normal flora or is frequently found in the environment.

Direct microscopy is clearly useful in diagnosing fungal infection; however, both false-negative and false-positive results may occur. Microscopy is less sensitive than

TABLE 71–1. Body Sites, Specimen Collection, and Diagnostic Procedures for Selected Fungal Infections

Infection Site and Infecting Organism	Specimen Options	Collection Methods	Diagnostic Procedure
Blood			
Candida spp., *Cryptococcus neoformans, Histoplasma capsulatum, Fusarium* spp., *Aspergillus terreus, Penicillium marneffei*	Whole blood	Venipuncture (sterile)	Culture, broth Culture, lysis-centrifugation
	Serum	Venipuncture (sterile)	Antigen (*Candida, Cryptococcus* and *Histoplasma*); nucleic acid amplification
	Urine	Sterile	Antigen (*Histoplasma*)
Bone Marrow			
Histoplasma capsulatum, Penicillium marneffei	Aspirate	Sterile	Microscopic examination, culture
	Serum	Venipuncture (sterile)	Serology (*Histoplasma*), antigen, antibody
	Urine	Sterile	Antigen (*Histoplasma*)
Central Nervous System			
Candida spp., *Cryptococcus neoformans, Aspergillus* spp., *Scedosporium* spp., dematiaceous moulds	Spinal Fluid	Sterile	Microscopic examination, culture, antigen (*Cryptococcus*)
	Biopsy	Sterile, nonsterile to histopathology	Microscopic examination, culture (do not grind tissue)
	Serum	Sterile	Cryptococcal antigen
Bone and Joint			
Candida spp., *Fusarium* spp., *Aspergillus* spp., *Histoplasma capsulatum, Coccidioides immitis, Blastomyces dermatitidis, Penicillium marneffei, Sporothrix schenckii*	Aspirate	Sterile	Microscopic examination, culture
	Biopsy	Sterile, nonsterile to histopathology	Microscopic examination, culture (do not grind tissue)
	Serum	Venipuncture	Serology, antigen, antibody
Eye			
Fusarium spp., *Candida* spp., *Cryptococcus neoformans, Aspergillus* spp., zygomycetes	Cornea	Scraping or biopsy	Microscopic examination, culture
	Vitreous fluid	Sterile aspirate	Microscopic examination, culture
Urogenital System			
Candida spp., *Cryptococcus neoformans, Trichosporon, Rhodotorula,* Rarely: *Histoplasma capsulatum, Blastomyces dermatitidis, Coccidioides immitis*	Urine	Sterile	Microscopic examination, culture
	Vaginal, urethral, prostatic secretions or discharge	Saline swab	Microscopic examination Wet mount Calcofluor/KOH Culture
	Serum	Venipuncture	Serology (antibody)
	Biopsy	Sterile, nonsterile to histopathology	Microscopic examination, culture (do not grind tissue)
Respiratory Tract			
Cryptococcus neoformans, Aspergillus spp., *Fusarium* spp., *Zygomycetes, Scedosporium apiospermum,* dematiaceous moulds, endemic dimorphic fungi, *Pneumocystis jiroveci* (*carinii*)	Sputum	Induced, no preservative	Microscopic examination, culture
	Lavage	No preservative	Microscopic examination, culture
	Transbronchial	Aspirate or biopsy	Microscopic examination, culture
	Open lung biopsy	Sterile, nonsterile to histopathology	Microscopic examination, culture (do not grind tissue)
	Serum	Venipuncture	Serology, antigen, antibody, nucleic acid amplification
	Urine	Sterile	Antigen (*Histoplasma* spp.)

TABLE 71–1. Body Sites, Specimen Collection, and Diagnostic Procedures for Selected Fungal Infections—cont'd

Infection Site and Infecting Organism	Specimen Options	Collection Methods	Diagnostic Procedure
Skin and Mucous Membranes			
Candida spp., *Cryptococcus neoformans, Trichosporon* spp., *Aspergillus* spp., zygomycetes, *Fusarium* spp., dematiaceous moulds, endemic dimorphic fungi, *Sporothrix schenckii*	Biopsy	Sterile, nonsterile to histopathology	Microscopic examination, culture (do not grind tissue)
	Mucosal	Saline swab	Microscopic examination Wet mount, Calcofluor/KOH Culture
	Skin scraping	Non-sterile	Calcofluor/KOH
	Serum	Venipuncture	Serology Antigen, antibody Nucleic acid amplification
	Urine	Sterile	Antigen (*Histoplasma*)
Multiple Systemic Sites			
Candida spp., *Cryptococcus neoformans, Trichosporon,* hyaline moulds, dematiaceous moulds, endemic dimorphic fungi	Whole blood	Venipuncture (sterile)	Culture, broth Culture, lysis-centrifugation
	Serum	Venipuncture (sterile)	Serology Antigen, antibody Nucleic acid amplification
	Urine	Sterile	Antigen (*Histoplasma*)
	Biopsy	Sterile, nonsterile to histopathology	Microscopic examination, culture (do not grind tissue)

Adapted from Pfaller MA, McGinnis MR: The laboratory and clinical mycology. In Anaissie EJ, McGinnis MR, Pfaller MA: *Clinical mycology,* New York, 2003, Churchill Livingstone.

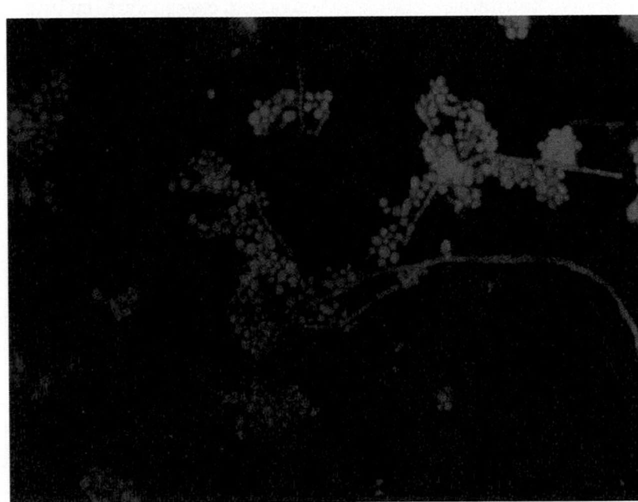

FIGURE 71–1. Calcofluor white stain demonstrating budding yeasts and pseudohyphae of *Candida albicans.*

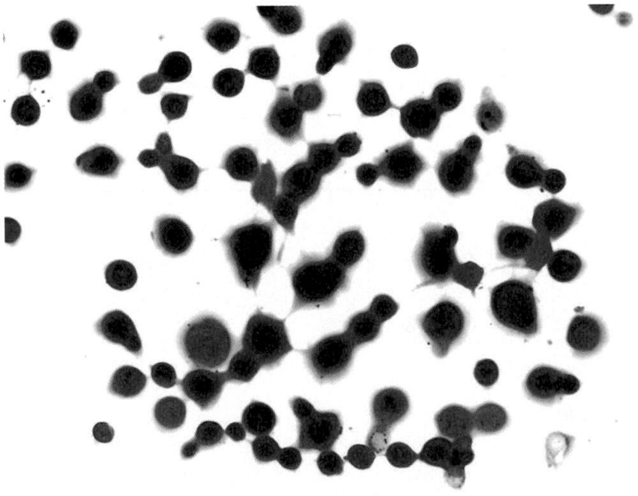

FIGURE 71–2. Gram stain of *Cryptococcus neoformans*. Variably sized, encapsulated budding yeasts showing a stippled pattern due to uneven retention of crystal violet stain.

culture, and a negative direct examination does not rule out a fungal infection.

A number of different stains and microscopic techniques can be used to detect and characterize fungi directly in clinical material (Table 71–2). The approaches used most often in the clinical mycology laboratory include the fluorescent reagent Calcofluor white or staining of smears and touch preparations with either Gram or Giemsa stains. The Calcofluor white stains the cell walls of fungi causing the fungi to fluoresce, allowing for easier and faster detection (Figure 71–1). The Gram stain is useful for detection of yeasts such as species of *Candida* or *Cryptococcus* (Figure 71–2), but it also stains hyphal elements of filamentous fungi such as *Aspergillus* (Figure 71–3). Fungi are typically gram positive but may appear speckled or gram negative (see Figures 71–2 and 71–3).

TABLE 71–2. Selected Methods and Stains Commonly Used for Direct Microscopic Detection of Fungal Elements in Clinical Specimens

Method/Stain	Use	Comments
Calcofluor white stain	Detection of all fungi including *Pneumocystis jiroveci* (*carinii*)	Rapid (1-2 min); detects fungal cell wall chitin by bright fluorescence. Used in combination with KOH. Requires fluorescent microscope with proper filters. Background fluorescence may make examination of some specimens difficult.
Fluorescent monoclonal antibody treatment	Examination of respiratory specimen for *P. jiroveci* (*carinii*)	Sensitive and specific method for detecting the cysts of *P. jiroveci* (*carinii*). Does not stain the extracystic (trophic) forms.
Giemsa stain	Examination of bone marrow, peripheral blood smears, touch preparations of tissue, and respiratory specimens	Detect intracellular *Histoplasma capsulatum* and both intracystic and trophic forms of *P. jiroveci* (*carinii*). Does not stain the cyst wall of *Pneumocystis* spp. Does stain organisms other than *Histoplasma* spp. and *Pneumocystis* spp.
Gram stain	Detection of bacteria and fungi	Commonly performed on clinical specimens. Will stain most yeasts and hyphal elements. Most fungi stain gram positive but some, such as *Cryptococcus neoformans,* exhibit stippling or appear gram negative.
Hematoxylin and eosin stain	General purpose histologic stain	Best stain to demonstrate host reaction in infected tissue. Stains most fungi but small numbers of organisms may be difficult to differentiate from background. Useful in demonstrating natural pigment in dematiaceous fungi.
Gomori methenamine silver stain	Detection of fungi in histologic sections and *P. jiroveci* (*carinii*) cysts in respiratory specimens	Best stain for detecting all fungi. Stains hyphae and yeast forms black against a green background. Usually performed in histopathology laboratory.
Mucicarmine stain	Histopathologic stain for mucin	Useful for demonstrating capsular material of *Cryptococcus neoformans.* May also stain the cell walls of *Blastomyces dermatitidis* and *Rhinosporidium sieberi.*
Periodic acid-Schiff (PAS) stain	Histologic stain for fungi	Stains both yeasts and hyphae in tissue. PAS-positive artifacts may resemble yeast cells.

Adapted from Pfaller MA, McGinnis MR: The laboratory and clinical mycology. In Anaissie EJ, McGinnis MR, Pfaller MA: *Clinical mycology,* New York, 2003, Churchill Livingstone.

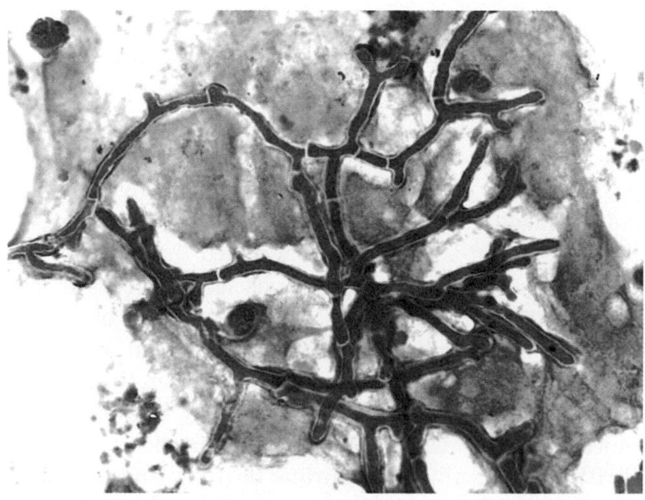

FIGURE 71–3. Gram stain of *Aspergillus*. This specimen did not retain the crystal violet stain and appears gram negative.

The Giemsa stain is especially useful for detecting the intracellular yeast forms of *H. capsulatum* in peripheral blood smears, bone marrow, or touch preparations of tissue (Figure 71–4).

The respiratory pathogen *P. jiroveci* (*carinii*) can be detected in induced sputum or specimens obtained by bronchoscopy. The cysts may be stained with Gomori methenamine silver (GMS) stain (Figure 71–5) or by a fluorescent monoclonal antibody, and the trophic and intracystic forms are stained with the Giemsa stain (Figure 71–6).

Stains such as hematoxylin and eosin (H&E), GMS, and periodic acid-Schiff (PAS) are performed in the cytology and/or histopathology laboratory and are used for detection of fungi in cytologic preparations, fine-needle aspirates, tissues, body fluids, and exudates (see Tables 71–1 and 71–2). These stains can detect fungi such as *B. dermatitidis, H. capsulatum, C. immitis, Candida* spp.,

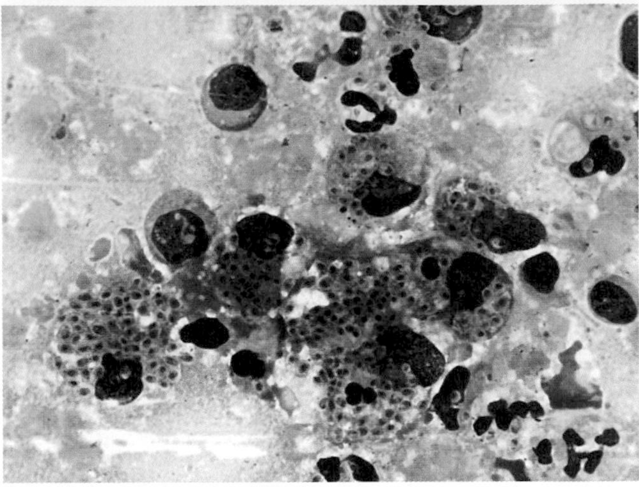

FIGURE 71–4. Giemsa stain showing intracellular yeast forms of *Histoplasma capsulatum.*

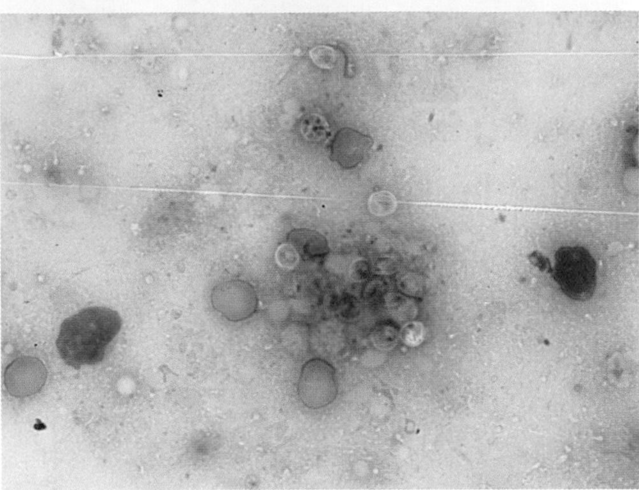

FIGURE 71–6. Giemsa stain showing intracystic and trophic forms of *Pneumocystis jiroveci* (*carinii*).

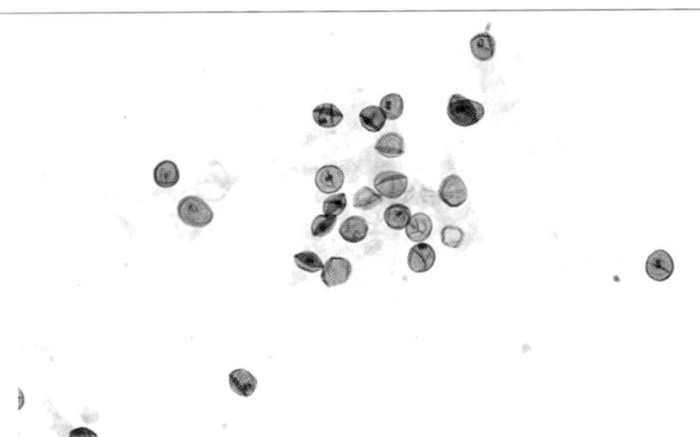

FIGURE 71–5. Silver stain of *Pneumocystis jiroveci* (*carinii*) cysts.

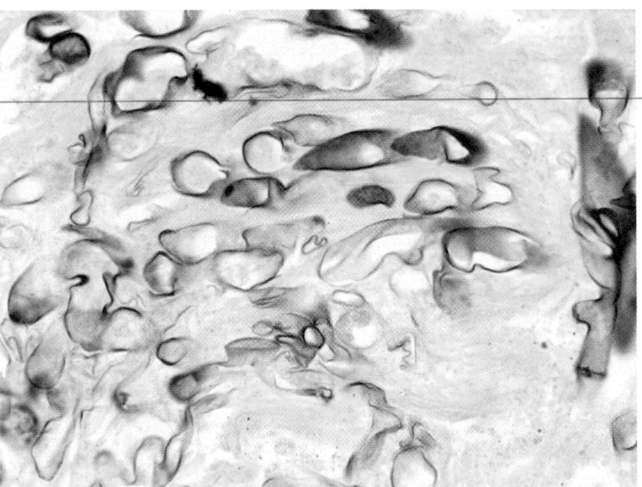

FIGURE 71–7. Silver stain of *Rhizopus.*

C. neoformans and the hyphae of zygomycetes (Figure 71–7), *Aspergillus,* and other moulds. Fungi can be visualized with the H&E stain, but small numbers of organisms may be missed. The more fungus-specific stains are the GMS and PAS stains. These are useful in detecting small numbers of organisms and for clearly defining characteristic features of fungal morphology. Histologic examination of fixed tissue provides the opportunity to determine whether the fungus is invading the tissue or is merely present superficially, information that is helpful in distinguishing between infection and colonization. The microscopic morphologic features of several of the more common fungal pathogens are presented in Table 71–3.

CULTURE

The most sensitive means of diagnosing a fungal infection is usually considered to be isolation of the fungus in culture. Culture is also necessary, in most instances, to identify the etiologic agents. Optimal recovery of fungi from clinical material depends on procurement of an adequate clinical specimen and then use of culture methods that will ensure the recovery of organisms that are usually present in small amounts and are slow growing. No single culture medium is sufficient to isolate all medically important fungi, and it is generally accepted that at least two types of media, selective and nonselective, be used. The nonselective medium will permit the growth of rapidly growing yeasts and moulds as well as the more slowly growing fastidious fungi. Fungi will grow in most media used for bacteria; however, growth may be slow, and a more enriched medium such as brain heart infusion (BHI) agar or SABHI (Sabouraud dextrose and BHI) agar is recommended. Fastidious dimorphic fungi such as *H. capsulatum* and *B. dermatitidis* usually require a blood-containing medium such as BHI with 5% to 10% sheep

TABLE 71–3. Characteristic Features of Selected Opportunistic and Pathogenic Fungi in Clinical Specimens and in Cultures

Fungus	Microscopic Morphologic Features in Clinical Specimens	Characteristic Morphologic Features in Culture		Additional Tests for Identification
		Macroscopic	Microscopic	
Candida spp.	Oval budding yeasts 2–6 µm in diameter. Hyphae and pseudohyphae may be present.	Variable morphology. Colonies usually pasty, white to tan, and opaque. May have smooth or wrinkled morphology.	Clusters of blastoconidia, pseudohyphae, and/or terminal chlamydospores in some species.	Germ tube production by *Candida albicans, Candida dubliniensis* and *Candida stellatoidea.* Carbohydrate assimilation. Morphology on corn meal agar.
Cryptococcus neoformans	Spherical budding yeasts of variable size, 2–15 µm. Capsule may be present. No hyphae or pseudohyphae.	Colonies are shiny, mucoid, dome shaped, and cream to tan in color.	Budding spherical cells of varying size. Capsule present. No pseudohyphae. Cells may have multiple narrow-based buds.	Tests for urease (+), phenoloxidase (+), and nitrate reductase (–). Latex agglutination or EIA test for polysaccharide antigen. Mucicarmine and melanin stains in tissue.
Aspergillus	Septate, dichotomously branched hyphae of uniform width (3–6 µm).	Varies with species. *A. fumigatus:* blue-green to gray; *A. flavus:* yellow-green; *A. niger:* black.	Varies with species. Conidiophores with enlarged vesicles covered with flask-shaped metulae or phialides. Hyphae are hyaline and septate.	Identification based on microscopic and colonial morphology.
Zygomycetes	Broad, thin- walled, pauci- septate hyphae, 6–25 µm with nonparallel sides and random branches. Hyphae stain poorly with GMS stain and often stain well with H&E stain.	Colonies are rapid growing, wooly, and gray-brown to gray-black in color.	Broad, ribbon-like hyphae with rare septa. Sporangium or sporangiola produced from sporangiophore. Rhizoids present in some species.	Identification based on microscopic morphologic features.
Dematiaceous moulds (see Table 7–3)	Pigmented (brown, tan, or black) hyphae, 2–6 µm wide. May be branched or un-branched. Often constricted at point of septation.	Colonies are usually rapidly growing, wooly, and gray, olive, black or brown in color.	Varies depending on genus and species. Hyphae are pigmented. Conidia may be single or in chains, smooth or rough and dematiaceous.	Identification based on microscopic and colonial morphology.
Histoplasma capsulatum	Small (2–4 µm) budding yeasts within macrophages.	Colonies are slow growing and white or buff-brown in color (25°C). Yeast phase colonies (37°C) are smooth, white, and pasty.	Thin septate hyphae that produce tuberculate macroconidia and smooth-walled microconidia (25°C). Small oval budding yeasts produced at 37°C.	Demonstration of temperature-regulated dimorphism by conversion from mould to yeast phase at 37°C. Exoantigen and nucleic acid probe tests allow identification without phase conversion.

EIA, Enzyme immunoassay; GMS, Gomori methenamine silver; H&E, hematoxylin and eosin.

TABLE 71–3. Characteristic Features of Selected Opportunistic and Pathogenic Fungi in Clinical Specimens and in Cultures—cont'd

Fungus	Microscopic Morphologic Features in Clinical Specimens	Characteristic Morphologic Features in Culture		Additional Tests for Identification
		Macroscopic	Microscopic	
Blastomyces dermatitidis	Large (8–15 μm) thick-walled, broad-based budding yeast.	Colonies vary from membranous yeast- like colonies to cottony white mould-like colonies at 25°C. When grown at 37°C, yeast phase colonies are wrinkled, folded and glabrous.	Hyaline, septate hyphae with one-celled smooth conidia (25°C). Large, thick-walled budding yeast at 37°C.	Demonstration of temperature-regulated dimorphism; exoantigen and nucleic acid probe tests.
Coccidioides immitis	Spherical, thick-walled spherules, 20–200 μm. Mature spherules contain small, 2–5 μm endospores.	Colonies initially appear moist and glabrous, rapidly becoming downy and gray-white with a tan or brown reverse.	Hyaline hyphae with rectangular arthroconidia separated by empty disjunctor cells.	Exoantigen and nucleic acid probe tests.
Sporothrix schenckii	Yeast-like cells of varying sizes. Some may appear elongated or "cigar-shaped." Tissue reaction forms asteroid bodies.	Colonies initially smooth, moist, and yeast-like becoming velvety as aerial hyphae develop (25°C). Tan to brown pasty colonies at 37°C.	Thin, branching septate hyphae. Conidia borne in rosette-shaped clusters at the end of the conidiophore (25°C). Variably sized budding yeasts produced at 37°C.	Demonstration of thermal dimorphism. Exoantigen and nucleic acid probe.
Penicillium marneffei	Oval intracellular yeast cells with septum.	Colonies produce diffusible red pigment at 25°C.	Septate hyphae with metulae, phialides with chains of conidia in a "paint brush" distribution (25°C). Yeast cells divide by fission (37°C).	Demonstration of thermal dimorphism.
Pneumocystis jiroveci (carinii)	Cysts are round, collapsed, or crescent shaped. Trophic forms seen on special stains.	Not applicable.	Not applicable.	Immunofluorescent stain, GMS, Giemsa, toluidine blue stains (see Table 71–2)

blood for optimal recovery from clinical material. Cycloheximide is often added to this medium to inhibit the more rapidly growing yeasts and moulds that may contaminate the specimen. Although cycloheximide does not affect the endemic dimorphic pathogens, it will inhibit the growth of many opportunistic pathogens (e.g., *Candida, Aspergillus*) that might also be the etiologic agent of infection. For this reason, one should always pair cycloheximide-containing media with complementary media without cycloheximide. Specimens that may be contaminated with bacteria should be inoculated onto selective media such as SABHI or BHI supplemented with antibiotics (penicillin plus streptomycin is often used). Specific fungi may require specialized media. For example, *Malassezia furfur,* an agent that causes superficial skin infections and infections of vascular catheters, requires a medium containing olive oil or another source of long-chain fatty acid for optimal recovery.

The detection of fungemia is an important measure in diagnosing invasive fungal infection. Although contamination of blood cultures with a fungus may take place, for the most part blood cultures with results positive for fungi are significant. Unfortunately, blood cultures often have negative results despite the presence of disseminated disease, especially when the infecting organism is a mould. Detection of fungemia has improved due to the development of continuous monitoring blood culture instruments with improved media formulations that take into account the growth requirements of fungi as well as bacteria. In addition to these broth-based systems, the agar-based lysis-centrifugation method provides a flexible and sensitive method for detection of fungemia caused by yeasts, moulds, and dimorphic pathogens (see Table 71–1).

Once inoculated, fungal cultures should be incubated in air at a proper temperature and for a sufficient period to ensure the recovery of fungi from clinical specimens. Most fungi grow optimally at 25° to 30°C, although most species of *Candida* can be recovered from blood cultures incubated at 35° to 37°C. Culture dishes should be sealed with gas-permeable tape to prevent dehydration. Specimens submitted for fungal culture are generally incubated for 2 weeks; however, most blood cultures become positive within 5 to 7 days. Determination of the clinical significance of a fungal isolate must be made in consultation with the responsible clinician in the context of the clinical setting of the patient.

IDENTIFYING CHARACTERISTICS OF VARIOUS FUNGI

Determination of the identity of the specific etiologic agent of mycotic disease may have a direct bearing on prognosis and therapeutic considerations. It is becoming clear that a single therapeutic approach, for example, using amphotericin B, is inadequate for many fungal infections (see Chapter 70). The identification of fungal pathogens may have additional diagnostic and epidemiologic implications. Knowing the genus and species of the infecting agent can also provide access to fungal registries and to the literature, where the experiences of others may serve as a guide to the clinical course of infection and response to therapy, especially for the more unusual opportunistic mycoses.

Distinguishing yeast-like fungi from moulds is the first step in identifying a fungal isolate. Gross colony morphology usually provides a good clue because yeast-like fungi form pasty opaque colonies and moulds form large filamentous colonies that vary in texture, color, and topography. Microscopic examination provides further delineation and often is all that is required for identification of many fungi (see Table 71–3). Identification to genus and species, depending on the fungus, requires more detailed microscopic study to delineate characteristic structures. Yeast identification usually requires additional biochemical and physiologic testing, whereas the identification of both yeasts and moulds may be enhanced by specialized immunologic and molecular characterization (see Table 71–3).

The identification of yeast-like fungi to the species level often requires the determination of the biochemical and physiologic profile of the organism in addition to the assessment of the microscopic morphology (see Table 71–3); however, the definitive identification of a mould is based almost entirely on its microscopic morphology. The important features include the shape, method of production, and arrangement of conidia or spores, as well as the size and appearance of the hyphae. The preparation of material for microscopic examination must be done in such a way that produces minimal disruption of the arrangement of the reproductive structures and their conidia or spores. Determination of the presence of melanin and thermal-regulated dimorphism are also important features. Immunologic and/or nucleic acid probe–based tests are often used to identify the endemic dimorphic pathogens, and nucleic aid sequencing is being applied as an aid in the identification of a variety of moulds. The characteristic features of several of the commonly isolated filamentous and dimorphic pathogens are listed in Table 71–3.

Immunologic, Molecular, and Biochemical Markers for Direct Detection of Invasive Fungal Infections

Rapid, sensitive, and specific diagnostic tests for serious fungal infections would allow for more timely and focused application of specific therapeutic measures. As such, tests for the detection of antibodies and antigens, metabolites, and fungus-specific nucleic acids have great appeal. Considerable progress has been made in several of these areas in recent years (Table 71–4) although, with few exceptions, such testing still remains confined to reference laboratories or the research setting.

Determination of antibody and/or antigen titers in serum may be useful in diagnosing fungal infections and, when performed in a serial fashion, also provide a means of monitoring the progression of disease and the patients' response to therapy. With the exception of antibody tests for histoplasmosis and coccidioidomycosis, however, most tests for antibodies lack both the sensitivity and the specificity for diagnosis of invasive fungal infections.

Detection of fungal cell wall and cytoplasmic antigens and metabolites in serum or other body fluids represents the most direct means of providing a serologic diagnosis of invasive fungal infection (see Table 71–4). The best examples of this approach are the commercially available tests for the detection of polysaccharide antigens of *C. neoformans* and *H. capsulatum*. These tests have proved to be of great value in the rapid diagnosis of cryptococcal meningitis and disseminated histoplasmosis, respectively. Immunoassays for detection of *Aspergillus* galactomannan and *Candida* mannan are now commercially available, although the clinical value of these tests remains unclear.

Another fungal-specific cell wall component is β-(1,3)-glucan. This material may be detected in the serum of patients infected with *Candida* and *Aspergillus* through its interaction in the limulus lysate assay. Studies of this test

TABLE 71–4. Antigenic, Biochemical, and Molecular Markers for Direct Detection of Invasive Fungal Infections

Organism	Cell Wall or Capsule Components	Cytoplasmic Antigens	Metabolites	Genomic DNA Sequences*
Candida	Mannans LA RIA EIA β-(1,3)-glucans Limulus test Chitin Spectrophotometry	Enolase EIA Immunoblot Antienolase antibody EIA 47-kD breakdown product of HSP-90 Enzyme-linked dot Immunobinding assay	D-Arabinitol Rapid enzymatic GLC/FID Mass spectroscopy/GLC	Actin gene Chitin synthase gene P450 gene ITS Ribosomal RNA genes
Cryptococcus neoformans	Capsular polysaccharide LA EIA		D-Mannitol Mass spectroscopy GLC	Ribosomal RNA genes ITS URA 5 gene
Aspergillus	Galactomannan LA EIA RIA β-(1,3)-glucans Limulus test Chitin Spectrophotometry		D-Mannitol GLC/FID Mass spectroscopy/GLC	P450 gene Ribosomal RNA genes ITS Alkaline protease gene Mitochondrial genes
Blastomyces dermatitidis	Cell wall RIA for 120-kD cell wall adhesion protein			Ribosomal RNA genes ITS
Histoplasma capsulatum	Cell wall RIA and EIA for polysaccharide antigen			Ribosomal RNA genes ITS
Penicillium marneffei	Cell wall mannoprotein EIA			ITS
Coccidioides immitis				Ribosomal RNA genes

Adapted from Mujeeb I et al: Fungi and fungal infections. In McClatchey KD, editor: *Clinical laboratory medicine,* ed 2, Philadelphia, 2002, Lippincott Williams & Wilkins.

EIA, enzyme immunoassay; FID, flame ionization detector; GLC, gas-liquid chromatography; ITS, internal transcribed spacer region; LA, latex agglutination; P450, C-14 lanosterol demethylase gene; RIA, radioimmunoassay.

*All sequences detected by polymerase chain reaction.

for β-glucan, which indicates the presence of fungi but does not identify the genus causing the infection, have been promising in certain highly selected patient populations.

The detection of fungal metabolites has potential for the rapid diagnosis of both candidiasis and aspergillosis (see Table 71–4). The detection of D-arabinitol in serum appears to be an indication of hematogenously disseminated candidiasis, whereas detection of elevated levels of D-mannitol in bronchoalveolar lavage fluid may be useful in the diagnosis of pulmonary aspergillosis. The diagnostic utility of metabolite detection remains uncertain due to the lack of a commercially available test and problems with method-dependent variability in sensitivity and specificity.

The application of the polymerase chain reaction (PCR) to detect fungal-specific nucleic acids directly in clinical material offers great promise for the rapid diagnosis of fungal infections. A variety of target sequences have been investigated and found to be of potential diagnostic value for most of the more common opportunistic and systemic fungal pathogens (see Table 71–4). Recent developments such as real-time PCR and gene chip technology will facilitate the broad use of this technology, although it is not yet available in most mycology laboratories.

In addition to detection of fungi in clinical material, immunologic and molecular methods have also proved useful in the identification of fungi in culture. Nucleic acid probes are useful in identifying the endemic dimorphic pathogens, and analysis of ribosomal DNA sequences is being applied to both common and uncommon opportunistic yeasts and moulds. Exoantigen immunodiffusion tests are widely applied to identify *H. capsulatum*, *B. dermatitidis*, and *C. immitis*, obviating the need to demonstrate thermal dimorphism in the identification of these agents (see Table 71–3).

QUESTIONS

1. Why is it important to know which fungus is causing a given infection?
2. The laboratory procedure used to identify yeasts differs from that for moulds. How and why?
3. Discuss the different ways that the endemic dimorphic pathogens are identified.
4. What are the advantages of direct microscopic examination of clinical material for the diagnosis of fungal infection?

Bibliography

Merz WG, Roberts GD: Algorithms for detection and identification of fungi. In Murray PR et al, editors: *Manual of clinical microbiology*, ed 8, Washington, 2003, American Society for Microbiology.

Mujeeb I et al: Fungi and fungal infections. In McClatchey KD, editor: *Clinical laboratory medicine*, ed 2, Philadelphia, 2002, Lippincott Williams & Wilkins.

Pfaller MA, McGinnis MR: The laboratory and clinical mycology. In Anaissie EJ, McGinnis MR, Pfaller MA: *Clinical mycology*, New York, 2003, Churchill Livingstone.

Yeo SF, Wong B: Current status of nonculture methods for diagnosis of invasive fungal infections, *Clin Microbiol Rev* 15: 465-484, 2002.

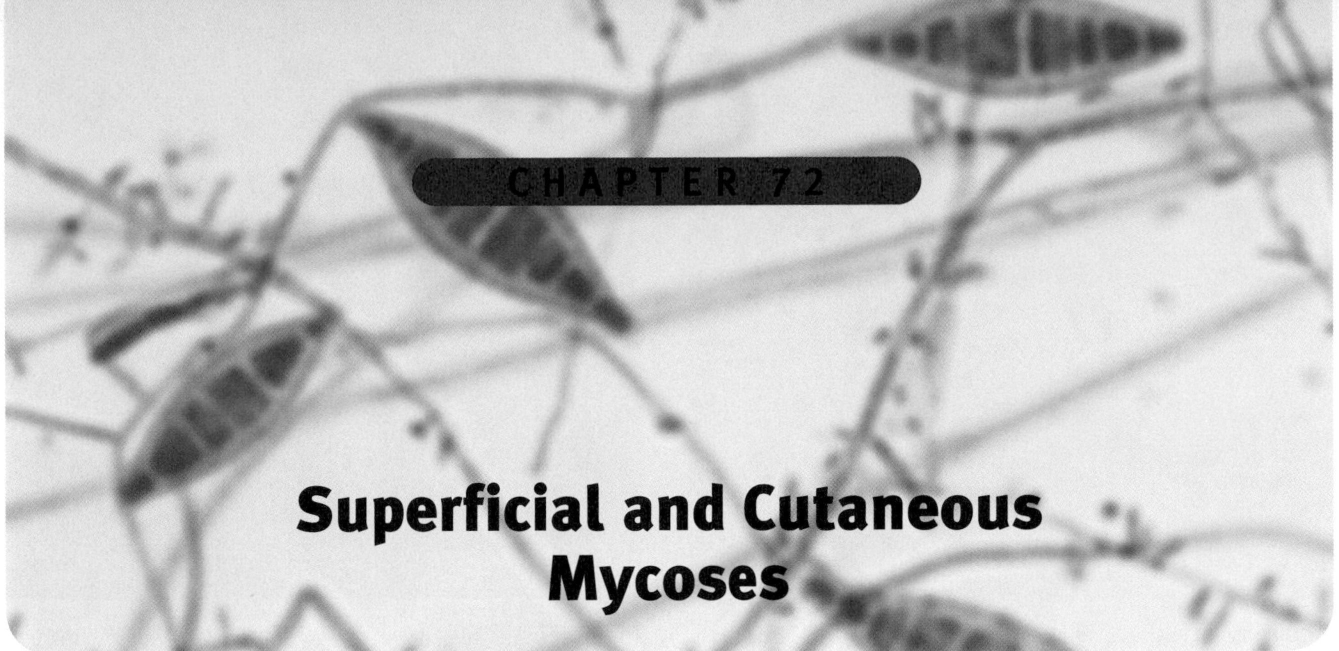

Superficial and Cutaneous Mycoses

Fungal infections of the skin and skin structures are extremely common. These infections are generally categorized by the structures that the fungi colonize or invade:

1. **Superficial mycoses** are limited to the outmost layers of the skin and hair.
2. **Cutaneous mycoses** are infections that involve the deeper layers of the epidermis and its integuments, the hair and nails.
3. **Subcutaneous mycoses** involve the dermis, subcutaneous tissues, muscle, and fascia.

The subcutaneous mycoses will be discussed separately in Chapter 73. This chapter will deal with the superficial and cutaneous mycoses.

Superficial Mycoses

Agents of superficial mycoses are fungi that colonize the keratinized outer layers of the skin, hair, and nails. Infections caused by these organisms elicit little or no host immune response and are nondestructive and thus asymptomatic. They are usually of cosmetic concern only and are easy to diagnosis and treat.

PITYRIASIS (TINEA) VERSICOLOR

Pityriasis versicolor is a common superficial fungal infection that is seen worldwide. In certain tropical environments, it may affect up to 60% of the population. It is caused by the lipophilic yeast *Malassezia furfur*.

Morphology

When viewed in skin scrapings, *M. furfur* appears as clusters of spherical or oval, thick-walled yeastlike cells that are 3 to 8 μm in diameter (Figure 72–1). The yeast cells may be mixed with short, infrequently branched hyphae that tend to orient end to end. The yeastlike cells represent phialoconidia and show polar bud formation with a "lip" or collarette around the point of bud initiation on the parent cell (Figure 72–2). In culture on standard media containing or overlaid with olive oil, *M. furfur* grows as cream-to-tan yeastlike colonies composed of budding yeastlike cells; hyphae are infrequently produced.

Epidemiology

Pityriasis versicolor is a disease of healthy persons that occurs worldwide but is most prevalent in tropical and subtropical regions. Young adults are most commonly affected. *M. furfur* is not found as a saprophyte in nature, and pityriasis versicolor has not been documented in animals. Human infection is thought to result from the direct or indirect transfer of infected keratinous material from one person to another.

Clinical Syndromes

The lesions of pityriasis versicolor are small hypopigmented or hyperpigmented macules. The upper trunk, arms, chest, shoulders, face, and neck are most often involved, but any part of the body can be affected (Figure 72–3). The lesions are irregular, well-demarcated patches of discoloration that can be raised and covered by a fine scale. Because *M. furfur* tends to interfere with melanin production, lesions are hypopigmented in dark-skinned persons. In persons who are light-skinned, the lesions are pink to pale brown and become more obvious when they fail to tan after exposure to sunlight. Little or no host reaction occurs and the lesions are asymptomatic, with the exception of mild pruritus in severe cases. Infection of the hair follicles, resulting in folliculitis, perifolliculitis, and dermal abscesses, is a rare complication of this disease.

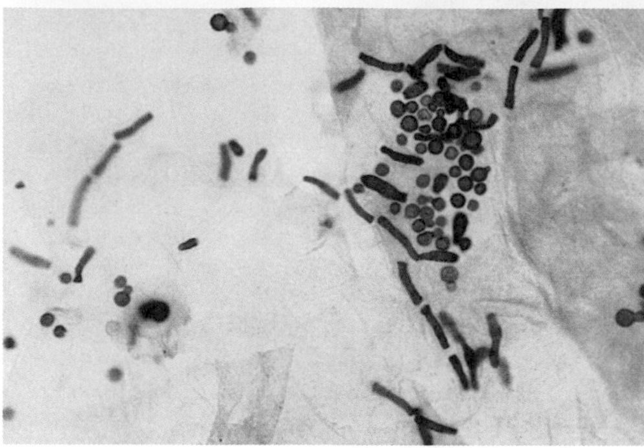

FIGURE 72–1. Pityriasis versicolor. Periodic acid-Schiff–stained skin scraping showing yeastlike cells and short, infrequently branched hyphae that are often oriented end to end (×100). (From Connor DH et al: *Pathology of infectious diseases,* Stamford, Conn, 1997, Appleton & Lange.).

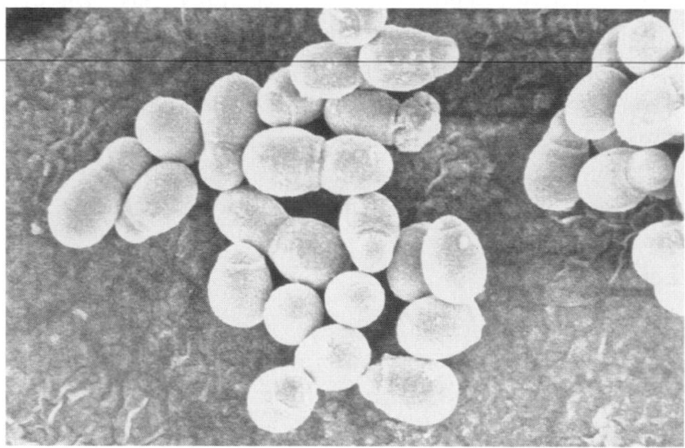

FIGURE 72–2. Scanning electron micrograph of *Malassezia furfur* demonstrating the liplike collarette around the point of bud initiation on the parent cell.

Laboratory Diagnosis

The laboratory diagnosis of pityriasis versicolor is made by the direct visualization of the fungal elements on microscopic examination of epidermal scales in 10% KOH with or without calcofluor white. The organisms are usually numerous and may also be visualized with hematoxylin and eosin (H&E) or periodic acid-Schiff (PAS) stains (see Figure 72–1). The lesions will also fluoresce with a yellowish color on exposure to a Wood's lamp.

Although not usually necessary for establishing the diagnosis, culture can be performed using synthetic mycologic media supplemented with olive oil as a source of lipid. Growth of yeastlike colonies appear after incubation at 30°C for 5 to 7 days. Microscopically, the colonies are composed of budding yeastlike cells with occasional hyphae.

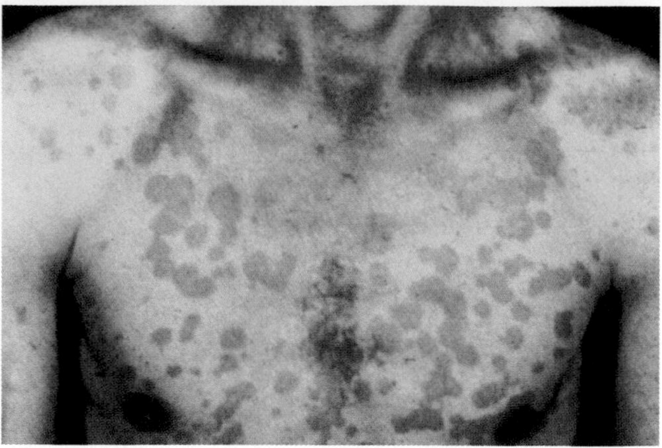

FIGURE 72–3. Pityriasis versicolor. Multiple, pale brown, hyperpigmented patches on chest and shoulders. (From Chandler FW, Watts JC: *Pathologic diagnosis of fungal infections,* Chicago, 1987, ASCP Press. Copyright 1987, American Society of Clinical Pathologists.)

Treatment

Although spontaneous cure has been reported, the disease is generally chronic and persistent. Treatment consists of the use of topical azoles or selenium sulfide shampoo. For more widespread infection, oral ketoconazole or itraconazole can be used.

TINEA NIGRA

Tinea nigra is a superficial phaeohyphomycosis caused by the black fungus, *Hortaea werneckii* (formerly, *Exophiala werneckii*).

Morphology

Microscopically, *H. werneckii* appears as dematiaceous, frequently branched septate hyphae, 1.5 to 3.0 μm wide. Arthroconidia and elongate budding cells are also present (Figure 72–4). *H. werneckii* also grows in culture on standard mycologic media at 25°C, where it is a black mould producing annelloconidia (conidia possessing annelids or rings), which often slide down the sides of the conidiophore.

Epidemiology

Tinea nigra is a tropical or subtropical condition. It is likely contracted by traumatic inoculation of the fungus into the superficial layers of the epidermis. It is most prevalent in Africa, Asia, and Central and South America. Children and young adults are most often affected, with a higher incidence in females.

Clinical Syndromes

Tinea nigra appears as a solitary irregular pigmented (brown to black) macule, usually on the palms or soles

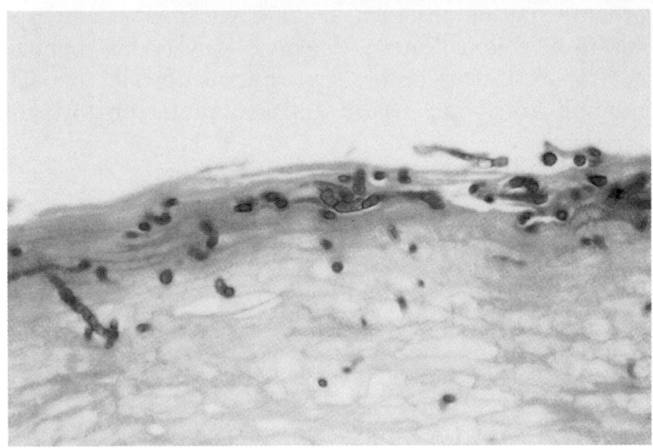

FIGURE 72–4. Tinea nigra. Dematiaceous hyphae of *Hortaea werneckii* (H&E, magnification 100X). (From Connor DH et al: *Pathology of infectious diseases,* Stamford, Conn, 1997, Appleton & Lange.)

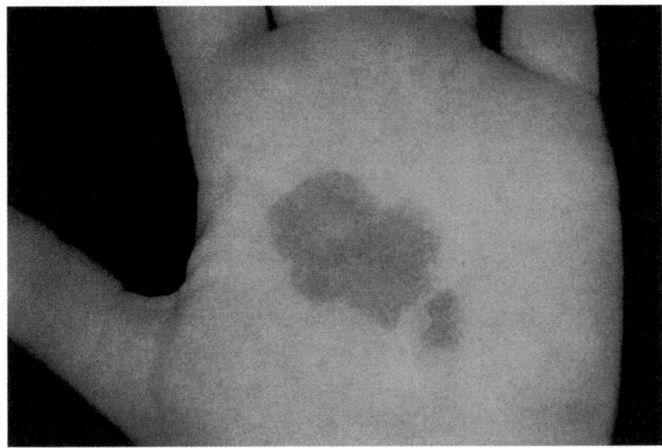

FIGURE 72–5. Tinea nigra. Darkly pigmented macules with irregular edges present on the palm. (From Chandler FW, Watts JC: *Pathologic diagnosis of fungal infections,* Chicago, 1987, ASCP Press. Copyright 1987, American Society of Clinical Pathologists.)

(Figure 72–5). There is no scaling or invasion of hair follicles and the infection is not contagious. Because of its superficial location, there is little or no discomfort or host reaction. Because the lesion grossly may resemble a malignant melanoma, biopsy or local excision may be considered. Such invasive procedures may be avoided by a simple microscopic examination of skin scrapings of the affected area.

Laboratory Diagnosis

Tinea nigra is easily diagnosed by microscopic examination of skin scrapings placed in 10% to 20% KOH. The pigmented hyphae and yeast forms are confined to the outer layers of the stratum corneum and are easily detected on H&E stained sections (see Figure 72–4). Once fungal elements are detected, skin scrapings should be placed on mycologic media with antibiotics. A dematiaceous yeastlike colony should appear within 3 weeks, becoming velvety with age. Microscopic examination reveals two-celled, cylindrical yeastlike cells and, depending on the age of the colony, toruloid hyphae.

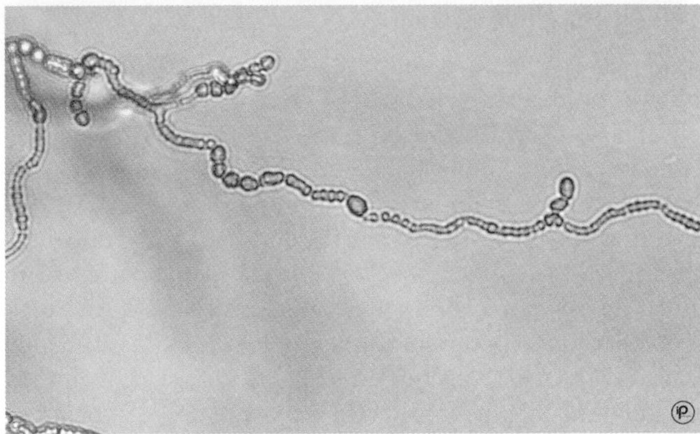

FIGURE 72–6. *Trichosporon* spp. Corn meal agar showing hyphae and arthroconidia (magnification 400X). (From Marler LM et al: *Mycology* CD-ROM, Indiana Pathology Images, 2004.)

Treatment

The infection responds well to topical therapy, including Whitfield's ointment, azole creams, and terbinafine.

WHITE PIEDRA

White piedra is a superficial infection of hair caused by yeastlike fungi of the genus *Trichosporon: T. inkin, T. asahii, T. beigelii,* or *T. mucoides.*

Morphology

Microscopic examination reveals hyphal elements, arthroconidia (rectangular cells resulting from the fragmentation of hyphal cells), and blastoconidia (budding yeast cells) (Figure 72–6).

Epidemiology

This condition occurs in tropical and subtropical regions and is related to poor hygiene.

Clinical Syndromes

White piedra affects the hairs of the groin and axillae. The fungus surrounds the hair shaft and forms a white to brown swelling along the hair strand. The swellings are soft and pasty and may be easily removed by running a section of the hair between the thumb and forefinger. The infection does not damage the hair shaft.

Laboratory Diagnosis

When microscopic examination reveals hyphal elements, arthroconidia, and/or budding yeast cells, infected hair should be placed on mycologic media without cycloheximide (cycloheximide will inhibit *Trichosporon* spp.). *Trichosporon* spp. will form cream-colored, dry, wrinkled colonies within 48 to 72 hours of incubation at room temperature. The various species of *Trichosporon* can be identified in the same manner as other yeast isolates. Sugar assimilations, potassium nitrate (KNO_3) assimilation (negative), urease production (positive) and morphology on corn meal agar (both arthroconidia and blastoconidia are present) should be determined.

Treatment

Treatment can be accomplished with topical azoles; however, improved hygiene and shaving of the infected hair are also effective and usually negate the necessity of medical treatment.

BLACK PIEDRA

Another condition affecting the hair, primarily the scalp, is black piedra. The causative agent of black piedra is *Piedraia hortae.*

Morphology

The organism grows as pigmented (brown to reddish-black) mould. As the culture ages, asci containing spindle-shaped ascospores are formed within specialized structures. These structures (asci and ascospores) are also produced within the rock hard hyphal mass that surrounds the hair shaft.

Epidemiology

Black piedra is uncommon and has been reported from tropical areas in Latin America and Central Africa. It is thought to be a condition of poor hygiene.

Clinical Syndromes

Black piedra presents as small dark nodules that surround the hair shafts. It is asymptomatic and generally involves the scalp. The hyphal mass is held together by a cementlike substance and contains asci and ascospores, the sexual phase of the fungus.

Laboratory Diagnosis

Examination of the nodule reveals branched, pigmented hyphae held together by a cementlike substance. *P. hortae* can be cultured on routine mycologic media. Very slow growth may be observed at 25°C and may begin as a yeastlike colony, later becoming velvety as hyphae develop. Asci can be observed microscopically, usually ranging from 4 to 30 µm and containing up to eight ascospores.

Treatment

Treatment of black piedra is easily accomplished by a haircut and proper regular washings.

Cutaneous Mycoses

The cutaneous mycoses include infections caused by dermatophytic fungi (dermatophytosis) and nondermatophytic fungi (dermatomycosis) (Table 72–1). Because of the overwhelming importance of dermatophytes as etiologic agents of cutaneous mycoses, the majority of this section will deal with those fungi. The nondermatophytic fungi will be discussed regarding their role in onychomycosis. The superficial and cutaneous infections caused by *Candida* spp. will be discussed in Chapter 75.

DERMATOPHYTOSES

The term *dermatophytosis* refers to a complex of diseases caused by any of several species of taxonomically related filamentous fungi in the genera *Trichophyton, Epidermophyton,* and *Microsporum* (Tables 72–1 to 72–3). These fungi are known collectively as the dermatophytes, and all possess the ability to cause disease in humans, animals, or both. All have in common the ability to invade the skin, hair, or nails. In each case, these fungi are keratinophilic and keratinolytic and so are able to break down the keratin surfaces of these structures. In the case of skin infections the dermatophytes invade only the upper, outermost layer of the epidermis, the stratum corneum. Penetration below the granular layer of the epidermis is rare. Likewise with hair and nails, being part of the skin, only the keratinized layers are invaded. The various forms of dermatophytosis are referred to as “tineas” or ringworm. Clinically, the tineas are classified according to the anatomic site or structure affected: (1) tinea capitis of the scalp, eyebrows, and eyelashes; (2) tinea barbae of the beard; (3) tinea corporis of the smooth or glabrous skin; (4) tinea cruris of the groin; (5) tinea pedis of the foot; (6) tinea unguium of the nails (also known as *onychomycosis*). The clinical signs and symptoms of dermatophytosis vary according to the etiologic agents, the host reaction, and the site of infection.

Morphology

Each genus of dermatophytic mould is characterized by a specific pattern of growth in culture and by the

TABLE 72–1. Common and Uncommon Agents of Superficial and Cutaneous Dermatomycoses and Dermatophytoses

Fungus	Type of Infection									
	TP	TCO	TCR	TCA	TBA	TVR	O	TN	BP	WP
Dermatophytic										
Trichophyton rubrum	X	X	X				X			
T. mentagrophytes	X	X	X	X			X			
T. tonsurans		X		X			X			
T. verrucosum		X		X	X					
T. equinum				X						
T. violaceum				X						
T. schoenleinii				X						
T. megninii							X			
Epidermophyton floccosum	X		X				X			
Microsporum canis		X		X						
M. audouinii				X						
Nondermatophytic										
Scopulariopsis brevicaulis							X			
Scytalidium spp.	X						X			
Malassezia spp.						X				
Candida albicans	X						X			
Aspergillus terreus							X			
Acremonium spp.							X			
Fusarium spp.							X			
Trichosporon spp.										X
Piedraia hortae									X	
Hortaea werneckii								X		

BP, Black piedra; O, onychomycosis; TBA, tinea barbae; TCA, tinea capitis; TCO, tinea corporis; TCR, tinea cruris; TN, tinea nigra; TP, tinea pedis; TVR, tinea versicolor; WP, white piedra; X, etiologic agents of.

production of macroconidia and microconidia (see Table 72–2). Further identification to species level requires consideration of colony morphology, spore production, and nutritional requirements in vitro.

Microscopically, the genus *Microsporum* is identified by observation of its macroconidia, whereas microconidia are the characteristic structures of the genus *Trichophyton* (see Table 72–2). *Epidermophyton floccosum* does not produce microconidia, but its smooth-walled macroconidia borne in clusters of two or three are quite distinctive (Figure 72–7). *Microsporum canis* produces characteristic large, multicellular (5 to 8 cells per conidium), thick- and rough-walled macroconidia (Figure 72–8). *Trichophyton rubrum* produces teardrop- or peg-shaped microconidia borne rough along the sides of hyphae (Figure 72–9), whereas *T. mentagrophytes* produces both single cigar-shaped macroconidia and grapelike clusters of spherical microconidia (Figure 72–10). *T. tonsurans* produces variably sized and shaped microconidia, with relatively large spherical conidia often located right alongside of small, parallel-walled conidia and other microconidia of various size and shapes (Figure 72–11).

In skin biopsies, all of the dermatophytes are morphologically similar and appear as hyaline septate hyphae, chains of arthroconidia, or dissociated chains of arthroconidia that invade the stratum corneum, hair follicles, and hairs. When the hair is infected, the pattern of fungal invasion can be either **ectothrix, endothrix,** or **favic**

TABLE 72–2. Characteristic In Vitro and In Vivo Features of Dermatophytes

Genus	In vitro		In vivo hair	
	Macroconidia	Microconidia	Invasion	Fluorescence*
Epidermophyton	Smooth-walled, borne in clusters of two or three	Absent	NA	NA
Microsporum	Numerous, large, thick- and rough-walled†	Rare	Ectothrix	+/–‡
Trichophyton	Rare, smooth, thin walled	Numerous, spherical, teardrop- or peg-shaped§	Endothrix‖	+/–¶

NA, Not applicable.
*Fluorescence with Wood's lamp.
†Except *M. audouinii.*
‡*M. gypseum* not fluorescent.
§Except *T. schoenleinii.*
‖*T. verrucosum*, ectothrix; *T. schoenleinii*, favic.
¶*T. schoenleinii* is fluorescent.

TABLE 72–3. Classification of Dermatophytes According to Ecologic Niche

Ecologic Niche	Species	Principal Hosts	Geographic Distribution	Prevalence
Anthropophilic	*Epidermophyton floccosum*		Worldwide	Common
	Microsporum audouinii		Worldwide	Common
	Microsporum ferrugineum		Africa, Asia	Endemic
	Trichophyton concentricum		Asia, Pacific Islands	Endemic
	Trichophyton megninii		Europe, Africa	Endemic
	Trichophyton mentagrophytes var *interdigitale*		Worldwide	Common
	Trichophyton rubrum		Worldwide	Common
	Trichophyton schoenleinii		Europe, Africa	Endemic
	Trichophyton soudanense		Africa	Endemic
	Trichophyton tonsurans		Worldwide	Common
	Trichophyton violaceum		Europe, Africa, Asia	Common
Zoophilic	*Microsporum canis*	Cat, dog, horse	Worldwide	Common
	Microsporum gallinae	Fowl	Worldwide	Rare
	Microsporum nanum	Swine	Worldwide	Rare
	Microsporum persicolor	Vole	Europe, USA	Rare
	Trichophyton equinum	Horse	Worldwide	Rare
	Trichophyton mentagrophytes			
	var *mentagrophytes*	Rodent	Worldwide	Common
	var *erinacei*	Hedgehog	Europe, New Zealand, Africa	Occasional
	var *quinckeanum*	Mouse	Worldwide	Rare
	Trichophyton simii	Monkey	India	Occasional
	Trichophyton verrucosum	Cow	Worldwide	Common
	Microsporum gypseum		Worldwide	Occasional
	Microsporum fulvum		Worldwide	Occasional

Adapted from Hiruma M, Yamaguchi H: Dermatophytes. In Anaissie EJ, McGinnis MR, Pfaller MA, editors: *Clinical mycology,* New York, 2003, Churchill Livingstone.

depending on the dermatophytic species (Figure 72–12). Septate hyphae may be seen within the hair shaft in all three patterns. In the ectothrix pattern, **arthroconidia** are formed on the outside of the hair (Figures 72–12 and 72–13); in the endothrix pattern, arthroconidia are formed inside the hair (see Figure 72–12); and in the favic pattern, hyphae, arthroconidia and empty spaces resembling air bubbles ("honeycomb" pattern) are formed inside the hair and at the root of the hair shaft (see Figure 72–12). The dermatophytes can usually be seen on H&E

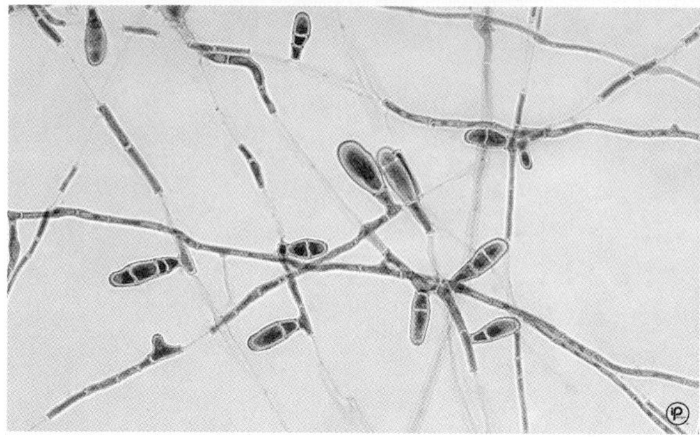

FIGURE 72–7. *Epidermophyton floccosum*, lactophenol cotton blue showing smooth-walled macroconidia (magnification 400×). (From Marler LM et al: *Mycology* CD-ROM, Indiana Pathology Images, 2004.)

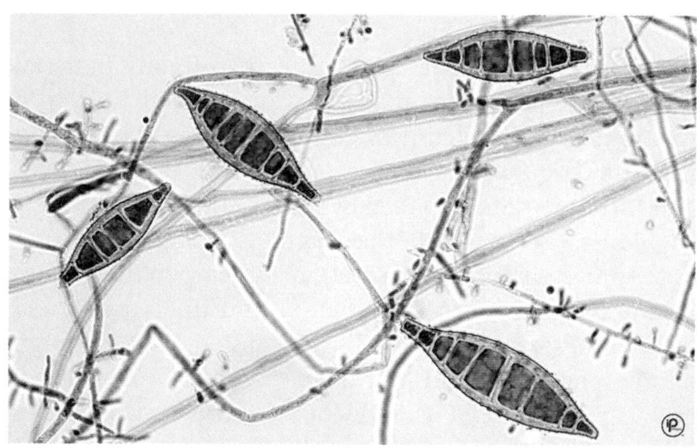

FIGURE 72–8. *Microsporum canis*, lactophenol cotton blue showing rough-walled macroconidia and microconidia (magnification 400×). (From Marler LM et al: *Mycology* CD-ROM, Indiana Pathology Images, 2004.)

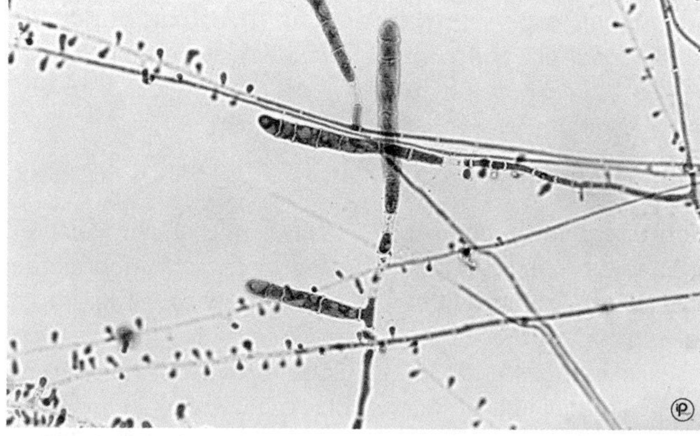

FIGURE 72–9. *Trichophyton rubrum*, lactophenol cotton blue showing teardrop- and peg-shaped microconidia and multicelled macrocondia (magnification 500×). (From Marler LM et al: *Mycology* CD-ROM, Indiana Pathology Images, 2004.).

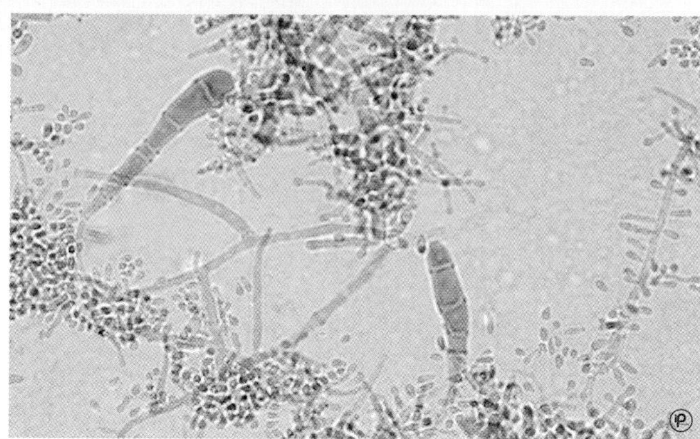

FIGURE 72–10. *Trichophyton mentagrophytes*, lactophenol cotton blue showing cigar-shaped macroconidia and grapelike clusters of microconidia (magnification 400×). (From Marler LM et al: *Mycology* CD-ROM, Indiana Pathology Images, 2004.)

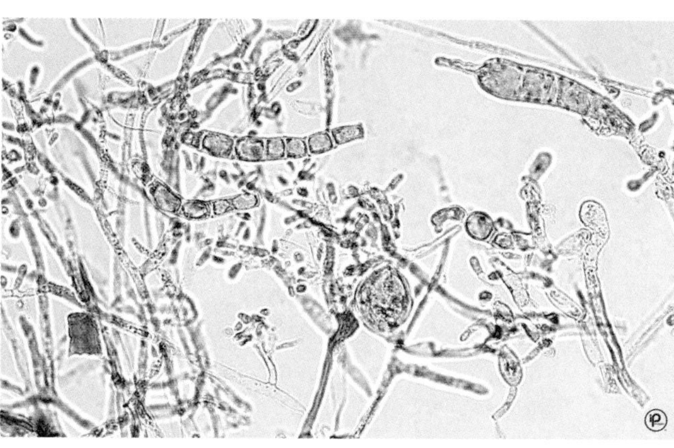

FIGURE 72–11. *Trichophyton tonsurans*, lactophenol cotton blue showing microconidia, macroconidia, and arthroconidia (magnification 400×). (From Marler LM et al: *Mycology* CD-ROM, Indiana Pathology Images, 2004.)

stain; however, they are best with special stains for fungi such as GMS and PAS (see Figure 72–13).

Ecology and Epidemiology

Dermatophytes can be classified into three different categories based on their natural habitat (see Table 72–3): (1) geophilic, (2) zoophilic, and (3) anthropophilic. The geophilic dermatophytes live in the soil and are occasional pathogens of both animals and humans. Zoophilic dermatophytes normally parasitize the hair and skin of animals but can be transmitted to humans. Anthropophilic dermatophytes generally infect humans and can be transmitted directly, or indirectly, from person to person. This classification is quite useful prognostically and emphasizes the importance of identifying the etiologic agent of dermatophytoses. Species of dermatophytes that are considered anthropophilic tend to cause chronic,

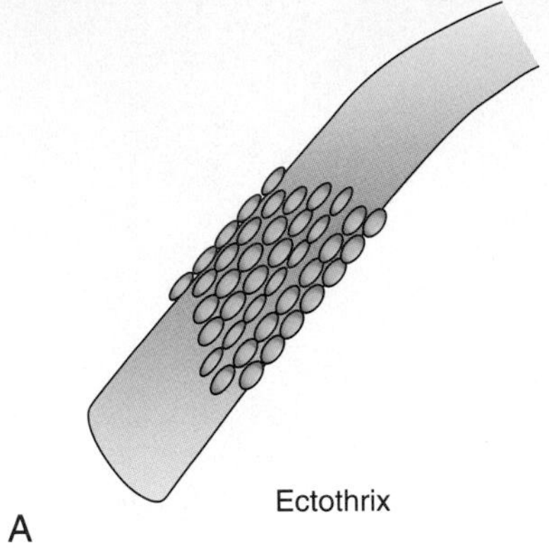

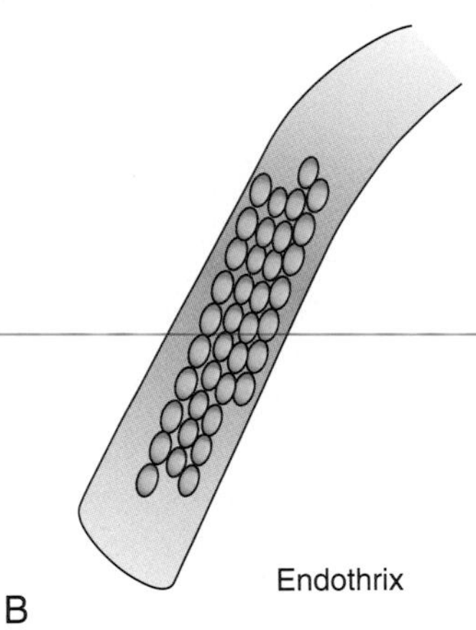

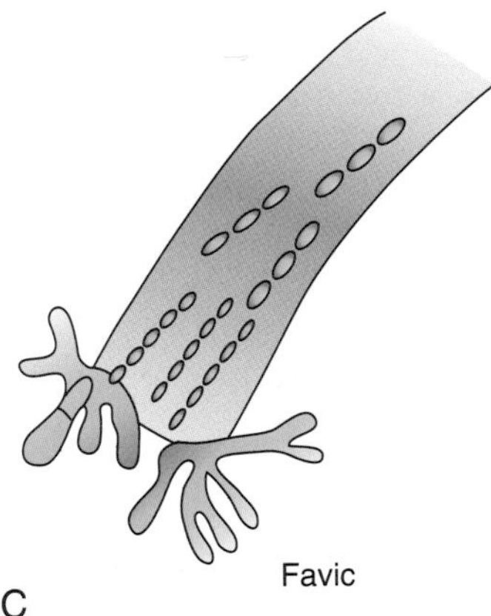

FIGURE 72–12. Schematic of **(A)** ectothrix hair infection, **(B)** endothrix hair infection, and **(C)** favic hair infection.

relatively noninflammatory infections that are difficult to cure. In contrast, the zoophilic and geophilic dermatophytes tend to elicit a profound host reaction causing lesions that are highly inflammatory and respond well to therapy. In some instances these infections heal spontaneously.

The dermatophytes are worldwide in distribution (see Table 72–3) and infection can be acquired from the transfer of arthroconidia or hyphae, or keratinous material containing these elements, from an infected host to a susceptible, uninfected host. Dermatophytes may remain viable in desquamated skin scales or hair for long periods, and infection can be either by direct contact or indirect via fomites. Persons of both sexes and all ages are susceptible to dermatophytosis; however, tinea capitis is more common in prepubescent children and tinea cruris and tinea pedis are primarily diseases of adult males. Although dermatomycoses occur worldwide, especially in tropical and subtropical regions, individual dermatophyte species may vary in their geographic distribution and in their virulence for humans (see Table 72–3). For example, *Trichophyton concentricum*, the cause of tinea imbricata, is confined to the islands of the South Pacific and Asia, whereas *T. tonsurans* has replaced *Microsporum audouinii* as the principal agent of tinea capitis in the United States. Infections caused by dermatophytes are generally endemic but may assume epidemic proportions in selected settings (e.g., tinea capitis in schoolchildren). On a worldwide scale, *T. rubrum* and *T. mentagrophytes* account for 80% to 90% of all dermatophytoses.

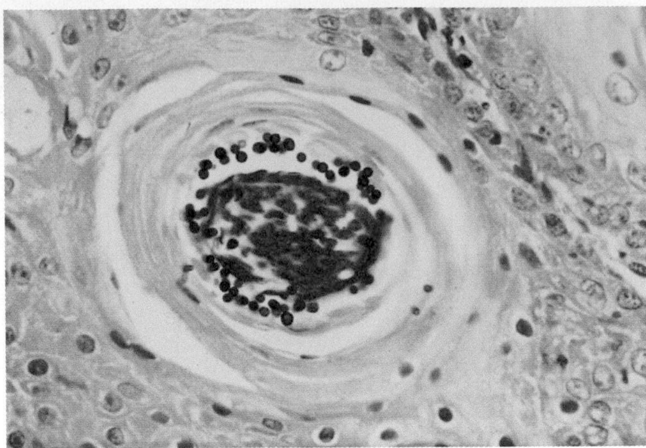

FIGURE 72–13. Arthroconidia surrounding a hair shaft. Ectothrix hair infection caused by *Microsporum canis* (GMS-H&E, magnification 160×). (From Connor DH et al: Pathology of infectious diseases. Stamford, Conn, 1997, Appleton & Lange.)

Clinical Syndromes

Dermatophytoses manifest a wide range of clinical presentations, which may be affected by factors such as the species of dermatophytes, the inoculum size, the site of infection, and the immune status of the host. Any given disease manifestation may result from several different species of dermatophytes as shown in Table 72–1.

The classic pattern of dermatophytosis is the "ringworm" pattern of a ring of inflammatory scaling with diminution of inflammation toward the center of the lesion. Tineas of hair-bearing areas often present as raised

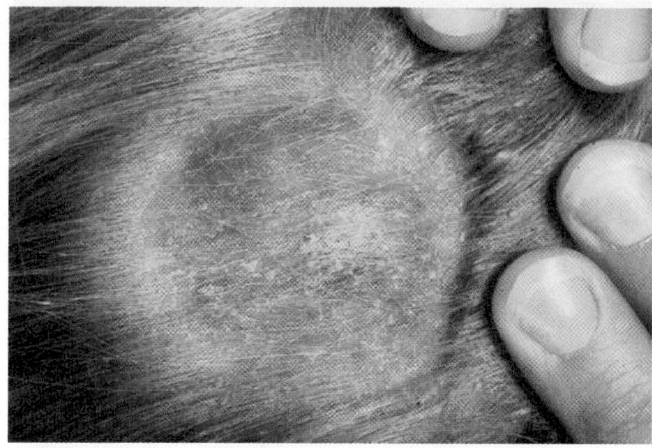

FIGURE 72–14. Tinea capitis caused by *Microsporum canis.* (From Hay RJ: Cutaneous and subcutaneous mycoses. In Anaissie EJ, McGinnis MR, Pfaller MA, editors: *Clinical mycology,* New York, 2003, Churchill Livingstone.)

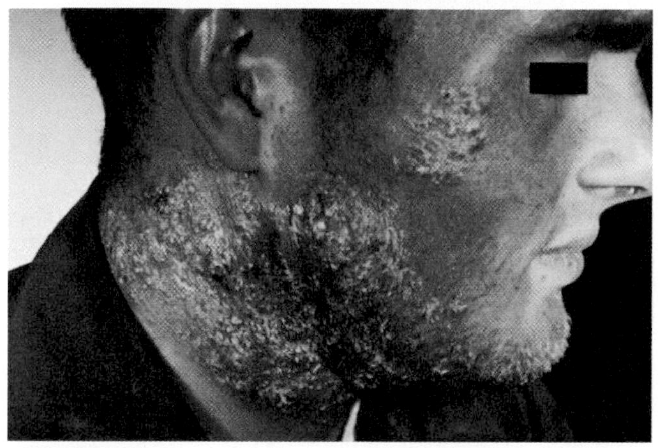

FIGURE 72–15. Tinea barbae caused by *Trichophyton verrucosum.* (From Chandler FW, Watts JC: *Pathologic diagnosis of fungal infections,* Chicago, 1987, ASCP Press. Copyright 1987, American Society of Clinical Pathologists.)

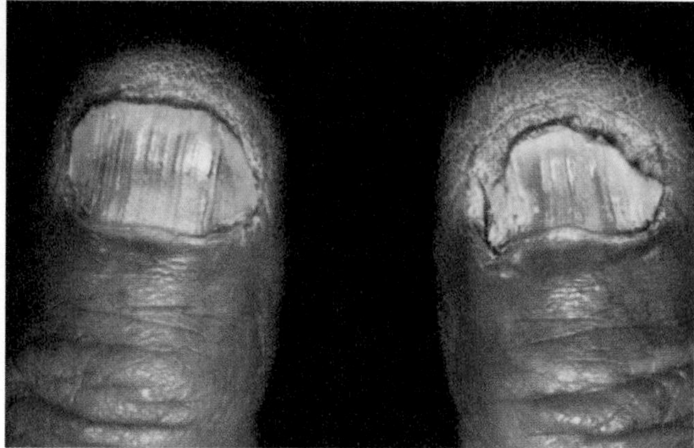

FIGURE 72–16. Onychomycosis caused by *Trichophyton rubrum.* (From Hay RJ: Cutaneous and subcutaneous mycoses. In Anaissie EJ, McGinnis MR, Pfaller MA, editors: *Clinical mycology,* New York, 2003, Churchill Livingstone.)

circular patches of alopecia with erythema and scaling (Figure 72–14) or as more diffusely scattered papules, pustules, vesicles, and kerions (severe inflammation involving the hair shaft) (Figure 72–15). Hairs infected with certain species, such as *M. canis, M. audouinii,* and *Trichophyton schoenleinii,* often fluoresce yellow-green when exposed to Wood's light (see Table 72–2). Infections of smooth skin commonly present as erythematous and scaling patches that expand in centripetal pattern with central clearing. Dermatophytoses of the foot and hand may often become complicated by onychomycosis (Figure 72–16), in which the nail plate is invaded and destroyed by the fungus. Onychomycosis is caused by a variety of dermatophytes (see Table 72–1) and is estimated to affect approximately 3% of the population in most temperate countries. It is a disease seen mostly in adults, with toenails affected more commonly than fingernails. The infection is usually chronic and the nails become thickened, discolored, raised, friable, and deformed (see Figure 72–16). *T. rubrum* is the most common etiologic agent in most countries. A rapidly progressive form of onychomycosis that originates from the proximal nailfold and involves the upper and under side of the nail is seen in AIDS patients.

Laboratory Diagnosis

The laboratory diagnosis of dermatophytoses relies on the demonstration of fungal hyphae by direct microscopy of skin, hair, or nail samples and the isolation of organisms in culture. Specimens are mounted in a drop of 10% to 20% KOH on a glass slide and examined microscopically. Filamentous, hyaline hyphal elements characteristic of dermatophytes may be seen in skin scrapings, nail scrapings, and hairs. Calcofluor white has been used in examining specimens for fungal elements with excellent results.

Cultures are always useful and can be obtained by scraping the affected areas and placing the skin, hair, or nail clippings onto standard mycologic media such as Sabouraud's agar, with and without antibiotics, or dermatophyte test medium. Colonies develop within 7 to 28 days. Their gross and microscopic appearance and nutritional requirements can be used in identification.

Treatment

Dermatophytic infections that are localized and do not affect hair or nails can usually be treated effectively with topical agents; all others require oral therapy. Topical agents include azoles (miconazole, clotrimazole, econazole, tioconazole, and itraconazole), terbinafine, and haloprogin. Whitfield's ointment (benzoic and salicylic acids) is an optional agent for dermatophytosis, but responses are usually slower than those seen with agents with specific antifungal activity.

Oral antifungal agents with systemic activity against dermatophytes include griseofulvin, itraconazole, fluconazole, and terbinafine. The azoles and terbinafine are more rapidly and broadly efficacious than griseofulvin, especially for the treatment of onychomycosis.

ONYCHOMYCOSIS CAUSED BY NONDERMATOPHYTIC FUNGI

A number of nondermatophytic moulds and *Candida* species have been associated with nail infections (see Table 72–1). These organisms include *Scopulariopsis brevicaulis, Scytalidium dimidiatum, Scytalidium hyalinum,* and a variety of others including *Aspergillus, Fusarium,* and *Candida* spp. Among these organisms, *S. brevicaulis* and *Scytalidium* spp. are proven nail pathogens. The other fungi certainly may be the cause of nail pathology; however, the interpretation of nail cultures with these organisms should be done with caution because they may simply represent saprophytic colonization of abnormal nail material. Criteria used to determine an etiologic role for these fungi include isolation on multiple occasions and the presence of abnormal hyphal or conidial structures on microscopic examination of nail material.

Infections caused by *S. brevicaulis, S. dimidiatum,* and *S. hyalinum* are notoriously difficult to treat because they are not usually susceptible to any antifungal agents. Partial surgical removal of infected nails coupled with oral itraconazole or terbinafine or intensive treatment with 5% amorolfine nail lacquer or Whitfield's ointment may be useful in achieving a clinical response.

CASE STUDY AND QUESTIONS

Darrell, a 24-year-old medical student, just loves his new bulldog puppy Delbert. He recently purchased Delbert from a local "backyard" breeder. Darrell has taken to giving Delbert frequent smooches on his muzzle, which Delbert loves because he knows a treat is soon to follow. After approximately 3 months of proud puppy ownership and smooching, Darrell noticed that his mustache began itching and his upper lip was beginning to swell. Over a 1-week period, his upper lip became swollen and inflamed, and small pustular areas became apparent among the sparse hairs of his moustache. Similar changes were also becoming apparent on Delbert's muzzle. This concerned Darrell, so he promptly took Delbert to the vet. The vet took one look at the pair, wrote a prescription for Delbert, and told Darrell that he should make a visit to the dermatologist.

1. What was the likely cause of Darrell/Delbert's affliction? Be specific.
2. How would you go about making a diagnosis?
3. How would you go about treating this infection?
4. Who gave what to whom?

Bibliography

Chandler FW, Watts JC: *Pathologic diagnosis of fungal infections,* Chicago, 1987, ASCP Press.

Hay RJ: Cutaneous and subcutaneous mycoses. In Anaissie EJ, McGinnis MR, Pfaller MA, editors: *Clinical mycology,* New York, 2003, Churchill Livingstone.

Hiruma M, Yamaguchi H: Dermatophytes. In Anaissie EJ, McGinnis MR, Pfaller MA, editors: *Clinical mycology,* New York, 2003, Churchill Livingstone.

Mujeeb I et al: Fungi and fungal infections. In McClatchy KD, editor: *Clinical laboratory medicine,* ed 2, Philadelphia, 2002, Lippincott Williams & Wilkins.

Richardson MD, Warnock DW, Campbell CK: Slide atlas of fungal infection, London, 1995, Blackwell Science, Ltd.

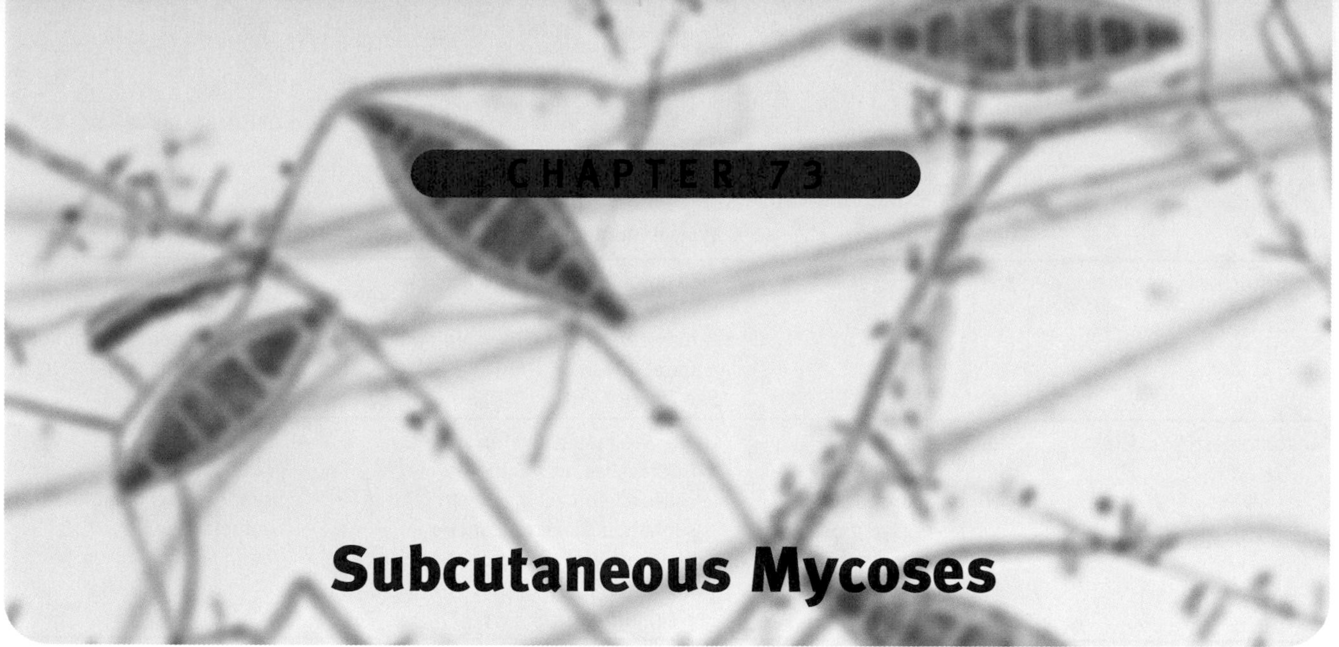

Subcutaneous Mycoses

Many fungal pathogens can produce subcutaneous lesions as part of their disease processes; however, certain fungi are commonly introduced traumatically through the skin and have a propensity to involve the deeper layers of the dermis, subcutaneous tissue, and bone. Although they may ultimately present clinically as lesions on the skin surface, they rarely spread to distant organs. In general, the clinical course is chronic and insidious, and, once established, the infections are refractory to most antifungal therapy. The main subcutaneous fungal infections include lymphocutaneous sporotrichosis, chromoblastomycosis, eumycotic mycetoma, subcutaneous zygomycosis, and subcutaneous phaeohyphomycosis. Two additional subcutaneous fungal or fungal-like processes, lobomycosis and rhinosporidiosis, are discussed separately in Chapter 76.

Although lymphocutaneous sporotrichosis is caused by a single fungal pathogen, *Sporothrix schenckii*, the other subcutaneous mycoses are clinical syndromes caused by multiple fungal etiologies (Table 73–1). The causative agents of subcutaneous mycoses are generally considered to have low pathogenic potential and are commonly isolated from soil, wood, or decaying vegetation. Exposure is largely occupational or related to hobbies (e.g., gardening, wood gathering). Infected patients generally have no underlying immune defect.

Lymphocutaneous Sporotrichosis

Lymphocutaneous sporotrichosis is caused by *S. schenckii*, a dimorphic fungus that is ubiquitous in soil and decaying vegetation. Infection with this organism is chronic and is characterized by nodular and ulcerative lesions that develop along lymphatics that drain the primary site of inoculation (Figure 73–1). Dissemination to the other sites such as bones, eyes, lungs, and central nervous system is extremely rare (<1% of all cases) and will not be discussed further here. At room temperature, *S. schenckii* grows as a mould (Figure 73–2) at 37°C and in tissue it is a pleomorphic yeast (Table 73–1 and Figure 73–3).

MORPHOLOGY

S. schenckii is thermally dimorphic. Mycelial form cultures grow rapidly and have a wrinkled membranous surface that gradually becomes tan, brown, or black. Microscopically, the mould form consists of narrow, hyaline, septate hyphae that produce abundant oval conidia (2×3 μm to 3×6 μm) borne on delicate sterigmata or in a rosette or "daisy petal" formation on conidiophores (see Figure 73–2). The yeast form consists of spherical, oval, or elongated ("cigar-shaped") yeast-like cells, 2 to 10 μm in diameter, with single or (rarely) multiple buds (see Table 73–1 and Figure 73–3). These forms are rarely seen on histopathologic examination of tissue.

EPIDEMIOLOGY

Sporotrichosis is usually sporadic and is most common in warmer climates. The major known areas of current endemicity are in Japan and in North and South America, especially Mexico, Brazil, Uruguay, Peru, and Colombia. Outbreaks of infection related to forest work, mining, and gardening have occurred. Classic infection is associated with traumatic inoculation of soil, vegetable, or organic matter contaminated with the fungus. Zoonotic transmission has been reported in armadillo hunters and in association with infected cats. A recent outbreak of cat-transmitted sporotrichosis involving 178 patients between 1998 and 2001 was reported from Rio de Janeiro, Brazil.

TABLE 73–1. Common Agents of Subcutaneous Mycoses

Disease	Etiologic Agent(s)	Typical Morphology in Tissue	Usual Host Reaction
Sporotrichosis	*Sporothrix schenckii*	Pleomorphic, spherical to oval or cigar-shaped yeasts, 2–10 µm diameter with single or multiple (rare) buds. See Figure 73–3.	Mixed suppurative and granulomatous Splendore-Hoeppli material surrounds fungus (asteroid body) See Figure 73–4.
Chromoblastomycosis	*Cladophialophora* (*Cladosporium*) *carrionii Fonsecaea compacta F. pedrosoi* *Phialophora verrucosa* *Rhinocladiella* sp. *Exophiala* spp.	Large, 6–12 µm diameter, spherical, thick-walled, brown muriform cells (sclerotic bodies) with septations along one or two planes; pigmented hyphae may be present. See Figure 73–6.	Mixed suppurative and granulomatous; pseudoepitheliomatous hyperplasia
Eumycotic mycetoma	*Acremonium* spp. *Fusarium* spp. *Aspergillus nidulans* *Scedosporium apiospermum* *Madurella* spp. *Exophiala jeanselmei* Among others	Granules, 0.2 to several mm diameter, composed of broad (2–6 µm), hyaline (pale granules) or dematiaceous (black granules) septate hyphae that branch and form chlamydoconidia See Figure 73–7.	Suppurative with multiple abscesses, fibrosis and sinus tracts; Splendore-Hoeppli material
Subcutaneous zygomycosis	*Basidiobolus ranarum* (*haptosporus*) *Conidiobolus coronatus*	Short, poorly stained hyphal fragments, 6–25 µm diameter, nonparallel sides, pausi-septate, random branches See Figure 73–10.	Eosinophilic abscesses and granulation tissue; Splendore-Hoeppli material around hyphae
Subcutaneous phaeohyphomycosis	*Exophiala jeanselmei* *Wangiella dermatitidis* *Bipolaris* spp. *Alternaria* spp. *Chaetomium* spp. *Curvularia* spp. *Phialophora* spp. Others	Pigmented (brown) hyphae, 2–6 µm diameter branched or unbranched, often constricted at prominent septations; yeast forms and chlamydoconidia may be present See Figure 73–11.	Subcutaneous cystic or solid granulomas; overlying epidermis rarely affected

Data from Chandler FW, Watts JC: *Pathologic diagnosis of fungal infections,* Chicago, 1987, ASCP Press; and Hay RJ: Cutaneous and subcutaneous mycoses. In Anaissie EJ, McGinnis MR, Pfaller MA, editors: *Clinical mycology,* New York, 2003, Churchill Livingstone.

CLINICAL SYNDROMES

Lymphangitic sporotrichosis classically appears after local trauma to an extremity. The initial site of infection appears as a small nodule that may ulcerate. Secondary lymphatic nodules appear about 2 weeks after the appearance of the primary lesion and consist of a linear chain of painless, subcutaneous nodules that extend proximally along the course of lymphatic drainage of the primary lesion (see Figure 73–1). With time, the nodules may ulcerate and discharge pus. Primary cutaneous lesions may remain "fixed" without lymphangitic spread. Clinically these lesions appear nodular, verrucous, or ulcerative and grossly may resemble a malignant process such as squamous cell carcinoma. Other infectious causes of lymphangitic and ulcerative lesions that must be ruled out include mycobacterial and nocardial infections.

LABORATORY DIAGNOSIS

Definitive diagnosis usually requires culture of infected pus or tissue. *S. schenckii* grows within 2 to 5 days on a variety of mycologic media and appears as a budding yeast at 35°C and as a mould at 25°C (see Figures 73–2 and 73–3). Laboratory confirmation can be established by converting the mycelial growth to the yeast form by subculture at 37°C or immunologically through the use of the exoantigen test. In tissue, the organism appears as a 2- to 10-µm pleomorphic budding yeast (see Figure 73–3) but

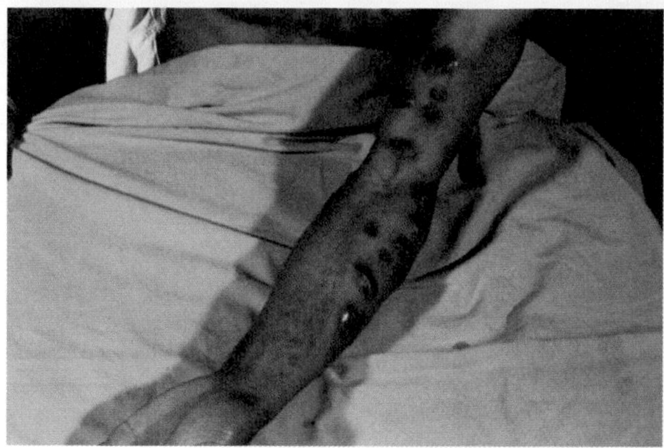

FIGURE 73–1. Classic lymphocutaneous form of sporotrichosis demonstrating a chain of subcutaneous nodules along the lymphatic drainage of the arm. (From Chandler FW, Watts JC: *Pathologic diagnosis of fungal infections,* Chicago, 1987, ASCP Press. Copyright 1987, American Society of Clinical Pathologists.)

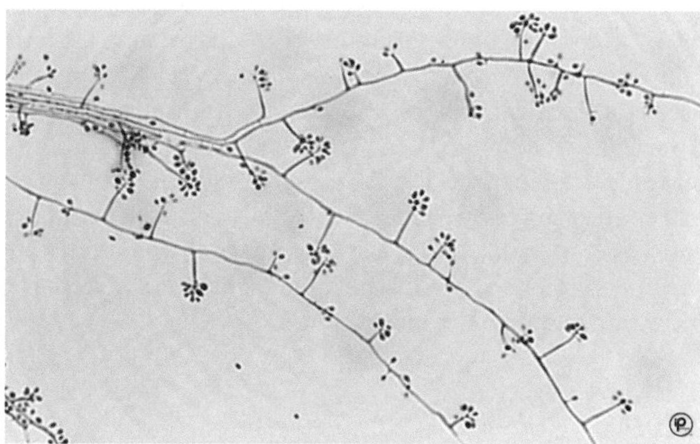

FIGURE 73–2. Mould phase of *Sporothrix schenckii.* (From Marler LM, Siders JA, Simpson AI, Allen SD: *Mycology* CD-Rom, Indiana Pathology Images, 2004.)

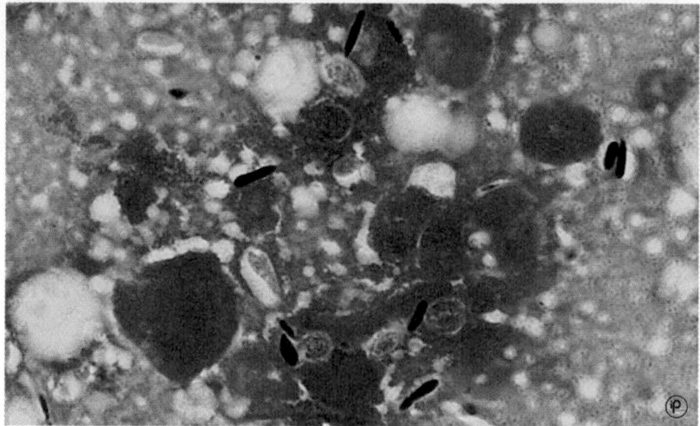

FIGURE 73–3. Yeast phase of *Sporothrix schenckii* in tissue (Gram stain, magnification 1000×). (From Marler LM, Siders JA, Simpson AI, Allen SD: *Mycology* CD-Rom, Indiana Pathology Images, 2004.)

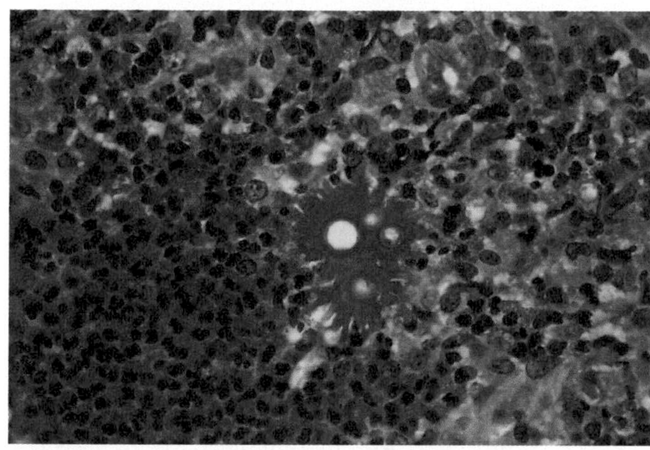

FIGURE 73–4. Asteroid body in sporotrichosis. Three spherical yeast-like cells are surrounded by Splendore-Hoeppli material (H&E, magnification 160×). (From Connor DH et al: *Pathology of infectious diseases,* Stamford, Conn, 1997, Appleton & Lange.)

is rarely observed in human lesions. The appearance of Splendore-Hoeppli material surrounding yeast cells (asteroid body) may be helpful (Figure 73–4) but is also seen in other types of infection (see Table 73–1).

TREATMENT

The classic treatment for lymphocutaneous sporotrichosis is oral potassium iodide in saturated solution. The efficacy and low cost of this medication make it a favored option, especially in developing countries; however, it must be given daily over 3 to 4 weeks and has frequent adverse effects (e.g., nausea, salivary gland enlargement). Itraconazole has been shown to be safe and highly effective at low doses and is the current treatment of choice. Spontaneous remission is rare but was seen in 13 of 178 cases in Brazil. The local application of heat has also been shown to be effective.

Chromoblastomycosis

Chromoblastomycosis (Chromomycosis) is a chronic fungal infection affecting skin and subcutaneous tissues characterized by the development of slow-growing verrucous nodules or plaques (Figure 73–5). Chromoblastomycosis is most commonly seen in the tropics, where the warm, moist environment coupled with the lack of protective footwear and clothing predisposes people to direct inoculation with infected soil or organic matter. The organisms most often associated with chromoblastomycosis are pigmented (dematiaceous) fungi of the genera

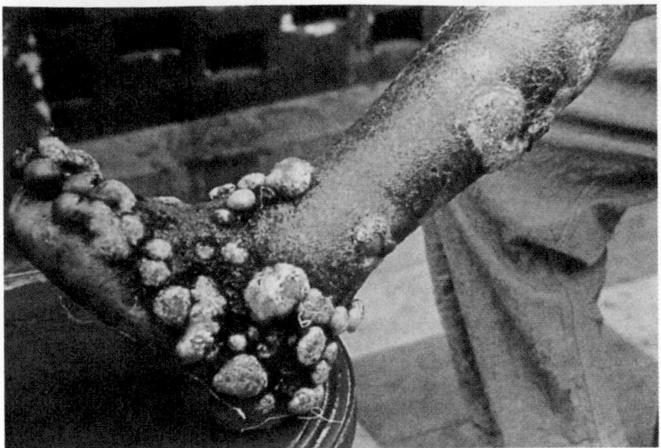

FIGURE 73–5. Chromoblastomycosis of the foot and leg. (From Connor DH et al: *Pathology of infectious diseases,* Stamford, Conn, 1997, Appleton & Lange.)

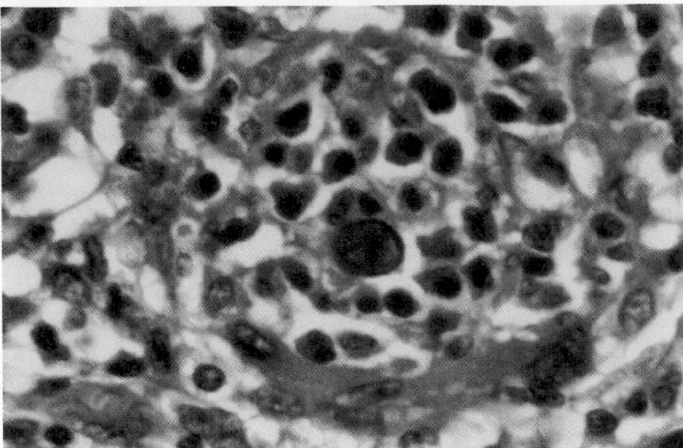

FIGURE 73–6. Brown-pigmented muriform cell or Medlar body of chromoblastomycosis (H&E, magnification 250×). (From Connor DH et al: *Pathology of infectious diseases,* Stamford, Conn, 1997, Appleton & Lange.)

Fonsecaea, Cladosporium, Exophiala, Cladophialophora, and *Phialophora* (see Table 73–1).

MORPHOLOGY

The fungi that cause chromoblastomycosis are all dematiaceous (naturally pigmented) moulds but are morphologically diverse, and most are capable of producing several different forms when grown in culture. For example, *Exophiala* species may grow as a mould and produce conidia-bearing cells called *annelids* and also as a yeast-like form that may appear in freshly isolated colonies. Although the basic form of these organisms is a pigmented septate mould, the different mechanisms of sporulation produced in culture make specific identification difficult.

In contrast to the diverse morphology seen in culture, in tissue the fungi that cause chromoblastomycosis all characteristically form muriform cells (i.e., sclerotic bodies, Medlar bodies) that are chestnut brown due to the melanin in their cell walls (Table 73–1 and Figure 73–6). Muriform cells divide by internal septation and appear as cells with vertical and horizontal lines within the same or different planes. In addition to muriform cells, pigmented hyphae may also be present. The fungal cells may be free within the tissue but most often are contained within macrophages or giant cells.

EPIDEMIOLOGY

Chromoblastomycosis generally affects persons working in rural areas of the tropics. The etiologic agents grow on woody plants and in the soil. Most infections have been in men and involve legs and arms, likely due to occupational exposure. Other body sites include shoulders, neck, trunk, buttocks, face, and ears. Local climatic factors may influence the distribution of different infections and different etiologic agents. For example, in Madagascar, infections caused by *Fonsecaea pedrosoi* are seen in areas of high rainfall (200 to 300 cm annually) whereas in the same island, infections caused by *Cladophialophora carrionii* occur in areas of low rainfall (50 to 60 cm annually). In the Americas, *F. pedrosoi* is the principal cause of chromoblastomycoses and the lesions most often involve the lower extremities. In contrast, in Australia the most common cause is *C. carrionii,* and the lesions are most frequently on the upper limbs, especially the hands. There are no reports of person-to-person transmission.

CLINICAL SYNDROMES

Chromoblastomycosis tends to be chronic, pruritic, progressive, indolent, and resistant to treatment. In most instances, patients do not present until the infection is well established. Early lesions are small warty papules and usually enlarge only slowly. There are different morphologic forms of the disease ranging from verrucous lesions to flat plaques. Established infections appear as multiple large warty "cauliflower-like" growths that are usually clustered within the same region (see Figure 73–5). Satellite lesions may occur secondary to autoinoculation. Plaquelike lesions often show central scarring as they enlarge. Ulceration and cyst formation may occur. Large lesions are hyperkeratotic, and the limb is grossly distorted due to fibrosis and secondary lymphedema (see Figure 73–5). Secondary bacterial infection may also occur and contribute to regional lymphadenitis, lymph stasis, and eventual elephantiasis.

LABORATORY DIAGNOSIS

The clinical presentation (see Figure 73–5), histopathologic findings of chestnut brown muriform cells (see

Figure 73–6), and isolation in culture of one of the causal fungi (see Table 73–1) confirm the diagnosis. Scrapings obtained from the surface of the warty lesions where small dark dots are observed may result in the demonstration the characteristic cells when mounted in 20% potassium hydroxide (KOH). Biopsy specimens stained with hematoxylin and eosin stain (H&E) will also show the organism present in the epidermis or in microabscesses containing macrophages and giant cells. The inflammatory reaction is both suppurative and granulomatous, with dermal fibrosis and pseudoepitheliomatous hyperplasia. The organisms are easily cultured from the lesions, although identification may be difficult. There are no serologic tests available for chromoblastomycosis.

TREATMENT

Treatment with specific antifungal therapy is often ineffective due to the advanced stage of infection at the time of presentation. Itraconazole and terbinafine appear to be most effective. These agents are often combined with flucytosine in refractory cases. Attempts are often made to shrink larger lesions with local heat or cryotherapy before administering antifungal agents in an effort to improve the response. Surgery is not indicated due to the risk of recurrences developing within the scar. Squamous cell carcinomas may develop in longstanding lesions, and those with atypical areas or fleshy outgrowths should be biopsied to rule out this complication.

Eumycotic Mycetoma

Eumycotic mycetomas are those caused by true fungi as opposed to actinomycotic mycetomas, which are caused by aerobic actinomycetes (bacteria). This section will deal only with the eumycotic mycetomas.

As with chromoblastomycosis, most eumycotic mycetomas are seen in the tropics. A mycetoma is defined clinically as a localized, chronic, granulomatous, infectious process involving cutaneous and subcutaneous tissues. It is characterized by the formation of multiple granulomas and abscesses, which contain large aggregates of fungal hyphae known as *granules* or *grains.* These grains contain cells that have marked modifications of internal and external structure, ranging from reduplications of the cell wall to the formation of a hard, cementlike extracellular matrix. The abscesses drain externally through the skin, often with extrusion of granules. The process may be quite extensive and deforming with destruction of muscle, fascia, and bone. The etiologic agents of eumycotic mycetoma encompass a wide range of fungi, including *Acremonium, Fusarium, Madurella, Exophiala,* and *Scedosporium* spp. (see Table 73–1).

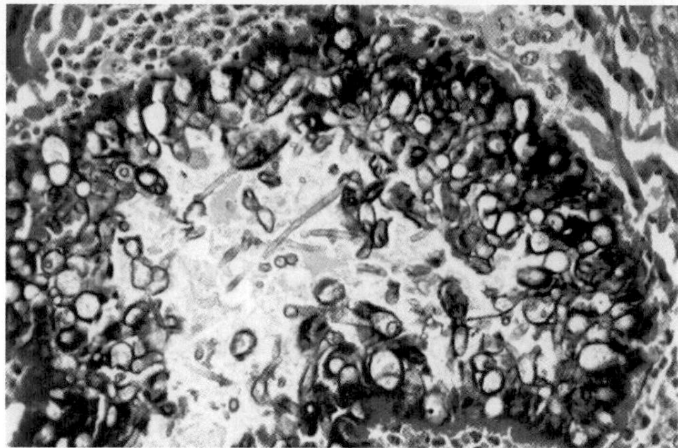

FIGURE 73–7. Mycetoma granule of *Curvularia geniculata.* Compact dematiaceous hyphae and chlamydoconidia embedded in cementlike substance (H&E, magnification 100×). (From Chandler FW, Watts JC: *Pathologic diagnosis of fungal infections,* Chicago, 1987, ASCP Press. Copyright 1987, American Society of Clinical Pathologists.)

MORPHOLOGY

The granules of eumycotic mycetomas are composed of septate, fungal hyphae that are 2 to 6 μm or greater in width, and they are either dematiaceous (black grain) or hyaline (pale or white grain) depending on the etiologic agent (Figure 73–7). The hyphae are frequently distorted and bizarre in form and size. Large, spherical, thick-walled chlamydoconidia are often present. The hyphae may be embedded in an amorphous cementlike substance. Splendore-Hoeppli material often interdigitates among the mycelial elements at the periphery of the granule. Eumycotic granules can be differentiated from actinomycotic granules based on morphologic (branched filaments versus septate hyphae and chlamydoconidia) and staining (gram-positive beaded rods versus periodic acid-Schiff [PAS]- and Gomori methenamine silver [GMS]-positive hyphae) characteristics. Culture is usually necessary for definitive identification of the fungus (or actinomycete) involved.

EPIDEMIOLOGY

Mycetomas are primarily seen in tropical areas with low rainfall. Eumycotic mycetomas are more frequently encountered in Africa and the Indian subcontinent but also may be seen in Brazil, Venezuela, and the Middle East. All patients are infected from sources in nature via traumatic percutaneous implantation of the etiologic agent into exposed parts of the body. The foot and hand are most common, but back, shoulders, and chest wall infections are also seen. Men are more often affected than women. The fungi that cause eumycotic mycetomas differ from country to country, and the agents that are common in one region are rarely reported from others. Mycetomas are not contagious.

CLINICAL SYNDROMES

Similar to chromoblastomycosis, patients with eumycotic mycetoma most commonly present with longstanding infection. The earliest lesion to appear is a small, painless, subcutaneous nodule or plaque that increases slowly, but progressively, in size. As the mycetoma develops, the affected area gradually enlarges and becomes disfigured as a result of chronic inflammation and fibrosis. With time, sinus tracts appear on the skin surface and drain serosanguineous fluid that often contains grossly visible granules. The infection commonly breaches tissue planes and destroys muscle and bone locally. Hematogenous or lymphatic spread from a primary focus to distant sites or viscera is extremely rare.

LABORATORY DIAGNOSIS

The key to the diagnosis of eumycotic mycetoma is the demonstration of grains or granules. Grains may be grossly visible in draining sinus tracts or may be expressed onto a glass slide. Material can also be obtained by deep surgical biopsy.

Grains can be visualized microscopically by mounting in 20% KOH. The hyphae are usually clearly visible, as is the presence or absence of pigmentation. Grains can be washed and then cultured or fixed and sectioned for histopathology.

Grains are easily visualized in tissue stained with H&E (see Figure 73–7). Special stains such as PAS and GMS may also be helpful. Although the color, shape, size, and microscopic morphology can be characteristic of a specific causal agent, culture is usually necessary for definitive identification of the organism. Most organisms will grow on standard mycologic medium; however, inclusion of an antibiotic such as penicillin may be useful to inhibit contaminating bacteria that may overgrow the fungus.

TREATMENT

Treatment of eumycotic mycetoma is usually unsuccessful. Response of the various etiologic agents to amphotericin B, terbinafine, ketoconazole, or itraconazole is variable and often poor, although such therapy may slow the course of infection. Local excision is usually ineffective or not possible, and amputation is the only definitive treatment. Because these infections are usually slowly progressive, and may be slowed further by specific antifungal therapy, the decision to amputate should take into account the rate of progression, the symptomatology, the availability of adequate prosthesis, and the individual circumstances of the patient. For all of these reasons, it is imperative to differentiate eumycotic mycetoma from actinomycotic mycetoma. Medical therapy is usually effective in cases of actinomycotic mycetoma.

Subcutaneous Zygomycosis

Subcutaneous zygomycosis, also known as entomophthoromycosis, is caused by Zygomycetes of the order Entomophthorales: *Conidiobolus coronatus* and *Basidiobolus ranarum (haptosporus)* (see Table 73–1). Both of these fungi cause a chronic subcutaneous form of zygomycosis that occurs sporadically as a result of traumatic implantation of the fungus that is present in plant debris in tropical environments. They differ in that they cause infections with different anatomic locations: *B. ranarum* causes subcutaneous infection of the proximal limbs in children, whereas *C. coronatus* infection is localized to the facial area predominantly in adults (see Figures 73–8 and 73–9).

MORPHOLOGY

The appearance of the agents of subcutaneous zygomycosis in tissue differs from that of the mucoraceous zygomycetes. The hyphal elements are sparse and often appear as hyphal fragments surrounded by intensely eosinophilic Splendore-Hoeppli material (Figure 73–10). The inflammatory response is granulomatous and rich

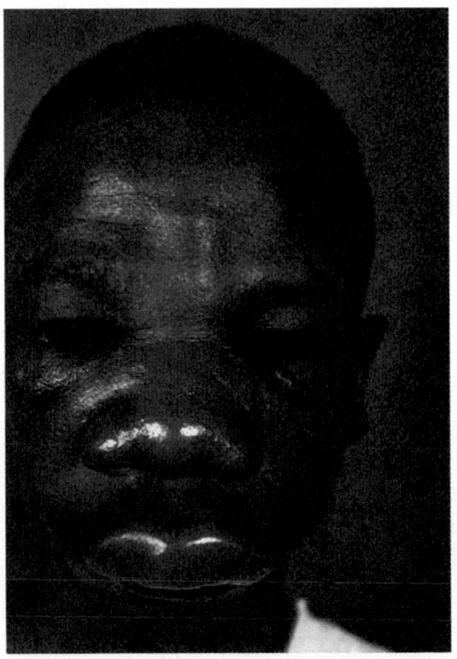

FIGURE 73–8. Subcutaneous zygomycosis caused by *Conidiobolus coronatus*. (From Chandler FW, Watts JC: *Pathologic diagnosis of fungal infections*, Chicago, 1987, ASCP Press. Copyright 1987, American Society of Clinical Pathologists.)

in eosinophils. The hyphal fragments are thin walled and poorly staining. Although septae are infrequent, they are more prominent than those seen with Mucoraceae. The hyphae of the Entomophthoraceae are not angioinvasive.

EPIDEMIOLOGY

Both types of subcutaneous zygomycosis are seen most commonly in Africa and, to a lesser extent, in India. Infection caused by *B. ranarum* has also been reported from the Middle East, Asia, and Europe, whereas that caused by *C. coronatus* has been reported from Latin America, Africa, and India. Both fungi are saprophytes that are present in leaf and plant debris. *B. ranarum* has also been found in the intestinal contents of small reptiles and amphibians. Both are rare diseases without known predisposing factors (e.g., acidosis or immunodeficiency). Infection caused by *B. ranarum* is thought to occur after traumatic implantation of the fungus into the subcutaneous tissues of the thighs, buttocks, and trunk. This form of subcutaneous zygomycosis occurs mainly in children (80% younger than the age of 20 years) with a male:female ratio of 3:1. *C. coronatus* infections occur after inhalation of the fungal spores which then invade the tissues of the nasal cavity, the paranasal sinuses, and facial soft tissues. There is a 10:1 male : female ratio, and the disease is seen predominantly among young adults. Infection among children is rare.

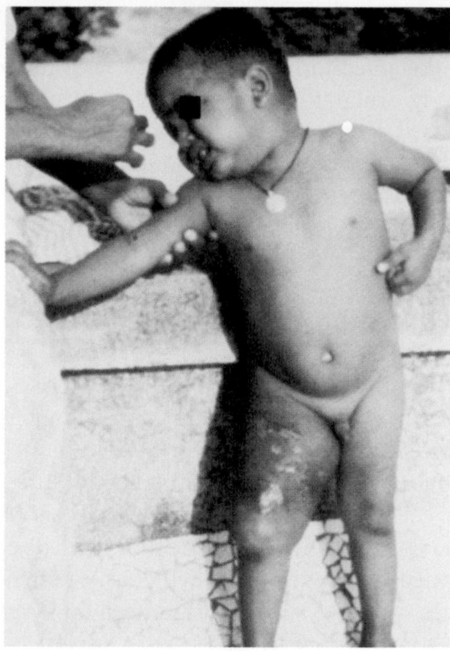

FIGURE 73–9. Subcutaneous zygomycosis caused by *Basidiobolus ranarum*. The right thigh is extensively swollen and indurated. (From Chandler FW, Watts JC: *Pathologic diagnosis of fungal infections,* Chicago, 1987, ASCP Press. Copyright 1987, American Society of Clinical Pathologists.)

CLINICAL SYNDROMES

Patients infected with *B. ranarum* have disk-shaped, rubbery, movable masses that may be quite large and are localized to the shoulder, pelvis, hips, and thighs (Figure 73–9). The masses may expand locally and eventually ulcerate. Dissemination or involvement of deeper structures is rare. Gastrointestinal basidiobolomycosis has recently been reported in the Southwestern United States.

C. coronatus infection is confined to the rhinofacial area and often does not come to medical attention until there is a noticeable swelling of the upper lip or face (Figure 73–8). The swelling is firm and painless and may progress slowly to involve the nasal bridge and the upper and lower face, including the orbit. The facial deformity can be quite dramatic (see Figure 73–8); however, because of the lack of angioinvasion, intracranial extension does not occur.

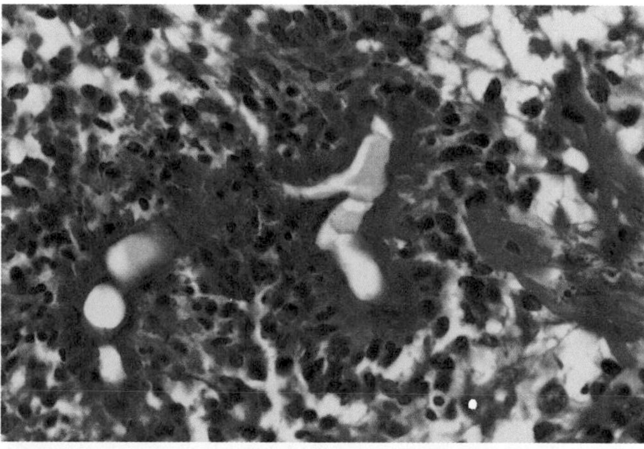

FIGURE 73–10. Subcutaneous zygomycosis. Broad hyphal fragments surrounded by eosinophilic Splendore-Hoeppli material (H&E, magnification 160×). (From Chandler FW, Watts JC: *Pathologic diagnosis of fungal infections,* Chicago, 1987, ASCP Press. Copyright 1987, American Society of Clinical Pathologists.)

LABORATORY DIAGNOSIS

Both types of subcutaneous zygomycosis require biopsy for diagnosis despite the characteristic clinical features of the infections. The histopathologic picture is the same for both organisms (see Figure 73–10) marked by focal clusters of inflammation with eosinophils and typical zygomycotic hyphae often surrounded by eosinophilic Splendore-Hoeppli material. The organisms can be cultured from clinical material on standard mycologic medium.

TREATMENT

Both types of infection can be treated with itraconazole. Alternatively, oral potassium iodide, in saturated solution, has been used. Facial reconstructive surgery may be necessary in the case of *C. coronatus* infection because the extensive fibrosis remains after eradication of the fungus.

Subcutaneous Phaeohyphomycosis

Phaeohyphomycosis is a term used to describe a heterogeneous array of fungal infections caused by pigmented, or dematiaceous, fungi that are present in tissue as irregular hyphae (Figure 73–11) rather than the sclerotic muriform cells seen in chromoblastomycosis (see Table 73–1 and Figure 73–6). These infections can be caused by a wide range of fungi, all of which exist in nature as saprophytes of soil, wood, and decaying vegetation. Phaeohyphomycotic processes may be superficial, subcutaneous, or deeply invasive or disseminated. The superficial (Chapter 72) and deeply invasive (Chapter 75) forms are discussed in their respective chapters. The subcutaneous form is discussed in this section.

MORPHOLOGY

The agents of subcutaneous phaeohyphomycosis are numerous and diverse (see Table 73–1), but all grow as black moulds in culture and appear as dark-walled, irregular hyphal and yeastlike forms in tissue (see Figure 73–11). The hyphae vary from 2 to 6 μm in width, can be branched, and are septate and often constricted at the point of septation. Bizarre, thick-walled, vesicular swellings that can be as large as 25 μm in diameter may be present, as can budding yeastlike structures. Cell wall pigmentation ranges from light to dark and may require special stains such as the Fontana-Masson melanin stain to confirm the dematiaceous nature of the fungus. In culture, the different fungi grow as black or brown moulds and are identified by their characteristic mode of sporulation.

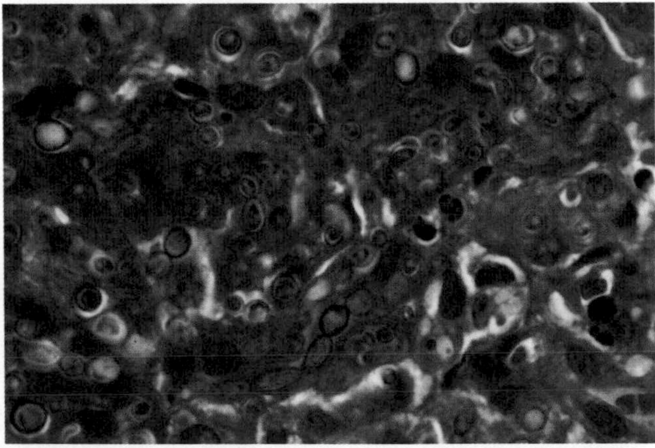

FIGURE 73–11. Subcutaneous phaeohyphomycosis. Dematiaceous yeast-like cells and septate hyphae of *Exophiala spinifera.* (H&E, magnification 250×). (From Chandler FW, Watts JC: *Pathologic diagnosis of fungal infections,* Chicago, 1987, ASCP Press. Copyright 1987, American Society of Clinical Pathologists.)

EPIDEMIOLOGY

More than 20 different dematiaceous fungi have been cited as causes of subcutaneous phaeohyphomycosis. The most frequent etiologic agents have been *Exophiala jeanselmei, Wangiella dermatitidis,* and *Bipolaris* spp. (see Table 73–1). Because these fungi are found in soil and plant debris, the route of infection is thought to result from traumatic implantation of the fungus. Indeed, wood splinters have been found in histopathologic material, suggesting both the mode of inoculation and possibly that the formation of the characteristic phaeohyphomycotic cyst is a reaction to implantation. There is no explanation for why some organisms produce phaeohyphomycotic cysts and others develop into mycetomas.

CLINICAL SYNDROMES

Most commonly, subcutaneous phaeohyphomycosis presents as a solitary inflammatory cyst. The lesions generally occur on the feet and legs, although the hands and other body sites may be involved. The lesions grow slowly and expand over a period of months or years. They may be firm or fluctuant and are usually painless. If located near a joint, they may be mistaken for a synovial cyst and may become large enough to interfere with movements. Other manifestations include the formation of pigmented plaquelike lesions that are indurated but not tender.

LABORATORY DIAGNOSIS

The diagnosis is made when the cyst is surgically excised. On histopathologic examination, the appearance is of an inflammatory cyst with a fibrous capsule, granulomatous reaction, and central necrosis. Individual and clustered dematiaceous fungal elements are seen within giant cells and extracellularly amid the necrotic debris (see Figure 73–11). Generally, the pigmentation is easily seen on examination of H&E-stained tissue. The organisms can be grown in culture and identified by their pattern of sporulation.

TREATMENT

The main treatment is surgical excision. Plaquelike lesions may not be amenable to this approach and generally respond to treatment with itraconazole.

CASE STUDY AND QUESTIONS

A 40-year-old ecotourist was on an extended trip to the jungles of Costa Rica. During this time she camped, climbed trees, waded in streams, slogged through mud, and endured drenching rains. She lost her shoes about 2 weeks into the adventure and continued to hike about barefoot for another 2 weeks, during which time she sustained minor cuts and abrasions to both feet. Approximately 6 months after returning home to the Midwest United States, she noticed mild swelling of her right foot. There was no pain, inflammation, or drainage from the foot. She comes to you for medical advice.

1. What is the differential diagnosis of this process?
2. What types of fungi might cause this infection?
3. How will you proceed with establishing the diagnosis?
4. What are the therapeutic options and the likelihood that they will be successful?

Bibliography

Basto de Lima Barros M et al: Cat-transmitted sporotrichosis epidemic in Rio de Janeiro, Brazil: Description of a series of cases, *Clin Infect Dis* 38:529-535, 2004.

Chandler FW, Watts JC: *Pathologic diagnosis of fungal infections,* Chicago, 1987, ASCP Press.

Connor DH et al: *Pathology of infectious diseases,* Stamford, Conn, 1997, Appleton & Lange.

Hay RJ: Cutaneous and subcutaneous mycoses. In Anaissie EJ, McGinnis MR, Pfaller MA, editors: *Clinical mycology,* New York, 2003, Churchill Livingstone.

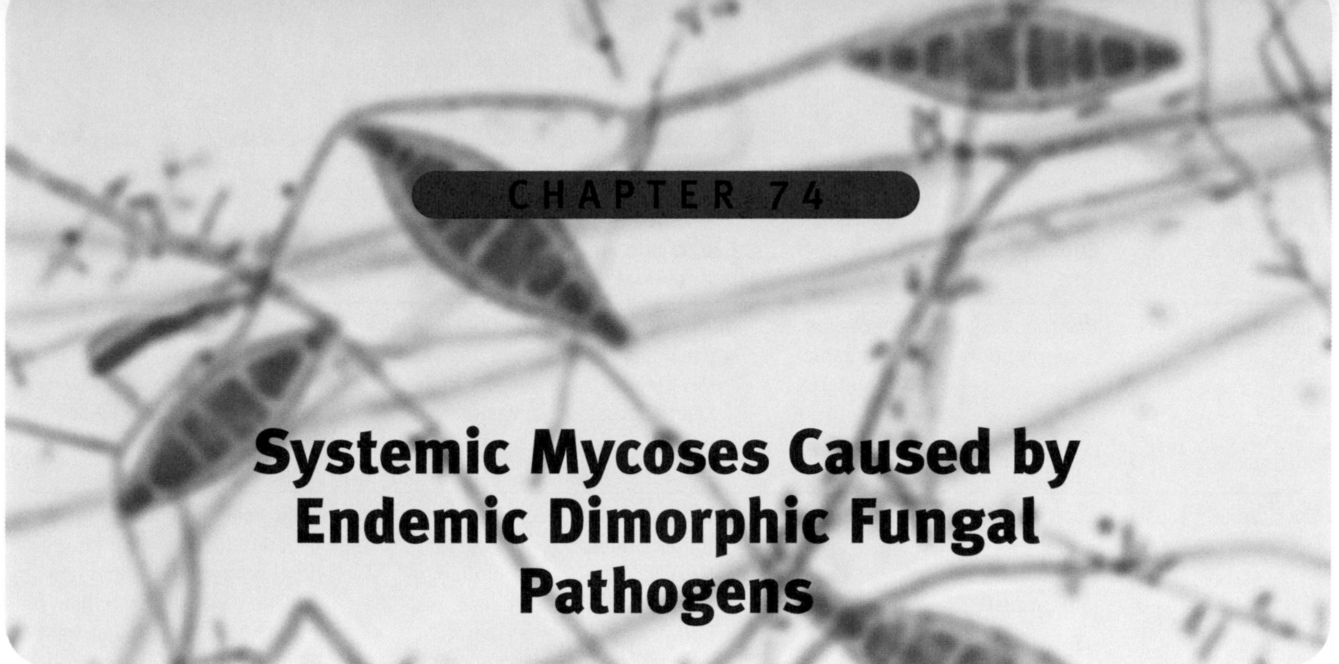

Systemic Mycoses Caused by Endemic Dimorphic Fungal Pathogens

The **dimorphic** fungal pathogens are organisms that exist in a mould form in nature or in the laboratory at 25° to 30°C and in a yeast or spherule form in tissues or when grown on enriched medium in the laboratory at 37°C (Figure 74–1). The organisms in this group are considered primary **systemic** pathogens due to their ability to cause infection in both "normal" and immunocompromised hosts and for their propensity to involve the deep viscera after dissemination of the fungus from the lungs after its inhalation from nature. The dimorphic pathogens include *Blastomyces dermatiditis, Coccidioides immitis, Coccidioides posadasii, Histoplasma capsulatum* var *capsulatum, H. casulatum* var *duboisii, Paracoccidioides brasiliensis,* and *Penicillium marneffei* (Table 74–1). These organisms are also known as **endemic** pathogens in that their natural habitat is delimited to specific geographic regions (Figure 74–2) and infection due to a particular fungus is acquired by inhalation of spores from that specific environment and geographic location (see Table 74–1). *H. capsulatum, C. immitis (C. posadasii),* and *P. marneffei* have emerged as major opportunistic pathogens in persons with acquired immune deficiency syndrome (AIDS) and other forms of immunosuppression. Recognition of these endemic mycoses may be complicated by the fact that they can become manifest only after the patient has left the area of endemicity. Often the infection may be quiescent, only to reactivate when the patient becomes immunosuppressed and is living in an area where the fungus is not endemic.

Blastomycosis

Blastomycosis is a systemic fungal infection caused by the dimorphic pathogen *Blastomyces dermatitidis.* Like other endemic mycoses, this infection is confined to specific geographic regions; most infections originate in the Mississippi River basin, around the Great Lakes, and in the southeast region of the United States (see Figure 74–2). Cases have also been diagnosed in other parts of the world including Africa, Europe, and the Middle East.

MORPHOLOGY

As a thermally dimorphic fungus, *B. dermatitidis* produces nonencapsulated yeastlike cells in tissue and in culture on enriched media at 37°C and white-to-tan filamentous mould colonies on standard mycologic media at 25°C. The mould form produces round to oval or pear-shaped conidia (2 to 10 μm) located on long or short terminal hyphal branches (Figure 74–3). Older cultures may also produce thick-walled chlamydospores 7 to 18 μm in diameter. This form of *B. dermatitidis* is not diagnostic and may not be distinguishable from the monomorphic *Chrysosporium* spp. or from an early culture of *H. capsulatum.*

The yeast form of *B. dermatitidis* is seen in tissue and in culture at 37°C. This form is quite distinctive (Figure 74–4). The yeast cells are spherical, hyaline, 8 to 15 μm in diameter, multinucleated, and have thick "double-contoured" walls. The cytoplasm is often retracted from the rigid cell wall as a result of shrinkage during the fixation process. The yeast cells reproduce by the formation of buds or **blastoconidia.** The buds are usually single and attached to the parent cell by broad bases (see Figure 74–4).

The yeast forms may be visualized in tissue stained with hematoxylin and eosin (H&E); however, the fungal stains Gomori methenamine silver (GMS) and periodic acid-Schiff (PAS) help locate the organisms and delineate their morphology.

TABLE 74–1. Characteristics of Endemic Dimorphic Mycoses

Mycosis	Etiology	Ecology	Geographic Distribution	Morphology in Tissue	Clinical Manifestation
Blastomycosis	*Blastomyces dermatitidis*	Decaying organic material	North America (Ohio and Mississippi River Valleys) Africa	Broad-based budding yeasts (8–15 µm in diameter)	Pulmonary disease (<50%); extrapulmonary: skin, bone, genitourinary, central nervous system; disseminated disease in immunocompromised patients
Coccidioidomycosis	*Coccidioides immitis* *Coccidioides posadasii*	Soil, dust	Southwestern United States, Mexico, Central and South America	Spherules (20–60 µm) containing endospores (2–4 µm)	Asymptomatic pulmonary infection (60%) in normal host; progressive pulmonary infection and dissemination (skin, bone, joints, meninges) in immunocompromised patients
Histoplasmosis capsulatum	*Histoplasma capsulatum* var *capsulatum*	Soil with high nitrogen content (bird/bat droppings)	North America (Ohio and Mississippi River valleys), Mexico, Central and South America	Small (2–4 µm) oval, narrow-based budding yeasts (intracellular)	Asymptomatic pulmonary infection (90%) in normal host and low-intensity exposure; disseminated disease in immunocompromised host and in children
Histoplasmosis duboisii	*Histoplasma capsulatum* var *duboisii*	Soil with high nitrogen content	Tropical areas of Africa	Larger (8–15 µm), thick-walled budding yeast; prominent isthmus and bud scar	Low rate of pulmonary disease; higher frequency of skin and bone involvement
Paracoccidioido-mycosis	*Paracoccidioides brasiliensis*	Likely soil associated	South and Central America	Thin to moderately thick walled, multiply budding yeast (15–30 µm; pilot wheel)	Self-limited pulmonary disease; progressive pulmonary infection and dissemination (skin, mucosa, bones, lymph nodes, viscera and meninges) more common in children and immunocompromised patients
Penicilliosis marneffei	*Penicillium marneffei*	Soil; bamboo rat	Southeast Asia	Globose to elongated sausage-shaped yeasts (3–5 µm) that are intracellular and divide by fission	Disseminated infection (skin, soft tissues, viscera) more common in those with AIDS; resembles histoplasmosis, cryptococcosis, or tuberculosis

Adapted from Perea S, Patterson TF: Endemic mycoses. In Anaissie EJ, McGinnis MR, Pfaller MA, editors: *Clinical mycology,* New York, 2003, Churchill Livingstone.

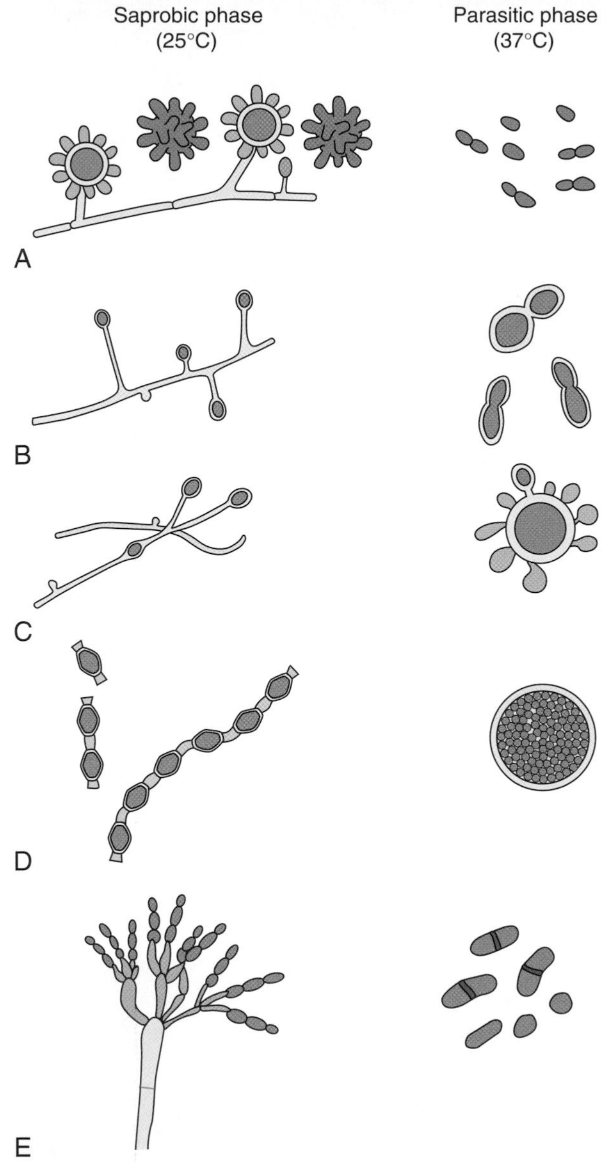

FIGURE 74–1. Saprobic and parasitic phases of endemic dimorphic fungi. **A,** *Histoplasma capsulatum;* **B,** *Blastomyces dermatitidis;* **C,** *Paracoccidioides brasiliensis;* **D,** *Coccidioides immitis.* **E,** *Penicillium marneffei.*

EPIDEMIOLOGY

The ecologic niche of *B. dermatitidis* appears to be in decaying organic matter. Studies in humans and animals indicate that infection is acquired after the inhalation of aerosolized conidia produced by the fungus growing in soil and leaf litter (Figure 74–5). Outbreaks of infection have been associated with occupational or recreational contact with soil, and infected individuals include all ages and both sexes. Blastomycosis is not transmitted from patient to patient; however, laboratory-acquired primary cutaneous and pulmonary blastomycosis has been reported.

In North America, the area of endemicity overlaps that of histoplasmosis (see Figure 74–2) and includes the southeastern and south central states, especially those bordering the Ohio and Mississippi River basins; the Midwest states and Canadian provinces bordering the Great Lakes; and an area in New York and Canada along the St. Lawrence River. Blastomycosis is also endemic in Africa. It is estimated that one to two cases of symptomatic blastomycosis requiring therapy occur per 100,000 population per year in areas with endemic disease. Among animals, dogs are most susceptible; the infection rate is estimated to be 10 times that for humans.

CLINICAL SYNDROMES

The usual route of infection in blastomycosis is inhalation of conidia (see Figure 74–5). As with most of the endemic mycoses, the severity of symptoms and the course of disease are dependent on the extent of exposure and the immune status of the exposed person. Based largely on studies of blastomycosis outbreaks, it appears that symptomatic disease occurs in fewer than half of infected persons. Clinical illness caused by *B. dermatitidis* may present as pulmonary disease or an extrapulmonary disseminated disease. Among those patients with extrapulmonary dissemination, two thirds exhibit involvement of skin and bones. Other sites of hematogenous dissemination include prostate, liver, spleen, kidney, and central nervous system.

Pulmonary blastomycosis may be asymptomatic or present as a mild flulike illness. More severe infection resembles bacterial pneumonia with acute onset, high fever, lobar infiltrates, and cough. Progression to fulminant adult respiratory distress syndrome with high fever, diffuse infiltrates, and respiratory failure may occur. A more subacute or chronic respiratory form of blastomycosis may resemble tuberculosis or lung cancer with radiographic presentation of pulmonary mass lesions or fibronodular infiltrates.

A classic form of blastomycosis is that of chronic cutaneous involvement. The cutaneous form of blastomycosis is almost always the result of hematogenous dissemination from the lung, in most instances without evident pulmonary lesions or systemic symptoms. The lesions may be papular, pustular, or indolent, and ulcerative-nodular and verrucous with crusted surfaces and raised serpiginous borders. They are usually painless and are localized to exposed areas such as the face, scalp, neck, and hands. They may be mistaken for squamous cell carcinoma. Left untreated, cutaneous blastomycosis takes on a chronic course with remissions, exacerbations, and gradual increase in the size of lesions.

Blastomycosis is relatively uncommon among persons with AIDS or other immunocompromising conditions. However, when it occurs in these persons it tends to be

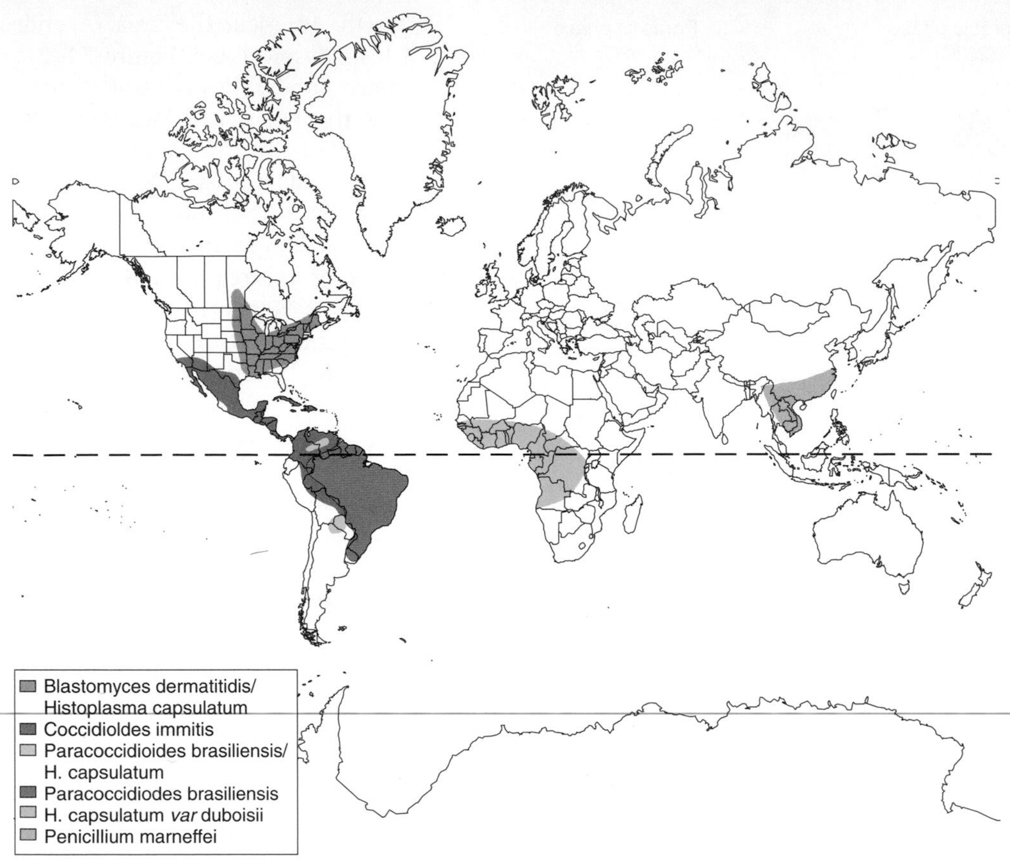

FIGURE 74–2. Major geographic regional distribution of the endemic mycoses.

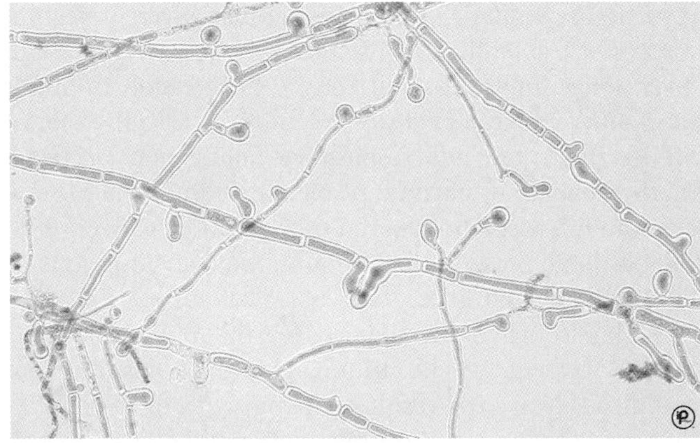

FIGURE 74–3. *Blastomyces dermatitidis* mould phase. (Reprinted from Indiana Pathology Images.)

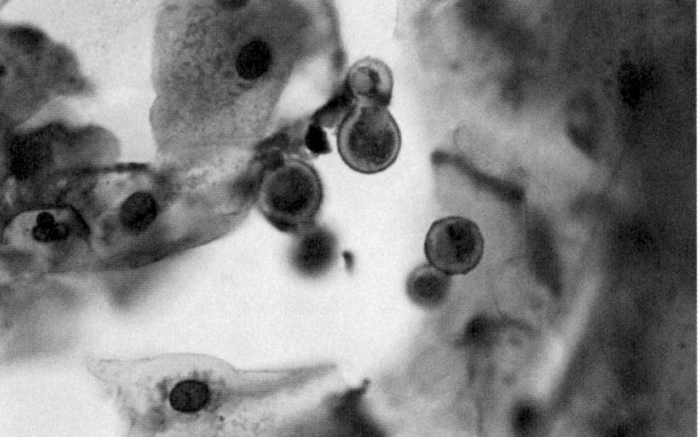

FIGURE 74–4. Giemsa stain of *Blastomyces dermatitidis* showing broad-based budding yeast.

acute, involve the central nervous system, and have a much poorer prognosis.

LABORATORY DIAGNOSIS

The diagnosis of blastomycosis rests with microscopic detection of the fungus in tissue or other clinical material with confirmation by culture (Table 74–2). The most useful specimens for the diagnosis of pulmonary blastomycosis include sputum, bronchoalveolar lavage, or lung biopsy. Direct examination of material stained with GMS, PAS, Papanicolaou, or Giemsa stains should be performed. Likewise, fresh wet preparations of sputum, cerebrospinal fluid, urine, pus, skin scrapings, and tissue impression smears may be examined directly using calcofluor white and fluorescence microscopy to detect the

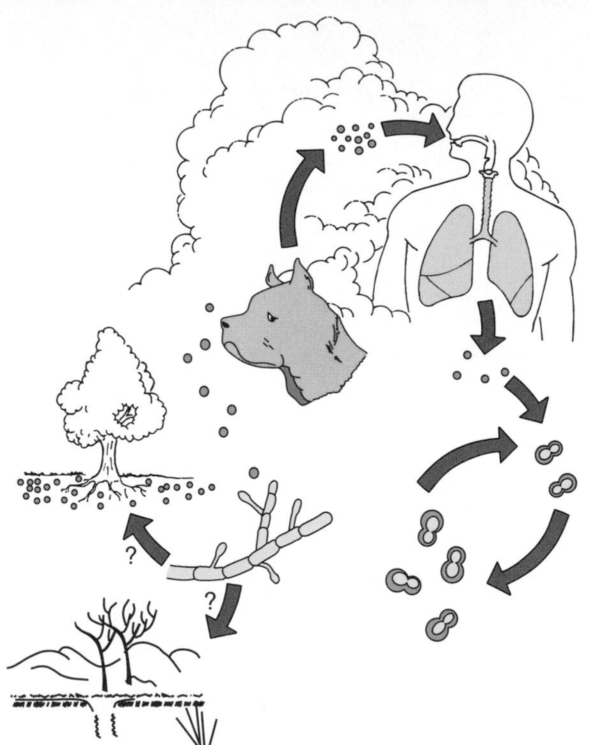

FIGURE 74–5. Natural history of the mould (saprobic) and yeast (parasitic) cycle of *Blastomyces dermatitidis.*

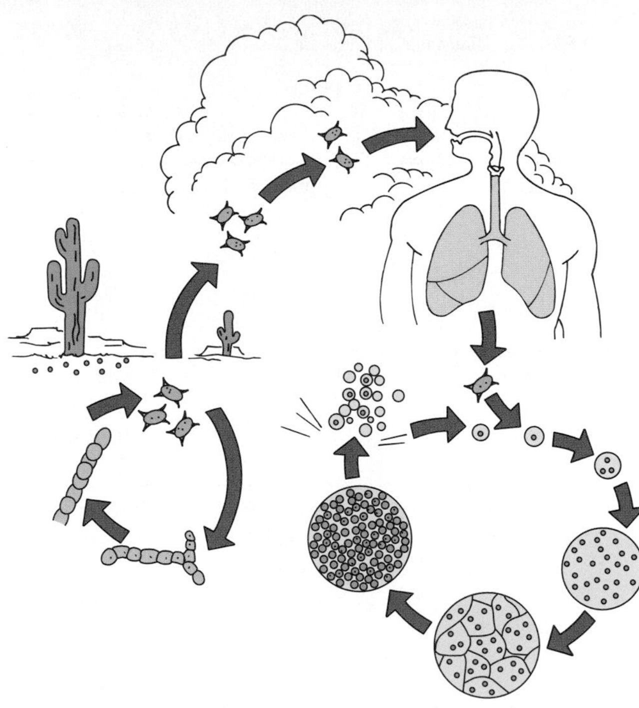

FIGURE 74–6. Natural history of the mould (saprobic) and spherule (parasitic) cycle of *Coccidioides immitis.*

characteristic yeast forms. When typical broad-based budding yeast forms are present, a definitive diagnosis can be made.

Culture of clinical material on selective and nonselective mycologic media incubated at both 25° to 30°C and at 37°C should be performed. The mycelial form of the fungus is easily cultured at 25° to 30°C; however, growth is slow, often requiring 4 weeks or more. The mycelial form (see Figure 74–3) is not diagnostic, and the identity must be confirmed by conversion to the yeast form at 37°C, by exoantigen testing (immunologic detection of cell-free antigen A), or by nucleic acid probe hybridization. Care should be taken to handle the culture in an appropriate biosafety cabinet because the conidia are infectious.

Although serologic tests to detect antibodies directed at *B. dermatitidis* antigens are available (see Table 74–2), they are neither sensitive nor specific and are of little use in diagnosis. A test to detect antigen in urine is commercially available, but its performance characteristics are not well described and it is unclear what role it will play in diagnosis.

TREATMENT

The decision to treat patients with blastomycosis must take into consideration the clinical form and severity of disease and the immune status of the patient and the toxicity of antifungal agents. Clearly, pulmonary blastomycosis in immunocompromised patients and those with progressive pulmonary disease should be treated. Likewise, all patients with evidence of hematogenous dissemination (e.g., skin, bone, all nonpulmonary sites) require antifungal therapy. Amphotericin B is the agent of choice for the treatment of life-threatening or meningeal disease. Mild or moderate disease can be treated with itraconazole. Fluconazole may be an alternative for those patients unable to tolerate itraconazole. Depending on the severity of the disease and the status of the host, therapeutic success rates with amphotericin B or azole therapy range from 70% to 95%. Survival for patients with AIDS and other immunocompromised patients is about half of this figure. The latter patients may require long-term suppressive therapy with itraconazole in an effort to avoid relapses of the infection.

Coccidioidomycosis

Coccidioidomycosis is an endemic mycosis caused by either of two indistinguishable species, *C. immitis* and *C. posadasii.* The disease is caused by the inhalation of infectious arthroconidia (Figure 74–6) and can range from an asymptomatic infection (in most people) to progressive infection and death. The two species differ in geographic distribution and genotype: *C. immitis* is localized to

TABLE 74–2. Diagnosis of Endemic Dimorphic Mycoses

Mycosis	Culture	Morphology in Culture		Histopathology	Serology
		25°C	37°C		
Blastomycosis	Sputum, BAL, lung tissue, skin biopsy	Mould, round to oval or pear-shaped conidia (2–10 μm diameter)	Thick-walled broad-based budding yeast (8–15 μm)	Broad-based budding yeast	Antibody: CF, ID, EIA (poor sensitivity and specificity) Antigen: urine (performance undefined)
Coccidioidomycosis	Sputum, BAL, tissue	Mould with barrel-shaped arthroconidia (3–6 μm)	NA	Spherules (20–60 μm) containing endospores	Antibody: TP, CF, ID, LP (diagnostic and prognostic)
Histoplasmosis capsulatum	Sputum, BAL, blood, bone marrow, tissue	Mould with tuberculate macroconidia (8–15 μm) and small, oval microconidia (2–4 μm)	Small (2–4 μm) budding yeast	Intracellular budding yeast	Antibody: CF, ID Antigen: serum and urine (92% sensitive in disseminated disease)
Paracoccidioidomycoses	Sputum, BAL, tissue	Mould, round microconidia (2–3 μm) and intercalary chlamydospores	Large (15–30 μm) multiple budding yeast	Large multiply budding yeasts	Antibody: ID, CF (variable specificity, CF useful for monitoring response)
Penicilliosis marneffei	Blood, bone marrow, tissue	Mould with diffusible red pigment; conidiophores terminating in conspicuous penicillus bearing ellipsoidal, smooth conidia	Pleomorphic elongated yeast (1–8 μm) with transverse septae	Intracellular elongated yeast with transverse septae	Under development

BAL, Bronchoalveolar lavage; CF, complement fixation; EIA, enzyme immunoassay; ID, immunodiffusion; LP, latex particle agglutination; NA, not applicable; TP, tube precipitin.

California and *C. posadasii* accounts for the majority of infections outside of California. Aside from these differences, there does not appear to be any additional differences in phenotype or pathogenicity. As such, the more familiar name *C. immitis* will be used in this chapter.

Like syphilis and tuberculosis, coccidioidomycosis causes a wide variety of lesions and has been called "the great imitator." Synonyms for coccidioidomycosis include *coccidioidal granuloma* and *San Joaquin Valley fever*, among others.

MORPHOLOGY

C. immitis (C. posadasii) is a dimorphic fungus that exists as a mould in nature and when cultured in the laboratory at 25°C and as an endosporulating spherule in tissue and under very specific conditions in vitro (Table 74–2 and Figures 74–1, 74–7, and 74–8). A variety of mould morphologies can be seen in culture at 25°C. Initial growth is white to gray, moist, and glabrous and occurs within 3 to 4 days. It rapidly develops abundant aerial mycelia, and the colony enlarges into a circular "bloom." Mature colonies usually become tan to brown or lavender.

Microscopically, the vegetative hyphae give rise to fertile hyphae that produce alternating (separated by disjunctor cells) hyaline arthroconidia (see Figure 74–7). When released, the infectious conidia are typically barrel shaped and have an annular frill at both ends. As the culture ages, the vegetative hyphae also fragment into arthroconidia.

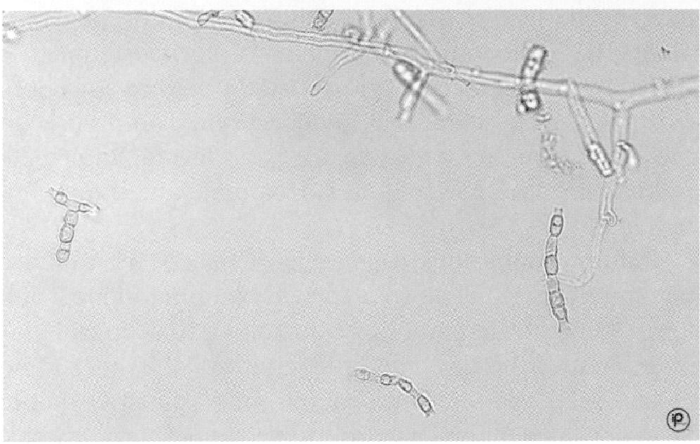

FIGURE 74–7. *Coccidioides immitis* mould phase. (From Marler LM, Siders JA, Simpson AI, Allen SD: *Mycology* CD-ROM, Indiana Pathology Images, 2004.)

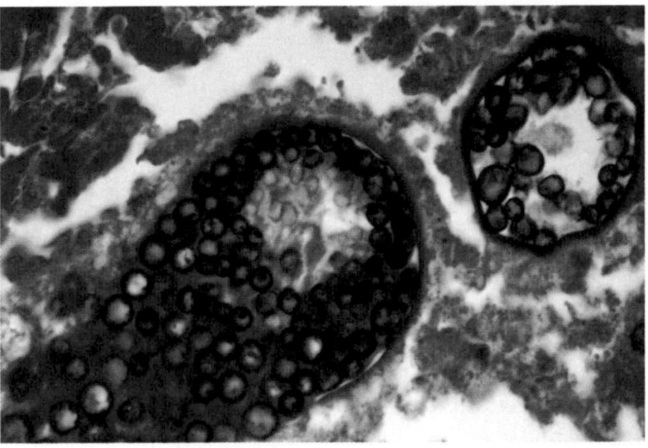

FIGURE 74–8. *Coccidioides immitis* spherule. (From Chandler FW, Watts JC: *Pathologic diagnosis of fungal infections,* Chicago, 1987, ASCP Press. Copyright 1987, American Society of Clinical Pathologists.)

Upon inhalation, the arthroconidia (2.5 to 4 μm wide) become rounded as they convert to spherules in the lung (see Figure 74–8). At maturity, the spherules (20 to 60 μm in diameter) produce endospores by a process known as "progressive cleavage." Rupture of the spherule walls releases the endospores, which in turn form new spherules (see Figure 74–6). In approximately 10% to 30% of pulmonary cavities associated with coccidioidomycosis, branched, septate hyphae and arthroconidia may be produced.

EPIDEMIOLOGY

Coccidioidomycosis is endemic to the desert southwestern United States, northern Mexico, and scattered areas of Central and South America (see Figure 74–2). *C. immitis* is found in soil, and the growth of the fungus in the environment is enhanced by bat and rodent droppings. Exposure to the infectious arthroconidia is greatest in late summer and fall, when dusty conditions prevail. Cycles of drought and rain enhance dispersion of the organism because heavy rains facilitate the growth of the organism in the nitrogenous soil wastes, and subsequent drought and windy conditions favor aerosolization of arthroconidia (see Figure 74–6). Acquisition of coccidioidomycosis occurs principally by inhalation of arthroconidia, and in endemic areas infection rates may be 16% to 42% by early adulthood. The incidence of coccidioidomycosis is approximately 15 cases per 100,000 population annually in the endemic area; however, it is know to disproportionally affect persons aged 65 years and older (~36 per 100,000) and those with HIV infection (~20 per 100,000).

CLINICAL SYNDROMES

C. immitis is probably the most virulent of all human mycotic pathogens. The inhalation of only a few arthroconidia produces primary coccidioidomycosis, which may include asymptomatic pulmonary disease (~60% of patients) or a self-limited flulike illness marked by fever, cough, chest pain, and weight loss. Patients with primary coccidioidomycosis may have a variety of allergic reactions (~10%) as a result of immune complex formation, including an erythematous macular rash, erythema multiforme, and erythema nodosum.

Primary disease usually resolves without therapy and confers a strong, specific immunity to reinfection, which is detected by the coccidioidin skin test. In patients symptomatic for 6 weeks or longer, the disease progresses to secondary coccidioidomycosis, which may include nodules, cavitary disease, or progressive pulmonary disease (5% of cases); single- or multisystem dissemination follows in approximately 1% of this population. Extrapulmonary sites of infection include skin, soft tissues, bones, joints, and meninges. Persons in certain ethnic groups (e.g., Filipino, African American, Native American, Hispanic) run the highest risk of dissemination, with meningeal involvement a common sequela (Table 74–3). In addition to ethnicity, males (9 : 1), women in the third trimester of pregnancy, persons with a cellular immunodeficiency (including AIDS and organ transplantation), and persons at the extremes of age are at high risk for disseminated disease (see Table 74–3). The mortality in disseminated disease exceeds 90% without treatment, and chronic infection is common.

LABORATORY DIAGNOSIS

The diagnosis of coccidioidomycosis involves the use of histopathologic examination of tissue or other clinical material, isolation of the fungus in the culture, and serologic testing (see Table 74–2). Direct microscopic

TABLE 74–3. Risk Factors for Disseminated Coccidioidomycosis

Risk Factor	Highest Risk
Age	Infants and elderly
Sex	Male
Genetics	Filipino > African American > Native American > Hispanic > Asian
Serum CF antibody titer	>1 : 32
Pregnancy	Late pregnancy and postpartum
Skin test	Negative
Depressed cell-mediated immunity	Malignancy, chemotherapy, steroid treatment, HIV infection

Reprinted from Mitchell TG: Systemic fungi. In Cohen J, Powderly WG, editors: *Infectious diseases,* ed 2, Philadelphia, 2004, Elsevier.
CF, complement fixation.

visualization of endosporulating spherules in sputum, exudates, or tissue is sufficient to establish the diagnosis (see Figure 74–8) and is preferred over culture because of the highly infectious nature of the mould when grown in culture. Clinical exudates should be examined directly in 10% to 20% potassium hydroxide (KOH) with calcofluor white, and tissue from biopsy can be stained with H&E or specific fungal stains such as GMS or PAS (see Figure 74–8).

Clinical specimens may be cultured on routine mycologic media at 25°C. Colonies of *C. immitis* develop within 3 to 5 days, and typical sporulation can be seen in 5 to 10 days. Because of the highly infectious nature of the fungus, all plates or tubes should be sealed using gas-permeable tape (plates) or screw caps (tubes) and only examined within a suitable biosafety cabinet. The identification of *C. immitis* from culture can be accomplished by using the exoantigen immunodiffusion test or nucleic acid hybridization. Conversion of the mould into spherules in vitro is not usually attempted outside of a research setting.

Several serologic procedures exist for initial screening, confirmation, or prognostic evaluation (see Table 74–2). For initial diagnosis, the combined use of the immunodiffusion test and the latex particle agglutination test detects approximately 93% of cases. The complement fixation and tube precipitin tests can also be used for diagnosis and prognosis. Prognostic studies frequently use serial complement fixation titers: rising titers are a bad prognostic sign and falling titers indicate improvement.

TREATMENT

Most persons with primary coccidioidomycosis do not require specific antifungal therapy. For those with concurrent risk factors (see Table 74–3) such as organ transplant, HIV infection, or high doses of corticosteroids, or when there is evidence of unusually severe infection, treatment is necessary. Primary coccidioidomycosis in the third trimester of pregnancy or during immediate postpartum therapy requires treatment with amphotericin B.

Immunocompromised patients or others with diffuse pneumonia should be treated with amphotericin B followed by an azole (either fluconazole or itraconazole) as maintenance therapy. The total length of therapy should be at least 1 year. Immunocompromised patients should be maintained on an oral azole as secondary prophylaxis.

Chronic cavitary pneumonia should be treated with an oral azole for at least 1 year. In cases in which the response is suboptimal, the alternatives are to switch to another azole (e.g., from itraconazole to fluconazole), increase the dose of the azole in the case of fluconazole, or switch to amphotericin B. Surgical treatment is required in the event of rupture of a cavity into the pleural space, hemoptysis, or localized refractory lesions.

The treatment of nonmeningeal extrapulmonary disseminated infections is based on oral azole therapy with either fluconazole or itraconazole. In the case of vertebral involvement or inadequate clinical response, treatment with amphotericin B is recommended along with appropriate surgical débridement and stabilization.

Meningeal coccidioidomycosis is managed with the administration of fluconazole or itraconazole (secondary choice due to poor CNS penetration) indefinitely. Intrathecal administration of amphotericin B is recommended only in the event of failure of azole therapy because of its toxicity when administered by this route.

Histoplasmosis

Histoplasmosis is caused by two varieties of *Histoplasma capsulatum: H. capsulatum* var *capsulatum* and *H. capsulatum* var *duboisii* (see Table 74–1). *H. capsulatum* var *capsulatum* causes pulmonary and disseminated infections in the eastern half of the United States and most of Latin America, whereas *H. capsulatum* var *duboisii* causes predominately skin and bone lesions and is restricted to the tropical areas of Africa (see Figure 74–2).

MORPHOLOGY

Both varieties of *H. capsulatum* are thermally dimorphic fungi existing as a hyaline mould in nature and in culture at 25°C and as an intracellular budding yeast in tissue and in culture at 37°C (Table 74–2 and Figures 74–9, 74–10 and 74–11). In culture, the mould forms of *H. capsulatum* var *capsulatum* and var *duboisii* are indistinguishable

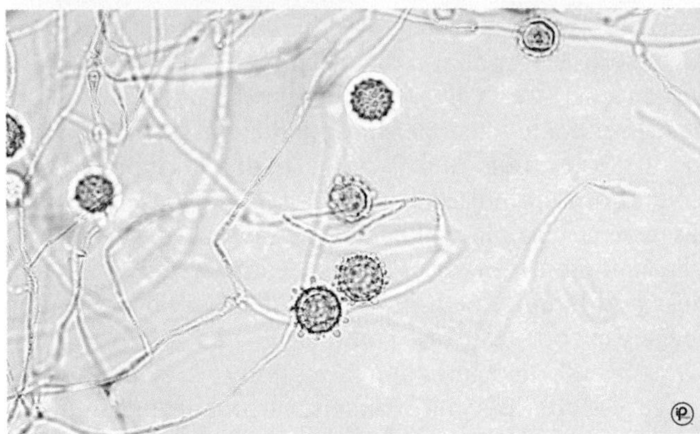

FIGURE 74–9. *Histoplasma capsulatum* mould phase showing tuberculate macroconidia. (From Marler LM et al: *Mycology* CD-ROM, Indiana Pathology Images, 2004.)

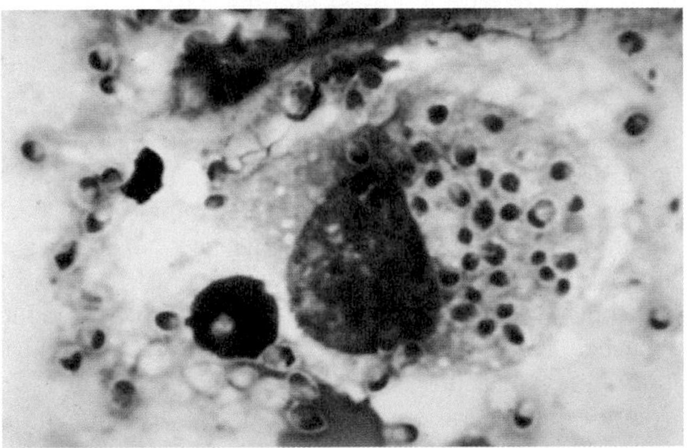

FIGURE 74–10. Giemsa-stained preparation showing intracellular yeast forms of *Histoplasma capsulatum* var *capsulatum*.

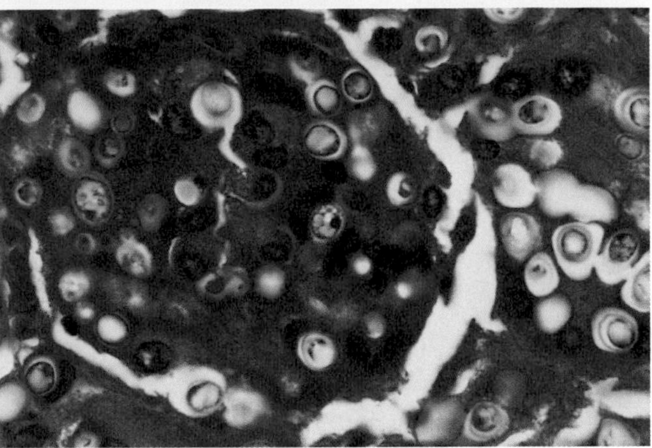

FIGURE 74–11. H&E-stained tissue section showing intracellular yeast forms of *Histoplasma capsulatum* var *duboisii.* (From Connor DH et al: *Pathology of infectious diseases,* Stamford, Conn, 1997, Appleton & Lange.)

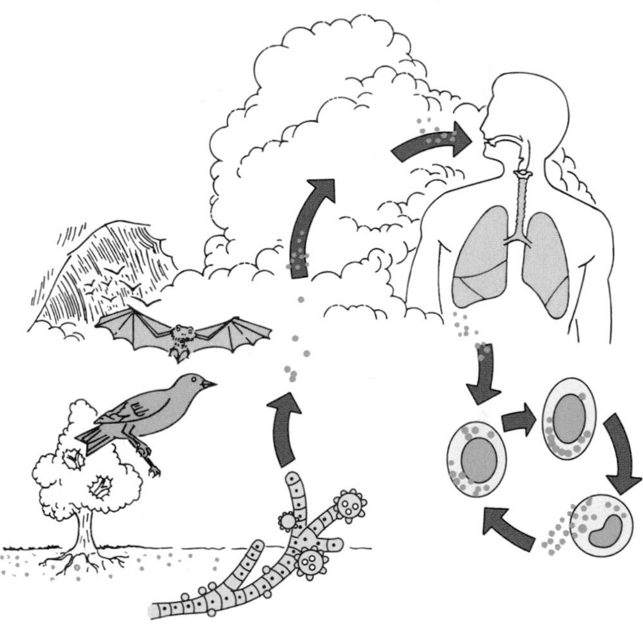

FIGURE 74–12. Natural history of the mould (saprobic) and yeast (parasitic) cycle of *Histoplasma capsulatum.*

macroscopically and microscopically. The mould colonies grow slowly and develop as white or brown hyphal colonies after several days to a week. The mould form produces two types of conidia: (1) large (8 to 15 µm), thick-walled spherical macroconidia with spikelike projections (tuberculate macroconidia) that arise from short conidiophores (see Figures 74–1 and 74–9) and (2) small, oval microconidia (2 to 4 µm) with smooth or slightly rough walls that are sessile or on short stalks (see Figure 74–1 and Figure 74–9). The yeast cells are thin walled, oval, and measure 2 to 4 µm (var *capsulatum*) (see Figure 74–10) or are thicker walled and 8 to 15 µm (var *duboisii*) (see Figure 74–11). The yeast cells of both varieties of *H. capsulatum* are intracellular in vivo and are uninucleate (see Figures 74–10 and 74–11).

EPIDEMIOLOGY

Histoplasmosis capsulatum is localized to the broad regions of the Ohio and Mississippi River valleys in the United States and occurs throughout Mexico and Central and South America (see Figure 74–2 and Table 74–1). Histoplasmosis duboisii, or African histoplasmosis, is confined to the tropical areas of Africa, including Gabon, Uganda, and Kenya (see Figure 74–2 and Table 74–1).

The natural habitat of the mycelial form of both varieties of *H. capsulatum* is soil with a high nitrogen content, such as that found in areas contaminated with bird or bat droppings. Outbreaks of histoplasmosis have been associated with exposure to bird roosts, caves, and decaying buildings or urban renewal projects involving excavation and demolition. Aerosolization of microconidia and hyphal fragments in the disturbed soil with subsequent inhalation by exposed persons is considered to be the basis for these outbreaks (see Figure 74–12). Although attack rates may reach 100% in certain of these exposures, most cases remain asymptomatic and are detected only by skin testing. Immunocompromised persons and children are more prone to develop symptomatic disease with either variety of *Histoplasma.* Reactivation of the disease and dissemination is common among immunosuppressed persons, especially those with AIDS.

CLINICAL SYNDROMES

The usual route of infection for both varieties of histoplasmosis is via inhalation of microconidia, which in turn germinate into yeasts within the lung and may remain localized or disseminate hematogenously or by the lymphatic system (Figure 74–12). The microconidia are rapidly phagocytosed by pulmonary macrophages and neutrophils, and it is thought that conversion to the parasitic yeast form takes place intracellularly.

Histoplasmosis Capsulatum

The clinical presentation of histoplasmosis caused by *H. capsulatum* var *capsulatum* depends on the intensity of exposure and immunologic status of the host. Asymptomatic infection occurs in 90% of persons after a low-intensity exposure. In the event of an exposure to a heavy inoculum, however, most individuals exhibit some symptoms. The self-limited form of acute pulmonary histoplasmosis is marked by a flulike illness with fever, chills, headache, cough, myalgias, and chest pain. Radiographic evidence of hilar or mediastinal adenopathy and patchy pulmonary infiltrates may be seen. Most acute infections resolve with supportive care and do not require specific antifungal treatment. In rare instances, usually after very heavy exposure, acute respiratory distress syndrome may be seen. In approximately 10% of patients, inflammatory sequelae such as persistent lymphadenopathy with bronchial obstruction, arthritis, arthralgias, or pericarditis may be seen. Another rare complication of histoplasmosis is a condition known as mediastinal fibrosis in which persistent host response to the organism may result in massive fibrosis and constriction of mediastinal structures including the heart and great vessels.

Progressive pulmonary histoplasmosis may follow acute infection in approximately 1 in 100,000 cases per year. Chronic pulmonary symptoms are associated with apical cavities and fibrosis and are more likely to occur in patients with prior underlying pulmonary disease. These lesions generally do not heal spontaneously, and persistence of the organism leads to progressive destruction and fibrosis secondary to the immune response to the organism.

Disseminated histoplasmosis follows acute infection in 1 in 2000 adults and is much higher in children and immunocompromised adults. Disseminated disease may assume a chronic, subacute, or acute course. Chronic disseminated histoplasmosis is characterized by weight loss and fatigue, with or without fever. Oral ulcers and hepatosplenomegaly are common.

Subacute disseminated histoplasmosis is marked by fever, weight loss, and malaise. Oropharyngeal ulcers and hepatosplenomegaly are prominent. Bone marrow involvement may produce anemia, leukopenia, and thrombocytopenia. Other sites of involvement include the adrenals, cardiac valves, and the central nervous system. Untreated subacute disseminated histoplasmosis will result in death within 2 to 24 months.

Acute disseminated histoplasmosis is a fulminant process that is most commonly seen in severely immunosuppressed individuals including those with AIDS, organ transplant recipients, and those receiving steroids or other immunosuppressive chemotherapy. In addition, children younger than 1 year and adults with debilitating medical conditions are also at risk given sufficient exposure to the fungus. In contrast to the other forms of histoplasmosis, acute disseminated disease may present with a septic shocklike picture with fever, hypotension, pulmonary infiltrates, and acute respiratory distress. Oral and gastrointestinal ulcerations and bleeding, adrenal insufficiency, meningitis, and endocarditis may also be present. If untreated, acute disseminated histoplasmosis is fatal within days to weeks.

Histoplasmosis Duboisii

In contrast to classic histoplasmosis, pulmonary lesions are uncommon in African histoplasmosis. The localized form of histoplasmosis duboisii is a chronic disease characterized by regional lymphadenopathy with lesions of skin and bone. Skin lesions are papular or nodular and eventually progress to abscesses which then ulcerate. About one third of patients will exhibit osseous lesions characterized by osteolysis and involvement of contiguous joints. The cranium, sternum, ribs, vertebrae, and long bones are most frequently involved, often with overlying abscesses and draining sinuses.

A more fulminant disseminated form of histoplasmosis duboisii may be seen in profoundly immunodeficient individuals. Hematogenous and lymphatic dissemination to bone marrow, liver, spleen, and other organs occurs and is marked by fever, lymphadenopathy, anemia, weight loss, and organomegaly. This form of the disease is uniformly fatal unless promptly diagnosed and treated.

TABLE 74–4. Laboratory Tests for Histoplasmosis

Test	Sensitivity (% true positives) in Disease States		
	Disseminated	Chronic Pulmonary	Self-limited*
Antigen	92	21	39
Culture	85	85	15
Histopathology	43	17	9
Serology	71	100	98

Reprinted from Wheat LJ: Endemic mycoses. In Cohen J, Powderly WG, editors: *Infectious diseases,* ed 2, Philadelphia, 2004, Elsevier.
*Includes acute pulmonary histoplasmosis, rheumatologic syndrome, and pericarditis.

LABORATORY DIAGNOSIS

The diagnosis of histoplasmosis may be made by direct microscopy, culture of blood, bone marrow, or other clinical material and by serology including antigen detection in blood and urine (Table 74–2 and 74–4). The yeast phase of the organism can be detected in sputum, bronchoalveolar lavage fluid, peripheral blood films, bone marrow, and tissue stained with Giemsa, GMS, or PAS stains (see Figure 74–10). In tissue sections, cells of *H. capsulatum* var *capsulatum* are yeastlike, hyaline, spherical to oval, 2 to 4 μm in diameter and uninucleate and have single buds attached by a narrow base. The cells are usually intracellular and clustered together. The cells of *H. capsulatum* var *duboisii* are also intracellular, yeastlike and uninucleate but are much larger (8 to 15 μm) and have thick "doubly contoured" walls. They are usually in macrophages and giant cells (see Figure 74–11).

Cultures of respiratory specimens, blood, bone marrow, and tissue are of value in patients with disseminated disease due to the high organism burden. They are less useful in self-limited or localized disease (see Table 74–4). Growth of the mycelial form in culture is slow, and once isolated, the identification must be confirmed by conversion to the yeast phase or by use of exoantigen testing or nucleic acid hybridization. As with the other dimorphic pathogens, cultures of *Histoplasma* must be handled with care in a biosafety cabinet.

Serologic diagnosis of histoplasmosis involves tests for both antigen and antibody detection (see Table 74–2). Antibody detection assays include a complement fixation assay and immunodiffusion test. These tests are usually used together to maximize sensitivity and specificity, but neither is useful in the acute setting and both often have negative results in immunocompromised patients with disseminated infection.

Detection of histoplasma antigen in serum and urine by enzyme immunoassay has become very useful, particularly in diagnosing disseminated disease (see Table 74–2 and 74–4). The sensitivity of antigen detection is greater in urine specimens than in blood and ranges from 21% in chronic pulmonary disease to 92% in disseminated disease. Serial measurements of antigen may be used to assess response to therapy and for establishing relapse of the disease.

TREATMENT

Since most patients with histoplasmosis recover without therapy, the first decision must be whether specific antifungal therapy is necessary. Some immunocompetent patients with more severe infection may exhibit prolonged symptoms and may benefit from treatment with itraconazole. In cases of severe acute pulmonary histoplasmosis with hypoxemia and acute respiratory distress syndrome, amphotericin B should be administered followed by oral itraconazole to complete a 12-week course.

Chronic pulmonary histoplasmosis also warrants treatment because it is known to progress if left untreated. Treatment with amphotericin B followed by itraconazole for 12 to 24 months is recommended.

Disseminated histoplasmosis usually responds well to amphotericin B therapy. Once stabilized, the patient may be switched to oral itraconazole to be administered over 6 to 18 months. Patients with AIDS may require lifelong therapy with itraconazole.

Histoplasmosis of the central nervous system is universally fatal if not treated. The therapy of choice is amphotericin B followed by fluconazole for 9 to 12 months.

Patients with severe obstructive mediastinal histoplasmosis require amphotericin B therapy. Itraconazole can be used for outpatient therapy.

Paracoccidioidomycosis

Paracoccidioidomycosis is a systemic fungal infection caused by the dimorphic pathogen *Paracoccidioides brasiliensis.* This infection is also known as South American blastomycosis and is the major dimorphic endemic fungal infection in Latin America countries. Primary paracoccidioidomycosis usually appears in young people as a self-limited pulmonary process. At this stage, it rarely displays a progressive acute or subacute course. Reactivation of a primary quiescent lesion may occur years later, resulting in chronic progressive pulmonary disease with or without involvement of other organs.

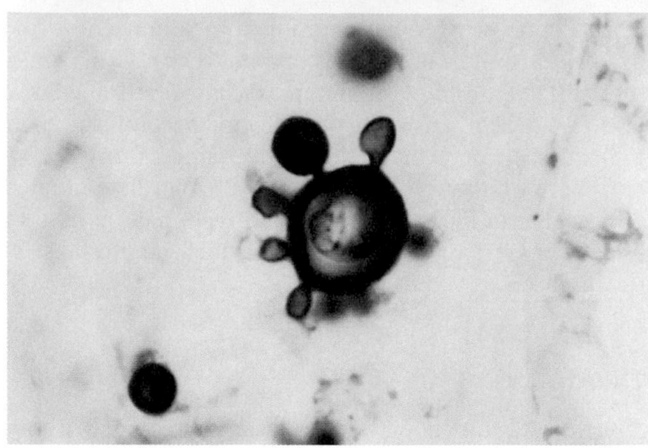

FIGURE 74–13. GMS-stained yeast form of *Paracoccidioides brasiliensis* showing multiple budding "pilots wheel" morphology. (From Connor DH et al: *Pathology of infectious diseases*, Stamford, Conn, 1997, Appleton & Lange.)

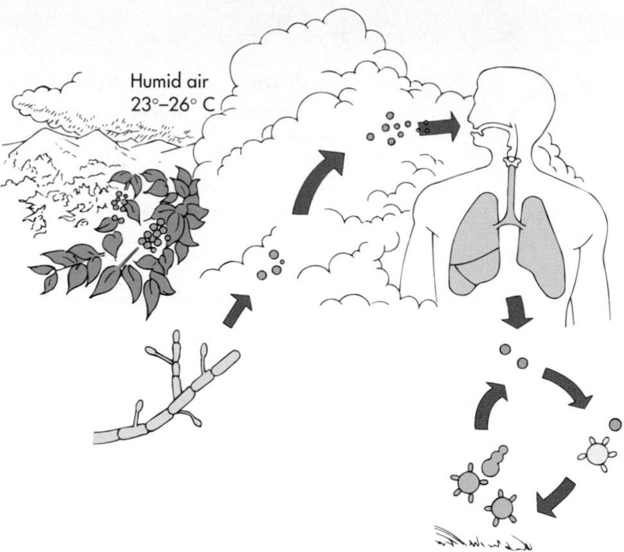

FIGURE 74–14. Natural history of the mould (saprobic) and yeast (parasitic) cycle of *Paracoccidioides brasiliensis.*

MORPHOLOGY

The mould phase of *P. brasiliensis* grows slowly in vitro at 25°C. White colonies become apparent in 3 to 4 weeks, eventually taking on a velvety appearance. Glabrous, wrinkled, brownish colonies may also be seen. The mycelial form is nondescript and nondiagnostic: hyaline, septate hyphae with intercalated chlamydoconidia. Specific identification requires conversion to the yeast form or exoantigen testing.

The characteristic yeast form is seen in tissue and in culture at 37°C. Variably sized (3 to 30 μm or more in diameter), oval to round yeastlike cells with double refractile walls and single or multiple buds (blastoconidia) are characteristic of this fungus (Figure 74–13). The blastoconidia are connected to the parent cell by a narrow isthmus and six or more of various sizes may be produced from a single cell: the so-called "mariners" or "pilot wheel" morphology. The variability in size and number of blastoconidia and their connection to the parent cell are identifying features (see Figure 74–13). These features are best disclosed by the GMS stain but may also be seen in H&E-stained tissues or in KOH mounts of clinical material.

EPIDEMIOLOGY

Paracoccidioidomycosis is endemic throughout Latin America, but it is more prevalent in South America than in Central America (see Figure 74–2). The highest incidence is seen in Brazil, followed by Colombia, Venezuela, Ecuador, and Argentina. All patients diagnosed outside of Latin America had previously lived in Latin America. The ecology of the endemic areas includes high humidity, rich vegetation, moderate temperatures, and acid soil. These conditions are found along rivers from the Amazon jungle to small indigenous forests in Uruguay. *P. brasiliensis* has been recovered from soil in these areas; however, its ecologic niche is not well established. The portal of entry is thought to be either by inhalation or traumatic inoculation (Figure 74–14), although even this is poorly understood. Natural infection has only been documented in armadillos.

Although infection occurs in children (peak incidence, 10 to 19 years), overt disease is uncommon in both children and adolescents. In adults, disease is more common in men aged 30 to 50 years. Most patients with clinically apparent disease live in rural areas and have close contact with the soil. There are no reports of epidemics or human-to-human transmission. Depression of cell-mediated immunity correlates with the acute progressive form of the disease.

CLINICAL SYNDROMES

Paracoccidioidomycosis may be subclinical or progressive with acute or chronic pulmonary forms or acute, subacute, or chronic disseminated forms of the disease. Most primary infections are self-limited; however, the organism may become dormant for long periods of time and reactivate to cause clinical disease concomitant with impaired host defenses. A subacute disseminated form is seen in younger patients and immunocompromised individuals with marked lymphadenopathy, organomegaly, bone marrow involvement, and osteoarticular manifestations mimicking osteomyelitis. Recurrent fungemia results in dissemination and frequent skin lesions. Pulmonary and mucosal lesions are not seen in this form of the disease.

Adults most often present with a chronic pulmonary form of the disease marked by respiratory problems, often as the sole manifestation. The disease progresses slowly over months to years with persistent cough, purulent sputum, chest pain, weight loss, dyspnea, and fever. Pulmonary lesions are nodular, infiltrative, fibrotic, and cavitary.

Although 25% of patients exhibit only pulmonary manifestations of the disease, the infection can disseminate to extrapulmonary sites in the absence of diagnosis and treatment. Prominent extrapulmonary locations include skin and mucosa, lymph nodes, adrenal glands, liver, spleen, central nervous system, and bones. The mucosal lesions are painful and ulcerated and usually are confined to the mouth, lips, gums, and palate. More than 90% of those affected are male.

LABORATORY DIAGNOSIS

The diagnosis is established by the demonstration of the characteristic yeast forms on microscopic examination of sputum, bronchoalveolar lavage fluid, scrapings or biopsy of ulcers, pus draining from lymph nodes, cerebrospinal fluid, or tissue (see Table 74–2). The organism can be visualized by a variety of staining methods including calcofluor fluorescence, H&E, GMS, PAS, or Papanicolaou stains (see Figure 74–13). The presence of multiple buds distinguish *P. brasiliensis* from *Cryptococcus neoformans* and *B. dermatitidis.*

Isolation of the organism in culture requires confirmation by demonstration of thermal dimorphism or exoantigen testing (detection of exoantigen 1, 2, and 3). Cultures should be manipulated in a biosafety cabinet.

Serologic testing using either immunodiffusion or complement fixation to demonstrate antibody may be helpful in suggesting the diagnosis and in evaluating response to therapy (see Table 74–2).

TREATMENT

Itraconazole is the treatment of choice for most forms of the disease and generally must be given for at least 6 months. More severe or refractory infections may require amphotericin B therapy followed by either itraconazole or sulfonamide therapy. Relapses are common with sulfonamide therapy, and both dose and duration require adjustment based on clinical and mycologic parameters. Fluconazole has some activity against this organism, although frequent relapses have limited its use for the treatment of this disease.

Penicilliosis Marneffei

Penicilliosis marneffei is a disseminated mycosis caused by the dimorphic fungus *Penicillium marneffei.* This infection involves the mononuclear phagocytic system and occurs primarily in HIV-infected persons in Thailand and Southern China (see Figure 74–2).

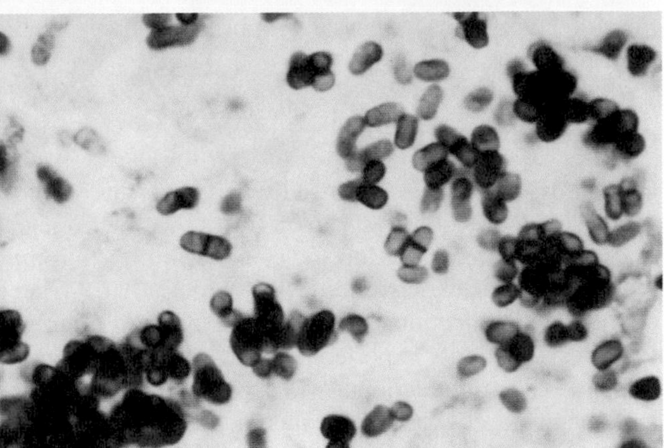

FIGURE 74–15. GMS-stained yeast forms of *Penicillium marneffei,* including forms with single, wide, transverse septa (center). (From Connor DH et al: *Pathology of infectious diseases,* Stamford, Conn, 1997, Appleton & Lange.)

MORPHOLOGY

P. marneffei is the only species of *Penicillium* that is a pathogenic dimorphic fungus. In its mould phase in culture at 25°C, it exhibits sporulating structures that are typical of the genus (see Figure 74–1). Identification is aided by the formation of a soluble red pigment that diffuses into the agar (see Table 74–3).

At 37°C in culture and in tissue, *P. marneffei* grows as a yeastlike organism that divides by fission and exhibits a transverse septum (Figure 74–15). The yeast form is intracellular in vivo and in this way resembles *H. capsulatum,* although it is somewhat more pleomorphic and elongated and does not bud (see Table 74–2 and Figures 74–10 and 74–15).

EPIDEMIOLOGY

P. marneffei has emerged as a prominent mycotic pathogen among HIV-infected individuals in Southeast Asia (see Figure 74–2). Imported cases have been reported in Europe and the United States. Although infection has been seen in immunocompetent hosts, the vast majority of infections since 1987 have been in patients with AIDS or in other immunocompromised hosts residing in, or who have visited, Southeast Asia or Southern China. Penicilliosis marneffei has become an early indicator of HIV infection in that part of the world. *P. marneffei* has been isolated from bamboo rats and occasionally from soil. Laboratory-acquired infection has been reported in an immunocompromised person exposed to the mycelial form in culture.

CLINICAL SYNDROMES

Penicilliosis marneffei is caused when a susceptible host inhales conidia of *P. marneffei* from the environment and disseminated infection develops. The infection may mimic tuberculosis, leishmaniasis, and other AIDS-related opportunistic infections such as histoplasmosis and cryptococcosis. Patients experience fever, cough, pulmonary infiltrates, lymphadenopathy, organomegaly, anemia, leukopenia, and thrombocytopenia. Skin lesions reflect hematogenous dissemination and appear as molluscum contagiosum-like lesions on the face and trunk.

LABORATORY DIAGNOSIS

P. marneffei is readily recovered from clinical specimens including blood, bone marrow, bronchoalveolar lavage specimens, and tissue. Isolation of a mould in culture at 25° to 30°C that exhibits typical *Penicillium* morphology and a diffusible red pigment is highly suggestive. Conversion to the yeast phase at 37°C is confirmatory. Microscopic detection of the elliptical fission yeasts inside phagocytes in smears of bone marrow, ulcerative skin lesions, or lymph nodes or buffy coat preparations is diagnostic (see Figure 74–15). Serologic tests are under development.

TREATMENT

Amphotericin B with or without flucytosine is the treatment of choice. Administration of amphotericin B for 2 weeks should be followed by itraconazole for another 10 weeks. AIDS patients may require lifelong treatment with itraconazole to prevent relapses of the infection. Fluconazole therapy has been associated with a high rate of failure and is not recommended.

CASE STUDY AND QUESTIONS

Jane and Joan were two women in their mid-30s who avidly participated in outdoor activity. In the past 5 years they had been spelunking in southern Missouri, backpacking in northern Wisconsin, and camping in Arizona. Most recently, they had been renovating an old farmhouse in rural Iowa and in the process had to tear down an old chicken coop that was attached to the back of the house. About 1 week into the process, they both suffered from a "flulike" illness, and Jane developed a cough and shortness of breath. They went to the family practice clinic to get examined. At the clinic, Joan appeared fine but Jane was noted to be quite short of breath and appeared to be ill. The doctor thought it would be a good idea to perform a chest x-ray on Jane. Joan got one too "just in case." The results of Jane's chest x-ray showed a diffuse bilateral pneumonia. Although Joan's radiograph did not show pneumonia, it was noted that she had a solitary nodule in the right upper lobe.

1. To what dimorphic fungal pathogens were Jane and Joan exposed?
2. What constitutes a dimorphic fungus?
3. Aside from dimorphism, what feature is common to all of the endemic mycoses?
4. Describe the life cycles of the six dimorphic endemic pathogens.
5. What do you think is the cause of Jane's pneumonia? How would you make the diagnosis? How would you treat her pneumonia?
6. What do you think accounts for Joan's lung nodule? How would you make the diagnosis? How would you treat her?

Bibliography

Connor DH et al: *Pathology of infectious diseases*, Stamford, Conn, 1997, Appleton & Lange.

Mitchell TG: Systemic fungi. In Cohen J, Powderly WG, editors: *Infectious diseases*, ed 2, Philadelphia, 2004, Elsevier.

Perea S, Patterson TF: Endemic mycoses. In Anaissie EJ, McGinnis MR, Pfaller MA, editors: *Clinical mycology*, New York, 2003, Churchill Livingstone.

Wheat LJ: Endemic mycoses. In Cohen J, Powderly WG, editors: *Infectious diseases*, ed 2, Philadelphia, 2004, Elsevier.

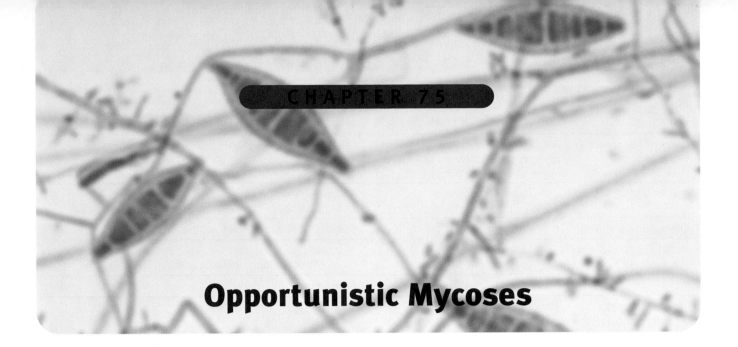

CHAPTER 75

Opportunistic Mycoses

The frequency of invasive mycoses due to opportunistic fungal pathogens has increased significantly over the past two decades (see Table 7–2). This increase in infections is associated with excessive morbidity and mortality (see Table 7–1) and is directly related to increasing patient populations at risk for the development of serious fungal infections, which includes persons undergoing blood and marrow transplantation (BMT), solid organ transplantation, and major surgery (especially gastrointestinal [GI] tract surgery), those with AIDS, neoplastic disease, immunosuppressive therapy, advanced age, and those born in a premature birth (Table 75–1). The most well known causes of opportunistic mycoses include *Candida albicans*, *Cryptococcus neoformans*, and *Aspergillus fumigatus* **(Box 75–1).** The estimated annual incidence of invasive mycoses due to these pathogens is 72 to 228 infections per million population for *Candida*, 30 to 66 per million for *C. neoformans* and 12 to 34 per million for *Aspergillus* (see Table 7–2). In addition to these agents, of increasing importance is the growing list of "other" opportunistic fungi (see Box 75–1). New and emerging fungal pathogens include species of *Candida* and *Aspergillus* other than *C. albicans* and *A. fumigatus*, opportunistic yeastlike fungi such as *Trichosporon* spp., *Malassezia* spp., *Rhodotorula* spp., and *Geotrichum capitatum (Blastoschizomyes capitatus)*, the Zygomycetes, hyaline moulds such as *Fusarium*, *Acremonium*, *Scedosporium*, *Scopulariopsis*, *Paecilomyces*, and *Trichoderma* species, and a wide variety of demateaceous fungi (see Box 75–1). Infections caused by these organisms range from catheter-related fungemia and peritonitis to more localized infections involving lung, skin, and paranasal sinuses to widespread hematogenous dissemination. Many of these fungi were previously thought to be non-pathogenic and now are recognized causes of invasive mycoses in compromised patients. Estimates of the annual incidence of the less common mycoses have been virtually non-existent; however, data from a population-based survey conducted by the Centers for Disease Control (CDC) indicate that zygomycosis occurs at a rate of 1.7 infections per million per year, hyalohyphomycosis (*Fusarium*, *Acremonium* etc) at 1.2 infections per million per year and phaeohyphomycosis (demateaceous moulds) at 1.0 infection per million per year (see Table 7–1).

Given the complexity of the patients at risk for infection and the diverse array of fungal pathogens, opportunistic mycoses pose a considerable diagnostic and therapeutic challenge. Diagnosis depends on a heightened clinical suspicion (think "FUNGUS") and obtaining appropriate material for culture and histopathology. Isolation and identification of the infecting organisms is very important in properly managing infections due to the less common opportunistic fungi. Some of these organisms are inherently nonsusceptible to standard azole or polyene therapy (see Chapter 70) and may require the use of alternative antifungal agents in addition to surgical management and reversal of the underlying impairment of host defenses.

Candidiasis

It is clear that the most important group of opportunistic fungal pathogens are the *Candida* species. *Candida* spp. are the fourth most common cause of nosocomial (hospital-acquired) bloodstream infections (BSI), exceeding that of any individual gram-negative pathogen (Table 75–2). Between 1980 and the present time, the frequency of *Candida* BSI has risen steadily in hospitals of all sizes and in all age groups (see Table 7–2).

Although more than 100 species of *Candida* have been described, only a few have been implicated in clinical infections (see Box 75–1). *C. albicans* is the species most commonly isolated from clinical material and generally

TABLE 75–1. Predisposing Factors for Opportunistic Mycoses

Factor	Possible Role in Infection	Major Opportunistic Pathogens
Antimicrobial agents Number Duration	Promote fungal colonization Provide intravascular access	*Candida* spp., other yeastlike fungi
Adrenal corticosteroid	Immunosuppression	*Cryptococcus neoformans,* *Aspergillus* spp., Zygomycetes, other moulds, *Pneumocystis*
Chemotherapy	Immunosuppression	*Candida* spp., *Aspergillus* spp., *Pneumocystis*
Hematologic/solid organ malignancy	Immunosuppression	*Candida* spp., *Aspergillus* spp., spp., Zygomycetes, other moulds and yeastlike fungi, *Pneumocystis*
Previous colonization	Translocation across mucosa	*Candida* spp.
Indwelling catheter Central venous, Pressure transducer, Swan-Ganz	Direct vascular access Contaminated product	*Candida* spp., other yeastlike fungi
Total parenteral nutrition	Direct vascular access Contamination of infusate	*Candida* spp., *Malassezia* spp., other yeastlike fungi
Neutropenia (WBC <500/mm^3)	Immunosuppression	*Aspergillus* spp., *Candida* spp., other moulds and yeastlike fungi
Extensive surgery or burns	Route of infection Direct vascular access	*Candida* spp., *Fusarium* spp., Zygomycetes
Assisted ventilation	Route of infection	*Candida* spp., *Aspergillus* spp.
Hospitalization or intensive care unit stay	Exposure to pathogens Exposure to additional risk factors	*Candida* spp., other yeastlike fungi, *Aspergillus* spp.
Hemodialysis or peritoneal dialysis	Route of infection Immunosuppression	*Candida* spp., *Rhodotorula* spp., other yeastlike fungi
Malnutrition	Immunosuppression	*Pneumocystis, Candida* spp., *Cryptococcus neoformans*
HIV infection/AIDS	Immunosuppression	*Cryptococcus neoformans, Pneumocystis, Candida* spp.
Extremes of age	Immunosuppression Numerous comorbidities	*Candida* spp.

TABLE 75–2. Nosocomial Bloodstream Infections: Most Frequent Associated Pathogens—SCOPE Surveillance Program

Rank	Pathogen	% of Isolates*
1	Coagulase-negative staphylococci	32.3
2	*Staphylococcus aureus*	16.7
3	*Enterococcus* spp.	11.7
4	*Candida* spp.	8.0
5	*Escherichia coli*	6.4
6	*Klebsiella* spp.	5.3
7	*Pseudomonas aeruginosa*	5.0
8	*Enterobacter* spp.	4.9
9	Other *Streptococcus* spp.	2.9
10	*Serratia marcescens*	1.4

Adapted from Pfaller MA et al: *Diagn Microbiol Infect Dis* 31:327-332, 1998.
*Percent of a total of 4525 infections.

accounts for 90% to 100% of mucosal isolates and 50% to 70% of isolates from BSI (Table 75–3). Approximately 95% of all *Candida* BSI are accounted for by four species: *C. albicans, C. glabrata, C. parapsilosis,* and *C. tropicalis.* Among these common species, only *C. glabrata* can be said to be truly "emerging" as a cause of BSI, due in part to its intrinsic and acquired resistance to azoles and other commonly used antifungal agents. The remaining 5% of *Candida* BSI encompasses 12 to 14 different species including *C. krusei, C. lusitaniae, C. dubliniensis,* and *C. rugosa* among others (see Box 75–1). Although these species must be considered "rare" causes of candidiasis, several have been observed to occur in nosocomial clusters or to exhibit innate or acquired resistance to one or more established antifungal agents.

MORPHOLOGY

All *Candida* species exist as oval yeastlike forms (3 to 5 μm) that produce buds or blastoconidia. Species of *Candida*

TABLE 75–3. Species Distribution of *Candida* Bloodstream Infection Isolates by Year: Data from the Global Antifungal Surveillance Program, 1992-2003

Species	% of isolates by year (no. tested)					
	1992 (235)	**1995 (332)**	**1997 (413)**	**1999 (320)**	**2001 (2770)**	**2003 (1715)**
C. albicans	44.3	53.3	54.0	54.7	59.8	65.1
C. glabrata	16.6	20.5	15.3	15.3	16.4	14.2
C. parapsilosis	21.7	9.0	18.9	10.3	10.7	9.3
C. tropicalis	11.9	11.4	7.0	11.9	7.9	6.9
C. krusei	2.6	4.2	1.7	2.8	2.7	2.7
C. lusitaniae	2.1	0.6	0.0	2.2	1.3	0.4
C. guilliermondii	0.4	0.4	1.9	0.9	0.6	0.3

Adapted from Pfaller MA, Diekema DJ: *Clin Microbiol Infect* 10[Suppl. 1]:11-23, 2004.

BOX 75–1. Agents of Opportunistic Mycoses*

***Candida* Species**
C. albicans
C. glabrata
C. parapsilosis
C. tropicalis
C. krusei
C. lusitaniae
C. guilliermondii
C. dubliniensis
C. rugosa

***Cryptococcus neoformans* and Other Opportunistic Yeastlike Fungi**
Cryptococcus neoformans
Malassezia spp.
Trichosporon spp.
Rhodotorula spp.
Geotrichum capitatum

***Aspergillus* Species**
A. fumigatus
A. flavus
A. niger
A. versicolor
A. terreus

Zygomycetes
Rhizopus spp.
Mucor spp.
Rhizomucor spp.
Absidia spp.
Cunninghamella spp.

Other Hyaline Moulds
Fusarium spp.
Acremonium spp.
Scedosporium spp.
Paecilomyces spp.
Trichoderma spp.
Scopulariopsis spp.

Dematiaceous Moulds
Alternaria spp.
Bipolaris spp.
Cladophialophora spp.
Curvularia spp.
Exophiala spp.
Exserohilum spp.
Wangiella spp.

Pneumocystis jiroveci

*List is not all-inclusive.

other than *C. glabrata* also produce pseudohyphae and true hyphae (Figure 75–1; also see Chapter 7, Figure 7–2A and Chapter 71, Figure 71-1). In addition, *C. albicans* forms germ tubes (Figure 7–2) and terminal, thick-walled chlamydoconidia (Figure 75–2). *C. glabrata*, the second most common species of *Candida* in many settings, is incapable of forming pseudohyphae, germ tubes, or true

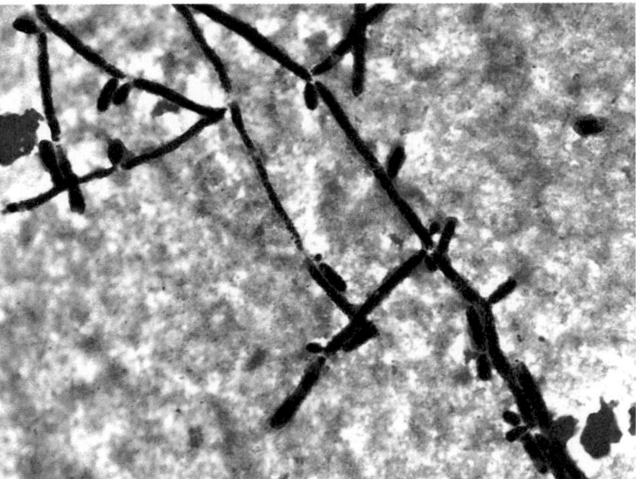

FIGURE 75–1. *Candida tropicalis* blastoconidia and pseudohyphae (Gram stain, magnification 1000×).

hyphae under most conditions. In histologic sections, all *Candida* spp. stain poorly with hematoxylin and eosin (H&E) and well with the periodic-acid Schiff (PAS), Gomori methenamine silver (GMS), and Gridley fungus stains.

In culture, most *Candida* spp. form smooth, white, creamy, domed colonies. *C. albicans* and other species may also undergo phenotypic switching in which a single strain of *Candida* may change reversibly among several different morphotypes, ranging from the typical smooth white colony composed of predominantly budding yeast-like cells to very "fuzzy" or "hairy" colonies composed primarily of pseudohyphal and hyphal forms. The frequency of the switching phenomenon is too high to result from gene mutations and too low to be attributable to mass conversion whereby all cells in the population change their phenotype in response to signals from the environment. It

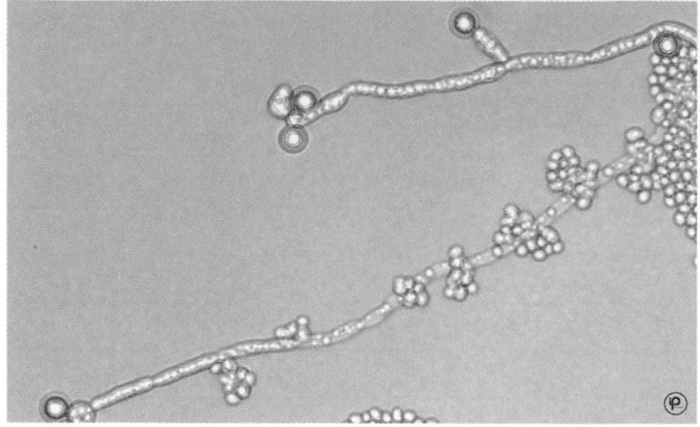

FIGURE 75–2. *Candida albicans,* microscopic morphology in corn meal agar showing large chlamydospores, blastoconidia, hyphae, and pseudohyphae (magnification 400×). (From Marler LM et al: *Mycology* CD-ROM, Indiana Pathology Images, 2004.)

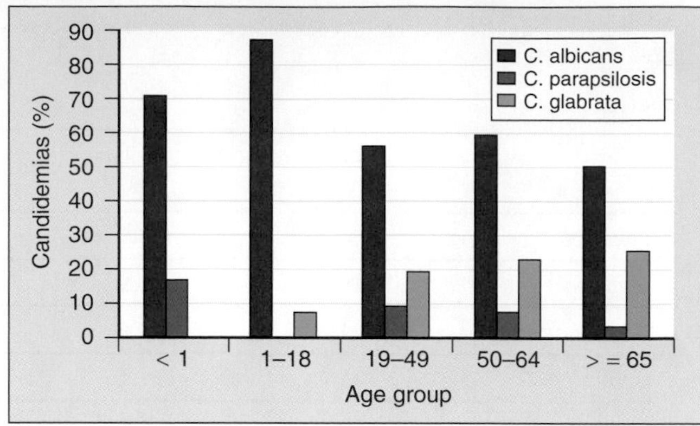

FIGURE 75–3. Percentage of all candidemias caused by selected *Candida* spp. in each age group. (Data from the Emerging Infections and the Epidemiology of Iowa Organisms Survey, 1998 to 2001. Reprinted from Pfaller MA, Diekema DJ: *J Clin Microbiol* 40:3551-3557, 2002.)

is likely that switching serves as some type of master system in *C. albicans*, and other species, for rapid response at the level of individual cells to changes in the local microenvironment. It has been postulated that phenotypic switching explains the ability of *C. albicans* to survive in many different environmental microniches within the human host.

EPIDEMIOLOGY

Candida spp. are known colonizers of humans and other warm-blooded animals. As such, they are found in humans and in nature worldwide. The primary site of colonization is the GI tract from mouth to rectum. They may also be found as commensals in the vagina and urethra, on the skin, and under the fingernails and toenails. *C. albicans*, the most common etiologic agent of human disease, has also been found apart from humans and animals in air, water, and soil.

It is estimated that 25% to 50% of healthy subjects carry *Candida* as part of the normal flora of the mouth, with *C. albicans* accounting for 70% to 80% of isolates. Oral carriage rates are increased substantially in children, hospitalized patients, those with HIV infection, dentures, diabetes, patients receiving antineoplastic chemotherapy, and those receiving antibiotics. Virtually all humans may carry one or more *Candida* species throughout their GI tract, and the levels of carriage may increase to that detectable in illness or other circumstances in which the host's microbial suppression mechanisms become compromised.

The predominant source of infection caused by *Candida* spp.—from superficial mucosal and cutaneous disease to hematogenous dissemination—is the patient. That is, most types of candidiasis represent **endogenous** infection in which the normally commensal host flora take advantage of the "opportunity" to cause infection. To do so, there must be a lowering of a host anti-*Candida* barrier. In the case of *Candida* BSI, transfer of the organism from the GI mucosa to the bloodstream requires prior overgrowth of the numbers of yeasts in their commensal habitat coupled with a breach in the integrity of the GI mucosa.

Exogenous transmission of *Candida* may also account for a proportion of certain types of candidiasis. Examples include the use of contaminated irrigation solutions, parenteral nutrition fluids, vascular pressure transducers, cardiac valves, and corneas. Transmission of *Candida* spp. from health care workers to patients and from patient to patient has been well documented, especially in the intensive care unit environment. The hands of health care workers serve as potential reservoirs for nosocomial transmission of *Candida* spp.

Among the various species of *Candida* capable of causing human infection (see Box 75–1 and Table 75–3), *C. albicans* predominates in most types of infection. Infections of genital, cutaneous, and oral sites almost always involve *C. albicans*. A wider array of *Candida* spp. is seen causing BSI, and although *C. albicans* usually predominates (see Table 75–3), the frequency with which this and other species of *Candida* are isolated from blood varies considerably according to the age of the patient (Figure 75–3) and the local, regional, or global setting (Table 75–4). Whereas *C. albicans* and *C. parapsilosis* predominate as causes of BSI among infants and children, a decrease in *C. albicans* and *C. parapsilosis* infections and a prominent increase in *C. glabrata* infections are seen among older persons (see Figure 75–3). Likewise, although *C. albicans* is the dominant species causing BSI in the Asia-Pacific region of the world, it is seen at a lower frequency in Latin America, where *C. parapsilosis* and *C. tropicalis* are more common (see Table 75–4). The differences in the number

TABLE 75–4. Species Distribution of *Candida* Bloodstream Infection Isolates by Geographic Region

Region	Number of Hospitals	Number of Isolates	% of Isolates by Species					
			CA	CG	CP	CT	CK	Other
Asia-Pacific	17	441	73.5	10.2	8.4	3.9	3.2	0.8
Europe	40	775	57.6	12.9	14.1	7.5	3.4	4.5
Latin America	18	560	46.6	7.5	17.1	21.3	3.6	3.3
Canada	8	623	58.9	20.1	10.3	5.9	2.4	2.4
United States	167	3683	54.4	18.3	13.2	9.6	2.1	2.4
Total	250	6082	55.9	16.2	13.1	9.6	2.5	2.7

Adapted from Pfaller MA, Diekema DJ: *Clin Microbiol Infect* 10[Suppl 1]:11-23, 2004.
CA, *Candida albicans;* CG, *Candida glabrata;* CK, *Candida krusei;* CP, *Candida parapsilosis;* CT, *Candida tropicalis.*

and types of *Candida* spp. causing infections may be influenced by numerous factors including patient age, increased immunosuppression, antifungal drug exposure, or differences in infection control practices. Each one of these factors, alone or in combination, can affect the prevalence of different *Candida* spp. in each institution. For example, the use of azoles (e.g., fluconazole) for antifungal prophylaxis may increase the likelihood of infections caused by *C. glabrata* and *C. krusei,* two species with decreased susceptibility to this class of antifungal agents. Likewise, breaks in infection control precautions and in the proper care of vascular catheters can lead to more infections with *C. parapsilosis,* the predominant species isolated from the hands of health care workers and a frequent cause of catheter-related fungemia.

The consequences of *Candida* BSI in the hospitalized patient are severe. Hospitalized patients with candidemia have been shown to be at a two-fold greater risk of death in hospital than those with non-candidal BSI. Among all patients with nosocomial BSI, candidemia was found to be an independent predictor of death in hospital. Although estimates of mortality can be confounded by the serious nature of the underlying diseases in many of these patients, matched cohort studies have confirmed that the mortality directly attributable to the fungal infection is quite high (Table 75–5). Notably, the excess or attributable mortality due to candidemia has not decreased from that observed in the mid-1980s to that observed in 2001 despite the introduction of new antifungal agents with good activity against most species of *Candida.*

More is known about the epidemiology of nosocomial candidemia than any other fungal infection. The accumulated evidence allows one to propose a general view of nosocomial candidemia (Figure 75–4). Certain hospitalized individuals are clearly at increased risk of acquiring candidemia during hospitalization as a result of their underlying medical condition: patients with hematologic malignancies or neutropenia, those undergoing GI surgery, and both premature infants and those older than 70 years of age (see Table 75–1 and Figure 75–4). Compared to control subjects without the specific risk factors or exposures, the likelihood of these already high-risk patients contracting candidemia in hospital is approximately 2 times greater for each class of antibiotics they receive, 7 times greater if they have a central venous catheter, 10 times greater if *Candida* has been found to be colonizing other anatomic sites, and 18 times greater if the patient has undergone acute hemodialysis. Hospitalization in the intensive care unit setting provides the opportunity for transmission of *Candida* among patients and has been shown to be an additional independent risk factor.

TABLE 75–5. Excess Mortality Attributable to Nosocomial Infections with *Candida* and *Aspergillus*

Type of Mortality Rate	Percent Mortality		
	*Candida**		*Aspergillus*†
	1988	2001	1991
Crude mortality			
Cases	57	61	95
Control subjects	19	12	10
Attributable mortality	38	49	85

*Patients with candidemia. (Data from Wey SB et al: *Arch Intern Med* 148:2642-2645, 1988; and Gudlagson O et al: *Clin Infect Dis* 37:1172-1177, 2003).

†Bone marrow transplant patients with invasive pulmonary aspergillosis. (Data from Pannuti CS et al: *J Clin Oncol* 9:1-5, 1991.)

The available epidemiologic data indicates that between 5 and 10 of every 1000 high-risk patients exposed to the above risk factors will contract BSI caused by *Candida* spp. (8% to 10% of all nosocomial BSI; Table 75–2). Approximately 49% of these patients will die as a result of their infection, 12% will die of their underlying disease, and 39% will survive hospitalization (see

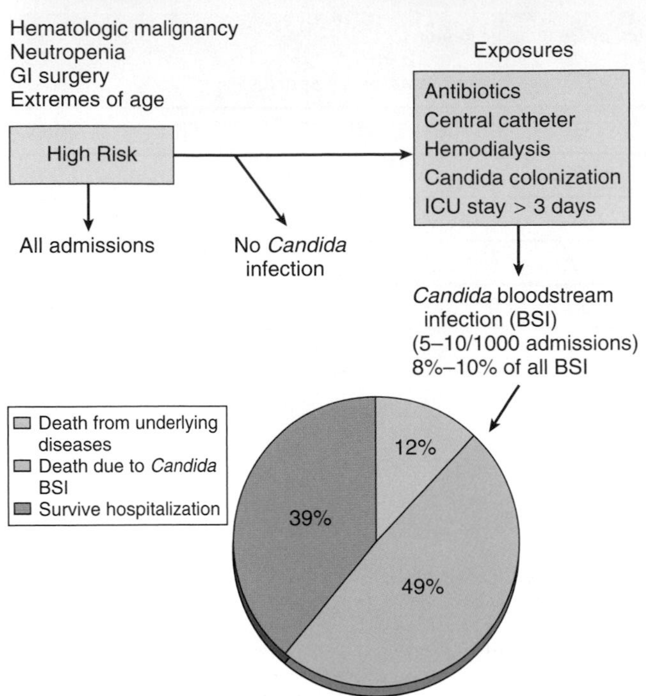

FIGURE 75–4. Global view of hospital-acquired candidemia. GI, Gastrointestinal; ICU, intensive care unit. (Adapted from Pfaller MA, Wenzel RP: The epidemiology of fungal infections. In Anaissie EJ, McGinnis MR, Pfaller MA, editors: *Clinical mycology,* New York, 2003, Churchill Livingstone.)

Figure 75–4). This picture has not changed and may even be worse than that seen in the mid 1980s. The outcome for almost half of those patients with candidemia could be improved by more effective means of prevention, diagnosis, and therapy. Clearly the most desirable of these is prevention, which is best approached by rigorous control of the exposures especially limiting the use of broad-spectrum antibiotics and improved catheter care and adherence to infection control practices.

CLINICAL SYNDROMES

Given the right setting, *Candida* spp. can cause clinically apparent infection of virtually any organ system (Table 75–6). Infections range from superficial mucosal and cutaneous candidiasis to widespread hematogenous dissemination involving target organs such as the liver, spleen, kidney, heart, and brain. In the latter situation, the mortality directly attributable to the infectious process approaches 50% (see Table 75–5 and Figure 75–4).

Mucosal infections caused by *Candida* spp. (known as "thrush") may be limited to the oropharynx or extend to the esophagus and the entire gastrointestinal tract. In women, the vaginal mucosa is also a common site of infection. These infections are generally seen in persons with local or generalized immunosuppression or those settings in which candidal overgrowth is favored (see Table 75–6).

TABLE 75–6. Types of *Candida* Infection and Associated Predisposing Factors

Type of Disease	Predisposing Factors
Oropharyngeal infection	Age extremes Denture wearers Diabetes mellitus Antibiotic use Radiotherapy for head and neck cancer Inhaled and systemic steroids Cytotoxic chemotherapy HIV infection Hematologic malignancies Stem cell or solid organ transplantation
Esophagitis	Systemic corticosteroids AIDS Cancer Stem cell or solid organ transplantation
Vulvovaginal infection	Oral contraceptives Pregnancy Diabetes mellitus Systemic corticosteroids HIV infection Antibiotic use
Infections of the skin and nails	Local moisture and occlusion Immersion of hands in water Peripheral vascular disease
Chronic mucocutaneous candidiasis	T-lymphocyte defects
Urinary tract infection	Indwelling urinary catheter Urinary obstruction Urinary procedures Diabetes mellitus
Pneumonia	Aspiration
Endocarditis	Major surgery Previous valvular disease Prosthetic valve Intravenous drug use Long-term central venous catheter
Pericarditis	Thoracic surgery Immunosuppression
Central nervous system (CNS) infection	CNS surgery Ventriculoperitoneal shunt Ocular surgery
Ocular infection	Trauma Surgery
Bone and joint infection	Trauma Intraarticular injections Diabetic foot
Abdominal infection	Perforation Abdominal surgery Anastomotic leaks Pancreatitis Continuous ambulatory peritoneal dialysis
Hematogenous infection	Solid organ transplantation Colonization Prolonged antibiotic use Abdominal surgery Intensive care support Total parenteral nutrition Hemodialysis Immunosuppression Extremes of age Stem cell transplantation

Adapted from Dignani MC, Solomkin JS, Anaissie EJ: *Candida.* In Anaissie EJ, McGinnis MR, Pfaller MA, editors: *Clinical mycology,* New York, 2003, Churchill Livingstone.

These infections usually present as white "cottage cheese"-like patches on the mucosal surface. Other presentations include the pseudomembranous type, which reveals a raw bleeding surface when scraped; the erythematous type, which are flat, red, occasionally sore areas; candidal leukoplakia, nonremovable white thickening of epithelium caused by *Candida* spp.; and angular chelitis, sore fissures at the corners of the mouth.

Candida spp. may cause localized skin infection in areas where the skin surface is occluded and moist (e.g., groin, axillae, toe webs, breast folds). These infections present as a pruritic rash with erythematous vesiculopustular lesions.

Onychomycosis and paronychia may occur in the setting of a mixed microbial flora including *Candida*. The species most commonly involved are *C. albicans, C. parapsilosis,* and *C. guilliermondii.*

Skin lesions may also appear during the course of hematogenous dissemination. These lesions are of major diagnostic importance because they can be directly biopsied and thus provide an etiologic diagnosis of a systemic process.

Chronic mucocutaneous candidiasis is a rare condition marked by a deficiency in T-lymphocyte responsiveness to *Candida* spp. These patients suffer from severe unremitting mucocutaneous *Candida* lesions including extensive nail involvement and vaginitis. The lesions may become quite large, with a disfiguring granulomatous appearance.

Urinary tract involvement with *Candida* spp. ranges from asymptomatic bladder colonization to renal abscesses secondary to hematogenous seeding. Bladder colonization with *Candida* spp. is essentially not seen unless a patient requires an indwelling bladder catheter, has diabetes, suffers from urinary obstruction or has had prior urinary procedures. Benign colonization of the bladder is most common in these settings but urethritis or cystitis may occur. Hematogenous seeding of the kidney may result in renal abscess, papillary necrosis, or fungal ball of the ureter or renal pelvis.

Candida peritonitis may be seen in the setting of chronic ambulatory peritoneal dialysis or after GI surgery, anastomotic leak, or intestinal perforation. These infections may remain localized to the abdomen, involve adjacent organs, or lead to hematogenous candidiasis.

Hematogenous candidiasis may be acute or chronic and usually results in seeding of deep tissues including the abdominal viscera, heart, eyes, bones and joints, and brain. Chronic hepatosplenic candidiasis can occur after either overt or occult fungemia and presents as an indolent process marked by fever, elevated alkaline phosphatase, and multiple lesions in the liver and spleen.

Central nervous system (CNS) candidiasis can occur as a result of hematogenous disease or associated with neurosurgical procedures and ventriculoperitoneal shunts. This process may mimic bacterial meningitis or the course may be indolent or chronic.

Most cardiac involvement with *Candida* spp. is the result of hematogenous seeding of a prosthetic or damaged heart valve, the myocardium, or the pericardial space. Implantation of heart valves contaminated with *C. parapsilosis* has been reported. The clinical presentation resembles bacterial endocarditis with fever and a new or changing heart murmur. The vegetations are classically large and friable, and embolic events are more common with endocarditis caused by *Candida* spp. than with bacterial endocarditis.

The eye is frequently involved in patients with hematogenous candidiasis, presenting as chorioretinitis and endophthalmitis. For this reason, all patients at risk for candidemia should receive careful and frequent ophthalmologic examinations. Traumatic keratitis may also be seen.

Bone and joint infections caused by *Candida* spp. are almost always sequelae of candidemia. Often these infections will appear several months after successful treatment of candidemia. Similarly occult or "transient" candidemia may result in seeding of a skeletal focus that becomes clinically apparent at a later time. Vertebral osteomyelitis is a frequent presentation with local pain and low-grade fever.

Although hematogenous candidiasis is most often an endogenous infection arising from the GI or genitourinary tract, it may also result from the contamination of an indwelling catheter. Organisms transferred to the hub or lumen of the catheter may form a biofilm within the lumen of the catheter with subsequent spread into the circulation. Although such infections are no less serious than those arising from an endogenous source, they may be dealt with somewhat more successfully since removal of the catheter essentially removes the nidus of infection. Of course if the infected catheter resulted in the seeding of distant organs, the consequences and problems in treating the infection would be the same as that arising from an endogenous source.

LABORATORY DIAGNOSIS

The laboratory diagnosis of candidiasis involves the procurement of appropriate clinical material followed by direct microscopic examination and culture (see Chapter 71). Scrapings of mucosal or cutaneous lesions may be examined directly following treatment with 10% to 20% potassium hyroxide (KOH) containing calcofluor white. The budding yeastlike forms and pseudohyphae are easily detected on examination with a fluorescence microscope (see Figure 71–1). Culture on standard mycologic medium will allow the isolation of the organism for subsequent identification to species. Increasingly, such specimens are plated directly on a selective chromogenic medium such as

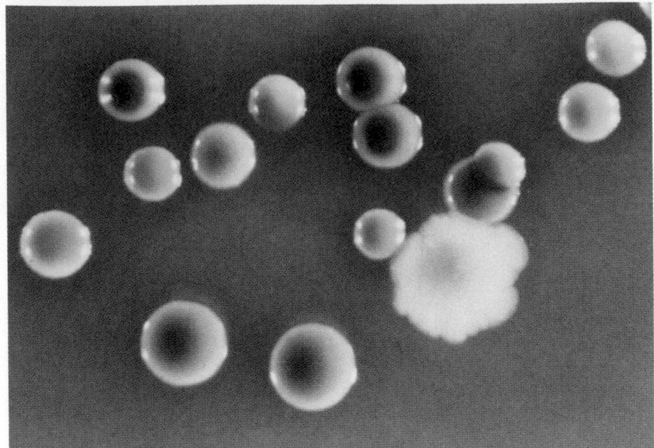

FIGURE 75–5. Differentiation of *Candida* species by isolates on CHROMagar *Candida*. The green colonies are *C. albicans;* the blue-gray colonies are *C. tropicalis*, and the large rough pale pink colony is *C. krusei*. The smooth pink or mauve colonies are another yeast species (only *C. albicans, C. tropicalis*, and *C. krusei* can be reliably recognized on this media; other species have colonies ranging from white, to pink, to mauve). (From Anaissie EJ, McGinnis MR, Pfaller MA, editors: *Clinical mycology*, New York, 2003, Churchill Livingstone.)

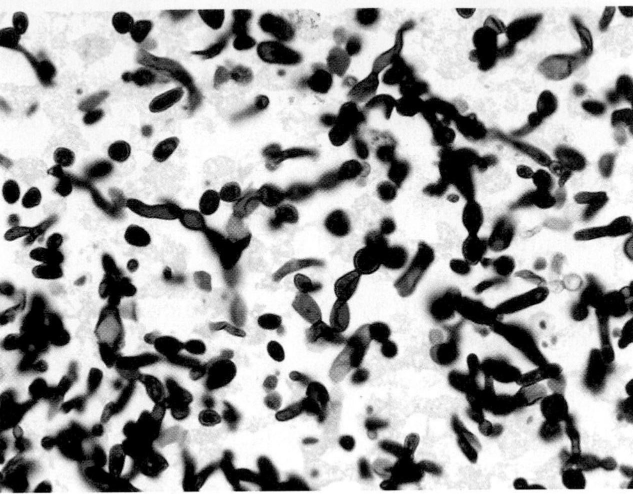

FIGURE 75–6. *Candida* stained with GMS demonstrating budding yeasts and pseudohyphae (magnification 1000×).

CHROMagar, which allows the detection of mixed species of *Candida* within the specimen and the rapid identification of *C. albicans* (green colonies) and *C. tropicalis* (blue colonies) based on their morphologic appearance (Figure 75–5).

All other types of infection require culture for diagnosis unless tissue can be obtained for histopathologic examination (see Chapter 71). Whenever possible, skin lesions should be biopsied and histologic sections stained with GMS or another fungal-specific stain. Visualization of characteristic budding yeasts and pseudohyphae is sufficient for the diagnosis of candidiasis (Figure 75–6). Cultures of blood, tissue, and normally sterile body fluids should also be performed. Identification of *Candida* isolates to species level is important given the differences in response to the various antifungal agents (see Chapter 70). This can be accomplished as described in Chapter 71 using the germ-tube test *(C. albicans)*, various chromogenic media/tests (see Figure 75–5), and commercially available sugar assimilation panels.

Immunologic, biochemical, and molecular markers for the diagnosis of candidiasis are described in Chapter 71. Unfortunately, these methods are not yet suitable for use in routine clinical diagnosis.

TREATMENT, PREVENTION, AND CONTROL

There are a wide variety of treatment options for candidiasis (see Chapter 70). Mucosal and cutaneous infections can be treated with a number of different topical creams, lotions, ointments, and suppositories containing various azole antifungal agents (see Table 70–1). Oral systemic therapy of these infections can also be accomplished with either fluconazole or itraconazole.

Bladder colonization or cystitis can be treated with either instillation of amphotericin B directly into the bladder (bladder wash) or by oral administration of fluconazole. Both of these measures will likely be unsuccessful if the bladder catheter cannot be removed.

More deep-seated infections require systemic therapy, the choice of which depends on the type of infection, the infecting species, and the overall status of the host. In many instances, oral fluconazole can be quite effective in treating candidiasis. It may be used in the treatment of peritonitis and in more long-term maintenance therapy of invasive disease after an initial intravenous course of therapy. Fluconazole is efficacious when administered intravenously for the treatment of candidemia in nonneutropenic patients. Those patients who become candidemic while taking fluconazole prophylaxis or those with documented infection caused by *C. krusei* or fluconazole-resistant *C. glabrata* require treatment with either amphotericin B (conventional or lipid formulation) or caspofungin. In those clinical settings in which *C. glabrata* or *C. krusei* are plausible etiologic agents (e.g., prior fluconazole therapy/prophylaxis or an endemic situation), initial therapy with either caspofungin or an amphotericin B formulation is advised with a switch to fluconazole or voriconazole (less toxic than amphotericin B, less expensive, and orally available versus caspofungin) based on final species identification and susceptibility test results. In every instance, care should be taken to remove the nidus of infection if possible. Thus, vascular catheters should be removed or changed, abscesses should be drained, and other potentially infected implanted materials should be removed to the fullest extent possible. Likewise, efforts should be directed toward immune reconstitution.

As in most infectious diseases, prevention is clearly preferable to the treatment of an established candidal infection. Avoidance of broad-spectrum antimicrobial agents, meticulous catheter care, and rigorous adherence to infection control precautions are a must. Decreased colonization achieved by fluconazole prophylaxis has been shown to be efficacious when used in *specific* high-risk groups such as patients receiving BMT or liver transplant. Such prophylaxis carries with it the potential for selecting for, or creating, strains or species that are resistant to the agent administered. This in fact has been seen with the emergence of fluconazole-resistant *C. glabrata* and *C. krusei* in certain institutions, but the overall benefit in high-risk patient groups outweighs the risk. Transfer of this approach to other patient groups, however, is fraught with problems and should not be undertaken without careful study and risk-stratification to identify those persons most likely to benefit from antifungal prophylaxis.

Opportunistic Mycoses Caused by *Cryptococcus neoformans* and Other Non-Candidal Yeastlike Fungi

In the same manner that *Candida* species have taken advantage of immunocompromising conditions, indwelling devices and broad-spectrum antibiotic use, so too have a number of non-*Candida* yeastlike fungi found an "opportunity" to colonize and infect immunocompromised patients. These organisms may occupy environmental niches or be found in food and water and can be normal human microbial flora. The list of these opportunistic yeasts is long, but we will limit this discussion to one major pathogen, *C. neoformans*, and four genera that pose particular problems as opportunistic pathogens: *Malassezia* spp., *Trichosporon* spp., *Rhodotorula* spp., and *Geotrichum capitatum* (formerly *Blastoschizomyces capitatus;* teleomorph, *Dipodascus capitatus*).

CRYPTOCOCCOSIS

Cryptococcosis is a systemic mycosis caused by the encapsulated, basidiomycetous, yeastlike fungus *C. neoformans*. The fungus is worldwide in distribution and is found as a ubiquitous saprophyte of soil, especially that enriched with pigeon droppings. There are five serotypes (A, B, C, D, and AD) and two varieties: *C. neoformans* var *neoformans* (serotypes A, D, and AD) and *C. neoformans* var *gatti* (serotypes B and C).

Morphology

Microscopically, *C. neoformans* is a spherical to oval, encapsulated, yeastlike organism that is 2 to 20 µm in diameter. Replication occurs via budding from a relatively narrow base. Single buds are usually formed, but multiple buds and chains of budding cells are sometimes present (Figure 75–7). Germ tubes, hyphae, and pseudohyphae are usually absent in clinical material.

In tissue, and on staining with india ink, the cells are variable in size; spherical, oval, or elliptical; and surrounded by optically clear, smoothly contoured, spherical zones or "halos" that represent the extracellular polysaccharide capsule (Figure 75–8). The capsule is a distinctive marker that may have a diameter of up to five times that of the fungal cell and is readily detected with mucin stain such as Mayer's mucicarmine (Figure 75–9). The organism stains poorly with H&E but is easily detected with PAS and GMS stains. The cell wall of *C. neoformans* contains melanin, which can be demonstrated by staining with the Fontana-Masson stain.

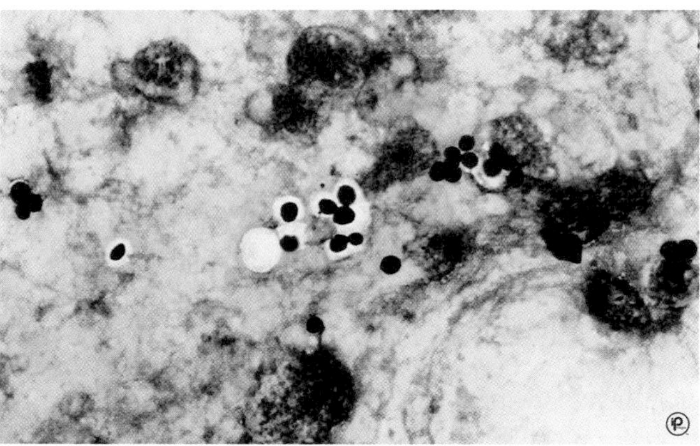

FIGURE 75–7. *Cryptococcus neoformans,* microscopic morphology (GMS, magnification 1000×). (From Marler LM et al: *Mycology* CD-ROM, Indiana Pathology Images, 2004.)

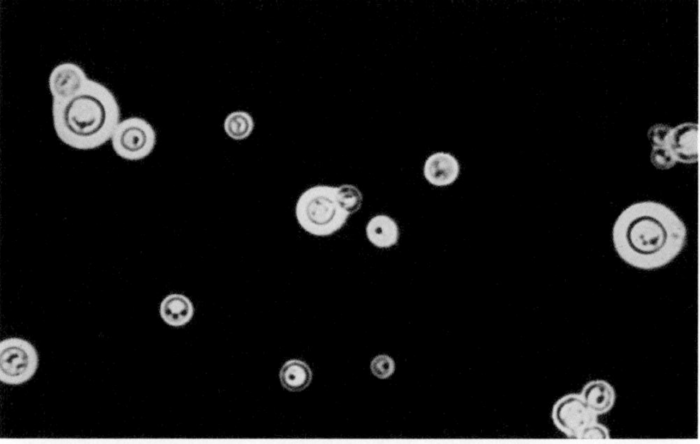

FIGURE 75–8. *Cryptococcus neoformans* India ink preparation demonstrating the large capsule surrounding budding yeast cells (magnification 1000×).

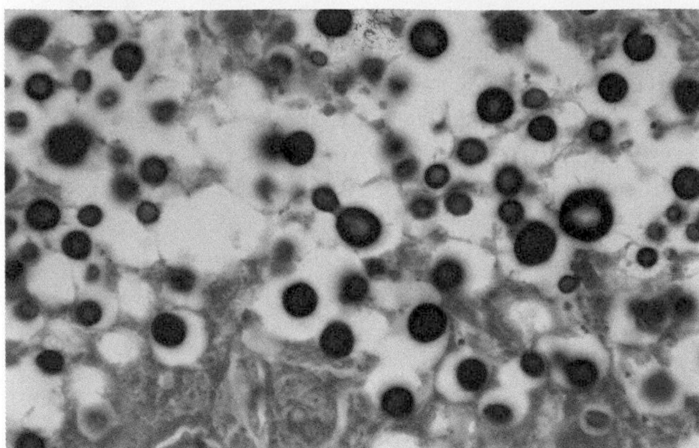

FIGURE 75–9. *Cryptococcus neoformans* stained with mucicarmine (magnification 1000×).

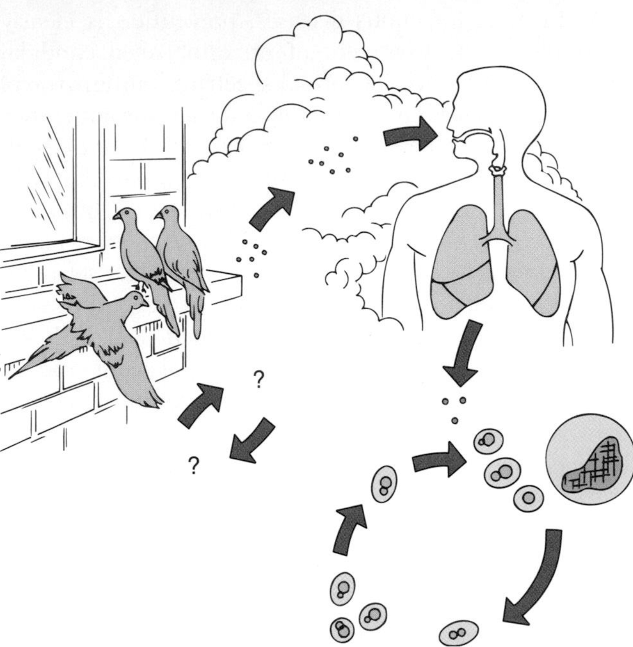

FIGURE 75–10. Natural history of saprobic and parasitic cycle of *Cryptococcus neoformans.*

Epidemiology

Cryptococcosis is usually acquired by inhaling aerosolized cells of *C. neoformans* from the environment (Figure 75–10). Subsequent dissemination from the lungs, usually to the CNS, produces clinical disease in susceptible individuals. Primary cutaneous cryptococcosis can occur after transcutaneous inoculation but is rare.

Although *C. neoformans* is pathogenic for immunecompetent individuals, it is most often encountered as an opportunistic pathogen. It is the most common cause of fungal meningitis and tends to occur in patients with defective cellular immunity.

Whereas *C. neoformans* var *neoformans* is found worldwide in association with soil contaminated with avian excreta, *C. neoformans* var *gattii* is found in tropical and subtropical climates in association with *Eucalyptus* trees. Both varieties cause a similar disease, although var *gattii* infections tend to occur in immunocompetent individuals and has a lower associated mortality but more severe neurologic sequelae due to CNS granuloma formation.

C. neoformans var *neoformans* is a major opportunistic pathogen of patients with AIDS. Those individuals with CD4+ lymphocyte counts of less than 200/mm^3 (usually <100/mm^3) are at high risk for CNS and disseminated cryptococcosis. The incidence of cryptococcosis seems to have peaked in the United States in the early 1990s (65.5 infections per million per year; see Table 7–2) and has progressively declined since then because of the widespread use of fluconazole and, more importantly, successful treatment of the HIV infection with new antiretroviral drugs.

Clinical Syndromes

Cryptococcosis may present as a pneumonic process or, more commonly, as a CNS infection secondary to hematogenous and lymphatic spread from a primary pulmonary focus. Less often, a more widely disseminated infection appears with cutaneous, mucocutaneous, osseous, and visceral forms of the disease.

Pulmonary cryptococcosis is variable in presentation from an asymptomatic process to a more fulminant bilateral pneumonia. Nodular infiltrates can be either unilateral or bilateral, becoming more diffuse in severe infections. Cavitation is rare.

C. neoformans is highly neurotropic, and the most common form of disease is cerebromeningeal. The course of disease is variable and can be quite chronic; however, it is inevitably fatal if untreated. Both meninges and the underlying brain tissue are involved and the clinical presentation is that of fever, headache, meningismus, visual disturbances, abnormal mental status, and seizures. The clinical picture is highly dependent on the patient's immune status and tends to be dramatically severe in AIDS patients and other severely compromised patients treated with steroids or other immunosuppressive agents.

Parenchymal lesions, or cryptococcomas, are uncommon in infections caused by *C. neoformans* var *neoformans* but are the most common presentation of CNS cryptococcosis in immunocompetent hosts infected with var *gattii.*

Other manifestations of disseminated cryptococcosis include skin lesions, which occur in 10% to 15% of patients and may mimic those of molluscum contagiosum; ocular infections, including chorioretinitis, vitritis, and ocular nerve invasion; osseous lesions involving the vertebrae and bony prominences; and prostatic involvement, which may be an asymptomatic reservoir of infection.

Laboratory Diagnosis

The diagnosis of infection caused by *C. neoformans* can be made by culture of blood, cerebrospinal fluid (CSF), or other clinical material (see Chapter 71). Microscopic examination of CSF may reveal the characteristic encapsulated budding yeast cells. The cells of *C. neoformans*, when present in CSF or other clinical material, can be visualized with Gram stain (see Figure 71–2) and with India ink (see Figure 75–8) or other stains (see Figure 75–7). Culture of clinical material on routine mycologic media will produce mucoid colonies comprised of round, urease-positive, encapsulated budding yeast cells within 3 to 5 days. Species identification can be accomplished by means of carbohydrate assimilation testing by growth on niger seed agar (*C. neoformans* colonies become brown to black in color), or by directly testing for phenoloxidase activity (positive).

Most commonly, however, the diagnosis of cryptococcal meningitis is made by direct detection of the capsular polysaccharide antigen in serum or CSF (Table 75–7). Detection of cryptococcal antigen is accomplished by using one of several commercially available latex agglutination or enzyme immunoassay kits. These assays have been shown to be rapid, sensitive, and specific for the diagnosis of cryptococcal disease (see Table 75–7).

Treatment

Cryptococcal meningitis and other disseminated forms of cryptococcosis are universally fatal if left untreated. All patients should receive amphotericin B plus flucytosine acutely for 2 weeks (induction therapy), followed by 8-week consolidation with either oral fluconazole (preferred) or itraconazole. AIDS patients generally require lifelong maintenance therapy with either fluconazole or itraconazole. In patients who do not have AIDS, treatment can be discontinued after the consolidation therapy; however, relapse may be seen in up to 26% of these patients within 3 to 6 months after discontinuation of therapy. Thus a prolonged consolidation treatment with an azole for up to 1 year may be advisable even in patients without AIDS.

Treatment of these patients should be followed up both clinically and mycologically. Mycologic follow-up requires repeat lumbar puncture to be performed (1) at the end of the 2-week induction therapy to ensure sterilization of the CSF; (2) at the end of the consolidation therapy; and (3) whenever indicated by a change in clinical status during follow-up. CSF samples collected during follow-up **must** undergo culture. Determination of CSF protein, glucose, cell count, and cryptococcal antigen titer are helpful in assessing the response to therapy but are not highly predictive of outcome. Failure to sterilize the CSF by day 14 of therapy is indicative of a much higher probability that the consolidation therapy will fail.

TABLE 75–7. Sensitivity of Antigen Detection, India Ink Microscopy, and Culture of Cerebral Spinal Fluid in the Diagnosis of Cryptococcal Meningitis

Test	% Sensitivity	
	AIDS Patients	Non-AIDS Patients
Antigen	100	86–95
India ink	82	50
Culture	100	90

Adapted from Viviani MA, Tortorano AM, Ajello L: Cryptococcus. In Anaissie EJ, McGinnis MR, Pfaller MA, editors: *Clinical mycology,* New York, 2003, Churchill Livingstone.

OTHER MYCOSES CAUSED BY YEASTLIKE FUNGI

Among the non-*Candida*, non-*Cryptococcus* yeastlike pathogens, nosocomial infections caused by *Malassezia* spp., *Trichosporon* spp., *Rhodotorula* spp., and *Geotrichum capitatum (Blastoschizomyces capitatus)* are most prominent either because they are difficult to detect or because they may pose particular problems with respect to antifungal resistance.

Malassezia Species

Infections caused by *Malassezia* spp. *(M. furfur* and *M. pachydermatis)* are usually catheter related and tend to occur in premature infants or in other patients receiving lipid infusions. Both of these organisms are budding yeasts (Figures 72–2 and 75–11). *M. furfur* is a common skin

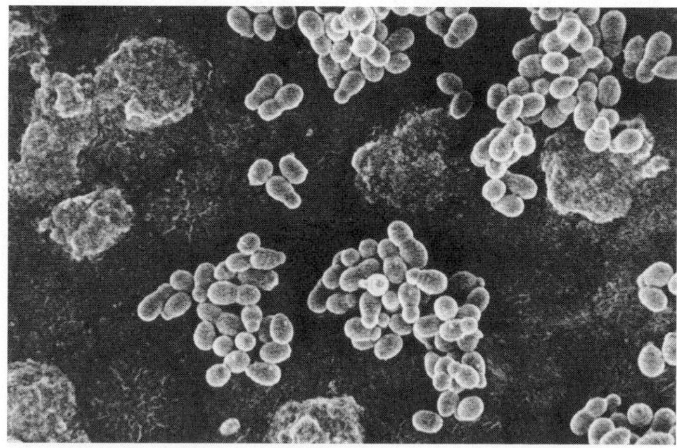

FIGURE 75–11. Scanning electron micrograph of *Malassezia furfur* adhering to the lumen of a central venous catheter. (Courtesy S.A. Messer.)

colonizer and is the etiologic agent of tinea (pityriasis) versicolor (see Chapter 72), whereas *M. pachydermatis* is a frequent cause of otitis in dogs and a human skin commensal.

Among the *Malassezia* spp., *M. furfur* is known for its requirement of exogenous lipid for growth. This growth requirement, plus its ecologic niche on skin, explains some of the epidemiology of *M. furfur* because nosocomial infections caused by this organism are directly related to the administration of intravenous lipid supplements through a central venous catheter. Although *M. pachydermatis* does not require exogenous lipids for growth, fatty acids do stimulate its growth, and infections due to this organism have been associated with parenteral nutrition and intravenous lipid administration. Although most infections with *Malassezia* spp. are sporadic, outbreaks of fungemia have been observed among infants receiving intravenous lipid supplementation. The growth of the organism is favored by the lipid-rich infusion, and the organism gains access via the catheter. One notable outbreak of *M. pachydermatis* fungemia was linked to nurses who owned dogs with *M. pachydermatis* otitis. The outbreak strain was found on the hands of the nurses and at least one of the affected dogs.

Malassezia spp. should be considered when yeasts are seen microscopically in blood culture bottles or clinical material but no organisms are recovered on routine agar medium. To isolate *Malassezia* spp. (especially *M. furfur*) on agar medium the plates must be inoculated and then overlaid with sterile olive oil. Olive oil provides the lipid requirement, and growth should be detected within 3 to 5 days.

Treatment of fungemia caused by *Malassezia* spp. does not usually require the administration of antifungal agents. The infection subsides once the lipid infusion is stopped and the intravascular lines are removed.

Trichosporon Species

The genus *Trichosporon* currently consists of six species: *T. asahii* and *T. mucoides* are known to cause deep invasive infections; *T. asteroides* and *T. cutaneum* cause superficial skin infections; *T. ovoides* causes white piedra of the scalp and *T. inkin* causes that of the pubic hair. Confusingly, most of the literature regarding deep-seated trichosporonosis refers to the older nomenclature of *T. beigelii*. Morphologically these organisms are similar and appear in clinical material as hyphae, arthroconidia, and budding yeast cells.

Trichosporon causes catheter-associated fungemia in neutropenic patients but also may gain entrance to the bloodstream via the respiratory or GI tract. Widespread hematogenous dissemination can manifest as positive blood cultures and multiple cutaneous lesions. Chronic hepatic trichosporonosis may mimic hepatic candidiasis and is seen upon recovery from neutropenia. *Trichosporon* has been reported as the most common cause of non-candidal yeast infection in patients with hematologic malignancies and carries a mortality in excess of 80%. Susceptibility to amphotericin B is variable, and this agent lacks fungicidal activity against *Trichosporon*. Clinical failures with amphotericin B, fluconazole, and combinations of the two have been reported and the outcome is generally dismal in the absence of neutrophil recovery.

Rhodotorula Species

Rhodotorula spp. are characterized by the production of carotenoid pigments (producing pink to red colonies) and variably encapsulated, multilateral budding yeast cells. Species of *Rhodotorula* include *R. glutinis, R. mucilaginosa, R. rubra,* and *R. minuta*. These yeastlike fungi are found as commensals on skin, nails, and mucous membranes as well as in cheese and milk products and environmental sources including air, soil, shower curtains, bathtub grout, and toothbrushes. *Rhodotorula* spp. are emerging as important human pathogens in immunocompromised patients and those with indwelling devices. *Rhodotorula* has been implicated as a cause of central venous catheter infection and fungemia, ocular infections, peritonitis, and meningitis. Amphotericin B performs well against *Rhodotorula* and, coupled with catheter removal, is an optimal approach to infections with this organism. Flucytosine has excellent activity as well but should not be considered for monotherapy. Neither fluconazole, nor the echinocandins, should be used to treat infections due to *Rhodotorula* spp. and the role of the new extended-spectrum triazoles (e.g., voriconazole and posaconazole) is uncertain pending clinical data.

Geotrichum capitatum

Among the emerging opportunistic yeastlike pathogens, *Geotrichum capitatum* (formerly *Blastoschizomyces capitatus*, teleomorph *Dipodascus capitatus*) is a rarely described fungus that produces severe systemic infection in immunocompromised patients, especially those with hematologic malignancies. This organism produces hyphae and arthroconidia, is widely distributed in nature, and can be found as part of the normal skin flora. Infection with *G. capitatum* presents similar to that with *Trichosporon* in neutropenic patients, with frequent fungemia and multiorgan (including brain) dissemination and a mortality rate of 60% to 80%. Blood cultures usually yield positive results. As with *Trichosporon*, a chronic disseminated form, similar to chronic disseminated candidiasis, may be seen on resolution of neutropenia.

The optimal approach to therapy of infections caused by *G. capitatum* is not yet defined. Some clinicians feel that *G. capitatum* has decreased susceptibility to amphotericin

B. The excellent in vitro activity of voriconazole suggest that it may be a useful agent for treatment of infections due to this organism. Rapid removal of central venous catheters, adjuvant immunotherapy, and novel antifungal therapies (e.g., either voriconazole or high-dose fluconazole plus amphotericin B) are recommended for treatment of this rare but devastating infection.

Aspergillosis

Aspergillosis encompasses a broad spectrum of diseases caused by members of the genus *Aspergillus* (Box 75–2). Exposure to *Aspergillus* in the environment can cause allergic reactions in hypersensitized hosts or destructive, invasive pulmonary and disseminated disease in highly immunosuppressed individuals. Although approximately 19 species of *Aspergillus* have been documented as agents of human disease, the majority of infections are caused by *A. fumigatus, A. flavus, A. niger* and *A. terreus.*

MORPHOLOGY

Aspergillus spp. grows in culture as a hyaline mould. Grossly the colonies of *Aspergillus* may be black, brown, green, yellow, white, or other colors depending on the species and the growth conditions. Colonial appearance may provide an initial suggestion as to the species of *Aspergillus*, but definitive identification requires microscopic examination of the hyphae and the structure of the conidial head.

Aspergilli grow as branched, septate hyphae that produce conidial heads when exposed to air in culture and in tissue. A conidial head consists of a conidiophore with a terminal vesicle, on which are borne one or two layers of phialides, or sterigmata (see Figure 7–3*B*). The elongated phialides in turn produce columns of spherical conidia, which are the infectious propagules from which the mycelial phase of the fungus develops. Identification of individual species of *Aspergillus* depends, in part, on difference of their conidial heads, including the arrangement and morphology of the conidia (Figures 75–12 and 75–13).

In tissue, the hyphae of *Aspergillus* spp. stain poorly with H&E but are well visualized by the PAS, GMS, and Gridley fungal stains. The hyphae are homogeneous and uniform in width (3 to 6 μm), with parallel contours, regular septations, and a progressive, tree-like pattern of branching (Figure 75–14). The branches are dichotomous and usually arise at acute (~45 degrees) angles. The hyphae can be seen within blood vessels (angioinvasion) causing thrombosis. The conidial heads are rarely seen in tissue but may arise within a cavity (Figure 75–15). The important species *A. terreus* can be identified in tissue by its spherical or oval aleurioconidia that develop from the lateral walls of the mycelium (Figure 75–16). Otherwise, the hyphae of pathogenic *Aspergillus* spp. are morphologically indistinguishable from one another.

BOX 75–2. Spectrum of Diseases Caused by Aspergillus Species

Allergic Reactions	**Limited Invasive Infections**
Nasal cavity	Bronchi
Paranasal sinuses	Pulmonary parenchyma
Lower respiratory tract	Mildly immunodeficient patients
Colonization	
Obstructed paranasal sinuses	**Frankly Invasive Pulmonary Infection**
Bronchi	Severely immunodeficient patients
Preformed pulmonary cavities	Systemic dissemination
Superficial Cutaneous Infections	Death

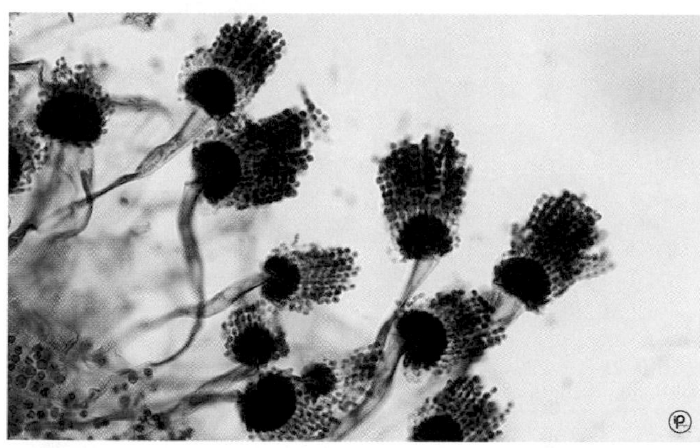

FIGURE 75–12. *Aspergillus fumigatus,* lactophenol cotton blue preparation showing conidial head (magnification 400×). (From Marler LM et al: *Mycology* CD-ROM, Indiana Pathology Images, 2004.)

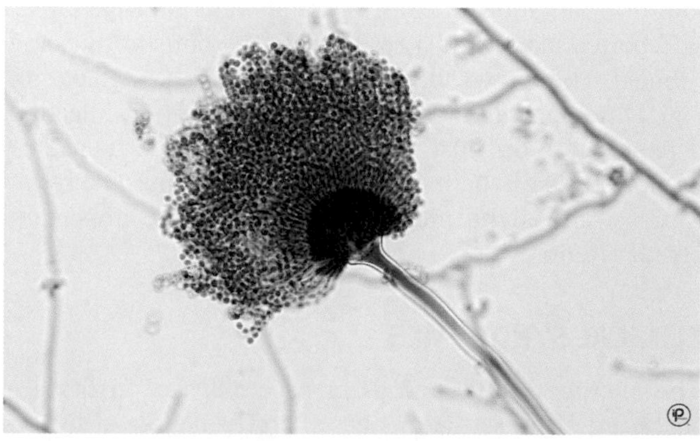

FIGURE 75–13. *Aspergillus terreus,* lactophenol cotton blue preparation showing conidial head (magnification 400×). (From Marler LM et al: *Mycology* CD-ROM, Indiana Pathology Images, 2004.)

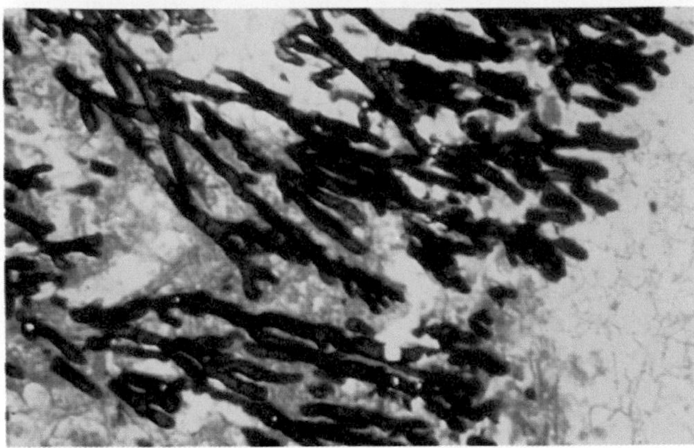

FIGURE 75–14. *Aspergillus* in tissue showing acute angle branching, septate hyphae (GMS, magnification 1000×).

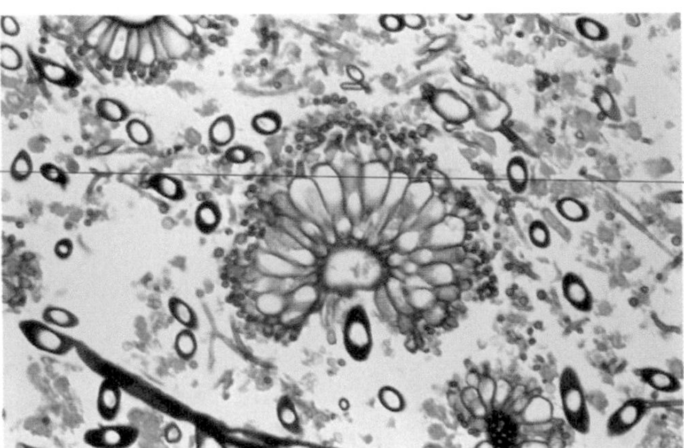

FIGURE 75–15. *Aspergillus niger* in a cavitary lung lesion showing both hyphae and conidial head (GMS, magnification 1000×).

EPIDEMIOLOGY

Aspergillus spp. are common throughout the world. Their conidia are ubiquitous in air, soil, and decaying matter. Within the hospital environment *Aspergillus* spp. can be found in air, showerheads, hospital water storage tanks, and potted plants. As a result, they are constantly being inhaled. The type of host reaction, the associated pathologic findings, and the ultimate outcome of infection depend more on host factors than on the virulence or pathogenesis of the individual *Aspergillus* spp. The respiratory tract is the most frequent and most important portal of entry.

CLINICAL SYNDROMES

The allergic manifestations of aspergillosis constitute a spectrum of presentations based on the degree of hypersensitivity to *Aspergillus* antigens. In the bronchopulmonary form, asthma, pulmonary infiltrates, peripheral eosinophilia, elevated serum immunoglobulin E levels,

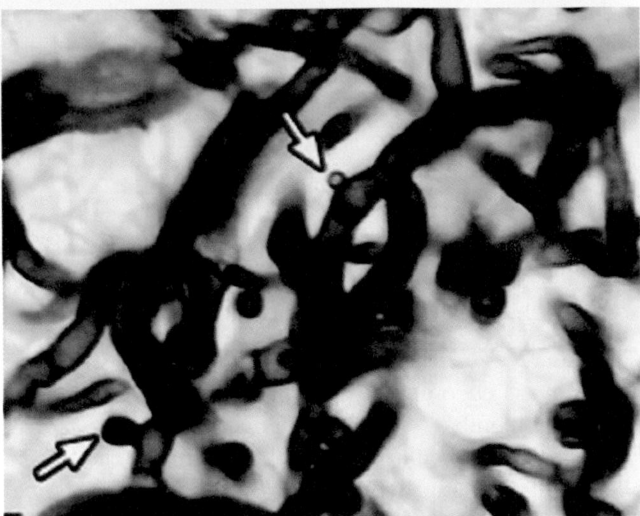

FIGURE 75–16. *Aspergillus terreus* in tissue. Arrows point to aleurioconidia (GMS, magnification 1000×). (Taken from Walsh et al: *J Infect Dis* 188:305-319, 2003.)

and evidence of hypersensitivity to *Aspergillus* antigens (skin test) may be seen. Allergic sinusitis shows laboratory evidence of hypersensitivity to go along with upper respiratory symptoms of nasal obstruction and discharge, headache, and facial pain.

Both the paranasal sinuses and the lower airways can become colonized with *Aspergillus* spp., resulting in obstructive bronchial aspergillosis and true aspergilloma ("fungus ball"). Obstructive bronchial aspergillosis usually occurs in the setting of underlying pulmonary disease such as cystic fibrosis, chronic bronchitis, or bronchiectasis. The condition is marked by the formation of bronchial casts or plugs composed of hyphal elements and mucinous material. The symptoms remain those of the underlying disease, no tissue injury results, and no treatment is necessary. An aspergilloma can form either in the paranasal sinuses or in a preformed pulmonary cavity secondary to old tuberculosis or other chronic cavitary lung disease. Aspergillomas can be seen on radiographic examination but usually are asymptomatic. Treatment is generally not warranted unless pulmonary hemorrhage occurs. In the event of pulmonary hemorrhage, which may be severe and life-threatening, surgical excision of the cavity and fungus ball is indicated. Likewise, radical débridement of the paranasal sinuses may be necessary to alleviate any symptomatology or hemorrhage due to a fungus ball of the sinuses.

Forms of invasive aspergillosis run the gamut from superficially invasive disease that may occur in the setting of mild immunosuppression (e.g., low-dose steroid therapy, collagen vascular disease, or diabetes) to destructive locally invasive pulmonary or disseminated aspergillosis. The more limited forms of invasion generally include necrotizing pseudomembranous bronchial aspergillosis and chronic necrotizing pulmonary aspergillosis. Bronchial aspergillosis may cause wheezing, dyspnea, and hemoptysis. Most patients with chronic necrotizing pulmonary aspergillosis have underlying structural pulmonary disease that can be treated with low-dose corticosteroids. This is a chronic infection that can be locally destructive, with the development of infiltrates and fungus balls seen on radiographic examination. It is not associated with vascular invasion or dissemination. Surgical resection of affected areas and administration of antifungal therapy are efficacious in treating this condition.

Invasive pulmonary aspergillosis and disseminated aspergillosis are devastating infections seen in severely neutropenic and immunodeficient patients. The major predisposing factors for this infectious complication include neutrophil count less than $500/mm^3$, cytotoxic chemotherapy, and corticosteroid therapy. Patients present with fever and pulmonary infiltrates often accompanied by pleuritic chest pain and hemoptysis. Definitive diagnosis is often delayed because sputum and blood cultures usually have negative results. The mortality of this infection, despite specific antifungal therapy, is quite high, usually exceeding 70% (see Table 75–5). Hematogenous dissemination of infection to extrapulmonary sites is common due to the angioinvasive nature of the fungus. Sites most often involved include brain, heart, kidneys, GI tract, liver, and spleen.

LABORATORY DIAGNOSIS

As with other ubiquitous fungi, the diagnosis of aspergillosis necessitates caution when evaluating the isolation of an *Aspergillus* species from clinical specimens. Recovery from surgically removed tissue or sterile sites, accompanied by positive histopathology (moniliaceous, septate, dichotomously branching hyphae) should always be considered significant; isolation from normally contaminated (e.g., respiratory) sites requires closer scrutiny.

Most etiologic agents of aspergillosis grow readily on routine mycologic media lacking cycloheximide. Species-level identification of the major human pathogens can be made by observing cultural and microscopic characteristics from growth on potato dextrose agar. Microscopic morphology (e.g., conidiophores, vesicles, metulae, phialides, conidia) is best observed with a slide culture and is necessary for species identification.

Invasive aspergillosis caused by *A. fumigatus*, and most other species, is rarely documented by positive blood cultures. In fact, most bloodstream isolates of *Aspergillus* spp. have been shown to represent pseudofungemia or terminal events at autopsy. Notably *A. terreus*, among all species of *Aspergillus*, has been shown to cause true aspergillemia. Similar to other angioinvasive filamentous fungi (e.g., *Fusarium, Scedosporium* spp.), *A. terreus* is capable of adventitious sporulation in which yeastlike spores, or aleurioconidia, are formed in tissue and blood and are more likely to be detected in blood obtained for culture (see Figure 75–16). Recognition of these aleurioconidia on microscopic examination of tissue, fine needle aspirates, or bronchoscopy specimens can allow a rapid, presumptive identification of *A. terreus*.

The rapid diagnosis of invasive aspergillosis has been advanced by the development of immunoassays for the *Aspergillus* galactomannan antigen in serum. This test uses an enzyme immunoassay format and is available as a commercial kit or from reference laboratories. This test appears to be reasonably specific but exhibits variable sensitivity. It is best used on serial specimens from high-risk patients (primarily neutropenic and BMT patients) as an early indication to begin empiric or preemptive antifungal therapy and to more aggressively pursue a definitive diagnosis.

TREATMENT AND PREVENTION

Prevention of aspergillosis in high-risk patients is paramount. Neutropenic and other high-risk patients are generally housed in facilities where the air is filtered so as to minimize exposure to *Aspergillus* conidia.

Specific antifungal therapy of aspergillosis usually involves the administration of amphotericin B or one of its lipid-based formulations. It is important to realize that *A. terreus* is considered resistant to amphotericin B and should be treated with an alternative agent such as voriconazole. The recent introduction of voriconazole provides a treatment option that is more efficacious and less toxic than amphotericin B (see Chapter 70). Concomitant efforts to decrease immunosuppression and/or reconstitute host immune defenses are important components of the treatment of aspergillosis. Likewise, surgical resection of involved areas, if possible, are recommended.

Zygomycosis

Zygomycosis refers to diseases caused by fungi of the class Zygomycetes. The principal human pathogens in the class Zygomycetes are encompassed by two orders: Mucorales and Entomophthorales. The order Entomophthorales contains two pathogenic genera, *Conidiobolus* and *Basidiobolus*. These agents generally incite a chronic, granulomatous infection of subcutaneous tissues and are discussed in Chapter 73.

In the order Mucorales, pathogenic genera include *Rhizopus, Mucor, Absidia, Rhizomucor, Saksenaea, Cunninghamella, Syncephalastrum*, and *Apophysomyces*. Infections due to the zygomycetes are rare, occurring at an annual rate of 1.7 infections per million population in the United

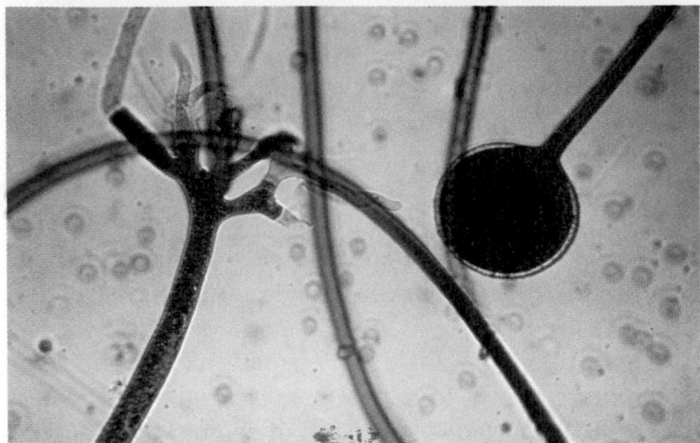

FIGURE 75–17. *Rhizopus* sp. showing sporangium and rhizoids.

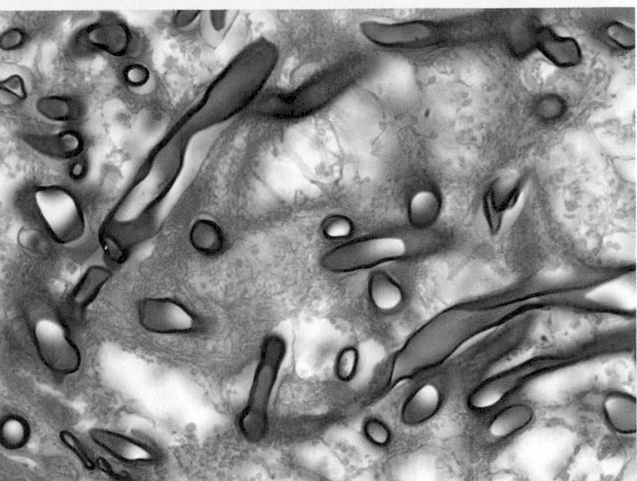

FIGURE 75–18. *Rhizopus* sp. in tissue showing broad, ribbony, aseptate hyphae (H&E, magnification 1000×).

States. Unfortunately when they do occur, infections due to these agents are generally acute and rapidly progressive, with mortality rates of 70% to 100%.

MORPHOLOGY

Macroscopically, the pathogenic Mucorales grow rapidly, producing gray to brown wooly colonies within 12 to 18 hours. Further identification to the genus and species level is based on microscopic morphology. Microscopically, the zygomycetes are moulds with broad, hyaline, sparsely septate, coenocytic hyphae. The asexual spores of the order Mucorales are contained within a sporangium and are referred to as *sporangiospores.* The sporangia are borne at the tips of stalk-like sporangiophores that terminate in a bulbous swelling called the *columella* (Figure 7–3*A* and 75–17). The presence of root-like structures, called rhizoids, is helpful in identifying specific genera within the Mucorales order.

In tissue, the zygomycetes (order Mucorales) are seen as ribbon-like, aseptate or sparsely septate moniliaceous (nonpigmented) hyphae (see Figure 75–18). In contrast to *Aspergillus* spp. and other hyaline moulds, the diameter of the hyphae often exceeds 10 μm and the hyphae are irregularly contoured and pleomorphic, often folding and twisting back on themselves. The pattern of hyphal branching is haphazard and nonprogressive, and branches typically arise from the parent hyphae at right angles. The walls of the hyphae are thin, stain weakly with GMS and other fungal stains, and are often more easily detected with H&E (Figure 75–18). The zygomycetes are typically angioinvasive.

EPIDEMIOLOGY

Zygomycosis is a sporadic disease that occurs worldwide. *Rhizopus arrhizus* is the most common cause of human zygomycosis; however, additional species of *Rhizopus, Rhizomucor, Absidia,* and *Cunninghamella* are known to cause invasive disease in hospitalized persons. The organisms are ubiquitous in soil and decaying vegetation, and infection can be acquired by inhalation, ingestion, or contamination of wounds with sporangiospores from the environment. As with *Aspergillus* spp., nosocomial spread of zygomycetes may occur by way of air-conditioning systems, particularly during construction. Focal outbreaks of zygomycosis have also been associated with the use of contaminated adhesive bandages or tape in surgical wound dressings resulting in primary cutaneous zygomycosis.

Invasive zygomycosis occurs in immunocompromised patients and is similar clinically to aspergillosis. It is estimated that zygomycetes may cause infection in 1% to 9% of solid organ transplants, especially those with underlying diabetes mellitus. Risk factors include corticosteroid and deferoxamine therapy, diabetic ketoacidosis, renal failure, hematologic malignancy, myelosuppression, and exposure to hospital construction activity. Recently, zygomycoses has been seen after BMT in patients receiving antifungal prophylaxis with voriconazole, an agent that is not active against the zygomycetes.

CLINICAL SYNDROMES

There are several clinical forms of zygomycosis caused by members of the order Mucorales. Rhinocerebral zygomycosis is an acute invasive infection of the nasal cavity, paranasal sinuses, and orbit that involves the facial structures and extends into the CNS involving the meninges and the brain. Most of these infections occur in patients with metabolic acidosis, particularly diabetic ketoacidosis, and those with hematologic malignancies.

Pulmonary zygomycosis occurs as a primary infection in neutropenic patients and may be misdiagnosed as invasive aspergillosis. The pulmonary lesions are infarctive as a result of hyphal invasion and subsequent thrombosis of large pulmonary vessels. Chest radiographs show a rapidly progressive bronchopneumonia, segmented or lobar consolidation, and signs of cavitation. Fungus ball formation mimicking aspergilloma may be seen. Pulmonary hemorrhage with fatal hemoptysis may be seen as a result of vascular invasion by the fungus.

The angioinvasive nature of the mucoraceous zygomycetes often produces disseminated infection with tissue infarction of various organs. Presenting symptoms point to neurologic, pulmonary, or GI tract involvement. Involvement of the GI tract often results in massive hemorrhage or perforation.

Cutaneous zygomycosis may be a sign of hematogenous dissemination. Lesions tend to be nodular with an ecchymotic center. Primary cutaneous zygomycosis may occur following traumatic injury, in surgical dressings, or colonization of burn wounds. The infection may be superficial or extend rapidly into the subcutaneous tissues.

LABORATORY DIAGNOSIS

Because of the extremely poor prognosis of zygomycosis, every effort should be made to obtain tissue for direct microscopic examination, histologic study, and culture. As the zygomycetes are an extremely ubiquitous group of fungi, demonstration of characteristic fungal elements in tissue merits considerably more importance than simple isolation in culture.

Appropriate specimens include scrapings of nasal mucosa, aspirates of sinus contents, bronchial alveolar lavage fluid, and biopsy of any and all necrotic infected tissue. Direct examination of material mounted in KOH with calcofluor white may reveal the broad, aseptate hyphae. Histopathologic sections stained with H&E or PAS are most useful (see Figure 75–18). Broad irregularly branched, pausiseptate twisted hyphae can be observed.

Tissue for culture should be minced, not homogenized, and placed on standard mycologic media without cycloheximide. Negative culture results are common, occurring about 40% of the time despite the microscopic demonstration of hyphae in tissue. The diagnosis of zygomycosis cannot be established or rejected based on culture alone. It depends on a panel of evidence gathered by both the clinician and microbiologist. Unfortunately, there are no widely available serologic or molecular tests specific for the zygomycetes yet available (see Chapter 71).

TREATMENT

Amphotericin B remains the first-line therapy for zygomycosis, often supplemented by surgical débridement and immune reconstitution. Most of the zygomycetes appear quite susceptible to amphotericin B and are generally not susceptible to the azoles or echinocandins (see Chapter 70). Among the extended-spectrum triazoles, however, posaconazole stands out in that it appears to be active against most of the zygomycetes. Posaconazole has documented efficacy in murine models of zygomycosis and in limited experience in the treatment of infections in humans. In contrast, voriconazole is inactive against these agents, and breakthrough zygomycosis has been reported in BMT patients receiving voriconazole prophylaxis.

Mycoses Caused by Other Hyaline Moulds

The list of hyaline moulds, also known as hyalohyphomycetes, is quite long and it is well beyond the scope of this chapter to discuss them all (see Box 75–1). The taxonomically diverse agents of hyalohyphomycosis (infection caused by nonpigmented moulds) do share several characteristics in that many exhibit decreased susceptibility to a number of antifungal agents and when present in tissue they appear as hyaline (nonpigmented), septate, branching filamentous fungi that may be indistinguishable from *Aspergillus*. Culture is necessary to identify these agents and may be critical in determining the most appropriate therapy.

Although infections caused by most of these fungi are relatively uncommon, they appear to be increasing in incidence. Most disseminated infections are thought to be acquired by the inhalation of spores or by the progression of previously localized cutaneous lesions. In this chapter, the discussion of specific genera is limited to selected clinically important hyaline moulds: *Fusarium* spp., *Scedosporium* spp., *Acremonium* spp., *Paecilomyces* spp., *Trichoderma* spp., and *Scopulariopsis* spp. These organisms tend to cause infections in neutropenic patients, often disseminated in nature, and are almost uniformly fatal in the absence of immune reconstitution. Several of these organisms are capable of adventitious conidiation (i.e., generation of spores in tissue) with concomitant hematogenous dissemination, positive blood cultures, and multiple cutaneous lesions.

Fusarium spp. have been recognized with increased frequency as causes of disseminated infection in immunocompromised patients. The most common species isolated from clinical specimens include *Fusarium moniliforme*, *Fusarium solani*, and *Fusarium oxysporum*. The hallmark of disseminated fusariosis is the appearance of multiple purpuric cutaneous nodules with central necrosis. Biopsy of these nodules generally reveals branching, hyaline, septate hyphae invading dermal blood vessels (Figure 75–19). Cultures of biopsy material and of blood are useful in establishing the diagnosis of *Fusarium* infection.

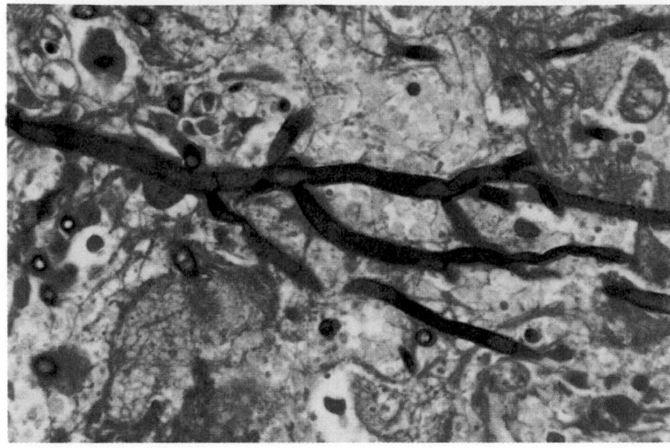

FIGURE 75–19. *Fusarium* sp. in tissue showing acute angle branching, septate hyphae that are indistinguishable from that of *Aspergillus* spp. (From Chandler FW, Watts JC, editors: *Pathologic diagnosis of fungal infections,* Chicago, 1987, ASCP Press. Copyright 1987, American Society of Clinical Pathologists.)

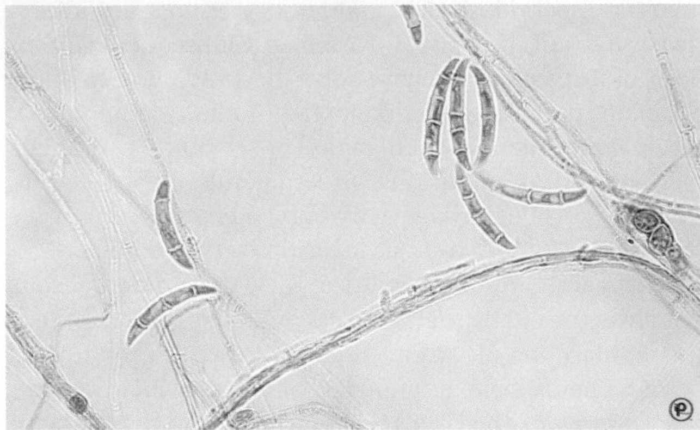

FIGURE 75–20. *Fusarium oxysporum,* lactophenol cotton blue preparation showing sickle-shaped or canoe-shaped macroconidia (magnification 400×). (From Marler LM et al: *Mycology* CD-ROM, Indiana Pathology Images, 2004.)

Although blood cultures virtually always have negative results in invasive infections caused by *Aspergillus* spp., approximately 75% of patients with fusariosis will have positive blood cultures. In culture, colonies of *Fusarium* spp. are rapidly growing, cottony to wooly, flat, and spreading. Colors may include blue-green, beige, salmon, lavender, red, violet, and purple. Microscopically, *Fusarium* spp. are characterized by the production of both macroconidia and microconidia. Microconidia are single- or double-celled, ovoid to cylindrical, and generally borne as mucous balls or short chains. Macroconidia are fusiform or sickle shaped and comprise many cells (Figure 75–20). *Fusarium* spp. often appears resistant to amphotericin B in vitro, and breakthrough infections occur frequently in patients treated with this agent. Voriconazole has been used successfully in some patients with amphotericin B–refractory fusariosis. Primary therapy with either a lipid formulation of amphotericin B or voriconazole plus vigorous efforts at immune reconstitution are recommended for treatment of fusariosis.

Within the genus *Scedosporium, S. apiospermum* (teleomorph *Pseudallescheria boydii*) and *S. prolificans* represent two important antifungal-resistant opportunistic pathogens. *S. apiospermum* may be readily isolated from soil and is an occasional cause of mycetoma worldwide; however, it is also the cause of serious disseminated and localized infection in immunocompromised patients. In addition to widespread disseminated disease, *S. apiospermum* has been reported to cause corneal ulcers, endophthalmitis, sinusitis, pneumonia, endocarditis, meningitis, arthritis, and osteomyelitis. *S. apiospermum* is indistinguishable from *Aspergillus* spp. and other agents of hyalohyphomycosis on histopathologic examination. Such distinction is important clinically because *S. apiospermum* is resistant to amphotericin B and susceptible to voriconazole and posaconazole. In culture, colonies are wooly to cottony

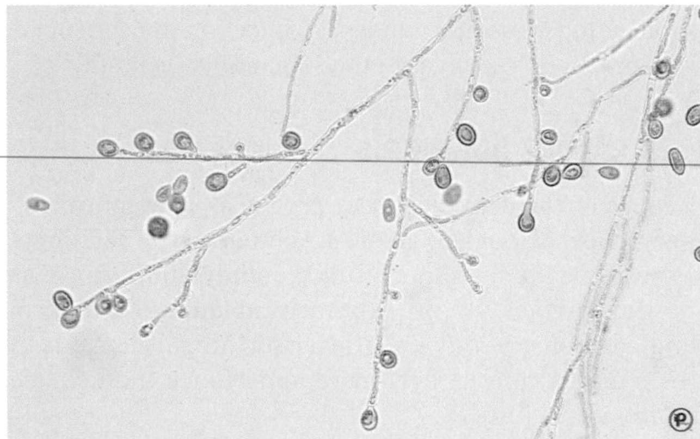

FIGURE 75–21. *Scedosporium apiospermum (Pseudallescheria boydii),* lactophenol cotton blue preparation showing conidia and septate hyphae (magnification 400×). (From Marler LM et al: *Mycology* CD-ROM, Indiana Pathology Images, 2004.)

and are initially white, becoming smoky brown to green. Microscopically, conidia are one-celled, elongate, and pale brown and are borne singly or in balls on either short or long conidiophores (Figure 75–21).

S. prolificans (formerly *S. inflatum*) is a potentially virulent and highly aggressive emerging agent of hyalohyphomycosis. Although far less important than *Fusarium* spp. or *S. apiospermum,* infections caused by *S. prolificans* are associated with soft tissue trauma and are characterized by widespread local invasion, tissue necrosis, and osteomyelitis. *S. prolificans* resembles *S. apiospermum* in macroscopic and microscopic morphology. The formation by *S. prolificans* of annelloconidia in wet clumps at the apices of annellides with swollen bases is the most useful characteristic in differentiating this organism from *S. apiospermum*. *S. prolificans* is considered to be resistant to virtually all of the systemically active antifungal agents including the extended spectrum triazoles and the echinocandins. Surgical resection remains the only definitive therapy for infection by *S. prolificans.*

Invasive infections caused by *Acremonium* spp. are almost exclusively seen in patients with neutropenia, transplantation, or other immunodeficiency and present in a manner similar to that of *Fusarium* with hematogenously disseminated skin lesions and positive blood cultures. Species of *Acremonium* are commonly found in soil, decaying vegetation, and decaying food. Colonies of *Acremonium* spp. are white-gray or rose with a velvety to cottony surface. The conidia may be single-celled, in chains, or in a conidial mass arising from short, unbranched, tapered phialides. The optimal treatment for infections caused by *Acremonium* spp. has not been established. Resistance is seen to amphotericin B, itraconazole, and the echinocandins. A recent report of successful treatment of a pulmonary infection caused by *Acremonium strictum* with posaconazole suggests that the new triazoles may be useful in treatment of *Acremonium* infections.

Although uncommon, *Paecilomyces* spp. may cause invasive disease in organ and hematopoietic stem cell recipients, persons with AIDS, and other immunocompromised patients. The portal of entry is often through breaks in the skin or intravascular catheters and dissemination, possibly aided by adventitious conidiation in tissue, is common. The two most common species are *Paecilomyces lilacinus* and *Paecilomyces variotii*. Microscopically, the *Paecilomyces* spp. conidia form chains and are unicellular and ovoid to fusiform. Phialides have a swollen base and a long tapered neck. Susceptibility to amphotericin B is variable, with resistance seen with *P. lilacinus*. Voriconazole has been used successfully to treat both severe cutaneous infection and disseminated disease.

Trichoderma spp. are excellent examples of fungi previously labeled as nonpathogenic that have emerged as important opportunistic pathogens in immunocompromised patients and in patients undergoing peritoneal dialysis. Fatal disseminated disease caused by *Trichoderma longibrachiatum* occurs in patients with hematologic malignancies, after BMT, or solid organ transplantation. Most *Trichoderma* spp. show decreased susceptibility to amphotericin B, itraconazole, fluconazole, and flucytosine. Voriconazole appears to be active against the few isolates tested.

Scopulariopsis spp. are ubiquitous soil saprobes that have been rarely implicated in invasive human disease. *Scopulariopsis brevicaulis* is the most frequently isolated species. Infection is usually confined to the nails; however, serious deep infection has been noted in neutropenic leukemia patients and after BMT. Both local and disseminated infections have been described with involvement of the nasal septum, skin and soft tissues, blood, lungs, and brain. Diagnosis is made by culture and histopathology. *Scopulariopsis* spp. grow moderately to rapidly on standard mycologic media. Colonies are initially smooth, becoming granular to powdery with age. Conidiophores are simple or branched; the conidiogenous cells are annellides that form singly or in clusters or may form a broom-like structure, or scopula, similar to that seen with *Penicillium* spp. The annelloconidia are smooth initially, become rough at maturity, are shaped like light bulbs, and form basipetal chains. *Scopulariopsis* spp. are usually resistant to itraconazole and moderately susceptible to amphotericin B. Invasive infections may require surgical and medical treatment and are often fatal.

Phaeohyphomycosis

Phaeohyphomycosis is defined as tissue infection caused by dematiaceous (pigmented) hyphae, yeasts, or both. Infections due to dematiaceous fungi constitute a significant and increasingly prevalent group of opportunistic fungal diseases and may take the form of disseminated disease or become localized to the lung, paranasal sinuses, or CNS. Primary inoculation, resulting in localized subcutaneous infection, occurs commonly in underdeveloped countries and has been discussed in Chapter 73.

The dematiaceous fungi that have been documented to cause human infection encompass a large number of different genera; however, the more common causes of human infection include *Alternaria, Bipolaris, Cladosporium, Curvularia,* and *Exserohilum* species. Additionally, several of the dematiaceous fungi appear to be neurotropic: *Cladophialophora bantiana, Bipolaris spicifera, Exophiala* spp., *Wangiella dermatitidis, Ramichloridium obovoideum,* and *Chaetomium atrobrunneum*. Brain abscess is the most common CNS presentation. *Bipolaris* spp. and *Exserohilum* spp. infections may present initially as sinusitis that then extends into the CNS.

In tissue, hyphae with or without yeast forms are present. Most often the pale brown to dark melanin-like pigment within the cell wall is apparent in H&E- or Papanicolaou-stained tissue (Figure 75–22). Staining with the Fontana-Masson technique (a melanin-specific stain) may help visualize the dematiaceous elements.

The dematiaceous fungi differ considerably in the clinical spectrum of infection and response to therapy. Furthermore, the different genera are not readily distinguished on histopathologic examination. Thus an accurate microbiologic diagnosis based on culture of the infected tissue is important for optimal clinical management of infections due to these fungi.

Alternaria spp. are important causes of paranasal sinusitis in both healthy and immunocompromised individuals. Other sites of infection include skin and soft tissue, cornea, lower respiratory tract, and peritoneum. *Alternaria alternata* is the best-documented human pathogen in this genus. In culture, *Alternaria* colonies are rapidly growing, cottony, and gray to black. The conidiophores are usually solitary and simple or branched. The

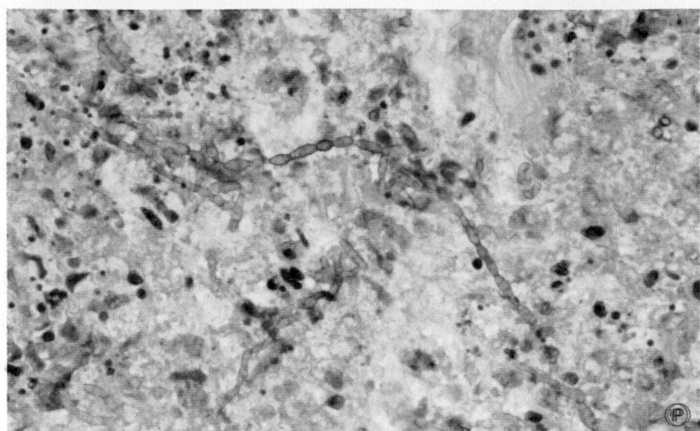

FIGURE 75–22. *Cladophialophora bantiana* in tissue showing pigmented hyphae (H&E, magnification 400×). (From Marler LM et al: *Mycology* CD-ROM, Indiana Pathology Images, 2004.)

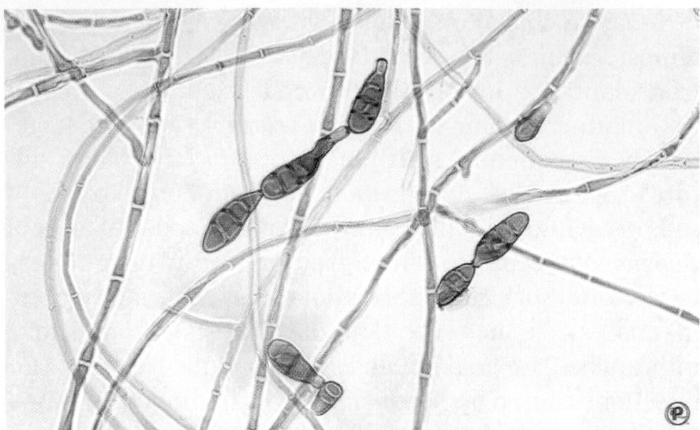

FIGURE 75–23. *Alternaria* sp., lactophenol cotton blue preparation showing darkly pigmented chains of muriform conidia (magnification 400×). (From Marler LM et al: *Mycology* CD-ROM, Indiana Pathology Images, 2004.)

conidia develop in branching chains and are dematiaceous, muriform, and smooth or rough and taper toward the distal end with a short beak at their apices (Figure 75–23).

Cladosporium spp. usually cause superficial cutaneous infections but may cause deep infections as well. These fungi are rapidly growing with a velvety, olive gray to black colony. The conidiophores arise from the hyphae and are dematiaceous, tall and branching. The conidia may be smooth or rough and single- to several-celled and form branching chains at the apex of the conidiophore.

Curvularia spp. are ubiquitous inhabitants of the soil and have been implicated in both disseminated and local infections. Sites of infection include endocarditis, local catheter site infections, nasal septum and paranasal sinuses, lower respiratory tract, skin and subcutaneous tissues, bones, and cornea. In tissue, the hyphae may appear nonpigmented. Common species found to be etiologic agents of human infection include *Curvularia geniculata, Curvularia lunata, Curvularia pallescens,* and *Curvularia senegalensis*. In culture, colonies are rapidly growing, wooly, and gray to grayish black. Microscopically, the conidia are dematiaceous, solitary or in groups, septate, simple or branched, sympodial, and geniculate.

Infections caused by the genera *Bipolaris* and *Exserohilum* present similarly to those of *Aspergillus* spp., except that the disease progresses more slowly. Clinical presentations include dissemination with vascular invasion and tissue necrosis, involvement of the CNS and paranasal sinuses, and association with allergic bronchopulmonary disease. These organisms cause sinusitis in "normal" (atopic or asthmatic) hosts and more invasive disease in immunocompromised hosts. In culture, both *Bipolaris* and *Exserohilum* form rapidly growing, wooly, gray to black colonies. Microscopically, the conidiophores are sympodial and geniculate. The conidia are dematiaceous, oblong to cylindrical, and multicelled (Figure 75–24).

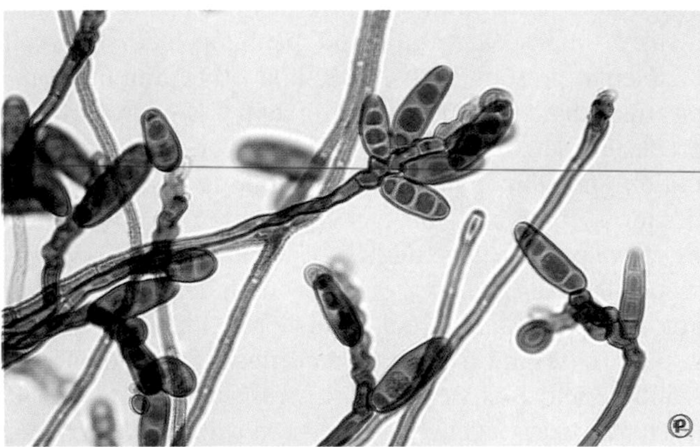

FIGURE 75–24. *Bipolaris* sp., lactophenol cotton blue preparation showing pigmented conidia borne on geniculate conidiophores (magnification 400×). (From Marler LM et al: *Mycology* CD-ROM, Indiana Pathology Images, 2004.)

The optimal treatment of deep-seated phaeohyphomycosis has not yet been established, although it most often includes early administration of amphotericin B and aggressive surgical excision. Despite these efforts, phaeohyphomycosis does not respond well to treatment and relapses are common. Posaconazole has been used successfully to treat disseminated infection caused by *Exophiala spinifera*. In those patients with brain abscesses, complete excision of the lesion has been associated with improved survival. Long-term triazole (posaconazole or voriconazole) therapy coupled with repeated surgical excision may prevent recurrences.

Pneumocystosis

Pneumocystis jiroveci (formerly *Pneumocystis carinii*) is an organism that causes infection almost exclusively in debilitated and immunosuppressed patients, especially those

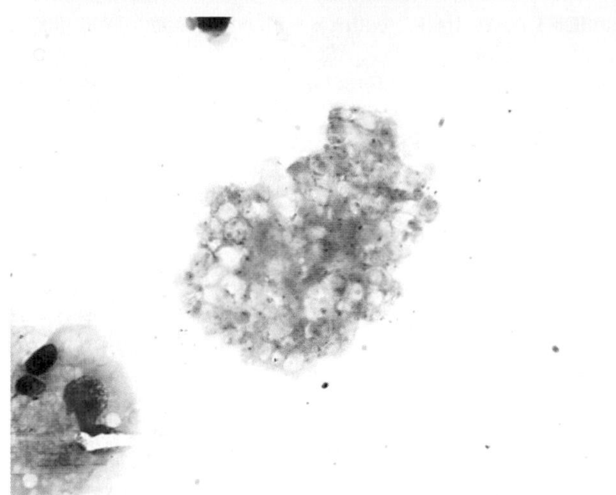

FIGURE 75–25. *Pneumocystis jiroveci* in bronchoalveolar lavage fluid. Giemsa stain shows intracystic forms (magnification 1000×).

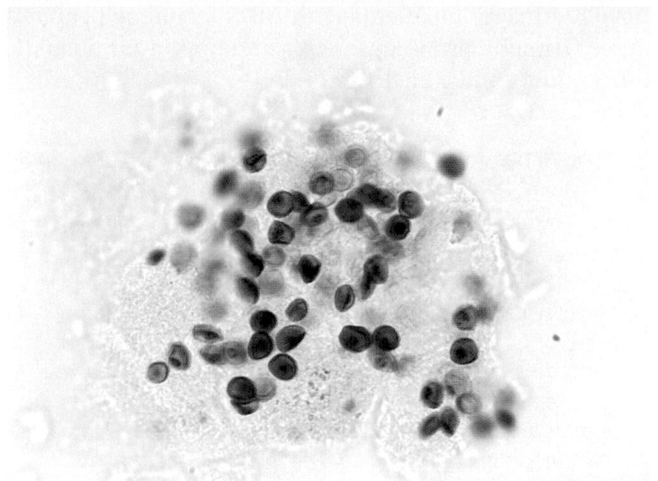

FIGURE 75–26. *Pneumocystis jiroveci* in bronchoalveolar lavage fluid. GMS stain shows typical intact and collapsed cysts (magnification 1000×).

with HIV infection. It is the most common opportunistic infection among persons with AIDS; however, the incidence has decreased considerably in recent years with the use of highly active antiretroviral therapy (HAART). Although previously considered to be a protozoan parasite, recent molecular and genetic evidence place it among the fungi (see Chapter 7).

The life cycle of *P. jiroveci* includes both sexual and asexual components. During the course of human infection, *P. jiroveci* may exist as free trophic forms (1.5 to 5 μm in diameter), as a uninucleate sporocyst (4 to 5 μm), or as a cyst (5 μm) containing up to eight ovoid to fusiform intracystic bodies (Figure 75–25). After rupture of the cyst, the cyst wall may be seen as an empty collapsed structure (Figure 75–26).

The reservoir for *P. jiroveci* in nature is unknown. Although airborne transmission has been documented experimentally among rodents, the rodent strains are genetically distinct from those of humans, making it unlikely that rodents serve as a zoonotic reservoir for human disease.

The respiratory tract is the main portal of entry for *P. jiroveci* in humans. Pneumonia is clearly the most common presentation of pneumocystosis, although extrapulmonary manifestations can be seen among AIDS patients. Involvement of lymph nodes, spleen, bone marrow, liver, small bowel, genitourinary tract, eyes, ears, skin, bone, and thyroid have been reported. Recent evidence suggests that both reactivation of quiescent old infection and primary infection can occur. Malnourished, debilitated, and immunosuppressed patients, especially AIDS patients with low CD4 counts ($<200/mm^3$), are at high risk of infection.

The hallmark of *P. jiroveci* infection is an interstitial pneumonitis with a mononuclear infiltrate composed predominantly of plasma cells. The onset of disease is insidious with signs and symptoms including dyspnea, cyanosis, tachypnea, nonproductive cough, and fever. The radiographic appearance is typically one of diffuse interstitial infiltrates with a ground glass appearance extending from the hilar region, but it may appear normal or show nodules or cavitation. The mortality rate is high among untreated patients, and death is caused by respiratory failure.

Histologically, a foamy exudate is seen within the alveolar spaces with an intense interstitial infiltrate composed predominantly of plasma cells. Other possible patterns include diffuse alveolar damage, noncaseating granulomatous inflammation, and infarct-like coagulative necrosis.

The diagnosis of *P. jiroveci* infection is almost entirely based on microscopic examination of clinical material including bronchial alveolar lavage fluid, bronchial brushing, induced sputum, and transbronchial or open lung biopsy specimens. Examination of bronchial alveolar lavage fluid has been shown to have a sensitivity of 90% to 100% and usually precludes the need for transbronchial or open lung biopsy. Microscopic examination of induced sputum may be useful in AIDS patients with a very high organism load; however, it has a 20% to 25% false-negative rate. A variety of histologic and cytologic stains have been used to detect *P. jiroveci* including GMS, Giemsa, PAS, toluidine blue, calcofluor, and immunofluorescence. The Giemsa stain demonstrates the trophic forms but does not stain the cyst wall (see Figure 75–25), whereas the GMS stain is specific for the cyst wall (see Figure 75–26). Immunofluorescent techniques stain both trophic forms and the cyst wall.

The cornerstone for both prophylaxis and treatment is trimethoprim-sulfamethoxazole. Alternative therapies have been used in patients with AIDS including pentamidine, trimethoprim-dapsone, clindamycin-primaquine, atovaquone, and trimetrexate.

CASE STUDY AND QUESTIONS

George is a 45-year-old man who underwent an allogeneic stem cell transplant as part of his treatment for acute leukemia. The transplant went well and after engraftment George was discharged from the hospital. During the course of his transplant, George's physicians administered antifungal prophylaxis with voriconazole due to concerns regarding aspergillosis that had been a problem in the hospital over the past few years. After discharge, George did well and his antifungal prophylaxis was continued; however, on a clinical visit on day 140 posttransplant he was noted to have a rash and elevated liver function studies. About 1 week later he began having bloody diarrhea, and his physician became concerned about graft-versus-host disease (GVHD). A rectal biopsy was performed confirming GVHD and George's immunosuppressive regimen was increased, as was his daily dose of voriconazole. The signs and symptoms of GVHD continued and eventually George was readmitted to the hospital. He was found to be confused, febrile, and short of breath. A chest x-ray showed a wedge-shaped infiltrate in the right lower lung field, and imaging studies of his sinuses showed bilateral opacification.

1. What is the differential diagnosis of this process?
2. What fungal pathogens would you be concerned about in an immunosuppressed individual receiving voriconazole prophylaxis?
3. How would you go about making a diagnosis?
4. What course of therapy would you undertake?

Bibliography

Anaissie EJ, McGinnis MR, Pfaller MA, editors: *Clinical mycology*, New York, 2003, Churchill Livingstone.

Chandler FW, Watts JC, editors: *Pathologic diagnosis of fungal infections*, Chicago, 1987, ASCP Press.

Cohen J, Powderly WG, editors: *Infectious diseases*, ed 2, Philadelphia, 2004, Elsevier.

Connor DH et al, editors: *Pathology of infectious diseases*, Stamford, Conn., 1997, Appleton & Lange.

Dignani MC, Solomkin JS, Anaissie EJ: *Candida*, In Anaissie EJ, McGinnis MR, Pfaller MA, editors: *Clinical mycology*, New York, 2003, Churchill Livingstone.

Gudlagson O et al: Attributable mortality of nosocomial candidemia, revisited, *Clin Infect Dis* 37:1172-1177, 2003.

Pannuti CS et al: Nosocomial pneumonia in adult patients undergoing bone marrow transplantation: A 9-year study, *J Clin Oncol* 9:1-5, 1991.

Pfaller MA, Diekema DJ: Rare and emerging opportunistic fungal pathogens: Concern for resistance beyond *Candida albicans* and *Aspergillus fumigatus*, *J Clin Microbiol* 42:4419-4431, 2004.

Pfaller MA, Diekema DJ: The role of sentinel surveillance of candidemia: Trends in species distribution and antifungal susceptibility, *J Clin Microbiol* 40:3551-3557, 2002.

Pfaller MA, Diekema DJ: Twelve years of fluconazole in clinical practice: Global trends in species distribution and fluconazole susceptibility of bloodstream isolates of *Candida*, *Clin Microbiol Infect* 10 (Suppl. 1):11-23, 2004.

Pfaller MA, Wenzel RP: The epidemiology of fungal infections. In Anaissie EJ, McGinnis MR, Pfaller MA, editors: *Clinical mycology*, New York, 2003, Churchill Livingstone.

Pfaller MA et al: National surveillance of nosocomial blood stream infections due to *Candida albicans*: Frequency of occurrence and antifungal susceptibility in the SCOPE Program, *Diagn Microbiol Infect Dis* 31:327-332, 1998.

Viviani MA, Tortorano AM, Ajello L: Cryptococcus. In Anaissie EJ, McGinnis MR, Pfaller MA, editors: *Clinical mycology*, New York, 2003, Churchill Livingstone.

Walsh TJ et al: Experimental pulmonary aspergillosis due to *Aspergillus terreus*: pathogenesis and treatment of an emerging fungal pathogen resistant to amphotericin B, *J Infect Dis* 188:305-319, 2003.

Wey SB et al: Hospital acquired candidemia: Attributable mortality and excess length of stay, *Arch Intern Med* 148:2642-2645, 1988.

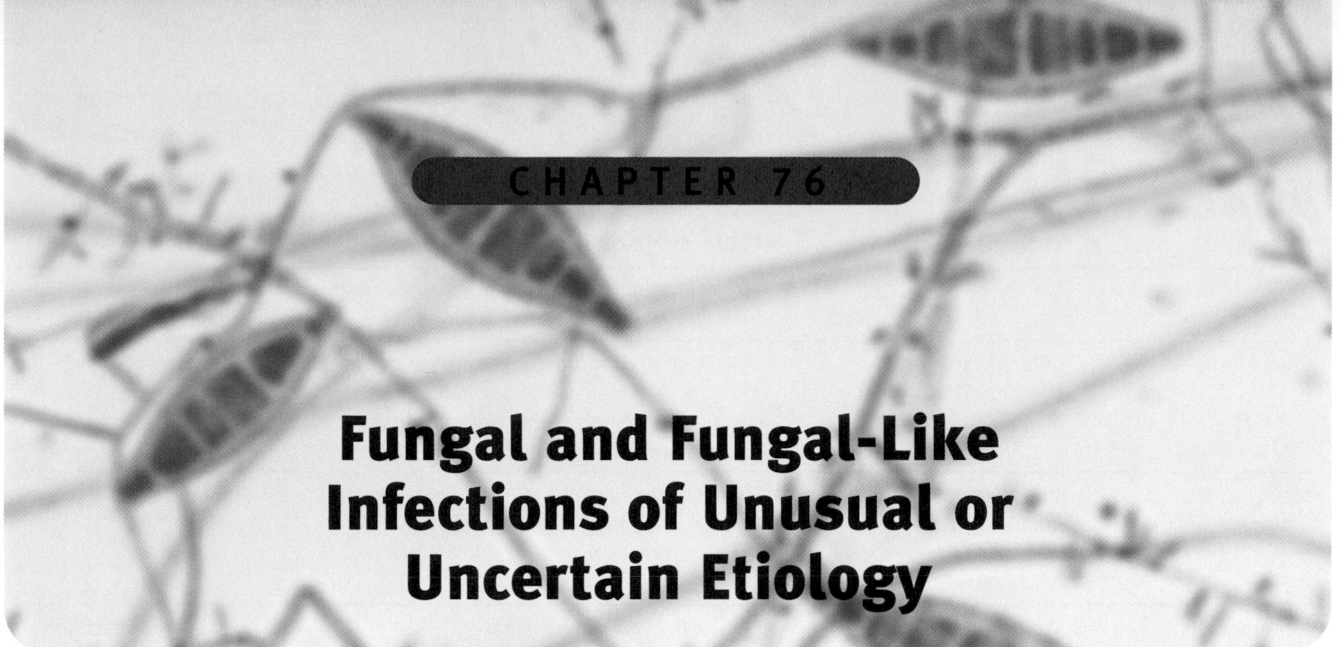

CHAPTER 76

Fungal and Fungal-Like Infections of Unusual or Uncertain Etiology

Thus far we have discussed mycotic processes caused by reasonably well characterized fungi that may serve as colonizers, opportunistic pathogens, or true pathogens. Although many of these organisms have undergone minor taxonomic reclassification over time, they all share the characteristics of the kingdom Fungi (see Chapter 7). One notable exception to this statement is *Pneumocystis jiroveci (carinii)*, an organism formerly considered to be a protozoan and now classified as a fungus of the class Archiascomycetes based on molecular evidence (see Chapters 7 and 75). The fact that *P. jiroveci* cannot be grown on artificial media has complicated its characterization and assignment to the proper taxonomic category. In this chapter we will discuss several infections that historically have been considered to represent fungal or "fungal-like" processes based on clinical and histopathologic presentation but, similar to *P. jiroveci*, have been difficult to classify because they cannot be grown on artificial media. In one instance, recent molecular evidence has suggested that an organism previously thought to be a fungus (*Rhinosporidium seeberi*) is in fact a protistan parasite. We also discuss two algal infections and an unusual infection due to the oomycete *Pythium insidiosum*. In addition to being both unusual and uncommon, these infections are all diagnosed based on detection of characteristic structures on histopathologic examination of tissue. A listing of the infections, the etiologic agents, and the typical morphology in tissue is provided in Table 76–1.

Adiaspiromycosis

In humans, adiaspiromycosis is a rare, self-limited pulmonary infection caused by inhalation of the asexual conidia of the soil saprophyte *Emmonsia crescens* (formerly *Chrysosporium parvum* var *crescens*). Synonyms include haplomycosis or adiaspirosis.

MORPHOLOGY

The fungus, *Emmonsia crescens,* grows as a mould in culture at room temperature and in nature. The hyphae are septate and branched. The small (2 to 4 μm) aleurioconidia are born on conidiophores that arise at right angles to the vegetative hyphae. On incubation at 40°C in vitro, or when introduced into the lungs, the conidia transform into spherical adiaconidia, which then undergo massive enlargement but show no evidence of replication (e.g., budding, endospore formation).

When mature, the adiaconidia are thick-walled spherules measuring 200 to 400 μm or more in diameter (Table 76–1 and Figure 76–1). The walls of the spherule are refractile, 20 to 70 μm thick, and, when stained with hematoxylin and eosin (H&E) stain, are composed of two layers: a narrow, outer, eosinophilic layer containing periodic fenestrations and a broad, hyaline, inner layer composed predominantly of chitin (see Figure 76–1). The conidial walls stain with Gomori methenamine silver (GMS), periodic acid-Schiff (PAS), and the Gridley fungus stains but not with mucicarmine (Table 76–2). In human lung tissue, the adiaconidia are usually empty but may contain small eosinophilic globules along the inner surface of the walls (see Figure 76–1).

EPIDEMIOLOGY

Although human adiaspiromycosis is uncommon, the infection is prevalent in rodents worldwide. Likewise, the fungus can be found in nature predominantly in temperate zones. Human disease has been reported from France, Czechoslovakia, Russia, Honduras, Guatemala,

TABLE 76–1. Morphologic Features of Fungal and Fungal-Like Infections of Unusual or Uncertain Etiology

Disease	Etiologic Agent(s)	Typical Morphology in Tissue	Usual Host Reaction
Adiaspiromycosis	*Emmonsia crescens*	Large adiaconidia, 200–400 μm diameter with thick (20–70 μm) walls. See Figure 76–1.	Granulomatous fibrotic and noncaseating
Chlorellosis	*Chlorella* sp. (chlorophyllous green algae)	Unicellular endosporulating, round organisms, 4–15 μm diameter, containing multiple cytoplasmic granules (chloroplasts). Lesions are green-pigmented. See Figure 76–2.	Pyogranulomatous
Lobomycosis	*Lacazia loboi* (*Loboa loboi*)	Spherical budding yeasts, 5–12 μm diameter, that form chains of cells connected by tube-like structures; secondary budding may be present. See Figure 76–3.	Granulomatous
Protothecosis	*Prototheca wickerhamii*, *P. zopfii* (achlorophyllous green algae)	Spherical, oval, or polyhedral spherules, 2–25 μm diameter, containing 2–20 endospores when mature. See Figure 76–5.	Variable; no reaction to granulomatous
Pythiosis insidiosi	*Pythium insidiosum* (not a true fungus; belongs to class Oomycetes)	Hyphae and short hyphal fragments that are hyaline, thin walled, pausiseptate, irregularly branched, 5–7 μm wide, non-parallel contours; angioinvasive. See Figure 76–6.	Granulomatous, necrotizing, suppurative, arteritis
Rhinosporidiosis	*Rhinosporidium seeberi* (aquatic protistan parasite of the Mesomycetozoan clade)	Large sporangia, 100–350 μm diameter, with thin walls (3–5 μm) that enclose numerous endospores, 6–8 μm diameter, with a zonal distribution. See Figures 76–7 and 76–8.	Nonspecific chronic inflammatory or granulomatous

Data from Chandler FW, Watts JC: *Pathologic diagnosis of fungal infections,* Chicago, 1987, ASCP Press; and Connor DH et al: *Pathology of infectious diseases,* vol II, Stamford, Conn., 1997, Appleton & Lange.

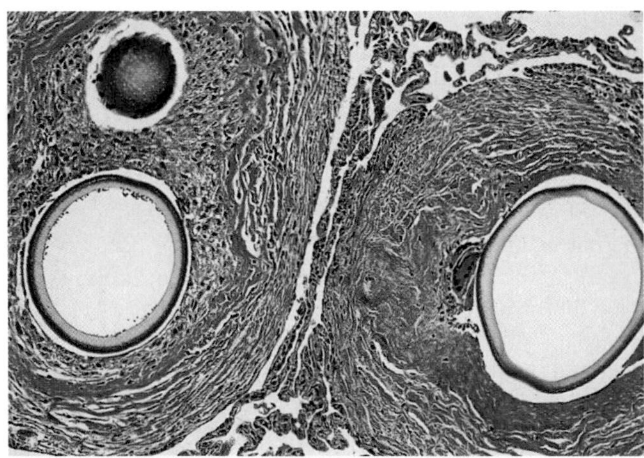

FIGURE 76–1. Pulmonary adiaspiromycosis. The hematoxylin and eosin (H&E) stain defines three layers in the wall of the adiaconidium. Each adiaconidium has evoked a fibrogranulomatous response (H&E, magnification 40×). (From Connor DH et al: *Pathology of infectious diseases,* vol II, Stamford, Conn, 1997, Appleton & Lange.)

Venezuela, and Brazil. Rodents may serve as a zoonotic reservoir for the disease, although the fungus causing disease in rodents, *E. parva* (formerly *C. parvum* var *parvum*), has rarely been known to infect humans. The likely mode of infection is by inhalation of fungal conidia aerosolized by contaminated soil.

CLINICAL SYNDROMES

As with many fungal infections, most cases of documented adiaspiromycosis have been asymptomatic. Pulmonary nodules can be detected radiographically or incidentally at autopsy or in surgical specimens of lung removed for another reason.

Three forms of human adiaspiromycosis have been recognized: solitary granuloma, localized granulomatous disease, and diffuse, disseminated granulomatous disease. Patients with the disseminated granulomatous form of pulmonary adiaspiromycosis may experience fever, cough, and progressive dyspnea due to compression and displacement of distal airways and alveolar parenchyma by the expanding granulomas. Fungal replication in the lungs does not occur, and dissemination to extrapulmonary sites has not been reported. The severity of the disease appears to be entirely a result of the number of conidia inhaled.

LABORATORY DIAGNOSIS

The diagnosis of adiaspiromycosis is established by histopathologic examination of the affected lung and identification of the characteristic adiaconidia. Each adiaconidium is surrounded by an epithelioid and giant cell

TABLE 76–2. Comparative Morphologic Features of Fungi and Fungal-Like Organisms That Appear as Large Spherules in Tissue

Feature	Organisms		
	Coccidioides immitis	***Rhinosporidium seeberi****	***Emmonsia crescens***†
External diameter of spherule (μm)	20-200	10-350	200-400
Thickness of spherule wall (μm)	1-2	3-5	20-70
Diameter of endospores (μm)	2-5	6-10‡	None
Pigmentation	None	None	None
Hyphae or arthroconidia	Rare	None	None
Host reaction	**Necrotic granulomas**	**Mucosal polyps with acute and chronic inflammation**	**Fibrotic granulomas**
Growth in culture	+	–	±§
Special stain reactions			
GMS	+	+	+
PAS	+	+	+
Mucicarmine	–	+	–

Data from Chandler FW, Watts JC: *Pathologic diagnosis of fungal infections,* Chicago, 1987, ASCP Press.
GMS, Gomori methenamine silver; PAS, periodic acid-Schiff.
*Not a fungus. Newly classified as an aquatic protistan parasite of the Mesomycetozoan clade.
†Adiaconidia.
‡Endospores arranged in characteristic zonal distribution. Mature endospores contain distinctive eosinophilic globules.
§Grows as a mould on agar medium. Organism not recoverable from tissue.

granulomatous response, which is further encompassed by a dense capsule of fibrous tissue (see Figure 76–1). All of the granulomas are at a similar stage of development, reflecting a one-time exposure without subsequent replication within the lung.

The spherules represented by the adiaconidia should not be confused with those of *Coccidioides immitis* or *R. seeberi,* two other organisms that produce large spherules in tissue (see Table 76–2). In contrast to *C. immitis,* the adiaconidia of *Emmonsia crescens* are much larger, have a thicker wall, and do not contain endospores. The sporangia of *R. seeberi* are distinguished by the zonation of the sporangiospores and the distinctive eosinophilic globules seen within the mature sporangiospores (see Table 76–2). No other fungus of medical importance has walls as thick as those of the adiaconidia of *E. crescens.* Culture of infected tissue is not useful because the adiaconidia do not represent a replicative form of the fungus.

TREATMENT

Human pulmonary adiaspiromycosis is a self-limited infection. Specific antifungal therapy is not necessary.

Chlorellosis

Chlorellosis is an infection of humans and animals caused by a unicellular green algae of the genus *Chlorella.* In contrast to *Prototheca* spp., another algae that causes human infection, *Chlorella* spp. contain chloroplasts that give the lesions of chlorellosis a distinct green color. Most infections with this organism occur in sheep and cattle. A single human infection has been reported thus far.

MORPHOLOGY

Chlorella spp. are unicellular, ovoid, spherical, or polygonal, and 4 to 5 μm in diameter, and they reproduce by endosporulation. The organisms contain numerous green chloroplasts that appear as cytoplasmic granules. The chloroplasts contain starch granules that stain intensely with GMS, PAS, and Gridley fungal stains. The cell walls may appear doubly contoured (Figure 76–2 and Table 76–1). *Chlorella* spp. reproduce asexually by internal septation and cytoplasmic cleavage, producing up to 20 daughter cells (sporangiospores) within the sporangium (parent cell). On maturation, the outer wall of the sporangium ruptures and releases the

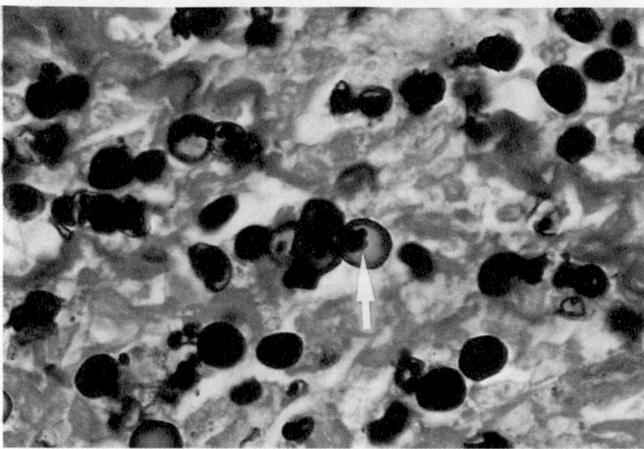

FIGURE 76–2. *Chlorella* sp. showing intracellular chloroplasts and doubly contoured cell wall (GMS, magnification 400×). (From Connor DH et al: *Pathology of infectious diseases,* vol II, Stamford, Conn, 1997, Appleton & Lange.)

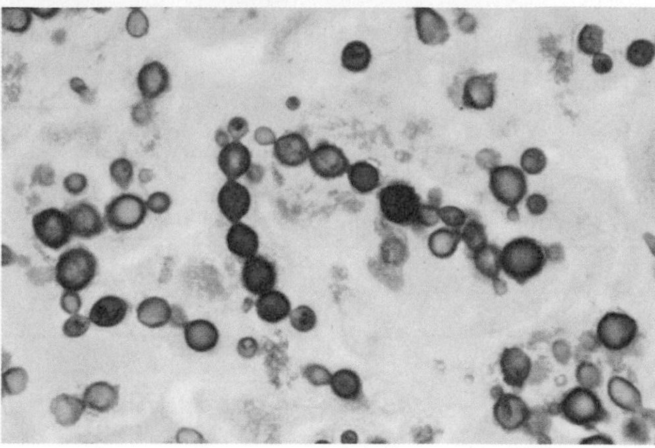

FIGURE 76–3. *Lacazia loboi.* The fungi form a single chain with individual cells joined by tubelike bridges (Gridley, magnification 400×). (From Chandler FW, Watts JC: *Pathologic diagnosis of fungal infections,* Chicago, 1987, ASCP Press. Copyright 1987, American Society of Clinical Pathologists.)

sporangiospores, each of which goes on to produce sporangiospores of their own.

EPIDEMIOLOGY

The single human case of chlorellosis took place in Nebraska and resulted from exposure of a surgical wound to river water. Infections in domestic (e.g., sheep and cattle) and wild animals (e.g., beaver) range from lymph node and deep organ involvement to cutaneous and subcutaneous lesions, presumably related to exposure to water containing the organism.

CLINICAL SYNDROMES

As noted previously, the human case of chlorellosis involved a healing surgical wound contaminated with river water. The wound subsequently drained a greenish-yellow exudate. The infection was cured by repeated surgical débridement over a 10-month period. In animals, fresh lesions in liver, lymph nodes, and subcutaneous tissue are green in color on gross examination, and smears reveal organisms that contain green refractile granules (chloroplasts).

LABORATORY DIAGNOSIS

Infections caused by *Chlorella* spp. may be diagnosed by culture and by histopathologic examination of infected tissue. The organism grows well on most solid media, producing bright green colonies. Wet mounts of wound exudate or touch preparations of infected tissue reveal ovoid, endosporulating cells with characteristic green cytoplasmic granules representing chloroplasts. In tissue the cells stain well with GMS and PAS, but not H&E, stains. They may be distinguished histopathologically from *Prototheca* spp. by the intracellular chloroplasts.

TREATMENT

Treatment in the only human case of chlorellosis consisted of repeat débridement, irrigation with Dakin's solution, and gauze packing and removal for drainage and granulation. Alternatively amphotericin B therapy combined with administration of tetracycline has proved efficacious in the treatment of protothecosis and may be useful for chlorellosis as well.

Lobomycosis

Lobomycosis is a chronic fungal infection of the skin caused by *Lacazia loboi* (formerly *Loboa loboi*). The disease is seen primarily in the South and Central American tropics. Natural infection occurs only in humans and dolphins, although it has been reproduced experimentally by injecting infected tissue into hamsters and armadillos. The organism has never been cultured in vitro.

MORPHOLOGY

L. loboi is spherical to oval and yeastlike in appearance. The fungi are 6 to 12 μm in diameter and have a thick double refractile cell wall. It reproduces by sequential budding and usually forms chains of cells connected by a narrow tubelike bridges (Figure 76–3). Some of the cells may have one or two secondary buds and may be mistaken for the "mariners wheel" form of *Paracoccidioides brasiliensis. L. loboi* is usually intracellular, although extracellular forms exist.

EPIDEMIOLOGY

The human disease is endemic in the tropical regions of Central and South America and has been reported in central and western Brazil, Bolivia, Columbia, Costa Rica, Ecuador, Guyana, French Guiana, Mexico, Panama, Peru, Surinam, and Venezuela. Isolated cases have been reported from Holland, and a single case has been reported recently in the United States in a patient with a history of travel to Venezuela.

L. loboi is believed to be a saprophyte of soil or vegetation, and lobomycosis predominates in tropical regions with thick vegetation, such as the Amazon rain forests. Cutaneous trauma is believed to be the mode of infection. A plant reservoir has not been identified.

Given the fact that lobomycosis occurs in marine dolphins and in freshwater dolphins, an aquatic habitat is likely as well. Infection among dolphins has been reported for Florida, the Texas coast, the Spanish-French coast, the South Brazilian coast, and the Surinam River estuary. One instance of dolphin-to-human transmission has been reported; however, there is no evidence of human-to-human transmission.

Lobomycosis occurs primarily in men or in women who are involved in farming and jungle clearing. Farmers, miners, hunters, and rubber plant workers have an increased incidence of disease. There is no racial predilection and lobomycosis affects all age groups, with the peak age of onset at 20 to 40 years.

CLINICAL SYNDROMES

Lobomycosis is characterized by slowly developing cutaneous nodules of varying size and shape (Figure 76–4). The dermal lesions are polymorphic, ranging from macules, papules, keloidal nodules, and plaques, to verrucous and ulcerated lesions, all of which may be present in a single patient. The nodular keloidlike lesion is the most common. The disease is characterized by a long dormancy period of months to years. The increase in the number and size of lesions is also a slow process, progressing over a period of 40 to 50 years. Lesions tend to arise on traumatized areas of skin, such as the face, ears, arms, legs, and feet. The disease does not involve mucous membranes or internal organs. Local cutaneous spread can occur through autoinoculation. Aside from occasional pruritus and hypesthesia or anesthesia of the affected area, patients are asymptomatic. There are no systemic manifestations of the disease.

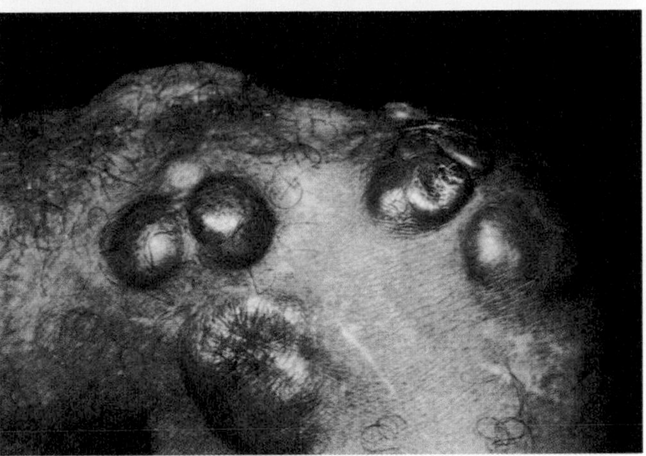

FIGURE 76–4. Multiple keloidlike lesions of lobomycosis. (From Chandler FW, Watts JC: *Pathologic diagnosis of fungal infections,* Chicago, 1987, ASCP Press. Copyright 1987, American Society of Clinical Pathologists.)

LABORATORY DIAGNOSIS

Diagnosis is based on demonstrating the presence of the characteristic yeast cells in lesion exudate or tissue sections. Biopsy reveals a dispersed granulomatous infiltrate along with numerous fungal forms in the dermis and subcutaneous tissue. The granuloma consists primarily of giant cells, macrophages, and epithelioid cells. Both the giant cells and macrophages contain fungi that have been phagocytosed.

L. loboi stains intensely with both GMS and PAS stains. H&E stain reveals the thick doubly contoured hyaline cell wall and one or more hematoxylinophilic nuclei.

Although the lesions of lobomycosis grossly resemble keloids, microscopically keloids have marked fibrosis, which is not the case with lobomycosis. Similarly, keloids lack granulomas and fungal elements. The morphology and pattern of budding of *L. loboi* are distinctive and should not be confused with that of *P. brasiliensis* (i.e., multiple buds, variable size), *Blastomyces dermatitidis* and *Histoplasma capsulatum* var *duboisii* (i.e., no chains of cells), or *Sporothrix schenckii* and *H. capsulatum* var *capsulatum* (both smaller, 2 to 8 μm versus 5 to 12 μm). The later fungi will also grow in culture, whereas *L. loboi* has never been cultured in vitro.

TREATMENT

Surgical excision of localized lesions is the optimal therapy. More widespread disease usually recurs when treated surgically and does not respond to antifungal therapy. Clofazimine has been used in these situations, but at this time medical treatment of lobomycosis is not satisfactory.

Protothecosis

Protothecosis is an infection of humans and animals caused by achlorophyllous algae of the genus *Prototheca.* These organisms belong to the same family as the green algae of the genus *Chlorella.* Two species, *Prototheca wickerhamii* and *Prototheca zopfii,* are known to cause infection. Three forms of human protothecosis have been described: cutaneous, olecranon bursitis, and disseminated.

MORPHOLOGY

The protothecae are unicellular, oval or spherical organisms that reproduce asexually by internal septation and irregular cleavage within a hyaline sporangia. Each sporangium contains between two and 20 sporangiospores arranged in a "morula" configuration (Figure 76–5). The sporangiospores are released after rupture of the sporangium and in turn develop into mature endosporulating forms. The cells measure 3 to 30 μm in diameter and differ from those of *Chlorella* by the lack of chloroplasts. Protothecae differ from fungi by the lack of glucosamine in their cell walls. The two species of *Prototheca* that cause human disease differ from one another in size: *P. wickerhamii* measures 3 to 15 μm in diameter and *P. zopfii*'s diameter measures 7 to 30 μm. Both species are readily stained with PAS, GMS, and the Gridley fungus stain (see Figure 76–5) and are gram positive.

EPIDEMIOLOGY

Prototheca spp. are ubiquitous environmental saprobes that have been isolated from grass, soil, water, and both wild and domestic animals. Human protothecosis has been reported on all continents with the exception of Antarctica.

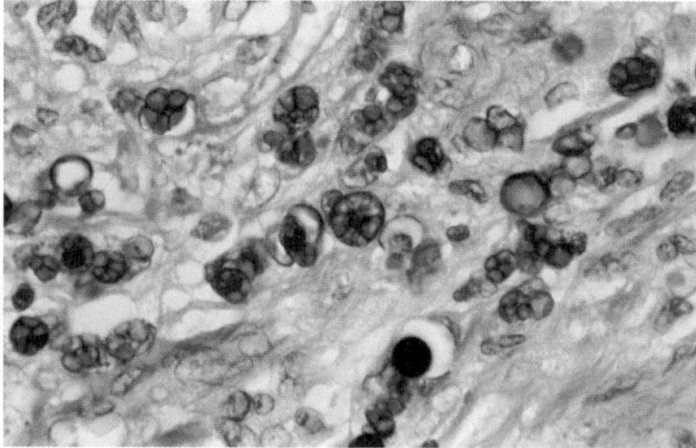

FIGURE 76–5. *Prototheca wickerhamii.* Single and endosporulating algal cells that are readily demonstrated with the PAS stain. A classic "morula" form is present (magnification 1000×).

CLINICAL SYNDROMES

At least half of all cases of protothecosis are simple cutaneous infections. For the most part, these infections occur in patients who are immunocompromised due to immunosuppressive therapy, AIDS, malnutrition, renal or hepatic disease, cancer, or autoimmune disorders. Lesions usually arise in areas exposed to traumatic implantation and present in an indolent fashion as nodules, papules, or as an eczematoid eruption.

Those persons presenting with olecranon bursitis are usually not immunocompromised but report some sort of penetrating or nonpenetrating trauma to the affected elbow. Signs and symptoms of olecranon bursitis usually occur several weeks after the trauma and include mild induration of the bursa accompanied by tenderness, erythema, and production of a variable amount of serosanguineous fluid.

Disseminated protothecosis is rare but has been reported in persons with no known immunologic deficiency. One patient with visceral protothecosis presented with abdominal pain and abnormal liver function studies that were initially considered to be due to cholangitis. The patient had multiple peritoneal nodules that resembled metastatic cancer but were in fact manifestations of protothecosis. Another patient presented with protothecal lesions on the forehead and nose.

LABORATORY DIAGNOSIS

Prototheca spp. grow easily on a wide variety of solid media at 30° to 37°C. Colonies are yeastlike, white, and creamy in appearance and consistency. A wet mount of the culture material may be stained with lactophenol cotton blue to reveal the characteristic sporangia and sporangiospores. The organisms are quite metabolically active and may be identified to species using one of several commercially available yeast identification panels to determine the carbohydrate assimilation profile.

On histopathologic examination of infected tissue, *Prototheca* spp. appear as sporangiospores that are wedge shaped and arranged in a radial or "morula" pattern within the sporangium (see Figure 75–5). The organisms are best visualized by stains used to demonstrate fungi in tissue: the GMS, PAS, and Gridley fungus procedures. In addition to the size differences noted above, the two species of *Prototheca* differ in that *P. wickerhamii* tends to form very symmetrical morula forms that are rare with *P. zopfii,* the latter exhibiting more random internal divisions. The inflammatory response in protothecosis is predominantly granulomatous.

TREATMENT

Treatment of olecranon bursitis usually involves bursectomy. Repeated drainage has failed; however, drainage coupled with local instillation of amphotericin B was curative in one patient. Treatment of cutaneous protothecosis with a variety of topical and systemic antibacterial, antifungal, and antiprotozoal agents has been unsuccessful. Local excision coupled with topical amphotericin B, systemic tetracycline, and systemic ketoconazole has proved useful despite ketoconazole–related hepatotoxicity. Disseminated protothecosis has been treated with systemic antifungal agents; both amphotericin B and ketoconazole have been used.

Pythiosis Insidiosi

Pythiosis insidiosi is a "fungal-like" infection of humans and animals caused by the oomycete *Pythium insidiosum*. Although described as an aquatic fungus, this organism is not a true fungus. It belongs to the kingdom Stramenopila, phylum Oomycota, class Oomycetes, and family Pythiaceae. In humans, pythiosis is a cutaneous and subcutaneous vascular process marked by rapidly developing granulomatous lesions leading to progressive arterial insufficiency, tissue infarction, aneurisms, and occasionally, death. In animals (e.g., cats, dogs, horses, cattle), it is an osseous, subcutaneous, or pulmonary infection. Dogs and horses can also present with intestinal infection.

MORPHOLOGY

P. insidiosum grows as white colonies with submerged vegetative hyphae and short aerial hyphae on solid culture medium. Because this organism is a plant pathogen, it requires water cultures containing the appropriate leaves to produce zoosporangia and zoospores in vitro. In nature, it produces biflagellate zoospores that attach and penetrate the leaves of various grasses and water lilies. The zoospores have a strong tropism for skin and hair as well as water lily and grass leaves. If zoospores contact injured tissue, they encyst, form germ tubes that produce hyphae, and cause invasive disease.

In tissue, *P. insidiosum* exists as hyaline, pausiseptate, thin-walled hyphae or hyphal fragments that branch infrequently. The hyphal elements are 5 to 7 µm wide with nonparallel contours that superficially resemble those of zygomycetes (Figure 76–6). Like the zygomycetes, *P. insidiosum* is angioinvasive and stains poorly with GMS and other special stains for fungi.

EPIDEMIOLOGY

P. insidiosum grows in aquatic to wet environments in tropical to subtropical regions. Reports of pythiosis have come from Australia, Costa Rica, India, Japan, New Guinea, Thailand, and the United States.

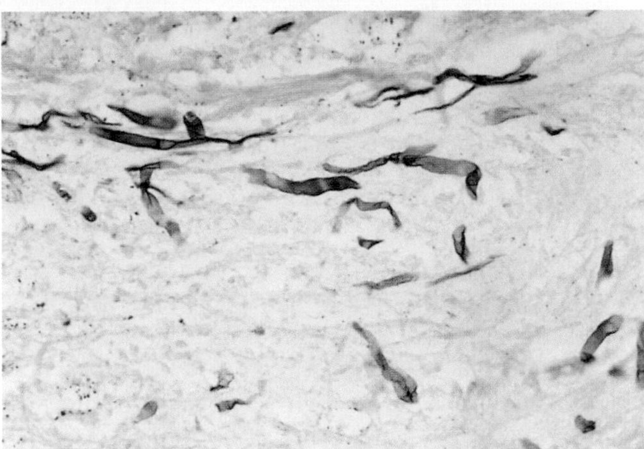

FIGURE 76–6. *Pythium insidiosum* invading an arterial wall. Infrequently septate, weakly stained hyphae and hyphal fragments resemble those of zygomycetes (GMS, magnification 160×). (From Connor DH et al: *Pathology of infectious diseases,* vol II, Stamford, Conn, 1997, Appleton & Lange.)

CLINICAL SYNDROMES

Human disease caused by *P. insidiosum* has occurred in patients with thalassemia who developed pythiosis of the lower limbs. The disease process was marked by progressive ischemia of the lower limbs, necrosis, thrombosis of major arteries due to fungal invasion, gangrene, aneurism formation, and ultimately fatal hemorrhage. Less serious forms of the infection include keratitis and localized cutaneous infections following injury.

In horses, pythiosis presents as localized inflammation of the legs and lower abdomen with necrotic cores. Septic arthritis, osteitis, and tenosynovitis are also common.

LABORATORY DIAGNOSIS

The organism may be isolated from fresh clinical material seeded onto mycologic medium such as Sabouraud's glucose agar. Demonstration of biflagellate zoospores may be accomplished using water cultures with grass or lily bait incubated at 37°C for 1 hour.

Histopathologic examination of infected tissue shows a necrotizing arteritis and thrombosis. Vascular invasion by sparsely septate, irregularly branched hyphae is seen (see Figure 76–6). The acute perivascular inflammatory reaction is eventually replaced by granulomas that contain sparse hyphae and hyphal fragments. Pythiosis insidiosi in humans must be differentiated from cutaneous and subcutaneous zygomycosis, sporotrichosis, mycetoma, and neoplasms.

TREATMENT

Although potassium iodide has been used to treat cutaneous infections, medical treatment of pythiosis insidiosi is generally not effective. Surgical débridement and excision of infected tissue has been used with some success. There is some evidence that azole antifungal agents such as fluconazole, ketoconazole, and miconazole exhibit in vitro activity against this organism.

Rhinosporidiosis

Rhinosporidiosis is a granulomatous disease of humans and animals that is characterized by the development of polyps that primarily affect the nasopharynx and the ocular conjunctiva of infected persons. The disease is caused by *R. seeberi,* an organism with a confusing taxonomic history. This organism has been considered to be a protozoan, a fungus, and most recently has been placed in a novel clade of aquatic protistan parasites, the Mesomycetozoa. Since *R. seeberi* will not grow in synthetic media, this reclassification was based on sequence analysis of the 18S small-subunit ribosomal DNA (rDNA) of this organism. This analysis placed *R. seeberi* among the Mesomycetozoa (formerly DRIP; *Dermocystidium,* rosette agent, *Ichthyophonus,* and *Psorospermium*), a clade of fish parasites that form a branch of the evolutionary tree near the animal-fungal divergence.

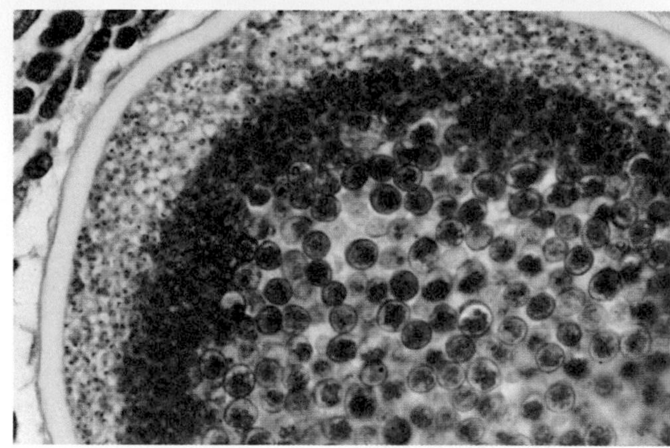

FIGURE 76–7. Mature sporangium of *Rhinosporidium seeberi* showing the zonal arrangement of immature, maturing, and fully mature sporangiospores (H&E, magnification 480×). (From Connor DH et al: *Pathology of infectious diseases,* vol II, Stamford, Conn, 1997, Appleton & Lange.)

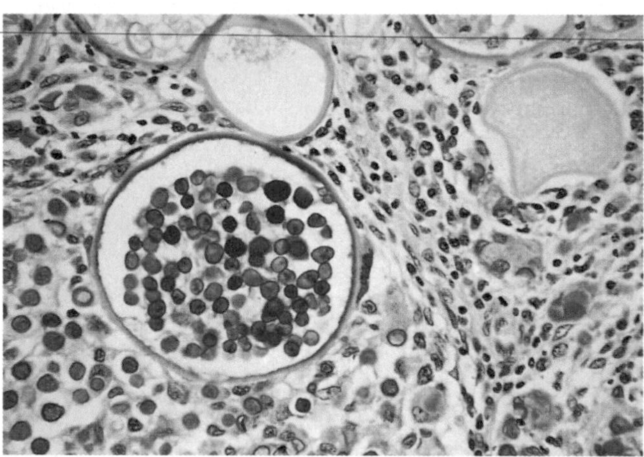

FIGURE 76–8. Mature sporangium of *R. seeberi.* The walls of the mature sporangiospores are carminophilic (Mayer's mucicarmine, magnification 100×). (From Connor DH et al: *Pathology of infectious diseases,* vol II, Stamford, Conn, 1997, Appleton & Lange.)

MORPHOLOGY

Given the fact that *R. seeberi* will not grow on artificial media, the morphologic descriptions are entirely based on the organism as it appears in infected tissue. Two developmental forms of *R. seeberi* are seen in tissue: the large spherical form, or sporangia, and the smaller trophocyte. The sporangium is considered the mature form of the organism and measures 100 to 350 μm in diameter. The sporangial wall is 3 to 5 μm thick and is composed of an inner hyaline layer and thin outer eosinophilic layer. The sporangium contains numerous sporangiospores (endospores) that are arranged in a characteristic zonal formation whereby the small, flattened, uninucleate immature sporangiospores (1 to 2 μm) form a crescentic mass at the periphery of one wall of the sporangiospore with the larger maturing and mature sporangiospores arranged sequentially toward the center (Figure 76–7). The mature sporangiospores range in size from 5 to 10 μm in diameter and contain multiple refractile cytoplasmic globules. This zonal arrangement of immature, maturing, and fully mature sporangiospores is diagnostic of this pathogen and distinguishes it from other spherical endosporulating organisms in the tissue (see Table 76–2).

The trophocytes are considered to develop directly from sporangiospores that have been released from the sporangium. The trophocytes range in size from 10 to 100 μm in diameter and have refractile eosinophilic walls (2 to 3 μm thick), granular cytoplasm, and a round pale nucleus with a prominent nucleolus. Ultimately, the trophocytes enlarge and transform into mature sporangia through a process of endosporulation.

The walls of both the sporangia and sporangiospores stain with both GMS and PAS fungal stains. In addition, the walls of the sporangiospores and the inner wall of the sporangium stain positively with the mucin stain, mucicarmine (Figure 76–8 and Table 76–2).

EPIDEMIOLOGY

Approximately 90% of all known cases of rhinosporidiosis occur in India and Sri Lanka. The disease also occurs in the Americas, Europe, and Africa. The natural habitat and the extent of distribution of *R. seeberi* in nature is unknown. The disease occurs primarily in young men (20 to 40 years old) and appears to be associated with both rural and aquatic environments. There is no evidence that rhinosporidiosis is contagious.

CLINICAL SYNDROME

Rhinosporidiosis manifests as slow-growing polypoid or tumorlike masses, usually of the nasal mucosa or conjunctiva. Lesions may also be seen in the paranasal sinuses, larynx, and external genitalia. Secondary spread to surrounding skin is thought to result from autoinoculation by scratching. In most patients, the disease remains localized and symptoms are primarily nasal obstruction and bleeding as a result of polyp formation. Limited systemic dissemination has been reported but is rare.

LABORATORY DIAGNOSIS

The diagnosis of rhinosporidiosis is made by histopathologic examination of the affected tissue. The distinctive appearance of the trophocytes and sporangia in routine H&E-stained sections is diagnostic (see Figure 76–7). Although other organisms that occur in tissue in the form of large spherules may be mistaken for *R. seeberi*, they are usually easily differentiated from this organism by consideration of the tissue involved and the morphologic and staining characteristics of the spherule and the endospores (see Table 76–2).

TREATMENT

The only effective form of treatment is surgical excision of the lesions. Recurrences are common, especially in mucosal sites such as the oropharynx and paranasal sinuses, where complete excision is often difficult to achieve.

CASE STUDY AND QUESTIONS

Jim is a 50-year-old ex-smoker who went to his family physician for an annual physical examination. In the process, a chest x-ray was performed, revealing a nodule in the left upper lobe of the lung. Because of his age and prior smoking history, Jim underwent a thoracotomy and the nodule was excised. Pathologic examination revealed fibrosis and several large spherical structures but no evidence of cancer.

1. What is the differential diagnosis of a solitary lung nodule?
2. Describe how one can differentiate the spherules of *Rhinosporidium seeberi* from those of *Coccidioides immitis* and *Emmonsia crescens*.
3. Describe the disease process of adiaspiromycosis.
4. Which of the following agents can be identified using commercially available yeast identification systems?
   a. *Lacazia loboi*
   b. *Pythium insidiosum*
   c. *Rhinosporidium seeberi*
   d. *Prototheca wickerhamii*
5. How are the agents of chlorellosis and protothecosis different from one another? How are they similar?

Bibliography

Burns RA et al: Report of the first human case of lobomycosis in the United States, *J Clin Microbiol* 38:1283-1285, 2000.

Chandler FW, Watts JC: *Pathologic diagnosis of fungal infections*, Chicago, 1987, ASCP Press.

Connor DH, et al: *Pathology of infectious diseases*, vol II, Stamford, Conn, 1997, Appleton & Lange.

Fredericks DN et al: *Rhinosporidium seeberi:* A human pathogen from a novel group of aquatic protistan parasites, *Emerg Infect Dis* 6:273-282, 2000.

Herr RA et al: Phylogenetic analysis of *Rhinosporidium seeberi's* 18S small-subunit ribosomal DNA groups this pathogen among members of the protoctistan Mesomycetozoa clade, *J Clin Microbiol* 37:2750-2754, 1999.

Taborda PR et al: *Lacazia loboi* gen. nov., comb. nov., the etiologic agent of lobomycosis, *J Clin Microbiol* 37:2031-2033, 1999.

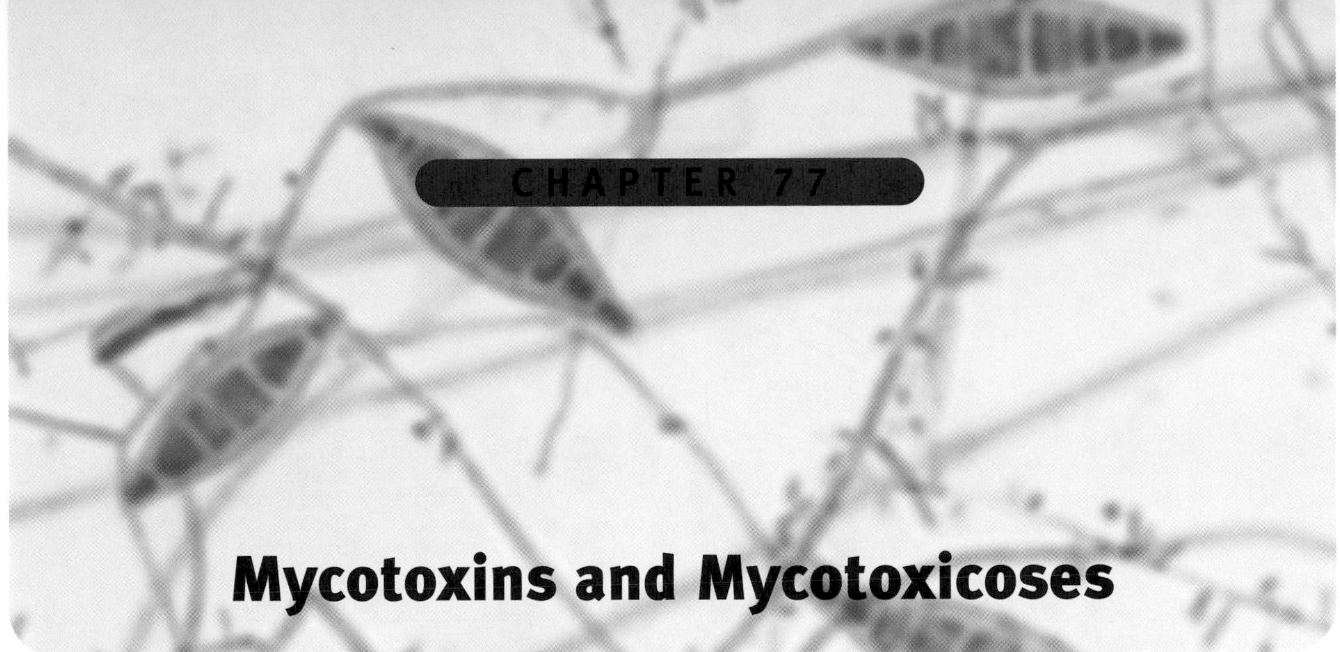

Mycotoxins and Mycotoxicoses

In addition to their role as opportunistic pathogens, filamentous fungi can produce toxins that have been implicated in a variety of illnesses and clinical syndromes in humans and in animals. These mycotoxins are secondary fungal metabolites that cause diseases, known collectively as mycotoxicoses, after ingestion, inhalation, or direct contact with the toxin (Figure 77–1). Mycotoxicoses may be manifest as acute or chronic disease ranging from rapid death to tumor formation. In this regard, mycotoxicoses are analogous to the pathologies caused by other "poisons" such as pesticides or heavy metal residues. The presenting symptoms and severity of a mycotoxicosis depend on the type of mycotoxin; the amount and duration of exposure; the route of exposure; and the age, sex, and health of the exposed person. In addition, a variety of other circumstances, such as malnutrition, alcohol abuse, infectious disease status, and other toxin exposures, may act synergistically to compound the effect and severity of mycotoxin poisoning.

There are more than 100 toxigenic fungi and more than 300 compounds now recognized as mycotoxins. The number of people affected by mycotoxicoses, however, is unknown. The majority of mycotoxicoses result from eating contaminated foods. The occurrence of mycotoxins in foods is most commonly caused by preharvest contamination of the material by toxigenic fungi that are plant pathogens. In addition, stored grains can be damaged by insects or moisture providing a portal of entry for toxigenic fungi present in the storage environment. Mycotoxicoses are more common in undeveloped countries where methods of food handling and storage are inadequate, malnutrition is prevalent, and there are few regulations designed to protect exposed populations.

Some mycotoxins are dermonecrotic, and cutaneous or mucosal contact with mould-infected substrates can result in disease. Likewise, inhalation of spore-borne toxins also constitutes an important form of exposure. Aside from supportive therapy, there are almost no treatments for mycotoxin exposure. Fortunately, mycotoxicoses are not communicable from person to person.

Among fungal plant pathogens, the elaboration of mycotoxins plays a role in causing or exacerbating the plant disease. Despite the fact that mycotoxins can be poisonous to humans and some may have potent immunosuppressive properties, there is very little evidence that mycotoxins enhance the ability of the fungus to grow and cause disease in vertebrate hosts. Those fungi, such as *Aspergillus fumigatus*, which are both important opportunistic pathogens and are capable of producing gliotoxins (inhibitors of T-cell activation and proliferation), generally do not produce the toxin in significant amounts during the course of human disease to have an effect on the disease process. Whereas an opportunistic fungus must be able to grow at human body temperature (37°C) to cause disease, the optimum temperature for biosynthesis of most mycotoxins is much lower (20° to 30°C). For these and other reasons, the importance of mycotoxin exposure during the course of a mycotic infection with a toxigenic fungus is largely unknown.

In the remainder of this chapter we will discuss those mycotoxins that have been implicated in human disease and metabolites that are produced by moulds that may be associated with human foods or living/working environments. Although mushroom poisoning is a form of mycotoxicosis, it will not be discussed herein. A listing of mycotoxicoses in which there is considerable evidence for the involvement of a specific mycotoxin is provided in Table 77–1.

Aflatoxins

The aflatoxins are produced primarily by *Aspergillus flavus* and *Aspergillus parasiticus*, but many other species of *Aspergillus* produce aflatoxins as well. *A. flavus* is the most

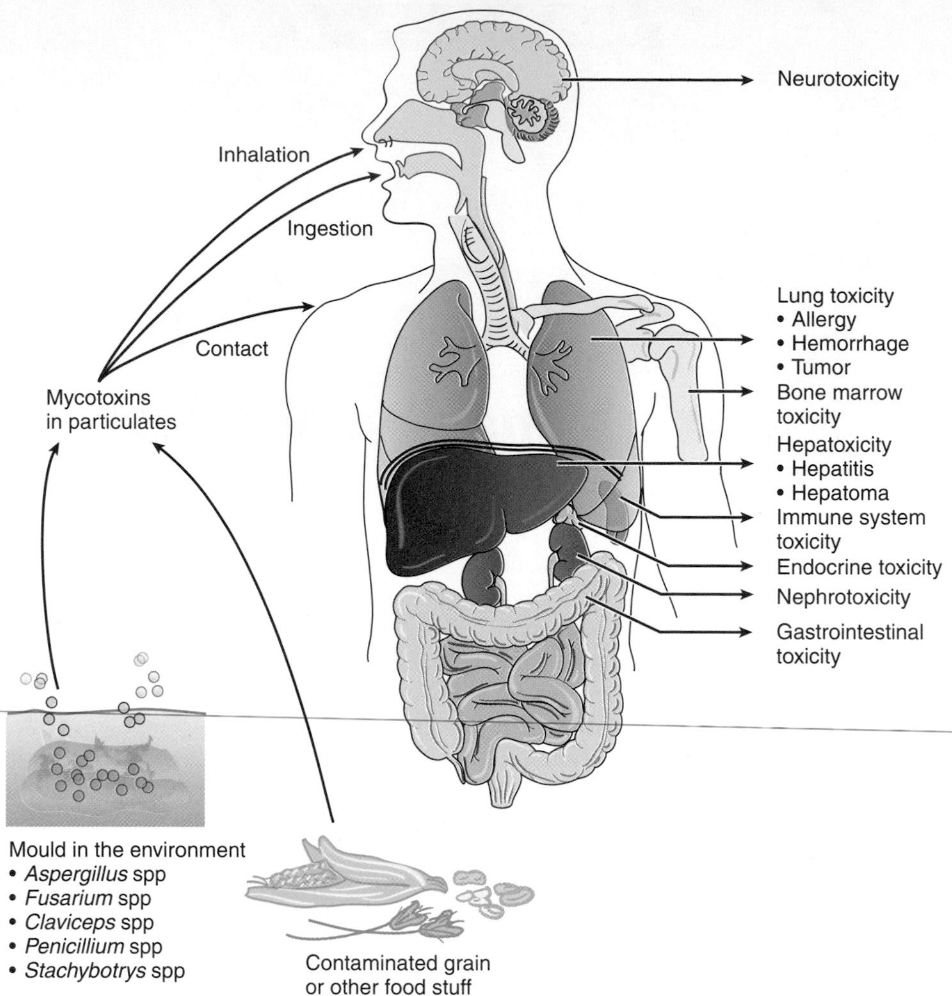

FIGURE 77–1. Various exposures and influences of mycotoxins. (Adapted from Richard JL: Mycotoxins and human disease. In Anaissie EJ, McGinnis MR, Pfaller MA, editors: *Clinical mycology*, New York, 2003, Churchill Livingstone.)

common aflatoxin-producing species found in agriculture and may produce as much as 10^6 mg/kg. The commodities most often affected in the United States are corn, cottonseed, peanuts, and certain tree nuts. Aflatoxin B_1 is the most potent natural carcinogen known and is the major aflatoxin produced by toxigenic strains; however, there are more than a dozen other aflatoxins that have been described.

Aflatoxin is associated with both toxicity and carcinogenicity in human and animal populations. Acute aflatoxicosis results in death, whereas chronic aflatoxicosis results in more prolonged pathologic changes including cancer and immunosuppression. The liver is the primary target organ, and liver damage has been documented in rodents, poultry, and nonhuman primates after ingestion of aflatoxin B_1. Acute aflatoxicosis has been manifested in humans as acute hepatitis. An outbreak of hepatitis occurred in India in 1974 in which 100 people died after consumption of maize that was heavily contaminated with aflatoxin. Aflatoxin B_1 was detected in high concentration in the livers of those persons who died.

It has been hypothesized that both kwashiorkor, a severe malnutrition disease, and Reye's syndrome, marked by encephalopathy and fatty degeneration of the viscera, represent forms of pediatric aflatoxicosis. Although aflatoxins have been found in the livers of children with kwashiorkor and in Reye's syndrome patients, a strong cause-and-effect relationship between aflatoxin exposure and these disease states has not been established.

Chronic low-level exposure to aflatoxins in the diet is considered a risk factor for the development of hepatocellular carcinoma. Such exposure has been shown experimentally to produce cancer in many animal species. Hepatocellular carcinoma is one of the leading causes of cancer mortality in Asia and Africa, and several epidemiologic investigations have shown that increased aflatoxin ingestion correlates with increased risk.

TABLE 77–1. Mycotoxin-Related Illnesses Postulated to Affect Humans Based on Analytic or Epidemiologic Data

Disease	Toxin	Substrate	Fungus	Clinical Presentation
Akakabi-byo (red mould disease)	*Fusarium* metabolites	Wheat, barley, oats, rice	*Fusarium* spp.	Headaches, vomiting, diarrhea
Alimentary toxic aleukia (ATA)	Trichothecenes (T-2 toxin, DAS)	Cereal grains (toxic bread)	*Fusarium* spp.	Vomiting, diarrhea, angina, skin inflammation
Balkan endemic nephropathy (BEN)	Ochratoxin	Cereal grains	*Aspergillus* spp. *Penicillium* spp.	Chronic nephritis
Cardiac beriberi	Citreoviridin	Rice	*Penicillium* spp.	Palpitations, vomiting, mania, respiratory failure
Ergotism (gangrenous and convulsive)	Ergot alkaloids	Rye, cereal grains	*Claviceps purpurea* *Claviceps fusiformis*	Gangrenous: vasoconstriction, edema, pruritus, and necrosis of extremities Convulsive: numbness, tingling, pruritus, cramps, seizures, hallucinations
Esophageal cancer	Fumonisins	Corn	*Fusarium moniliforme*	Dysphagia, pain, hemorrhage
Hepatitis and hepatic cancer	Aflatoxins	Cereal grains, peanuts	*Aspergillus flavus* *A. parasiticus*	Acute and chronic hepatitis, liver failure
Kodua poisoning	Cyclopiazonic acid	Millet	*Penicillium* spp. *Aspergillus* spp.	Somnolence, tremors, giddiness
Mouldy sugarcane poisoning	3-Nitropropionic acid	Sugarcane	*Arthrinium* spp.	Dystonia, seizures, carpopedal spasms, coma
Onyalai disease	*Fusarium* metabolites	Millet	*Fusarium* spp.	Thrombocytopenia, purpura
Stachybotryotoxicosis	Trichothecenes (T-2 toxin, DAS)	Hay, cereal grains, fodder (skin contact, inhaled hay dust)	*Stachybotrys, Fusarium, Myrothecium, Trichoderma, Cephalosporium* spp.	Tremors, loss of vision, dermonecrosis, gastrointestinal bleeding (horses and cattle), nasal inflammation, dermatitis, headache, fatigue, respiratory symptoms (humans), idiopathic pulmonary hemorrhage of infants (?)
Yellow rice disease	Citrinin	Wheat, oats, barley, rice	*Penicillium* spp. *Aspergillus* spp.	Nephropathy

Data from Kuhn DM, Ghannoum MA: Indoor mold, toxigenic fungi, and *Stachybotrys chartarum*: Infectious disease perspective, *Clin Microbiol Rev* 16:144-172, 2003; Richard JL: Mycotoxins and human disease. In Anaissie EJ, McGinnis MR, Pfaller MA, editors: *Clinical mycology,* New York, 2003, Churchill Livingstone; Bennett JW, Klich M: Mycotoxins, *Clin Microbial Rev* 16:497-516, 2003.

The primary mode of human exposure to aflatoxins is the consumption of contaminated foods such as peanuts and cereal grains. Aflatoxins can be aerosolized and have been detected in air near farm sources and in dust. Aflatoxin is a pulmonary carcinogen in experimental animals; however, the evidence that airborne aflatoxin exposure leads to cancer in humans is generally weak.

The mechanism of aflatoxin-induced carcinogenesis is thought to involve tumor promotion or progression. There is evidence that aflatoxin is involved in the activation of proto-oncogenes (C-*myc*, C-Ha-*ras*, Ki-*ras*, and N-*ras*) and also may cause mutations in the tumor suppressor gene p53. Aflatoxin exposure and p53 mutations have been tightly linked in epidemiologic studies in Africa and China. Specifically, aflatoxin has been linked to a p53 mutation whereby there occurs a G-to-T transversion at codon 249. This particular mutation has been called the first example of a "carcinogen-specific" biomarker that remains fixed in the human tissue. This biomarker has been used in epidemiologic studies to establish the link between aflatoxins and hepatic cancer and to show that cofactors such as infection with hepatitis B virus increase the risk of hepatocellular cancer substantially.

Significant aflatoxin exposure is uncommon among those living in developed countries where sufficient amounts of food are available and regulations exist to monitor the level of aflatoxin in those foods. Notably, liver cancer incidence rates are 2 to 10 times higher in developing countries than in developed countries. In those countries where food supplies are limited and people are facing starvation, or where regulations are nonexistent or not enforced, routine ingestion of aflatoxin can occur.

Citrinin

Citrinin is produced by several species of *Penicillum* and *Aspergillus*, including strains used to produce cheese *(Penicillum camemberti)* and sake *(Aspergillus oryzae)*. Citrinin acts as a potent nephrotoxin in all animal species tested and has been associated with yellow rice disease in Japan (see Table 77–1). Citrinin may act synergistically with another nephrotoxin, ochratoxin A. Citrinin is regularly associated with human foods including wheat, oats, rye, corn, barley, and rice; however, its significance as a cause of human disease is unknown.

Ergot Alkaloids

The ergot alkaloids constitute a family of compounds that are derived from a tetracyclic ergoline ring system. Lysergic acid is a structure common to all ergot alkaloids and the hallucinogen lysergic acid diethylamide (LSD) was discovered as a result of research with these compounds.

Mixtures of these alkaloids are produced within the sclerotia, or "ergots," of common grass pathogens of the genus *Claviceps*. The ergots are hardened masses of fungal tissue (sclerotia) that are formed when the fungus invades the floret and replaces the grain of wheat, barley, or rye. The ergots are ingested when the contaminated grain is used to make bread or cereals. The two forms of ergotism, convulsive and gangrenous (see Table 77–1), are thought to be caused by different modes of action of the various alkaloids produced by different species of *Claviceps*. The gangrenous form, marked by peripheral vasoconstriction and necrosis of the distal extremities, is associated primarily with the ingestion of wheat and rye contaminated with *Claviceps purpurea* and containing alkaloids of the ergotamine group. In addition to tissue infarction and necrosis, the gangrenous form of ergotism is associated with edema, pruritus, and sensations varying from pricking to severe muscle pain.

Convulsive ergotism has been associated with the ingestion of millet contaminated by *C. fusiformis*. Neurologic or convulsive ergotism is marked by muscle spasms, seizures, and hallucinations. The ergot of pearl millet implicated in an outbreak of convulsive ergotism in India in 1974 contained alkaloids of the clavine group.

Apparently, different species of *Claviceps* produce different alkaloids, although it is likely that the substrate also plays a role in the composition of the secondary metabolites. Although modern methods of grain cleaning have virtually eliminated ergotism as a human disease, it is still an important veterinary problem. Cattle, pigs, sheep, and poultry are the animals at highest risk. Clinical symptoms of ergotism among these animals include gangrene, abortion, seizures, and ataxia.

Fumonisins

Fumonisins are produced by a number of *Fusarium* species. The major species of economic importance is *F. moniliforme* (*F. verticilloides*), a corn pathogen. Fumonsins, especially fumonsin B1, interfere with sphingolipid metabolism and cause leukoencephalomalacia (severe necrotizing brain disease) in horses; pulmonary edema and hydrothorax in pigs; and hepatotoxic and carcinogenic effects in the liver of rats. Fumonisin B1 has been associated with a higher incidence of esophageal cancer in people living in South Africa, China, and Italy. It may be isolated in high concentrations in corn meal and corn grits. Although this evidence is intriguing, multiple factors, including other mycotoxins, have been implicated in the etiology of human esophageal cancer.

Acute intoxication with fumonisin B1 has been observed in India, where consumption of unleavened bread made from mouldy corn caused transient abdominal pain and diarrhea. Fumonisins have also been shown to cause neural tube defects in experimental animals and may have a role in human cases. Fumonisins have been classified as group 2B carcinogens (probably carcinogenic) by the International Agency for Research on Cancer.

Ochratoxin

Ochratoxin belongs to a group of secondary metabolites produced by *Aspergillus* and *Penicillium* spp., found on cereals, coffee, bread, and foods of animal origin (e.g., pork). Ochratoxin A (OA) is the most common and most toxic chemical in its class. OA is nephrotoxic, teratogenic, and carcinogenic in all animals tested. It has been implicated in porcine nephropathy and urinary tract tumors and may cause cholinergic responses such as bronchospasm, vasodilation, and smooth muscle contraction.

Ochratoxin has been linked to a disease known as Balkan endemic nephropathy (BEN), which is a chronic progressive nephritis seen in populations living in areas bordering the Danube River in parts of Romania, Bulgaria, and the former Yugoslavia. In addition, persons with BEN also suffer from a high frequency of renal tumors. Ochratoxin contamination of food and the presence of OA in human serum have been shown to be more common in families with BEN and those with urinary tract tumors than in unaffected families. Despite this evidence, a number of other factors such as genetics, heavy metals, and possible occult infectious agents may also contribute to this disease. Although much of the evidence for the cause of BEN leans toward ochratoxin, the evidence is not conclusive. Regardless, its acute nephrotoxicity, immunosuppressive action, and teratogenic effects in animals, together with its propensity to be carried through the food chain, merit concern and further investigation.

Trichothecenes

The trichothecenes are all tricyclic sesquiterpinoid metabolites that are produced by a number of fungi including *Fusarium, Myrothecium, Stachybotrys, Trichoderma,* and *Cephalosporium* spp. (see Table 77–1). There are more than 148 natural trichothecenes of which at least 40 are mycotoxins. Trichothecenes act by inhibiting various aspects of protein synthesis in eukaryotic cells. The most potent of these mycotoxins are T-2 toxin, diacetoxyscirpenol (DAS), deoxynivalenol (vomitoxin), and fusarenon-X. These mycotoxins are commonly found as food and feed contaminants, and consuming them can result in gastrointestinal hemorrhage and vomiting; direct contact causes dermatitis.

So-called mouldy grain intoxication of humans and animals is well documented in Japan. Such intoxications have been attributed to *Fusarium* mycotoxins. Akakabibyo toxicosis or red mould disease is believed to be caused by ingestion of grain contaminated with *Fusarium graminearum* (see Table 77–1).

T-2 toxin, DAS, and deoxynivalenol are the most widely studied of the fusarial trichothecenes. The symptoms produced by these agents include effects on almost every system of the vertebrate body. T-2 toxin and DAS appear to be the most potent and exhibit both cytotoxic and immunosuppressive activity. They cause a wide range of gastrointestinal, dermatologic, and neurologic symptoms and also decrease host resistance to infection with various microbes. Deoxynivalenol is a common contaminant of grains used in animal feed and, when ingested in high doses, causes vomiting and diarrhea; at lower doses farm animals exhibit weight loss and food refusal.

Both T-2 toxin and DAS have been implicated in a human disease known as alimentary toxic aleukia (ATA). The most important outbreak of ATA occurred in Russia during World War II. Thousands of people became sick after eating overwintered grain contaminated with *Fusarium sporotrichioides* and *Fusarium poae.* The disease was characterized by several stages with initial oral mucosal ulceration and gastroenteritis followed by pancytopenia; bleeding from the nose, mouth, and vagina; hypotension; and vertigo. The high acute mortality rate was augmented by opportunistic bacterial infections during the later neutropenic stages of the disease.

Despite the fact that the two species of *Fusarium* that were isolated from the mouldy grain were subsequently shown to be able to produce T-2 toxin and other trichothecenes, no attempt was made to document the presence of these mycotoxins in the grain or the affected people. Almost all signs of ATA have been documented in animals given T-2 toxin; however, the association between the toxin and human disease remains merely speculative.

Stachybotryotoxicosis is a well-described disease among horses and cattle consuming mouldy straw and hay contaminated with *Stachybotrys.* Equine stachybotryotoxicosis is characterized by acute neurologic signs, such as tremors, incoordination, and loss of vision, and more chronic manifestations such as dermonecrosis, leukopenia, and gastrointestinal bleeding. Humans handling mouldy hay have exhibited contact dermatitis, mucosal inflammation, fever, chest pain, and leukopenia resulting from inhalation of dust from the hay. Macrocyclic trichothecenes were isolated from the contaminated hay.

Given these findings, and because *Stachybotrys* grows well on wet building materials such as ceiling tiles, wood fiber boards, and dust-lined air conditioning ducts, toxins from this fungus have become suspect in illnesses of humans living or working in *Stachybotrys*-contaminated buildings. Complaints of pulmonary irritation, headaches, fatigue, malaise, and diarrhea have been registered by residents and workers in buildings contaminated with *Stachybotrys chartarum. Stachybotrys* has also been associated with idiopathic pulmonary hemorrhage of infants; however, a cause-and-effect relationship has not been proved. Critical evaluation of the available literature has failed to find supportive evidence for serious human illness caused by *Stachybotrys* exposure in the contemporary human environment.

Other Mycotoxins and Purported Mycotoxicoses

Given the wide variety of environmental moulds that have been shown to be capable of producing mycotoxins, it is not surprising that there is a vast amount of literature describing the potential role of these agents in human and animal disease states. Unfortunately, much of this literature is quite flawed, and critical review almost always finds it to be lacking in rigorous proof of a cause-and-effect relationship between mycotoxins and human disease.

Cyclopiazonic acid is an indole tetramic acid that is a specific inhibitor of calcium-dependent ATPase and induces alterations in ion transport across cell membranes. It is produced by many species of *Penicillium* and *Aspergillus*, including *A. flavus*. Consumption of millet that was heavily contaminated with moulds and contained high levels of cyclopiazonic acid produced a condition known as kodua poisoning, characterized by giddiness and nausea (see Table 77–1).

Cardiac beriberi, a condition seen in Japan and other Asian countries in the early 20th century, has been associated with the yellow rice toxins, citreoviridin, citrinin, and related compounds. This disease is characterized by palpitations, nausea, vomiting, respiratory distress, hypotension, and violent mania leading to respiratory failure and death. The neurologic symptoms and respiratory failure have been reproduced in animals given citreoviridin.

Several rare and obscure diseases have been purported to be mycotoxicosis, often with minimal objective evidence. These include Kashin-Beck disease in Russia, onyalai disease in Africa, and mouldy sugar cane disease in China (see Table 77–1).

It is difficult to prove that a disease is a mycotoxicosis. Even known toxigenic moulds can be present in foods or the environment and not produce toxin. The mere isolation of mould from cultures of a given substrate is not the same as detection of a specific mycotoxin. Likewise, even when mycotoxins are detected, it is difficult to prove conclusively that they are the cause of specific acute or chronic disease states. Regardless, valid concerns do exist with respect to the relationship between mycotoxins and human disease. Examples of certain fungus-disease associations are reasonably well documented in the literature including ATA from *Fusarium*, liver disease from *Aspergillus*, and ergotism from *Claviceps* spp. Beyond these examples, the evidence is tenuous. It is likely that mycotoxins do pose an important danger to the health of humans and animals, the extent of which can only be determined by rigorous well-designed clinical and laboratory studies.

CASE STUDY AND QUESTIONS

1. Which of the following mycotoxins is the most potent natural carcinogen?
   a. Ochratoxin A
   b. Fumonisin
   c. Cyclopiazonic acid
   d. Aflatoxin B1
2. Describe the different mycotoxicoses caused by aflatoxin.
3. Describe the different presentations of ergotism.
4. What is the relationship between *Stachybotrys chartarum* and idiopathic pulmonary hemorrhage of infancy?

Bibliography

Bennett JW, Klich M: Mycotoxins, *Clin Microbial Rev* 16:497-516, 2003.

Kuhn DM, Ghannoum MA: Indoor mold, toxigenic fungi, and *Stachybotrys chartarum:* Infectious disease perspective, *Clin Microbiol Rev* 16:144-172, 2003.

Richard JL: Mycotoxins and human disease. In Anaissie EJ, McGinnis MR, Pfaller MA, editors: *Clinical mycology*, New York, 2003, Churchill Livingstone.

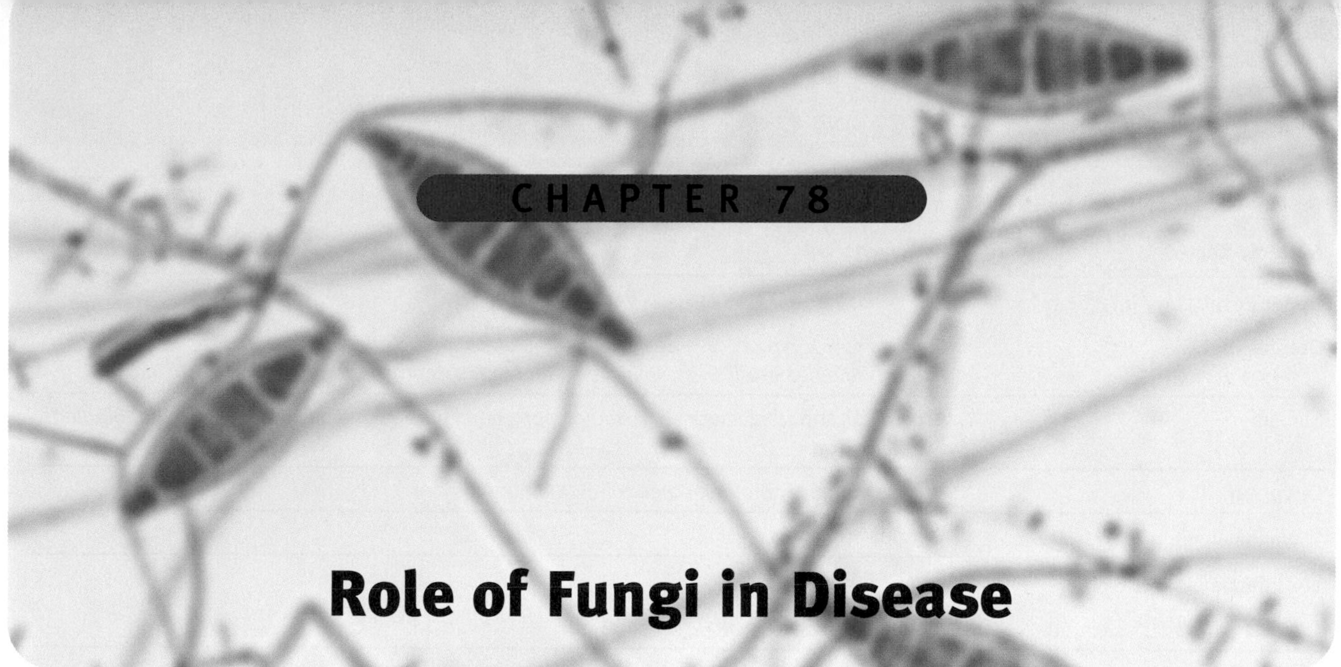

Role of Fungi in Disease

A summary of fungi (yeasts and moulds) most commonly associated with human disease is presented in this chapter. Mycotic diseases in humans develop as pathogenic processes in one or more organ systems. The affected systems may be as superficial as the outer layers of the skin or as deep as the heart, central nervous system, or abdominal viscera. Although a single fungus may be more commonly associated with infection involving a single organ system (e.g., *Cryptococcus neoformans* and the central nervous system), more often several different organisms can produce a similar disease syndrome. Because the management of a given infection can differ according to the etiologic agent, it is useful to establish a differential diagnosis that includes the most likely fungal pathogens to guide subsequent diagnostic and therapeutic efforts.

Because the development of a fungal infection depends on factors that often outweigh the virulence potential of the infecting organism, one must take into account numerous factors, such as the immune status of the host, the opportunity for interaction between host and fungus (e.g., is the fungus **endogenous** to the patient or **exogenous**), and the potential infectious dose (e.g., in the case of an endemic dimorphic fungus), in determining the possibility of a fungal infection, the significance of the microbiologic data (e.g., culture results), and the necessity to treat and with what agent. Fungal infections often occur in very sick patients and it is not possible to summarize here the incredibly complex interactions that ultimately lead to the establishment of infection and disease in each organ system. Instead, this chapter provides a very broad listing of the various fungi commonly associated with infections at specific body sites and/or specific clinical manifestations (Table 78–1). This information is meant to be used in conjunction with that in Table 71–1 as an aid in establishing a differential diagnosis and for the selection of the most likely clinical specimens that will help establish a specific etiologic diagnosis. Other factors that may be important in determining the relative frequency with which specific fungi cause disease (e.g., age, comorbidities, host immunity, epidemiologic exposures and risk factors) are covered in the individual chapters in this text or in the more comprehensive infectious disease texts cited in this and other chapters.

Bibliography

Anaisse EJ, McGinnis MR, Pfaller MA, editors: *Clinical mycology*, New York, 2003, Churchill Livingstone.

Chandler FW, Watts JC, editors: *Pathologic diagnosis of fungal infections*, Chicago, 1987, ASCP Press.

Cohen J, Powderly WG, editors: *Infectious diseases*, ed 2, Philadelphia, 2004, Elsevier.

Connor DH et al, editors: *Pathology of infectious diseases*, Stamford, Conn, 1997, Appleton & Lange.

Murray PR et al, editors: *Manual of clinical microbiology*, ed 8, Washington DC, 2003, American Society for Microbiology.

Mujeeb I et al: Fungi and fungal infections. In McClatchey KD, editor: *Clinical laboratory medicine*, ed 3, Philadelphia, 2002, Lippincott Williams & Wilkins.

TABLE 78–1. Summary of Fungi Associated with Human Disease

System Affected	Pathogens
Upper Respiratory Infections	
Oropharyngeal	*Candida* spp., *Cryptococcus neoformans, Histoplasma capsulatum, Blastomyces dermatitidis, Paracoccidioides brasiliensis, Penicillium marneffei, Geotrichum candidum*
Sinusitis	*Aspergillus* spp., Zygomycetes, *Fusarium* spp., dematiaceous moulds (e.g., *Alternaria, Bipolaris, Exophiala* spp.)
Laryngeal	*H. capsulatum, Sporothrix schenckii, B. dermatitidis*
Esophageal	*Candida* spp.
Ear Infections	
External otitis	*Aspergillus niger, Candida* spp.
Eye Infections	
Endophthalmitis	*Candida* spp., *Aspergillus* spp., *B. dermatitidis, Coccidioides immitis, Fusarium* spp., *H. capsulatum, C. neoformans*
Keratitis	*Candida* spp., *Fusarium* spp., dematiaceous moulds, *Scedosporium* spp., *Paecilomyces lilacinus*
Sino-orbital	Zygomycetes, *Aspergillus* spp.
Dacryocystitis and canaliculitis	*Candida albicans, A. niger*
Pleuropulmonary and Bronchial Infections	
Bronchitis	*Aspergillus* spp., *C. neoformans*
Pneumonia	*Aspergillus* spp., Zygomycetes, *Fusarium* spp., *Scedosporium apiospermum, Trichosporon* spp., dematiaceous moulds, *C. neoformans, H. capsulatum, B. dermatitidis, C. immitis, P. brasiliensis, P. marneffei, Pneumocystis jiroveci, Candida* spp. (rare)
Fungus ball	*Aspergillus* spp., Zygomycetes, *S. apiospermum, Fusarium* spp., *Candida* spp.
Empyema	*Aspergillus* spp., Zygomycetes, *S. apiospermum, Fusarium* spp., *Candida* spp., *C. immitis*
Genitourinary Tract Infections	
Vulvovaginal	*Candida* spp., *Saccharomyces cerevisiae*
Cystitis and pyelonephritis	*Candida* spp. (most common), *C. neoformans, Aspergillus* spp., *C. immitis, H. capsulatum, B. dermatitidis* (rare), *Trichosporon* spp. (rare), *Geotrichum capitatum* (rare), *Rhodotorula* spp. (rare)
Epididymitis and orchitis	*Candida* spp., *C. neoformans, Aspergillus* spp., *C. immitis, H. capsulatum, B. dermatitidis* (all rare)
Prostatitis	*Candida* spp. (common), *C, neoformans* (common), *B. dermatitidis* (common), *H. capsulatum, Aspergillus* spp. (rare), *C. immitis* (rare)
Intraabdominal Infections	
Peritonitis	*Candida* spp., *Rhodotorula* spp., *Trichosporon* spp., *Aspergillus* spp. (rare)
Visceral abscesses	*Candida* spp., *Trichosporon* spp., *G. capitatum*
Cardiovascular Infections	
Endocarditis	*Candida* spp., *Trichosporon* spp., *Rhodotorula* spp., *Aspergillus* spp., other hyaline hyphomycetes (e.g., *Fusarium, Acremonium*), demateacious moulds
Pericarditis	*Candida* spp., *Aspergillus* spp., *H. capsulatum, C. immitis*

TABLE 78–1. Summary of Fungi Associated with Human Disease—cont'd

System Affected	Pathogens
Central Nervous System	
Meningitis	*Candida* spp., *C, neoformans, Aspergillus* spp., Zygomycetes (rare), *C. immitis, H. capsulatum, B. dermatitidis* (rare), *Rhodotorula* spp., *G. capitatum, P. marneffei*
Brain abscess	*Candida* spp., *C. neoformans, Aspergillus* spp., Zygomycetes, *S. apiospermum, Trichosporon* spp., *Trichoderma* spp., dematiaceous moulds (especially *Cladophialophora bantiana* and *Bipolaris hawaiiensis*), endemic dimorphic fungi (rare)
Skin and Soft Tissue Infections	
Superficial and cutaneous	Dermatophytes, *Candida* spp., *Scytalidium* spp., *Scopulariopsis* spp., *Aspergillus* spp., *Malassezia* spp., *P. lilacinus*
Subcutaneous	Dematiaceous moulds, *Fusarium* spp., *Acremonium* spp., *S. apiospermum, S. schenckii, Basidiobolus* sp., *Conidiobolus* sp.
Wounds (surgical or traumatic)	*Candida* spp., Zygomycetes, *Aspergillus* spp., *Fusarium* spp., *Trichosporon* spp., *Rhodotorula* spp., *Scedosporium prolificans*
Cutaneous nodules (hematogenous)	*Candida* spp., *Aspergillus* spp., Zygomycetes, *C. neoformans, Trichosporon* spp., *B. dermatitidis, C. immitis, P. marneffei, Fusarium* spp., *Acremonium* spp., dematiaceous moulds (rare), *H. capsulatum* var *duboisii*
Bone and Joint Infections	
Osteomyelitis	*B. dermatitidis, C. immitis, Candida* spp., *C. neoformans, Aspergillus* spp., Zygomycetes, dematiaceous moulds (mycetoma), other hyaline hyphomycetes (e.g., *Scedosporium* spp., *Trichosporon*), *H. capsulatum* var *duboisii*
Arthritis	*C. immitis, B. dermatitidis, C. neoformans, Candida* spp., *Aspergillus* spp., dematiaceous moulds (mycetoma; rare), *H. capsulatum* (rare), *P. brasiliensis* (rare), *S. schenckii* (rare)
Prosthetic Joint	*Candida* spp., all others very rare
Hematogenous Dissemination	*Candida* spp., *H. capsulatum, B. dermatitidis, C. immitis, C. neoformans, P. brasiliensis, S. schenckii, Aspergillus* spp., *Fusarium* spp., *Trichosporon* spp., *Malassezia* spp., *G. capitatum, P. marneffei*, others (e.g., *Rhodotorula, Acremonium, Saccharomyces* spp. in neutropenic or transplant patients)

SECTION VII

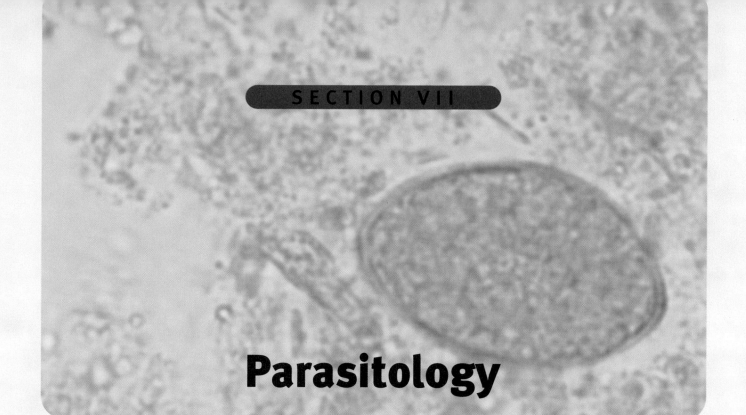

Parasitology

CHAPTER 79

Pathogenesis of Parasitic Disease

Given the wide diversity that exists among human parasites, it is not surprising that the pathogenesis of protozoan and helminthic disease is highly variable. Although the various human parasites exhibit a wide range of direct pathogenic mechanisms, in most instances the organisms themselves are not highly virulent, are unable to replicate within the host, or have both reactions. Thus the severity of illness caused by many parasites is related to the infecting dose and the number of organisms acquired over time. Unlike many bacterial and viral infections, parasitic infections are often chronic, lasting months to years. Repeated exposures result in an ever-increasing parasite burden. When infection with a particular organism is associated with a strong immune response, there is undoubtedly a considerable immunopathologic contribution to the disease manifestations attributed to the infection.

Important factors to consider when discussing parasite pathogenicity are listed in Box 79–1. Parasites are almost always exogenous to the human host and thus must enter the body through ingestion or direct penetration of anatomic barriers. Inoculum size and duration of exposure greatly influence the disease-causing potential of an organism. Likewise, the route of exposure is critical for most organisms. For example, pathogenic strains of *Entamoeba histolytica* are unlikely to cause disease on exposure to intact skin but may cause severe dysentery after oral ingestion. Many parasites have active, self-directed means of invading the human host. Once they have invaded, parasites attach to specific host cells or organs, avoid immune detection, replicate (most protozoa and some helminths), produce toxic substances that destroy tissue, and cause disease secondary to the host's own immunologic response (see Box 79–1). In addition, some parasites physically obstruct and damage organs and tissues because of their size alone. This chapter discusses factors that are important for parasite pathogenicity and provide examples of organisms and disease processes related to each factor.

Exposure and Entry

Although many infectious diseases are caused by **endogenous** organisms that are part of the normal flora of the human host, this is not the case with most diseases caused by protozoan and helminthic parasites. These organisms are virtually always acquired from an **exogenous** source and as such have evolved numerous ways to enter the body of the human host. The most common modes of entry are oral ingestion or direct penetration through the skin or other surfaces (Table 79–1). Transmission of parasitic diseases is frequently facilitated by environmental contamination with human and animal wastes. This is most applicable to diseases transmitted by the fecal-oral route but also applies to helminthic infections such as hookworm disease and strongyloidiasis, which rely on larval penetration of the skin.

Many parasitic diseases are acquired via the bites of **arthropod** vectors. Transmission of disease in this manner is extraordinarily effective, as evidenced by the widespread distribution of diseases such as malaria, trypanosomiasis, and filariasis. Examples of parasites and their ports of entry are listed in Table 79–1. This compilation should not be considered exhaustive; rather, the list provides examples of some of the more common parasites and the means by which they enter the human body.

Additional factors that determine the outcome of the interaction between parasite and host are route of **exposure** and **inoculum** size. Most human parasites have a limited range of organs or tissues in which they can replicate or survive. For example, simple skin contact with most intestinal protozoa does not result in disease; rather, the organisms must be ingested for the disease process to be initiated. Likewise, a minimum number of organisms is required to establish infection. Although some parasitic diseases may be acquired by the ingestion or inoculation of only a few organisms, a sizable inoculum is usually required. Whereas an individual may acquire malaria by a single bite of an infected female mosquito, large inocula are usually necessary to produce diseases such as amebiasis in humans.

Adherence and Replication

Most infections are initiated by the attachment of the organism to host tissues, followed by replication to establish colonization. The life cycle of a parasite is based on species and **tissue tropisms**, which determine the organs or tissues of the host in which a parasite can survive. The attachment of the parasite to host cells or tissue can be relatively nonspecific, can be mediated by mechanical or biting mouthparts, or can result from the interaction between structures on the parasite surface known as adhesins and specific glycoprotein or glycolipid receptors found on some cell types but not on others. Specific surface structures that facilitate parasite adhesion include surface **glycoproteins** such as glycophorin A and B, complement receptors, adsorbed components of the complement cascade, fibronectin, and N-acetylglucosamine conjugates. Examples of some of the adherence mechanisms identified in human parasites are listed in Table 79–2.

E. histolytica is a good model for the importance of **adhesins** in virulence. The pathogenesis of invasive amebiasis requires adherence of amoebae to the colonic mucous layer, parasite attachment to and lysis of colonic epithelium and acute inflammatory cells, and resistance of the amoebic trophozoites to host humoral and cell-mediated immune defense mechanisms. Amoebic adherence to colonic mucins, epithelial cells, and leukocytes is

BOX 79–1. Factors Associated with Parasite Pathogenicity

- Infective dose and exposure
- Penetration of anatomic barriers
- Attachment
- Replication
- Cell and tissue damage
- Disruption, evasion, and inactivation of host defenses

TABLE 79–1. Parasite Ports of Entry

Route	Examples
Ingestion	*Giardia* spp., *Entamoeba histolytica*, *Cryptosporidium* spp., cestodes, nematodes
Direct Penetration	
Arthropod bite	Malaria, *Babesia* spp., filaria, *Leishmania* spp., trypanosomes
Transplacental penetration	*Toxoplasma gondii*
Organism-directed penetration	Hookworm, *Strongyloides* spp., schistosomes

TABLE 79–2. Examples of Parasitic Adherence Mechanisms

Organism	Disease	Target	Mechanism of attachment and receptor
Plasmodium vivax	Malaria	Red blood cell	Merozoite (non–complement-mediated attachment), Duffy antigen
Plasmodium falciparum	Malaria	Red blood cell	Merozoite and glycophorin A and B
Babesia spp.	Babesiosis	Red blood cell	Complement-mediated C3b receptor
Giardia lamblia (duodenalis)	Diarrhea	Duodenal and jejunal epithelium	Trypsin-activated *G. lamblia* lectin and mannose 6-phosphate, *G. lamblia* adherence molecule–1 on disk
Entamoeba histolytica	Dysentery	Colonic epithelium	Lectin and N-acetylglucosamine conjugates
Trypanosoma cruzi	Chagas' disease	Fibroblast	Penetrin, fibronectin, and fibronectin receptor
Leishmania major	Leishmaniasis	Macrophage	Adsorbed C3bi and CR3
Leishmania mexicana	Leishmaniasis	Macrophage	Surface glycoprotein (gp63) and CR2
Necator americanus *Ancylostoma duodenale*	Hookworm	Intestinal epithelium	Mechanical and biting mouthparts

mediated by a surface lectin inhibitable by galactose (gal) or N-acetyl-D-galactosamine (GalNAc). Binding of the galactose-inhibitable adherence lectin to carbohydrates on the host cell surface is required for *E. histolytica* trophozoites to exert their cytolytic activity. The presence of the galactose-inhibitable adherence lectin is one feature that distinguishes pathogenic from nonpathogenic strains of *E. histolytica*.

Various attachment mechanisms have been associated with specific infections. For example, the **Duffy blood group antigen** acts as an attachment site for *Plasmodium vivax*. Red blood cells from most West Africans, in contrast to those from Europeans, lack the Duffy antigen. Accordingly, malaria resulting from *P. vivax* is almost unknown in West Africa. The physical structures of parasites may interact with adhesion molecules to promote attachment to host cells. *Giardia lamblia (duodenalis)* is a protozoan parasite that uses a ventral disk to attach to the intestinal epithelium by a clasping or suction-like mechanism. Two recently identified adhesins, trypsin-activated *G. lamblia* lectin (taglin) and *G. lamblia* adherence molecule–1 (GLAM-1), may also be important in attachment to enterocytes. It is believed that initial contact of the parasite with the intestinal surface is facilitated by taglin, which is distributed over the surface of the parasite, and that the disk-specific GLAM-1 is responsible for the avid attachment of the disk to the enterocyte surface.

After attachment to the specific cell or tissue type, the parasite may undergo replication as the next step in establishing infection. Most protozoan parasites replicate intracellularly or extracellularly in the human host, whereas replication is generally not observed with the helminths capable of establishing human infection.

Temperature may also play an important role in the ability of parasites to infect a host and cause disease. This is well illustrated by the *Leishmania* species. *Leishmania donovani* replicates well at 37°C and causes visceral leishmaniasis involving the bone marrow, liver, and spleen. In contrast, *L. tropica* grows well at 25° to 30°C but poorly at 37°C and causes an infection of the skin without involvement of deeper organs.

Cell and Tissue Damage

Although some microorganisms may cause disease by localized multiplication and elaboration of potent microbial **toxins**, most organisms initiate the disease process by invading normally sterile tissue with subsequent replication and destruction. Parasitic protozoa and helminths are generally not known to produce toxins with potencies comparable to those of classic bacterial toxins such as anthrax toxin and botulinum toxin; however, parasitic disease can be established by the elaboration of toxic products, mechanical tissue damage, and immunopathologic reactions (Table 79–3).

TABLE 79–3. Some Pathologic Mechanisms in Parasitic Diseases

Mechanism	Examples
Toxic Parasite Products	
Hydrolytic enzymes, proteinases, collagenase, elastase	Schistosomes (cercariae), *Strongyloides* spp., hookworm, *Entamoeba histolytica*, African trypanosomes, *Plasmodium falciparum*
Amoebic ionophore	*E. histolytica*
Endotoxins	African trypanosomes, *P. falciparum*
Indole catabolites	Trypanosomes
Mechanical Tissue Damage	
Blockage of internal organs	*Ascaris* spp., tapeworms, schistosomes, filaria
Pressure atrophy	*Echinococcus* spp., *Cysticercus* spp.
Migration through tissue	Helminthic larvae
Immunopathology	
Hypersensitivity	See Table 79–4
Autoimmunity	See Table 79–4
Protein-losing enteropathies	Hookworm, tapeworm, *Giardia* spp., *Strongyloides* spp.
Metaplastic changes	*Opisthorchis* spp. (liver flukes), schistosomes

Numerous authors have suggested that toxic products elaborated by parasitic protozoa are responsible for at least some aspects of pathology (see Table 79–3). **Proteases** and **phospholipases** may be secreted and are released on the destruction of the parasites. These enzymes can cause host cell destruction, inflammatory responses, and gross tissue pathology. For example, the intestinal parasite *E. histolytica* produces proteinases that can degrade epithelial basement membrane and cell-anchoring proteins, disrupting epithelial cell layers. Furthermore, the amoebae produce phospholipases and an ionophore-like protein that lyse the responding host neutrophils, resulting in the release of neutrophil constituents that are toxic to host tissues. The expression of certain proteinases increases relative to the virulence of the strain of *E. histolytica*. In contrast to the protozoan parasites, many of the pathogenic consequences of helminthic infections are related to the size, movement, and longevity of the parasites. The host is exposed to long-term damage and immune stimulation, as well as the sheer physical consequences of being inhabited by large foreign bodies. The most obvious forms of direct damage from helminthic parasites are those resulting from mechanical blockage of internal organs or from the effects of pressure exerted by growing parasites. Large adult *Ascaris* organisms can physically block the intestine and the bile ducts. Likewise, blockage of lymph flow, leading to elephantiasis, is associated with the presence of adult *Wuchereria* organisms in the lymphatic system. Some neurologic manifestations of cysticercosis are due to the pressure exerted by the slowly expanding larval cysts of *Taenia solium* on the central nervous system (CNS) and eyes. Migration of helminths (usually larval forms) through body tissues such as the skin, lungs, liver, intestines, eyes, and CNS can damage the tissues directly and initiate hypersensitivity reactions.

As with many infectious agents, the manifestations of parasitic disease are due not only to the mechanical or chemical tissue damage produced by the parasite, but also to the host responses to the presence of the parasite. Cellular hypersensitivity is observed in protozoan and helminthic disease (Table 79–4). During a parasitic infection, host cell products such as cytokines and lymphokines are released from activated cells. These mediators influence the action of other cells and may contribute directly to the pathogenesis of parasite infections. **Immunopathologic reactions** range from acute anaphylactic reactions to cell-mediated delayed hypersensitivity reactions (see Table 79–4). The fact that many parasites are long-lived means that many inflammatory changes become irreversible, producing functional changes in tissues. Examples include hyperplasia of the bile ducts resulting from the presence of liver flukes and extensive fibrosis leading to genitourinary and hepatic dysfunction in chronic schistosomiasis. Migration of larval helminths through tissues such as the skin, lungs, liver, intestine, CNS, and eyes produces immune-mediated inflammatory changes in these structures. Finally, chronic inflammatory changes around parasites such as *Opisthorchis sinensis* and *Schistosoma haematobium* have been linked to the induction of carcinomatous changes in the bile ducts and the bladder, respectively.

Disruption, Evasion, and Inactivation of Host Defenses

Although the processes of cell and tissue destruction are often sufficient to initiate clinical disease, the parasite must be able to evade the host's immune defense system

TABLE 79–4. Immunopathologic Reactions to Parasitic Disease

Reaction	Mechanism	Result	Example
Type 1: anaphylactic	Antigen + immunoglobulin E antibody attached to most cells: histamine release	Anaphylactic shock, bronchospasm, local inflammation	Helminth infection, African trypanosomiasis
Type 2: cytotoxic	Antibody + antigen on cell surface: complement activation or antibody-dependent cellular cytotoxicity	Lysis of cell-bearing microbial antigens	*Trypanosoma cruzi* infection
Type 3: immune complex	Antibody + extracellular antigen complex	Inflammation and tissue damage; complex deposition in glomeruli, joints, skin vessels, brain; glomerulonephritis, and vasculitis	Malaria, schistosomiasis, trypanosomiasis
Type 4: cell-mediated (delayed)	Sensitized T-cell reaction with antigen, liberation of lymphokines, triggered cytotoxicity	Inflammation, mononuclear accumulation, macrophage activation; tissue damage	Leishmaniasis, schistosomiasis, trypanosomiasis

(Modified from Mims C et al: *Mims' pathogenesis of infectious disease*, ed 4, London, 1995, Academic Press.)

TABLE 79–5. Microbial Interference with or Avoidance of Immune Defenses

Type of Interference or Avoidance	Mechanism	Examples
Antigenic variation	Variation of surface antigens within the host	African trypanosomes, *Plasmodium* spp., *Babesia* spp., *Giardia* spp.
Molecular mimicry	Microbial antigens mimicking host antigens, leading to poor antibody response	*Plasmodium* spp., trypanosomes, schistosomes
Concealment of antigenic site (masking)	Acquisition of coating of host molecules	Hydatid cyst, filaria, schistosomes, trypanosomes
Intracellular location	Failure to display microbial antigen on host cell surface	*Plasmodium* spp. (RBC), trypanosomes, *Leishmania* spp., *Toxoplasma* spp.
	Inhibition of phagolysosomal fusion	*Toxoplasma* spp.
	Escape from phagosome into cytoplasm with subsequent replication	*Leishmania* spp., *Trypanosoma cruzi*
Immunosuppression	Suppression of parasite-specific B- and T-cell responses; degradation of immunoglobulins	Trypanosomes, *Plasmodium* spp.; schistosomes

for the disease process to be maintained. Like other organisms, parasites elicit humoral and cell-mediated immune responses; however, parasites are particularly adept at interfering with or avoiding these defense mechanisms (Table 79–5).

Organisms can shift antigenic expression, such as that observed with the African trypanosomes. Rapid variation of expression of antigens in the glycocalyces of these organisms occurs each time the host exhibits a new humoral response. Similar changes have been observed with *Plasmodium*, *Babesia*, and *Giardia* spp. Some organisms may produce antigens that mimic host antigens **(mimicry)** or acquire host molecules that conceal the antigenic site **(masking)**, thus preventing immune recognition by the host.

Many protozoan parasites evade the immune response by assuming an intracellular location in the host. The organisms that reside in macrophages have developed a variety of mechanisms to avoid intracellular killing. These include prevention of phagolysosome fusion, resistance to killing after exposure to lysosomal enzymes, and escape of phagocytosed cells from the phagosome into the cytoplasm with subsequent replication of the organism (see Table 79–5).

Immunosuppression of the host is often observed during the course of parasitic infections. The immunosuppression may be parasite specific or generalized, involving a response to various nonparasite and parasite antigens. Proposed mechanisms include antigen overload, antigenic competition, induction of suppressor cells, and production of lymphocyte-specific suppressor factors. Certain helminths such as *Schistosoma mansoni* may also produce proteinases that can degrade immunoglobulins.

QUESTIONS

1. What are the most common modes of entry of parasites into the human host?
2. Name two factors that determine the outcome of the interaction between parasite and host.
3. Give an example of an adhesin that is directly related to the virulence of a parasite.
4. Name three pathologic mechanisms thought to be important in parasitic diseases.
5. How can parasites resist immunologic clearance? Give at least one example of each mechanism.
6. Name the four types of immunopathologic reactions that occur in parasitic diseases and provide examples of each.

Bibliography

Chen Q, Schlichtherle M, Wahlgren M: Molecular aspects of severe malaria, *Clin Microbiol Rev* 13:439-450, 2000.

Choi BI et al: Clonorchiasis and cholangiocarcinoma: Etiologic relationship and imaging diagnosis, *Clin Microbiol Rev* 17:540-552, 2004.

Clark IA et al: Pathogenesis of malaria and clinically similar conditions, *Clin Microbiol Rev* 17:509-539, 2004.

Cunningham MW, Fujinami RS, editors: *Molecular mimicry, microbes, and autoimmunity*, Washington, DC, 2000, ASM Press.

Espinosa-Cantellano M, Martinez-Palomo A: Pathogenesis of intestinal amebiasis: From molecules to disease, *Clin Microbiol Rev* 13:318-331, 2000.

Hall LR, Pearlman E: Pathogenesis of onchocercal keratitis (River Blindness), *Clin Microbiol Rev* 12:445-453, 1999.

Van Velthuysen M-LF, Florquin S: Glomerulopathy associated with parasitic infections, *Clin Microbiol Rev* 13:55-66, 2000.

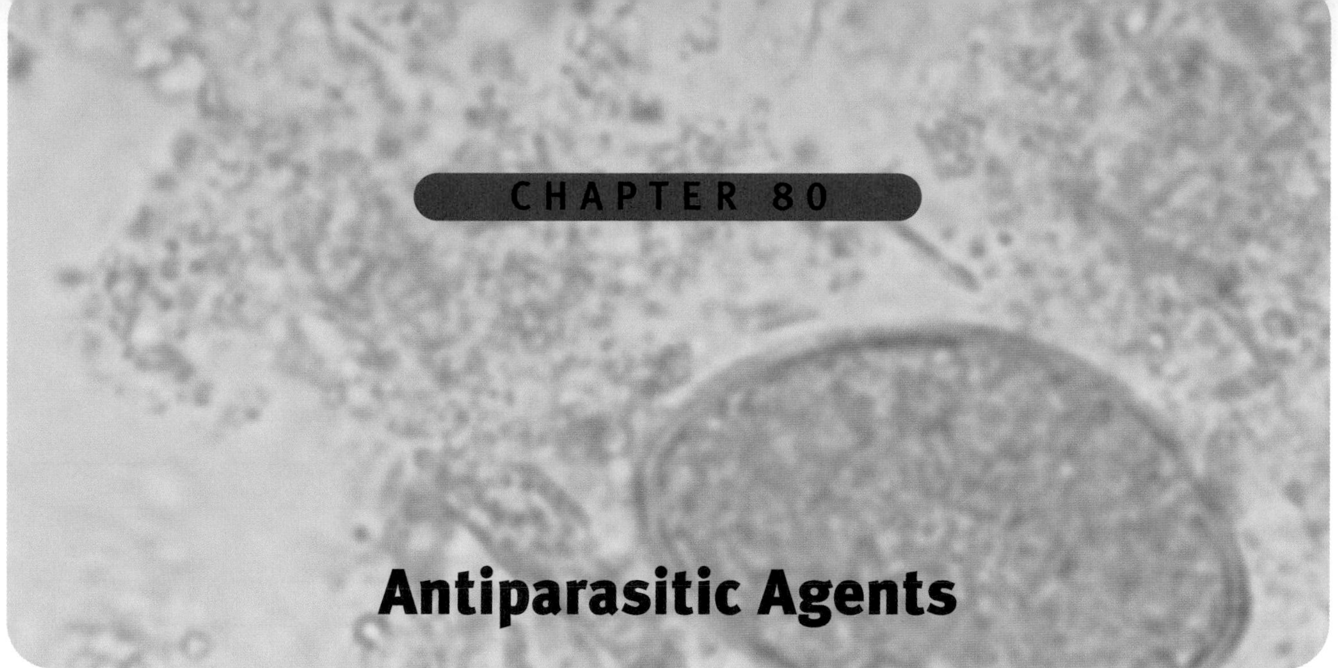

Antiparasitic Agents

The chemotherapeutic approach to the management of infectious diseases has clearly changed the face of medicine. Unfortunately, few of the antiinfective agents that have proved so successful against bacterial pathogens have been effective against parasites. In many instances, clinicians continue to rely on antiparasitic agents from the preantibiotic era. These and some newer agents remain limited in effectiveness and are relatively toxic. Many antiparasitic agents require prolonged or parenteral administration and may be effective only in certain disease states. Fortunately, in the last 5 to 10 years, several new agents have appeared that constitute significant advances in the treatment of parasitic diseases. In each case, the previously available drugs were toxic and often ineffective.

In large part, the difficulties in the treatment of parasitic diseases stem from the fact that parasites are **eukaryotic** organisms and thus are more similar to the human host than the more successfully treated prokaryotic bacterial pathogens. Furthermore, the chronic and prolonged course of infection and the complex life cycles and multiple developmental stages of many parasites add to the difficulties of effective chemotherapeutic intervention. Additional complicating factors in developing countries, where the majority of parasitic diseases occurs, include (1) the presence of multiple infections and the high probability of reinfection, (2) the large number of persons immunocompromised by malnutrition and human immunodeficiency virus infection, and (3) the overwhelming influence of poverty and poor sanitation, which facilitate the transmission of many parasitic infections. Although chemotherapeutic approaches can be used effectively to treat and prevent many parasitic infections, some agents have adverse effects or eventually meet with resistance (microbial and social). Most antiparasitic agents are too expensive for widespread use in developing countries. Thus the global approach to the prevention and treatment of parasitic diseases must involve several strategies, including improved hygiene and sanitation, control of the disease vector, use of **vaccinations** if available (largely unavailable for parasitic diseases), and prophylactic and therapeutic administration of safe and effective chemotherapy. These strategies now must also include efforts to decrease the transmission of infection by the human immunodeficiency virus.

Targets for Antiparasite Drug Action

As mentioned previously, parasites are eukaryotic organisms and thus have more similarities than differences with the human host. Consequently, many antiparasitic agents act on pathways (nucleic acid synthesis, carbohydrate metabolism) or targets (neuromuscular function) shared by both the parasite and the host. For this reason, developing safe and effective antiparasitic drugs based on biochemical differences between the parasite and host has been difficult. **Differential toxicity** is commonly achieved by preferential uptake, metabolic alteration of the drug by the parasite, or differences in the susceptibility of functionally equivalent sites in the parasite and host. Fortunately, as our understanding of the basic biology and biochemistry of parasites and the mechanism of action of antimicrobial agents has improved, so has our recognition of potential parasite-specific targets for chemotherapeutic attack. Examples of the chemotherapeutic strategies that exploit the differences between parasite and host are provided in Table 80–1. These are discussed in greater detail as we deal with the specific agents.

TABLE 80–1. Chemotherapeutic Strategies that Exploit Differences Between Parasite and Host

Unique Site of Attack	Drug	Organism
Drug-concentrating mechanism unique to parasite	Chloroquine	*Plasmodium* spp.
Folic acid pathway (parasite unable to use exogenous folate)	Pyrimethamine or trimethoprim-sulfamethoxazole	*Plasmodium* or *Toxoplasma* spp.
Inhibitor of trypanothione-dependent mechanisms for reducing oxidized thiol groups	Arsenicals, difluoromethylornithine	Trypanosomes
Interference with neuromediators unique to parasites	Pyrantel pamoate, piperazine	*Ascaris* spp.
Inhibitors of GABA-mediated conduction in peripheral nervous system of parasites	Ivermectin	Filaria
Interaction with tubulin unique to parasites	Benzimidazoles	Many helminths
Inhibition of topoisomerase II	Pentamidine	Trypanosomes

Drug Resistance

Resistance to antimicrobial agents is an important consideration in the treatment of infections resulting from bacteria and fungal pathogens and certainly plays a role in the chemotherapy of parasitic diseases. Unfortunately, our understanding of the molecular and genetic basis for resistance to most antiparasitic agents is quite limited. Most of the information regarding the molecular mechanisms of drug resistance in parasites has come from studies in plasmodia. Resistance to chloroquine, a major antimalarial agent, is most likely caused by the presence of an active chloroquine efflux mechanism similar to that producing the rapid efflux of anticancer drugs observed in multidrug-resistant mammalian cancer cells. In addition, the development of plasmodial resistance to antifolate compounds such as pyrimethamine is due to a series of mutations in the parasite's combined dihydrofolate reductase–thymidylate synthetase enzyme. Further insights into the mechanisms of action and resistance to antiparasitic agents are necessary to optimize the effectiveness of antiparasite chemotherapy.

Antiparasitic Agents

Although the number of effective antiparasitic agents is small relative to the vast array of antibacterial agents, the list is expanding (Table 80–2). Certainly in many cases the goal of antiparasitic therapy is similar to that of antibacterial therapy: to eradicate the organism rapidly and completely. In many cases, however, the agents and treatment regimens used for parasitic diseases are designed simply to decrease the parasite burden, to prevent the systemic complications of chronic infection, or both. Thus the goals of antiparasitic therapy, particularly as applied in endemic areas, may be quite different from those usually considered for therapy of microbial infection in the United States or other developed countries. Given the significant toxicity of many of these agents, in every case the need for treatment must be weighed against the toxicity of the drug. A decision to withhold therapy may often be correct, particularly when the drug can cause severe adverse effects.

Immunocompromised persons pose a particular problem with respect to antiparasitic chemotherapy. On the one hand, **prophylaxis,** such as that administered for toxoplasmosis, may be effective in preventing infection. However, once infection is established, radical cure may not be possible, and long-term **suppressive** therapy may be indicated. In some diseases, such as cryptosporidiosis and microsporidiosis, effective (curative) therapy is not available, and care must be taken to avoid unnecessary toxicity while providing supportive care for the patient.

The remainder of this chapter provides an overview of the major classes of antiprotozoal and antihelminthic agents. These and additional antiparasitic agents, their mechanisms of action, and their clinical indications are listed in Table 80–2. Treatment of specific infections is discussed in the chapters that deal with the parasites. This chapter's bibliography lists several excellent reviews for more complete information and for discussions of the antiparasitic agents that are available.

ANTIPROTOZOAL AGENTS

Similar to antibacterial and antifungal agents, the antiprotozoal agents are generally targeted at relatively rapidly proliferating, young, growing cells. Most commonly, these agents target nucleic acid synthesis, protein synthesis, or specific metabolic pathways (e.g., folate metabolism) unique to the protozoan parasites.

TABLE 80–2. Mechanisms of Action and Clinical Indications for the Major Antiparasitic Agents

Drug Class	Mechanism of Action	Examples	Clinical Indications
Antiprotozoal Agents			
Heavy metals: arsenicals and antimonials	Inactivate sulfhydryl groups	Melarsoprol, sodium stibogluconate, meglumine antimonite	Trypanosomiasis, leishmaniasis
Aminoquinoline analogues	Accumulate in parasitized cells, interfere with DNA replication, bind to ferriprotoporphyrin IX, raise intravesicular pH, interfere with hemoglobin digestion	Chloroquine, mefloquine, quinine, primaquine	Malaria prophylaxis and therapy, radical cure (exoerythrocytic-primaquine only)
Folic acid antagonists	Inhibit dihydropteroate synthetase and dihydrofolate reductase	Sulfonamides, pyrimethamine, trimethoprim	Toxoplasmosis, malaria, cyclosporiasis
Inhibitors of protein synthesis	Block peptide synthesis at level of ribosome	Clindamycin, spiramycin, paromomycin, tetracycline, doxycycline	Malaria, babesiosis, amebiasis, cryptosporidiosis
Diamidines	Bind DNA, interfere with uptake and function of polyamines	Pentamidine	Leishmaniasis, trypanosomiasis
Nitroimidazoles	Unclear; interact with DNA, inhibit metabolism of glucose and interfere with mitochondrial function	Metronidazole, benzimidazole, tinidazole	Amebiasis, giardiasis, trichomoniasis
Quinolones	Inhibit DNA gyrase	Ciprofloxacin	Malaria
Sesquiterpenes	React with heme, causing free-radical damage to parasite membranes	Artemisinin	Malaria
Ornithine analogue	Inhibits ornithine decarboxylase, interferes with polyamine metabolism	Difluoromethylornithine	African trypanosomiasis
Inhibitors of nucleic acid synthesis	Inhibit enzymes in purine salvage pathway	Allopurinol	Leishmaniasis
Acetanilide	Unknown	Diloxanide furoate	Intestinal amebiasis
Sulfated naphthylamine	Inhibits *sn*-glycerol phosphate oxidase and glycerol 3-phosphate dehydrogenase, causing decreased ATP synthesis	Suramin	African trypanosomiasis
Phenanthrenemethanols	Bind to ferriprotoporphyrin IX, affect mitochondria	Halofantrine	Malaria
Antihelminthic agents			
Benzimidazoles	Inhibit fumarate reductase, inhibit glucose transport, disrupt microtubular function	Mebendazole, thiabendazole, albendazole	Broad-spectrum antihelminthics: nematodes, cestodes
Tetrahydropyrimidine	Blocks neuromuscular action, inhibits fumarate reductase	Pyrantel pamoate	Ascariasis, pinworm, hookworm

ATP, Adenosine triphosphate.

TABLE 80–2. Mechanisms of Action and Clinical Indications for the Major Antiparasitic Agents—cont'd

Drug Class	Mechanism of Action	Examples	Clinical Indications
Piperazines	Serve as GABA agonists, cause neuromuscular paralysis, stimulate phagocytic cells	Piperazine, diethylcarbamazine	Ascaris and pinworm infections
Avermectins	Block neuromuscular action, serve as GABA antagonists, inhibit filarial reproduction	Ivermectin	Filarial infections
Pyrazinoisoquinoline	Serves as a calcium agonist, causes tetanic muscular contractions, causes tegumental disruption provides synergy with host defenses	Praziquantel	Broad-spectrum antihelminthics: cestodes, trematodes
Phenol	Uncouples oxidative phosphorylation	Niclosamide	Intestinal tapeworm
Quinolone	Alkylates DNA, inhibits DNA, RNA, and protein synthesis	Bithionol, oxamniquine	Paragonimiasis, schistosomiasis
Organophosphate	Is anticholinesterase; blocks neuromuscular action	Metrifonate	Schistosomiasis
Sulfated naphthylamidine	Inhibits glycerophosphate oxidase and dehydrogenase	Suramin	Onchocerciasis

GABA, γ-aminobutyric acid.

Heavy Metals

The heavy metals used for the treatment of parasitic infections include arsenical (melarsoprol) and antimonial compounds (sodium stibogluconate, meglumine antimonate). These agents are thought to oxidize sulfhydryl groups of enzymes, which are essential catalysts in carbohydrate metabolism. Melarsoprol inhibits parasite pyruvate kinase, causing decreased concentrations of adenosine triphosphate (ATP), pyruvate, and phosphoenolpyruvate. Arsenicals also inhibit sn-glycerol 3-phosphate oxidase, which is needed for the regeneration of nicotinamide adenine dinucleotide in trypanosomes but is not found in mammalian cells. The antimonials, sodium stibogluconate and meglumine antimonate, inhibit the glycolytic enzyme phosphofructokinase and certain Krebs cycle enzymes in *Leishmania* organisms. In each instance, the inhibition of parasite metabolism is **parasiticidal**. Unfortunately, the heavy metal compounds are toxic to the host, as well as the parasite. The toxicity is greatest on cells that are most metabolically active, such as neuronal, renal tubular, intestinal, and bone marrow stem cells. Their differential toxicity and therapeutic value are largely related to enhanced uptake by the parasite and its intense metabolic activity.

Melarsoprol is the drug of choice for trypanosomiasis involving the central nervous system. It can penetrate the blood-brain barrier and is effective in all stages of trypanosomiasis. The antimonial compounds are restricted to the management of leishmaniasis. Meglumine antimonate and sodium stibogluconate are important agents for the treatment of leishmaniasis and are active against all forms of the disease. Prolonged therapy is usually required for disseminated leishmaniasis, and relapses are common.

Aminoquinoline Analogues

The aminoquinoline analogues include the 4-aminoquinolines (chloroquine), the 8-aminoquinolines (primaquine), and the 4-quinolinemethanols (mefloquine). Additional quinoline analogues include quinine, quinidine, quinacrine, and amodiaquine. These compounds all have antimalarial activity and accumulate preferentially in parasitized red blood cells. Several potential mechanisms of action have been proposed, including (1) binding to DNA and interfering with DNA replication; (2) binding to ferriprotoporphyrin IX released from hemoglobin in infected erythrocytes, producing a toxic complex; and (3) raising the pH of the parasite's intracellular acid vesicles, thus interfering with its ability to degrade hemoglobin. Quinine, the 4-aminoquinolines, and 4-quinolinemethanols rapidly destroy the erythrocytic stage of malaria and thus may be used **prophylactically** to suppress clinical illness or **therapeutically** to terminate an acute attack. The 8-aminoquinolines (e.g., primaquine) accumulate in tissue cells and destroy the extraerythrocytic (hepatic) stages of malaria, resulting in a radical cure of the infection.

Chloroquine remains the drug of choice for the prophylaxis and treatment of susceptible malaria strains. Chloroquine is active against all four *Plasmodium* species (i.e., *P. falciparum, P. vivax, P. ovale, P. malariae*) and is well tolerated, inexpensive, and effective orally. Unfortunately, resistance of *P. falciparum* to chloroquine is widespread in Asia, Africa, and South America, greatly limiting the use of this agent. Resistance of *P. vivax* to chloroquine has also been reported from Papua New Guinea, the Solomon Islands, Indonesia, and Brazil.

Quinine is used primarily to treat chloroquine-resistant *P. falciparum* infection. Presumably, it is active against the rare chloroquine-resistant strains of *P. vivax* as well. Quinine is used orally only to treat mild attacks and by the intravenous route to treat acute attacks of multidrug-resistant *P. falciparum*. Quinine is quite toxic and not rapidly parasiticidal; thus it is never used alone but is often used with a sulfonamide or tetracycline antibiotic with antimalarial activity.

Mefloquine is a 4-quinolinemethanol antimalarial agent used for the prophylaxis and treatment of falciparum malaria. It displays a high level of activity against most chloroquine-resistant parasites. Unfortunately, mefloquine-resistant strains of falciparum malaria have been reported from Southeast Asia and Africa.

Folic Acid Antagonists

Similar to other organisms, protozoan parasites require folic acid for the synthesis of nucleic acids and ultimately DNA. Protozoa are unable to absorb exogenous folate and thus are susceptible to drugs that inhibit folate synthesis. The folic acid **antagonists** that are useful in treating protozoan infections include the diaminopyrimidines (pyrimethamine and trimethoprim) and the sulfonamides. These compounds block separate steps in the folic acid pathway. The sulfonamides inhibit the conversion of aminobenzoic acid to dihydropteroic acid. The diaminopyrimidines inhibit dihydrofolate reductase, which effectively blocks the synthesis of tetrahydrofolate, a precursor necessary for the formation of purines, pyrimidines, and certain amino acids. These agents are effective at concentrations far below those needed to inhibit the mammalian enzyme, so selectivity can be attained. When a diaminopyrimidine is used with a sulfonamide, a **synergistic** effect is achieved via the blockade of two steps in the same metabolic pathway, resulting in very effective inhibition of protozoan growth.

The diaminopyrimidine trimethoprim is used with sulfamethoxazole to treat toxoplasmosis. Another diaminopyrimidine, pyrimethamine, has a high affinity for sporozoan dihydrofolate reductase and has been very effective when combined with a sulfonamide in the treatment of malaria and toxoplasmosis. Resistance to antifolates is due to specific point mutations at the active site of the parasite's dihydrofolate reductase and has been largely confined to species of *Plasmodia.*

Inhibitors of Protein Synthesis

Several antibiotics that inhibit protein synthesis in bacteria also exhibit antiparasitic activity in vitro and in vivo. These agents include clindamycin, spiramycin, tetracycline, and doxycycline.

Clindamycin and the tetracyclines are active against *Plasmodium* spp., *Babesia* spp., and amoebae. Doxycycline is used for the chemoprophylaxis of chloroquine-resistant *P. falciparum* malaria, and tetracycline can be used with quinine for the treatment of chloroquine-resistant *P. falciparum* infection. Clindamycin may be useful in the treatment of central nervous system toxoplasmosis. Spiramycin is recommended as an alternative to the antifolates in the treatment of toxoplasmosis. Although spiramycin appears active against *Cryptosporidium* spp. in vitro, it has not been shown to be effective clinically for human cryptosporidiosis. Recent studies suggest that paromomycin, an older aminoglycoside, may be at least partially effective in treating cryptosporidiosis. Paromomycin, which is not systemically absorbed, is also used as a secondary drug in amebiasis and in giardiasis.

Diamidines

Pentamidine, a diamidine, is a relatively toxic agent. Pentamidine is a polycation and may interact with DNA, or it may interfere with the uptake and function of polyamines.

Pentamidine is effective in treating the tissue forms of leishmania and the early (pre–central nervous system) forms of African trypanosomiasis. Pentamidine does not penetrate the central nervous system and therefore is not useful in the late stages of infection with *Trypanosoma brucei gambiense*. Recent information suggests that pentamidine may inhibit kinetoplast topoisomerase II activity and may act against trypanosomes in part by this mechanism.

Nitroimidazoles

The nitroimidazoles include the well-known antibacterial agent metronidazole as well as benzimidazole and tinidazole. The mechanism of action of these compounds is unclear. It has been suggested that they inhibit DNA and

RNA synthesis and also inhibit the metabolism of glucose and interfere with mitochondrial function. Metronidazole binds to parasite guanine and cytosine residues, causing the loss of helical structure and breakage of DNA strands.

The nitroimidazoles have excellent penetration into body tissues and therefore are particularly effective for the treatment of disseminated amebiasis. Metronidazole is the drug of choice for trichomoniasis and is effective in the treatment of giardiasis. Tinidazole appears to be more effective and less mutagenic than metronidazole; however, it is not yet available for use in the United States.

Sesquiterpenes

The sesquiterpenes are antimicrobial agents that are represented by the artemisinins, artemether and artesunate. These agents react with the heme moiety, causing **free-radical** damage to parasite membranes. The artemisinins are the most active of the available antimalarial compounds and produce a fractional reduction in parasite biomass of approximately 10^4 per asexual cycle. Artemisinins have efficacy against small ring forms and maturing schizonts of both *P. vivax* and *P. falciparum*, stages that are less susceptible to quinolines or quinine. The earlier stage ring forms are immediately cleared (within 6 to 12 hours) after exposure to artemisinins. The artemisinin derivatives also have the advantage of reducing gametocyte carriage and thus transmission. These agents are highly effective when used in combination with mefloquine, halofantrine, and lumefantrine in the treatment of severe malaria, including that due to multidrug-resistant *P. falciparum*.

Other Antiprotozoal Agents

A number of additional agents used in therapy, their mechanism of action (if known), and clinical use are listed in Table 80–2.

ANTIHELMINTHIC AGENTS

The strategy for the use of antihelminthic drugs is quite different from that for the use of drugs for treating most protozoal infections. Most antihelminthic drugs are targeted at **nonproliferating** adult organisms, whereas with protozoa the targets are generally younger, more rapidly proliferating cells. The helminthic life cycle is frequently quite complex, and the adaptation to survival in the human host depends strongly on (1) neuromuscular coordination for feeding movements and for maintenance of a favorable location of the worm within the host; (2) carbohydrate metabolism as the major source of energy, with glucose the primary substrate; and (3) microtubular integrity, since egg laying and hatching, larval development, glucose transport, and enzyme activity and secretion are impaired when microtubules are modified. Most antihelminthic agents are targeted at one of these biochemical functions in the adult organism.

The mechanisms of action and clinical indications for common antihelminthic agents are listed in Table 80–2.

Benzimidazoles

The benzimidazoles are broad-spectrum antihelminthic agents and include mebendazole, thiabendazole, and albendazole. The basic structure of these agents consists of linked imidazole and benzene rings. Three mechanisms of action have been proposed for the benzimidazoles: (1) inhibition of fumarate reductase; (2) inhibition of glucose transport, resulting in glycogen depletion, cessation of ATP formation, and paralysis or death; and (3) disruption of microtubular function. Benzimidazoles block the assembly of tubulin dimers into tubulin polymers in a process mimicked by colchicine, a powerful antimitotic and embryotoxic drug. Because tubulin is important for parasite motility, drugs such as the benzimidazoles, which bind to parasite tubulin, are thought to act against nematode parasites by reducing or eliminating their motility.

The benzimidazoles have a wide spectrum of activity, including intestinal nematodes *(Ascaris, Trichuris, Necator*, and *Ancylostoma* spp.; *Enterobius vermicularis)* and a number of cestodes (*Taenia, Hymenolepis*, and *Echinococcus* spp.). Thiabendazole acts against larval and adult nematodes and is useful in the management of cutaneous larval migrans, trichinosis, and most intestinal nematode infections. Mebendazole is active against the intestinal nematodes and the cestodes previously listed. Albendazole has a spectrum similar to that of mebendazole and may have greater activity against *Echinococcus* spp. In addition to its broad-spectrum antihelminthic activity, albendazole also has activity against *Giardia* spp. and appears promising in the treatment of intestinal microsporidiosis in patients with acquired immunodeficiency syndrome.

Tetrahydropyrimidines

Pyrantel pamoate, a tetrahydropyrimidine, is a cholinergic agonist that has a powerful effect on nematode muscle cells by binding to cholinergic receptors, which results in cell depolarization and muscle contraction. This **paralytic** action on intestinal nematodes leads to expulsion of the worm from the host intestinal tract.

Pyrantel pamoate is not readily absorbed from the intestine and is active against *Ascaris* spp., pinworm, and hookworm. An analogue of pyrantel, oxantel, may be used with pyrantel to provide effective therapy for the three major soil-transmitted nematodes: *Ascaris* species, hookworm, and *Trichuris* spp.

Piperazines

The piperazine antihelmintics include piperazine and diethylcarbamazine. Piperazine is thought to act by hyperpolarization of the muscle membrane, producing a flaccid paralysis. The current hypothesis is that piperazine acts against nematodes as a low-potency γ-aminobutyric acid (GABA) agonist. Diethylcarbamazine may act by stimulating cholinergic receptors and depolarizing muscle cells, with subsequent paralysis of the worms. However, additional evidence suggests that it enhances the adherence of leukocytes to microfilariae and thus may act by altering the parasite surface membrane or by directly stimulating phagocytic cells.

The piperazines are active against *Ascaris* spp. and pinworm *(E. vermicularis)*. In addition, diethylcarbamazine is active against the filariae that produce river blindness *(Onchocerca volvulus)* and lymphatic filariasis *(Wuchereria bancrofti* and *Brugia malayi)*. Unfortunately, destruction of the microfilariae in the tissues may increase the pathology because of the host inflammatory response to the parasite antigens released on exposure to diethylcarbamazine. Recent information suggests that single-dose treatment with diethylcarbamazine may produce antiparasitic effects similar to those obtained with 14- to 21-day courses without the severe side effects observed with the multidose regimens.

Avermectins

Ivermectin, an avermectin, acts by interacting with the chloride channel on the helminth GABA receptor complex, thus inhibiting GABA-ergic synapses in the peripheral nervous system of nematode parasites. As a result, the parasites become paralyzed and can be eliminated by the host. The drug also inhibits the reproductive function of the adult female *O. volvulus* and alters the ability of the *O. volvulus* microfilariae to evade the host immune system.

Although ivermectin is used extensively to control gut-dwelling nematode infections in domestic and farm animals, its use in humans is limited primarily to treating ocular and lymphatic filariasis. Ivermectin is effective in the treatment of strongyloidiasis and several common intestinal parasitic nematodes including *Ascaris, Trichuris,* and *Enterobius* spp. When used to treat filariasis, ivermectin has fewer side effects than diethylcarbamazine, and a single dose can eliminate microfilariae for up to 6 months. Ivermectin has a dramatic effect on the tissue-dwelling microfilariae of *O. volvulus* and reduces the severity of the ocular pathology seen in onchocerciasis. Because of its ability to markedly reduce the number of microfilariae in the skin of people with onchocerciasis, ivermectin has been effective in reducing the transmission of onchocerciasis in endemic areas.

Pyrazinoisoquinolines

Praziquantel, a pyrazinoisoquinoline, is an antihelminthic active used against a broad spectrum of trematodes and cestodes. The drug is rapidly taken up by susceptible helminths in which it acts as a **calcium agonist.** The entry of calcium into various cells results in elevated intracellular calcium levels, tetanic muscular contraction, and destruction of the tegument. Praziquantel appears to act with the host immune system to produce a synergistic antihelminthic effect. The drug causes disruption of the parasite surface and tegument, allowing antibodies to attack parasite antigens not normally exposed on the surface (Figure 80–1). Irreversible damage to the parasite probably occurs when complement or host leukocytes are recruited to the sites where antibody is bound.

Praziquantel has extremely broad-spectrum activity against trematodes including *Fasciolopsis, Clonorchis, Opisthorchis, Paragonimus,* and *Schistosoma* spp. It is also active against cestodes including *Echinococcus, Taenia,* and *Dipylidium* spp. Praziquantel is the drug of choice for the treatment of schistosomiasis, clonorchiasis, opisthorchiasis, and neurocysticercosis. There is now reliable evidence that praziquantel reduces hepatosplenomegaly and portal

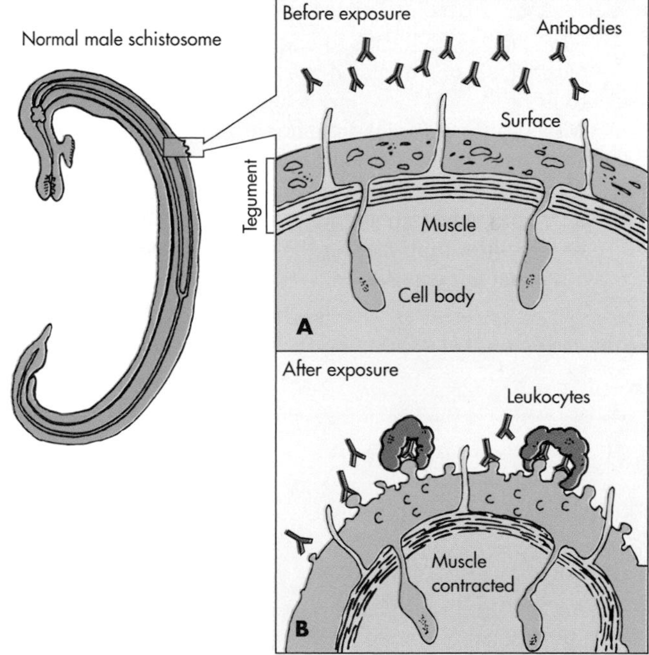

FIGURE 80–1. Before exposure to praziquantel, the schistosome is capable of avoiding the numerous antibodies directed toward surface and internally located antigens. **A,** Cross section of the dorsal surface of a normal male schistosome. Within 1 to 2 seconds after exposure to praziquantel, the muscles of the schistosome contract because of a drug-induced influx of calcium ions into the schistosome tegument. **B,** The change in permeability of the schistosome surface toward external ions initiates the appearance of small holes and balloonlike structures, making the parasite vulnerable to antibody-mediated adherence of host leukocytes that kill the helminth. (From Wingard LB Jr et al: *Human pharmacology: Molecular to clinical,* St Louis, 1991, Mosby.)

hypertension in schistosomiasis. Effective activity has also been demonstrated against other common trematode and cestode infections.

Phenols

Niclosamide, a phenol, is a nonabsorbable antihelminthic agent with selective activity against intestinal tapeworms. The drug is absorbed by gut-dwelling cestodes but not by nematodes. It acts by uncoupling oxidative phosphorylation in mitochondria, resulting in a loss of helminth ATP that ultimately immobilizes the parasite so that it is expelled with the feces. Niclosamide is effective in the treatment of intestinal tapeworms in humans and animals.

Other Antihelminthic Agents

Additional antihelminthic agents, including oxamniquine, metrifonate, and suramin, are described in Table 80–2. These agents are generally considered secondary agents for the treatment of trematode (oxamniquine and metrifonate) and filarial (suramin) infections.

QUESTIONS

1. What are the obstacles to effective treatment and prophylaxis of parasitic diseases in developing countries?
2. What are the goals of antiparasitic therapy, and how are they different from antibacterial therapy?
3. What is the importance of aminoquinoline analogues?
4. How does the strategy for the use of antihelminthic agents differ from that for the use of drugs for protozoal infections?

Bibliography

Abiose A: Onchocercal eye disease and the impact of Mectizan treatment, *Ann Trop Med Parasitol* 92:S11-S22, 1998.

Doenhoff MJ et al: Resistance of *Schistosoma mansoni* to prazquantel: Is there a problem? *Trans R Soc Trop Med Hyg* 96:465-469, 2002.

Edwards G, Krishna S: Pharmacokinetic and pharmacodynamic issues in the treatment of parasitic infections, *Eur J Clin Microbiol Infect Dis* 23:233-242, 2004.

Faubert G: Immune response to *Giardia duodenalis*, *Clin Microbiol Rev* 13:35-54, 2000.

Gardner TB, Hill DR: Treatment of giardiasis, *Clin Microbiol Rev* 14:114-128, 2001.

Geertz S, Gryseels B: Drug resistance in human helminthes: Current situation and lesions from livestock, *Clin Microbiol Rev* 13:207-222, 2000.

Gilbert DN et al, editors: *The Sanford guide to antimicrobial therapy*, ed 34, Hyde Park, Vt, 2004, Antimicrobial Therapy Inc.

Talisuna AO, Bloland P, D'Alessandro U: History, dynamics, and public health importance of malaria parasite resistance, *Clin Microbiol Rev* 178:235-254, 2004.

Wingard LB Jr et al, editors: *Human pharmacology: Molecular to clinical*, St Louis, 1991, Mosby.

CHAPTER 81

Laboratory Diagnosis of Parasitic Diseases

The diagnosis of parasitic infections may be very difficult, particularly in the nonendemic setting. The clinical manifestations of parasitic diseases are seldom specific enough to raise the possibility of these processes in the mind of the clinician, and routine laboratory tests are seldom helpful. Although peripheral **eosinophilia** is widely recognized as a useful indicator of parasitic disease, this phenomenon is characteristic only of helminthic infection and even in these cases is frequently absent. Thus the physician must maintain a heightened index of suspicion and must rely on detailed travel, food intake, transfusion, and socioeconomic history to raise the possibility of parasitic disease. Proper diagnosis requires that (1) the physician consider the possibility of parasitic infection, (2) appropriate specimens be obtained and transported to the laboratory in a timely fashion, (3) the laboratory competently perform the appropriate procedures for the recovery and identification of the etiologic agent, (4) the laboratory results be effectively communicated to the physician, and (5) the results be correctly interpreted by the physician and applied to the care of the patient. In addition, for most parasitic diseases, appropriate test selection and interpretation is based on an understanding of the **life cycle** of the parasite and the **pathogenesis** of the disease process in humans.

Numerous methods for diagnosing parasitic diseases have been described (Box 81–1). Some are useful in detecting a wide variety of parasites, and others are particularly useful for one or a few parasites. Although the mainstay of diagnostic clinical microbiology is the isolation of the causative pathogen in culture, the diagnosis of parasitic diseases is accomplished almost entirely by morphologic (usually microscopic) demonstration of parasites in clinical material. Occasionally, demonstration of a specific antibody response (serodiagnosis) helps in establishing the diagnosis. The detection of parasite antigens in serum, urine, or stool now provides a rapid and sensitive means of diagnosing infection with certain organisms. Likewise, the development of nucleic acid probe–based assays may prove to be an excellent means of detecting and identifying a number of parasites in biologic samples such as blood, stool, urine, sputum, and tissue biopsies obtained from infected patients. In general, it is better for the laboratory to offer a limited number of competently performed procedures than to offer a wide variety of infrequently and poorly performed tests.

This chapter provides a general description of the principles of specimen collection and processing necessary to diagnose most parasitic infections. Specific details of these and other procedures of general and limited usefulness may be found in several reference texts listed in the bibliography.

Parasite Life Cycle as a Diagnostic Aid

Parasites may have complex life cycles involving single or multiple hosts. Understanding the life cycle of parasitic organisms is a key to understanding important features of geographic distribution, transmission, and pathogenesis of many parasitic diseases. The life cycles of parasites often suggest useful clues for diagnosis as well. For example, in the life cycle of filariae that infect humans, certain species such as *Wuchereria bancrofti* have a **"nocturnal periodicity,"** in which greater numbers of microfilariae are found in the peripheral blood at night. Sampling the blood of such patients during daytime hours may fail to detect the microfilariae, whereas blood specimens collected between 10 PM and 4 AM may demonstrate many microfilariae. Likewise, intestinal nematodes such as *Ascaris lumbricoides* and hookworm, which reside in the lumen of the intestine, produce large numbers of eggs that can be detected easily in the stool of an infected patient. In

BOX 81–1. Laboratory Methods for Diagnosing Parasitic Disease

- Macroscopic examination
- Microscopic examination
  - Wet mount
  - Permanent stains
  - Stool concentrates
- Serologic examination
  - Antibody response
  - Antigen detection
- Nucleic acid hybridization
  - Probes and amplification techniques
  - Detection
  - Identification
- Culture
- Animal inoculation
- Xenodiagnosis

contrast, another intestinal nematode, *Strongyloides stercoralis,* lays its eggs in the bowel wall rather than in the intestinal lumen. As a result, the eggs are rarely seen on stool examination; to make the diagnosis, the parasitologist must be alert for the presence of larvae. Finally, parasites may cause clinical symptoms at a time when diagnostic forms are not yet present in the usual site. For example, in certain intestinal nematode infections the **migration** of larvae through the tissues may cause intense symptomatology weeks before the characteristic eggs are present in the feces.

General Diagnostic Considerations

The importance of appropriate specimen collection, the number and timing of specimens, timely transport to the laboratory, and prompt examination by an experienced microscopist cannot be overemphasized. Because the majority of parasitologic examinations and identifications are based entirely on recognizing the characteristic morphology of the organisms, any condition that may obscure or distort the morphologic appearance of the parasite may result in an erroneous identification or missed diagnosis. As noted previously and in Box 81–1, there may be alternatives to microscopy for the detection and identification of certain parasites. These tests (e.g., antigen detection, nucleic acid probes), although presently uncommon, may become more widely applied in the future. They offer the promise of more rapid, sensitive, and specific diagnostic testing for parasitic diseases. These diagnostic test options may expand the testing capabilities of many laboratories, allowing laboratories with limited proficiency in parasitology to offer diagnostic testing for certain parasitic diseases. A list of common and uncommon diagnostic procedures and specimens to be collected for selected parasitic infections is provided in Table 81–1.

Parasitic Infections of the Intestinal and Urogenital Tract

Protozoa and helminths may colonize or infect the intestinal and urogenital tract of humans. Most commonly these parasites are amoebae, flagellates, or nematodes (Table 81–2). However, infection with trematodes, cestodes, or ciliate, coccidian, or microsporidian parasites may also be encountered.

In intestinal and urogenital infections, a simple wet mount or stained smear is often inadequate. Repeated specimen collection and testing are often necessary to optimize the detection of organisms that are shed intermittently or in fluctuating numbers. Concentration of specimens by sedimentation or flotation techniques may be required to detect low numbers of ova (worms) or cysts (protozoa) in fecal specimens.

Occasionally, specimens other than stool or urine must be examined (see Table 81–1). Optimal detection of small bowel pathogens, such as *Giardia lamblia (duodenalis)* and *S. stercoralis,* may require the aspiration of duodenal contents or even small bowel biopsy. Likewise, the detection of colonic parasites such as *Entamoeba histolytica* and *Schistosoma mansoni* may necessitate proctoscopic or sigmoidoscopic examination with aspiration or biopsy of mucosal lesions. Sampling of the perianal skin is a useful means of recovering the eggs of *Enterobius vermicularis* (pinworm) or *Taenia* species (tapeworm).

FECAL SPECIMEN COLLECTION

Patients, clinicians, and laboratory personnel must be properly instructed on collection and handling of specimens. Fecal specimens should be collected in clean, wide-mouthed, waterproof containers with a tight-fitting lid to ensure and maintain adequate moisture. Specimens must not be contaminated with water, soil, or urine because water and soil may contain free-living organisms that can be mistaken for human parasites and urine can destroy motile trophozoites and may cause helminth eggs to hatch. Stool specimens should not contain barium, bismuth, or medications containing mineral oil, antibiotics, antimalarials, or other chemical substances because such specimens compromise the detection of intestinal parasites. Specimen collection should be delayed for 5 to 10 days to allow barium to clear and for at least 2 weeks to allow intestinal parasites to recover from the toxic (but not curative) effects of antibiotics such as tetracycline.

Purged specimens may be collected when organisms are not detected in normally passed fecal specimens; however, only certain purgatives (sodium sulfate and buffered sodium biphosphate [Phospho-Soda]) are

TABLE 81–1. Body Sites, Specimen Collection, and Diagnostic Procedures for Selected Parasitic Infections

Infecting Organism	Specimen Options	Collection Methods	Diagnostic Procedure
Blood			
Plasmodium species, *Babesia* species, filaria	Whole blood, anticoagulated	Venipuncture	Microscopic examination (Giemsa stain) or acridine orange fluorescent stain Thin film Thick film Blood concentration (filaria) Serology Antibody Antigen
Bone Marrow			
Leishmania species	Aspirate Serum	Sterile Venipuncture	Microscopic examination (Giemsa stain) Culture Serology (antibody)
Central Nervous System			
Acanthamoeba species, *Naegleria* species, trypanosomes *Angiostrongylus cantonensis*	Spinal fluid Serum	Sterile Venipuncture	Microscopic examination Wet mount Permanent stain Culture Serology (antibody)
Cutaneous Ulcers			
Leishmania species	Aspirate Biopsy Serum	Sterile plus smears Sterile, nonsterile to histology Venipuncture	Microscopic examination (Giemsa stain) Culture Serology (antibody)
Eye			
Acanthamoeba species	Corneal scrapings Corneal biopsy	Sterile saline, air-dried smear Sterile saline	Microscopic examination Wet mount Permanent stain Culture
Intestinal Tract			
Entamoeba histolytica	Fresh stool Preserved stool Sigmoidoscopy material Serum	Waxed container Formalin, PVA Fresh, PVA Schaudinn's smears Venipuncture	Microscopic examination Wet mount Permanent stains Serology Antigen (stool) Antibody (serum) Culture
Giardia species	Fresh stool Preserved stool Duodenal contents	Waxed container Formalin, PVA Entero-Test or aspirate	Microscopic examination Wet mount Permanent stains Antigen IFA EIA Culture
Cryptosporidium species	Fresh stool Preserved stool Biopsy	Waxed container Formalin, PVA Saline	Microscopic examination (acid-fast) Antigen IFA EIA

TABLE 81–1. Body Sites, Specimen Collection, and Diagnostic Procedures for Selected Parasitic Infections—cont'd

Infecting Organism	Specimen Options	Collection Methods	Diagnostic Procedure
Microsporidia	Fresh stool Preserved stool Duodenal contents Biopsy	Waxed container Formalin, PVA Aspirate Saline	Microscopic Giemsa stain Gram stain Chromotrope stain
Pinworm	Anal impression smear	Cellophane tape	Macroscopic examination Microscopic examination (eggs)
Helminths	Fresh stool Preserved stool Serum	Waxed container Formalin, PVA Venipuncture	Macroscopic examination (adults) Microscopic examination (larvae and eggs) Serology (antibody) Culture (*Strongyloides* species)
Liver, Spleen			
E. histolytica, Leishmania species	Aspirates Biopsy Serum	Sterile, collected in four separate aliquots (liver) Sterile; nonsterile to histology Venipuncture	Microscopic examinatione Wet mount Permanent stains Serology Antigen Antibody Culture
Lung			
Rarely: amoebae, (*E. histolytica*), trematodes (*Paragonimus westermani*), larvae (*Strongyloides stercoralis*), or cestode hooklets	Sputum Lavage Transbronchial aspirate Brush biopsy Open lung biopsy	Induced, no preservative No preservative Air-dried smears Same as above Fresh squash preparation Nonsterile to histology	Microscopic examination Giemsa stain Gram stain Hematoxylin and eosin Antigen IFA EIA Serum (antibody)
Muscle			
Trichinella spiralis *Trypanosoma cruzi*	Biopsy Serum	Nonsterile to histology Venipuncture	Microscopic examination (permanent stains) Serology Antibody Antigen
Skin			
Onchocerca volvulus, Leishmania species	Scrapings Skin snip Biopsy	Aseptic, smear, or vial No preservative Nonsterile to histology	Microscopic examination Wet mount Permanent stains
Cutaneous larval migrans	Serum	Venipuncture	Serology (antibody) Culture (*Leishmania* species)
Urogenital System			
Trichomonas vaginalis	Vaginal discharge Prostatic secretions Urethral discharge	Saline swab, culture medium Same as above	Microscopic examination Wet mount Permanent stains Antigen (IFA) Culture (*T. vaginalis*) Serology (antibody) Nucleic acid probes (*T. vaginalis*)
Schistosoma haematobium	Urine Biopsy	Single unpreserved specimen Nonsterile to histology	Microscopic examination

EIA, Enzyme immunoassay; IFA, immunofluorescent assay; PVA, polyvinyl alcohol.

TABLE 81–2. Most Commonly Identified Intestinal Parasites in U.S. Laboratories

Organism	% of Total Positive Specimens (n = 1537)
Giardia lamblia (duodenalis)	58.3
Cryptosporidium parvum	7.4
Dientamoeba fragilis	6.6
Ascaris lumbricoides	4.7
Entamoeba histolytica	4.3
Trichuris trichiura	3.8
Hookworm	3.4
Enterobius vermicularis	3.4
Strongyloides stercoralis	3.3
Hymenolepis nana	1.5
Isospora species	0.8
Microsporidia	0.5
Clonorchis or *Opisthorchis* species	0.3
Other helminths	1.7

Modified from Valenstein P et al: *Arch Pathol Lab Med* 120:206-211, 1996.

TABLE 81–3. Number of Specimens Required to Detect Intestinal Parasites

Number of Specimens per Patient	Percentage of Infected Patients Detected*
1	91.9
2	97.6
3	99.8
4	99.9

Modified from Valenstein P et al: Arch Pathol Lab Med 120:206-211, 1996.
*n, 1159.

satisfactory. One series of purged specimens may be examined in place of, or in addition to, a series of normally passed specimens.

Unpreserved formed fecal specimens should arrive in the laboratory within 2 hours after passage. If the stool is liquid and thus more likely to contain trophozoites, it should reach the laboratory for examination within 30 minutes. Soft or loose stools should be examined within 1 hour of passage. All fresh fecal samples should be placed into preservatives, such as 10% formalin, polyvinyl alcohol (PVA), merthiolate-iodine-formalin, or sodium acetate–formalin (SAF) if examination is not possible within the recommended time limits. Fecal specimens may be stored at 4°C but should not be incubated or frozen.

The number of specimens required to demonstrate intestinal parasites varies depending on the quality of the specimen submitted, the accuracy of the examination performed, the severity of the infection, and the purpose for which the examination is made. If the physician is interested only in determining the presence or absence of helminths, one or two examinations may suffice, provided that concentration methods are used. For a routine parasitic examination, a total of three fecal specimens is recommended. The examination of three specimens using a combination of techniques ensures detection of more than 99% of infections. In a survey conducted in the United States, examination of three specimens detected 99.8% of infected patients, and examination of four specimens detected an additional 0.1% (Table 81–3).

It is inappropriate for multiple specimens to be collected on the same patient on the same day. It is also not recommended for the three specimens to be submitted, one each day for 3 consecutive days. The series of three specimens should be collected within no more than 10 days. Many parasites do not appear in fecal specimens in consistent numbers on a daily basis; therefore collection of specimens on alternate days tends to yield a higher percentage of positive findings.

It has become apparent that in the United States, submission of stool for parasitologic examination from patients with hospital-acquired diarrhea (onset more than 3 days after admission) is usually inappropriate. This is because the frequency of acquisition of protozoan or helminthic parasites in a hospital is vanishingly rare. A request for stool examination for ova and parasites in a hospitalized patient should be accompanied by a clear statement of clinical indications and only after the more common causes of hospital-acquired diarrhea (e.g., antibiotic induced) have been ruled out.

TECHNIQUES OF STOOL EXAMINATION

A competent microscopist should systematically examine specimens for helminth eggs and larvae and intestinal protozoa. For optimal detection of these various infectious agents a combination of several techniques of examination is required.

Macroscopic Examination

The fecal specimen should be examined for consistency and for the presence of blood, mucus, worms, and proglottids.

Direct Wet Mount

Fresh stools should be examined under the microscope using the saline and iodine wet-mount technique to detect motile trophozoites or larvae (*Strongyloides* species). The saline and iodine wet mounts are also used to detect helminth eggs, protozoan cysts, and host cells, such as leukocytes and red blood cells. This approach is also useful in examining material from sputum, urine, vaginal swabs, duodenal aspirates, sigmoidoscopy, abscesses, and tissue biopsies.

Concentration

All fecal specimens should be placed in 10% formalin to preserve parasite morphology and should be concentrated using a procedure such as formalin–ethyl acetate (or formalin-ether) sedimentation or zinc sulfate flotation. These methods separate protozoan cysts and helminth eggs from the bulk of fecal material and thus enhance the ability to detect small numbers of organisms usually missed by the use of only a direct smear. After concentration, the material is stained with iodine and examined microscopically.

Permanently Stained Slides

The detection and correct identification of intestinal protozoa often depend on the examination of the permanently stained smear. These slides provide a permanent record of the protozoan organisms that are identified. The cytologic detail revealed by one of the permanent staining methods is essential for accurate identification, and most identification should be considered tentative until confirmed by the permanently stained slide. The common permanent stains used are trichrome, iron hematoxylin, and phosphotungstic acid–hematoxylin. Slides are made either by preparing smears of fresh fecal material and placing them in Schaudinn's fixative solution or by fixing a small amount of fecal material in PVA fixative.

COLLECTION AND EXAMINATION OF SPECIMENS OTHER THAN STOOL

Frequently, specimens other than fecal material must be collected and examined to diagnose infections caused by intestinal pathogens. These specimens include perianal samples, sigmoidoscopic material, aspirates of duodenal contents and liver abscesses, sputum, urine, and urogenital specimens.

Perianal Specimens

The collection of perianal specimens is often necessary to diagnose pinworm *(E. vermicularis)* and, occasionally, *Taenia* (tapeworm) infections. The methods include the preparation of a clear cellulose tape slide or an anal swab. The cellulose tape slide preparation is the method of choice for the detection of pinworm eggs. Specimens collected by either method should be obtained in the morning before the patient bathes or goes to the bathroom. The tape method requires that the adhesive surface of the tape be pressed firmly against the right and left perianal folds and then spread onto the surface of a microscope slide. Likewise, the anal swab should be rubbed gently over the perianal area and transported to the laboratory for microscopic examination. With either collection method the slides or swabs should be kept at 4°C if transport to the laboratory is to be delayed.

Sigmoidoscopic Material

Material from sigmoidoscopy can be helpful in the diagnosis of *E. histolytica* infection that has not been detected by routine fecal examinations. The specimens consist of scraped or aspirated material from the mucosal surface. At least six areas should be sampled. After collection, the material should be placed in a tube containing 0.85% saline and should be kept warm during transport to the laboratory. The specimens should be examined immediately for motile trophozoites.

Duodenal Aspirates

Sampling and examination of duodenal contents is a means of recovering *Strongyloides* larvae; the eggs of *Clonorchis, Opisthorchis,* and *Fasciola* species; and other small bowel parasites, such as *Giardia, Isospora,* and *Cryptosporidium* organisms. Specimens may be obtained by endoscopic intubation or by the use of the enteric capsule or string test (Entero-Test). Endoscopic biopsy of the small intestinal mucosa may reveal *Giardia* organisms, *Cryptosporidium* organisms, and microsporidia, as well as *Strongyloides* larvae. Specimens should be collected in saline and transported directly to the laboratory for microscopic examination.

Liver Abscess Aspirate

Suppurative lesions of the liver and subphrenic spaces may be caused by *E. histolytica* (extraintestinal amebiasis). Extraintestinal amebiasis may occur in the absence of any history of symptomatic intestinal infection. The specimen should be collected from the liver abscess margin instead of the necrotic center. The first portion removed is usually yellowish white in appearance and seldom contains amoebae. Later portions, which are reddish, are more likely to contain organisms. A minimum of two separate portions of exudative material should be removed. After aspiration, the collapse of the abscess and the subsequent inflowing of blood often release amoebae from the tissue. Subsequent aspirations may have a greater chance of revealing organisms. The aspirated material should be transported immediately to the laboratory.

Sputum

Occasionally, intestinal parasites may be detected in sputum. These organisms include the larvae of *Ascaris* species, *Strongyloides* species, and hookworm; cestode hooklets; and intestinal protozoa, such as *E. histolytica* and *Cryptosporidium* species. The specimen should be a deep sputum rather than primarily saliva, and it should be delivered immediately to the laboratory. Microscopic examination should include saline wet-mount and permanent stain preparations.

Urine

Examination of urine specimens may be useful in diagnosing infections caused by *Schistosoma haematobium* (occasionally other species as well) and *Trichomonas vaginalis*. Detection of eggs in urine can be accomplished using direct detection or concentration using the sedimentation centrifugation technique. Eggs may be trapped in mucus or pus and are more frequently present in the last few drops of the specimen rather than the first portion. The production of *Schistosoma* eggs fluctuates; therefore examinations should be performed over several days. *T. vaginalis* may be found in the urinary sediment of male and female patients.

Urogenital Specimens

Urogenital specimens are collected if infection with *T. vaginalis* is suspected. Identification is based on wet-mount preparation examinations of vaginal and urethral discharges, prostatic secretions, or urine sediment. Specimens should be placed in a container with a small amount of 0.85% saline and sent immediately to the laboratory for examination. If no organisms are detected by direct wet mounts, culture may be used.

Parasitic Infections Of Blood and Tissue

Parasites localized within the blood or tissues of the host are more difficult to detect than intestinal and urogenital parasites. Microscopic examination of blood films is a direct and useful means of detecting malarial parasites, trypanosomes, and microfilariae. Unfortunately, the concentration of organisms often fluctuates; thus the collection of multiple specimens over several days is required. The preparation of both wet mounts (microfilariae and trypanosomes) and permanently stained thick and thin blood films is the mainstay of diagnosis. Examination of sputum may reveal helminth ova (lung flukes) or larvae (*Ascaris* and *Strongyloides* species) after appropriate concentration techniques. Biopsy of skin (onchocerciasis) or muscle (trichinosis) may be required for the diagnosis of certain nematode infections (see Table 81–1).

BLOOD FILMS

The clinical diagnosis of parasitic diseases such as malaria, leishmaniasis, trypanosomiasis, and filariasis largely rests on the collection of appropriately timed blood samples and the expert microscopic examination of properly prepared and stained thick and thin blood films. The optimal time for obtaining blood for parasitologic examination varies with the particular parasite expected.

Because malaria is one of the few parasitic infections that can be life threatening, blood collection and examination of blood films should be performed immediately as soon as the diagnosis is suspected. Laboratories offering this service should be prepared to do so on a 24-hour basis, 7 days a week. Because the levels of parasitemia may be low or fluctuating, it is recommended that repeat blood films be obtained and examined at 6, 12, and 24 hours after the initial sample. Detection of trypanosomes in blood is occasionally possible during the early acute phase of the disease. *Trypanosoma cruzi* (Chagas' disease) may also be detected during subsequent febrile periods. After several months to a year, the trypomastigotes of African trypanosomiasis (*Trypanosoma brucei rhodesiense* and *T. b. gambiense*) are better demonstrated in spinal fluid than in blood. Blood films for the detection of nocturnal microfilariae (*W. bancrofti* and *Brugia malayi*) should be prepared between 10 PM and 4 AM, whereas for the diurnal *Loa loa*, films are prepared at noon.

Two types of blood films are prepared for the diagnosis of blood parasite infections: thin films and thick films. Although wet-mount preparations of blood films can be examined for motile parasites (microfilariae and trypanosomes), most laboratories proceed directly to the preparation of thick and thin films for staining. In the thin film the blood is spread over the slide in a thin (single-cell) layer, and the red blood cells remain intact after staining. In the thick film the red cells are lysed before staining, and only the white blood cells, platelets, and parasites (if present) are visible. Thick films allow a larger amount of blood to be examined, which increases the possibility of detecting light infections. Unfortunately, increased distortion of the parasites makes species identification using the thick film particularly difficult. Proper use of this technique usually requires a great deal of expertise and experience.

Occasionally, other blood-concentration procedures may be used to detect light infections. Alternative concentration methods for detecting blood parasites include the use of microhematocrit centrifugation, the examination of buffy coat preparations, a triple centrifugation technique for the detection of low numbers of trypanosomes, and a membrane filtration technique for the detection of microfilariae.

Once prepared, blood films must be stained. The most dependable staining of blood parasites is obtained with Giemsa stain buffered to pH 7.0 to 7.2, although special stains may be occasionally used to identify species of microfilariae. Giemsa stain is particularly useful for the staining of protozoa (malaria and trypanosomes); however, the sheath of microfilariae may not always stain with Giemsa. In this case, hematoxylin-based stains may be used.

SPECIMENS OTHER THAN BLOOD

Examination of tissue and body fluids other than blood may be necessary based on clinical presentation and epidemiologic considerations. Smears and concentrates of cerebrospinal fluid are necessary to detect trophozoites of *Naegleria* species, trypanosomes, and larvae of *Angiostrongylus cantonensis* within the central nervous system. Cerebrospinal fluid must be promptly examined because the trophozoite forms of these parasites are very labile (trypanosomes) or tend to round up and become nonmotile (*Naegleria* species). Examination of tissue impression smears of lymph nodes, liver biopsy material, spleen, or bone marrow stained with Giemsa stain is very useful in detecting **intracellular** parasites, such as *Leishmania* and *Toxoplasma* species. Likewise, biopsies of various tissues are an excellent means of detecting localized or disseminated infections caused by protozoan and helminthic parasites. Saline mounts of superficial skin snips are very useful in detecting the microfilariae of *Onchocerca volvulus*. Examination of sputum (induced) is indicated when there is a question of pulmonary paragonimiasis (lung fluke) or abscess formation with *E. histolytica*. *Strongyloides* larvae may be detected in sputum in hyperinfection syndrome.

Alternatives to Microscopy

In the majority of cases the diagnosis of parasitic disease is made in the laboratory by microscopic detection and morphologic identification of the parasite in clinical specimens. In some cases the parasite cannot be detected, despite a careful search, because of low or absent levels of organisms in readily available clinical material. In such cases the clinician may need to rely on alternative methods based on the detection of parasite-derived material (antigens or nucleic acids) or by the host response to parasitic invasion (antibodies). Additional approaches used in selected infections include culture, animal inoculation, and xenodiagnosis.

IMMUNODIAGNOSTICS

Immunodiagnostic methods have long been used as aids in the diagnosis of parasitic diseases. The majority of these serologic tests are based on the detection of specific antibody responses to the presence of the parasite. The analytical approaches include the use of classical agglutination, complement fixation, and gel-diffusion methods and more recently include immunofluorescence, enzyme immunoassay (EIA), and Western blot assays. Antibody detection is useful and indicated in the diagnosis of many protozoan diseases (e.g., extraintestinal amebiasis, South American trypanosomiasis, leishmaniasis, transfusion-acquired malaria, toxoplasmosis) and helminthic diseases (e.g., clonorchiasis, cysticercosis, hydatidosis, lymphatic filariasis, schistosomiasis, trichinellosis, toxocariasis). There is a problem with the detection of antibody as a means of diagnosis: Because of the persistence of antibody for months to years after the acute infection, demonstration of antibody can rarely differentiate between acute and chronic infection.

In contrast to antibody detection, the measurement of circulating parasite antigen in serum, urine, or feces may provide a more appropriate marker for the presence of active infection and may also indicate parasite load. Likewise, demonstrations of specific **parasite antigen** in lesion fluid, such as material from an amoebic abscess or fluid from a hydatid cyst, may provide a definitive diagnosis of the infecting organism. Most common antigen-detection assays use an EIA format; however, immunofluorescence, radioimmunoassay, and immunoblot methods have also proved useful. Several commercial assays for the detection of parasite antigens are now available in kits. These include EIA and immunochromatographic assays for the detection of *Giardia*, *E. histolytica*, *Entamoeba dispar* and *Cryptosporidium* species in stool, EIA for the detection of *T. vaginalis* in urogenital specimens, and immunofluorescent assays for the detection of *Giardia*, *Cryptosporidium*, and *Trichomonas* species. The reported sensitivity and specificity for most of these kits are quite good. The advantages to these approaches are labor savings and a potential increase in sensitivity. The disadvantages are the loss of parasitologic expertise and the fact that in some instances the available assay tests are for only a single organism, whereas conventional microscopic examination provides the opportunity to recognize many different parasites. Although antigen-detection assays have been described for many other parasites, they are not widely available. The availability of a broad panel of antigen-detection assays makes the use of an antigen screen a viable alternative to tedious microscopic examination.

MOLECULAR DIAGNOSTIC APPROACHES

In addition to immunodiagnostic methods, the diagnosis of parasitic diseases has been enhanced considerably by the application of molecular diagnostic methods based on **nucleic acid hybridization**. This approach takes advantage of the fact that all organisms contain nucleic acid sequences that may be used in a hybridization assay to distinguish among strains, species, and genera. Thus, parasites may be simultaneously detected and identified in clinical material, depending on the specificity of the nucleic acid probe used. Another advantage of nucleic acid–based detection systems is that they are independent of the patients' immunologic status or previous infection history, thereby identifying active infection. Finally, the development of target amplification techniques, such as the polymerase chain reaction (PCR), provides exquisite sensitivity, allowing the detection of as little as one organism in a biologic sample (Table 81–4).

Nucleic acid probes can be used to detect parasites not only in clinical samples of blood, stool, or tissue from infected patients but also in their natural vector. The application of DNA "fingerprinting" allows precise identification of the parasite or vector to the subspecies or strain level and has considerable value in epidemiologic studies. Assay formats using nucleic acid probes range from dot blot and Southern hybridization methods to in situ hybridization in tissue to PCR amplification coupled with solid or solution phase hybridization. The use of nonisotopic DNA labeling techniques greatly expands the potential applicability of these assays worldwide. Diagnostic kits based on these methods are not widely available; however, several are under development and may be available for clinical use in the near future. A simple nucleic acid probe assay for *T. vaginalis* in urogenital specimens is now available commercially in kit form for use in clinics and physicians' offices.

Irrespective of the assay format, nucleic acid probes and amplification techniques are now being used on a research basis for the detection and identification of numerous species and strains, including *Plasmodium* species, *Leishmania* species, *T. cruzi*, *E. histolytica*, and *Toxoplasma gondii* (see Table 81–4). It must be understood that the application of nucleic acid hybridization methods to the diagnosis of parasitic diseases is still in its infancy. The widespread use of these techniques requires further development of simple procedures for sample handling and preparation and will require extensive clinical and field testing before they can be applied broadly to aid in clinical diagnosis.

CULTURE

Although culture is the standard for the diagnosis of most infectious diseases, it is not commonly used in the parasitology laboratory. Certain protozoan parasites such as *T. vaginalis*; *E. histolytica*; *Acanthamoeba*, *Naegleria*, and *Leishmania* species; *T. cruzi*, and *Toxoplasma* species can be cultured with relative ease. However, culture of other parasites has not been successful or is too difficult or cumbersome to be of practical value in routine diagnostic efforts.

TABLE 81–4. Examples of Techniques for Detection of Parasitic Infections Based on PCR Analysis

Organism	Gene	Target Sensitivity (%)	Comment
Plasmodium vivax	Circumsporozoite gene	91–96	Dried blood–spotted filter paper samples are used.
Leishmania species	kDNA minicircle sequence	87–100	Results are compared to culture and microscopy of biopsy specimens.
Trypanosoma cruzi	kDNA minicircle sequence	100	Results are compared to serology and xenodiagnosis of blood samples.
Toxoplasma gondii	B1 repetitive gene p30 major surface antigen Recombinant DNA sequences	46–99	PCR of BAL, blood, cerebrospinal fluid, and amniotic fluid show great potential for diagnosis of toxoplasmosis.
Entamoeba histolytica	p145 tandem repeat sequence	96	Results are compared to microscopic diagnosis of stool samples. Test may distinguish pathogenic from nonpathogenic strains.

BAL, Bronchoalveolar lavage; PCR, polymerase chain reaction.

ANIMAL INOCULATION

Animal inoculation is a sensitive means of detecting infection caused by blood and tissue parasites, such as *T. b. gambiense, T. b. rhodesiense, T. cruzi, Leishmania* species, and *T. gondii*. Although useful, this approach is not practical for most diagnostic laboratories and is largely confined to research settings.

XENODIAGNOSIS

The technique of xenodiagnosis uses laboratory-raised arthropod vectors to detect low levels of parasites in infected individuals. Classically, this approach was used to diagnose Chagas' disease by allowing an uninfected reduviid bug to feed on an individual suspected of having the disease. Subsequently, the bug was dissected and examined microscopically for evidence of developmental stages of *T. cruzi*. Although this technique may be used in endemic areas, it is obviously not practical for most diagnostic laboratories.

QUESTIONS

1. Why is it important to understand the life cycle of parasites when diagnosing parasitic diseases?
2. What factors may confound the use of microscopy in the diagnosis of parasitic disease?
3. Describe the important considerations in collecting and submitting a fecal specimen for parasitologic examination.
4. Which parasites can be detected in blood?
5. What are the alternatives to microscopy for the diagnosis of parasitic infections?

Bibliography

Connor DH et al, editors: *Pathology of infectious diseases*, vol II, Stamford, Conn, 1997, Appleton & Lange.

Garcia LS, editor: *Diagnostic medical parasitology*, ed 4, Washington, 2001, ASM Press.

Garcia LS, Schimizu RY, Bernard CN: Detection of *Giardia lamblia, Entamoeba histolytica/Entamoeba dispar*, and *Cryptosporidium parvum* antigens in human fecal specimens using the Triage Parasite Panel enzyme immunoassay, *J Clin Microbiol* 38:3337-3340, 2000.

Hague R et al: Diagnosis of amebic liver abscess and intestinal infection with the Tech Lab *Entamoeba histolytica* II antigen detection and antibody tests, *J Clin Microbiol* 38:3235-3239, 2000.

Marshall MM et al: Waterborne protozoan pathogens, *Clin Microbiol Rev* 10:67-85, 1997.

Moody A: Rapid diagnostic tests for malaria parasites, *Clin Microbiol Rev* 15:66-78, 2002.

Tanyuksel M, Petri WA Jr: Laboratory diagnosis of amebiasis, *Clin Microbiol Rev* 16:713-729, 2003.

Valenstein P, Pfaller M, Yungbluth M: The use and abuse of routine stool microbiology: A College of American Pathologists Q-Probes study of 601 institutions, *Arch Pathol Lab Med* 120:206-211, 1996.

Weiss JB: DNA probes and PCR for diagnosis of parasitic infections, *Clin Microbiol Rev* 8:113-130, 1995.

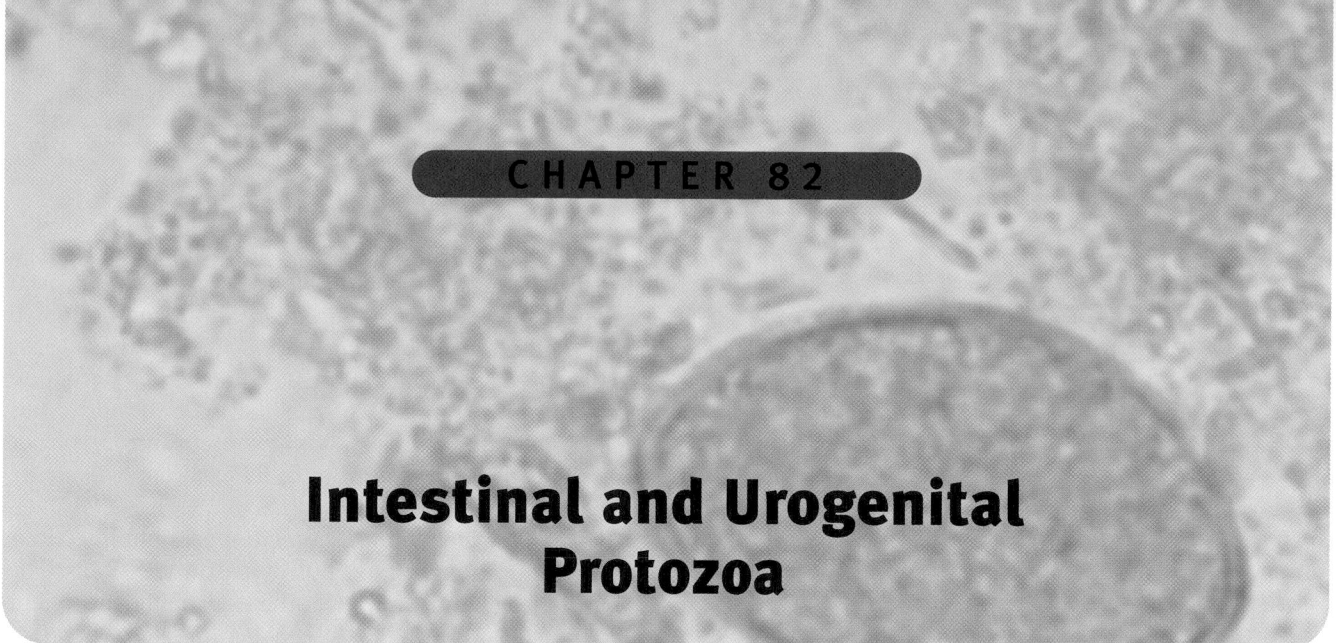

Intestinal and Urogenital Protozoa

Protozoa may colonize and infect the oropharynx, duodenum and small bowel, colon, and urogenital tract of humans. The majority of these parasites belong to the amoebae and flagellates; however, infection with ciliate, coccidian, or microsporidian parasites may also be encountered (see Table 81–2). These organisms are transmitted by the **fecal-oral route.** In the United States, transmission of intestinal protozoa is particularly problematic in daycare centers, where several outbreaks of diarrhea caused by *Giardia* or *Cryptosporidium* species have been documented. In other parts of the world, the spread of enteric protozoal infections may be controlled in part by improved sanitation and by chlorination and filtration of water supplies; however, this may be difficult or impossible in many developing countries.

Amoebae

The amoebae are primitive **unicellular** microorganisms. Their life cycle is relatively simple and divided into two stages: the actively motile feeding stage (trophozoite) and the quiescent, resistant, infective stage (cyst). Replication is accomplished by binary fission (splitting the trophozoite) or by the development of numerous trophozoites within the mature multinucleated cyst. Motility is accomplished by extension of a **pseudopod** ("false foot") with extrusion of the cellular ectoplasm and then drawing up of the rest of the cell in a snail-like movement to meet this pseudopod. The amoebic trophozoites remain actively motile as long as the environment is favorable. The cyst form develops when the environmental temperature or moisture level drops.

Most amoebae found in humans are **commensal** organisms (*Entamoeba coli, Entamoeba hartmanni, Entamoeba dispar, Entamoeba gingivalis, Endolimax nana, Iodamoeba bütschlii*). However, *Entamoeba histolytica* is an important human pathogen. Other amoebae, particularly *Entamoeba polecki*, can cause human disease but are rarely detected. The pathogenicity of *Blastocystis hominis* is still controversial. Some free-living amoebae (*Naegleria fowleri, Acanthamoeba* species) are present in soil and in warm freshwater ponds or swimming pools and can be opportunistic human pathogens, causing meningoencephalitis or keratitis.

ENTAMOEBA HISTOLYTICA

Physiology and Structure

Cyst and trophozoite forms of *E. histolytica* are detected in fecal specimens from infected patients (Figure 82–1). Trophozoites can also be found in the crypts of the large intestine. In freshly passed stools, actively motile trophozoites can be seen, whereas in formed stools the cysts are usually the only form recognized. For the diagnosis of amebiasis, distinguishing between the *E. histolytica* trophozoites and cysts and those of commensal amoebae is important.

Pathogenesis

After ingestion, the cysts pass through the stomach, where exposure to gastric acid stimulates the release of the pathogenic trophozoite in the duodenum. The trophozoites divide and produce extensive local necrosis in the large intestine. The basis for this tissue destruction is incompletely understood, although it is attributed to production of a **cytotoxin.** Attachment of *E. histolytica* trophozoites to host cells via a galactose-inhibitable adherence protein is required for cytolysis and tissue necrosis to occur. The lysis of colonic epithelial cells, human neutrophils, lymphocytes, and monocytes by

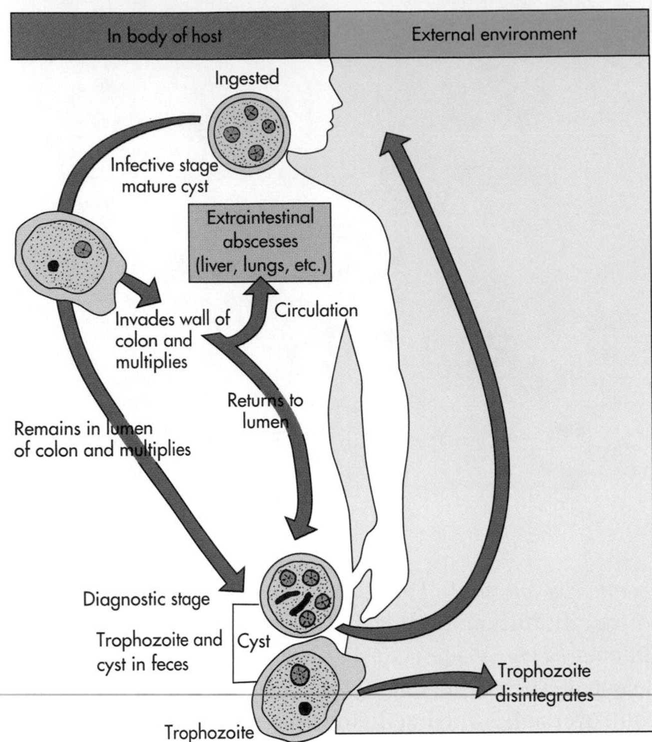

FIGURE 82–1. Life cycle of *Entamoeba histolytica.*

trophozoites is associated with a lethal alteration of host cell membrane permeability, resulting in an irreversible increase in intracellular calcium levels. The release of toxic neutrophil constituents after the lysis of neutrophils may contribute to the tissue destruction. Flask-shaped ulcerations of the intestinal mucosa are present with inflammation, hemorrhage, and secondary bacterial infection. Invasion into the deeper mucosa with extension into the peritoneal cavity may occur. This can lead to secondary involvement of other organs, primarily the liver but also the lungs, brain, and heart. Extraintestinal amebiasis is associated with trophozoites. Amoebae are found only in environments that have a low oxygen pressure, because the protozoa are killed by ambient oxygen concentrations.

Recently, lectin binding, zymodeme analysis, genome deoxyribonucleic acid (DNA) analysis, and staining with specific monoclonal antibodies have been used as markers to identify invasive strains of *E. histolytica.* It is now recognized that the ameba morphologically identified as *E. histolytica* is actually two distinct species. The pathogenic species is *E. histolytica*, and the nonpathogenic species is *E. dispar.* The zymodeme profiles and biochemical, molecular and immunogic differences are stable and support the existence of two species.

Epidemiology

E. histolytica has a worldwide distribution. Although it is found in cold areas such as Alaska, Canada, and Eastern Europe, its incidence is highest in tropical and subtropical regions that have poor sanitation and contaminated water. The average prevalence of infection in these areas is 10% to 15%, with as many as 50% of the population infected in some areas. Many of the infected individuals are asymptomatic carriers, who represent a reservoir for the spread of *E. histolytica* to others. The prevalence of infection in the United States is 1% to 2%.

Patients infected with *E. histolytica* pass noninfectious trophozoites and the infectious cysts in their stools. The trophozoites cannot survive in the external environment or in transport through the stomach if ingested. Therefore the main source of water and food contamination is the asymptomatic carrier who passes cysts. This is a particular problem in hospitals for the mentally ill, military and refugee camps, prisons, and crowded daycare centers. Flies and cockroaches can also serve as vectors for the transmission of *E. histolytica* cysts. Sewage containing cysts can contaminate water systems, wells, springs, and agricultural areas where human waste is used as fertilizer. Finally, cysts can be transmitted by oral-anal sexual practices, with amebiasis prevalent in homosexual populations. Direct trophozoite transmission in sexual encounters can produce cutaneous amebiasis.

Clinical Syndromes

The outcome of infection may result in a carrier state, intestinal amebiasis, or extraintestinal amebiasis. If the strain of *E. histolytica* has a low virulence, if the inoculum is low, or if the patient's immune system is intact, the organisms may reproduce, and cysts may be passed in stool specimens with no clinical symptoms. Although infections with *E. histolytica* may be asymptomatic, most asymptomatic individuals are infected with the noninvasive *E. dispar* as characterized by specific isoenzyme profiles (zymodemes), their susceptibility to complement-mediated lysis, and their failure to agglutinate in the presence of the lectin concanavalin A. Detection of carriers of *E. histolytica* in areas with a low endemicity is important for epidemiologic purposes.

Patients with intestinal amebiasis develop clinical symptoms related to the localized tissue destruction in the large intestine. These include abdominal pain, cramping, and colitis with diarrhea. Numerous bloody stools per day are characteristic of more severe disease. Systemic signs of infection (fever, leukocytosis, rigors) are present in patients with extraintestinal amebiasis. The liver is primarily involved because trophozoites in the blood are removed as they pass through this organ. Abscess formation is common. The right lobe is most commonly involved. Pain over the liver with hepatomegaly and elevation of the diaphragm is observed.

Laboratory Diagnosis

The identification of *E. histolytica* trophozoites (Figure 82–2) and cysts in stools and trophozoites in tissue is diagnostic of amoebic infection. Care must be taken to distinguish between these amoebae and commensal amoebae, as well as between these amoebae and polymorphonuclear leukocytes. Microscopic examination of stool specimens is inherently insensitive because the protozoa are not usually distributed homogeneously in the specimen and the parasites are concentrated in the intestinal ulcers and at the margins of the abscess, not in the stool or the necrotic center of the abscess. For this reason, multiple stool specimens should be collected. Extraintestinal amebiasis is sometimes diagnosed using scanning procedures for the liver and other organs. Specific serologic tests, together with microscopic examination of the abscess material, can confirm the diagnosis. Virtually all patients with hepatic amebiasis and most patients (more than 80%) with intestinal disease have positive serologic findings at the time of clinical presentation. This may be less useful in endemic areas where the prevalence of positive serologic results is higher. Examinations of stool specimens are often negative in extraintestinal disease. In addition to conventional microscopic and serologic tests, researchers have developed several immunologic tests for the detection of fecal antigen, as well as polymerase chain reaction and DNA-probe assays for the detection of pathogenic strains of *E. histolytica* (versus nonpathogenic *E. dispar*). These newer diagnostic approaches are promising and are commercially available.

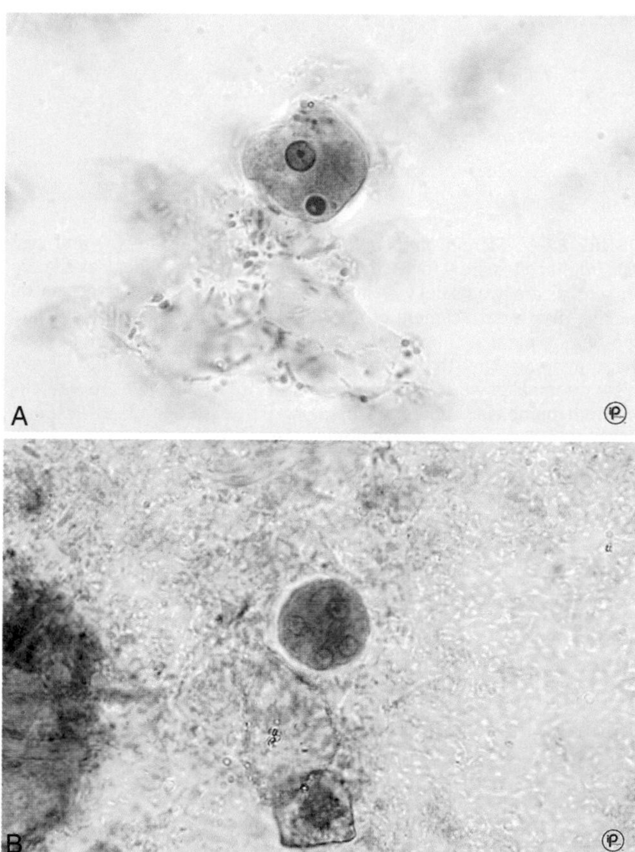

FIGURE 82–2. *Entamoeba histolytica* trophozoite **(A)** and cyst **(B)**. Trophozoites are motile and vary in size from 12 to 60 μm (average, 15 to 30 μm). The single nucleus in the cell is round with a central dot (karyosome) and an even distribution of chromatin granules around the nuclear membrane. Ingested erythrocytes may be in the cytoplasm. The cysts are smaller (10 to 20 μm, with an average size of 15 to 20 μm) and contain one to four nuclei (usually four). Round chromatoidal bars may be present in the cytoplasm. (From Marler LM et al: *Parasitology* CD-Rom, Indiana Pathology Images, 2003.)

Treatment, Prevention, and Control

Acute, fulminating amebiasis is treated with metronidazole followed by iodoquinol. Asymptomatic carriage can be eradicated with iodoquinol, diloxanide furoate, or paromomycin. As already noted, human infection results from the ingestion of food or water contaminated with human feces or as a result of specific sexual practices. The elimination of the cycle of infection requires the introduction of adequate sanitation measures and education about the routes of transmission. The chlorination and filtration of water supplies may limit the spread of these and other enteric protozoal infections but are not possible in many developing countries. Physicians should alert travelers to developing countries of the risks associated with the consumption of water (including ice cubes), unpeeled fruits, and raw vegetables. Water should be boiled and fruits and vegetables thoroughly cleaned before consumption.

OTHER INTESTINAL AMOEBAE

Other amoebae that can parasitize the human gastrointestinal tract include *E. coli, E. hartmanni, E. polecki, E. nana, I. bütschlii*, and *B. hominis*. *E. polecki*, which is primarily a parasite of pigs and monkeys, can cause human disease, a mild, transient diarrhea. The diagnosis of *E. polecki* infection is confirmed by the microscopic detection of cysts in stool specimens. Treatment is the same as for *E. histolytica* infections.

B. hominis, previously regarded as a nonpathogenic yeast, is now the center of considerable controversy concerning its taxonomic position and its pathogenicity. The organism is found in stool specimens from asymptomatic individuals and from persons with persistent diarrhea. It has been suggested that the presence of large numbers of

TABLE 82–1. Morphologic Identification of *Entamoeba histolytica* and *Entamoeba coli*

	E. histolytica	*E. coli*
Size (diameter; μm)		
Trophozoite	12–50 μm	20–30 μm
Cyst	10–20 μm	10–30 μm
Pattern of peripheral nuclear chromatin	Fine, dispersed ring	Coarse, clumped
Karyosome	Central, sharp	Eccentric, coarse
Ingested erythrocytes	Present	Absent
Cyst structure		
No. of nuclei	1–4	1–8
Chromatoidal bars	Rounded ends	Splintered, frayed ends

these parasites (five or more per oil-immersion microscopic field) in the absence of other intestinal pathogens indicates disease. Other investigators have concluded that "symptomatic blastocystosis" is attributable to an undetected pathogen or functional bowel problems. The organism may be detected in wet mounts or trichrome-stained smears of fecal specimens. Treatment with iodoquinol or metronidazole has been successful in eradicating the organisms from the intestine and alleviating symptoms. However, the definitive role of this organism in disease remains to be demonstrated.

The nonpathogenic intestinal amoebae are important because they must be differentiated from *E. histolytica*, *E. polecki*, and *B. hominis*. This is particularly true for *E. coli*, which is frequently detected in stool specimens collected from patients exposed to contaminated food or water. Accurate identification of intestinal amoebae requires careful microscopic examination of the cyst and trophozoite forms present in stained and unstained stool specimens (Table 82–1). Likewise, differentiation of *E. dispar* is now possible using specific immunologic reagents.

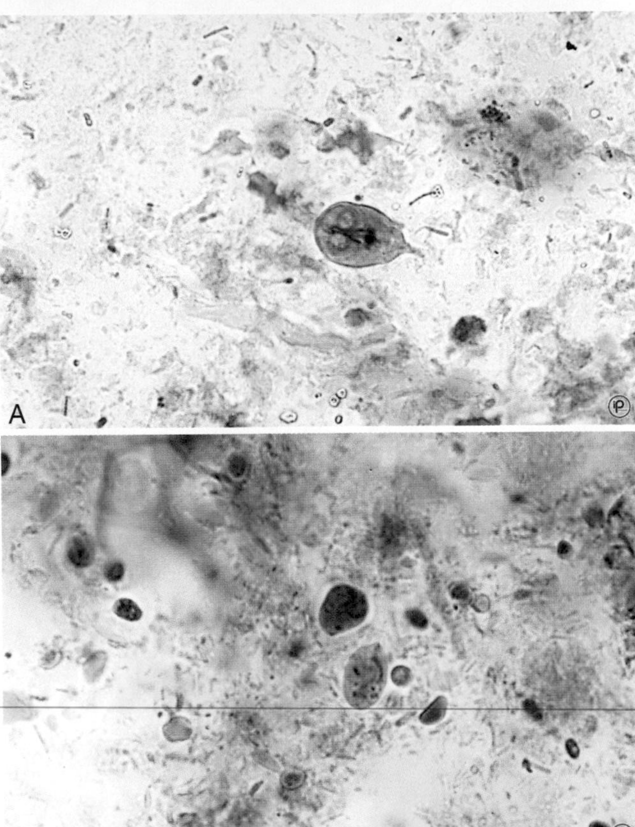

FIGURE 82–3. *Giardia lamblia (duodenalis)* trophozoite **(A)** and cyst **(B)**. Trophozoites are 9 to 12 μm long and 5 to 15 μm wide. Flagella are present, as are two nuclei with large central karyosomes, a large ventral sucking disk for attachment of the flagellate to the intestinal villi, and two oblong parabasal bodies below the nuclei. The morphology gives the appearance that the trophozoites are looking back at the viewer. Cysts are smaller—8 to 12 μm long and 7 to 10 μm wide. Four nuclei and four parabasal bodies are present. (From Marler LM et al: *Parasitology* CD-Rom, Indiana Pathology Images, 2003.)

Flagellates

The flagellates of clinical significance include *Giardia lamblia (duodenalis)*, *Dientamoeba fragilis*, and *Trichomonas vaginalis*. Nonpathogenic commensal flagellates such as *Chilomastix mesnili* (enteric) and *Trichomonas tenax* (oral) may also be observed. *Giardia* organisms, like *E. histolytica*, have cyst and trophozoite stages in their life cycles. In contrast, no cyst stage has been observed for *Trichomonas* or *Dientamoeba* species. Unlike the amoebae, most flagellates move by the lashing of flagella that pull the organisms through fluid environments. Diseases produced by flagellates are primarily the result of mechanical irritation and inflammation. For example, *G. lamblia (duodenalis)* attaches to the intestinal villi with an adhesive disk, resulting in localized tissue damage. The tissue invasion with extensive tissue destruction, as seen with *E. histolytica*, is rare with flagellates.

GIARDIA LAMBLIA (DUODENALIS)

Physiology and Structure

Both cyst and trophozoite forms of *G. lamblia* (*duodenalis*) are detected in fecal specimens from infected patients (Figure 82–3).

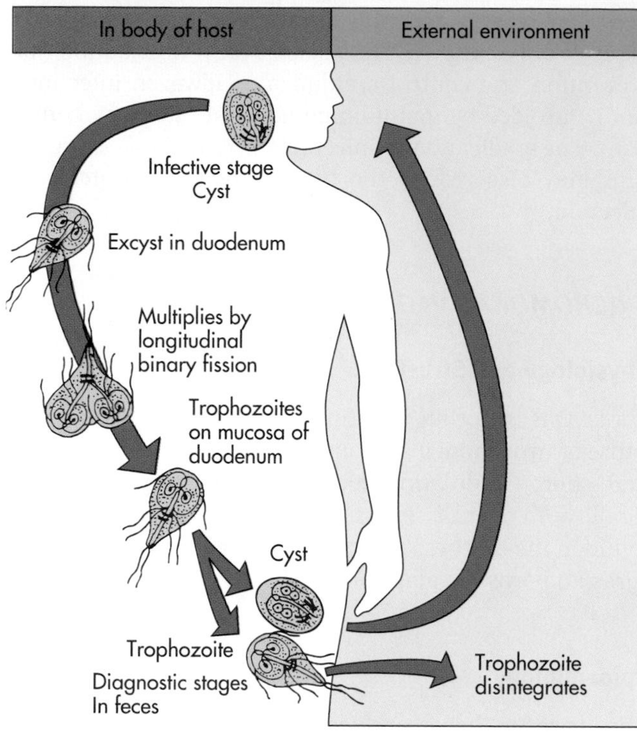

FIGURE 82–4. Life cycle of *Giardia lamblia (duodenalis).*

Pathogenesis

Infection with *G. lamblia (duodenalis)* is initiated by ingestion of cysts (Figure 82–4). The minimum infective dose for humans is estimated to be 10 to 25 cysts. Gastric acid stimulates excystation with the release of trophozoites in the duodenum and jejunum, where the organisms multiply by **binary fission.** The trophozoites can attach to the intestinal villi by a prominent ventral sucking disk. Although the tips of the villi may appear flattened and inflammation of the mucosa with hyperplasia of lymphoid follicles may be observed, frank tissue necrosis does not occur. In addition, metastatic spread of disease beyond the gastrointestinal tract is very rare.

Epidemiology

Giardia species has a worldwide distribution, and this flagellate has a sylvatic or "wilderness" distribution in many streams, lakes, and mountain resorts. This sylvatic distribution is maintained in reservoir animals, such as beavers and muskrats. Giardiasis is acquired by the consumption of inadequately treated contaminated water, ingestion of contaminated uncooked vegetables or fruits, or person-to-person spread by the fecal-oral or oral-anal route. The cyst stage is resistant to chlorine concentrations (1 to 2 parts per million) used in most water-treatment facilities. Thus adequate water treatment should include chemicals with filtration.

Risk factors associated with *Giardia* infections include poor sanitary conditions, travel to known endemic areas, consumption of inadequately treated water (e.g., from contaminated mountain streams), daycare centers, and oral-anal sexual practices. Infections may occur in outbreak and endemic forms within daycare centers and other institutional settings and among family members of infected children. Scrupulous attention to hand washing and treatment of all infected individuals are important in controlling the spread of infection in these settings.

Clinical Syndromes

Giardia infection can result in either asymptomatic carriage (observed in approximately 50% of infected individuals) or symptomatic disease ranging from mild diarrhea to a severe malabsorption syndrome. The incubation period before symptomatic disease develops ranges from 1 to 4 weeks (average, 10 days). The onset of disease is sudden, with foul-smelling, watery diarrhea; abdominal cramps; flatulence; and steatorrhea. Blood and pus are rarely present in stool specimens, which is consistent with the absence of tissue destruction. Spontaneous recovery generally occurs after 10 to 14 days, although a more chronic disease with multiple relapses may develop. This is particularly a problem for patients with immunoglobulin A deficiency or intestinal diverticula.

Laboratory Diagnosis

With the onset of diarrhea and abdominal discomfort, stool specimens should be examined for cysts and trophozoites (see Figure 82–3). *Giardia* species may occur in "showers," with many organisms present in the stool on a given day and few or none detected the next day. For this reason the physician should never accept the results of a single negative stool specimen as evidence that the patient is free of intestinal parasites. One stool specimen per day for 3 days should be examined. If stools remain persistently negative in a patient in whom giardiasis is highly suspected, additional specimens can be collected by duodenal aspiration, Entero-Test or string test, or biopsy of the upper small intestine. In addition to conventional microscopy, several immunologic tests for the detection of **fecal antigen** are available commercially. These tests include countercurrent immunoelectrophoresis, enzyme immunoassay, an immunochromatographic assay, and indirect immunofluorescent staining. Reported sensitivities range from 88% to 98% and specificities from 87% to 100%.

Treatment, Prevention, and Control

It is important to eradicate *Giardia* species from asymptomatic carriers and diseased patients. The drug of choice is metronidazole, with furazolidone, tinidazole, or quinacrine all acceptable alternatives. The prevention and control of giardiasis involves the avoidance of contaminated water and food, especially by travelers and outdoorsmen. Protection is afforded by boiling drinking water from streams and lakes or in countries with a high incidence of endemic disease. Maintenance of properly functioning filtration systems in municipal water supplies is also required because cysts are resistant to standard chlorination procedures. Public health efforts should be made to identify the reservoir of infection to prevent spread of disease. In addition, high-risk sexual behavior should be avoided.

DIENTAMOEBA FRAGILIS

Physiology and Structure

D. fragilis was initially classified as an amoeba; however, the internal structures of the trophozoite are typical of a flagellate. No cyst stage has been described.

Epidemiology

D. fragilis has a worldwide distribution. The transmission of the delicate trophozoite is not completely understood. Some observers believe the organism can be transported from person to person inside the protective shell of worm eggs, such as *E. vermicularis,* the pinworm. Transmission by the fecal-oral and oral-anal routes does occur.

Clinical Syndromes

Most infections with *D. fragilis* are asymptomatic, with colonization of the cecum and upper colon. However, some patients may develop symptomatic disease with abdominal discomfort, flatulence, intermittent diarrhea, anorexia, and weight loss. There is no evidence of tissue invasion with this flagellate, although irritation of the intestinal mucosa occurs.

Laboratory Diagnosis

Infection is confirmed by the microscopic examination of stool specimens in which typical trophozoites can be seen. The trophozoite is small (5 to 12 mm), with one or two nuclei. The central karyosome consists of four to six discrete granules. The excretion of the parasite may fluctuate markedly from day to day, and thus collection of several stool samples may be necessary. Examination of a purged stool sample may also be useful.

Treatment, Prevention, and Control

The therapy of choice for *D. fragilis* infection is iodoquinol, with tetracycline and paromomycin acceptable alternatives. The reservoir for this flagellate and the organism's life cycle are unknown. Thus specific recommendations for prevention and control are difficult. However, infections can be avoided by maintaining adequate sanitary conditions. The eradication of infections with *Enterobius* organisms may also reduce the transmission of *Dientamoeba* infection.

TRICHOMONAS VAGINALIS

Physiology and Structure

T. vaginalis is not an intestinal protozoan but rather the cause of urogenital infections. The flagellate's four flagella and short, undulating membrane are responsible for motility. *T. vaginalis* exists only as a trophozoite and is found in the urethras and vaginas of women and the urethras and prostate glands of men.

Epidemiology

This parasite has worldwide distribution, with sexual intercourse as the primary mode of transmission (Figure 82–5). Occasionally, infections have been transmitted by fomites (toilet articles, clothing), although this transmission is limited by the lability of the trophozoite form. Infants may be infected by passage through the mother's infected birth canal. The prevalence of this flagellate in developed countries is reported to be 5% to 20% in women and 2% to 10% in men.

Clinical Syndromes

Most infected women are asymptomatic or have a scant, watery vaginal discharge. Vaginitis may occur with more extensive inflammation and erosion of the epithelial lining that is associated with itching, burning, and painful urination. Men are primarily asymptomatic carriers who serve as a reservoir for infections in women. However, men occasionally experience urethritis, prostatitis, and other urinary tract problems.

Laboratory Diagnosis

The microscopic examination of vaginal or urethral discharge for characteristic trophozoites is the diagnostic method of choice (Figure 82–6). Stained (Giemsa, Papanicolaou) or unstained smears can be examined. The diagnostic yield may be improved by culturing the organism (93% sensitivity) or using monoclonal fluorescent antibody staining (86% sensitivity). A nucleic acid probe assay is also available commercially. Serologic tests may be useful in epidemiologic surveillance.

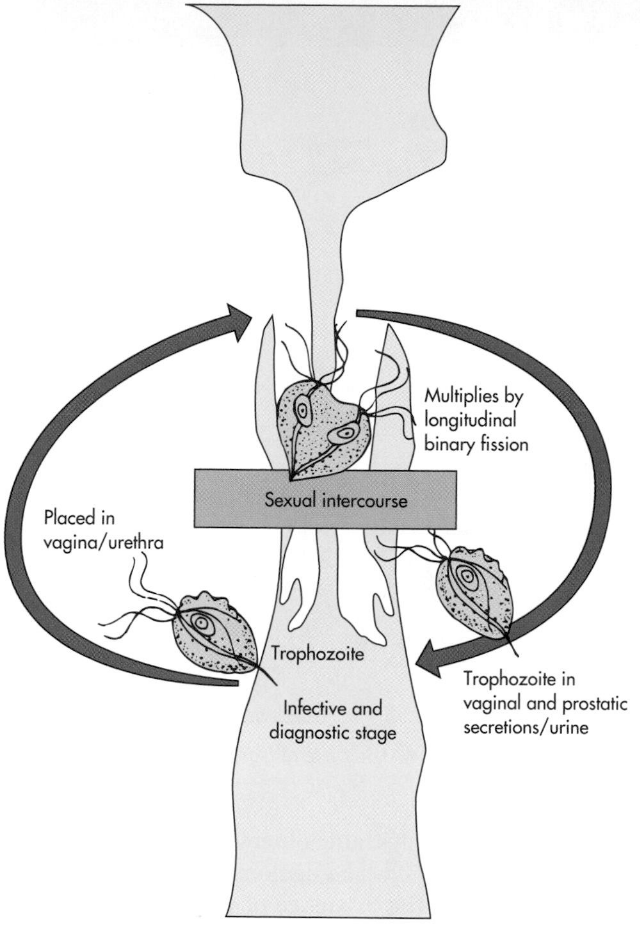

FIGURE 82–5. Life cycle of *Trichomonas vaginalis.*

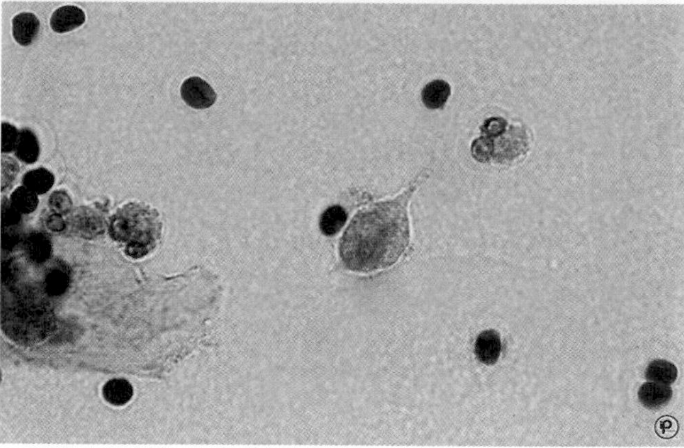

FIGURE 82–6. *Trichomonas vaginalis* trophozoite. The trophozoite is 7 to 23 μm long and 6 to 8 μm wide (average, 13 by 7 μm). The flagella and a short, undulating membrane are present at one side, and an axostyle extends through the center of the parasite. (From Marler LM et al: *Parasitology* CD-Rom, Indiana Pathology Images, 2003.)

Treatment, Prevention, and Control

The drug of choice is metronidazole. Both male and female sex partners must be treated to avoid reinfection. Resistance to metronidazole has been reported and may require retreatment with higher doses. Personal hygiene, avoidance of shared toilet articles and clothing, and safe sexual practices are important preventive actions. Elimination of carriage in men is critical for the eradication of disease.

Ciliates

The intestinal protozoan *Balantidium coli* is the only member of the ciliate group that is pathogenic for humans. Disease produced by *B. coli* is similar to amebiasis because the organisms elaborate proteolytic and cytotoxic substances that mediate tissue invasion and intestinal ulceration.

BALANTIDIUM COLI

Physiology and Structure

The life cycle of *B. coli* is simple, involving ingestion of infectious cysts, excystation, and invasion of trophozoites into the mucosal lining of the large intestine, cecum, and terminal ileum (Figure 82–7). The trophozoite is covered with rows of hairlike cilia that aid in motility. Morphologically more complex than amoebae, *B. coli* has a funnel-like primitive mouth called a **cytostome,** a large and a small nucleus involved in reproduction, food vacuoles, and two contractile vacuoles.

Epidemiology

B. coli is distributed worldwide. Swine and (less commonly) monkeys are the most important reservoirs. Infections are transmitted by the fecal-oral route; outbreaks are associated with contamination of water supplies with pig feces. Person-to-person spread, including through food handlers, has been implicated in outbreaks. Risk factors associated with human disease include contact with swine and substandard hygienic conditions.

Clinical Syndromes

As with other protozoan parasites, asymptomatic carriage of *B. coli* can exist. Symptomatic disease is characterized by abdominal pain and tenderness, tenesmus, nausea, anorexia, and watery stools with blood and pus. Ulceration of the intestinal mucosa, as with amebiasis, can be seen; a secondary complication caused by bacterial invasion into the eroded intestinal mucosa can occur. Extraintestinal invasion of other organs is extremely rare in balantidiasis.

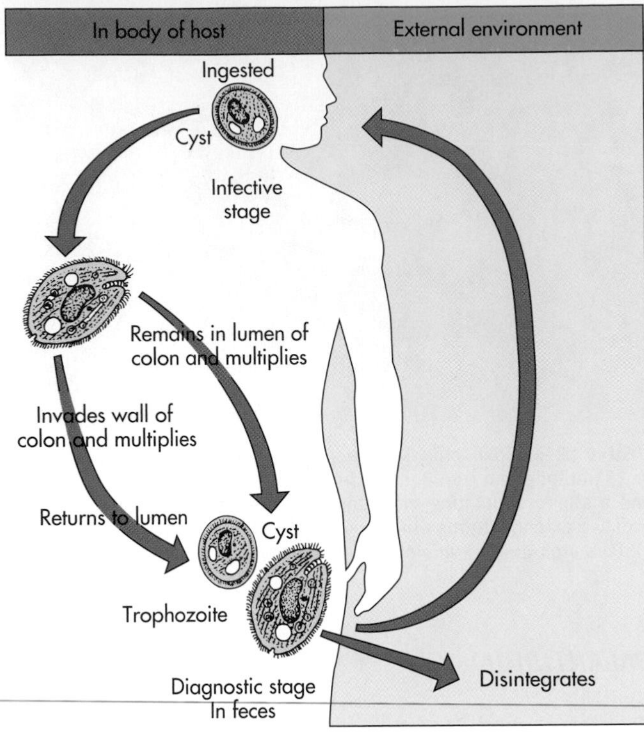

FIGURE 82–7. Life cycle of *Balantidium coli.*

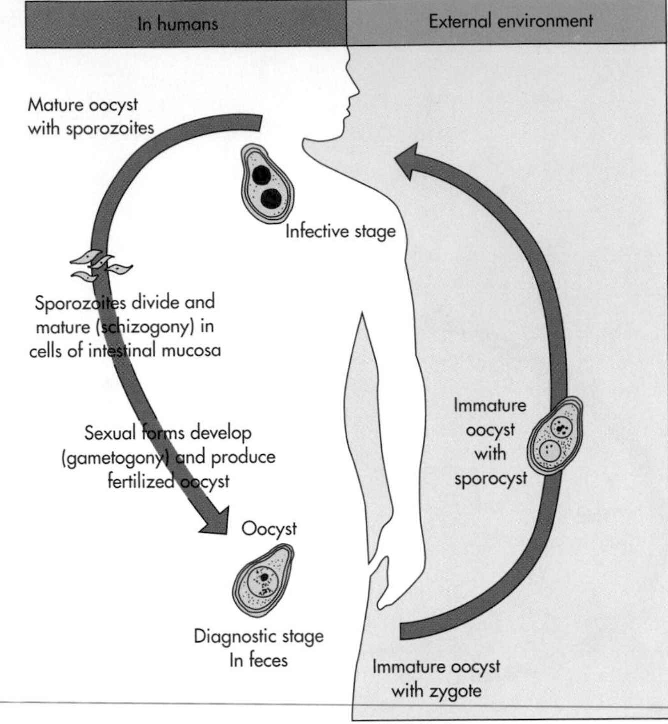

FIGURE 82–8. Life cycle of *Isospora* species.

Laboratory Diagnosis

Microscopic examination of feces for trophozoites and cysts is performed. The trophozoite is very large, varying in length from 50 to 200 µm and in width from 40 to 70 µm. The surface is covered with cilia, and the prominent internal structure is a **macronucleus.** A **micronucleus** is also present. Two pulsating, contractile vacuoles are also seen in fresh preparations of the trophozoites. The cyst is smaller (40 to 60 µm in diameter), is surrounded by a clear refractile wall, and has a single nucleus in the cytoplasm. *B. coli* is a large organism compared with other intestinal protozoa and is readily detected in fresh, wet microscopic preparations.

Treatment, Prevention, and Control

The drug of choice is tetracycline; iodoquinol and metronidazole are alternative antimicrobials. Actions for prevention and control are similar to those for amebiasis. Appropriate personal hygiene, maintenance of sanitary conditions, and the careful monitoring of pig feces are all important preventive measures.

Coccidia

Coccidia constitute a very large group called Apicomplexa, some members of which are discussed in this section with the intestinal parasites and others with the blood and tissue parasites. All *coccidia* demonstrate typical characteristics, especially the existence of asexual (schizogony) and sexual (gametogony) reproduction. Most members of the group also share alternative hosts; for example, in malaria, mosquitoes harbor the sexual cycle and humans the asexual cycle. *Coccidia* discussed in this chapter are *Isospora, Sarcocystis, Cryptosporidium,* and *Cyclospora* species.

ISOSPORA BELLI

Physiology and Structure

I. belli is a coccidian parasite of the intestinal epithelium. Both sexual and asexual reproduction can occur in the intestinal epithelium, resulting in tissue damage (Figure 82–8). The end product of gametogenesis is the oocyst, which is the diagnostic stage present in fecal specimens.

Epidemiology

Isospora organisms are distributed worldwide but are infrequently detected in stool specimens. Recently, however, this parasite has been reported with increasing frequency in healthy and immunocompromised patients. This is probably a result of the increased awareness of disease caused by *Isospora* species in patients with acquired immune deficiency syndrome (AIDS). Infection with this organism follows ingestion of contaminated food or water or oral-anal sexual contact.

Clinical Syndromes

Infected individuals may be asymptomatic carriers or suffer mild to severe gastrointestinal disease. Disease most commonly mimics giardiasis, with a malabsorption syndrome characterized by loose, foul-smelling stools. Chronic diarrhea with weight loss, anorexia, malaise, and fatigue can be seen, although it is difficult to separate this presentation from the patient's underlying disease.

Laboratory Diagnosis

Careful examination of concentrated stool sediment and special staining with iodine or a modified acid-fast procedure reveal the parasite (Figure 82–9). Small bowel biopsy has been used to establish the diagnosis when the results of tests on stool specimens are negative.

Treatment, Prevention, and Control

The drug of choice is trimethoprim-sulfamethoxazole, with the combination of pyrimethamine and sulfadiazine an acceptable alternative. Prevention and control are effected by maintaining personal hygiene and highly sanitary conditions and by avoiding oral-anal sexual contact.

SARCOCYSTIS SPECIES

Physician awareness of the genus *Sarcocystis* is important only in recognizing that it can be detected in stool specimens. *Sarcocystis* species can be isolated from pigs and cattle and are identical in all aspects to *Isospora* species with one exception: *Sarcocystis* oocysts rupture before passage in stool specimens, and only sporocysts are present.

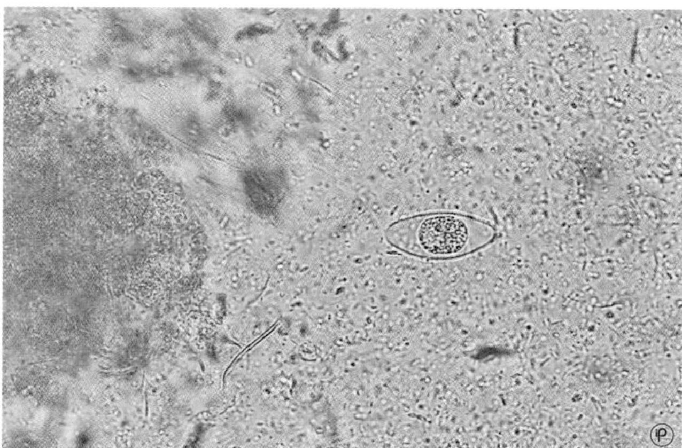

FIGURE 82–9. Immature oocyst of *Isospora* species. Oocysts are ovoid (approximately 25 µm long and 15 µm wide) with tapering ends. A developing sporocyst is seen within the cytoplasm. (From Marler LM et al: *Parasitology* CD-Rom, Indiana Pathology Images, 2003.)

CRYPTOSPORIDIUM SPECIES

Physiology and Structure

The life cycle of *Cryptosporidium* species is typical of coccidians, as is the intestinal disease, but this species differs in the intracellular location in the epithelial cells. In contrast to the deep intracellular invasion observed with *Isospora* species, *Cryptosporidium* organisms are found just within the brush border of the intestinal epithelium. The coccidia attach to the surface of the cells and replicate by a process that involves **schizogony** (Figure 82–10). *C. parvum* is the most common species of *Cryptosporidium* infecting humans. Other species, including *C. meleagridis, C. felis,* and *C. muris,* have also been isolated from infested immunocompromised individuals.

Epidemiology

Cryptosporidium species are distributed worldwide. Infection is reported in a wide variety of animals, including mammals, reptiles, and fish. Waterborne transmission of cryptosporidiosis is well documented as an important route of infection. The massive outbreak of cryptosporidiosis in Milwaukee (approximately 300,000 individuals infected) was linked to contamination of the municipal water supply. Cryptosporidia are resistant to the usual water-purification procedures (chlorination and ozone), and it is believed that runoff of local waste and surface water into municipal water supplies is an important source of contamination. Zoonotic spread from animal reservoirs to humans, as well as person-to-person spread by fecal-oral and oral-anal routes, is also common means of infection. Veterinary personnel, animal handlers, and homosexuals are at particularly high risk for infection. Many outbreaks have now been described in daycare centers where fecal-oral transmission is common.

CLINICAL SYNDROMES

As with other protozoan infections, exposure to *Cryptosporidium* organisms may result in asymptomatic carriage. Disease in previously healthy individuals is usually a mild, self-limiting **enterocolitis** characterized by watery diarrhea without blood. Spontaneous remission after an average of 10 days is characteristic. In contrast, disease in immunocompromised patients (e.g., patients with AIDS), characterized by 50 or more stools per day

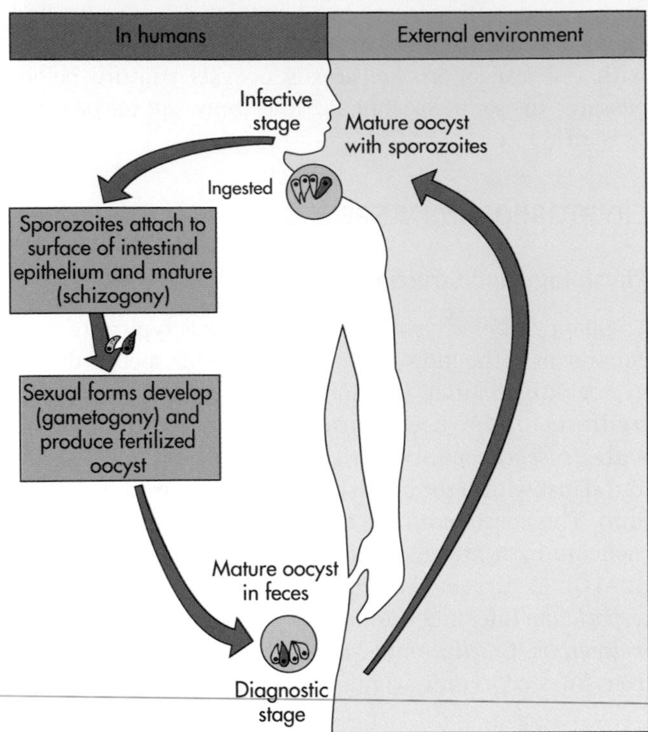

FIGURE 82–10. Life cycle of *Cryptosporidium* species.

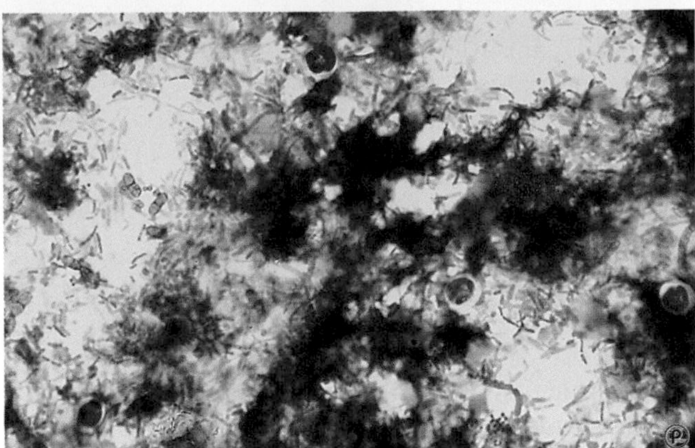

FIGURE 82–11. Acid-fast stained (red) *Cryptosporidium* oocysts (approximately 5 to 7 μm in diameter). (From Marler LM et al: *Parasitology* CD-Rom, Indiana Pathology Images, 2003.)

and tremendous fluid loss, can be severe and last for months to years. In some patients with AIDS, disseminated *Cryptosporidium* infections have been reported.

LABORATORY DIAGNOSIS

Cryptosporidium may be detected in large numbers in unconcentrated stool specimens obtained from immunocompromised individuals with diarrhea. Oocysts may be concentrated with the modified zinc sulfate centrifugal flotation technique or by Sheather's sugar flotation procedure. Specimens may be stained using the modified **acid-fast** method (Figure 82–11) or by an indirect immunofluorescence assay. Both an enzyme immunoassay and an immunochromatographic assay for detecting fecal antigen are commercially available. The number of oocysts shed in stool may fluctuate; therefore a minimum of three specimens should be examined. Serologic procedures for diagnosing and monitoring infections are under investigation but are not yet widely available.

TREATMENT, PREVENTION, AND CONTROL

Unfortunately, no broadly effective therapy has been developed for managing *Cryptosporidium* infections in immunocompromised patients. Therapeutic information is largely based on isolated reports and anecdotal information. Spiramycin may help control the diarrhea in some patients in the early stages of AIDS who have cryptosporidiosis, but it is ineffective in patients who have progressed to the later stages of AIDS. Spiramycin was no more effective than placebo in treating cryptosporidial diarrhea in infants. Recently, nitazoxanide was approved by the Food and Drug Administration (FDA) for the treatment of cryptosporidiosis in children ages 1 to 11 years. Reports concerning efficacy of azithromycin and paromomycin are promising, but these need confirmation. Therapy consists primarily of supportive measures to restore the tremendous fluid loss from the watery diarrhea.

Because of the widespread distribution of this organism in humans and other animals, preventing infection is difficult. The same methods of improved personal hygiene and sanitation used for other intestinal protozoa should be maintained for this disease. Contaminated water supplies should be treated with chlorination and filtration. In addition, avoidance of high-risk sexual activities is critical.

CYCLOSPORA SPECIES

Physiology and Structure

Cyclospora is a coccidian parasite that is taxonomically related to *Isospora* species, *Cryptosporidium parvum* and *Toxoplasma gondii.* A single species infecting humans, *Cyclospora cayetanensis,* has been identified thus far.

Although the details of its life cycle have yet to be determined, *Cyclospora* organisms are similar to *Isospora* in that oocysts are excreted unsporulated and require a period of time outside the host for maturation to occur. The pathogenic mechanisms by which *Cyclospora* species causes clinical illness are unknown; however, the organism usually infects the upper small bowel and causes pronounced histopathologic changes. The organism is found within vacuoles in the cytoplasm of jejunal epithelial cells, and its presence is associated with inflammatory changes, villous atrophy, and crypt hyperplasia.

The morphologic characteristics of *Cyclospora* species are similar to those of *Isopora* species and *C. parvum*, with a few exceptions. The oocysts of *Cyclospora* species are spherical and are 8 to 10 µm in diameter as opposed to the smaller oocysts of *C. parvum* (4 to 6 µm) and the much larger elliptical oocysts of *Isospora* species (15 to 25 µm). The oocysts of *Cyclospora* species contain two sporocysts, each of which contain two sporozoites, which in turn contain a membrane-bound nucleus and micronemes characteristic of the apicomplexans. In contrast, the *Cryptosporidium* oocyst contains four naked, or nonencysted, sporozoites, whereas the *Isospora* oocyst contains two sporocysts, each containing four sporozoites.

Epidemiology

As with *Cryptosporidium*, *Cyclospora* species is widely distributed throughout the world and infects a variety of reptiles, birds, and mammals. Although direct animal-to-human or person-to-person transmission has not been documented, there is now compelling evidence that *Cyclospora* infection is acquired through contaminated water. In areas of endemicity, such as Nepal, studies have documented an annual surge of cyclosporiasis that coincides with the rainy season. The prevalence of infection (symptomatic and asymptomatic) ranges from 2% to 18% in endemic areas and is estimated at 0.1% to 0.5% in developed countries. Recent outbreaks in the United States have occurred during the summer months, and although no source has been identified, transmission via contaminated water has been suggested. Like *Cryptosporidium*, *Cyclospora* species is resistant to chlorination and is not readily detected by methods used currently to ensure the safety of supplies of drinking water.

Clinical Syndromes

The clinical manifestations of cyclosporiasis resemble those of cryptosporidiosis and include mild nausea, anorexia, abdominal cramping, and watery diarrhea. Fatigue, malaise, flatulence, and bloating have also been reported. In immunocompetent hosts, diarrhea is self-limited but may be prolonged and last for weeks. Among immunocompromised people, specifically patients infected with the human immunodeficiency virus (HIV), clinical illness is typically prolonged and severe and is associated with a high rate of recurrence. Biliary tract infection with *Cyclospora* infection has been reported in two patients with AIDS.

Laboratory Diagnosis

The diagnosis of cyclosporiasis is based on the microscopic detection of oocysts in stool. Oocysts may be detected by light microscopic examination of unstained fecal material (wet mount), where they appear as nonrefractile, spherical to oval, slightly wrinkled bodies measuring 8 to 10 µm in diameter; they have an internal cluster of membrane-bound globules (Figure 82–12). In fresh specimens, *Cyclospora* organisms fluoresce when examined with an ultraviolet fluorescence microscope fitted with a 365-nm excitation filter.

Cyclospora oocysts may be concentrated with the modified zinc sulfate centrifugal flotation technique or by Sheather's sugar flotation procedure. Organisms are acid-fast and thus can be detected using one of the many acid-fast staining techniques, including the modified Ziehl-Neelsen stain or the Kinyoun acid-fast stain (Figure 82–13). A distinguishing feature of *Cyclospora* species is its variable appearance on acid-fast staining, which ranges from unstained to mottled pink to deep red.

The relative sensitivity, specificity, and predictive value of the various methods for diagnosing *Cyclospora* infection are not known. Currently, there are no immunodiagnostic techniques to aid in the diagnosis and monitoring of these infections. The rudimentary nature of the available diagnostic techniques and the incomplete understanding of the disease process may contribute to underrecognition of *Cyclospora* infection.

Treatment, Prevention, and Control

The effectiveness of trimethoprim-sulfamethoxazole has been demonstrated in anecdotal reports; in a large, open-label study of patients infected with HIV; and in a placebo-controlled trial. In HIV-infected patients, it appears that the high rate of recurrence can be attenuated with long-term suppressive therapy with trimethoprim-sulfamethoxazole. Although numerous additional agents,

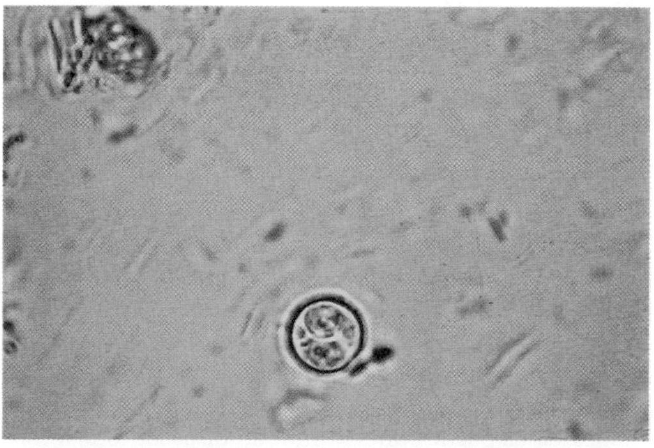

FIGURE 82–12. Sporulated oocyst of *Cyclospora cayetanensis*. The oocysts measure 8 to 10 µm in diameter and contain two sporocysts with two sporozoites. (Saline wet mount, magnification 900×.) (Courtesy Mr. J Williams; from Peters W, Giles HM: *Color atlas of tropical medicine and parasitology*, ed 4, London, 1995, Mosby-Wolfe.)

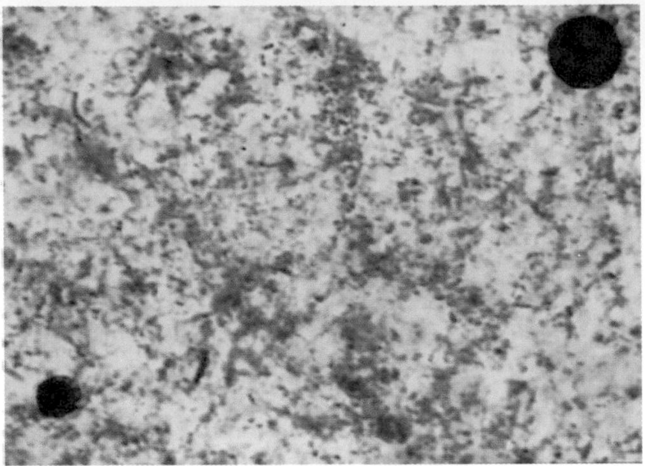

FIGURE 82–13. Oocysts of *Cryptosporidium parvum (lower left)* and *Cyclospora cayetanensis (upper right)*. Both parasites stain red with Ziehl-Neelsen stain; however, *Cyclospora* organisms typically take up variable amounts of the stain, and the oocysts are larger (8 to 10 μm compared with 4 to 6 μm). (Courtesy Mr. J Williams; from Peters W, Giles HM: *Color atlas of tropical medicine and parasitology*, ed 4, London, 1995, Mosby-Wolfe.)

including metronidazole, norfloxacin, quinacrine, nalidixic acid, tinidazole, and diloxanide furoate, have been used in various trials, the effectiveness of any one of these agents has not been proved.

As with *Cryptosporidium* species, prevention of *Cyclospora* infection is difficult. Although *Cyclospora* organisms appear resistant to chlorination, the treatment of water supplies with chlorination and filtration remains a reasonable practice. In addition, the same methods of improved personal hygiene and sanitation used for other intestinal protozoa should be used as preventive measures for this disease.

Microsporidia

PHYSIOLOGY AND STRUCTURE

Microsporidia are obligate intracellular pathogens belonging to the phylum Microspora. They are considered to be primitive eukaryotic organisms because they lack mitochondria, peroxisomes, Golgi membranes, and other typically eukaryotic organelles. The parasites are characterized by the structure of their spores, which have a complex tubular extrusion mechanism used for injecting the infective material (sporoplasma) into cells. Microsporidia have been detected in human tissues and implicated as participants in human disease. To date, six genera of Microsporidia *(Encephalitozoon, Pleistophora, Nosema, Vittaforma, Trachipleistophora,* and *Enterocytozoon)* and unclassified *Microsporidium* species have been reported in humans.

PATHOGENESIS

Infection with Microsporidia is initiated by the ingestion of spores. After ingestion the spores pass into the duodenum, where the sporoplasm with its nuclear material is injected into an adjacent cell in the small intestine. Once inside a suitable host cell the Microsporidia multiply extensively either within a **parasitophorous** vacuole or free within the cytoplasm. The intracellular multiplication includes a phase of repeated divisions by binary fission **(merogony)** and a phase culminating in spore formation **(sporogony).** The parasites spread from cell to cell, causing cell death and local inflammation. Although some species are highly selective in the cell type that they invade, collectively the microspora are capable of infecting every organ of the body, and disseminated infections have been described in severely immunocompromised individuals. After sporogony the mature spores containing the infective sporoplasm may be excreted into the environment, thus continuing the cycle.

EPIDEMIOLOGY

Microsporidia are distributed worldwide and have a wide host range among invertebrate and vertebrate animals. *Enterocytozoon bieneusi* and *Encephalitozoon (Septata) intestinalis* have gained increasing attention as causes of chronic diarrhea in patients with AIDS. Both *Encephalitozoon*-like and *Enterocytozoon*-like organisms have been reported in the tissues of AIDS patients with hepatitis and peritonitis. *Trachipleistophora* and *Nosema* are known to cause myositis in immunocompromised patients. *Nosema* species has caused localized keratitis and disseminated infection in a child with severe combined immunodeficiency. *Microsporidium* species and *Encephalitozoon hellem* have caused infection of the human cornea.

Although the reservoir for human infection is unknown, transmission is likely accomplished by ingestion of spores that have been shed in the urine and feces of infected animals or individuals. As with cryptosporidial infection, individuals with AIDS and other cellular immune defects appear to be at increased risk for infection with microsporidia.

CLINICAL SYNDROMES

Clinical signs and symptoms of microsporidiosis are quite variable in the few human cases reported. Intestinal infection caused by *E. bieneusi* in patients with AIDS is marked by persistent and debilitating diarrhea similar to that seen in patients with cryptosporidiosis, cyclosporiasis, or isosporiasis. The clinical presentation of infection with other species of *Microspora* depends on the organ system involved and ranges from localized ocular pain and loss of vision (*Microsporidium* and *Nosema* species) to neurologic disturbances and hepatitis *(Encephalitozoon cuniculi)* to a

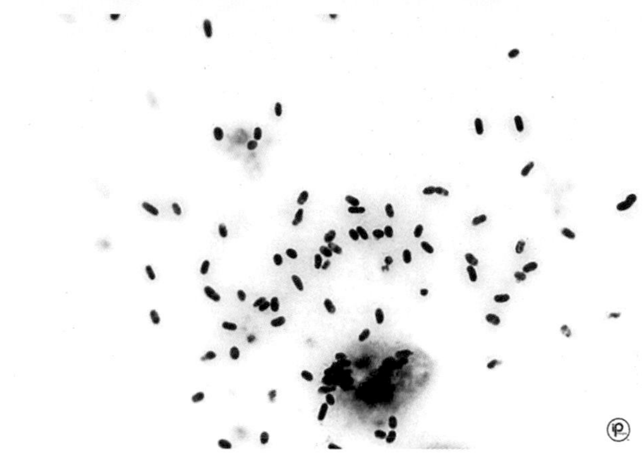

FIGURE 82–14. Gram-positive spores of *Encephalitozoon* species. (From Marler LM et al: *Parasitology* CD-Rom, Indiana Pathology Images, 2003.)

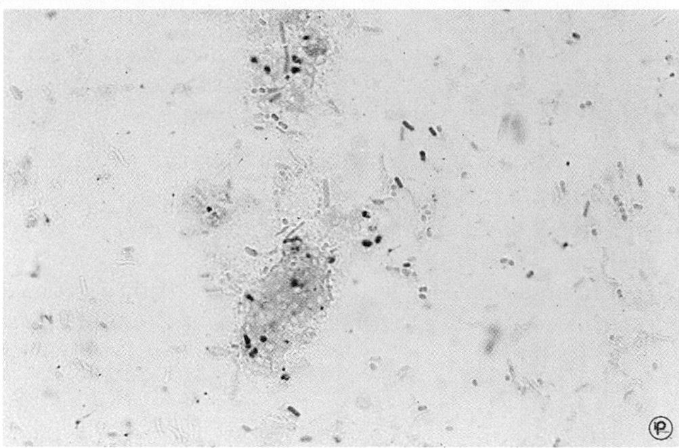

FIGURE 82–15. Smear of formalin-fixed stool specimen showing pinkish-red–stained microsporidia spores. Bacteria are stained a faint green. (Chromotrope-based stain, magnification 1000X.) (From Marler LM et al: *Parasitology* CD-Rom, Indiana Pathology Images, 2003.)

more generalized picture of dissemination with fever, vomiting, diarrhea, and malabsorption (*Nosema* species). In a report of disseminated infection with *Nosema connori*, the organism was observed involving the muscles of the stomach, bowel, arteries, diaphragm, and heart and the parenchymal cells of the liver, lungs, and adrenal glands.

LABORATORY DIAGNOSIS

Diagnosis of microsporidia infection may be made by detection of the organisms in biopsy material and by light microscopic examination of cerebrospinal fluid and urine. Spores measuring between 1 and 2 μm may be visualized by Gram (gram-positive), acid-fast, periodic acid–Schiff, immunochemical, and Giemsa staining techniques (Figure 82–14). A chromotrope-based staining tech-nique for light-microscopic detection of *E. bieneusi* and *Encephalitozoon (Septata) intestinalis* spores in stool and duodenal aspirates has also been described (Figure 82–15). Electron microscopy is considered the gold standard for diagnostic confirmation of microsporidiosis; however, its sensitivity is unknown. Additional diagnostic techniques, including polymerase chain reaction, culture, and serologic testing, are under investigation. These techniques are not yet considered reliable enough for routine diagnosis.

TREATMENT, PREVENTION, AND CONTROL

There is no completely effective treatment for microsporidian infections. Treatment with albendazole has resulted in clinical cure of HIV-associated encephalitozoonosis. Likewise, some patients treated with sulfa drugs have survived. Oral fumagillin administration has resulted in transient improvement in a small study of HIV-associated diarrhea caused by *E. bieneusi*. Albendazole is the current drug of choice for ocular *(E. hellem, E. cuniculi, Vitaforma corneae [Nosema corneum])*, intestinal *(E. bieneusi, Encephalitazoon [Septata] intestinalis)* and disseminated (*E. hellem, E. cuniculi, E. intestinalis, Pleistophora* spp.) microsporidiosis.

As with *Cryptosporidium*, preventing microsporidian infection is difficult. The same methods of improved personal hygiene and sanitation used for other intestinal protozoa should be maintained with this disease.

CASE STUDY AND QUESTIONS

A 31-year-old female veterinarian complained of diarrhea that she had experienced for 2 weeks. The diarrhea was described as thin, watery, and nonbloody. The patient described 10 to 14 diarrheal stools per day, the frequency of which was not influenced by a variety of over-the-counter antidiarrheal medications.

Physical examination revealed a well-developed, well-nourished woman who appeared somewhat fatigued and mildly dehydrated. The workup included a negative HIV serologic test, a normal flexible sigmoidoscope examination, and a negative stool culture for bacterial pathogens. A microscopic examination of the stool for white blood cells was negative, as was a test for Clostridium difficile *toxin. A stool specimen was sent for ova and parasite examination and, after appropriate concentration measures, demonstrated acid-fast oocysts.*

1. Which parasite was found in the patient's stool?
2. What was the likely source of this individual's infection?
3. If this individual were HIV positive, what other intestinal pathogens would have been considered?
4. Other than conventional microscopy, what other methods could have been used to diagnose this infection?
5. Should this patient have received specific antimicrobial therapy? If so, what would have been prescribed? If not, why not?

Bibliography

Adam RD: Biology of *Giardia lamblia, Clin Microbiol Rev* 14:447-475, 2001.

Clark DP: New insights into human cryptosporidiosis, *Clin Microbiol Rev* 12:554-563, 1999.

Connor DH et al, editors: *Pathology of infectious diseases,* vol II, Stamford, Conn, 1997, Appleton & Lange.

Espinosa-Cantellano M, Martinez-Palomo A: Pathogenesis of intestinal amebiasis: From molecules to disease, *Clin Microbiol Rev* 13:318-331, 2000.

Faubert G: Immune response to *Giardia duodenalis, Clin Microbiol Rev* 13:35-54, 2000.

Garcia LS, editor: *Diagnostic medical parasitology,* ed 4, Washington, 2001, ASM Press.

Gardner TB, Hill DR: Treatment of giardiasis, *Clin Microbiol Rev* 14:114-128, 2001.

Hunter PR, Nichols G: Epidemiology and clinical features of *Cryptosporidium* infection in immunocompromised patients, *Clin Microbiol Rev* 15:145-154, 2002.

Leber AL, Novak SM: Intestinal and urogenital amebae, flagellates, and ciliates. In Murray PR et al, editors: *Manual of clinical microbiology,* ed 8, Washington, 2003, American Society for Microbiology.

Ortega YR, Arrowood M: *Cryptosporidium, Cyclospora,* and *Isospora.* In Murray PR et al, editors: *Manual of clinical microbiology,* ed 8, Washington, 2003, American Society for Microbiology.

Peters W, Giles HM: *Color atlas of tropical medicine and parasitology,* ed 4, London, 1995, Mosby-Wolfe.

Schwartz DA et al: Pathology of microsporidiosis: Emerging parasitic infections in patients with acquired immunodeficiency syndrome, *Arch Pathol Lab Med* 120:173-188, 1996.

Soave R: Cyclospora: An overview, *Clin Infect Dis* 23:429-437, 1996.

Tanyuksel M, Petri WA Jr: Laboratory diagnosis of amebiasis, *Clin Microbiol Rev* 16:713-729, 2003.

Weber R, Canning EU: Microsporidia. In Murray PR et al, editors: *Manual of clinical microbiology,* ed 8, Washington, 2003, American Society for Microbiology.

Wittner M, Weiss LM, editors: The microsporidia and microsporidiosis, Washington, 1999, ASM Press.

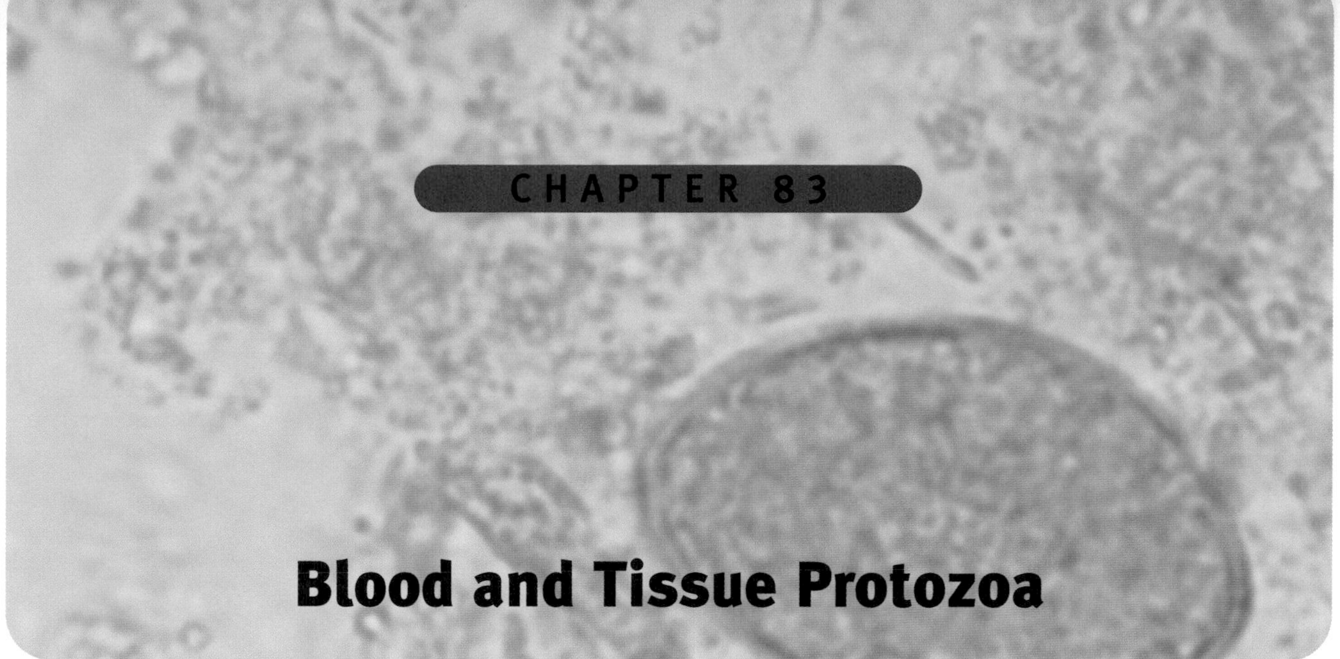

CHAPTER 83

Blood and Tissue Protozoa

The protozoa of blood and tissues are closely related to the intestinal protozoan parasites in practically all aspects except for their sites of infection (Box 83–1). The malaria parasites *(Plasmodium* species*)* infect both blood and tissues.

Plasmodium Species

Plasmodia are coccidian or sporozoan parasites of blood cells, and as seen with other coccidia, they require two hosts: the mosquito for the sexual reproductive stages and humans and other animals for the asexual reproductive stages. Infection with *Plasmodium* spp. (i.e., malaria) accounts for 1 to 5 billion febrile episodes and 1 to 3 million deaths annually, 85% of which are in Africa.

The four species of plasmodia that infect humans are *Plasmodium vivax, Plasmodium ovale, Plasmodium malariae,* and *Plasmodium falciparum* (Table 83–1). These species share a common life cycle, as illustrated in Figure 83–1. Human infection is initiated by the bite of an *Anopheles* mosquito, which introduces infectious plasmodia **sporozoites** via its saliva into the circulatory system. The sporozoites are carried to the parenchymal cells of the liver, where asexual reproduction **(schizogony)** occurs. This phase of growth is termed the **exoerythrocytic** cycle and lasts 8 to 25 days, depending on the plasmodial species. Some species (e.g., *P. vivax, P. ovale*) can establish a dormant hepatic phase in which the sporozoites (called **hypnozoites** or sleeping forms) do not divide. The presence of these viable plasmodia can lead to the relapse of infections months to years after the initial clinical disease (relapsing malaria). The hepatocytes eventually rupture, liberating the plasmodia (termed **merozoites** at this stage), which in turn attach to specific receptors on the surface of erythrocytes and enter the cells, thus initiating the erythrocytic cycle.

Asexual replication progresses through a series of stages (ring, trophozoite, schizont) that culminates in the rupture of the erythrocyte, releasing up to 24 merozoites, which initiates another cycle of replication by infecting other erythrocytes. Some merozoites also develop within erythrocytes into male and female **gametocytes.** If a mosquito ingests mature male and female gametocytes during a blood meal, the sexual reproductive cycle of malaria can be initiated, with the eventual production of sporozoites infectious for humans. This sexual reproductive stage within the mosquito is necessary for the maintenance of malaria within a population.

Most malaria seen in the United States is acquired by visitors or residents of countries with endemic disease (imported malaria). However, the appropriate vector *Anopheles* mosquito is found in several sections of the United States, and domestic transmission of disease has been observed (introduced malaria). In addition to transmission by mosquitoes, malaria can also be acquired by blood transfusions from an infected donor (transfusion malaria). This type of transmission can also occur among narcotic addicts who share needles and syringes ("mainline" malaria). Congenital acquisition, although rare, is also a possible mode of transmission (congenital malaria).

PLASMODIUM VIVAX

Physiology and Structure

P. vivax (Figure 83–2) is selective in that it invades only young, immature erythrocytes. In infections caused by *P. vivax,* infected red blood cells are usually enlarged and contain numerous pink granules or **Schüffner's dots,** the trophozoite is ring shaped but amoeboid in appear-

BOX 83–1. Medically Important Blood and Tissue Protozoa

Plasmodium species
Babesia species
Toxoplasma species
Sarcocystis species
Acanthamoeba species
Balamuthia species
Naegleria species
Leishmania species
Trypanosoma species

TABLE 83–1. Human Malarial Parasites

Parasite	Disease
Plasmodium vivax	Benign tertian or vivax malaria
P. ovale	Benign tertian or ovale malaria
P. malariae	Quartan or malarial malaria
P. falciparum	Malignant tertian or falciparum malaria

FIGURE 83–1. Life cycle of *Plasmodium* species.

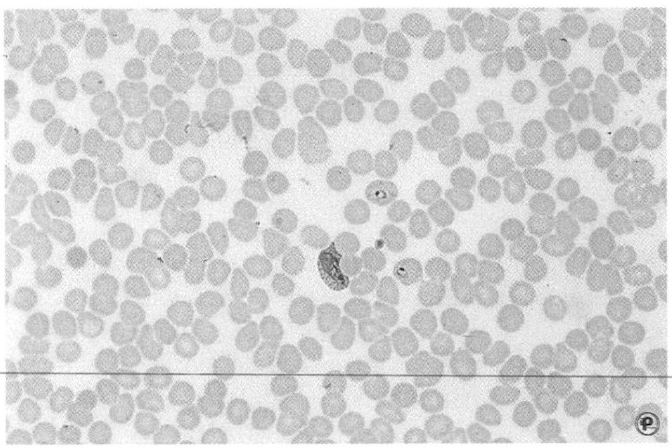

FIGURE 83–2. *Plasmodium vivax* ring forms and young trophozoites. Note the multiple stages of the parasite (rings and trophozoite) seen in the peripheral blood smear, the enlarged parasitized erythrocytes, and the presence of Schüffner's dots with the trophozoite form. These are characteristic of *P. vivax* infections. (From Marler LM et al: *Parasitology* CD-Rom, Indiana Pathology Images, 2003.)

ance, more mature trophozoites and erythrocytic schizonts containing up to 24 merozoites are present, and the gametocytes are round. These characteristics are helpful in identifying the specific plasmodial species, which is important for the treatment of malaria.

Epidemiology

P. vivax is the most prevalent of the human plasmodia, with the widest geographic distribution, including the tropics, subtropics, and temperate regions.

Clinical Syndromes

After an incubation period (usually 10 to 17 days) the patient experiences vague influenza-like symptoms with headache, muscle pains, photophobia, anorexia, nausea, and vomiting.

As the infection progresses, increased numbers of rupturing erythrocytes liberate merozoites and toxic cellular debris and hemoglobin into the circulation. Together, these produce the typical pattern of chills, fever, and malarial rigors. These **paroxysms** usually reappear periodically (generally every 48 hours) as the cycle of infection, replication, and cell lysis progresses. The paroxysms may remain relatively mild or progress to severe attacks, with hours of sweating, chills, shaking, persistently high temperatures (103° to 106°F [39° to 41°C]), and exhaustion.

P. vivax causes "benign tertian malaria," which refers to the cycle of paroxysms every 48 hours (in untreated patients) and the fact that most patients tolerate the attacks and can survive for years without treatment. If left untreated, however, chronic *P. vivax* infections can lead to brain, kidney, and liver damage as a result of the malarial pigment, cellular debris, and capillary plugging of these organs by masses of adherent erythrocytes.

Laboratory Diagnosis

Microscopic examination of thick and thin films of blood is the method of choice for confirming the clinical diagnosis of malaria and identifying the specific species responsible for disease. The thick film is a concentration method and may be used to detect the presence of organisms. With training, thick films may be used to diagnose the species as well. The thin film is most useful for establishing species identification. Blood films can be taken at any time over the course of the infection, but the best time is midway between paroxysms of chills and fever, when the greatest numbers of intracellular organisms are present. It may be necessary to take repeated films at intervals of 4 to 6 hours.

Serologic procedures are available, but they are used primarily for epidemiologic surveys or for screening blood donors. Serologic findings usually remain positive for approximately a year, even after complete treatment of the infection.

Treatment, Prevention, and Control

The treatment of *P. vivax* infection involves a combination of supportive measures and chemotherapy. Bed rest, relief of fever and headache, regulation of fluid balance, and in some cases, blood transfusion, are supportive therapies.

The chemotherapeutic regimens are as follows:

1. Suppressive—aimed at avoiding infection and clinical symptoms (i.e., a form of prophylaxis)
2. Therapeutic—aimed at eradicating the erythrocytic cycle
3. Radical cure—aimed at eradicating the exoerythrocytic cycle in the liver
4. Gametocidal—aimed at destroying erythrocytic gametocytes to prevent mosquito transmission

Chloroquine is the drug of choice for the suppression and therapeutic treatment of *P. vivax*, followed by primaquine for radical cure and elimination of gametocytes. Chloroquine-resistant forms of *P. vivax* have emerged in Indonesia, the Solomon Islands, New Guinea, and Brazil. Patients infected with chloroquine-resistant *P. vivax* may be treated with other agents, including mefloquine ± artesunate, quinine, pyrimethamine-sulfadoxine (Fansidar), and doxycycline. Primaquine is especially effective in preventing a relapse from the latent forms of *P. vivax* in the liver. Because antimalarial drugs are potentially toxic, it is imperative that physicians carefully review the recommended therapeutic regimens.

Chemoprophylaxis and prompt eradication of infections are critical in breaking the mosquito-human transmission cycle. Control of mosquito breeding and protection of individuals by screening, netting, protective clothing, and insect repellents are also essential. Immigrants from and travelers to endemic areas must be carefully screened, using blood films or serologic tests to detect possible infection. The development of vaccines to protect persons living in or traveling to endemic areas is under investigation.

PLASMODIUM OVALE

Physiology and Structure

P. ovale is similar to *P. vivax* in many respects, including its selectivity for young, pliable erythrocytes. As a consequence, the host cell becomes enlarged and distorted, usually in an oval form. Schüffner's dots appear as pale-pink granules, and the cell border is frequently fimbriated or ragged. The schizont of *P. ovale*, when mature, contains approximately half the number of merozoites seen in *P. vivax*.

Epidemiology

P. ovale is distributed primarily in tropical Africa, where it is often more prevalent than *P. vivax*. It is also found in Asia and South America.

Clinical Syndromes

The clinical picture of tertian attacks for *P. ovale* (benign tertian or ovale malaria) infection is similar to that for *P. vivax*. Untreated infections last only approximately a year instead of the several years for *P. vivax*. Both relapse and recrudescence phases are similar to *P. vivax*.

Laboratory Diagnosis

As with *P. vivax*, thick and thin blood films are examined for the typical oval host cell with Schüffner's dots and a ragged cell wall. Serologic tests reveal cross-reaction with *P. vivax* and other plasmodia.

Treatment, Prevention, and Control

The treatment regimen, including the use of primaquine to prevent relapse from latent liver forms, is similar to that used *for P. vivax* infections. Preventing *P. ovale* infection involves the same measures as for *P. vivax* and other plasmodia.

PLASMODIUM MALARIAE

Physiology and Structure

In contrast with *P. vivax* and *P. ovale*, *P. malariae* can infect only mature erythrocytes with relatively rigid cell membranes. As a result, the parasite's growth must conform to the size and shape of the red blood cell. This produces no red cell enlargement or distortion, as seen in *P. vivax* and *P. ovale*, but it does result in distinctive shapes of the parasite seen in the host cell: "band and bar forms," as well as very compact, dark-staining forms. The schizont of *P. malariae* shows no red cell enlargement or distortion and is usually composed of eight merozoites appearing in a rosette. Occasionally, reddish granules called Ziemann's dots appear in the host cell.

Unlike for *P. vivax* and *P. ovale*, hypnozoites of *P. malariae* are not found in the liver, and relapse does not occur. Recrudescence does occur, and attacks may develop after apparent abatement of symptoms.

Epidemiology

P. malariae infection occurs primarily in the same subtropical and temperate regions as the other plasmodia but is less prevalent.

Clinical Syndromes

The incubation period for *P. malariae* is the longest of the plasmodia, usually 18 to 40 days, but possibly several months to years. The early symptoms are influenza-like, with fever patterns of 72 hours (quartan or malarial malaria) in periodicity. Attacks are moderate to severe and last several hours. Untreated infections may last as long as 20 years.

Laboratory Diagnosis

Observing the characteristic bar and band forms and the rosette schizont in thick and thin films of blood establishes the diagnosis of *P. malariae* infection. As already noted, serologic tests cross-react with other plasmodia.

Treatment, Prevention, and Control

Treatment is similar to that for *P. vivax* and *P. ovale* infections and must be undertaken to prevent recrudescent infections. Treatment to prevent relapse caused by latent liver forms is not required because these forms do not develop with *P. malariae*. Preventive and controlling mechanisms are as discussed for *P. vivax* and *P. ovale*.

PLASMODIUM FALCIPARUM

Physiology and Structure

P. falciparum demonstrates no selectivity in host erythrocytes and invades any red blood cell at any stage in its existence. Also, multiple sporozoites can infect a single erythrocyte. Thus three or even four small rings may be seen in an infected cell (Figure 83–3). *P. falciparum* is often seen in the host cell at the very edge or periphery of the cell membrane, appearing almost as if it were "stuck" on the outside of the cell (see Figure 83–3). This is called the **appliqué** or **accolé** position and is distinctive for this species.

Growing trophozoite stages and schizonts of *P. falciparum* are rarely seen in blood films because their forms

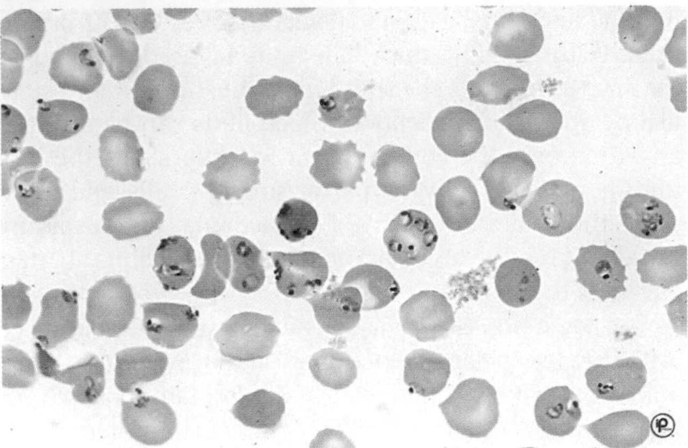

FIGURE 83–3. Ring forms of *Plasmodium falciparum*. Note the multiple ring forms within the individual erythrocytes, which is characteristic of this organism. (From Marler LM et al: *Parasitology* CD-Rom, Indiana Pathology Images, 2003.)

are sequestered in the liver and spleen. Only in very heavy infections are they found in the peripheral circulation. Thus, peripheral blood smears from patients with *P. falciparum* malaria characteristically contain only young ring forms and, occasionally, gametocytes. The typical crescentic gametocytes are diagnostic for the species (Figure 83–4). Infected red blood cells do not enlarge and become distorted, like they do with P. *vivax* and *P. ovale*. Occasionally, reddish granules known as **Maurer's dots** are observed in *P. falciparum*.

P. falciparum, like *P. malariae*, does not produce hypnozoites in the liver. Relapses from the liver are not known to occur.

Epidemiology

P. falciparum occurs almost exclusively in tropical and subtropical regions.

Clinical Syndromes

The incubation period of *P. falciparum* is the shortest of all the plasmodia, ranging from 7 to 10 days, and does not extend for months to years. After the early influenza-like symptoms, *P. falciparum* rapidly produces daily **(quotidian)** chills and fever, as well as severe nausea, vomiting, and diarrhea. The periodicity of the attacks then becomes tertian (36 to 48 hours), and fulminating disease develops. The term **malignant tertian** malaria is appropriate for this infection. Because the symptoms of this type of malaria are similar to those of intestinal infections, the nausea, vomiting, and diarrhea have led to the observation that malaria is "the malignant mimic."

Although any malaria infection may be fatal, *P. falciparum* is the most likely to result in death if left untreated. The increased numbers of erythrocytes infected and destroyed result in toxic cellular debris, adherence of red blood cells to vascular endothelium and to adjacent red blood cells, and formation of capillary plugging by masses of red blood cells, platelets, leukocytes, and malarial pigment.

Involvement of the brain (cerebral malaria) is most often seen in *P. falciparum* infection. Capillary plugging from an accumulation of malarial pigment and masses of cells can result in coma and death.

Kidney damage is also associated with *P. falciparum* malaria, resulting in an illness called **blackwater fever.** Intravascular hemolysis with rapid destruction of red blood cells produces a marked hemoglobinuria and can result in acute renal failure, tubular necrosis, nephrotic syndrome, and death. Liver involvement is characterized by abdominal pain, vomiting of bile, severe diarrhea, and rapid dehydration.

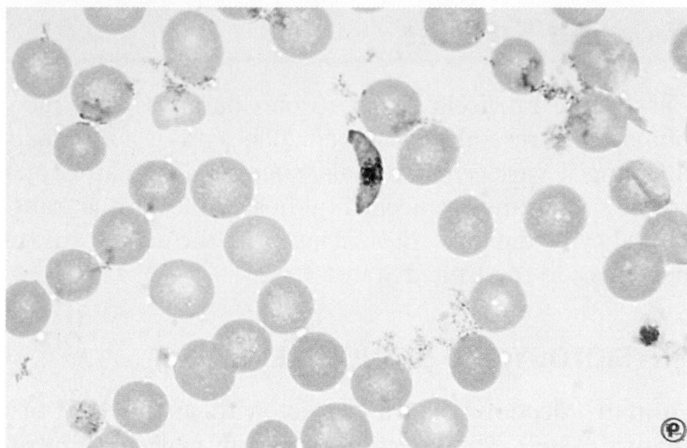

FIGURE 83–4. Mature gametocyte of *P. falciparum*. The presence of this sausage-shaped form is diagnostic of *P. falciparum* malaria. (From Marler LM et al: *Parasitology* CD-Rom, Indiana Pathology Images, 2003.)

Laboratory Diagnosis

Thick and thin blood films are searched for the characteristic rings of *P. falciparum*, which frequently occur in multiples within a single cell, as well as in the accolé position (see Figure 83–3). The distinctive crescentic gametocytes are also diagnostic (see Figure 83–4).

Laboratory personnel must perform a thorough search of the blood films because mixed infections can occur with any combination of the four species, but most often the combination is *P. falciparum* and *P. vivax*. The detection and proper reporting of a mixed infection directly affects the treatment chosen.

Treatment, Prevention, and Control

The treatment of malaria is based on the history regarding travel to endemic areas, prompt clinical review and differential diagnosis, accurate and rapid laboratory work, and correct use of antimalarial drugs.

Because chloroquine-resistant strains of *P. falciparum* are present in many parts of the world, physicians must review all current protocols for the proper treatment of *P. falciparum* infections, noting particularly where chloroquine resistance is known to occur. If the patient's history indicates that the origin is not from a chloroquine-resistant area, the drug of choice is either chloroquine or parenteral quinine. Patients infected with chloroquine-resistant *P. falciparum* (or *P. vivax*) may be treated with other agents, including atovaquone + proguanil (Malarone), mefloquine ± artesunate, quinine, quinidine, pyrimethamine-sulfadoxine (Fansidar), and doxycycline. Because quinine and pyrimethamine-sulfadoxine are potentially toxic, they are used more often for treatment than prophylaxis. Amodiaquine, an analogue of chloroquine, is effective against chloroquine-resistant *P. falciparum;* however, toxicity limits its use. Newer agents with excellent activity against multple-drug-resistant strains of *P. falciparum* include the phenanthrene methanols, halofantrine and lumafantrine, and the artemesinins, artemether and artesunate, both sesquiterpene derivatives.

Combinations of the rapid-acting artemesinins with an existing or newly introduced antimalarial compound have been shown to be highly effective in both treatment and control of malaria caused by *P. falciparum*. The rapid reduction in parasite biomass (approximately 10^8-fold within 3 days) produced by the artemesinins, leaves a relatively small number of organisms for the second agent (usually mefloquine or lumafantrine) to clear. This reduces considerably the exposure of the parasite population to mefloquine or lumafantrine, thus reducing the chance of an escape-resistant mutant arising from the infection. Combinations of artesunate and mefloquine and of artemether and lumafantrine have both been well tolerated and highly efficacious in the treatment of multidrug-resistant falciparum malaria in semi-immune and nonimmune individuals.

When there is uncertainty whether the *P. falciparum* is chloroquine resistant, it is advisable to assume that the strain is resistant and treat the patient accordingly. If the laboratory reports a mixed infection involving *P. falciparum* and *P. vivax*, the treatment must eradicate not only *P. falciparum* from the erythrocytes but also the liver stages of *P. vivax* to avoid relapses. Failure on the part of the laboratory to detect and report such a mixed infection can result in inappropriate treatment and unnecessary delay in accomplishing a complete cure.

P. falciparum infection can be prevented and controlled exactly as for *P. vivax* and the other human malarias. Chloroquine resistance complicates the management of these patients but can be overcome by the physician's awareness of appropriate regimens.

Babesia Species

Babesia are intracellular sporozoan parasites that morphologically resemble plasmodia. Babesiosis is a **zoonosis** infecting a variety of animals, such as deer, cattle, and rodents; humans are accidental hosts. Infection is transmitted by Ixodid ticks. *Babesia microti* is the usual cause of babesiosis in the United States.

PHYSIOLOGY AND STRUCTURE

Human infection follows contact with an infected tick (Figure 83–5). The infectious pyriform bodies are introduced into the bloodstream and infect erythrocytes. The intraerythrocytic trophozoites multiply by binary fission, forming tetrads, and then lyse the erythrocyte, releasing the merozoites. These can reinfect other cells to maintain the infection. Infected cells can also be ingested by feeding ticks, in which additional replication can take place. Infection in the tick population can also be maintained by transovarian transmission. The infected cells in humans resemble the ring forms of *P. falciparum*, but malarial pigment or other stages of growth characteristically seen with plasmodial infections are not seen with careful examination of blood smears (Figure 83–6).

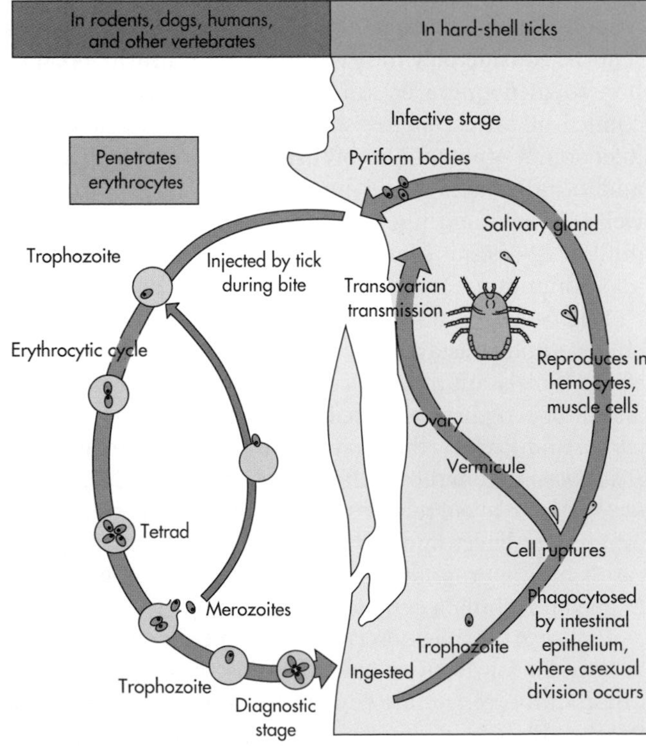

FIGURE 83–5. Life cycle of *Babesia* species.

EPIDEMIOLOGY

More than 70 different species of *Babesia* are found in Africa, Asia, Europe, and North America, with *B. microti* responsible for disease along the northeastern seaboard of the United States (e.g., Nantucket Island, Martha's Vineyard, Shelter Island). *Ixodes dammini* is the tick vector responsible for transmitting babesiosis in this area, and the natural reservoir hosts are field mice, voles, and other small rodents. Serologic studies in endemic areas have demonstrated a high incidence of past exposure to *Babesia*. Presumably, most infections are asymptomatic or mild. *Babesia divergens*, which has been reported more frequently from Europe, causes severe, often fatal infections in people who have undergone splenectomies. Although most infections follow tick bites, transfusion-related infections have been demonstrated.

CLINICAL SYNDROMES

After an incubation period of 1 to 4 weeks, symptomatic patients experience general malaise, fever without periodicity, headache, chills, sweating, fatigue, and weakness. As the infection progresses with increased destruction of erythrocytes, hemolytic anemia develops, and the patient may experience renal failure. Hepatomegaly and splenomegaly can develop in advanced disease. Low-grade parasitemia may persist for weeks. Splenectomy or functional asplenia, immunosuppression, and advanced age increase a person's susceptibility to infections and more severe disease.

LABORATORY DIAGNOSIS

Examination of blood smears is the diagnostic method of choice. Laboratory personnel must be experienced in dif-

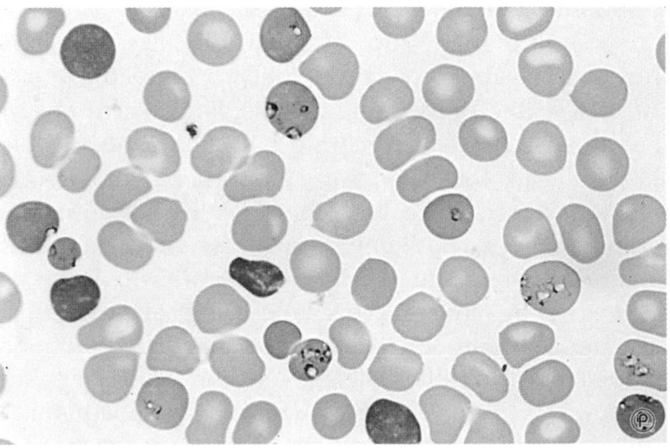

FIGURE 83–6. Ring forms of *Babesia microti*. Note the multiple ring forms within the individual erythocytes and the similarity to that of *P. falciparum* in Figure 83–3. (From Marler LM et al: *Parasitology* CD-Rom, Indiana Pathology Images, 2003.)

ferentiating *Babesia* and *Plasmodium* species. *Babesia* may mimic *P. falciparum* with red blood cells multiply infected with small ring forms (see Figure 83–6). Infected patients may have negative smears because of the low-grade parasitemia. These infections can be diagnosed by inoculating samples of blood into hamsters, which are highly susceptible to infection. Serologic tests are also available for diagnostic use.

TREATMENT, PREVENTION, AND CONTROL

The drugs of choice are clindamycin combined with quinine. Other antiprotozoal regimens, including chloroquine and pentamidine, have been used with variable results. However, most patients with mild disease recover without specific therapy. Exchange blood transfusion has also been successful in patients who have had splenectomies and have severe infections caused by *B. microti* or *B. divergens*. The use of protective clothing and insect repellents can minimize tick exposure in endemic areas, which is critical for the prevention of disease. Ticks must feed on humans for several hours before the organisms are transmitted, so prompt removal of ticks can be protective.

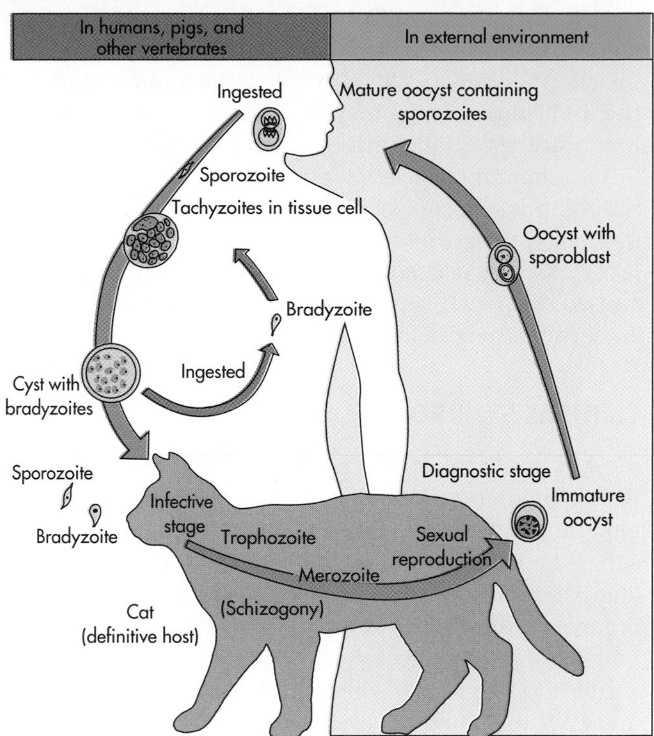

FIGURE 83–7. Life cycle of *Toxoplasma gondii.*

Toxoplasma gondii

T. gondii is a typical coccidian parasite related to *Plasmodium*, *Isospora*, and other members of the phylum Apicomplexa. *T. gondii* is an intracellular parasite, and it is found in a wide variety of animals, including birds and humans. Only one species exists, and there appears to be little strain-to-strain variation. The essential reservoir host of *T. gondii* is the common house cat and other felines.

PHYSIOLOGY AND STRUCTURE

Organisms develop in the intestinal cells of the cat, as well as during an extraintestinal cycle with passage to the tissues via the bloodstream (Figure 83–7). The organisms from the intestinal cycle are passed in cat feces and mature into infective cysts within 3 to 4 days in the external environment. These oocysts are similar to those of *Isospora belli*, the human intestinal protozoan parasite, and can be ingested by mice and other animals (including humans) and produce acute and chronic infection of various tissues, including brain. Infection in cats is established when the tissues of infected rodents are eaten.

Some infective forms, or trophozoites, from the oocyst develop as slender, crescentic types, called tachyzoites. These rapidly multiplying forms are responsible for the initial infection and the tissue damage. Slow-growing, shorter forms called bradyzoites also develop and form cysts in chronic infections.

EPIDEMIOLOGY

Human infection with *T. gondii* is ubiquitous; however, it is increasingly apparent that certain immunocompromised individuals (patients with acquired immune deficiency syndrome [AIDS]) are more likely to have severe manifestations. The wide variety of animals that harbor the organism—carnivores and herbivores, as well as birds—accounts for the widespread transmission.

Humans become infected from two sources: (1) ingestion of improperly cooked meat from animals that serve as intermediate hosts and (2) the ingestion of infective oocysts from contaminated cat feces. Serologic studies show an increased prevalence in human populations where the consumption of uncooked meat or meat juices is popular. It is noteworthy that serologic tests of human and rodent populations are negative in the few geographic areas where cats have not existed. Outbreaks of toxoplasmosis in the United States are usually traced to poorly cooked meat (e.g., hamburgers) and contact with cat feces.

Transplacental infection can occur in pregnancy, either from infection acquired from meat and meat juices or from contact with cat feces. Transfusion infection via contaminated blood can occur but is not common. Transplacental infection from an infected mother has a devastating effect on the fetus.

Although the rate of seroconversion is similar for individuals within a geographic location, the rate of severe infection is dramatically affected by the immune status of the individual. Patients with defects in cell-mediated immunity, especially those who are infected with the human immunodeficiency virus (HIV) or who have had an organ transplant or immunosuppressive therapy, are most likely to have disseminated or central nervous system (CNS) disease. It is believed that illness in this setting is caused by reactivation of previously latent infection rather than new exposure to the organism.

CLINICAL SYNDROMES

Most *T. gondii* infections are benign and asymptomatic, with symptoms occurring as the parasite moves from the blood to tissues, where it becomes an intracellular parasite. When symptomatic disease occurs, the infection is characterized by cell destruction, reproduction of more organisms, and eventual cyst formation. Many tissues may be affected; however, the organism has a particular predilection for cells of the lung, heart, lymphoid organs, and CNS, including the eye.

Symptoms of acute disease include chills, fever, headaches, myalgia, lymphadenitis, and fatigue; the symptoms occasionally resemble those of infectious mononucleosis. In chronic disease the signs and symptoms include lymphadenitis, occasionally a rash, evidence of hepatitis, encephalomyelitis, and myocarditis. In some of the cases, chorioretinitis appears and may lead to blindness.

Congenital infection with *T. gondii* also occurs in infants born to mothers infected during pregnancy. If infection occurs in the first trimester, the result is spontaneous abortion, stillbirth, or severe disease. Manifestations in the infant infected after the first trimester include epilepsy, encephalitis, microcephaly, intracranial calcifications, hydrocephalus, psychomotor or mental retardation, chorioretinitis, blindness, anemia, jaundice, rash, pneumonia, diarrhea, and hypothermia. Infants may be asymptomatic at birth, only to develop disease months to years later. Most often these children develop chorioretinitis with or without blindness or other neurologic problems, including retardation, seizures, microcephaly, and hearing loss.

A different spectrum of disease is seen in immunocompromised older patients. Reactivation of latent toxoplasmosis is a special problem for these people. The presenting symptoms of *Toxoplasma* infection in immunocompromised patients are usually neurologic, most frequently consistent with diffuse encephalopathy, meningoencephalitis, or cerebral mass lesions. Reactivation of cerebral toxoplasmosis has emerged as a major cause of encephalitis in patients with AIDS. The disease is usually multifocal, with more than one mass lesion appearing in the brain at the same time. Symptoms are related to the location of the lesions and may include hemiparesis, seizures, visual impairment, confusion, and lethargy. Other sites of infection that have been reported include the eye, lung, and testes. Although disease is seen predominantly in patients with AIDS, it may also occur with similar manifestations in other immunocompromised patients, in particular those undergoing solid organ transplantation.

LABORATORY DIAGNOSIS

Serologic testing is required for the diagnosis of acute active infection; the diagnosis is established by the finding of increasing antibody titers documented in serially collected blood specimens. Because contact with the organism is common, attention to increasing titers is essential to differentiate acute, active infection from previous asymptomatic or chronic infection. Currently the enzyme-linked immunosorbent assay (ELISA) for detecting immunoglobulin (Ig) M antibodies appears to be the most reliable procedure because of its simplicity and rapidity in documenting acute infections. The test is not generally satisfactory in AIDS patients with latent or reactivated infections, because they fail to produce an IgM response or increasing IgG titer.

Demonstration of these organisms as trophozoites and cysts in tissue and body fluids is the definitive method of diagnosis (Figure 83–8). Biopsy specimens from lymph nodes, brain, myocardium, or other suspected tissue, as well as body fluids, including cerebrospinal fluid, amniotic fluid, or bronchoalveolar lavage fluid, can be directly examined for the organisms. Newer monoclonal antibody–based fluorescent stains may facilitate direct detection of *T. gondii* in tissue. Culture methods for *T. gondii* are largely experimental and not usually

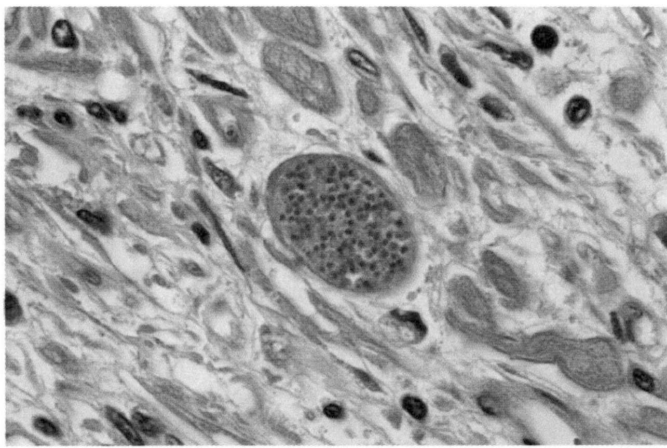

FIGURE 83–8. Cyst of *T. gondii* in tissue. Hundreds of organisms may be present in the cyst, which may become active and initiate disease with decreased host immunity (e.g., immunosuppression in transplant patients and in diseases such as AIDS).

available in clinical laboratories. The two methods available are to inoculate potentially infected material into either mouse peritoneum or tissue culture. Advances in developing polymerase chain reaction–based detection methods are promising and may provide rapid and sensitive approaches for detecting the organism in blood, cerebrospinal fluid, amniotic fluid, and other clinical specimens.

TREATMENT, PREVENTION, AND CONTROL

The therapy for toxoplasmosis depends on the nature of the infectious process and the immunocompetence of the host. Most mononucleosis-like infections in normal hosts resolve spontaneously and do not require specific therapy. In contrast, disseminated or CNS infection in immunocompromised people must be treated. Before the association of *T. gondii* with HIV infection, immunocompromised patients with toxoplasmosis were treated for 4 to 6 weeks. In the setting of HIV infection, discontinuing therapy after 4 to 6 weeks is associated with a relapse rate of 25%. Such patients are currently treated with an initial high-dose regimen of pyrimethamine plus sulfadiazine and then continued on lower doses of both drugs indefinitely. Although this drug combination is the regimen of choice, toxicity (rash and bone marrow suppression) may necessitate changes to alternative agents. Clindamycin plus pyrimethamine is the best-studied alternative. Atovaquone and azithromycin (each alone or with pyrimethamine) also have some activity, although their efficacy and safety compared with those of clindamycin-pyrimethamine need to be assessed. Trimethoprim-sulfamethoxazole is another alternative to pyrimethamine-sulfadiazine for treatment of disseminated or CNS toxoplasmosis. The use of corticosteroids is indicated as part of therapy of cerebral edema and ocular infections that involve or threaten the macula.

Infections in the first trimester of pregnancy are difficult to manage because of the teratogenicity of pyrimethamine in laboratory animals. Both clindamycin and spiramycin have been substituted with apparent success. Spiramycin does not appear to be effective for the treatment of toxoplasmosis in immunocompromised patients.

As more immunocompromised patients at risk for disseminated infection are identified, greater emphasis is placed on preventive measures and specific prophylaxis. Routine serologic screening of patients before organ transplantation and early in the course of HIV infection is now being performed. Individuals with positive serologic tests are at much higher risk for the development of disease and are now being considered for prophylaxis. Trimethoprim-sulfamethoxazole, which is also used as prophylaxis to prevent *Pneumocystis jiroveci* infections, also appears to be effective at preventing infections with *T. gondii.* Additional preventive measures for pregnant women and immunocompromised hosts should include avoiding the consumption and handling of raw or undercooked meat and avoiding exposure to cat feces.

Sarcocystis lindemanni

S. lindemanni is a typical coccidian closely related to the intestinal forms *Sarcocystis suihominis, Sarcocystis bovihominis,* and *Isospora belli* and the blood and tissue parasite *T. gondii. S. lindemanni* occurs worldwide in various animals, especially sheep, cattle, and pigs. Humans are accidentally infected only as the result of eating meat from these animals. Most infections are asymptomatic, but occasionally an infection may cause myositis, swelling of muscle, dyspnea, and eosinophilia. Infection of the myocardium has been observed but is extremely rare. There is no specific treatment for the muscle infection.

Free-Living Amoebae

Naegleria species, *Acanthamoeba* species, *Balamuthia* species, and other free-living amoebae are found in soil and in contaminated lakes, streams, and other water environments. Most human infections with these amoebae are acquired during the warm summer months by people exposed to the amoebae while swimming in contaminated water. Inhalation of cysts present in dust may account for some infections, whereas ocular infections with *Acanthamoeba* species are associated with the contamination of contact lenses with nonsterile cleaning solutions.

CLINICAL SYNDROMES

Naegleria, Acanthamoeba and *Balamuthia* organisms are opportunistic pathogens. Although colonization of the nasal passages is usually asymptomatic, these amoebae can invade the nasal mucosa and extend into the brain. Acute primary amebic **meningoencephalitis** is most commonly caused by *Naegleria fowleri.* Destruction of brain tissue is characterized by a fulminant, rapidly fatal meningoencephalitis. Symptoms include intense frontal headache, sore throat, fever, blocked nose with altered senses of taste and smell, stiff neck, and Kernig's sign. The cerebrospinal fluid is purulent and may contain many erythrocytes and motile amoebae. Clinically, the course of the disease is rapid, with death usually occurring within 4 or 5 days. Postmortem findings show *Naegleria* trophozoites present in the brain but no evidence of cysts (Figure 83–9). Although all cases were fatal before 1970, survival has since been reported in a few cases in which the disease was rapidly diagnosed and treated.

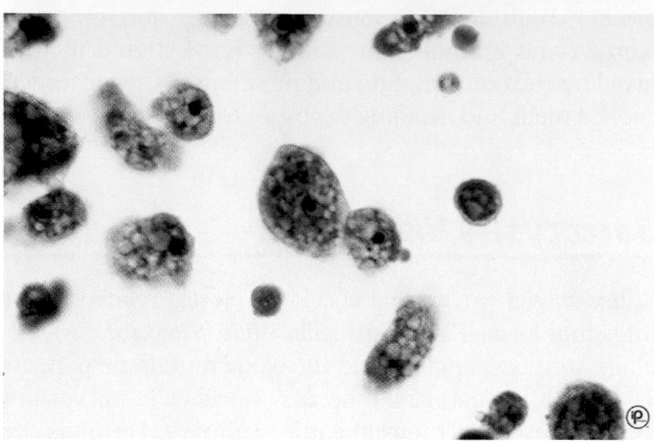

FIGURE 83–9. Numerous *Naegleria* trophozoites in brain tissue from a patient with amoebic meningoencephalitis. (From Marler LM et al: *Parasitology* CD-Rom, Indiana Pathology Images, 2003.)

In contrast to *Naegleria, Acanthamoeba* and *Balamuthia* organisms produce granulomatous amoebic encephalitis and single or multiple brain abscesses primarily in immunocompromised individuals. The course of the disease is slower, with an incubation period of at least 10 days. The resulting disease is a chronic granulomatous encephalitis with edema of the brain tissue.

Eye and skin infection caused by *Acanthamoeba* organisms may also occur. Keratitis is usually associated with eye trauma that occurred before contact with contaminated soil, dust, or water. The use of improperly cleaned contact lenses is also associated with this disease. Invasion by *Acanthamoeba* species produces corneal ulceration and severe ocular pain. Cases of apparent disseminated cutaneous and subcutaneous infection with *Acanthamoeba* and *Balamuthia* organisms recently have been described in patients with AIDS. These infections include multiple soft tissue nodules, which on biopsy contain amoebae. CNS or deep tissue involvement may also be present with this form of infection.

LABORATORY DIAGNOSIS

For the diagnosis of *Naegleria, Acanthamoeba,* and *Balamuthia* infections, nasal discharge, cerebrospinal fluid, and in the case of eye infections, corneal scrapings, should be collected. The specimens should be examined using a saline wet preparation and iodine-stained smears. *Naegleria* and *Acanthamoeba* species are difficult to differentiate except by experienced microscopists. However, the observation of an amoeba in a normally sterile tissue is diagnostic (see Figure 83–9). In *Naegleria* infection, only the **amoeboid trophozoites** are found within the tissue, whereas with *Acanthamoeba* and *Balamuthia* infection, both trophozoites and cysts are found in tissues. The clinical specimens can be cultured on agar plates seeded with live gram-negative enteric bacilli. Amoebae present in the specimens use the bacteria as a nutritional source and can be detected within 1 or 2 days by the presence of the trails that form on the agar surface as the amoebae move. *Balamuthia* do not grow on agar plates used for *Naegleria* and *Acanthamoeba* but have been recovered in tissue culture using mammalian cell lines.

TREATMENT, PREVENTION, AND CONTROL

Treatment of free-living amoebic infections is largely ineffective. Amoebic meningoencephalitis caused by either *Naegleria, Acanthamoeba,* or *Balamuthia* is unresponsive to most antimicrobial agents. The treatment of choice for *Naegleria* infections is amphotericin B combined with miconazole and rifampin. *Acanthamoeba* infections may be treated with pentamidine, ketoconazole and flucytosine, whereas *Balamuthia* infections have been treated with clarithromycin, fluconazole, sulfadiazine, and flucytosine. Amoebic keratitis and cutaneous infections may respond to topical miconazole, chlorhexidine gluconate, or propamidine isethionate. Treatment of amoebic keratitis may require repeated corneal transplantation or, rarely, enucleation of the eye. The wide distribution of these organisms in fresh and brackish waters makes the prevention and control of infection difficult. It has been suggested that known sources of infection be off-limits to bathing, diving, and water sports, although this is generally difficult to enforce. Swimming pools with cracks in the walls, allowing soil seepage, should be repaired to avoid creation of a source of infection.

Leishmania

The hemoflagellates are flagellated, insect-transmitted protozoa that infect blood and tissues. Three species of *Leishmania,* a protozoan **hemoflagellate,** produce human disease: *Leishmania donovani, Leishmania tropica,* and *Leishmania braziliensis* (Table 83–2). The diseases are distinguished by the ability of the organism to infect deep tissues (visceral leishmaniasis) or replicate only in cooler superficial tissues (cutaneous or mucocutaneous leishmaniasis). The reservoir hosts and geographic distribution differ for the three species, but transmission by sandflies (belonging to the genera *Phlebotomus* or *Lutzomyia*) is common to all leishmanial species.

LEISHMANIA DONOVANI

Physiology and Structure

The life cycles of all leishmanial parasites differ in epidemiology, tissues affected, and clinical manifestations

TABLE 83–2. Leishmaniasis in Humans

Parasite	Disease
Leishmania donovani	Visceral leishmaniasis (kala-azar, dumdum fever)
Leishmania tropica	Cutaneous leishmaniasis (Oriental sore, Delhi boil)
Leishmania braziliensis	Mucocutaneous leishmaniasis (American leishmaniasis, espundia, chiclero ulcer)

(Figure 83–10). The **promastigote** stage (long, slender form with a free flagellum) is present in the saliva of infected sandflies. Human infection is initiated by the bite of an infected sandfly, which injects the promastigotes into the skin, where they lose their flagella, enter the **amastigote** stage, and invade reticuloendothelial cells. Reproduction occurs in the **amastigote** stage, and as cells rupture, destruction of specific tissues (e.g., cutaneous tissues, visceral organs such as the liver and spleen) develops. The amastigote stage (Figure 83–11) is diagnostic for leishmaniasis, as well as the infectious stage for sandflies. Ingested amastigotes transform in the sandfly into the promastigote stage, which multiplies by binary fission in the fly midgut. After development, this stage migrates to the fly proboscis, where new human infection can be introduced during feeding.

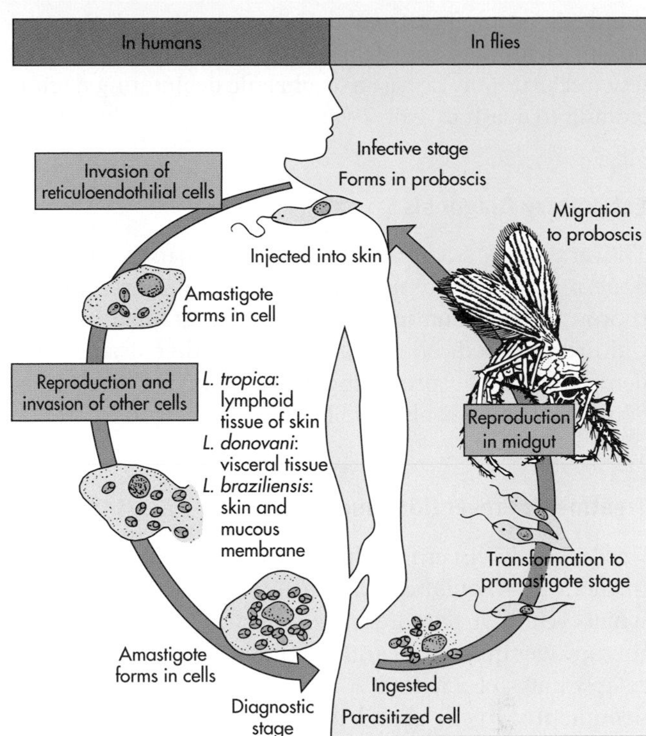

FIGURE 83–10. Life cycle of *Leishmania* species.

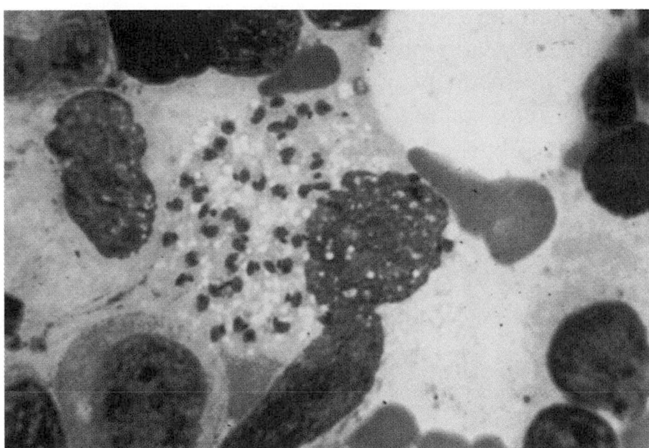

FIGURE 83–11. Giemsa-stained amastigotes (Leishman-Donovan bodies) of *L. donovani* present in a touch preparation of spleen. A small, dark-staining kinetoplast can be seen next to the spherical nucleus in some parasites. (From Connor DH et al, editors: *Pathology of infectious disease,* vol II, Stamford, Conn, 1997, Appleton & Lange.)

Epidemiology

L. donovani infection of the classic **kala-azar** or **dumdum fever** type **(visceral leishmaniasis)** occurs at a rate of approximately 500,000 new cases per year, 90% of which are localized to Bangladesh, Brazil, India, Nepal, and the Sudan. Except for some rodents in Africa, there are few reservoir hosts. The vector is the *Phlebotomus* sandfly. Variants of *L. donovani* are also recognized. *L. donovani infantum* is present in countries along the Mediterranean basin (European, Near Eastern, and African) and is found in parts of China and the former Soviet Union. Reservoir hosts of this organism include dogs, foxes, jackals, and porcupines. The vector is also the *Phlebotomus* sandfly. *L. donovani chagasi* is found in South and Central America, especially Mexico and the West Indies. Reservoir hosts are dogs, foxes, and cats, and the vector is the *Lutzomyia* sandfly.

Clinical Syndromes

The incubation period for visceral leishmaniasis may be from several weeks to a year, with a gradual onset of fever, diarrhea, and anemia. Chills and sweating that may resemble malaria symptoms are common early in the infection. As organisms proliferate and invade cells of the liver and spleen, marked enlargement of these organs, weight loss, and emaciation occur. Kidney damage may also occur as cells of the glomeruli are invaded. With persistence of the disease, deeply pigmented, granulomatous areas of skin, referred to as post–kala-azar dermal leishmaniasis, occur. If untreated, visceral leishmaniasis develops into a fulminating, debilitating, and lethal disease in a few weeks or may persist as a chronic debilitating disease, leading to death in 1 or 2 years.

Laboratory Diagnosis

The amastigote stage can be demonstrated in tissue biopsy, bone marrow examination, lymph node aspiration, and thorough examination of properly stained smears. Culture of blood, bone marrow, and other tissues often demonstrates the promastigote stage of the organisms. Serologic testing is also available.

Treatment, Prevention, and Control

Until recently, visceral leishmainasis was treated with pentavalent antimonial compounds, such as stibogluconate, which required parenteral administration. This form of therapy was quite toxic and not uniformly successful, with relapse rates of 2% to 8%. Remarkable success has been documented in the past 3 to 5 years with an oral agent, miltefosine (hexadecylphosphocholine). This drug is considered the first-choice treatment for immunocompetent patients of all ages in India based on its efficacy (>95% cure rate), tolerability, and the oral route of administration. Alternative approaches include the addition of allopurinol, or treatment with pentamidine or amphotericin B. Prompt treatment of human infections and control of reservoir hosts, along with insect control, help eliminate transmission of disease. Protection from sandflies by screening and insect repellents is also essential.

LEISHMANIA TROPICA

Physiology and Structure

The life cycle of *L. tropica* is illustrated in Figure 83–10.

Epidemiology

Cutaneous leishmaniasis produced by *L. tropica* is present in many parts of Asia, Africa, Mediterranean Europe, and the southern region of the former Soviet Union. In these regions, the reservoir hosts are dogs, foxes, and rodents, and the vector is the sandfly *Phlebotomus.* Two related species are also recognized. *Leishmania aethiopica* is endemic in Ethiopia, Kenya, and Yemen, with dogs and rodents as reservoir hosts and the *Phlebotomus* sandfly the vector. *Leishmania mexicana* occurs in South and Central America, especially in the Amazon basin, with sloths, rodents, monkeys, and raccoons as reservoir hosts. The vector is the *Lutzomyia* sandfly.

Clinical Syndromes

The incubation period after a sandfly bite may be as short as 2 weeks or as long as 2 months. The first sign, a red papule, appears at the site of the fly's bite. This lesion becomes irritated, with intense itching, and begins to enlarge and ulcerate. Gradually the ulcer becomes hard and crusted and exudes a thin, serous material. At this stage, secondary bacterial infection may complicate the disease. The lesion may heal without treatment in a matter of months but usually leaves a disfiguring scar. A disseminated nodular type of cutaneous leishmaniasis has been reported from Ethiopia, probably caused by an allergy to *L. aethiopica* antigens. A viscerotropic form of *L. tropica* has been described in people returning from the Persian Gulf.

Laboratory Diagnosis

Demonstration of the amastigotes in properly stained smears from touch preparations or ulcer biopsy specimens and cultures of ulcer tissue determines the diagnosis. Serologic tests are also available. Recently, deoxyribonucleic acid probes have been developed for the direct examination of cutaneous lesions. There are no commercially available products for these tests, and careful studies to determine the accuracy of testing procedures have not yet been performed.

Treatment, Prevention, and Control

The drug of choice is stibogluconate, with an alternative treatment of applying heat directly to the lesion. Recently, both fluconazole and miltefosine have been shown to be efficaceous. Protection from sandfly bites with the use of screening, protective clothing, and a repellent is essential. Prompt treatment and eradication of the ulcers to prevent transmission, along with control of sandflies and reservoir hosts, reduce the incidence of human infection.

LEISHMANIA BRAZILIENSIS

Physiology and Structure

The life cycle of *L. braziliensis* is illustrated in Figure 83–10.

Epidemiology

Mucocutaneous leishmaniasis produced by *L. braziliensis* is seen from the Yucatan peninsula into Central and South America, especially in rain forests where workers are exposed to sandfly bites while harvesting the chicle sap for chewing gum (thus the name chiclero ulcer). There are many jungle reservoir hosts, and domesticated dogs also serve as reservoirs. The vector is the

Lutzomyia sandfly. The variant *L. braziliensis panamensis* is similar in all respects to *L. braziliensis* except for its more frequent occurrence in Panama and slight difference in growth in cultures. Reservoir hosts and the vector are similar to *L. braziliensis*.

Clinical Syndromes

The incubation period and appearance of ulcers for *L. braziliensis* are similar to those of *L. tropica*, requiring a few weeks to months for the papule to appear. The essential difference in clinical disease is the involvement and destruction of mucous membranes and related tissue structures. This is often combined with edema and secondary bacterial infection to produce severe and disfiguring facial mutilation.

Laboratory Diagnosis

The diagnostic tests are similar for all *Leishmania* infections. Organisms are demonstrated in ulcers or cultured tissue. Serologic testing is also performed.

Treatment, Prevention, and Control

The drug of choice is stibogluconate; an alternative is amphotericin B. As with all the other *Leishmania* complexes, screening, protective clothing, insect repellents, and prompt treatment are needed to prevent transmission and control disease. The protection of forest and construction workers in endemic areas is most difficult, and disease in those places may be effectively controlled only by vaccination. Work to develop a vaccine is under way.

Trypanosomes

Trypanosoma, another hemoflagellate, causes two distinctly different forms of disease (Table 83–3). One is called **African trypanosomiasis**, or **sleeping sickness**, and is produced by *Trypanosoma brucei gambiense* and *Trypanosoma brucei rhodesiense*. It is transmitted by tsetse flies. The second infection is called **American trypanosomiasis**, or **Chagas' disease**, produced by *T. cruzi*. It is transmitted by true bugs (triatomids, reduviids, also called kissing bugs).

TABLE 83–3. *Trypanosoma* Species Responsible for Human Diseases

Parasite	Vector	Disease
Trypanosoma brucei gambiense and *Trypanosoma brucei rhodesiense*	Tsetse fly	African trypanosomiasis (sleeping sickness)
Trypanosoma cruzi	Reduviids	American trypanosomiasis (Chagas' disease)

TRYPANOSOMA BRUCEI GAMBIENSE

Physiology and Structure

The life cycle of the African forms of trypanosomiasis is illustrated in Figure 83–12. The infective stage of the organism is the **trypomastigote**, which is present in the salivary glands of transmitting tsetse flies. The organism in this stage has a free **flagellum** and an **undulating membrane** running the full length of the body (Figure 83–13). The trypomastigotes enter the wound created by the fly bite and find their way into blood and lymph, eventually invading the CNS. Reproduction of the trypomastigotes in blood, lymph, and spinal fluid is by binary or longitudinal fission. These trypomastigotes in blood are then infective for biting tsetse flies, where further reproduction occurs in the midgut. The organisms then migrate to the salivary glands, where an **epimastigote** form (with a free flagellum but only a partial undulating membrane) continues reproduction to the infective trypomastigote stage. Tsetse flies become infective 4 to 6 weeks after feeding on blood from a diseased patient.

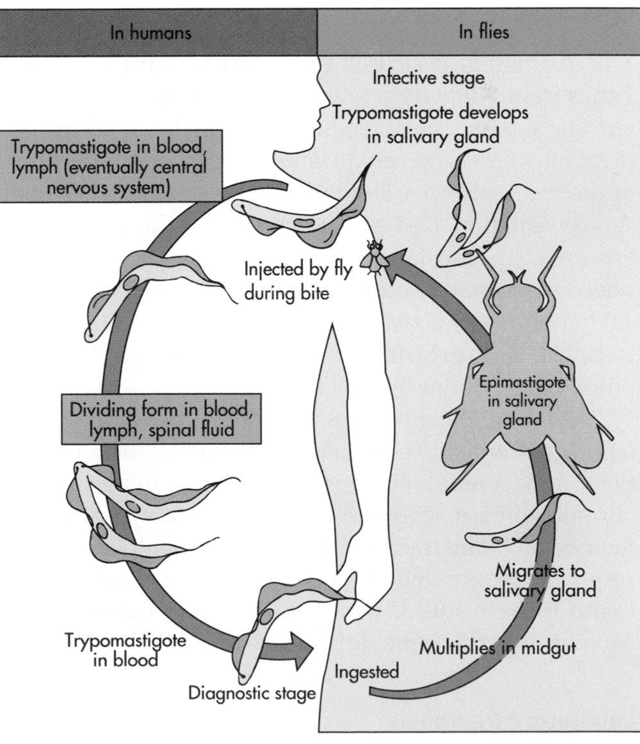

FIGURE 83–12. Life cycle of *Trypanosoma brucei*.

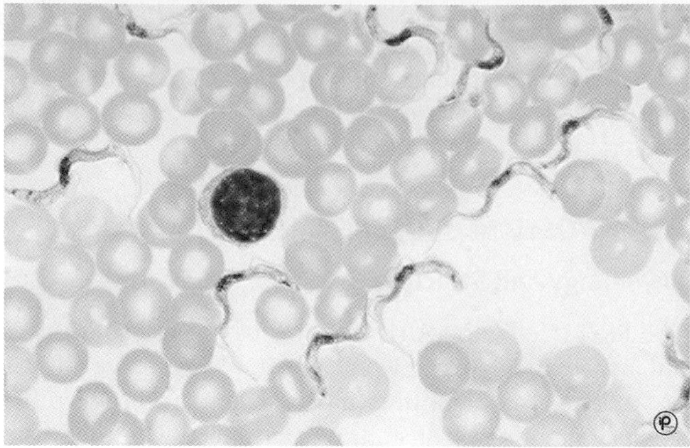

FIGURE 83–13. Trypomastigote stage of *T. b. gambiense* in a blood smear. (From Marler LM et al: *Parasitology* CD-Rom, Indiana Pathology Images, 2003.)

Epidemiology

T. b. gambiense is limited to tropical West and Central Africa, correlating to the range of the tsetse fly vector. The tsetse flies transmitting *T. b. gambiense* prefer shaded stream banks for reproduction and proximity to human dwellings. Persons who work in such areas are at greatest risk of infection. An animal reservoir has not been proved, although several species of animals have been infected experimentally.

Clinical Syndromes

The incubation period of **Gambian sleeping sickness** varies from a few days to weeks. *T. b. gambiense* produces chronic disease, often ending fatally, with CNS involvement after several years' duration. One of the earliest signs of disease is an occasional ulcer at the site of the fly bite. As reproduction of organisms continues, the lymph nodes are invaded, and fever, myalgia, arthralgia, and lymph node enlargement result. Swelling of the posterior cervical lymph nodes is characteristic of Gambian disease and is called **Winterbottom's sign.** Patients in this acute phase often exhibit hyperactivity.

Chronic disease progresses to CNS involvement with lethargy, tremors, meningoencephalitis, mental retardation, and general deterioration. In the final stages of chronic disease, convulsions, hemiplegia, and incontinence occur, and the patient becomes difficult to arouse or respond, eventually progressing to a comatose state. Death is the result of CNS damage and other infections, such as malaria or pneumonia.

Laboratory Diagnosis

Organisms can be demonstrated in thick and thin blood films, in concentrated anticoagulated blood preparations, and in aspirations from lymph nodes and concentrated spinal fluid (see Figure 83–13). Methods for concentrating parasites in blood may be helpful. Approaches include centrifugation of heparinized samples and anion-exchange chromatography. Levels of parasitemia vary widely, and several attempts to visualize the organism over a number of days may be necessary. Preparations should be fixed and stained immediately to avoid disintegration of the trypomastigotes. Serologic tests are also useful diagnostic techniques. Immunofluorescence, ELISA, precipitin, and agglutination methods have been used. Most reagents are not available commercially.

Treatment, Prevention, and Control

In the acute stages of the disease, the drug of choice is suramin, with pentamidine as an alternative. In chronic disease with CNS involvement, the drug of choice is melarsoprol; alternatives are tryparsamide combined with suramin. Difluoromethylornithine has also been introduced and holds promise for the treatment of all stages of disease.

The most essential elements are control of breeding sites of the tsetse flies by clearing brush, using insecticides, and treating human cases to reduce transmission to flies. People going into known endemic areas should wear protective clothing and use screening, bed netting, and insect repellents.

TRYPANOSOMA BRUCEI RHODESIENSE

Physiology and Structure

The life cycle of *T. b. rhodesiense* is similar to that of *T. b. gambiense* (see Figure 83–12), with both trypomastigote and epimastigote stages and transmission by tsetse flies.

Epidemiology

The organism is found primarily in East Africa, especially the cattle-raising countries where tsetse flies breed in the brush rather than along stream banks. *T. b. rhodesiense* also differs from *T. b. gambiense* in that domestic animal hosts (cattle and sheep) and wild game animals act as reservoir hosts. This transmission and vector cycle makes the organism more difficult to control than *T. b. gambiense.*

Clinical Syndromes

The incubation period for *T. b. rhodesiense* is shorter than that for *T. b. gambiense.* Acute disease (fever, rigors, and myalgia) occurs more rapidly and progresses to a fulminating, rapidly fatal illness. Infected persons are usually dead within 9 to 12 months if left untreated.

This more virulent organism also develops in greater numbers in the blood. Lymphadenopathy is uncommon. CNS invasion occurs early in the infection with lethargy, anorexia, and mental disturbance. The chronic stages described for *T. b. gambiense* are not often seen because in addition to rapid CNS disease, the organism produces kidney damage and myocarditis, leading to death.

Laboratory Diagnosis

Examination of blood and spinal fluid is carried out as for *T. b. gambiense.* Serologic tests are available; however, the marked variability of the surface antigens of trypanosomes limits the diagnostic usefulness of this approach.

Treatment, Prevention, and Control

The same treatment protocol applies as for *T. b. gambiense,* with early treatment for the more rapid neurologic manifestations. Similar prevention and control measures are needed: tsetse fly control and use of protective clothing, screens, netting, and insect repellent. In addition, early treatment is essential to control transmission, detect infection, and determine treatment in domestic animals. Control of infection in game animals is difficult, but infection can be reduced if measures to control the tsetse fly population, specifically eradication of brush and grassland breeding sites, are applied.

TRYPANOSOMA CRUZI

Physiology and Sturcture

The life cycle of *T. cruzi* (Figure 83–14) differs from *T. brucei* with the development of an additional form called an amastigote (Figure 83–15). The amastigote is an intracellular form with no flagellum and no undulating membrane. It is smaller than the trypomastigote, is oval, and is found in tissues. The infective trypomastigote, which is present in the feces of a **reduviid** bug **("kissing bug"),** enters the wound created by the biting, feeding bug. The bugs have been called kissing bugs because they often bite people around the mouth and in other facial sites. They are notorious for biting, feeding on blood and tissue juices, and then defecating into the wound. The organisms in the feces of the bug enter the wound; penetration is usually aided when the patient rubs or scratches the irritated site.

The trypomastigotes then migrate to other tissues (e.g., cardiac muscle, liver, brain), lose the flagellum and undulating membrane, and become the smaller, oval, intracellular amastigote form. These intracellular amastigotes multiply by binary fission and eventually destroy the host cells. Then they are liberated to enter new host tissue as intracellular amastigotes or to become trypomastigotes infective for feeding reduviid bugs. Ingested trypomastigotes develop into epimastigotes in the midgut of the insect and reproduce by longitudinal binary fission. The organisms migrate to the hindgut of the bug, develop into metacyclic trypomastigotes, and then leave the bug in the feces after biting, feeding, and defecating, initiating a new human infection.

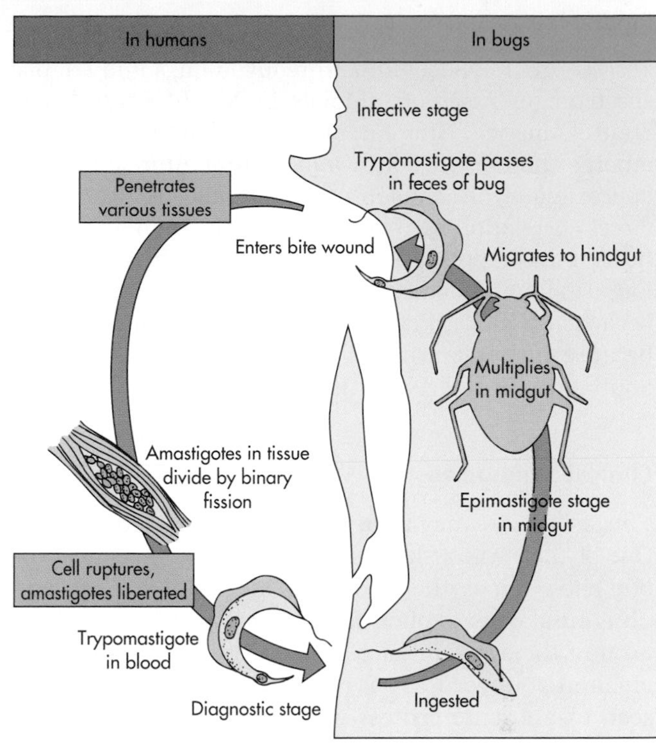

FIGURE 83–14. Life cycle of *Trypanosoma cruzi.*

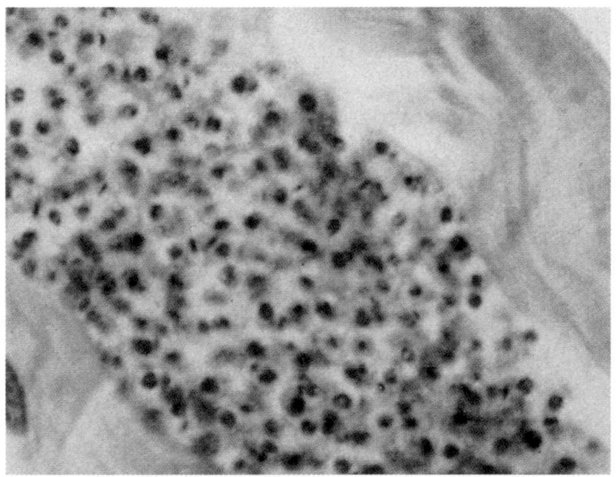

FIGURE 83–15. Amastigote stage of *T. cruzi* in skeletal muscle. (From Ash LR, Orihel TC: *Atlas of human parasitology,* ed 2, Chicago, 1984, American Society of Clinical Pathologists.)

Epidemiology

T. cruzi occurs widely in both reduviid bugs and a broad spectrum of reservoir animals in North, Central, and South America. Human disease is found most often among children in South and Central America, where approximately 12 million people are affected. There is a direct correlation between infected wild animal reservoir hosts and the presence of infected bugs whose nests are found in human homes. Cases are rare in the United States because the bugs prefer nesting in animal burrows and because homes are not as open to nesting as those in South and Central America.

Clinical Syndromes

Chagas' disease may be asymptomatic, acute, or chronic. One of the earliest signs is development at the site of the bug bite of an erythematous and indurated area, called a **chagoma.** This is often followed by a rash and edema around the eyes and face. The disease is most severe in children younger than 5 years of age and frequently is seen as an acute process with CNS involvement. Fever, chills, malaise, myalgia, and fatigue are also characteristics of acute infection. Parasites may be present in the blood during the acute phase; however, they are sparse in patients older than 1 year of age. Death may ensue a few weeks after an acute attack, the patient may recover, or the patient may enter the chronic phase as organisms proliferate and enter the heart, liver, spleen, brain, and lymph nodes.

Chronic Chagas' disease is characterized by hepatosplenomegaly, myocarditis, and enlargement of the esophagus and colon as a result of the destruction of nerve cells (e.g., Auerbach's plexus) and other tissues that control the growth of these organs.

Megacardia and electrocardiographic changes are commonly seen in chronic disease. Involvement of the CNS may produce granulomas in the brain with cyst formation and a meningoencephalitis. Death from chronic Chagas' disease results from tissue destruction in the many areas invaded by the organisms, and sudden death results from complete heart block and brain damage.

Laboratory Diagnosis

T. cruzi can be demonstrated in thick and thin blood films or concentrated anticoagulated blood early in the acute stage. As the infection progresses, the organisms leave the bloodstream and become difficult to find. Biopsy of lymph nodes, liver, spleen, or bone marrow may demonstrate the organisms in the amastigote stage. Culture of blood or inoculation into laboratory animals may be useful when the parasitemia is low. Serologic tests are also available. In endemic areas, xenodiagnosis is widely used. Gene amplification techniques, such as polymerase chain reaction, have been used to detect the organism in the bloodstream. These approaches are not widely available and have not been adapted for use in the field.

TREATMENT, PREVENTION, AND CONTROL

Treatment of Chagas' disease is limited by the lack of reliable agents. The drug of choice is nifurtimox. Although it has some activity against the acute phase of disease, it has little activity against tissue amastigotes and has a number of side effects. Alternative agents include allopurinol and benzimidazole. Education regarding the disease, its insect transmission, and the wild animal reservoirs is critical. Bug control, eradication of nests, and construction of homes to prevent nesting of bugs are also essential. The use of dichlorodiphenyltrichloroethane (DDT) in bug-infested homes has demonstrated a drop in the transmission of malaria and Chagas' disease. Screening of blood by serologic means or excluding blood donors from endemic areas prevents some infections that would otherwise be associated with transfusion therapy.

Development of a vaccine is possible because *T. cruzi* does not have the wide antigenic variation observed with the African trypanosomes.

CASE STUDY AND QUESTIONS

The patient, a 44-year-old heart transplant patient, complained to her primary physician about headache, nausea, and vomiting approximately 1 year after transplant. She had no skin lesions. A computed tomographic scan of the head demonstrated ring-enhancing lesions. A biopsy of the lesions was performed. All cultures (bacterial, fungal, viral) were negative. Special stains of the tissue revealed multiple cystlike structures of varying size.

1. What was the differential diagnosis of infectious agents in this patient? What was the most likely etiologic agent?
2. What other tests would have been done to confirm the diagnosis?
3. What aspects of the medical history might suggest a risk for infection with this agent?
4. What were the therapeutic options and the likelihood that therapy would be successful?

Bibliography

Connor DH et al, editors: *Pathology of infectious disease,* vol II, Stamford, Conn, 1997, Appleton & Lange.

Garcia LS, editors: *Diagnostic medical parasitology,* ed 4, Washington, 2001, American Society for Microbiology.

Handman E: Leishmaniasis: Current status of vaccine development. *Clin Microbiol Rev* 14:229-244, 2001.

Homer MJ et al: Babesiosis, *Clin Microbiol Rev* 13:451-469, 2000.

Marciano-Cabral F, Cabral G: *Acanthamoeba* spp. as agents of disease in humans. *Clin Microbiol Rev* 16:273-307, 2003.

Phillips RS: Current status of malaria and potential for control, *Clin Microbiol Rev* 14:208-226, 2001.

Shiff C: Integrated approach to malaria control, *Clin Microbiol Rev* 15:278-293, 2002.

Strickland GT, editor: *Hunter's tropical medicine and emerging infectious diseases,* ed 8, Philadelphia, 2000, WB Saunders.

Talisuna AO, Bloland P, D'Alessandro U: History, dynamics, and public health importance of malaria parasite resistance, *Clin Microbiol Rev* 17:235-254, 2004.

Visvesvara GS: Pathogenic and opportunistic free-living amebae. In Murray PR et al, editors: *Manual of clinical microbiology,* ed 8, Washington, 2003, American Society for Microbiology.

Zintl A et al: *Babesia divergens,* a bovine blood parasite of veterinary and zoonotic importance, *Clin Microbiol Rev* 16:622-636, 2003.

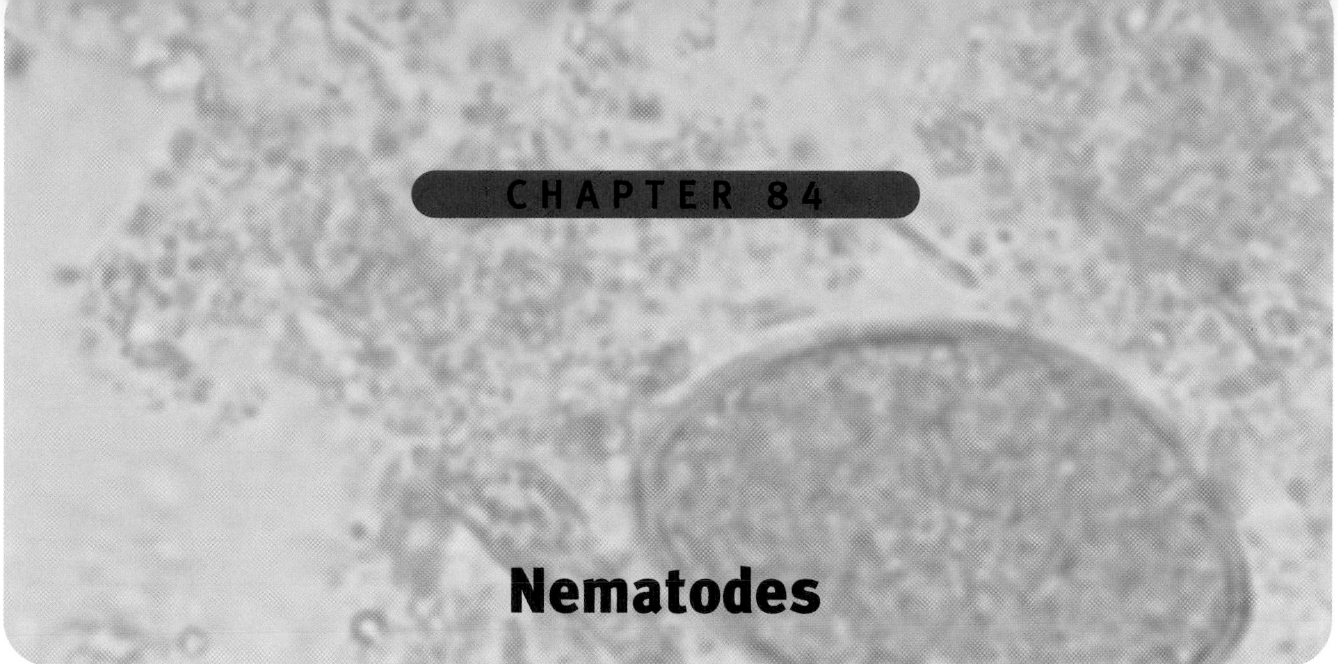

Nematodes

The most common helminths recognized in the United States are primarily intestinal nematodes, although in other countries nematode infections of blood and tissues can cause devastating disease. The nematodes are the most easily recognized form of intestinal parasite because of their large size and cylindrical, unsegmented bodies; hence the common name **roundworms.** These parasites live primarily as adult worms in the intestinal tract, and nematode infections are most commonly confirmed by detecting the characteristic eggs in feces. The identification of eggs should be approached in a systematic manner, taking into account the size and shape of the egg, the thickness of the shell, and the presence or absence of specialized structures, such as polar plugs, knobs, spines, and opercula. The presence and characteristics of larvae within the eggs may also be useful. The most common nematodes of medical importance are listed in Table 84–1.

The filariae are long, slender roundworms that are parasites of blood, lymph, subcutaneous, and connective tissues. All of these nematodes are transmitted by mosquitoes or biting flies. Most produce larval worms called microfilariae that are demonstrated in blood specimens or in subcutaneous tissues and skin snips.

Enterobius vermicularis

PHYSIOLOGY AND STRUCTURE

E. vermicularis, the **pinworm,** is a small, white worm that is familiar to parents who find them in the perianal folds or vagina of an infected child. Infection is initiated by ingestion of embryonated eggs (Figure 84–1). Larvae hatch in the small intestine and migrate to the large intestine, where they mature into adults in 2 to 6 weeks. Fertilization of the female by the male produces the characteristic asymmetrical eggs. The migrating female lays these eggs in the perianal folds. As many as 20,000 eggs are deposited on the perianal skin. The eggs rapidly mature and are infectious within hours.

EPIDEMIOLOGY

E. vermicularis occurs worldwide but is most common in the temperate regions, where person-to-person spread is greatest in crowded conditions, such as in daycare centers, schools, and mental institutions. An estimated 500 million cases of pinworm infection are reported worldwide, and this is the most common helminthic infection in North America.

Infection occurs when the eggs are ingested and the larval worm is free to develop in the intestinal mucosa. These eggs may be transmitted from hand to mouth by children scratching the perianal folds in response to the irritation caused by the migrating, egg-laying female worms, or the eggs may find their way to clothing and play objects in daycare centers. They can also survive long periods in the dust that accumulates over doors, on windowsills, and under beds in the rooms of infected people. Egg-laden dust can be inhaled and swallowed to produce infestation. In addition, **autoinfection ("retrofection")** can occur wherein eggs hatch in the perianal folds and the larval worms migrate into the rectum and large intestine. Infected individuals who handle food can also be a source of infection. No animal reservoir for *Enterobius* is known. Physicians should be aware of the related epidemiology of *Dientamoeba fragilis;* this organism correlates well with the presence of *E. vermicularis,* with *D. fragilis* transported in the pinworm eggshell.

CLINICAL SYNDROMES

Many children and adults show no symptoms and serve only as carriers. Patients who are allergic to the secretions

TABLE 84–1. Nematodes of Medical Importance

Parasite	Common Name	Disease
Enterobius vermicularis	Pinworm	Enterobiasis
Ascaris lumbricoides	Roundworm	Ascariasis
Toxocara canis	Dog ascaris	Visceral larva migrans
Toxocara cati	Cat ascaris	Visceral larva migrans
Trichuris trichiura	Whipworm	Trichuriasis
Ancylostoma duodenale	Old World hookworm	Hookworm infection
Necator americanus	New World hookworm	Hookworm infection
Ancylostoma braziliense	Dog or cat hookworm	Cutaneous larva migrans
Strongyloides stercoralis	Threadworm	Strongyloidiasis
Trichinella spiralis	—	Trichinosis
Wuchereria bancrofti	Bancroft's filariasis	Filariasis
Brugia malayi	Malayan filariasis	Filariasis
Loa loa	African eye worm	Loiasis
Mansonella species	Mansonelliasis	Filariasis
Onchocerca volvulus	River blindness	Onchocerciasis
Dirofilaria immitis	Dog heartworm	Filariasis
Dracunculus medinensis	Guinea worm	Dracunculosis

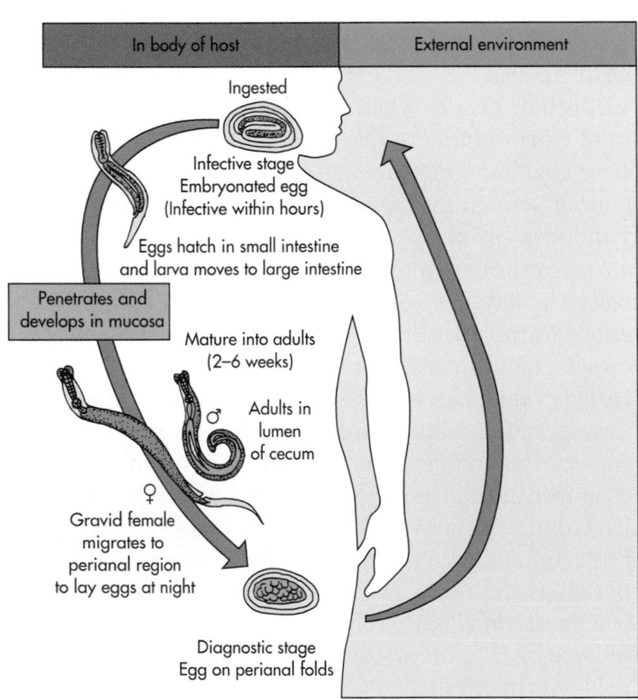

FIGURE 84–1. Life cycle of *Enterobius vermicularis*.

of the migrating worms experience severe pruritus, loss of sleep, and fatigue. The pruritus may cause repeated scratching of the irritated area and lead to secondary bacterial infection. Worms that migrate into the vagina may produce genitourinary problems and granulomas.

Worms attached to the bowel wall may produce inflammation and granuloma formation around the eggs. Although the adult worms may occasionally invade the appendix, there remains no proven relationship between pinworm invasion and appendicitis. Penetration through the bowel wall into the peritoneal cavity, liver, and lungs has been infrequently recorded.

LABORATORY DIAGNOSIS

The diagnosis of **enterobiasis** is usually suggested by the clinical manifestations and confirmed by detection of the characteristic eggs on the anal mucosa. Occasionally, laboratory personnel see the adult worms in stool specimens, but the method of choice for diagnosis involves use of an anal swab with a sticky surface that picks up the eggs (Figure 84–2) for microscopic examination. Sampling can be done with clear tape or commercially available swabs. The sample should be collected when the child arises and before bathing or defecation to pick up eggs laid by migrating worms during the night. Parents can collect the

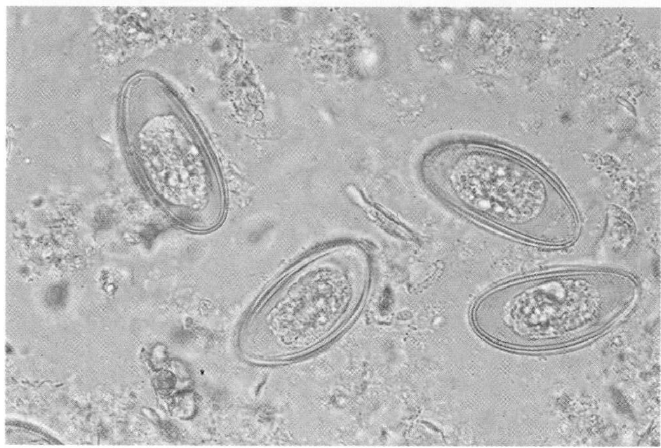

FIGURE 84–2. *E. vermicularis* egg. The thin-walled eggs are 50 to 60 μm × 20 to 30 μm, ovoid, and flattened on one side (not because children sit on them, but this is an easy way to correlate the egg morphology with the epidemiology of the disease).

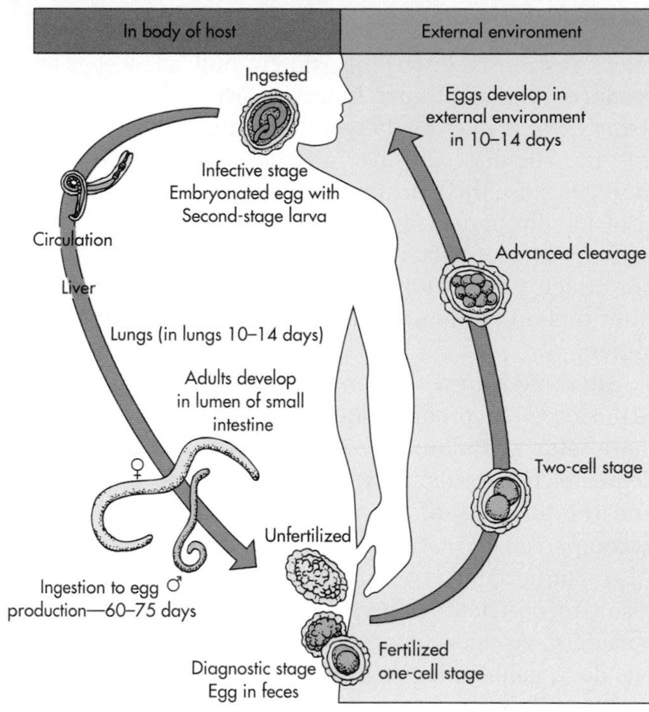

FIGURE 84–3. Life cycle of *Ascaris lumbricoides*.

specimen and deliver it to the physician for immediate microscopic examination. Three swabbings, one per day for 3 consecutive days, may be required to detect the diagnostic eggs. The eggs are rarely seen in fecal specimens. Systemic signs of infection such as eosinophilia are rare.

TREATMENT, PREVENTION, AND CONTROL

The drug of choice is pyrantel pamoate; as an alternative drug, mebendazole is used. To avoid reintroduction of the organism and reinfection in the family environment, it is customary to treat the entire family simultaneously. Although cure rates are high, reinfection is common. Repeat treatment after 2 weeks may be useful in preventing reinfection.

Personal hygiene, clipping of fingernails, thorough washing of bed clothes, and prompt treatment of infected individuals all contribute to control. When housecleaning is done in the home of an infected family, dusting under beds, on windowsills, and over doors should be done with a damp mop to avoid inhalation of infectious eggs.

Ascaris lumbricoides

PHYSIOLOGY AND STRUCTURE

A. lumbricoides are large (20- to 35-cm long), pink worms that have a more complex life cycle than *E. vermicularis* (Figure 84–3) but are otherwise typical of an intestinal roundworm.

The ingested infective egg releases a larval worm that penetrates the duodenal wall, enters the bloodstream, is carried to the liver and heart, and then enters the pulmonary circulation. The larvae break free in the alveoli of the lungs, where they grow and molt. In approximately 3 weeks, the larvae pass from the respiratory system to be coughed up, swallowed, and returned to the small intestine.

As the male and female worms mature in the small intestine (primarily jejunum), fertilization of the female by the male initiates egg production, which may amount to 200,000 eggs per day for as long as a year. Female worms can also produce unfertilized eggs in the absence of males. Eggs are found in the feces 60 to 75 days after the initial infection. Fertilized eggs become infectious after approximately 2 weeks in the soil.

EPIDEMIOLOGY

A. lumbricoides is prevalent in areas where sanitation is poor and where human feces are used as fertilizer. Because food and water are contaminated with *Ascaris* eggs, this parasite, more than any other, affects the world's population. Although no animal reservoir is known for *A. lumbricoides*, an almost identical species from pigs, *Ascaris suum*, can infect humans. This species is seen in swine growers and is associated with the use of pig manure for gardening. *Ascaris* eggs are quite hardy and can survive extreme temperatures and persist for several months in feces and sewage. Ascariasis is the most common helminthic infection worldwide, with an estimated 1 billion people infected.

CLINICAL SYNDROMES

Infections caused by the ingestion of only a few eggs may produce no symptoms; however, even a single adult *Ascaris* worm may be dangerous because it can migrate into the bile duct and liver and damage tissue. Furthermore, because the worm has a tough, flexible body, it can occasionally perforate the intestine, creating peritonitis with secondary bacterial infection. The adult worms do not attach to the intestinal mucosa but depend on constant motion to maintain their position within the bowel lumen.

After infection with many larvae, migration of worms to the lungs can produce pneumonitis resembling an asthmatic attack. Pulmonary involvement is related to the degree of hypersensitivity induced by previous infections and the intensity of the current exposure and may be accompanied by eosinophilia and oxygen desaturation. Also, a tangled bolus of mature worms in the intestine can result in obstruction, perforation, and occlusion of the appendix. As mentioned previously, migration into the bile duct, gallbladder, and liver can produce severe tissue damage. This migration can occur in response to fever, drugs other than those used to treat ascariasis, and some anesthetics. Patients with many larvae may also experience abdominal tenderness, fever, distention, and vomiting.

LABORATORY DIAGNOSIS

Examination of the sediment of concentrated stool reveals the knobby-coated, bile-stained, fertilized and unfertilized eggs. Eggs are oval, 55- to 75-mm long, and 50-mm wide. The thick-walled outer shell can be partially removed (**decorticated** egg). Occasionally, adult worms pass with the feces, which can be quite dramatic because of their large size (20- to 35-cm long). Roentgenologists may also visualize the worms in the intestine, and cholangiograms often disclose their presence in the biliary tract of the liver. The pulmonary phase of the disease may be diagnosed by the finding of larvae and eosinophils in sputum.

TREATMENT, PREVENTION, AND CONTROL

Treatment of symptomatic infection is highly effective. The drug of choice is mebendazole; pyrantel pamoate and piperazine are alternatives. Patients with mixed parasitic infections (*A. lumbricoides*, other helminths, *Giardia lamblia*, and *Entamoeba histolytica*) in the stool should be treated for ascariasis first to avoid provoking worm migration and possible intestinal perforation. Education, improved sanitation, and avoidance of human feces as fertilizer are critical. A program of mass treatment in highly endemic areas has been suggested, but this may not be economically feasible. Furthermore, eggs can persist in contaminated soil for 3 years or more. Certainly, improved personal hygiene among people who handle food is an important aspect of control.

Toxocara canis and *Toxocara cati*

PHYSIOLOGY AND STRUCTURE

T. canis and *T. cati* are ascarid worms, naturally parasitic in the intestines of dogs and cats, that accidentally infect humans, producing a disease called **visceral larval migrans** or **toxocariasis.** When ingested by humans, the eggs of these worms can hatch into larval forms that cannot follow the normal developmental cycle as in the natural dog or cat host. They can penetrate the human gut and reach the bloodstream and then migrate as larvae to various human tissues. They do not develop beyond the migrating larval form.

EPIDEMIOLOGY

Wherever infected dogs and cats are present, the eggs are a threat to humans. This is especially true for children who are exposed more readily to contaminated soil and who tend to put objects in their mouths.

CLINICAL SYNDROMES

The clinical manifestations of **toxocariasis** in humans are related to the migration of the larvae through tissues. The larvae may invade any tissue of the body, where they can induce bleeding, the formation of eosinophilic granulomas, and necrosis. Patients may be asymptomatic and have only eosinophilia, but they can also have serious disease directly related to the number and location of the lesions caused by the migrating larvae, as well as the degree to which the host is sensitized to the larval antigens. The organs most often involved are the lungs, heart, kidneys, liver, skeletal muscles, eyes, and central nervous system. Signs and symptoms include cough, wheezing, fever, rash, anorexia, seizures, fatigue, and abdominal discomfort. On examination, patients may have hepatosplenomegaly and nodular pruritic skin lesions. Death may result from respiratory failure, cardiac arrhythmia, or brain damage. Ocular disease can also occur with the movement of larvae through the eye and may be mistaken for malignant retinoblastoma. Prompt diagnosis is required to avoid unnecessary enucleation.

LABORATORY DIAGNOSIS

The diagnosis of **visceral larval migrans** is based on clinical findings, the presence of eosinophilia, known exposure to dogs or cats, and serologic confirmation. Enzyme-linked immunosorbent assays are readily available and appear to offer the best serologic marker for disease. The examination of feces from infected patients is not useful because egg-laying adults are not present. However, examination of fecal material from infected pets often supports the diagnosis. Tissue examination for larvae may provide a definitive diagnosis but may be negative because of sampling error.

TREATMENT, PREVENTION, AND CONTROL

Treatment is primarily symptomatic, because antiparasitic agents are not of proven benefit. The drug of choice is diethylcarbamazine or thiabendazole. Mebendazole is an acceptable alternative. Corticosteroid therapy may be life saving if the patient has serious pulmonary, myocardial, or central nervous system involvement, because a major component of the infection is an inflammatory response to the organism. This zoonosis can be greatly reduced if pet owners conscientiously eradicate worms from their animals and clean up pet fecal material from yards and school playgrounds. Children's play areas and sandboxes should be carefully monitored.

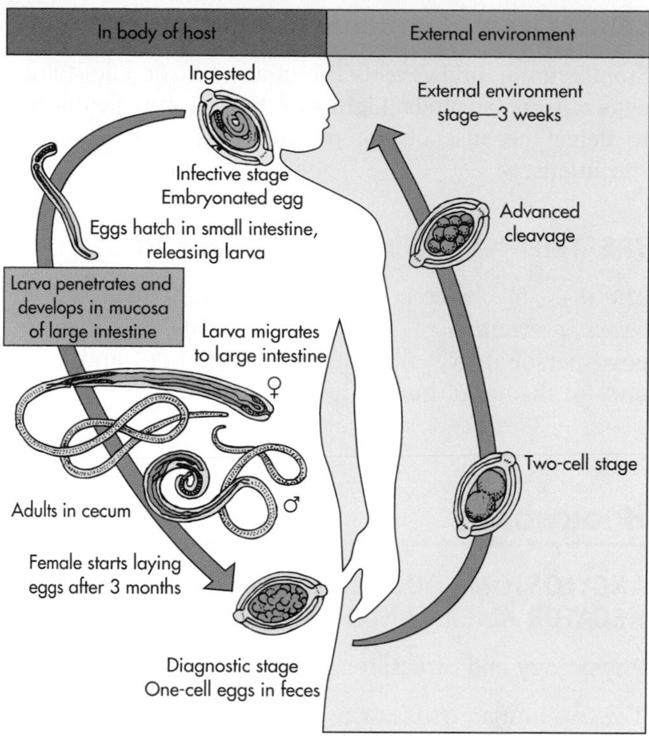

FIGURE 84–4. Life cycle of *T. trichiura.*

Trichuris trichiura

PHYSIOLOGY AND STRUCTURE

Commonly called **whipworm** because it resembles the handle and lash of a whip, *T. trichiura* has a simple life cycle (Figure 84–4). Ingested eggs hatch into a larval worm in the small intestine and then migrate to the cecum, where they penetrate the mucosa and mature to adults. Some 3 months after the initial infection, the fertilized female worm starts laying eggs and may produce 3000 to 10,000 eggs per day. Female worms can live for as long as 8 years. Eggs passed into the soil mature and become infectious in 3 weeks. *T. trichiura* eggs are distinctive, with dark bile staining, a barrel shape, and the presence of polar plugs in the egg shell (Figure 84–5).

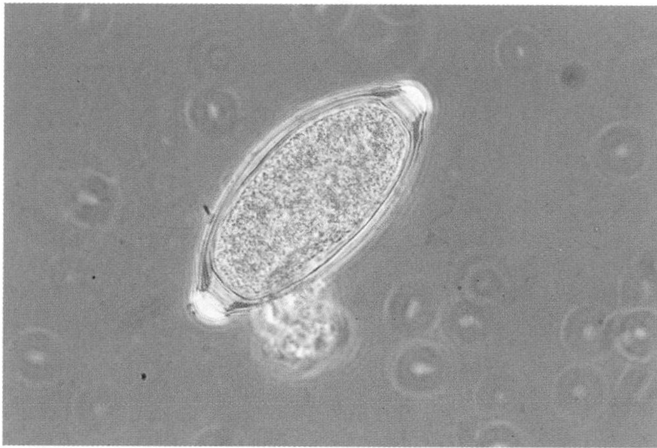

FIGURE 84–5. *Trichuris trichiura* egg. The eggs are barrel shaped, measuring 50 × 24 μm, with a thick wall and two prominent plugs at the ends. Internally, an unsegmented ovum is present.

EPIDEMIOLOGY

Like *A. lumbricoides, T. trichiura* has worldwide distribution and its prevalence is directly correlated with poor sanitation and the use of human feces as fertilizer. No animal reservoir is recognized.

CLINICAL SYNDROMES

The clinical manifestations of **trichuriasis** are generally related to the intensity of the worm burden. Most infections are with small numbers of *Trichuris* organisms and are usually asymptomatic, although secondary bacterial infection may occur because the heads of the worms penetrate deep into the intestinal mucosa. Infections with many larvae may produce abdominal pain and distention, bloody diarrhea, weakness, and weight loss. Appendicitis may occur as worms fill the lumen, and prolapse of the rectum is seen in children because of the irritation and straining during defecation. Anemia and eosinophilia are also seen in severe infections.

LABORATORY DIAGNOSIS

Stool examination reveals the characteristic bile-stained eggs with polar plugs. Light infestations may be difficult to detect because of the paucity of eggs in the stool specimens.

TREATMENT, PREVENTION, AND CONTROL

The drug of choice is mebendazole. As with *A. lumbricoides,* prevention of *T. trichiura* depends on education, good personal hygiene, adequate sanitation, and avoidance of the use of human feces as fertilizer.

Hookworms

ANCYLOSTOMA DUODENALE AND NECATOR AMERICANUS

Physiology and Structure

The two human hookworms are *A. duodenale* **(Old World hookworm)** and *N. americanus* **(New World hookworm).** Differing only in geographic distribution, structure of mouthparts, and relative size, these two species are discussed together as agents of hookworm infection. The human phase of the hookworm life cycle is initiated when a filariform (infective form) larva penetrates intact skin (Figure 84–6). The larva then enters the circulation; is carried to the lungs; and like *A. lumbricoides,* is coughed up, swallowed, and develops to adulthood in the small intestine. The adult *N. americanus* has a hooklike head, which accounts for the name commonly used. Adult worms lay as many as 10,000 to 20,000 eggs per day, which are released into feces. Egg laying is initiated 4 to 8 weeks after the initial exposure and can persist for as long as 5 years. On contact with soil, the **rhabditiform** (noninfective) larvae are released from the eggs and within 2 weeks develop into **filariform** larvae. The filariform larvae can then penetrate exposed skin (e.g., bare feet) and initiate a new cycle of human infection.

Both species have mouthparts designed for sucking blood from injured intestinal tissue. *A. duodenale* has chitinous teeth, and *N. americanus* has shearing chitinous plates.

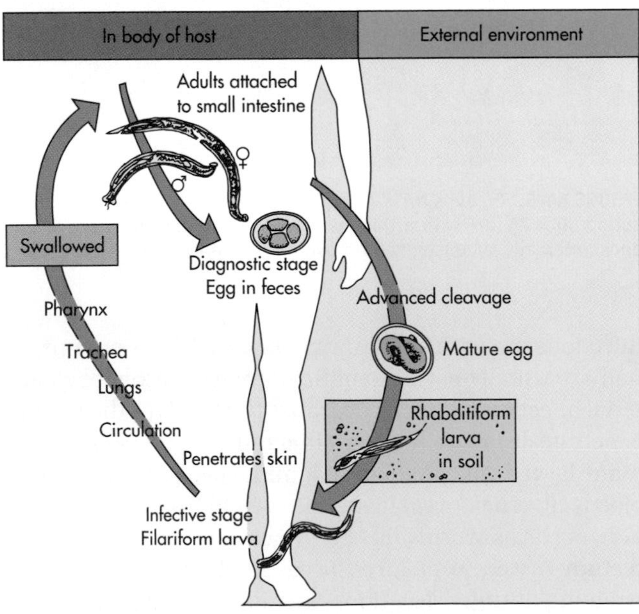

FIGURE 84–6. Life cycle of human hookworms.

Epidemiology

Transmission of hookworm infection requires the deposition of egg-containing feces on shady, well-drained soil and is favored by warm, humid (tropical) conditions. Hookworm infections are reported worldwide in places where direct contact with contaminated soil can lead to human disease, but they occur primarily in warm subtropical and tropical regions and in southern parts of the United States. It is estimated that more than 900 million individuals worldwide are infected with hookworms, including 700,000 in the United States.

Clinical Syndromes

Skin-penetrating larvae may produce an allergic reaction and rash at sites of entry, and larvae migrating in the lungs can cause pneumonitis. Adult worms produce the gastrointestinal symptoms of nausea, vomiting, and diarrhea. As blood is lost due to feeding worms, a microcytic hypochromic anemia develops. Daily blood loss is estimated at 0.15 to 0.25 ml for each adult *A. duodenale* and 0.03 ml for each adult *N. americanus.* In severe chronic infections, emaciation and mental and physical retardation may occur related to anemia from blood loss and nutritional deficiencies. Also, intestinal sites may be secondarily infected by bacteria when the worms migrate along the intestinal mucosa.

Laboratory Diagnosis

Stool examination reveals the characteristic non–bile-stained segmented eggs shown in Figure 84–7. Larvae are not found in stool specimens unless the specimen was left at ambient temperature for a day or more. The eggs of *A. duodenale* and *N. americanus* cannot be distinguished. The larvae must be examined to identify these hookworms specifically, although this is clinically unnecessary.

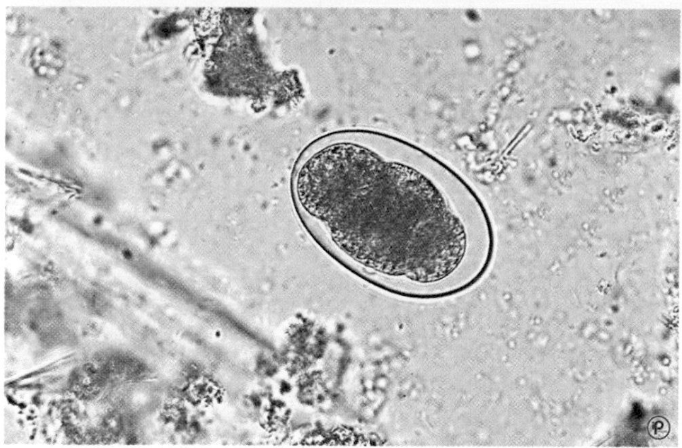

FIGURE 84–7. Human hookworm egg. The eggs are 60- to 75-µm long and 35- to 40-µm wide, are thin shelled, and enclose a developing larva. (From Marler LM et al: *Parasitology* CD-Rom, Indiana Pathology Images, 2003.)

Treatment, Prevention, and Control

The drug of choice is mebendazole; pyrantel pamoate is an alternative. In addition to eradication of the worms to stop blood loss, iron therapy is indicated to raise hemoglobin levels to normal. Blood transfusion may be necessary in severe cases of anemia. Education, improved sanitation, and controlled disposal of human feces are critical preventive measures. Wearing shoes in endemic areas helps reduce the prevalence of infection.

ANCYLOSTOMA BRAZILIENSE

Physiology and Structure

A. braziliense, a species of hookworm, is naturally parasitic in the intestines of dogs and cats and accidentally infects humans. It produces a disease properly called **cutaneous larva migrans** but also called **ground itch** and **creeping eruption.** The filariform larvae of this hookworm penetrate intact skin but can develop no further in humans. The larvae remain trapped in the skin of the wrong host for weeks or months, wandering through subcutaneous tissue and creating serpentine tunnels.

Epidemiology

Similar to the situation with *Ascaris* worms, the threat of infection with *A. braziliense* is greatest among children coming into contact with soil or sandboxes contaminated with animal feces that contains hookworm eggs. Infections are prevalent throughout the year on beaches in subtropical and tropical regions; in the summer, infection is reported as far north as the Canadian–U.S. border.

Clinical Syndromes

The migrating larvae may provoke a severe erythematous and vesicular reaction. Pruritus and scratching of the irritated skin may lead to secondary bacterial infection. Approximately half of patients develop transient pulmonary infiltrates with peripheral eosinophilia **(Loeffler's syndrome),** presumably resulting from pulmonary migration of the larvae.

Laboratory Diagnosis

Occasionally, larvae are recovered in skin biopsy or after freezing of the skin, but most diagnoses are based on the clinical appearance of the tunnels and a history of contact with dog and cat feces. The larvae are rarely found in sputum.

Treatment, Prevention, and Control

The drug of choice is thiabendazole. Antihistamines may be helpful in controlling pruritus. This zoonosis, as with animal *Ascaris* infection, can be reduced by educating pet owners to treat their animals for worm infections and to pick up pet feces from yards, beaches, and sandboxes. In endemic areas, shoes or sandals should be worn to prevent infection.

Strongyloides stercoralis

PHYSIOLOGY AND STRUCTURE

Although the morphology of these worms and epidemiology of their infections are similar to the hookworm, the life cycle of *S. stercoralis* (Figure 84–8) differs in three aspects: (1) Eggs hatch into larvae in the intestine and before they are passed in feces, (2) larvae can mature into filariforms in the intestine and cause autoinfection, and (3) a free-living, nonparasitic cycle can be established outside the human host.

In direct development, like the hookworm, a skin-penetrating *S. stercoralis* larva enters the circulation and follows the pulmonary course. It is coughed up and swallowed, and adults develop in the small intestine. Adult females burrow into the mucosa of the duodenum and reproduce parthenogenetically. Each female produces approximately a dozen eggs each day, which hatch within the mucosa and release **rhabditiform** larvae into the lumen of the bowel. The rhabditiform larvae are distinguished from the larvae of hookworms by their short buccal capsule and large genital primordium. The rhabditiform larvae are passed in the stool and may either continue the direct cycle by developing into infective

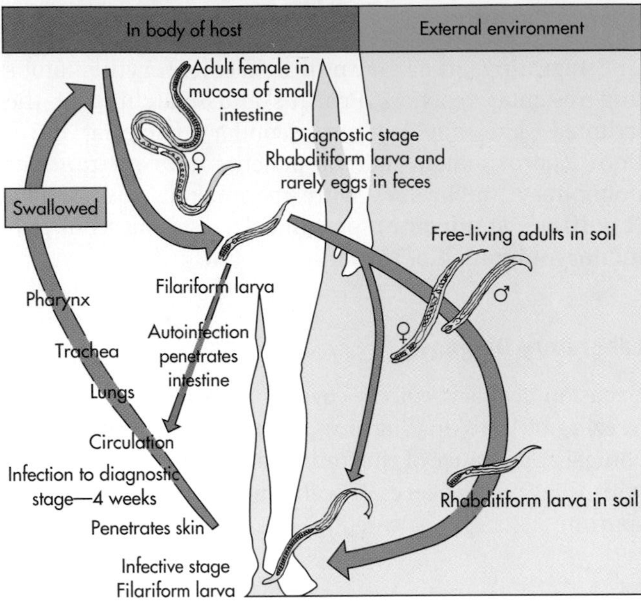

FIGURE 84–8. Life cycle of *Strongyloides stercoralis.*

filariform larvae or develop into free-living adult worms and initiate the indirect cycle.

In indirect development, the larvae in soil develop into free-living adults that produce eggs and larvae. Several generations of this nonparasitic existence may occur before new larvae become skin-penetrating parasites.

Finally, in **autoinfection,** rhabditiform larvae in the intestine do not pass with feces but become filariform larvae. These penetrate the intestinal or perianal skin and follow the course through the circulation and pulmonary structures, are coughed up, and then are swallowed; at this point they become adults, producing more larvae in the intestine. This cycle can persist for years and can lead to **hyperinfection** and massive or disseminated, often fatal infection.

EPIDEMIOLOGY

Similar to hookworms in its requirements for warm temperatures and moisture, *S. stercoralis* demonstrates low prevalence but a somewhat broader geographic distribution, including parts of the northern United States and Canada. Sexual transmission also occurs. Animal reservoirs, such as domestic pets, are recognized.

CLINICAL SYNDROMES

Individuals with **strongyloidiasis** frequently are afflicted with pneumonitis from migrating larvae similar to that seen in ascariasis and hookworm infection. The intestinal infection is usually asymptomatic. However, heavy worm loads may involve the biliary and pancreatic ducts, the entire small bowel, and the colon, causing inflammation and ulceration, leading to epigastric pain and tenderness, vomiting, diarrhea (occasionally bloody), and malabsorption. Symptoms mimicking peptic ulcer disease coupled with peripheral eosinophilia should strongly suggest the diagnosis of strongyloidiasis.

Autoinfection may lead to chronic strongyloidiasis that can last for years even in nonendemic areas. Although many of these chronic infections may be asymptomatic, as many as two thirds of patients have recurring episodic symptoms referable to the involved skin, lungs, and intestinal tract. Individuals with chronic strongyloidiasis are at risk of developing severe, life-threatening **hyperinfection syndrome** if the host-parasite balance is disturbed by any drug or illness that compromises the host's immune status. Hyperinfection syndrome is seen most commonly in individuals immunocompromised by malignancies (especially hematologic malignancies), corticosteroid therapy, or both. Hyperinfection syndrome has also been observed in patients who have undergone solid organ transplantation and in malnourished people. Loss of cellular immune function may be associated with the conversion of rhabditiform larvae to filariform larvae, followed by dissemination of the larvae via the circulation to virtually any organ. Most commonly, extraintestinal infection involves the lung and includes bronchospasm, diffuse infiltrates, and occasionally cavitation. Widespread dissemination that involves the abdominal lymph nodes, liver, spleen, kidneys, pancreas, thyroid, heart, brain, and meninges is common. Intestinal symptoms of hyperinfection syndrome include profound diarrhea, malabsorption, and electrolyte abnormalities. Notably, hyperinfection syndrome is associated with a mortality rate of approximately 86%. Bacterial sepsis, meningitis, peritonitis, and endocarditis secondary to larval spread from the intestine are frequent and often fatal complications of hyperinfection syndrome.

LABORATORY DIAGNOSIS

The diagnosis of strongyloidiasis may be difficult because of the intermittent passage of low numbers of first-stage larvae in stool. Examination of concentrated stool sediment reveals the larval worms (Figure 84–9), but in contrast with hookworm infections, eggs are generally not seen in *S. stercoralis* infections. Collecting samples from three stools, one per day for 3 days, as for *G. lamblia,* is recommended because *S. stercoralis* larvae may occur in "showers," with many present one day and few or none the next. Several authors favor the **Baermann funnel gauze method** of concentrating living *S. stercoralis* larvae from fecal specimens. This method uses a funnel with a stopcock and a gauze insert. The funnel is filled with lukewarm water to a level just covering the gauze, and a specimen of stool is placed on the gauze, partially in

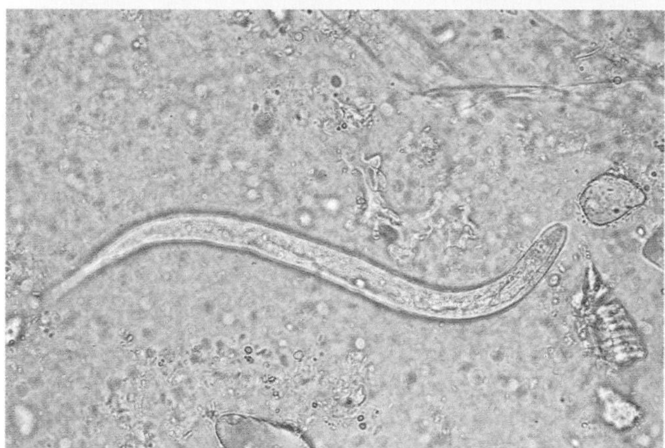

FIGURE 84–9. *S. stercoralis* larvae. The larvae are 180- to 380-μm long and 14- to 24-μm wide. They are differentiated from hookworm larvae by the length of the buccal cavity and esophagus and by the structure of the genital primordium.

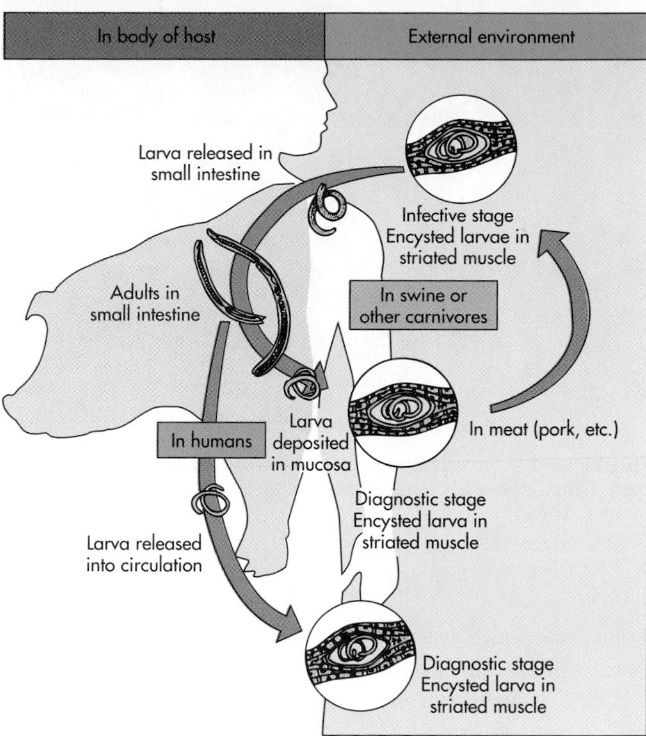

FIGURE 84–10. Life cycle of *Trichinella spiralis*.

contact with the water. The larvae in the stool migrate through the gauze into the water and then sediment into the neck of the funnel, where they may be detected by low-power microscopy. When absent from stool, larvae may be detected in duodenal aspirates or in sputum in the case of massive infection. Finally, culture of the larvae from stool using charcoal cultures or an agar plate method may be used, although these are not routine in most laboratories. Serologic tests are generally not available.

TREATMENT, PREVENTION, AND CONTROL

All infected patients should be treated to prevent autoinfection and potential dissemination (hyperinfection) of the parasite. The drug of choice is thiabendazole, with mebendazole as an alternative. Patients in endemic areas who are preparing to undergo immunosuppressive therapy should have at least three stool examinations to rule out *S. stercoralis* infection and thus avoid the risks of autoinfection. Strict infection-control measures should be enforced when clinicians care for patients with hyperinfection syndrome, because stool, saliva, vomitus, and body fluids may contain infectious filariform larvae. As with hookworm, control of *Strongyloides* species requires education, proper sanitation, and prompt treatment of existing infections.

Trichinella spiralis

PHYSIOLOGY AND STRUCTURE

T. spiralis is the etiologic agent of **trichinosis.** The adult form of this organism lives in the duodenal and jejunal mucosa of flesh-eating mammals worldwide. The infectious larval form is present in the striated muscles of carnivorous and omnivorous mammals. Among domestic animals, swine are most frequently involved. Figure 84–10 illustrates the simple, direct life cycle, which terminates in the musculature of humans, where the larvae eventually die and calcify.

The infection begins when meat that contains encysted larvae is digested. The larvae leave the meat in the small intestine and within 2 days develop into adult worms. A single fertilized female produces more than 1500 larvae in 1 to 3 months. These larvae move from the intestinal mucosa into the bloodstream and are carried in the circulation to various muscle sites throughout the body, where they coil in striated muscle fibers and become encysted (Figure 84–11). The muscles invaded most often include the extraocular muscles of the eye; the tongue; the deltoid, pectoral, and intercostal muscles; the diaphragm; and the gastrocnemius muscle. The encysted larvae remain viable for many years and are infectious if ingested by a new animal host.

EPIDEMIOLOGY

Trichinosis occurs worldwide in humans, and its greatest prevalence is associated with the consumption of pork products. In addition to its transmission from pigs, many carnivorous and omnivorous animals harbor the organism and are potential sources of human infection. Notably,

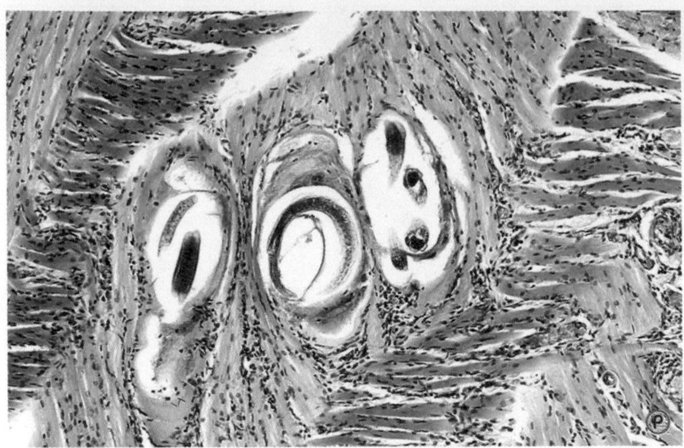

FIGURE 84–11. Encysted larva of *T. spiralis* in a muscle biopsy specimen. (From Marler LM et al: *Parasitology* CD-Rom, Indiana Pathology Images, 2003.)

polar bears and walruses in the Arctic account for outbreaks in human populations, especially with a strain of *T. spiralis* that is more resistant to freezing than the *T. spiralis* strains found in the continental United States and other temperate regions. It is estimated that more than 1.5 million Americans carry live *Trichinella* cysts in their musculature and that 150,000 to 300,000 acquire new infection annually.

CLINICAL SYNDROMES

Trichinosis is one of the few tissue parasitic diseases still seen in the United States. As with other parasitic infections, most patients have minimal or no symptoms. The clinical presentation depends largely on the tissue burden of organisms and the location of the migrating larvae. Patients in whom no more than 10 larvae are deposited per gram of tissue are usually asymptomatic; those with at least 100 generally have significant disease; and those with 1000 to 5000 have a very serious course that occasionally ends in death. In mild infections with few migrating larvae, patients may experience only an influenza-like syndrome with slight fever and mild diarrhea. With more extensive larval migration, persistent fever, gastrointestinal distress, marked eosinophilia, muscle pain, and periorbital edema occur. "Splinter" hemorrhages beneath the nails, a common finding, are probably caused by vasculitis resulting from toxic secretions of the migrating larvae. In heavy infections, severe neurologic symptoms, including psychosis, meningoencephalitis, and cerebrovascular accident, may occur.

Patients who survive the migration, muscle destruction, and encystment of larvae in moderate infections experience a decline in clinical symptoms in 5 or 6 weeks. Lethal trichinosis results when myocarditis, encephalitis, and pneumonitis combine; the patient dies 4 to 6 weeks after infection. Respiratory arrest often follows heavy invasion and muscle destruction in the diaphragm.

LABORATORY DIAGNOSIS

The diagnosis is usually established with clinical observations, especially when an outbreak can be traced to consumption of improperly cooked pork or bear meat. The laboratory may confirm the diagnosis if the encysted larvae are detected in the implicated meat or in a muscle biopsy specimen from the patient. Marked eosinophilia is characteristically present in patients with trichinosis. Serologic procedures are also available for confirmation of the diagnosis. Significant antibody titers are usually absent before the third week of illness but then may persist for years.

TREATMENT, PREVENTION, AND CONTROL

Treatment of trichinosis is primarily symptomatic because there are no good antiparasitic agents for tissue larvae. Treatment of the adult worms in the intestine with mebendazole may halt the production of new larvae. Steroids, along with thiabendazole or mebendazole, are recommended for severe symptoms. Education regarding disease transmission from pork and bear meat is essential, especially the recommendation that pork and bear meat be cooked until the interior is gray. Microwave cooking and smoking or drying meat do not kill all larvae.

Laws regulating the feeding of garbage to pigs help control transmission, as may regulations controlling the foraging of bears in garbage pits and public parks. Freezing pork, as conducted in federally inspected meat packing plants, has reduced transmission. Quick freezing of pork at −40°C effectively destroys the organisms, as does low-temperature storage at −15°C for 20 days or more.

Wuchereria bancrofti and *Brugia malayi*

PHYSIOLOGY AND STRUCTURE

Because of their many similarities, *W. bancrofti* and *B. malayi* are discussed together. Human infection is initiated by the introduction of infective larvae, which is present in the saliva of a biting mosquito, into a bite wound (Figure 84–12). Various species of *Anopheles, Aedes,* and *Culex* mosquitoes are vectors of **Bancroft's** and **Malayan filariasis.** The larvae migrate from the location of the bite to the lymphatic system, primarily in the arms, legs, or groin, where larval growth to adulthood occurs. From 3 to 12 months after the initial infection, the adult male

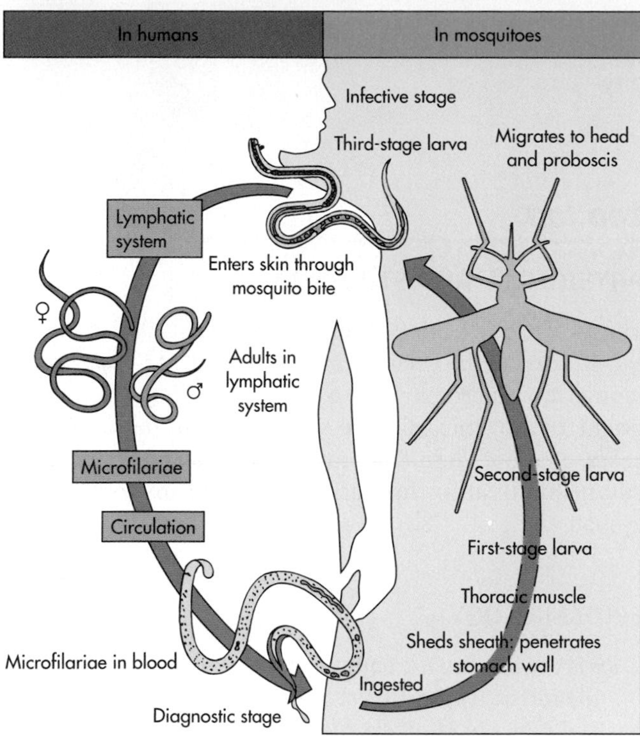

FIGURE 84–12. Life cycle of *Wuchereria bancrofti.*

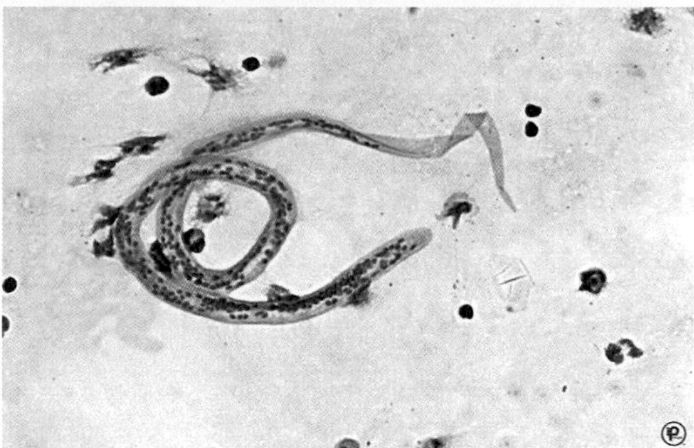

FIGURE 84–13. *W. bancrofti* microfilaria in blood smear. (From Marler LM et al: *Parasitology* CD-Rom, Indiana Pathology Images, 2003.)

worm fertilizes the female, which in turn produces the sheathed larval microfilariae that find their way into the circulation. The presence of **microfilariae** in blood is diagnostic for human disease and is infective for feeding mosquitoes. In the mosquito, the larvae move through the stomach and thoracic muscles in developmental stages and finally migrate to the proboscis. There, they become infective third-stage larvae and are transmitted by the feeding mosquito. The adult form in humans can persist for as long as 10 years.

EPIDEMIOLOGY

Infection with *W. bancrofti* occurs in tropical and subtropical areas and is endemic in central Africa, along the Mediterranean coast, and in many parts of Asia, including China, Korea, Japan, and the Philippines. It is also present in Haiti, Trinidad, Suriname, Panama, Costa Rica, and Brazil. No animal reservoir has been identified. *B. malayi* is found primarily in Malaysia, India, Thailand, Vietnam, and parts of China, Korea, Japan, and many Pacific islands. Animal reservoirs such as cats and monkeys are recognized.

CLINICAL SYNDROMES

In some patients, there is no sign of disease, even though blood specimens may show the presence of many microfilariae. In other patients, early acute symptoms are fever, lymphangitis and lymphadenitis with chills, and recurrent febrile attacks. The acute presentation is thought to result from the inflammatory response to the presence of molting adolescent worms and dead or dying adults within the lymphatic vessels. As the infection progresses, the lymph nodes enlarge, possibly involving many parts of the body, including the extremities, the scrotum, and the testes, with occasional abscess formation. This results from the physical obstruction of lymph in the vessels caused by the presence of adult worms and host reactivity in the lymphatic system. This process may be complicated by recurrent bacterial infections, which contribute to the tissue damage. The thickening and hypertrophy of tissues infected with the worms may lead to the enlargement of tissues, especially the extremities, progressing to filarial **elephantiasis.** Filariasis of this type is thus a chronic, debilitating, and disfiguring disease requiring prompt diagnosis and treatment. Occasionally, ascites and pleural effusions secondary to rupture of the enlarged lymphatic vessels into the peritoneal or pleural cavity may be observed.

LABORATORY DIAGNOSIS

Eosinophilia is usually present during acute inflammatory episodes; however, demonstration of microfilariae in the blood is required for definitive diagnosis. As with malaria, microfilariae can be demonstrated in Giemsa-stained blood films in infections with *W. bancrofti* and *B. malayi* (Figure 84–13). Concentration of anticoagulated blood specimens and urine specimens are also valuable procedures. Buffy coat films concentrate the white blood cells and are useful for the detection of microfilariae. The presence of small numbers of microfilariae in blood can be detected by a membrane-filtration technique in which anticoagulated blood is mixed with saline and forced

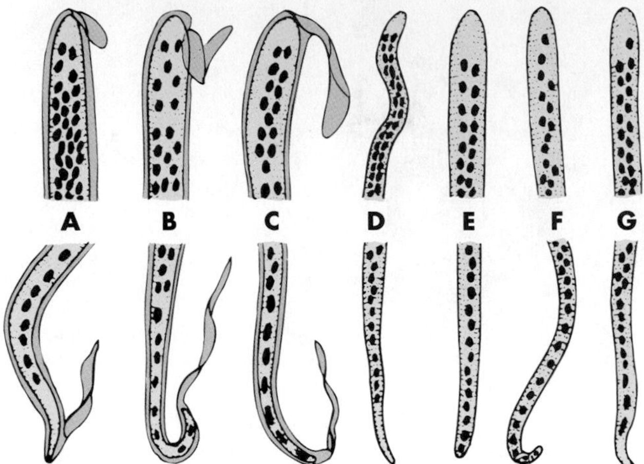

FIGURE 84–14. Differentiation of microfilariae. Identification of microfilariae is based on the presence of a sheath covering the larvae, as well as the distribution of nuclei in the tail region. A, *W. bancrofti;* B, *B. malayi;* C, *L. loa;* D, *O. volvulus;* E, *Mansonella perstans;* F, *Mansonella streptocerca;* G, *Mansonella ozzardi.*

through a 5-μm membrane filter. After several washes with saline or distilled water, the filter is examined microscopically for living microfilariae, or it is dried, fixed, and stained as for a thin blood film.

W. bancrofti and *B. malayi* have a periodicity in the production of microfilariae; it is called nocturnal periodicity. This results in greater numbers of microfilariae in blood at night. It is recommended that blood specimens be taken between 10 PM and 4 AM to detect infection.

W. bancrofti, B. malayi, and *Loa loa* demonstrate a sheath on their microfilariae. This can be the first step in identifying the specific types of filariasis. Further identification is based on study of head and tail structures (Figure 84–14). Clinically, an exact species identification is not critical because treatment for all the filarial infections, except *Onchocerca volvulus,* is identical.

Serologic testing is also available through reference laboratories so that a diagnosis can be reached. Detection of circulating filarial antigens is promising but not widely available as a diagnostic test.

TREATMENT, PREVENTION, AND CONTROL

Treatment is of little benefit in most cases of chronic lymphatic filariasis. The drug of choice for treatment of *W. bancrofti* and *B. malayi* infections is diethylcarbamazine. Ivermectin appears promising, although controlled studies have yet to be performed. Supportive and surgical therapy for lymphatic obstruction may be of some cosmetic help. Education regarding filarial infections, mosquito control, use of protective clothing and insect repellents, and treatment of infections to prevent further transmission is essential. Control of *B. malayi* infections is more difficult because of the presence of disease in animal reservoirs.

Loa loa

PHYSIOLOGY AND STRUCTURE

The life cycle of *L. loa* is similar to that illustrated in Figure 84–12, except the vector is a biting fly called *Chrysops,* the mango fly. Approximately 6 months after infection, the production of microfilariae starts and can persist for 17 years or more. Adult worms can migrate through subcutaneous tissues, through muscle, and in front of the eyeball.

EPIDEMIOLOGY

L. loa is confined to the equatorial rain forests of Africa and is endemic in tropical West Africa, the Congo basin, and parts of Nigeria. Monkeys in these areas serve as reservoir hosts in the life cycle, with mango flies as vectors.

CLINICAL SYNDROMES

Symptoms usually do not appear until a year or so after the fly bite because the worms are slow in reaching adulthood. One of the first signs of infection is the so-called fugitive or **Calabar swellings.** These swellings are transient and usually appear on the extremities, produced as the worms migrate through subcutaneous tissues, creating large, nodular areas that are painful and pruritic. Because eosinophilia (50% to 70%) is observed, Calabar swellings are believed to result from allergic reactions to the worms or their metabolic products.

Adult *L. loa* worms can also migrate under the conjunctiva, producing irritation, painful congestion, edema of the eyelids, and impaired vision. The presence of a worm in the eye can obviously cause anxiety in the patient. The infection may be long lived and in some cases asymptomatic.

LABORATORY DIAGNOSIS

The clinical observation of Calabar swellings or migration of worms in the eye, combined with eosinophilia, should alert the physician to consider infection with *L. loa.* The microfilariae can be found in the blood. In contrast to the other filariae, *L. loa* is primarily present during the daytime. Serologic testing can also be useful for confirming the diagnosis but is not readily available.

TREATMENT, PREVENTION, AND CONTROL

Diethylcarbamazine is effective against adults and microfilariae; however, destruction of the parasites may induce severe allergic reactions that require treatment with corticosteroids. The role of ivermectin remains undefined for this infection. Surgical removal of worms migrating across the eye or bridge of the nose can be accomplished by immobilizing the worm with instillation of a few drops of 10% cocaine. Education regarding the infection and its vector, especially for people entering the known endemic areas, is essential. Protection from fly bites by using screening, appropriate clothing, and insect repellents, along with treatment of cases, is also critical in reducing the incidence of infection. However, the presence of disease in animal reservoirs (e.g., monkeys) limits the feasibility of controlling this disease.

Mansonella Species

Filarial infections caused by *Mansonella* species are less important than those previously discussed, but physicians should be aware of the names because they may encounter patients with these infections. Infections caused by these organisms are generally asymptomatic but may cause dermatitis, lymphadenitis, hydrocele, and rarely, lymphatic obstruction resulting in elephantiasis.

All of the *Mansonella* species produce nonsheathed microfilariae in blood and subcutaneous tissues, and all are transmitted by biting midges (*Culicoides* species) or blackflies (*Simulium* species). As with previous filarial infections, infections from all of these species are treatable with diethylcarbamazine. Species identification, if desired, can be accomplished with blood smears, noting the structure of the microfilariae. Serologic tests are also available.

Prevention and control require measures involving insect repellents, screening, and other precautions as for all insect-transmitted diseases.

MANSONELLA PERSTANS

M. perstans occurs primarily in parts of tropical Africa and Central and South America. It may produce allergic skin reactions, edema, and Calabar swellings like those of *L. loa* infection. Reservoir hosts are chimpanzees and gorillas.

MANSONELLA OZZARDI

M. ozzardi is found primarily in Central and South America and the West Indies. It may produce swelling of the lymph nodes and occasional hydrocele. There are no known reservoir hosts.

MANSONELLA STREPTOCERCA

M. streptocerca occurs primarily in Africa, especially in the Congo basin. It may produce edema in the skin and, rarely, a form of elephantiasis. Monkeys serve as reservoir hosts.

Onchocerca volvulus

PHYSIOLOGY AND STRUCTURE

Infection occurs after the introduction of *O. volvulus* larvae through the skin during the biting and feeding of the *Simulium* or blackfly vector (Figure 84–15). The larval worms migrate from the skin to subcutaneous tissue and develop into adult male and female worms. The adults become encased in fibrous subcutaneous nodules within which they may remain viable for as long as 15 years. The female worm, after fertilization by the male, begins producing as many as 2000 nonsheathed microfilariae each day. The microfilariae exit the capsule and migrate to the skin, the eyes, and other body tissues. These nonsheathed

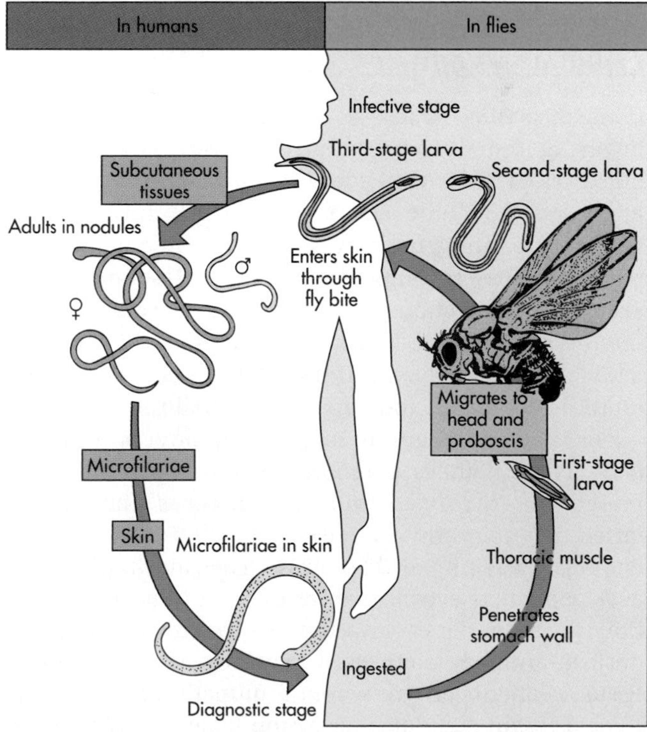

FIGURE 84–15. Life cycle of *Onchocerca volvulus.*

microfilariae appearing in skin tissue are infective for feeding blackflies.

EPIDEMIOLOGY

O. volvulus is endemic in many parts of Africa, especially in the Congo basin and the Volta River basin. In the western hemisphere, it occurs in many Central and South American countries. **Onchocerciasis** affects more than 18 million people worldwide and causes blindness in approximately 5% of infected people.

Several species of the blackfly genus *Simulium* serve as vectors but none so appropriately named as the principal vector, *Simulium damnosum* ("the damned blackfly"). These blackflies, or buffalo gnats, breed in fast-flowing streams, which makes control or eradication by insecticides almost impossible because the chemicals are rapidly washed away from the eggs and larvae.

There is a greater prevalence of infection in men than women in endemic areas because of their work in or near the streams where the blackflies breed. Studies in endemic areas in Africa have shown that 50% of men are totally blind before they reach 50 years of age. This accounts for the common term **river blindness,** which is applied to the disease onchocerciasis. This fear of blindness has created an additional problem in many parts of Africa because whole villages leave the area near streams and farmland that could produce food. The migrating populations then find themselves in areas where they face starvation.

CLINICAL SYNDROMES

Clinical onchocerciasis is characterized by infection involving the skin, subcutaneous tissue, lymph nodes, and eyes. The clinical manifestations of the infection are a result of the acute and chronic inflammatory reaction to antigens released by the microfilariae as they migrate through the tissues. The incubation period from infectious larvae to adult worms is several months to a year. The initial signs of disease are fever, eosinophilia, and urticaria. As the worms mature, copulate, and produce microfilariae, subcutaneous nodules begin to appear on any part of the body. These nodules are most dangerous when they are present on the head and neck because the microfilariae may migrate to the eyes and cause serious tissue damage, leading to blindness. The mechanisms for development of eye disease are thought to be a combination of both direct invasion by the microfilaria and antigen-antibody complex deposition within the ocular tissues. Patients progress from conjunctivitis with photophobia to punctate and sclerosing keratitis. Internal eye disease with anterior uveitis, chorioretinitis, and optic neuritis may also occur.

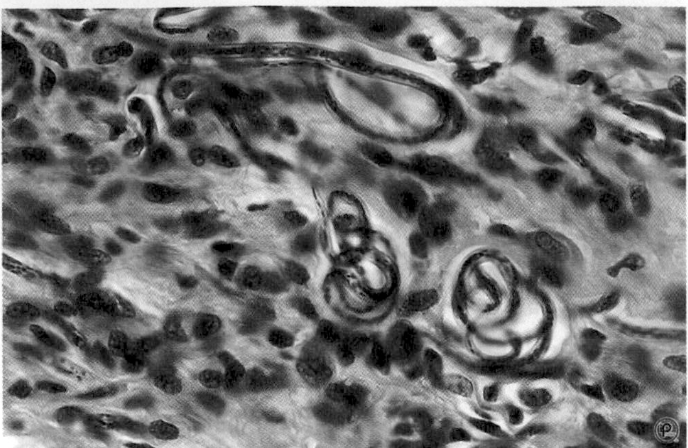

FIGURE 84–16. *O. volvulus* microfilariae in dermal tissue. (From Marler LM et al: *Parasitology* CD-Rom, Indiana Pathology Images, 2003.)

Within the skin the inflammatory process results in loss of elasticity and areas of depigmentation, thickening, and atrophy. A number of skin conditions, including pruritus, hyperkeratosis, and myxedematous thickening, are related to the presence of this parasite. A form of elephantiasis called **hanging groin** also occurs when the nodules are located near the genitalia.

LABORATORY DIAGNOSIS

The diagnosis of onchocerciasis is made by the demonstration of microfilariae in skin snip preparations from the infrascapular or gluteal region. A sample is obtained by raising the skin with a needle and shaving the epidermal layer with a razor. The specimen is incubated in saline for several hours and is then inspected with a dissecting microscope for the presence of nonsheathed microfilariae (Figure 84–16). In patients with ocular disease, the organism may also be seen in the anterior chamber with the aid of a slit lamp. Serologic and culture methods are not helpful, although efforts to develop serologic detection methods are ongoing.

TREATMENT, PREVENTION, AND CONTROL

Surgical removal of the encapsulated nodule is often performed to eliminate the adult worms and stop production of microfilariae (Figure 84–17). In addition, treatment with ivermectin is recommended. A single oral dose of ivermectin (150 mg/kg) greatly reduces the number of microfilariae in the skin and eyes, thus diminishing the likelihood of developing a disabling onchocerciasis. In endemic areas the dose of ivermectin can be repeated every 6 to 12 months to maintain suppression of dermal and ocular microfilariae. Suppression of dermal microfilariae reduces the transmission of this vector-borne

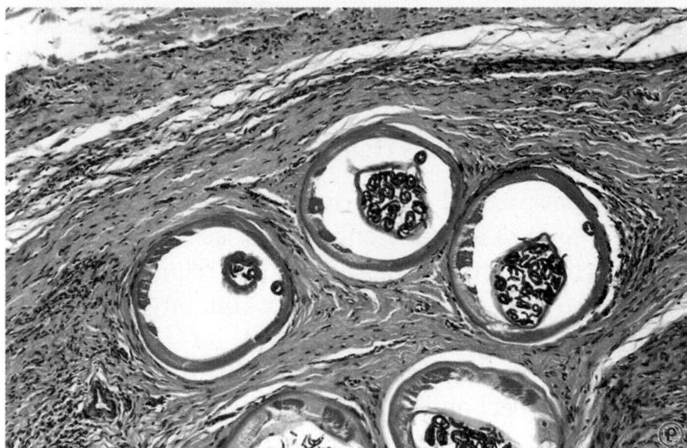

FIGURE 84–17. Cross-section of an adult female *O. volvulus* in an excised nodule showing numerous microfilariae. (From Marler LM et al: *Parasitology* CD-Rom, Indiana Pathology Images, 2003.)

disease, and thus mass chemotherapy may prove to be a successful strategy for the prevention of onchocerciasis. At present there is no firm evidence that *O. volvulus* is becoming resistant to ivermectin; however, whenever a single agent is used for disease control with varying doses over a long period, it is prudent to be on guard for the possibility of resistance developing.

Education regarding the disease and its transmission is essential. Protection from blackfly bites, through the use of protective clothing, screening, and insect repellents, as well as prompt diagnosis and treatment of infections to prevent further transmission, are critical.

Although control of blackfly breeding is difficult because insecticides wash away in the streams, some form of biologic control of this vector may reduce fly reproduction and disease transmission.

Dirofilaria immitis

Several mosquito-transmitted filariae infect dogs, cats, raccoons, and bobcats in nature and occasionally are found in humans. *D. immitis*, the **dog heartworm**, is notorious for forming a lethal worm bolus in the dog's heart. This nematode may also infect humans, producing a nodule called a **coin lesion** in the lung. Only very rarely have these worms been found in human hearts.

The coin lesion in the lung presents a problem for the radiologist and the surgeon because it resembles a malignancy requiring surgical removal. Unfortunately, no laboratory test can provide an accurate diagnosis of **dirofilariasis.** Peripheral eosinophilia is rare, and the radiographic features are insufficient to allow the clinician to distinguish pulmonary dirofilariasis from bronchogenic carcinoma. Serologic tests are not sufficiently sensitive or specific to preclude the surgical intervention. A definitive diagnosis is made when a thoracotomy specimen is examined microscopically, revealing the typical cross-sections of the parasite.

Transmission of the filarial infections can be controlled by mosquito control and the prophylactic use of the drug ivermectin in dogs.

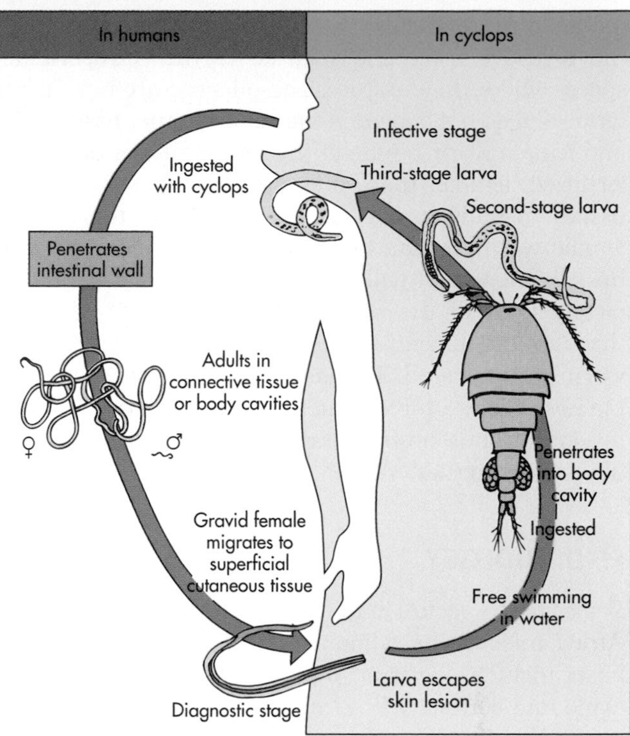

FIGURE 84–18. Life cycle of *Dracunculus medinensis.*

Dracunculus medinensis

The name *D. medinensis* means "little dragon of Medina." This is a very ancient worm infection thought by some scholars to be the "fiery serpent" noted by Moses with the Israelites at the Red Sea.

PHYSIOLOGY AND STRUCTURE

D. medinensis is not a filarial worm but a tissue-invading nematode of medical importance in many parts of the world. The worms have a very simple life cycle, depending on freshwater and a microcrustacean **(copepod)** of the genus *Cyclops* (Figure 84–18). When *Cyclops* species harboring larval *D. medinensis* are ingested in drinking water, the infection is initiated with liberation of the larvae in the stomach. These larvae penetrate the wall of the digestive tract and migrate to the retroperitoneal space, where they mature. These larvae are not microfilariae and do not appear in the blood or other tissues. Male and female worms mate in the retroperitoneum, and the fertilized female then migrates to the subcutaneous tissues, usually in the extremities. When the fertilized female worm becomes gravid, a vesicle is formed in the host tissue, which will ulcerate. When the ulcer is completely formed, the worm protrudes a loop of uterus through the ulcer. On contact with water, the larval worms are released. The larvae are then ingested by the *Cyclops* species in freshwater, where they are then infective for humans or animals drinking the water containing the *Cyclops* species.

EPIDEMIOLOGY

D. medinensis occurs in many parts of Asia and equatorial Africa, infecting an estimated 10 million people. Reservoir hosts include dogs and many fur-bearing animals that come into contact with drinking water containing infective *Cyclops* species.

Human infections usually result from ingestion of water from so-called step wells where people stand or bathe in the water, at which time the gravid female worm discharges larvae from lesions on the arms, legs, feet, and ankles to infect *Cyclops* species in the water. Ponds and standing water are occasionally the source of infection when humans use them for drinking water.

CLINICAL SYNDROMES

Symptoms of infection usually do not appear until the gravid female creates the vesicle and the ulcer in the skin for the liberation of larval worms. This occurs usually 1 year after initial exposure. At the site of the ulcer there are erythema and pain, as well as an allergic reaction to the worm. There is also the possibility of abscess formation and secondary bacterial infection, leading to further tissue destruction and inflammatory reaction with intense pain and sloughing of skin.

If the worm is broken in attempts to remove it, there may be toxic reactions, and if the worm dies and calcifies, there may be nodule formation and some allergic reaction. Once the gravid female worm has discharged all the larvae, it may retreat into deeper tissue, where it is gradually absorbed, or it may simply be expelled from the site.

LABORATORY DIAGNOSIS

Diagnosis is established by observing the typical ulcer and by flooding the ulcer with water to recover the larval worms when they are discharged. Occasionally, x-ray examination reveals worms in various parts of the body.

TREATMENT, PREVENTION, AND CONTROL

The ancient method of slowly wrapping the worm on a twig is still used in many endemic areas (Figure 84–19). Surgical removal is also a practical and reliable procedure for the patient. There is no evidence that any chemotherapeutic agents has a direct effect on *D. medinensis,* although various benzimidazoles may have an antiinflammatory effect and either eliminate the worm or make surgical removal easier. Treatment with mebendazole has been associated with aberrant migration of the worms, with the result that they were more likely to emerge at anatomic sites other than the lower limbs.

Education regarding the life cycle of the worm and avoidance of water contaminated with *Cyclops* species are critical. Protection of drinking water by prohibiting bathing and washing of clothing in wells is essential. Persons who live in or travel to endemic areas should boil water before drinking it. The treatment of water with chemicals and the use of fish that consume *Cyclops* species as food also help control transmission. Prompt diagnosis and treatment of cases also limit further transmission. These preventive measures have been incorporated into an ongoing global effort to eliminate dracunculiasis.

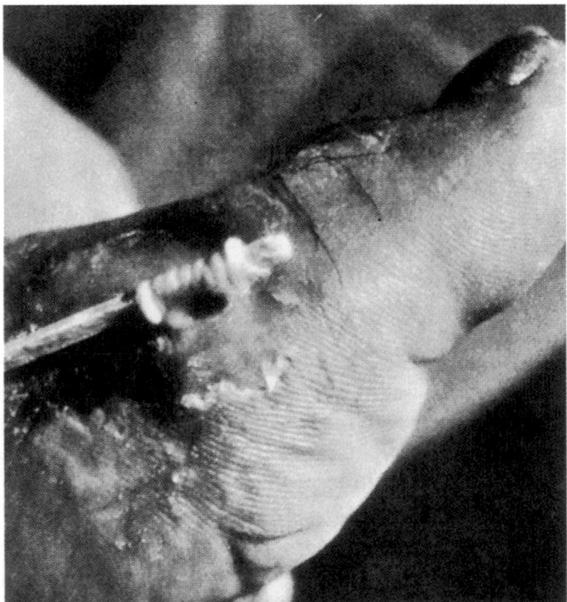

FIGURE 84–19. Removal of a *D. medinensis* adult from an exposed ulcer by winding the worm slowly around a stick. (From Binford CH, Conner DH: *Pathology of tropical and extraordinary diseases,* Washington, 1976, Armed Forces Institute of Pathology.)

CASE STUDY AND QUESTIONS

A 10-year-old boy was brought in by his father for evaluation of crampy abdominal pain, nausea, and mild diarrhea that had persisted for approximately 2 weeks. On the day before evaluation, the boy reported to his parents that he passed a large worm into the toilet during a bowel movement. He flushed the worm before the parents could see it. Physical examination was completely unremarkable. The boy had no fever, cough, or rash and did not complain of anal pruritus. His travel history was unremarkable. Examination of a stool specimen revealed the diagnosis.

1. Which intestinal parasites of humans are nematodes?
2. Which nematode was likely in this case? What organisms may be found in stool?
3. What was the most likely means of acquisition of this parasite?
4. Was this patient at risk of autoinfection?
5. Describe the life cycle of this parasite.
6. Can this parasite cause extraintestinal symptoms? What other organs may be invaded and what might stimulate extraintestinal invasion?

Bibliography

Cairncross S, Muller R, Zagaria N: Dracunculiasis (Guinea worm disease) and the eradication initiative, *Clin Microbiol Rev* 15:223-246, 2002.

Despommier D: Toxocariosis: Clinical aspects, epidemiology, medical ecology and molecular aspects, *Clin Microbiol Rev* 16:265-272, 2003.

Garcia LS, editor: *Diagnostic medical parasitology,* ed 4, Washington, 2001, ASM Press.

Hall LR, Pearlman E: Pathogenesis of onchocercal keratitis (River Blindness), *Clin Microbiol Rev* 12:445-453, 1999.

Keiser PB, Nutman TB: *Strongyloides stercoralis* in the immunocompromised population, *Clin Microbiol Rev* 17:208-217, 2004.

Strickland GT, editor: *Hunter's tropical medicine and emerging infectious diseases,* Philadelphia, 2000, WB Saunders.

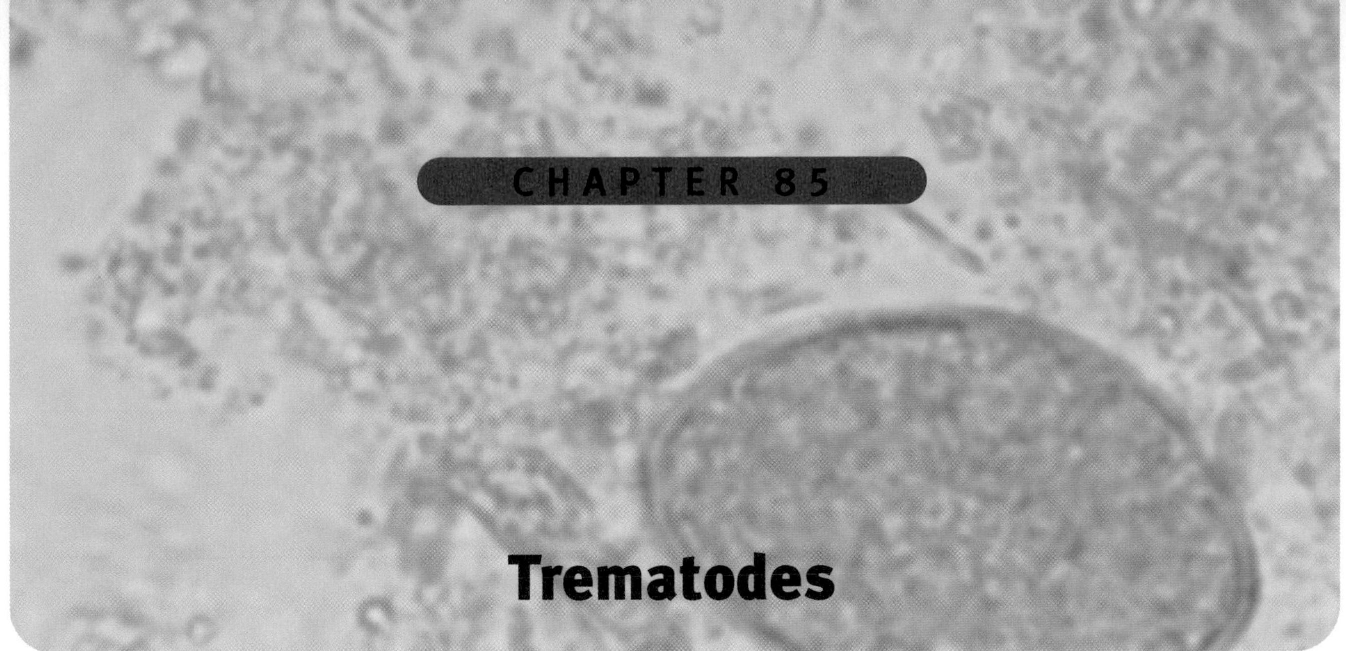

CHAPTER 85

Trematodes

The trematodes **(flukes)** are members of the phylum *Platyhelminthes* and are generally flat, fleshy, leaf-shaped worms. In general they are equipped with two muscular suckers: an oral type, which is the beginning of an incomplete digestive system, and a ventral sucker, which is simply an organ of attachment. The digestive system consists of lateral tubes that do not join to form an excretory opening. Most flukes are **hermaphroditic,** with both male and female reproductive organs in a single body. Schistosomes are the only exception; they have cylindrical bodies (like the nematodes), and separate male and female worms exist.

All flukes require intermediate hosts for the completion of their life cycles, and without exception the first intermediate hosts are mollusks (snails and clams). In these hosts, an asexual reproductive cycle is a type of germ cell propagation. Some flukes require various second intermediate hosts before reaching the final host and developing into adult worms. This variation is discussed in the sections on the individual species.

Fluke eggs are equipped with a "lid" at the top of the shell. Called an **operculum,** the lid opens to allow the larval worm to find its appropriate snail host. The schistosomes do not have an operculum; rather, the eggshell splits to liberate the larva. The medically significant trematodes are summarized in Table 85–1.

Fasciolopsis buski

A number of intestinal flukes are recognized, including *F. buski*, *Heterophyes heterophyes*, *Metagonimus yokogawai*, *Echinostoma ilocanum*, and *Gastrodiscoides hominis*. *F. buski* is the largest, most prevalent, and most important intestinal fluke. The other flukes are similar to *F. buski* in many respects (epidemiology, clinical syndromes, treatment) and are not discussed further. It is important only that physicians recognize the relationship among these different flukes.

PHYSIOLOGY AND STRUCTURE

This large intestinal fluke has a typical life cycle (Figure 85–1). Humans ingest the encysted larval stage **(metacercaria)** when they peel the husks from aquatic vegetation (e.g., water chestnuts) with the teeth. The metacercariae are scraped from the husk, swallowed, and develop into immature flukes in the duodenum. The fluke attaches to the mucosa of the small intestine with two muscular suckers, develops into an adult form, and undergoes self-fertilization. Egg production is initiated 3 months after the initial infection with the metacercariae. The operculated eggs pass in feces to water, where the operculum at the top of the eggshell pops open, liberating a free-swimming larval stage **(miracidium).** Glands at the pointed anterior end of the miracidium produce lytic substances that allow the penetration of the soft tissues of snails. In the snail tissue the miracidium develops through a series of stages by asexual germ cell propagation. The final stage **(cercaria)** in the snail is a free-swimming form that, after release from the snail, encysts on the aquatic vegetation, becoming the metacercariae, or infective stage.

EPIDEMIOLOGY

Because it depends on the distribution of its appropriate snail host, *F. buski* is found only in China, Vietnam, Thailand, parts of Indonesia, Malaysia, and India. Pigs, dogs, and rabbits serve as reservoir hosts in these endemic areas.

TABLE 85–1. Medically Significant Trematodes

Trematode	Common Name	Intermediate Host	Biologic Vector	Reservoir Host
Fasciolopsis buski	Giant intestinal fluke	Snail	Water plants (e.g., water chestnuts)	Pigs, dogs, rabbits, humans
Fasciola hepatica	Sheep liver fluke	Snail	Water plants (e.g., watercress)	Sheep, cattle, humans
Opisthorchis (Clonorchis) sinensis	Chinese liver fluke	Snail, freshwater fish	Uncooked fish	Dogs, cats, humans
Paragonimus westermani	Lung fluke	Snail, freshwater crabs, crayfish	Uncooked crabs, crayfish	Pigs, monkeys, humans
Schistosoma species	Blood fluke	Snail	None	Primates, rodents, domestic pets, livestock, humans

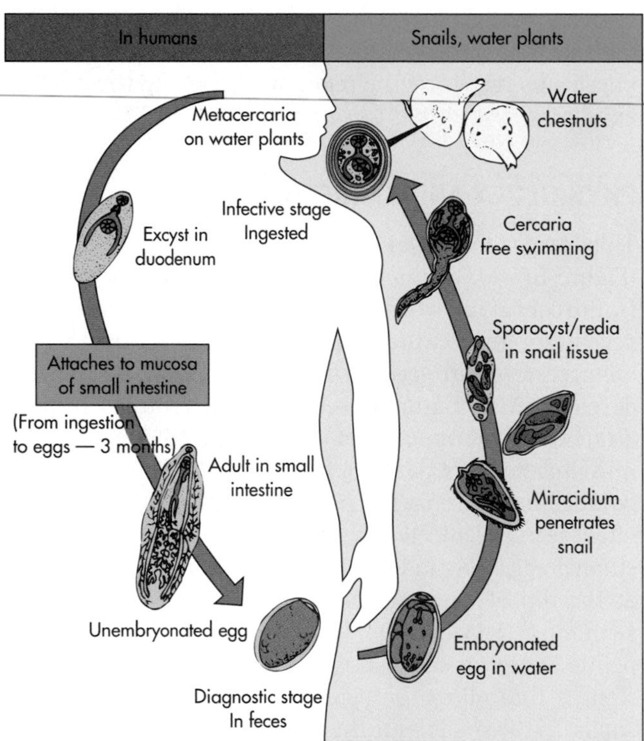

FIGURE 85–1. Life cycle of *Fasciolopsis buski* (giant intestinal fluke).

CLINICAL SYNDROMES

The symptomatology of *F. buski* infection relates directly to the worm burden in the small intestine. Attachment of the flukes in the small intestine can produce inflammation, ulceration, and hemorrhage. Severe infections produce abdominal discomfort similar to that of a duodenal ulcer, as well as diarrhea. Stools may be profuse, a malabsorption syndrome similar to giardiasis is common, and intestinal obstruction can occur. Marked eosinophilia is also present. Although death can occur, it is rare.

LABORATORY DIAGNOSIS

Stool examination reveals the large, golden, bile-stained eggs with an operculum on the top. The measurements and appearance of *F. buski* eggs are similar to that of the liver fluke *Fasciola hepatica,* and differentiation of the eggs of these species usually is not possible. Large (approximately 1.5×3.0 cm) adult flukes can rarely be found in feces or specimens collected at surgery.

TREATMENT, PREVENTION, AND CONTROL

The drug of choice is praziquantel, and the alternative is niclosamide. Education regarding the safe consumption of infective aquatic vegetation (particularly water chestnuts), proper sanitation, and control of human feces reduces the incidence of disease. In addition, the snail population may be eliminated with molluscacides. When infection occurs, treatment should be initiated promptly to minimize its spread. Control of the reservoir hosts also reduces transmission of the worm.

Fasciola hepatica

A number of liver flukes are recognized, including *F. hepatica, Opisthorchis sinensis, Opisthorchis felineus,* and *Dicrocoelium dendriticum.* Only *F. hepatica* and *O. sinensis* are discussed in this chapter, although the eggs of other flukes are occasionally detected in the feces of patients in other geographic areas.

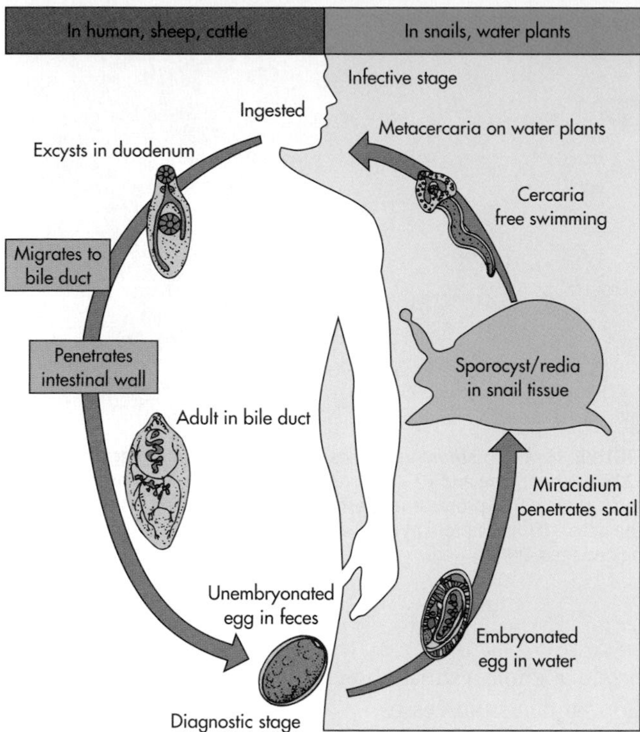

FIGURE 85–2. Life cycle of *Fasciola hepatica* (sheep liver fluke).

PHYSIOLOGY AND STRUCTURE

Commonly called the **sheep liver fluke,** *F. hepatica* is a parasite of herbivores (particularly sheep and cattle) and humans. Its life cycle (Figure 85–2) is similar to that of *F. buski*, with human infection resulting from the ingestion of watercress that harbors the encysted metacercariae. The larval flukes then migrate through the duodenal wall and across the peritoneal cavity, penetrate the liver capsule, pass through the liver parenchyma, and enter the bile ducts to become adult worms. Approximately 3 to 4 months after the initial infection the adult flukes start producing operculated eggs that are identical to those of *F. buski*, as seen in stool examination.

EPIDEMIOLOGY

Infections have been reported worldwide in sheep-raising areas, with the appropriate snail as an intermediate host. These areas include the former Soviet Union, Japan, Egypt, and many Latin American countries. Outbreaks are directly related to human consumption of contaminated watercress in areas where infected herbivores are present. Human infection is rare in the United States, but several well-documented cases have been reported in travelers from endemic areas.

CLINICAL SYNDROMES

Migration of the larval worm through the liver produces irritation of this tissue, tenderness, and hepatomegaly. Pain in the right upper quadrant, chills, and fever with marked eosinophilia are commonly observed. As the worms take up residence in the bile ducts, their mechanical irritation and toxic secretions produce hepatitis, hyperplasia of the epithelium, and biliary obstruction. Some worms penetrate eroded areas in the ducts and invade the liver to produce necrotic foci, referred to as liver rot. In severe infections, secondary bacterial infection can occur, and portal cirrhosis is common.

LABORATORY DIAGNOSIS

Stool examination reveals operculated eggs indistinguishable from the eggs of *F. buski*. Exact identification is a therapeutic problem because treatment is not the same for both infections. Whereas *F. buski* responds favorably to praziquantel, *F. hepatica* does not. When exact identification is desired, examination of a sample of the patient's bile differentiates the species; if the eggs are present in bile, they are *F. hepatica*, not *F. buski*, which is limited to the small intestine. Eggs may appear in stool samples from people who have eaten infected sheep or cattle liver. The spurious nature of this finding can be confirmed by having the patient refrain from eating liver and then rechecking the stool.

TREATMENT, PREVENTION, AND CONTROL

In contrast to *F. buski*, *F. hepatica* responds poorly to praziquantel. Treatment with bithionol or the benzimidazole compound triclabendazole has been effective. Preventive measures are similar to those for *F. buski* control; people who live in areas frequented by sheep and cattle should especially avoid ingestion of watercress and other uncooked aquatic vegetation.

Opisthorchis sinensis

PHYSIOLOGY AND STRUCTURE

O. sinensis, also referred to as *Clonorchis sinensis* in the older literature, is commonly called the **Chinese liver fluke.** Figure 85–3 illustrates its life cycle, which involves two intermediate hosts. This trematode differs from other fluke cycles because the eggs are eaten by the snail, then reproduction begins in the soft tissues of the snail. *O. sinensis* also requires a second intermediate host, freshwater fish, where the cercariae encyst and develop into infective metacercariae. When uncooked freshwater fish

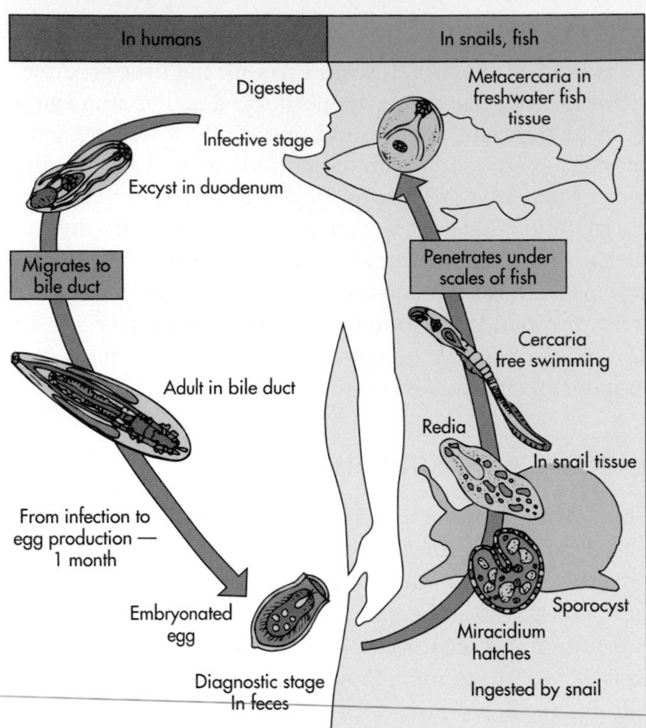

FIGURE 85–3. Life cycle of *Opisthorchis sinensis* (Chinese liver fluke).

harboring metacercariae are eaten, flukes develop first in the duodenum and then migrate to the bile ducts where they become adults. The adult fluke undergoes self-fertilization and begins producing eggs. *O. sinensis* may survive in the biliary tract for as long as 50 years, producing approximately 2000 eggs per day. These eggs pass with feces and are once again eaten by snails, reinitiating the cycle.

EPIDEMIOLOGY

O. sinensis is found in China, Japan, Korea, and Vietnam, where it is estimated to infect approximately 19 million people. It is one of the most frequent infections seen among Asian refugees, and it can be traced to the consumption of raw, pickled, smoked, or dried freshwater fish that harbor the viable metacercariae. Dogs, cats, and fish-eating mammals can also serve as reservoir hosts.

CLINICAL SYNDROMES

Infection in humans is usually mild and asymptomatic. Severe infections with many flukes in the bile ducts produces fever, diarrhea, epigastric pain, hepatomegaly, anorexia, and occasionally, jaundice. Biliary obstruction may occur, and chronic infection can result in adenocarcinoma of the bile ducts. Invasion of the gallbladder may produce cholecystitis, cholelithiasis, impaired liver function, and liver abscesses.

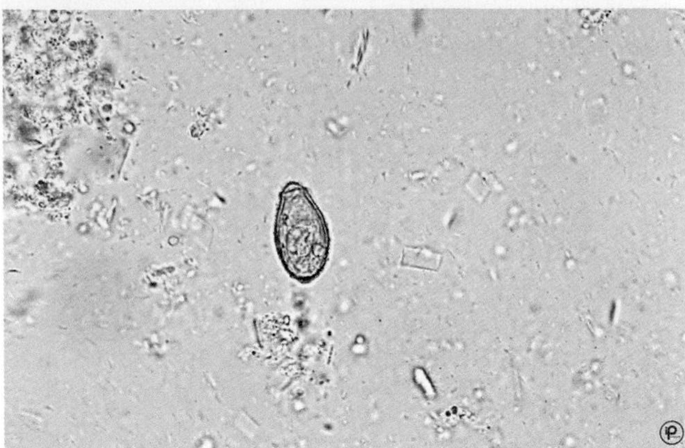

FIGURE 85–4. *Opisthorchis sinensis* egg. These ovoid eggs are small (22- to 30-μm long and 12- to 19-μm wide) and have a yellowish-brown, thick shell with a prominent operculum at one end and a small knob at the other. (From Marler LM et al: *Parasitology* CD-Rom, Indiana Pathology Images, 2003.)

LABORATORY DIAGNOSIS

The diagnosis is made by recovering the distinctive eggs from stool. The eggs measure 27 to 35 μm × 12 to 19 μm and are characterized by a distinct operculum with prominent shoulders and a tiny knob at the posterior (abopercular) pole (Figure 85–4). In mild infections, repeated examinations of stool or duodenal aspirates may be necessary. In acute symptomatic infection, there are usually eosinophilia and an elevation of serum alkaline phosphatase levels. Radiographic imaging procedures may detect abnormalities of the biliary tract.

TREATMENT, PREVENTION, AND CONTROL

The drug of choice is praziquantel. Prevention of infection is accomplished by not eating uncooked fish and by implementing proper sanitation policies, including the disposal of human, dog, and cat feces in adequately protected sites, so that they cannot contaminate water supplies with the intermediate snail and fish hosts.

Paragonimus westermani

PHYSIOLOGY AND STRUCTURE

P. westermani, commonly called the **lung fluke**, is one of several species of *Paragonimus* that infect humans and many other animals. Figure 85–5 shows a familiar fluke life cycle from egg to snail to infective metacercaria. The

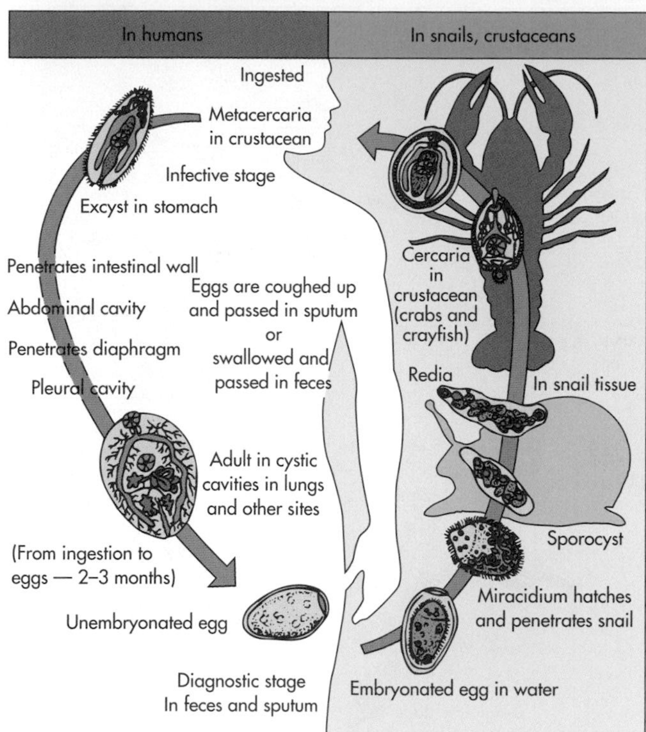

FIGURE 85–5. Life cycle of *Paragonimus westermani* (Oriental lung fluke).

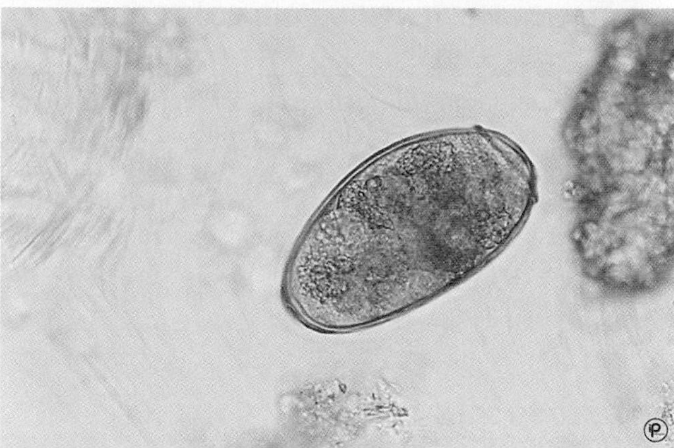

FIGURE 85–6. *Paragonimus westermani* egg. These large, ovoid eggs (80- to 120-µm long and 45- to 70-µm wide) have a thick, yellowish-brown shell and a distinct operculum. (From Marler LM et al: *Parasitology* CD-Rom, Indiana Pathology Images, 2003.)

infective stage occurs in a second intermediate host: the muscles and gills of freshwater crabs and crayfish. In humans who ingest infected meat, the larval worm hatches in the stomach and follows an extensive migration through the intestinal wall to the abdominal cavity, then through the diaphragm, and finally to the pleural cavity. Adult worms reside in the lungs and produce eggs that are liberated from ruptured bronchioles and appear in sputum or, when swallowed, in feces.

EPIDEMIOLOGY

Paragonimiasis occurs in many countries in Asia, Africa, India, and Latin America. It can be seen in refugees from Southeast Asia. Its prevalence is directly related to the consumption of uncooked freshwater crabs and crayfish. It is estimated that approximately 3 million people are infected with this lung fluke. As many as 1% of all Indochinese immigrants to the United States are infected with *P. westermani.* A wide variety of shore-feeding animals (e.g., wild boars, pigs, and monkeys) serve as reservoir hosts, and some human infections result from ingestion of meat containing migrating larval worms from these reservoir hosts. Human infections endemic to the United States are usually caused by a related species, *Paragonimus kellicotti,* which is found in crabs and crayfish in eastern and Midwestern waters.

CLINICAL SYNDROMES

The clinical manifestations of paragonimiasis may result from larvae migrating through tissues or from adults established in the lungs or other ectopic sites. The onset of disease coincides with larval migration and is associated with fever, chills, and high eosinophilia. The adult flukes in the lungs first produce an inflammatory reaction that results in fever, cough, and increased sputum. As the destruction of lung tissue progresses, cavitation occurs around the worms, sputum becomes blood tinged and dark with eggs (so-called rusty sputum), and patients experience severe chest pain. The resulting cavity may become secondarily infected with bacteria. Dyspnea, chronic bronchitis, bronchiectasis, and pleural effusion may be seen. Chronic infections lead to fibrosis in the lung tissue. The location of larvae, adults, and eggs in ectopic sites may produce severe clinical symptoms, depending on the site involved. The migration of larval worms may result in invasion of the spinal cord and brain, producing severe neurologic disease (visual problems, motor weakness, and convulsive seizures) referred to as cerebral paragonimiasis. Migration and infection may also occur in subcutaneous sites, the abdominal cavity, and the liver.

LABORATORY DIAGNOSIS

Examination of sputum and feces reveals golden-brown, operculated eggs (Figure 85–6). Pleural effusions, when present, should be examined for eggs. Results of chest x-ray films often show infiltrates, nodular cysts, and pleural effusion. Marked eosinophilia is common. Serologic procedures are available through reference laboratories and can be helpful, particularly in cases with extrapulmonary (e.g., central nervous system) involvement.

TREATMENT, PREVENTION, AND CONTROL

The drug of choice is praziquantel; bithionol is an alternative. Education regarding the consumption of uncooked freshwater crabs and crayfish, as well as the flesh of animals found in endemic areas, is critical. Pickling and wine soaking of crabs and crayfish do not kill the infective metacercarial stage. Proper sanitation and control of the disposal of human feces are essential.

Schistosomes

Schistosomiasis is a major parasitic infection of tropical areas, with some 200 million infections worldwide. The three schistosomes most frequently associated with human disease are *Schistosoma mansoni*, *Schistosoma japonicum*, and *Schistosoma haematobium*. They collectively produce the disease called **schistosomiasis,** also known as **bilharziasis** or **snail fever.** As discussed earlier, the schistosomes differ from other flukes: They are male and female rather than hermaphroditic, and their eggs do not have an operculum. They also are obligate intravascular parasites and are not found in cavities, ducts, and other tissues. The infective forms are skin-penetrating **cercariae** liberated from snails, and these differ from other flukes in that they are not eaten on vegetation, in fish, or in crustaceans.

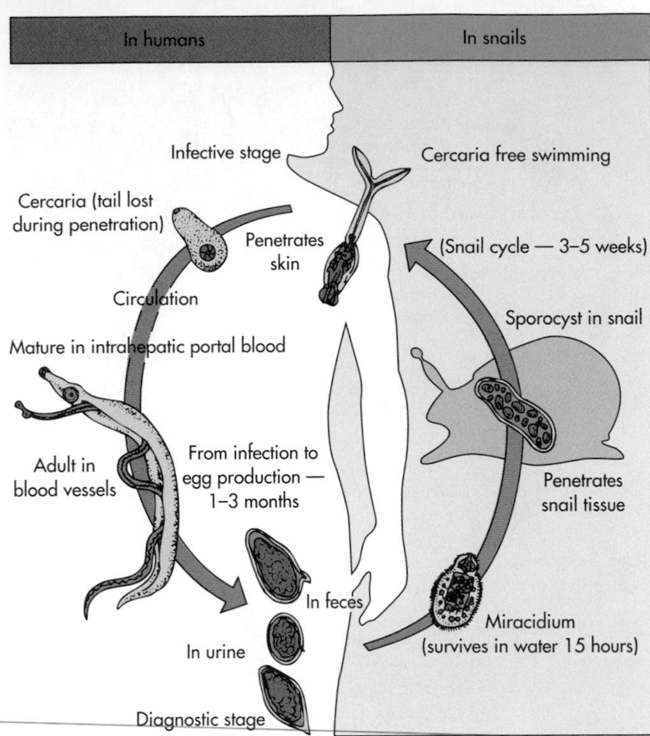

FIGURE 85–7. Life cycle of schistosomes.

Figure 85–7 illustrates the life cycle of the different schistosomes. Infection is initiated by ciliated, free-swimming cercaria in fresh water that penetrate intact skin, enter the circulation, and develop in the intrahepatic portal circulation (*S. mansoni* and *S. japonicum*) or in the vesical, prostatic, rectal, and uterine plexuses and veins (*S. haematobium*). The female has a long, slender, cylindrical body, whereas the shorter male, which appears cylindrical, is actually flat. The cylindrical appearance derives from folding the sides of the body to produce a groove, the gynecophoral canal, in which the female resides for fertilization. Both sexes have oral and ventral suckers and an incomplete digestive system, which is typical of a fluke.

As the worms develop in the portal circulation, they elaborate a remarkable defense against host resistance. They coat themselves with substances that the host recognizes as itself; consequently, there is little host response directed against their presence in blood vessels. This protective mechanism accounts for chronic infections that may last 20 to 30 years or longer.

After developing in the portal vein, the male and female adult worms pair up and migrate to their final locations, where fertilization and egg production begin. *S. mansoni* and *S. japonicum* are found in mesenteric veins and produce intestinal schistosomiasis; *S. haematobium* occurs in veins around the urinary bladder and causes vesicular schistosomiasis. On reaching the submucosal venules of their respective locations, the worms initiate oviposition, which may continue at the rate of 300 to 3000 eggs daily for 4 to 35 years. Although the host inflammatory response to the adult worms is minimal, the eggs elicit an intense inflammatory reaction with mononuclear and polymorphonuclear cellular infiltrates and the formation of microabscesses. In addition, the larvae inside the eggs produce enzymes that aid in tissue destruction and allow the eggs to pass through the mucosa and into the lumen of the bowel and bladder, where they are passed to the external environment in the feces and urine, respectively.

The eggs hatch quickly on reaching fresh water to release motile **miracidia.** The miracidia then invade the appropriate snail host, where they develop into thousands of infectious cercariae. The free-swimming cercariae are released into the water, where they are immediately infectious for humans and other mammals.

The infection is similar in all three species of human schistosomes in that disease results primarily from the host's immune response to the eggs. The very earliest signs and symptoms are caused by the penetration of the cercariae through the skin. Immediate and delayed hypersensitivity to parasite antigens result in an intensely pruritic papular skin rash.

The onset of oviposition results in a symptom complex known as **Katayama syndrome,** which is marked by fever, chills, cough, urticaria, arthralgias, lymphadenopathy, splenomegaly, and abdominal pain. This syndrome is typically seen 1 to 2 months after primary exposure and may persist for 3 months or more. It is thought to result from the massive release of parasite antigens with subsequent immune complex formation. Associated laboratory abnormalities include leukocytosis, eosinophilia, and polyclonal gammopathy.

The more chronic and significant phase of schistosomiasis is caused by the presence of eggs in various tissues and the resulting formation of granulomas and fibrosis. The retained eggs induce extensive inflammation and scarring, the clinical significance of which is directly related to the location and number of eggs.

Because of differences in some aspects of disease and epidemiology, these worms are discussed as separate species.

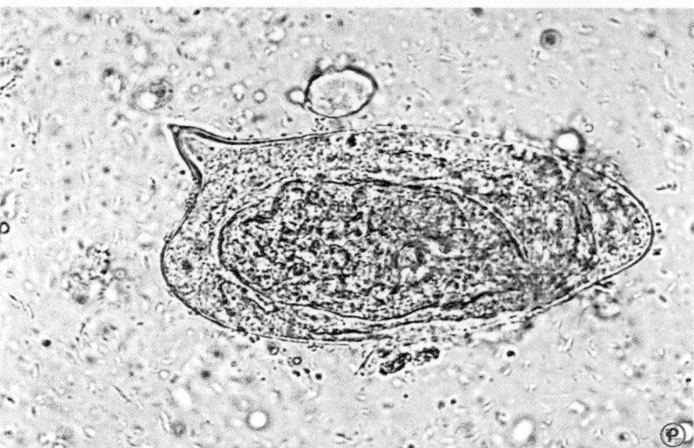

FIGURE 85–8. *Schistosoma mansoni* egg. These eggs are 115- to 175-µm long and 45- to 70-µm wide, contain a miracidium, and are enclosed in a thin shell with a prominent lateral spine. (From Marler LM et al: *Parasitology* CD-Rom, Indiana Pathology Images, 2003.)

SCHISTOSOMA MANSONI

Physiology and Structure

S. mansoni usually resides in the small branches of the inferior mesenteric vein near the lower colon. The species of *Schistosoma* can be differentiated by their characteristic egg morphology (Figures 85–8 to 85–10). The eggs of *S. mansoni* are oval, possess a sharp lateral spine, and measure 115 to 175 µm × 45 to 70 µm (see Figure 85–8).

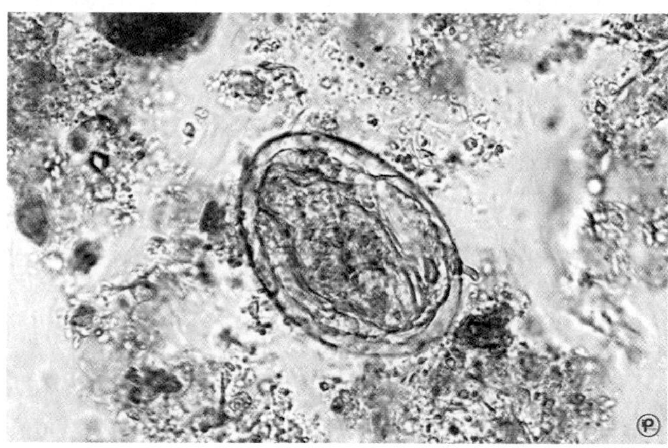

FIGURE 85–9. *Schistosoma japonicum* egg. These eggs are smaller than those of *Schistosoma mansoni* (70- to 100-µm long and 55- to 65-µm wide) and have a spine that is inconspicuous. (From Marler LM et al: *Parasitology* CD-Rom, Indiana Pathology Images, 2003.)

Epidemiology

The geographic distribution of the various species of *Schistosoma* depends on the availability of a suitable snail host. *S. mansoni* is the most widespread of the schistosomes and is endemic in Africa, Saudi Arabia, and Madagascar. It has also become well established in the western hemisphere, particularly in Brazil, Suriname Venezuela, parts of the West Indies, and Puerto Rico. Cases originating in these areas occur in the United States. In all of these areas there are also reservoir hosts, specifically primates, marsupials, and rodents. Schistosomiasis may be considered a disease of economic progress; the development of massive land irrigation projects in desert and tropical areas has resulted in the dispersion of infected humans and snails to previously uninvolved areas.

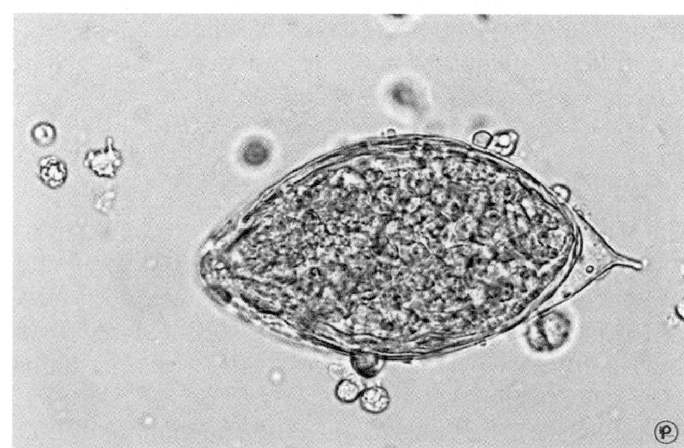

FIGURE 85–10. *Schistosoma haematobium* egg. These eggs are similar in size to those of *Schistosoma mansoni* but can be differentiated by the presence of a terminal spine. (From Marler LM et al: *Parasitology* CD-Rom, Indiana Pathology Images, 2003.)

Clinical Syndromes

As noted before, cercarial penetration of the intact skin may be seen as dermatitis with allergic reactions, pruritus, and edema. Migrating worms in the lungs may produce cough; as they reach the liver, hepatitis may appear.

Infections with *S. mansoni* may produce hepatic and intestinal abnormalities. As the flukes take up residence in the mesenteric vessels and begin laying eggs, fever, malaise, abdominal pain, and tenderness of the liver may be observed. Deposition of eggs in the bowel mucosa results in inflammation and thickening of the bowel wall with associated abdominal pain, diarrhea, and blood in the stool. Eggs may be carried by the portal vein to the liver, where inflammation can lead to periportal fibrosis and eventually to portal hypertension and its associated manifestations.

Chronic infection with *S. mansoni* produces a dramatic hepatosplenomegaly with large accumulations of ascitic fluid in the peritoneal cavity. On gross examination, the liver is studded with white granulomas (pseudotubercles). Although *S. mansoni* eggs are primarily deposited in the intestine, eggs may appear in the spinal cord, lungs, and other sites. A similar fibrotic process occurs at each site. Severe neurologic problems may follow when eggs are deposited in the spinal cord and brain. In fatal schistosomiasis caused by *S. mansoni*, fibrous tissue, reacting to the eggs in the liver, surrounds the portal vein in a thick, grossly visible layer **("clay pipestem fibrosis").**

Laboratory Diagnosis

The diagnosis of schistosomiasis is usually established by the demonstration of characteristic eggs in feces. Stool examination reveals the large golden eggs with a sharp lateral spine (see Figure 85–8). Concentration techniques may be necessary in light infections. Using rectal biopsy, the clinician can see the egg tracks laid by the worms in rectal vessels. Quantitation of egg output in stool is useful in estimating the severity of infection and in following the response to therapy. Serologic tests are also available but are largely of epidemiologic interest only. The development of newer tests using stage-specific antigens may allow the distinction of active from inactive disease and thus have greater clinical application.

Treatment, Prevention, and Control

The drug of choice is praziquantel, and the alternative is oxamniquine. Antihelminthic therapy may terminate oviposition but does not affect lesions caused by eggs already deposited in tissues. **Schistosomal dermatitis** and Katayama syndrome may be treated with the administration of antihistamines and corticosteroids. Education regarding the life cycles of these worms and control of snails using molluscacides are essential. Improved sanitation and control of human fecal deposits are critical. Mass treatment may one day be practical, and the development of a vaccine may be forthcoming.

SCHISTOSOMA JAPONICUM

Physiology and Structure

S. japonicum resides in branches of the superior mesenteric vein around the small intestine and in the inferior mesenteric vessels. *S. japonicum* eggs (see Figure 85–9) are smaller than those of *S. mansoni* and *S. haematobium*, are almost spherical, and possess a tiny spine. These eggs are produced in greater numbers than those of *S. mansoni* and *S. haematobium*. Because of the size, shape, and numbers of these eggs, they are carried to more sites in the body (liver, lungs, brain), and infection with a few *S. japonicum* adults can be more severe than infections involving similar numbers of *S. mansoni* or *S. haematobium*.

Epidemiology

This **Oriental blood fluke** is found only in China, Japan, the Philippines, and on the island of Sulawesi, Indonesia. Epidemiologic problems correlate directly with a broad range of reservoir hosts, many of which are domestic (cats, dogs, cattle, horses, and pigs).

Clinical Syndromes

The initial stages of infection with *S. japonicum* are similar to those of *S. mansoni*, with dermatitis, allergic reactions, fever, and malaise, followed by abdominal discomfort and diarrhea. Katayama syndrome associated with the onset of oviposition is observed more commonly with *S. japonicum* than with *S. mansoni*. In chronic *S. japonicum* infection, hepatosplenic disease, portal hypertension, bleeding esophageal varices, and accumulation of ascitic fluid are commonly seen. Granulomas that appear as pseudotubercles in and on the liver are common, along with the clay pipestem fibrosis, as described for *S. mansoni*.

S. japonicum frequently involves cerebral structures when eggs reach the brain and granulomas develop around them. The neurologic manifestations include lethargy, speech impairment, visual defects, and seizures.

Laboratory Diagnosis

Stool examination demonstrates the small, golden eggs with tiny spines; usually, rectal biopsy is similarly revealing. Serologic tests are available.

Treatment, Prevention, and Control

The drug of choice is praziquantel. Prevention and control may be achieved by measures similar to those for *S. mansoni*, especially education of populations in endemic areas regarding proper water purification, sanitation, and control of human fecal deposits. Control of *S. japonicum* must also involve the broad range of reservoir hosts and consider the fact that people work in rice paddies and on irrigation projects where infected snails are present. Mass treatment may offer help, and a vaccine may be developed someday.

SCHISTOSOMA HAEMATOBIUM

Physiology and Structure

After development in the liver, these blood flukes migrate to the vesical, prostatic, and uterine plexuses of the venous circulation; occasionally the portal bloodstream; and only rarely other venules.

Large eggs with a sharp terminal spine (see Figure 85–10) are deposited in the wall of the bladder and occasionally in the uterine and prostatic tissues. Those deposited in the bladder wall can break free and are found in urine.

Epidemiology

S. haematobium occurs throughout the Nile Valley and in many other parts of Africa, including islands off the eastern coast. It also appears in Asia Minor, Cyprus, southern Portugal, and India. Reservoir hosts include monkeys, baboons, and chimpanzees.

Clinical Syndromes

Early stages of infection with *S. haematobium* are similar to those of infections involving *S. mansoni* and *S. japonicum,* with dermatitis, allergic reactions, fever, and malaise. Unlike the other two schistosomes, *S. haematobium* produces hematuria, dysuria, and urinary frequency as early symptoms. Associated with hematuria, bacteriuria is often a chronic condition. Egg deposition in the walls of the bladder may eventually result in scarring with loss of bladder capacity and the development of obstructive uropathy.

Patients with *S. haematobium* infections involving many flukes frequently demonstrate squamous cell carcinoma of the bladder. It is commonly stated that the leading cause of cancer of the bladder in Egypt and other parts of Africa is *S. haematobium.* The granulomas and pseudotubercles seen in the bladder may also be present in the lungs. Fibrosis of pulmonary tissues caused by egg deposition leads to dyspnea, cough, and hemoptysis.

Laboratory Diagnosis

Examination of urine specimens reveals the large, terminally spined eggs. Occasionally, bladder biopsy is helpful in establishing the diagnosis. *S. haematobium* eggs may appear in stool if worms have migrated to mesenteric vessels. Serologic tests are also available.

Treatment, Prevention, and Control

The drug of choice is praziquantel. At present, education, possible mass treatment, and development of a vaccine are the best approaches to the control of *S. haematobium* disease. The basic problems of irrigation projects (e.g., dam building), migratory human populations, and multiple reservoir hosts make prevention and control extremely difficult.

CERCARIAL DERMATITIS

Several nonhuman schistosomes have cercariae that penetrate human skin, producing a severe dermatitis **("swimmer's itch"),** but these schistosomes cannot develop into adult worms in the human host. The natural hosts are birds and other shore-feeding animals from freshwater lakes throughout the world and a few marine beaches. The intense pruritus and urticaria from this skin penetration may lead to secondary bacterial infection from scratching the sites of infection.

Treatment consists of oral trimeprazine and topical applications of palliative agents. When indicated, sedatives may be given. Control is difficult because of bird migration and the transfer of live snails from lake to lake. Molluscicides such as copper sulfate have produced some reduction in the snail populations. Immediate drying of the skin when people leave such waters offers some protection.

CASE STUDY AND QUESTIONS

A 45-year-old Egyptian man was referred for evaluation of hematuria and urinary frequency of 2 months' duration. This individual had lived in the Middle East for most of his life but for the past year lived in the United States. He denied previous renal or urologic problems. His physical examination was unremarkable. A midstream urine specimen was grossly bloody.

1. What was the differential diagnosis of hematuria in this patient?
2. What was the etiologic agent of this patient's urologic process?
3. What exposures might put an individual at risk for this infection?
4. What are the major complications of this infection?
5. How is this disease treated?

Bibliography

Ash LR, Orihel TC: Intestinal helminths. In Murray PR et al, editors: *Manual of clinical microbiology,* ed 8, Washington, 2003, ASM Press.

Connor DH et al, editors: *Pathology of infectious diseases,* vol II, Stamford, Conn, 1997, Appleton & Lange.

Garcia LS, editor: *Diagnostic medical parasitology,* ed 4, Washington, 2001, ASM Press.

Markell EK, John DT, Krotoski WA, editors: *Markell and Voges' medical parasitology,* ed 8, Philadelphia, 1999, WB Saunders.

Strickland GT, editor: *Hunter's tropical medicine and emerging infectious diseases,* Philadelphia, 2000, WB Saunders.

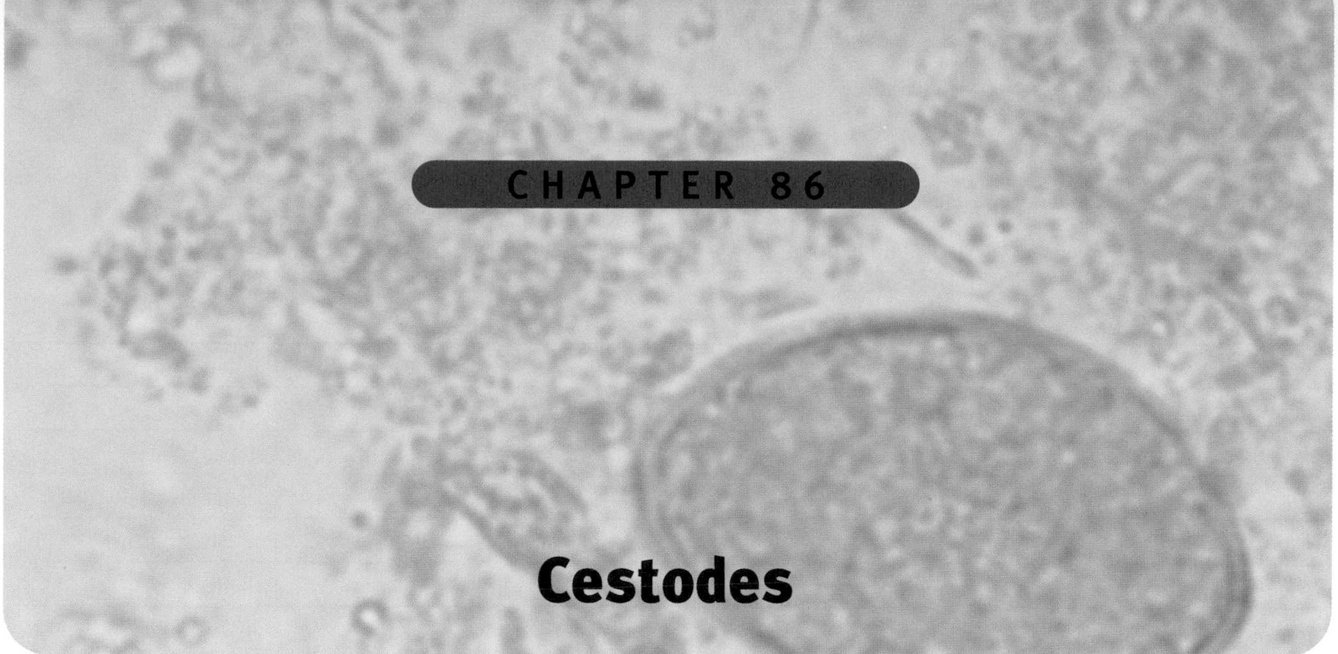

Cestodes

The bodies of cestodes, **tapeworms,** are flat and ribbonlike, and the heads are equipped with organs of attachment. The head, or **scolex,** of the worm usually has four muscular, cup-shaped suckers and a crown of hooklets. An exception is *Diphyllobothrium latum*, the fish tapeworm, whose scolex is equipped with a pair of long, lateral muscular grooves and lacks hooklets.

The individual segments of tapeworms are called **proglottids,** and the chain of proglottids is called a **strobila.**

All tapeworms are hermaphroditic, with male and female reproductive organs present in each mature proglottid. The eggs of most tapeworms are nonoperculated and contain a six-hooked **hexacanth embryo;** the one exception, *D. latum*, has an unembryonated, operculated egg similar to fluke eggs. Tapeworms have no digestive system, and food is absorbed from the host intestine through the soft body wall of the worm. Most tapeworms found in the human intestine have complex life cycles involving intermediate hosts, and in some instances (cysticercosis, echinococcosis, sparganosis) humans serve as a form of intermediate host that harbors larval stages. The presence of extraintestinal larvae are at times more serious than that of adult worms in the intestine. The most common cestodes of medical importance are listed in Table 86–1.

Taenia solium

PHYSIOLOGY AND STRUCTURE

After a person ingests pork muscle containing a larval worm called a **cysticercus ("bladder worm"),** attachment of the scolex with its four muscular suckers and crown of hooklets initiates infection in the small intestine (Figure 86–1). The worm then produces proglottids until a strobila of proglottids is developed, which may be several meters long. The sexually mature proglottids contain eggs, and as these proglottids leave the host in feces, they can contaminate water and vegetation ingested by swine. The eggs in swine become a six-hooked larval form called an oncosphere that penetrates the pig's intestinal wall, migrates in the circulation to the tissues, and becomes a cysticercus to complete the cycle.

EPIDEMIOLOGY

T. solium infection is directly correlated with eating insufficiently cooked pork and is prevalent in Africa, India, Southeast Asia, China, Mexico, Latin American countries, and Slavic countries. It is seen infrequently in the United States.

CLINICAL SYNDROMES

Adult *T. solium* in the intestine seldom causes appreciable symptoms. The intestine may be irritated at sites of attachment, and abdominal discomfort, chronic indigestion, and diarrhea may occur. Most patients become aware of the infection only when they see proglottids or a strobila of proglottids in their feces.

LABORATORY DIAGNOSIS

Stool examination may reveal proglottids and eggs, and treatment may produce the entire worm for identification. The eggs are spherical, are 30 to 40 μm in diameter, and possess a thick, radially striated shell containing a six-hooked hexacanth embryo (Figure 86–2). The eggs are identical to those of *Taenia saginata* **(beef tapeworm),** so eggs alone are not sufficient for species identification. Critical examination of the proglottids reveals their internal

TABLE 86–1. Medically Important Cestodes

Cestode	Common Name	Reservoir for Larvae	Reservoir for Adults
Taenia solium	Pork tapeworm Cysticercosis	Hogs Humans	Humans —
Taenia saginata	Beef tapeworm	Cattle	Humans
Diphyllobothrium latum	Fish tapeworm	Freshwater crustaceans and fish	Humans, dogs, cats, bears
Echinococcus granulosus	Unilocular hydatid cyst	Herbivores, humans	Canines
Echinococcus multilocularis	Alveolar hydatid cyst	Herbivores, humans	Foxes, wolves, dogs, cats
Hymenolepis nana	Dwarf tapeworm	Rodents, humans	Rodents, humans
Hymenolepis diminuta	Dwarf tapeworm	Insects	Rodents, humans
Dipylidium caninum	Pumpkin seed tapeworm	Fleas	Dogs, cats

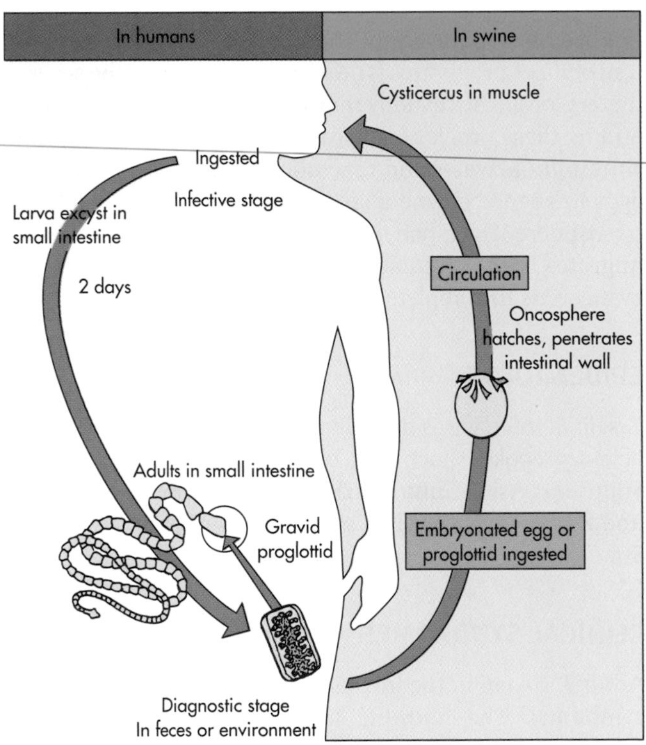

FIGURE 86–1. Life cycle of *Taenia solium* (pork tapeworm).

structure, which is important for the differentiation of *T. solium* and *T. saginata*. Gravid proglottids of *T. solium* are smaller than those of *T. saginata* and contain only seven to 13 lateral uterine branches versus 15 to 30 for the beef tapeworm.

TREATMENT, PREVENTION, AND CONTROL

The drug of choice is niclosamide; praziquantel, paromomycin, or quinacrine is an effective alternative. Prevention of **pork tapeworm** infections requires that pork be either cooked until the interior of the meat is gray or frozen at −20°C for at least 12 hours. Sanitation is critical; every effort must be made to keep human feces containing *T. solium* eggs out of water and vegetation ingested by pigs.

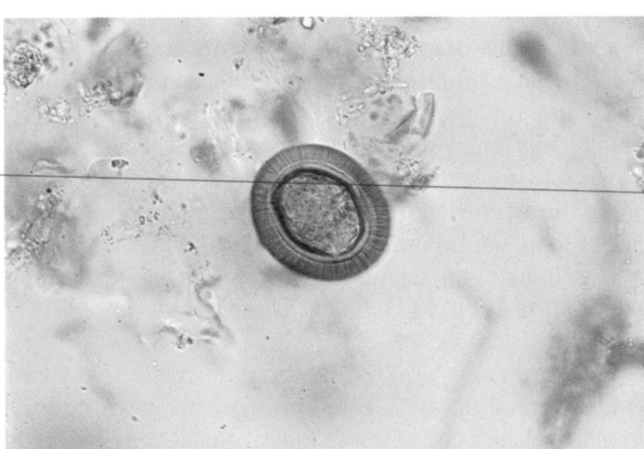

FIGURE 86–2. *Taenia* egg. The eggs are spherical, are 30 to 40 μm in diameter, and contain three pairs of hooklets internally. The eggs of the different *Taenia* species cannot be differentiated.

Cysticercosis

PHYSIOLOGY AND STRUCTURE

Cysticercosis involves infection of people with the larval stage of *T. solium*, the cysticerci, which normally infect pigs (Figure 86–3). Human ingestion of water or vegetation contaminated with *T. solium* eggs from human feces initiates the infection. Autoinfection may occur when eggs from a person infected with the adult worm are transferred from the perianal area to the mouth on contaminated fingers. Once ingested the eggs hatch in the stomach of the intermediate host, releasing the hexacanth embryo

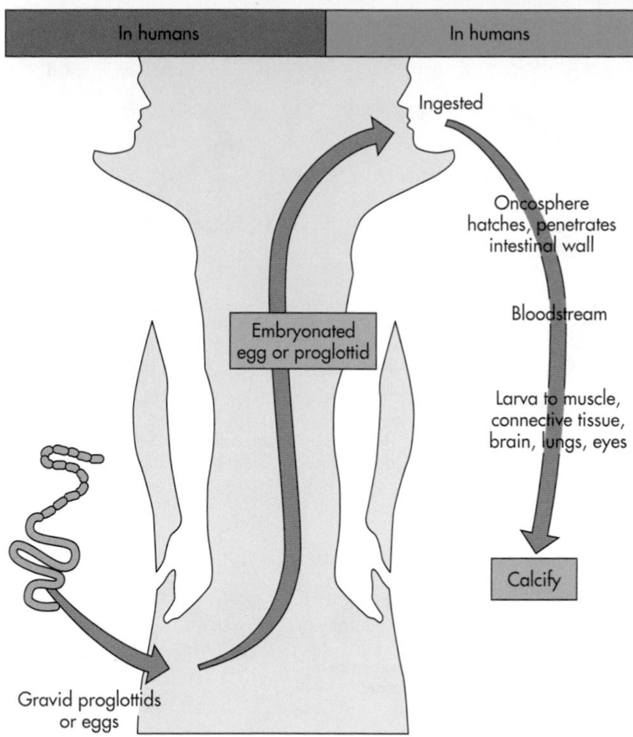

FIGURE 86–3. Development of human cysticercosis.

or **oncosphere.** The oncosphere penetrates the intestinal wall and migrates in the circulation to the tissues, where it develops into a cysticercus over 3 to 4 months. The cysticerci may develop in muscle, connective tissue, brain, lungs, and eyes and remain viable for as long as 5 years.

EPIDEMIOLOGY

Cysticercosis is found in the areas where *T. solium* is prevalent and is directly correlated with human fecal contamination. In addition to fecal-oral transmission, autoinfection may occur when a proglottid containing eggs is regurgitated from the small intestine into the stomach, allowing the eggs to hatch and release the infectious oncosphere.

CLINICAL SYNDROMES

A few cysticerci in nonvital areas (e.g., subcutaneous tissues) may not provoke symptoms, but serious disease may follow as the cysticerci lodge in vital areas, such as the brain and eyes. In the brain, they may produce hydrocephalus, meningitis, cranial nerve damage, seizures, hyperactive reflexes, and visual defects. In the eye, loss of visual acuity may occur, and if the larvae lodge along the optic tract, visual field defects result. Tissue reaction to viable larvae may be only moderate, thus minimizing symptoms. However, death of the larvae results in the release of antigenic material that stimulates a marked inflammatory reaction; exacerbation of symptoms can result in fever, muscle pains, and eosinophilia.

LABORATORY DIAGNOSIS

The presence of cysticerci is usually established by the appearance of calcified cysticerci in soft tissue roentgenograms, surgical removal of subcutaneous nodules, and visualization of cysts in the eye. Computed tomography, radioisotope scanning, or ultrasonography may detect central nervous system lesions. Serologic studies may be useful; false-positive results may occur in people with other helminthic infections.

TREATMENT, PREVENTION, AND CONTROL

The drug of choice for cysticercosis is either praziquantel or albendazole. Concomitant steroid administration may be necessary to minimize the inflammatory response to dying larvae. Surgical removal of cerebral and ocular cysts may be necessary. Critical to the prevention and control of human infection are the treatment of human cases harboring adult *T. solium* (to reduce egg transmission) and the controlled disposal of human feces. These measures also reduce the likelihood of infection in pigs.

Taenia saginata

PHYSIOLOGY AND STRUCTURE

The life cycle of *T. saginata*, the beef tapeworm, is similar to that of *T. solium* (Figure 86–4), with infection resulting after cysticerci are ingested in insufficiently cooked beef. After excystment, the larvae develop into adults in the small intestine and initiate egg production in maturing proglottids. The adult worm may parasitize the jejunum and small intestine of humans for as long as 25 years, attaining a length of 10 m. In contrast with *T. solium* infections, cysticercosis produced by *T. saginata* does not occur in humans. The adult *T. saginata* worm also differs from *T. solium* because it lacks a crown of hooklets on the scolex and has a different proglottid uterine branch structure. These facts are important in differentiating between the two tapeworms but do not affect therapy.

EPIDEMIOLOGY

T. saginata occurs worldwide and is one of the most common causes of cestode infections in the United States.

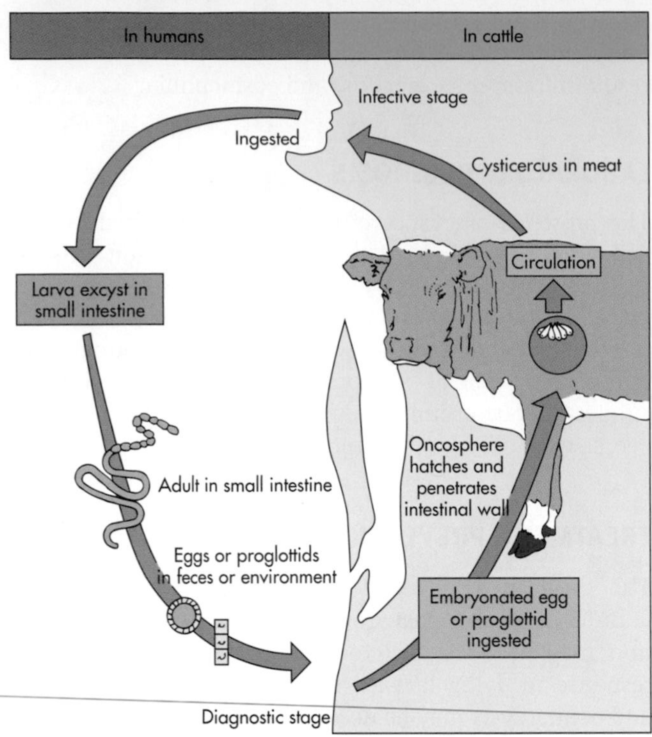

FIGURE 86–4. Life cycle of *Taenia saginata* (beef tapeworm).

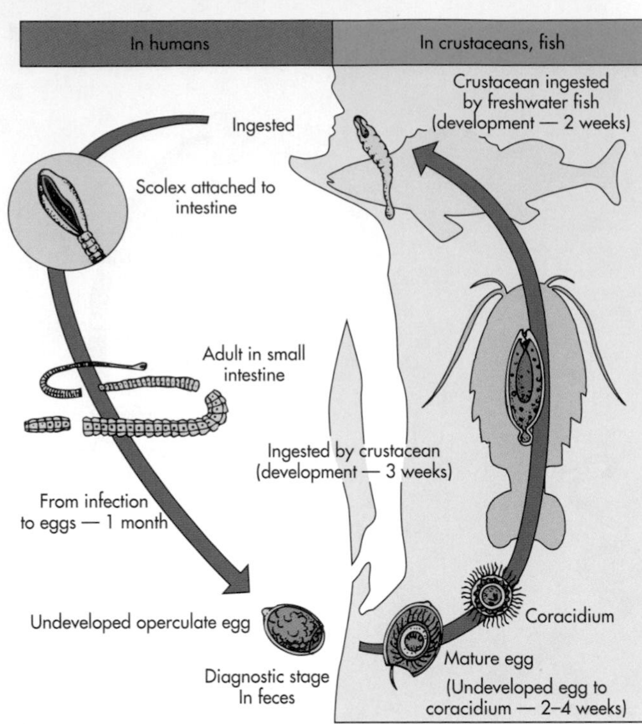

FIGURE 86–5. Life cycle of *Diphyllobothrium latum* (fish tapeworm).

Humans and cattle perpetuate the life cycle: Human feces contaminate water and vegetation with eggs, which are then ingested by cattle. The cysticerci in cattle produce adult tapeworms in humans when rare or insufficiently cooked beef is eaten.

CLINICAL SYNDROMES

The syndrome that results from *T. saginata* infection is similar to the intestinal infection with *T. solium*. Patients are generally asymptomatic or may complain of vague abdominal pains, chronic indigestion, and hunger pains. Proglottids may pass out of the anus directly.

LABORATORY DIAGNOSIS

The diagnosis of *T. saginata* infection is similar to that of *T. solium*, with recovery of proglottids and eggs or recovery of an entire worm whose scolex lacks hooklets. Study of the uterine branches in the proglottids differentiates *T. saginata* from *T. solium*.

TREATMENT, PREVENTION, AND CONTROL

Treatment is identical to that for the intestinal phase of *T. solium*. A single dose of niclosamide is highly effective in eliminating the adult worm. Education regarding cooking beef and controlling of the disposal of human feces is a critical measure.

Diphyllobothrium latum

PHYSIOLOGY AND STRUCTURE

One of the largest tapeworms (20 to 30 feet long), *D. latum* **(fish tapeworm)**, has a complex life cycle involving two intermediate hosts: freshwater crustaceans and freshwater fish (Figure 86–5). The ribbonlike larval worm in the flesh of freshwater fish is called a **sparganum.** Ingestion of this sparganum in raw or insufficiently cooked fish initiates infection. The scolex of *D. latum* is shaped like a lance and has long, lateral grooves **(bothria)** that serve as organs of attachment. The proglottids of *D. latum* are broad, have a central uterine structure resembling a rosette, and produce eggs with an operculum, like fluke eggs, and a knob on the shell at the bottom of the egg. The adult worms may produce eggs for months or years. More than 1 million eggs per day are released into the fecal stream. On reaching freshwater, the unembryonated, operculate eggs require a period of 2 to 4 weeks to develop a ciliated, free-swimming larval form called a **coracidium.** The fully developed coracidium leaves the egg via the operculum and is ingested by tiny crustaceans that are called copepods (e.g., *Cyclops* and *Diaptomus* species); then the coracidium develops into a **procercoid** larval form. The crustacean harboring the larval stage is then eaten by a fish, and the infectious **plerocercoid** or sparganum larvae develop in the musculature of the fish. If the fish is in turn eaten by another fish, the sparganum simply migrates into the muscles of the second fish. Humans are infected when they eat raw or undercooked fish containing the larval forms.

EPIDEMIOLOGY

D. latum infection occurs worldwide, most prevalently in cool lake regions where raw or pickled fish is popular. Insufficient cooking over campfires and tasting and seasoning "gefilte fish" account for many infections. A reservoir of infected wild animals, such as bears, minks, walruses, and members of the canine and feline families that eat fish, are also sources for human infections. The practice of dumping raw sewage into freshwater lakes contributes to the propagation of this tapeworm.

CLINICAL SYNDROMES

Clinically, as is the case with most adult tapeworm infections, most *D. latum* infections are asymptomatic. Occasionally, people complain of epigastric pain, abdominal cramping, nausea, vomiting, and weight loss. As many as 40% of *D. latum* carriers may have low serum levels of vitamin B_{12}, presumably because of the competition between the host and the worm for dietary vitamin B_{12}. A small percentage (0.1% to 2%) of people infected with *D. latum* develop clinical signs of vitamin B_{12} deficiency, including megaloblastic anemia and neurologic manifestations, such as numbness, paresthesia, and loss of vibration sense.

LABORATORY DIAGNOSIS

Stool examination reveals the bile-stained, operculated egg with its knob at the bottom of the shell (Figure 86–6). Typical proglottids with the rosette uterine structure may also be found in stool specimens. Concentration techniques are usually not necessary because the worms produce large numbers of ova.

TREATMENT, PREVENTION, AND CONTROL

The drug of choice is niclosamide; praziquantel and paromomycin are acceptable alternatives. Vitamin B_{12} supplementation may be necessary in people with evidence of clinical vitamin B_{12} deficiency. Avoiding the ingestion of insufficiently cooked fish; controlling the disposal of human feces, especially the proper treatment of sewage before disposal in lakes; and promptly treating infections reduce the prevalence of this infection.

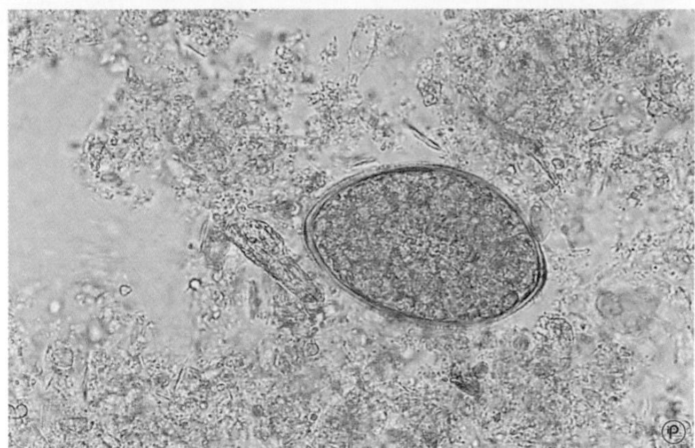

FIGURE 86–6. *D. latum* egg. Unlike other tapeworm eggs, *D. latum* eggs are operculated. They are 45 × 90 μm in size. (From Marler LM et al: *Parasitology* CD-Rom, Indiana Pathology Images, 2003.)

Sparganosis

PHYSIOLOGY AND STRUCTURE

The larval forms of several tapeworms closely related to *D. latum* (most often *Spirometra* species) can produce human disease in subcutaneous sites and in the eye. In these cases, humans act as the end-stage host for the larval stage, or **sparganum.** Infections are acquired primarily by drinking pond or ditch water that contains crustaceans (copepods) that carry a larval tapeworm. This larval form penetrates the intestinal wall and migrates to various sites in the body, where it develops into a sparganum. Infections may also occur if tadpoles, frogs, and snakes are ingested raw or if the flesh of these animals is applied to wounds as a poultice. The larval worm leaves the relatively cold flesh of the dead animal and migrates into the warm human flesh.

EPIDEMIOLOGY

Cases have been reported from various parts of the world, including the United States, but the infection is most prevalent in the Orient. Regardless of location, drinking contaminated water and eating raw tadpole, frog, and snake flesh lead to infection.

CLINICAL SYNDROMES

In subcutaneous sites, **sparganosis** can produce painful inflammatory tissue reactions and nodules. In the eye, the tissue reaction is intensely painful, and periorbital edema is common. Corneal ulcers may develop with ocular involvement. Ocular disease is frequently associated with the use of frog or snake flesh as a poultice over a wound near the eye.

LABORATORY DIAGNOSIS

Sections of tissue removed surgically show characteristic tapeworm features, including highly convoluted parenchyma and dark-staining calcareous corpuscles.

TREATMENT, PREVENTION, AND CONTROL

Surgical removal is the customary approach. The drug praziquantel may be used; however, no clinical data support its efficacy. Education regarding possible contamination of drinking water with crustaceans that harbor larval worms is essential, and contamination most likely occurs in pond and ditch water. Ingestion of raw frog and snake flesh, or their use as poultices over wounds, also should be avoided.

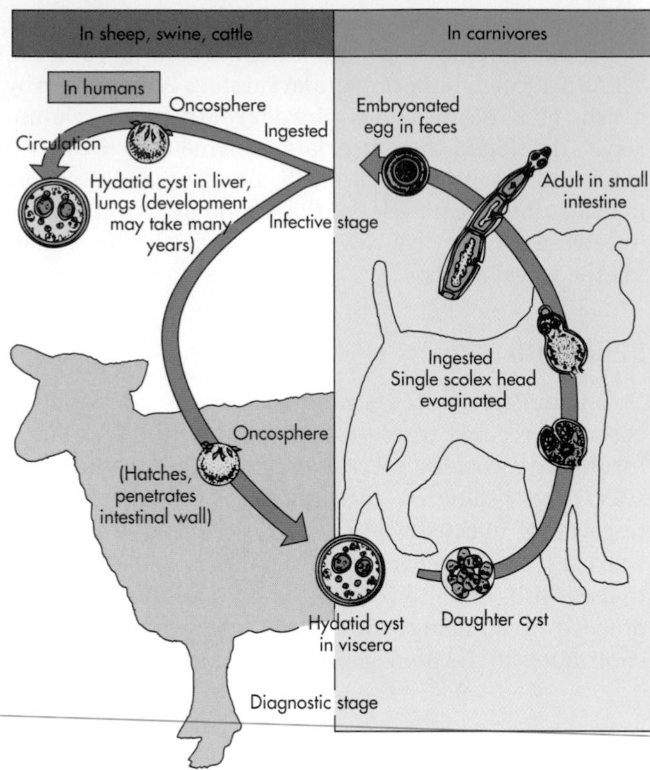

FIGURE 86–7. Life cycle of *Echinococcus granulosus.*

Echinococcus granulosus

PHYSIOLOGY AND STRUCTURE

Infection with *E. granulosus* is another example of accidental human infection, with humans serving as dead-end intermediate hosts in a life cycle that occurs naturally in other animals. *E. granulosus* adult tapeworms are found in nature in the intestines of canines (dog, fox, wolf, coyote, jackal, dingo); the larval cyst stage is present in the viscera of herbivores (sheep, cattle, swine, deer, moose, elk) (Figure 86–7). The worm consists of a *Taenia*-like scolex with four sucking disks and a double row of hooklets, as well as a strobila containing three proglottids: one immature, one mature, and one gravid. Adult tapeworms in the canine intestine produce infective eggs that pass in feces. The eggs are identical in appearance to those of the *Taenia* species. When these eggs are ingested by humans, a six-hooked larval stage called an oncosphere hatches. The oncosphere penetrates the human intestinal wall and enters the circulation to be carried to various tissue sites, primarily the liver and lungs but also the central nervous system and bone. This same cycle occurs in the viscera of herbivores. When the herbivore is killed by a canine predator or viscera is fed to canines, the ingestion of cysts produces adult tapeworms in the canine intestine to complete the cycle and initiate new egg production. Adult tapeworms do not develop in the intestines of herbivores or humans.

In humans, the larvae form a unilocular **hydatid cyst,** which is a slow-growing, tumorlike, space-occupying structure enclosed by a laminated germinative membrane. This membrane produces structures on its wall called **brood capsules,** where tapeworm heads **(protoscolices)** develop. Daughter cysts may develop in the original mother cyst and also produce brood capsules and protoscolices. The cysts and daughter cysts accumulate fluid as they grow. This fluid is potentially toxic; if spilled into body cavities, anaphylactic shock and death can result. Spillage and the escape of protoscolices can lead to the development of cysts in other sites because the protoscolices have the germinative potential to form new cysts. Eventually the brood capsules and daughter cysts disintegrate within the mother cyst, liberating the accumulated protoscolices. These become known as **hydatid sand.** This type of *Echinococcus* cyst is called a **unilocular cyst** to differentiate it from related cysts that grow differently. The unilocular cyst is approximately 5 cm in diameter, but some as large as 20 cm, containing almost 2 liters of cyst fluid, have been reported. The cyst may die and become calcified over long periods.

EPIDEMIOLOGY

Human infection with *E. granulosus* unilocular cyst is directly correlated with raising sheep in many countries in Europe, South America, Africa, Asia, Australia, and New Zealand. It occurs in Canada and in the United States, with cases reported from Alaska, Utah, New Mexico, Arizona, California, and the lower Mississippi valley. Human infection follows ingestion of contaminated water or vegetation, as well as hand-to-mouth transmission of canine feces carrying the infective eggs.

CLINICAL SYNDROMES

Because the unilocular cyst grows slowly, 5 to 20 years may pass before any symptoms appear. In many instances, it appears that the cyst is as old as its host. The pressure of the expanding cyst in an organ is usually the first sign of infection. In the majority of cases the cysts are located in the liver or lung. In the liver, the cyst may exert pressure on both bile ducts and blood vessels and create pain and biliary rupture. In the lungs, cysts may produce cough, dyspnea, and chest pains. Rupture of the cysts may occur in 20% of cases, producing fever, urticaria, and occasionally, anaphylactic shock and death, which are caused by the release of antigenic cyst contents. Cyst rupture may also lead to dissemination of infection resulting from the release of thousands of protoscolices. In bone, the cyst is responsible for erosion of the marrow cavity and the bone itself. In the brain, severe damage may occur as a result of the cyst's tumorlike growth into brain tissue.

LABORATORY DIAGNOSIS

The diagnosis of **hydatid disease** is difficult and depends primarily on clinical, radiographic, and serologic findings. Radiologic examination, scanning procedures, tomography, and ultrasound techniques all are valuable and may provide the first evidence of the cyst's presence. Aspiration of cyst contents may demonstrate the presence of the protoscolices (hydatid sand); however, it is contraindicated because of the risk of anaphylaxis and dissemination of the infection. Serologic testing may be useful, but results are negative in 10% to 40% of infections.

TREATMENT, PREVENTION, AND CONTROL

Surgical resection of the cyst is the treatment of choice. In some instances, the cyst is first aspirated to remove the fluid and hydatid sand, and then it is instilled with formalin to kill and detoxify remaining fluid; finally, it is rolled into a marsupial pouch and sewn shut. If the condition is inoperable because of the cyst's location, medical therapy with high-dose albendazole, mebendazole, or praziquantel may be considered. The most important factor in preventing and controlling **echinococcosis** is education regarding the transmission of infection and the role of canines in the life cycle. Proper personal hygiene and the washing of hands and cooking utensils in environments inhabited by dogs are critical. Dogs should not be allowed in the vicinity of animal slaughter and should never be fed the viscera of slain animals. In some areas the killing of stray dogs has reduced the incidence of infection.

Echinococcus multilocularis

PHYSIOLOGY AND STRUCTURE

Like infection with *E. granulosus*, human infection with *E. multilocularis* is accidental (Figure 86–8). Adult *E. multilocularis* tapeworms are primarily found in foxes and wolves, although farm dogs and cats harbor them in some rural environments. The intermediate hosts that harbor the cyst stage are rodents (mice, voles, shrews, and lemmings). Humans become infected with the cyst stage as a result of contact with fox, dog, or cat feces contaminated with eggs. Trappers and workers who handle fur pelts may become infected by inhaling fecal dust that carries eggs.

Infective eggs hatch in the intestinal tract, releasing oncospheres. These forms enter the circulation and take up residence primarily in the liver and lungs but also possibly in the brain.

The **alveolar hydatid cyst** develops as an alveolar or honeycombed structure that is not covered by a unilocular-limiting, mother cyst-laminated membrane. The cyst grows via exogenous budding, eventually resembling a carcinoma. In humans, individual cysts are said to be sterile and rarely produce protoscolices (hydatid sand).

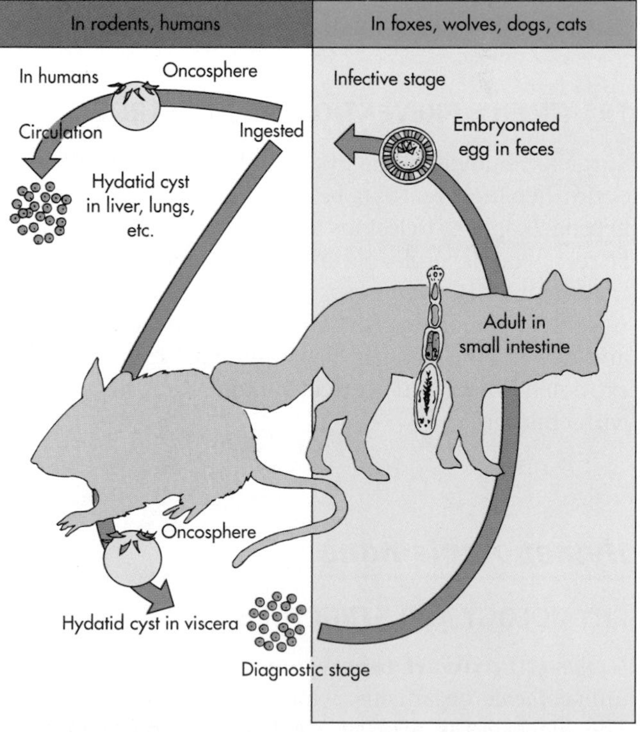

FIGURE 86–8. Life cycle of *Echinococcus multilocularis.*

EPIDEMIOLOGY

E. multilocularis is found primarily in northern areas such as Canada, the former Soviet Union, northern Japan, and Central Europe, and Alaska, Montana, North and South Dakota, Minnesota, and Iowa in the United States. There is evidence that the life cycle may be extending to other Midwestern states, where foxes and mice transmit the organism to dogs and cats and eventually to humans.

CLINICAL SYNDROMES

E. multilocularis, because of its slow growth, may be present in human tissues for many years before symptoms appear. In the liver, cysts eventually mimic a carcinoma, with liver enlargement and obstruction of biliary and portal pathways. Often the growth metastasizes to the lungs and brain. Malnutrition, ascites, and portal hypertension produced by *E. multilocularis* create the appearance of hepatic cirrhosis. Among all of the worm infections of humans, *E. multilocularis* is one of the most lethal. If left untreated, the mortality rate is approximately 70% of infected people.

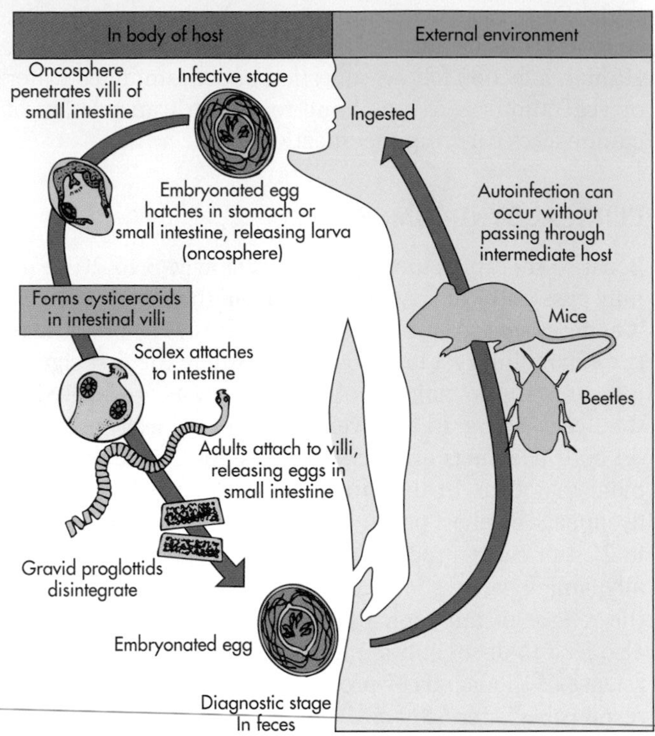

FIGURE 86–9. Life cycle of *Hymenolepis nana* (dwarf tapeworm).

LABORATORY DIAGNOSIS

Unlike *E. granulosus,* the tissue form of *E. multilocularis* presents no protoscolices, and the material so resembles a neoplasm that even pathologists mistake it for carcinoma. Radiologic procedures and scanning techniques are helpful, and serologic methods are available.

TREATMENT, PREVENTION, AND CONTROL

Surgical removal of the cyst is indicated, especially if an entire hepatic area can be resected. The same surgical approach applies to lesions in the lung wherein a lobe can be resected. Mebendazole and albendazole, as used for the treatment of *E. granulosus,* have produced clinical cures. As with *E. granulosus,* education, proper personal hygiene, and deworming of farm dogs and cats are critical. It is extremely important to treat animals that have contact with children.

Hymenolepis nana

PHYSIOLOGY AND STRUCTURE

H. nana, the **dwarf tapeworm,** is only 2 to 4 cm long, unlike *Taenia* organisms, which measure several meters. The life cycle is also simple and does not require an intermediate host (Figure 86–9), although mice and beetles may be infected and enter the cycle.

Infection begins when the embryonated eggs are ingested and develop in the intestinal villi into a larval cysticercoid stage. This cysticercoid larva attaches its four muscular suckers and crown of hooklets to the small intestine, and the adult worm produces a strobila of egg-laden proglottids. Eggs passing in the feces are then immediately and directly infective, initiating another cycle. Infection may also be acquired by ingesting infected insect intermediate hosts.

H. nana also can cause autoinfection, with a subsequent increased worm burden. Eggs are able to hatch in the intestine, develop into a cysticercoid larva, and then grow into adult worms without leaving the host. This can lead to hyperinfection with very heavy worm burdens and severe clinical symptoms.

EPIDEMIOLOGY

H. nana occurs worldwide in humans and is also a common parasite of mice. The most common tapeworm infection in North America, *H. nana* occasionally develops its cysticercoid stage in beetles; humans and mice may ingest these beetles in contaminated grain and flour. Children are especially at risk of infection, and because of the simple life cycle of the parasite, families with children in daycare centers experience problems in controlling the transmission of this organism.

CLINICAL SYNDROMES

With only a few worms in the intestine, there are no symptoms. In heavy infections, especially if autoinfection and hyperinfection occur, patients experience diarrhea, abdominal pain, headache, anorexia, and other vague complaints.

LABORATORY DIAGNOSIS

Stool examination reveals the characteristic *H. nana* egg, with its six-hooked embryo and polar filaments (Figure 86–10).

TREATMENT, PREVENTION, AND CONTROL

The drug of choice is praziquantel; an alternative is niclosamide. Treatment of cases, improved sanitation, and proper personal hygiene, especially in the family and institutional environments, are essential for controlling the transmission of *H. nana*.

Hymenolepis diminuta

PHYSIOLOGY AND STRUCTURE

H. diminuta, closely related to *H. nana*, is primarily a tapeworm of rats and mice, but it is also found in humans. It differs from *H. nana* in length, measuring 20 to 60 cm. The scolex lacks hooklets, and the egg is larger, is bile stained, and has no polar filaments. The life cycle of *H. diminuta* is more complex than that of *H. nana*, and it requires larval insects ("mealworms") to reach the infective cysticercoid stage.

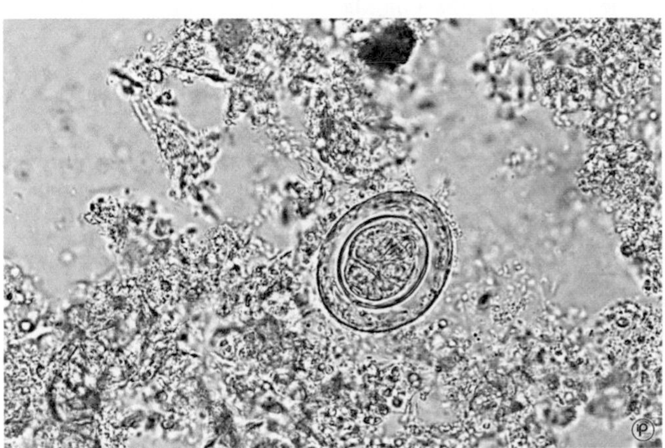

FIGURE 86–10. *H. nana* egg. The eggs are 30 to 45 μm in diameter and have a thin shell containing a six-hooked embryo. (From Marler LM et al: *Parasitology* CD-Rom, Indiana Pathology Images, 2003.)

EPIDEMIOLOGY

Infections have been found all over the world, including in the United States. Larval beetles and other larval insects become infected when they feed on rat feces that carry *H. diminuta* eggs. Humans are infected by ingesting the larval insects (mealworms) in contaminated grain products (e.g., flour, cereals).

CLINICAL SYNDROMES

Mild infections produce no symptoms, but heavier worm burdens produce nausea, abdominal discomfort, anorexia, and diarrhea.

LABORATORY DIAGNOSIS

Stool examination demonstrates the characteristic bile-stained egg that lacks polar filaments.

TREATMENT, PREVENTION, AND CONTROL

The drug of choice is niclosamide, with praziquantel an alternative. Rodent control in areas where grain products are produced or stored is essential. Thorough inspection of uncooked grain products to detect mealworms is also important.

Dipylidium caninum

PHYSIOLOGY AND STRUCTURE

D. caninum, a small tapeworm averaging about 15 cm in length, is primarily a parasite of dogs and cats, but it can infect humans, especially children whose mouths are licked by infected pets. The life cycle involves the development of larval worms in dog and cat fleas. These fleas, when crushed by the teeth of the infected pet, are carried on the tongue to the child's mouth when the child kisses the pet or the pet licks the child. Swallowing the infected flea leads to intestinal infection.

Because of the size and shape of the mature and terminal proglottids, *D. caninum* is often called the **pumpkin seed tapeworm**. The eggs are distinctive because they occur in packets covered with a tough, clear membrane. There may be as many as 25 eggs in a packet, and a single egg free of the packet is seldom seen.

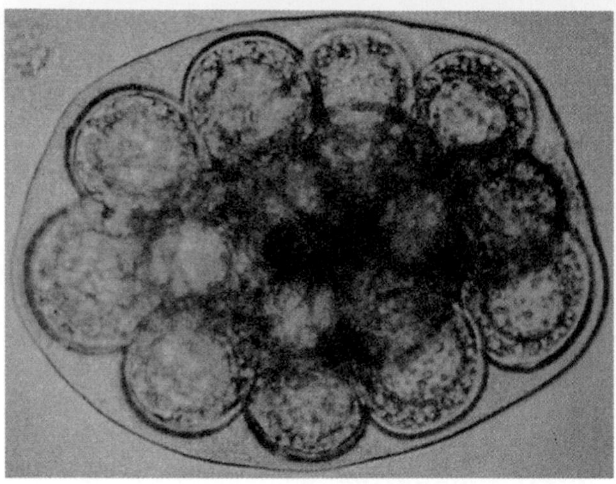

FIGURE 86–11. *Dipylidium caninum* eggs. Free eggs are rarely seen. Instead, egg packets that contain eight to 15 six-hooked oncospheres enclosed in a thin membrane are most commonly found in fecal specimens. (From Murray PR et al: *Manual of clinical microbiology,* ed 7, Washington, 1999, American Society for Microbiology.)

EPIDEMIOLOGY

D. caninum occurs worldwide, especially in children. Its distribution and transmission are directly correlated with dogs and cats infected with fleas.

CLINICAL SYNDROMES

Light infections are asymptomatic; heavier worm burdens produce abdominal discomfort, anal pruritus, and diarrhea. Anal pruritus results from the active migration of the motile proglottid.

LABORATORY DIAGNOSIS

Stool examination reveals the colorless egg packets (Figure 86–11), and proglottids may be in feces brought to physicians by patients.

TREATMENT, PREVENTION, AND CONTROL

The drug of choice is niclosamide; praziquantel and paromomycin are alternatives. Dogs and cats should be dewormed and not be allowed to lick the mouths of children. Pets should be treated to eradicate the fleas.

CASE STUDY AND QUESTIONS

A 30-year-old Hispanic man entered the emergency department after a focal neurologic seizure. The patient had recently emigrated from Mexico and was in his usual state of good health before the seizure. Neurologic examination revealed no focal findings. A computed tomographic scan of the head revealed multiple small cystic lesions in both cerebral hemispheres. Punctate calcification was noted in several of the lesions. A lumbar puncture revealed a glucose level of 65 mg/dl (normal) and a protein level of 38 mg/dl (normal) in cerebrospinal fluid. The white blood cell count was 20/mm^3 (abnormal) with a differential of 5% neutrophils, 90% lymphocytes, and 5% monocytes. A purified protein derivative skin test was negative with positive controls. Serologic test for human immunodeficiency virus was negative.

1. What was the differential diagnosis of this patient's neurologic process?
2. Which parasite or parasites may have caused this condition?
3. What diagnostic tests were available for this infection?
4. What were the therapeutic options for this patient?
5. How do people become infected with this parasite?
6. What tissue sites (besides the central nervous system) may be involved? How would these additional foci of infection be documented?

Bibliography

Ash LR, Orihel TC: Intestinal helminths. In Murray PR et al, editors: *Manual of clinical microbiology,* ed 8, Washington, 2003, ASM Press.

Eckert J, Deplazes P: Biological epidemiological, and clinical aspects of echinococcosis, a zoonosis of increasing concern, *Clin Microbiol Rev* 17:107-135, 2004.

Garcia HH et al: Current consensus guidelines for treatment of neurocysticercosis, *Clin Microbiol Rev* 15:747-756, 2002.

Garcia LS, editor: *Diagnostic medical parasitology,* ed 4, Washington, 2001, ASM Press.

Liu LX, Weller PF: Drug therapy: Antiparasitic drugs, *New Engl J Med* 334:1178-1184, 1996.

Markell EK, John DT, Krotoski WA, editors: *Markell and Voges medical parasitology,* ed 8, Philadelphia, 1999, WB Saunders.

Strickland GT, editor: *Hunter's tropical medicine and emerging infectious diseases,* Philadelphia, 2000, WB Saunders.

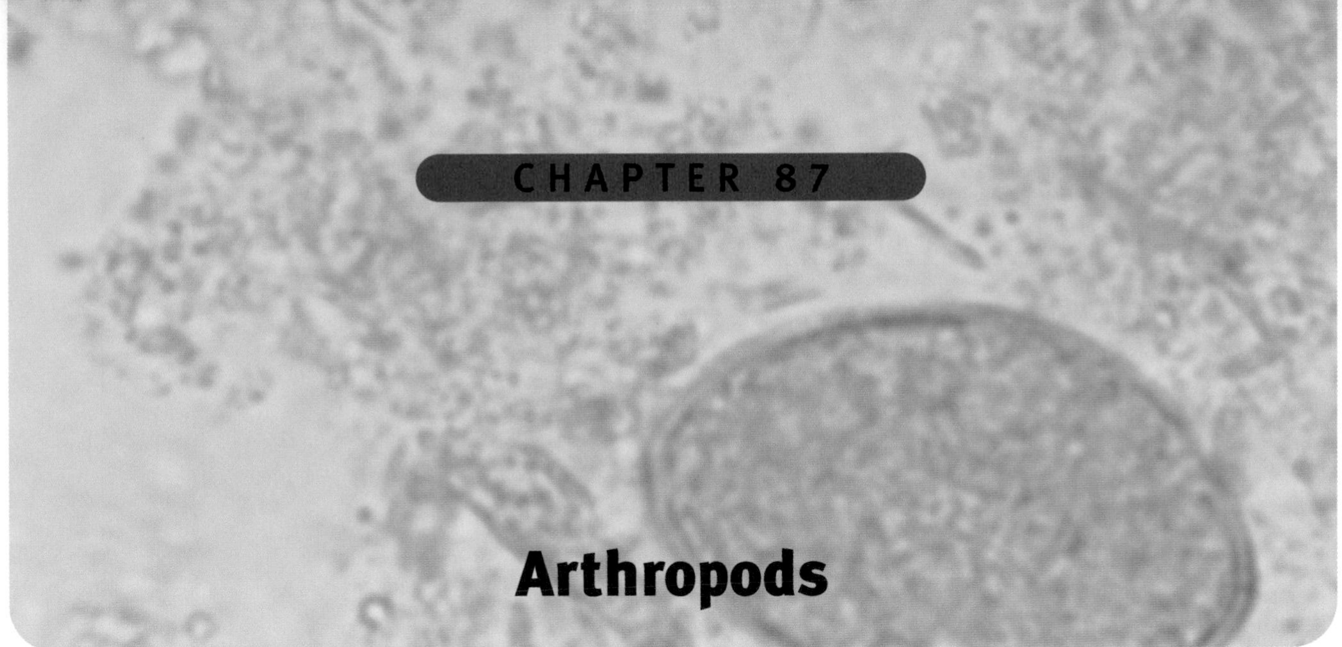

Arthropods

The arthropods are the largest of the animal phyla, with more than 1 million species. The phylum Arthropoda comprises invertebrate animals with a segmented body, several pairs of jointed appendages, bilateral symmetry, and a rigid, chitinous exoskeleton that is molted periodically as the animal grows. Characteristically, arthropods develop from egg to adult by a process known as **metamorphosis.** As they mature, the organisms pass through several distinct morphologic stages including egg, larvae or nymph, pupa (certain insects), and adult. Five classes of arthropods are of medical importance on the basis of the number or the severity of the illnesses they cause: the Chilopoda, Pentastomida, Crustacea, Arachnida, and Insecta (Table 87–1).

The arthropods or their larvae may affect human health in many ways. Most arthropods function indirectly in human disease; they transmit but do not produce disease. Arthropods may transmit disease mechanically, as when flies carry enteric bacterial pathogens from feces to human food. Of outstanding importance is the ability of many arthropods to act as biologic **vectors** and **intermediate hosts** in the transmission and developmental cycle of viruses, bacteria, protozoa, and metazoa (Table 87–2). Certain arthropods may inflict direct injury by their bites or stings. Other species, such as lice, scabies mites, and tissue-invading maggots, may act as true parasites. Still other species may function as both parasites and vectors of disease.

It is not the purpose of this chapter to consider medical entomology in detail. Rather, our purpose is to provide a brief overview of several of the more important aspects of arthropods and their relationship to human disease. More detailed information on arthropods of medical importance and the therapy and control of arthropod infestations may be found in the references listed in the bibliography.

Chilopoda

CENTIPEDES

Physiology and Structure

The centipedes are elongated, multisegmented (from 15 to more than 181 segments), many-legged, tracheate arthropods. They possess a distinct head and trunk. The body is dorsoventrally flattened, and each trunk segment bears a single pair of legs. **Maxillipeds** or poison claws are situated on the first segment and are used for capturing prey. The centipedes are sometimes classified with the millipedes; however, millipedes lack the poison claws of centipedes and have two pairs of legs per segment.

Epidemiology

Most centipedes are predaceous insectivores that are commonly found in dark, damp environments, such as the areas beneath logs, among rubbish, and inside old buildings. Bites in human are almost invariably the result of accidental exposure to the organism during outdoor activities.

Clinical Syndromes

Centipede bites may be extremely painful and cause swelling at the site of the bite. Reports of the effects of centipede bites on humans are conflicting. One species, *Scolopendra gigantea*, which is found in Central and South America and the Galapagos Islands, reportedly has caused several deaths. With the exception of *Scolopendra* and related tropical genera, the bite of most centipedes is harmless to humans.

TABLE 87–1. Medically Important Classes of Arthropods

Phylum	Class	Organisms
Arthrodpoda	Chilopoda	Centipedes
	Pentastomida	Tongue worms
	Crustacea	Copepods Decapods (crabs, crayfish)
	Arachnida	Spiders, scorpions, mites, ticks
	Insecta	Flies, mosquitoes, lice, fleas, bugs, stinging insects

Treatment, Prevention, and Control

Treatment of a centipede bite includes local measures, such as the application of compresses of sodium bicarbonate or solutions of Epsom salts. Control consists of removing rubbish near dwellings.

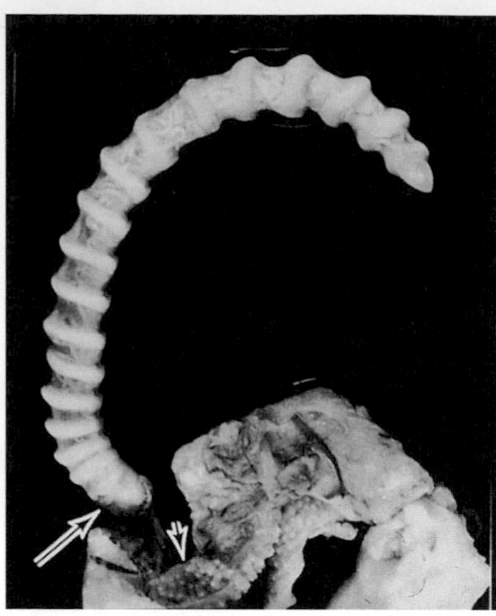

FIGURE 87–1. Adult female pentastome *(Armillifer armillatus)* attached to the respiratory surface of the lung *(short arrow)* of a rock python. Note the short cephalothorax *(long arrow)* and a long, annulated abdomen. (From Binford CH, Connor DH: *Pathology of tropical and extraordinary diseases,* vol 2, Washington, 1976, Armed Forces Institute of Pathology.)

Pentastomida

TONGUE WORMS

The pentastomids, or **tongue worms,** are bloodsucking endoparasites of reptiles, birds, and mammals. Their taxonomic status is uncertain. Some scientists include pentastomids among the arthropods because their larvae superficially resemble those of mites. Others consider them annelids, and still others place them in an entirely separate phylum. For purposes of this discussion they are considered with the arthropods.

Physiology and Structure

Tongue worms are degenerate, wormlike arthropods that live primarily in the nasal and respiratory passages of reptiles, birds, and mammals. Adult pentastomids are white, cylindrical or flattened parasites that possess two distinct body regions: an anterior head, or cephalothorax, and an abdomen. The adults are elongated and may attain a length of 1 to 10 cm. The head has a mouth and two pairs of hooks. Although the abdomen may appear annulated, it is not segmented (Figure 87–1). The pentastomids possess digestive and reproductive organs; however, they lack circulatory and respiratory systems.

The adult pentastomids are found in the lungs of reptiles and the nasal passages of mammals. Many vertebrates, including humans, may serve as intermediate hosts. The embryonated eggs are discharged in the feces or respiratory secretions of the infected definitive host and contaminate vegetation or water, which is in turn ingested by one of several possible intermediate hosts (fish, rodents, goats, sheep, or humans). The eggs hatch in the intestine, and the primary larvae penetrate the intestinal wall and attach to the peritoneum. The larvae mature in the peritoneum and develop into infective larvae, encyst in viscera, or die and become calcified. In tissue sections, encysted larvae can be identified by acidophilic glands, a chitinous cuticle, and prominent hooks, which are present in the anterior end of the organism. Subcuticular glands and striated muscle fibers may also be observed beneath the cuticle.

Humans may also become infected by ingesting the inadequately cooked flesh of infected reptiles or other definitive hosts or by eating the infected flesh of intermediate hosts (e.g., goats, sheep) containing infective larvae. In the latter instance, the infective larvae migrate from the stomach to the nasopharyngeal tissues, where they develop into adult pentastomids and produce the symptoms of the **halzoun syndrome** (see following section on clinical syndromes). In this case the human host is considered a temporary definitive host.

Epidemiology

Most tongue worm infections are reported in Europe, Africa, and South and Central America. The infection is common in Malaysia, where autopsy studies reveal **pentastomiasis** in up to 45% of people. As previously described, the infection is acquired by ingesting raw vegetables or water contaminated with pentastome eggs or by consuming raw or undercooked flesh of infected animals.

TABLE 87–2. Selected Human Illnesses Transmitted by Arthropods

Primary Vector or Intermediate Host	Disease	Etiologic Agent
Arachnida		
Mite: *Leptotrombidium* species	Scrub typhus (tsutsugamushi disease)	*Rickettsia tsutsugamushi*
Mite: *Liponyssoides sanguineus*	Rickettsial pox	*Rickettsia akari*
Tick: *Dermacentor* species	Tularemia	*Francisella tularensis*
Tick: *Dermacentor* species and other ixodid ticks	Rocky Mountain spotted fever	*Rickettsia rickettsii*
Tick: *Dermacentor, Boophilus* species	Q fever	*Coxiella burnetii*
Tick: *Dermacentor* species	Colorado tick fever	Orbivirus
Tick: *Ornithodoros* species	Relapsing fever	*Borrelia species*
Tick: *Ixodes* species	Babesiosis	*Babesia microti*
Tick: *Ixodes* species	Lyme disease	*Borrelia burgdorferi*
Tick: *Dermacentor variabilis, Amblyomma americanum*	Ehrlichiosis	*Ehrlichia risticii*
Crustacea		
Copepod: *Cyclops* species	Diphyllobothriasis	*Diphyllobothrium latum*
Copepod: *Cyclops* species	Dracunculiasis	*Dracunculus medinensis*
Crabs, crayfish: various freshwater species	Paragonimiasis	*Paragonimus westermani*
Insecta		
Lice: *Pediculus humanus*	Epidemic typhus	*Rickettsia prowazekii*
Lice: *Pediculus humanus*	Trench fever	*Rickettsia quintana*
Lice: *Pediculus humanus*	Louse-borne relapsing fever	*Borrelia recurrentis*
Flea: *Xenopsylla cheopis*, various other rodent fleas	Plague	*Yersinia pestis*
Flea: *Xenopsylla cheopis*	Murine typhus	*Rickettsia typhi*
Flea: Various species	Dipylidiasis	*Dipylidium caninum*
Bug: *Triatoma, Panstrongylus* species	Chagas' disease	*Trypanosoma cruzi*
Beetle: Flour beetle	Hymenolepiasis	*Hymenolepis nana*
Fly, gnat: *Glossina* species (tsetse fly)	African trypanosomiasis	*Trypanosoma brucei rhodesiense* and *Trypanosoma brucei gambiense*
Fly, gnat: *Simulium* species	Onchocerciasis	*Onchocerca volvulus*
Fly, gnat: *Chrysops* species	Tularemia	*Francisella tularensis*
Fly, gnat: *Phlebotomus* species, *Lutzomyia* species (sandfly)	Leishmaniasis	*Leishmania* species
Fly, gnat: *Phlebotomus* species	Bartonellosis	*Bartonella bacilliformis*
Mosquito: *Anopheles* species	Malaria	*Plasmodium* species
Mosquito: *Aedes aegypti*	Yellow fever	Flavivirus
Mosquito: *Aedes* species	Dengue fever	Flavivirus
Mosquito: *Culiseta melanura, Coquillettidia perturbans, Aedes vexans*	Eastern equine encephalitis	Alphavirus
Mosquito: *Aedes triseriatus*	La Crosse encephalitis	Bunyavirus
Mosquito: *Culex* species	St. Louis encephalitis	Flavivirus
Mosquito: *Culex* species	Venezuelan equine encephalitis	Alphavirus
Mosquito: *Culex tarsalis*	Western equine encephalitis	Alphavirus
Mosquito: Various species	Bancroftian filariasis	*Wuchereria bancrofti*
Mosquito: Various species	Malayan filariasis	*Brugia* species
Mosquito: Various species	Dirofilariasis	*Dirofilaria immitis*

Clinical Syndromes

In most cases, infection is asymptomatic and is discovered accidentally during roentgenographic examination (calcified larvae), at surgery, or at autopsy. Pneumonitis, pneumothorax, peritonitis, meningitis, nephritis, and obstructive jaundice have all been ascribed to pentastomid infections; however, definitive proof of a causal relationship between disease and the presence of the parasite is frequently lacking. Localized infection of the eye has been reported, presumably secondary to direct inoculation.

Halzoun syndrome, caused by the attachment of adult pentastomes to the nasopharyngeal tissues, is characterized by pharyngeal discomfort, paroxysmal coughing, sneezing, dysphagia, and vomiting. Asphyxiation has been rarely reported.

Laboratory Diagnosis

The diagnosis is made by identifying a pentastomid in a biopsy specimen obtained at surgery or at autopsy. Occasionally, calcified larvae may be observed on x-ray films of the abdomen or chest, providing a presumptive diagnosis. There are no useful serologic tests.

Treatment, Prevention, and Control

Treatment is not usually warranted. In symptomatic patients, surgical removal of free or encysted parasites should be attempted. Preventive measures include thorough cooking of meat and vegetables and avoidance of contaminated water.

Crustacea

The crustaceans are primarily gill-breathing arthropods of freshwater and saltwater. Those of medical importance are found in fresh water and serve as intermediate hosts of various worms (see Table 87–2).

The copepods, or water fleas, are represented by the genera *Cyclops* and *Diaptomus*. The larger crustaceans, called **decapods**, include crabs and crayfish. These crustaceans also serve as the second intermediate hosts of the lung fluke *Paragonimus westermani* (see Table 87–2).

COPEPODS

Physiology and Structure

Copepods are small, simple aquatic organisms. They lack a carapace, have one pair of maxillae, and have five pairs of biramous swimming legs. Free and parasitic forms exist. The genera *Diaptomus* and *Cyclops* are medically important.

Copepods are an intermediate host in the life cycle of several human parasites, including *Dracunculus medinensis* (dracunculiasis), *Diphyllobothrium latum* (diphyllobothriasis), *Gnathostoma spinigerum* (gnathostomiasis), and *Spirometra* species (sparganosis). Copepods have been associated with a single case of a perirectal abscess but generally are not considered a primary cause of human infection.

Epidemiology

Copepods have a worldwide distribution and serve as intermediate hosts for helminthic diseases in the United States, Canada, Europe, and the tropics. Human infection with these helminthic parasites results from ingesting water contaminated with copepods or from eating the raw or insufficiently cooked flesh of infected fish. Pseudooutbreaks of copepods present in human stool specimens submitted for ova and parasite examination have been reported from New York. As many as 40% of concentrated stools submitted for ova and parasite examination were found to contain copepods, presumably as a result of contamination of a hospital water supply. The single reported case of apparent human infection with copepods occurred in this hospital.

Clinical Syndromes

The clinical signs and symptoms associated with helminthic infections in which copepods serve as intermediate hosts are described in Chapters 84 and 86. The single case of apparent human infection with copepods occurred in a 22-year-old man with Crohn's disease who had a perirectal abscess. Drainage of the abscess revealed purulent material that on microscopic examination contained numerous copepods surrounded by leukocytes. It was hypothesized that the copepods were introduced into preexisting perirectal lesions during sitz baths, which were prepared with unfiltered tap water and may have contained copepods. Although the copepods contained within the abscess material were viable and may have been successfully feeding on body tissue, it was felt that the copepods were unlikely to have been the primary cause of the abscess.

Laboratory Diagnosis

The laboratory diagnosis of helminthic infections in which copepods serve as intermediate hosts are described in Chapters 84 and 86. In general, infection is demonstrated by detection of the infecting organism by microscopic examination of clinical material.

Treatment, Prevention, and Control

Specific treatment of copepod-associated helminthic infection is covered in Chapters 84 and 86. Prevention of these infections requires attention to standard public health measures, such as the chlorination and filtration of water and thorough cooking of all fish. Infected people must not be allowed to bathe in water used for drinking, and suspected water should be avoided.

DECAPODS

The decapods include the prawns, shrimps, lobsters, crayfish, and crabs. The cephalothorax of these animals is always covered by a carapace. They have three anterior pairs of thoracic appendages that are modified into biramous maxillipeds, and five posterior pairs that are developed into uniramous legs. Crabs and crayfish are medically important as the second intermediate hosts of the lung fluke *P. westermani.* The parasitic, epidemiologic, and clinical aspects of infection with *P. westermani* are described in Chapter 85. Thorough cooking of crabs and crayfish is the most effective means of preventing infection with *P. westermani.*

Arachnida

SPIDERS

Spiders have a number of characteristic features that permit easy identification. Specifically, they possess eight legs, no antennae, a body divided into two regions (cephalothorax and abdomen), and an unsegmented abdomen with posterior spinnerets. All true spiders produce venom and kill their prey by biting; however, few have fangs **(chelicerae)** powerful enough to pierce human skin or venom potent enough to produce more than a transitory local skin irritation. Venomous spiders may be classified as those that cause **systemic arachnidism** and those that cause **necrotic arachnidism.** This classification is based on the type of tissue damage produced.

Systemic arachnidism is primarily caused by tarantulas and black widow spiders. Tarantulas (family Theraphosidae) are large, hairy spiders of the tropics and subtropics. The tarantulas are of little importance because they are not very aggressive and avoid human habitations. Their bite causes intense pain and a phase of agitation, followed by stupor and somnolence. The black widow spider, *Latrodectus mactans,* is widespread through the southern and western United States. Related species of *Latrodectus* are found throughout temperate and tropical regions of all continents, but none is primarily domestic; thus their contact with humans is limited.

Necrotic arachnidism is produced by spiders that belong to the genus *Loxosceles.* The bites of these spiders may produce severe tissue reaction. *Loxosceles reclusa,* the brown recluse spider, is a medically important spider of this genus.

Black Widow Spiders

Physiology and Structure

The female black widow spider *(L. mactans)* is easily recognized by the presence of a globose, shiny, black abdomen bearing the characteristic orange or reddish hourglass marking on the ventral surface (Figure 87–2). Females vary from 5 to 13.5 mm in body length, but the males are much smaller.

The venom of the black widow spider is a potent peripheral neurotoxin, which is delivered by a pair of jawlike structures, or chelicerae. Only the female *Latrodectus* spider is dangerous to humans; the small, feeble male delivers an ineffective bite.

Epidemiology

These spiders frequent wood and brush piles, old wooden buildings, cellars, hollow logs, and privies. Given these locations, the bite is often located on the genitalia, buttocks, or extremities. Black widow spiders are common to the southern United States but are found throughout the temperate and tropical regions of both the New and Old World.

Clinical Syndromes

As is true with most cases of envenomation, the clinical picture depends on factors such as the amount of the venom injected, the location of the bite, and the age,

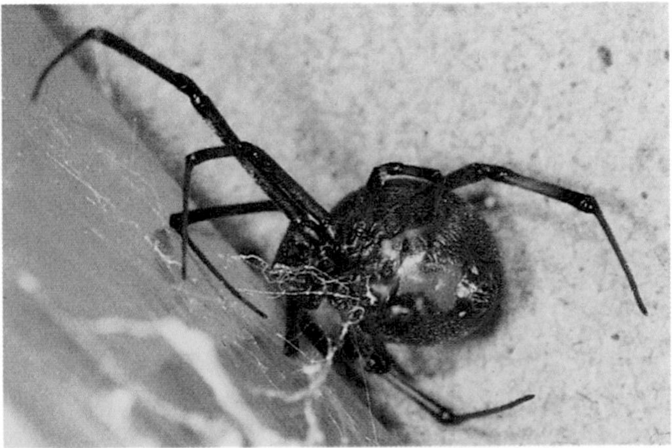

FIGURE 87–2. Female black widow spider *(L. mactans).* (From Peters W: *A colour atlas of arthropods in clinical medicine,* London, 1992, Wolfe.)

weight, and sensitivity of the patient. Shortly after the bite, there is a sharp pain but little or no immediate swelling. Local redness, swelling, and burning follow the pain. Systemic signs and symptoms generally occur within an hour of the bite and include muscular cramps, chest pains, nausea, vomiting, diaphoresis, intestinal spasms, and visual difficulties. Abdominal tetanic cramps producing a "boardlike" abdomen are highly characteristic and may mimic an acute surgical abdomen. The acute symptoms usually subside within 48 hours; however, in severe cases, paralysis and coma may precede cardiac or respiratory failure. Mortality from the bite of the black widow spider is estimated at 4% to 5%.

Treatment, Prevention, and Control

Healthy adults usually recover, but small children or weakened people suffer considerably from these bites and may die without treatment. Muscle spasms may be severe and may require the intravenous administration of calcium gluconate or other muscle relaxant agents. A specific antivenin is available and remains the treatment of choice. It is valuable if given shortly after the bite. Because it is prepared from the serum of hyperimmunized horses, patients must be tested for sensitivity to horse serum before administration. Hospitalization is advisable for the care of people with known or suspected bites.

Good housekeeping can be the simplest and most effective control for spiders in homes. This includes dusting webs and carefully removing debris from around homes and adjacent sheds. Children should be discouraged from playing on woodpiles and in woodsheds.

Brown Recluse Spiders

Physiology and Structure

Spiders producing necrotic arachnidism belong to the genus *Loxosceles.* These spiders are yellow to brown and are of medium size (5- to 10-mm long) with relatively long legs (Figure 87–3). They commonly display two distinguishing characteristics: a dark fiddle- or violin-shaped marking on the dorsal side of the cephalothorax, and six eyes arranged in three pairs that form a semicircle. The venom injected by the female or male spider is a necrotoxin that causes necrotic lesions with deep tissue damage; it may also have hemolytic properties.

Epidemiology

Four species of the genus *Loxosceles* are found in the Americas. *L. reclusa* is found in the south and central United States, *Loxosceles arizonica* is found in the western states, and *Loxosceles laeta* is found in South America. *L. reclusa* is found outdoors in woodpiles and debris in warmer climates and in basements or storage areas in cooler regions. *L. laeta* is found in closets and corners of rooms. Humans are bitten only when the spider is threatened or disturbed.

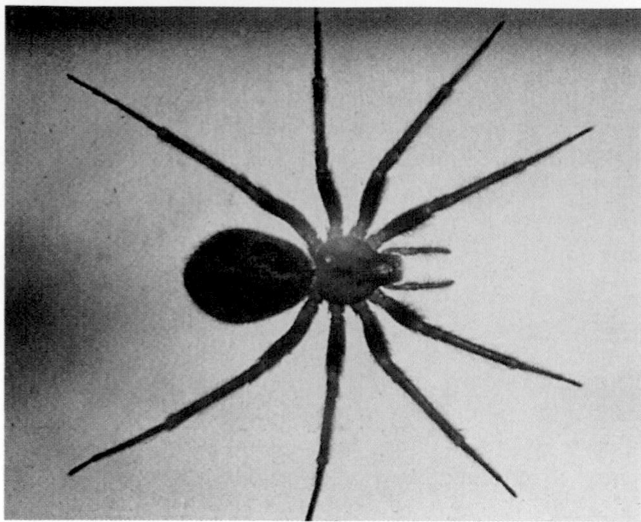

FIGURE 87–3. Female brown recluse spider *(L. laeta).* (Courtesy Professor H Schenone; from Peters W: *A colour atlas of arthropods in clinical medicine,* London, 1992, Wolfe.)

Clinical Syndromes

Initially, the bite of *Loxosceles* species tends to be painless; however, several hours later, itching, swelling, and soreness may develop in the area of the bite. Frequently, a vesicle or bleb may form at the site. General systemic symptoms are unusual but when present may include chills, headache, and nausea. Within 3 to 4 days the bleb sloughs and may be followed by ulceration and radiating necrosis, which does not heal but continues to spread for weeks or months.

Intravascular coagulation and hemolysis may occur and be accompanied by hemoglobinuria and cardiac and renal failure. This hemolytic syndrome may be life threatening and occurs more commonly after the bite of *L. laeta.* In South America, this syndrome is known as **visceral loxoscelism.**

Diagnosis

The discrimination of a species of spider is not possible from the appearance of the lesion alone; however, a working diagnosis is commonly based on the appearance of bleb formation around puncture marks and the nature of the developing lesion. The spider may be identified easily by the characteristic features previously described. An enzyme-linked immunosorbent assay has been developed to confirm the diagnosis of **brown recluse spider** bite but is not widely available.

Treatment, Prevention, and Control

The treatment of brown recluse spider bites is variable and based on the severity of the necrotic reaction. Most bites in the United States are inconsequential and require no specific therapy. Cleansing the bite wound and providing tetanus prophylaxis and antibiotics to prevent secondary infection may all be indicated. Healing is generally uncomplicated, and débridement or excision should not be performed for 3 to 6 weeks to allow natural healing to commence. Excision and skin grafting may be necessary for bites that have not healed in 6 to 8 weeks. Systemic therapy with corticosteroids may be useful in treating the hemolytic syndrome but are of little proven value in preventing or treating cutaneous necrosis. Although not available in the United States, an antivenin is used in South America for the treatment of visceral loxoscelism.

Preventive measures are similar to those recommended for black widow spiders. *Loxosceles* (and other) spiders may be controlled in dwellings with insecticide compounds.

SCORPIONS

Physiology and Structure

The typical scorpion is elongated, with conspicuous, pincherlike claws, or **pedipalps,** at the anterior end of the body; four pairs of walking legs; and a distinctly regimented abdomen that tapers to a curved, hollow, needlelike stinger (Figure 87–4). When the scorpion is disturbed, it uses the stinger for defense. Both male and female scorpions can sting. Venom is injected through the stinger from two venom glands in the abdomen. Most scorpions are unable to penetrate human skin or inject enough venom to cause real damage; however, a few species are capable of inflicting painful wounds that may cause death.

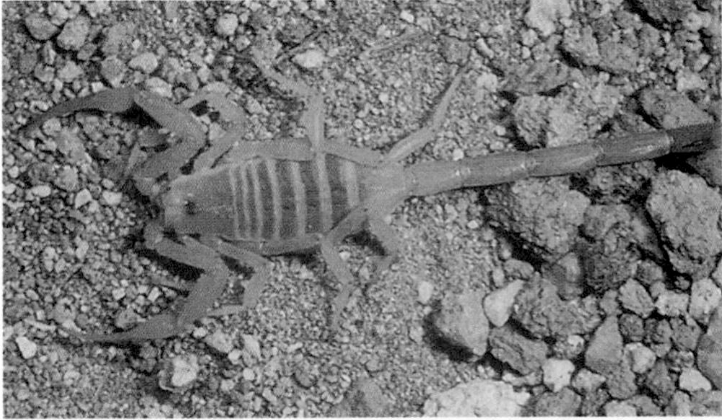

FIGURE 87–4. Scorpion (*Centruroides* species). (Courtesy Dr JC Cokendolpher; from Peters W: *A colour atlas of arthropods in clinical medicine*, London, 1992, Wolfe.)

Epidemiology

Scorpions considered dangerous may be found in the southwestern United States, Mexico, and Venezuela. This includes several species of the genus *Centruroides*, which accounts for as many as 1000 deaths annually. Several species of *Tityus*, found in Trinidad, Argentina, Brazil, Guyana, and Venezuela, are also important. Children under the age of 5 years are most likely to be fatally stung by scorpions.

Scorpions are nocturnal and during the day remain concealed under logs, rocks, and other dark, moist places. They invade human habitations at night, where they may hide in shoes, towels, clothing, and closets.

Clinical Syndromes

The effect of a scorpion sting in a patient is highly variable and depends on factors such as the species and age of the scorpion, the kind and amount of venom injected, and the age, size, and sensitivity of the person who was stung. Although the sting of many scorpions is relatively nontoxic and produces only local symptoms, other stings may be quite serious. Scorpions produce two types of venom: a neurotoxin and hemorrhagic or hemolytic toxin. The hemolytic toxin is responsible for local reactions at the site of the sting, including radiating, burning pain; swelling; discoloration; and necrosis. The neurotoxin produces minimal local reaction but rather severe systemic effects, including chills, diaphoresis, excessive salivation, difficulty speaking and swallowing, muscle spasm, tachycardia, and generalized seizures. In severe cases, death may result from pulmonary edema and respiratory paralysis.

Diagnosis

Local or systemic signs and symptoms coupled with physical evidence of a single point of skin penetration are usually sufficient to establish the diagnosis. The patient may have observed the scorpion or brought it in for identification. Although scorpions are relatively easy to identify, it is important to realize that other nonpoisonous arachnids strongly resemble scorpions. An entomologist or parasitologist should be consulted regarding taxonomic questions.

Treatment, Prevention, and Control

The management of scorpion stings varies. In the absence of systemic symptoms, palliative treatment may be all that is necessary. Pain may be relieved by analgesics or local injection of xylocaine; however, opiates appear to increase toxicity. Local cryotherapy may reduce swelling and retard the systemic absorption of the toxin. Hot packs produce vasodilatation and may accelerate toxin distribution systemically and are therefore contraindicated. Antivenin is available and is effective if administered soon after the sting. Very young children with systemic symptoms should be treated as medical emergencies. Systemic symptoms and shock should be treated supportively.

Preventive measures include the use of chemical pesticides to reduce scorpion populations. Removal of debris around dwellings can reduce hiding and breeding places.

MITES

Mites are small, eight-legged arthropods characterized by a saclike body and no antennae. A large number of mite species are free-living or are normally associated with other vertebrates (e.g., birds, rodents) and may cause dermatitis in humans on rare occasions. The number of mites that are considered true human parasites or present real medical problems is quite small and include the human itch mite *(Sarcoptes scabiei)*, the human follicle mite *(Demodex folliculorum)*, and the chigger mite. Mites affect humans in three ways: (1) by causing dermatitis, (2) by serving as vectors of infectious diseases, and (3) by acting as a source of allergens.

Itch Mites

Physiology and Structure

The itch mite *(S. scabiei)* causes an infectious skin disease variably known as **scabies,** mange, or the itch. The adult mites average 300 to 400 mm in length with an oval, saclike body in which the first and second pairs of legs are widely separated from the third and fourth pairs (Figure 87–5). The body has dorsal transverse parallel ridges, spines, and hairs. The ova measure 100 to 150 mm.

Adult mites enter the skin, creating serpiginous burrows in the upper layers of the epidermis. The female mite lays her eggs in the skin burrows, and the larval and nymph stages that develop also burrow in the skin. The female mites live and deposit eggs and feces in epidermal burrows for up to 2 months. Characteristically, the preferred sites of infestation are the interdigital and popliteal folds, the wrist and inguinal regions, and the inframammary folds. The presence of the mites and their secretions cause intense itching of the involved areas. The mite is an obligate parasite and can perpetuate itself in a single host indefinitely.

Epidemiology

Scabies is cosmopolitan in distribution, with an estimated global prevalence of approximately 300 million cases. The mite is an obligate parasite of domestic animals and humans; however, it may survive for hours to days away from the host, thus facilitating its spread. Transmission is accomplished by direct contact or by contact with contaminated objects such as clothing. Sexual transmission has been well documented. Scratching and manual transfer of the mite by the affected person accomplishes spread of the infection to other areas of the body. Scabies may occur in epidemic fashion among people in crowded conditions, such as daycare centers, nursing homes, military camps, and prisons.

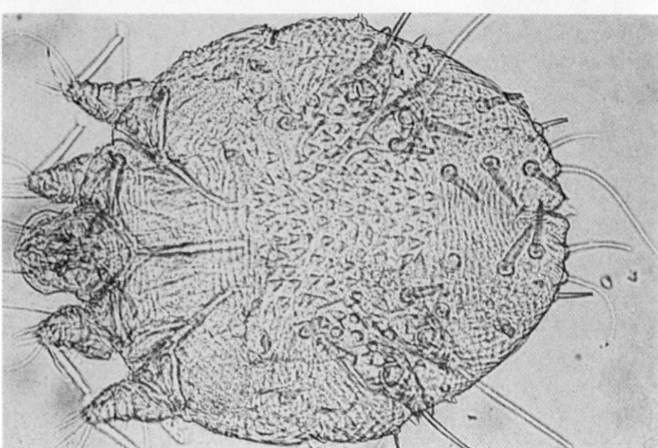

FIGURE 87–5. Scabies mite (*Sarcoptes* species). (From Peters W: *A colour atlas of arthropods in clinical medicine,* London, 1992, Wolfe.)

Clinical Syndromes

The outstanding clinical diagnostic symptom is intense itching, usually in the interdigital folds and sides of the fingers, buttocks, external genitalia, wrists, and elbows. The uncomplicated lesions appear as short, slightly raised cutaneous burrows. At the end of the burrow, there is often a vesicle containing the female mite. The intense pruritus usually leads to excoriation of the skin secondary to scratching, which in turn produces crusts and secondary bacterial infection. Patients experience their first symptoms within weeks to months after exposure; however, the incubation period may be as little as 1 to 4 days in persons sensitized by prior exposure. Host hypersensitivity (delayed or type IV) probably plays an important role in determining the variable clinical manifestations of scabies.

Some immunodeficient people may develop a variant of scabies, so-called **Norwegian scabies,** characterized by generalized dermatitis with extensive scaling and crusting and the presence of thousands of mites in the epidermis. This disease is highly contagious and suggests that host immunity also plays a role in suppressing *S. scabiei.*

Diagnosis

The clinical diagnosis of scabies is based on the characteristic lesions and their distribution. The definitive diagnosis of scabies depends on the demonstration of the mite in skin scrapings. Because the adult mite is most frequently found in the terminal portions of a fresh burrow, it is best to make scrapings in these areas. The scrapings are placed on a clean microscopic slide, cleared by the addition of 1 or 2 drops of a 20% solution of potassium hydroxide, covered with a coverslip, and examined under a low-power microscope. With experience, one may recognize the mite and ova. Skin biopsy may also reveal the mites and ova in tissue sections.

Treatment, Prevention, and Control

The standard, and very effective, treatment for scabies is 1% gamma benzene hexachloride (lindane) in a lotion base. One or two applications (head to toe) at weekly intervals is effective against scabies. Lindane is absorbed through the skin, and repeated applications may be toxic. For this reason, it is not advisable to use it in treating infants, small children, or pregnant or lactating women.

Recently, a 5% permethrin cream (Elimite) replaced lindane lotions as the treatment of choice for scabies. Clinical trials have shown permethrin to be more effective and less toxic than lindane. Other precautions used to treat scabies include crotamiton, sulfur (6%) preparations, benzyl benzoate, and tetraethylthiuram monosulfide. The last two preparations are not available in the United States.

Primary prevention of scabies is best achieved with good hygiene habits, personal cleanliness, and routine washing of clothing and bed linens. Secondary prevention includes the identification and treatment of infected people and possibly their household and sexual contacts. In an epidemic situation, simultaneous treatment of all affected people and their contacts may be necessary. This is followed by thorough cleansing of the environment (e.g., boiling clothing and linens) and ongoing surveillance to prevent reoccurrence.

Human Follicle Mites

Physiology and Structure

The human follicle mites include two species of the genus *Demodex*, *Demodex folliculorum* and *Demodex brevis*. These mites are minute (0.1- to 0.4-mm) organisms with a wormlike body, four pairs of stubby legs, and an annulate abdomen. *D. folliculorum* parasitizes the hair follicles of the face of most adult humans, whereas *D. brevis* is found in the sebaceous glands of the head and trunk.

Epidemiology

Organisms of the *Demodex* genus are obligate parasites of the human integument and are cosmopolitan in their distribution. Infestations are uncommon in young children and increase at the time of puberty. It is estimated that 50% to 100% of adults are infested with these mites.

Clinical Syndromes

The role of *Demodex* species in human disease is uncertain. They have been associated with acne, blackheads, blepharitis, abnormalities of the scalp, and truncal rashes. More recently, extensive papular folliculitis resulting from *Demodex* infestation has been described in people with acquired immuno deficiency syndrome. Factors such as poor personal hygiene, increased sebum production, mite hypersensitivity, and immunosuppression may increase host susceptibility and enhance the clinical presentation of *Demodex* infestation. Most people infested with these mites remain asymptomatic.

Diagnosis

Mites may be demonstrated microscopically in material expressed from an infested follicle. They may be seen as incidental findings in histologic sections of facial skin.

Treatment

Effective treatment consists of a single application of 1% gamma benzene hexachloride.

Chigger Mites

Physiology and Structure

Chiggers are the larvae of mites of the family Trombiculidae. The adult trombiculid mites infest grass and bushes, and their larvae (i.e., chiggers) attack humans and other vertebrates, producing severe dermatitis. The larvae have three pairs of legs and are covered with characteristic branched, featherlike hairs.

The larvae appear as minute, barely visible, reddish dots attached to the skin where they use their hooked mouthparts to ingest tissue fluids. Chiggers typically attach to the skin areas where clothing is tight or restricted, such as the wrists, ankles, armpits, groin, and waistline. After feeding, the engorged larvae fall to the ground, where they molt and undergo development into nymphs and adults.

Epidemiology

Chiggers that are important in North America include the larvae of *Eutrombicula alfreddugesi* and *Eutrombicula splendens*. In Europe, the important species is the harvest mite, *Trombicula autumnalis*. Chiggers are a particular problem for outdoor enthusiasts such as campers and picnickers. In Europe and the Americas, they are associated with intensely pruritic lesions; however, in Asia, Australia, and the western Pacific Rim, they serve as vectors of the rickettsial disease scrub typhus or tsutsugamushi fever *(Rickettsia tsutsugamushi)* (see Table 87–2).

Clinical Syndromes

Saliva injected into the skin at the time of mite attachment produces an intense pruritus and dermatitis. The skin lesions appear as small erythematous marks that progress to papules and may persist for weeks. Mite larvae may be visible in the center of the reddened, swollen area. The irritation may be so severe that it causes fever and sleep disruption. Secondary bacterial infection of the excoriated lesions may occur.

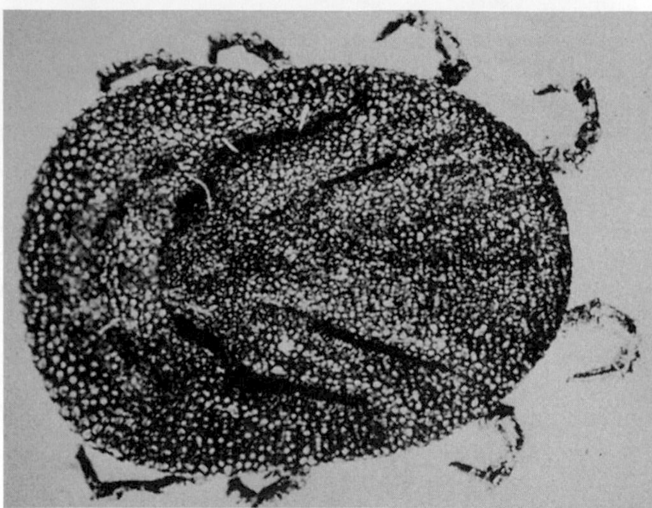

FIGURE 87–6. Soft tick (*Ornithodoros* species). (From Strickland GT: *Hunter's tropical medicine,* ed 7, Philadelphia, 1991, WB Saunders.)

Treatment, Prevention, and Control

Treatment for dermatitis caused by chiggers is largely symptomatic and consists of antipruritics, antihistamines, and steroids. The use of insect repellents such as N,N9-diethyl-m-toluamide (DEET) may be of some help in prevention for persons going into chigger-infested areas.

TICKS

Physiology and Structure

Ticks are bloodsucking ectoparasites of a number of vertebrates, including humans. Ticks are opportunistic rather than host specific and tend to suck blood from a number of large and small animals. Ticks have a four-stage life cycle that includes the egg, larva, nymph, and adult. Although the larva, nymph, and adults are all bloodsuckers, it is the adult tick that usually bites humans.

Ticks comprise two large families, the Ixodidae, or hard ticks, and the Argasidae, or soft ticks. Soft ticks have a leathery body that lacks a hard dorsal plate or scutum, and the mouthparts are located ventrally and are not visible from above (Figure 87–6). Hard ticks have a hard dorsal plate, and the mouthparts are clearly visible from above (Figure 87–7). Both hard and soft ticks serve as ectoparasites of humans. Soft ticks differ from hard ticks primarily in their feeding behavior. Soft ticks complete engorgement in a matter of minutes or at most a few hours; hard ticks feed slowly, taking 7 to 9 days to become engorged.

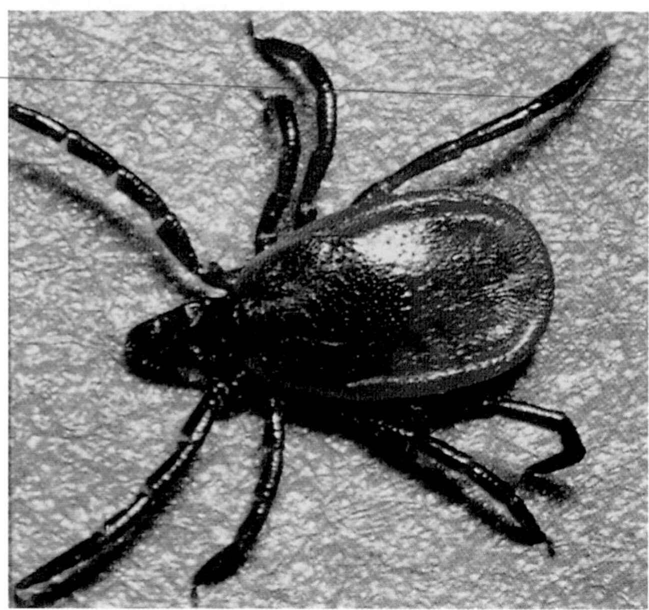

FIGURE 87–7. Hard Tick *(I. dammini)*. (Courtesy Professor A Spielman; from Peters W: *A colour atlas of arthropods in clinical medicine,* London, 1992, Wolfe.)

Epidemiology

Ticks are found in wooded and rural areas worldwide. In North America, the important species of hard ticks include *Dermacentor variabilis* (the American dog tick), *Dermacentor andersoni* (the Rocky Mountain wood tick), *Amblyomma americanum* (the lone star tick), *Rhipicephalus sanguineus* (the brown dog tick), and *Ixodes dammini* (the deer tick). These ticks are found variably throughout the United States and are important vectors of several infectious diseases, including Rocky Mountain spotted fever, tularemia, and Q fever (*Dermacentor* species); Lyme disease and babesiosis (*Ixodes* species); and ehrlichiosis (*D. variabilis* and *A. americanum*). Soft ticks of the genus *Ornithodoros* transmit relapsing fever spirochetes (*Borrelia* species) in limited areas in the Western United States (see Table 87–2). In general, people at risk for tick exposure are involved in outdoor activities in wooded areas. Tick exposure may also occur during stays in rural cabins inhabited by small rodents, which commonly serve as hosts for ticks and other ectoparasites.

Clinical Syndromes

Tick bites are generally of minor consequence and are limited to small erythematous papules. More serious consequences of tick bite include the development of a type of paralysis resulting from substances released by ticks during feeding, and transmission of a number of rickettsial, bacterial, viral, spirochetal, and protozoan diseases of humans and other animals.

Ticks may attach at any point on the body but typically favor the scalp hairline, ears, axillae, and groin. The initial bite is usually painless, and the presence of the tick may not be detected for several hours after contact. After the tick has dropped off or has been removed manually, the area may become reddened, painful, and pruritic. The wound may become secondarily infected and necrotic, particularly if the mouthparts remain attached after manual removal.

Three species of tick, *D. andersoni, D. variabilis,* and *A. americanum,* have all been reported to cause **tick paralysis.** This is characterized by an ascending flaccid paralysis, fever, and general intoxication, which may lead to respiratory compromise and death. The paralysis is caused by toxic substances released in the saliva of the tick and may be reversed by tick removal. Tick paralysis is observed more commonly in young children and when tick attachment is in opposition to the central nervous system (e.g., scalp, head, neck).

Ticks are also involved in the transmission of infections such as Lyme disease, Rocky Mountain spotted fever, ehrlichiosis, Colorado tick fever, relapsing fever, tularemia, Q fever, and babesiosis (see Table 87–2). Refer to the appropriate sections of this book for discussion of the clinical and microbiologic aspects of these infections.

Diagnosis

The diagnoses of tick bites and tick-borne diseases usually rest on the finding of a tick or a history of exposure to tick-infested areas. The identification of an organism as an adult tick is usually straightforward and based on the observations of an organism that is dorsoventrally flattened and possesses four pairs of legs and no visible segmentation (Figures 87–6 and 87–7). An entomologist or parasitologist should be consulted if further identification is desired. The diagnosis of specific tick-borne infectious diseases is covered in the respective sections of this book.

Treatment, Prevention, and Control

Early removal of attached ticks is of primary importance and may be accomplished by steady traction on the tick body, grasped with forceps as close to the skin as possible. Care should be taken to avoid twisting or crushing the tick, which may leave the mouthparts attached to the skin or inject potentially infectious material into the wound. Steady traction is superior to noxious stimuli or occlusive techniques for the removal of ticks. After removal, the wound should be cleansed and observed for secondary infection. Because ticks may harbor highly infectious agents, the clinician should use appropriate infection-control precautions (e.g., use of gloves, hand washing, proper disposal of ticks and contaminated material) during tick removal.

Preventive measures used in tick-infested areas include the wearing of protective clothing that fits snugly about the ankles, wrists, waist, and neck, so that ticks cannot gain access to the skin. Insect repellents such as DEET are generally effective. People and pets should be inspected for ticks after visits to tick-infested areas.

Insecta

The insects, or **hexapods,** constitute the largest and most important of all the classes of arthropods, accounting for approximately 70% of all known species of animals. Insects include animals such as mosquitoes, flies, fleas, lice, roaches, bees, wasps, beetles, and moths to name just a few. The insect body is divided into three parts—head, thorax, and abdomen—and is equipped with one pair of antennae, three pairs of appendages, and one or two pairs of wings or no wings at all. The medical significance of any insect is related to its way of life, particularly its mouthparts and feeding habits. Insects may serve as vectors for a number of bacterial, viral, protozoan, and metazoan pathogens. Certain insects may serve merely as mechanical vectors for the transmission of pathogens, whereas in other insects the pathogens undergo multiplication or cyclic development within the insect host. The methods by which the insects transmit pathogens vary and are discussed here. Insects can also be pathogens themselves by causing mechanical injury through bites, chemical injury through the injection of toxins, and allergic reactions to materials transmitted by bites or stings. There are more than 30 orders of insects, but only those of major medical importance are discussed in this section.

BLOODSUCKING DIPTERA

Diptera is the large order of flying insects. All dipterans have a single pair of functional membranous wings and various modifications of the mouthparts, which have been adapted for piercing the skin and sucking blood or tissue juices. Their most important feature is their role as mechanical or biologic vectors of a number of infectious diseases, including leishmaniasis, trypanosomiasis, malaria, filariasis, onchocerciasis, tularemia, bartonellosis, and the viral encephalitides (see Table 87–2). The bloodsucking flies include mosquitoes, sandflies, and blackflies, all of which are capable of transmitting diseases to humans. Other dipterans such as horseflies and stable flies are capable of inflicting painful bites but are not known to transmit human pathogens. Although the common housefly does not bite, it certainly is capable of mechanical transmission of a number of viral, bacterial, and protozoan infections to human hosts. The infectious diseases transmitted by bloodsucking flies are well covered in other chapters of this book. The following section deals only with injury resulting from the bite of these insects and the effects of salivary substances introduced into the human skin and tissues.

Mosquitoes

Physiology and Structure

Adult mosquitoes are small and have delicate legs, one pair of wings, long antennae, and greatly elongated mouthparts adapted for piercing and sucking. The two major families of mosquitoes (Culicidae), the Anophelinae and the Culicinae, share a number of similarities in their life cycles and development. They lay eggs on or near water, are good fliers, and feed on nectar and sugars. The females of most species also feed on blood, which they require for each clutch of 100 to 200 eggs. Females may take a blood meal every 2 to 4 days. In the act of feeding the female mosquito injects saliva, which produces mechanical damage to the host but also may transmit disease and produce immediate and delayed immune reactions.

Epidemiology

Within the family Anophelinae, the genus *Anopheles* contains the species responsible for the transmission of human malaria. In the tropics, these mosquitoes breed continually in relation to rainfall. These species vary in their capacity for the transmission of malaria, and within each geographic area the number of species that serves as malaria vectors is small. *A. gambiae* is an important vector of malaria in sub-Saharan Africa.

Mosquitoes from *Aedes*, the largest genus of the subfamily Culicinae, are found in all habitats ranging from the tropics to the Arctic. This species may develop overwhelming populations in marsh or tundra and pasture or floodwater and have a severe impact on wildlife, livestock, and humans. *Aedes aegypti*, the yellow fever mosquito, usually breeds in man-made containers (flower pots, gutters, cans) and is the primary vector of yellow fever and dengue in urban environments throughout the world.

Clinical Syndromes

Mechanical damage induced by the feeding mosquito is usually minor but may be accompanied by mild pain and irritation. The bite is usually followed within a few minutes by a small, flat wheal surrounded by a red flare. The delayed reaction consists of itching, swelling, and reddening of the wound region. Secondary infection may follow as a result of scratching.

Treatment, Prevention, and Control

Medical attention is usually not sought for a bite unless secondary infection occurs. Local anesthetics or antihistamines may be useful in treating reactions to mosquito bites.

Preventive measures in mosquito-infested areas include the use of window screens, netting, and protective clothing. Insect repellents such as DEET are generally effective. Mosquito-control measures that involve the use of insecticides have been effective in some areas.

Gnats and Biting Midges

Physiology and Structure

Ceratopogonids represent an assortment of tiny flies with names such as gnats, midges, and punkies. The majority of the flies that attack humans belong to the genus *Culicoides;* they are minute (0.5- to 4.0-mm long) and slender enough to pass through the fine mesh of ordinary window screens. The females suck blood and typically feed at dusk, when they may attack in large numbers.

Epidemiology

Biting midges may be important pests in beach and resort areas near salt marshes. Those of the genus *Culicoides* are the main vectors of filariasis in Africa and the New World tropics.

Clinical Syndromes

The mouthparts of biting midges are lancetlike and produce a painful bite. Bites may produce local lesions lasting hours or days.

Treatment, Prevention, and Control

Local treatment is palliative with lotions, anesthetics, and antiseptic measures. The treatment of breeding sites with pesticides and repellents may be useful against some of the common species of these pests.

Sandflies

Physiology and Structure

Sandflies, or moth flies, belong to a single subfamily of the Psychodidae, the Phlebotominae. They are small (1- to 3-mm), delicate, hairy, weak-flying insects that suck the blood of humans, dogs, and rodents. They transmit a number of infections, including leishmaniasis (see Table 87–2). Female flies become infected when they feed on infected people.

Epidemiology

Phlebotomine larvae develop in nonaquatic habitats such as moist soil, stone walls, and rubbish heaps. In many areas, sandflies cause problems as pests. They also serve as vectors of infectious diseases such as leishmaniasis in the Mediterranean, the Middle East, Asia, India, and Latin America.

Clinical Syndromes

The bite may be painful and pruritic around the local lesion. Sensitized people may have allergic reactions. Sandfly fever is characterized by severe frontal headaches, malaise, retroorbital pain, anorexia, and nausea.

Treatment, Prevention, and Control

Sandflies are very sensitive to insecticides, which should be applied to breeding sites and window screens. Various insect repellents may also be useful.

Blackflies

Physiology and Structure

Members of the family Simuliidae are commonly called **blackflies** or **buffalo gnats.** They are 1- to 5-mm long, are hump-backed, and have mouthparts consisting of six "blades" that are capable of tearing skin (Figure 87–8). Blackflies are bloodsucking insects and breed in fast-flowing streams and rivers. They are of major importance as vectors of onchocerciasis (see Table 87–2).

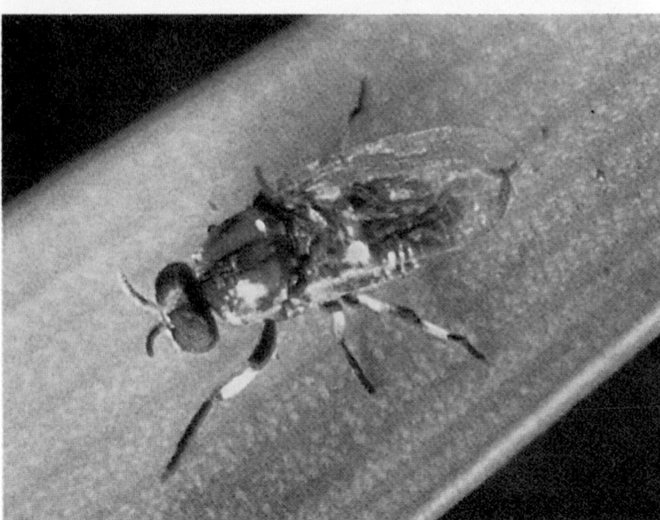

FIGURE 87–8. Blackfly (*Simulium* species), the vector of onchocerciasis. (Courtesy Dr S Meredith; from Peters W: *A colour atlas of arthropods in clinical medicine,* London, 1992, Wolfe.)

Epidemiology

Blackflies are common in Africa and South America, where they serve as vectors of onchocerciasis. In North America, they are common around the lake regions of Canada and the northern United States. They are pests to hunters and fisherman in these areas. In large numbers they may cause significant blood loss and pose a major threat to wild and domestic animals.

Clinical Syndromes

A variety of responses have been observed in humans after the bite of blackflies. The bite of the female can tear the skin surface and induce bleeding that continues for some time after the fly has departed. There is usually a distinct hemorrhagic spot at the site of the bite. Multiple bites may result in considerable blood loss. The bite is painful and is accompanied by local inflammation, itching, and swelling.

The local reaction may also be accompanied by a systemic response that varies according to the number of bites and the sensitivity of the person. This syndrome is known as blackfly fever and is marked by headache, fever, and adenitis. It usually subsides within 48 hours and is considered a hypersensitivity reaction to the salivary secretions of the fly.

In addition to local and systemic responses to blackfly bites, a hemorrhagic syndrome has been described after bites of blackflies in certain areas of Brazil. This syndrome resembles thrombocytopenic purpura and is characterized by local and disseminated cutaneous hemorrhages associated with mucosal bleeding. It is thought that this hemorrhagic syndrome may be produced by a hypersensitivity phenomenon or response to a toxin caused by multiple blackfly bites.

Diagnosis

The blackfly bite is marked characteristically by a point of dried blood and subcutaneous hemorrhage at the wound site. In people with the hemorrhagic syndrome, platelet counts are reduced; there is a prolonged bleeding time and poor clot retraction in approximately half of these patients.

Treatment, Prevention, and Control

Treatment includes the usual palliative measures (e.g., anesthetics, antihistamines, lotions) to relieve local pruritus and swelling. Patients with the hemorrhagic syndrome have shown marked improvement with corticosteroid therapy.

Preventive measures include protective clothing. In general, insect repellents are ineffective against blackflies. Some control is achieved by pouring insecticides into rivers and streams.

HORSEFLIES AND DEER FLIES

The family Tabanidae consists of species that attack animals, including horseflies, deer flies, gadflies, and mango flies. They are large, ranging in length from 7 to 30 mm. The males feed on plant juices, the females on blood. In the act of biting, the female fly leaves a deep wound, causing blood to flow, which the fly laps up. The fly may serve as a mechanical vector of infectious diseases when the fly's mouthparts become contaminated on one host and transfer organisms to the next. These flies are not considered important vectors of infectious disease in humans.

MUSCOID FLIES

Physiology and Structure

The muscoid flies include the important insects, the housefly, *Musca domestica;* the stable fly, *Stomoxys calcitrans;* and the **tsetse flies** of the genus *Glossina.* The stable fly, often mistaken for the housefly, is a true bloodsucker capable of serving as a short-term mechanical vector of a number of bacterial, viral, and protozoal infections. The tsetse fly (Figure 87–9) is also a biting fly and serves as the biologic vector and intermediate host for the agents of African trypanosomiasis, *Trypanosoma brucei rhodesiense,* and *Trypanosoma brucei gambiense.* The common housefly represents a host of genera that are nonpiercing or contaminating flies. Because of their living and feeding habits, they mechanically transmit diverse agents to humans.

Epidemiology

The tsetse fly is found in the eastern and central regions of Africa, where it is of major medical and veterinary importance as the intermediate host and biologic vector of a number of trypanosomes that infect humans and animals. The housefly and stable fly are cosmopolitan in distribution and serve as indicators of poor sanitation. The housefly, *M. domestica,* lays eggs on any matter that will serve as food for developing fly larvae, or maggots (feces, garbage, decaying plant matter). Stable flies commonly lay eggs in moist, decaying vegetable matter, such as grass clippings or compost heaps found in suburban communities.

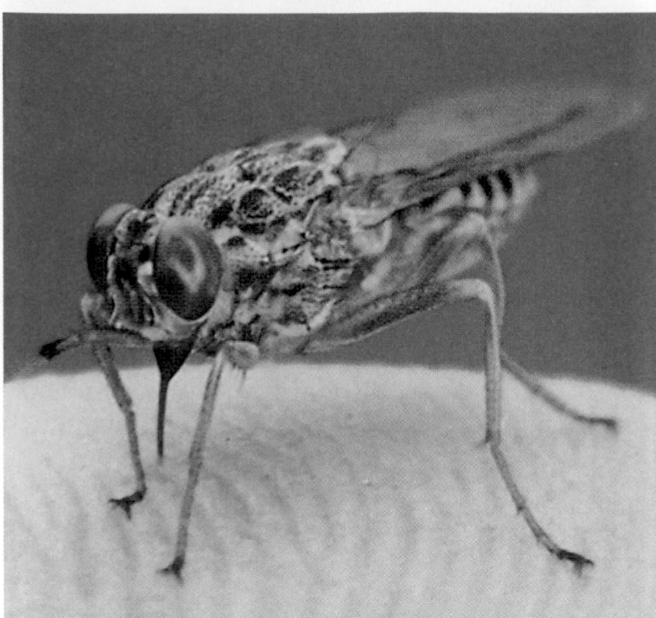

FIGURE 87–9. Tsetse fly, the vector of African trypanosomiasis. (Courtesy Wellcome Foundation, Ltd, Berkhamsted; from Peters W: *A colour atlas of arthropods in clinical medicine,* London, 1992, Wolfe.)

Prevention and Control

Control of tsetse fly populations has been problematic because of their widespread distribution in primarily rural and undeveloped areas. Insect repellents and insecticides may be effective against adult flies. Improved sanitation is important in controlling houseflies. Plant refuse should be protected from rain or destroyed.

MYIASIS-CAUSING FLIES

Myiasis is the term applied to the disease produced by maggots that live parasitically in human tissues. Clinically, myiasis may be classified according to the body part involved (e.g., nasal, intestinal, or urinary myiasis). The number of myiasis-producing flies and the diversity in lifestyle requirements are enormous. Only the host relations and sites of predilection of some of the more important species are covered in this section.

Specific myiasis refers to myiasis caused by flies that require a host for larval development. One important example is the human botfly, *Dermatobia hominis,* which is found in the humid regions of Mexico and Central and South America. The adult botfly attaches her eggs to the abdomen of bloodsucking flies or mosquitoes, which in turn distribute the eggs while obtaining a blood meal from an animal or human. The larvae enter the skin through the wound created by the biting insect. The larvae develop over 40 to 50 days, during which time a painful lesion known as a warble appears. When the larvae reach maturity, they leave the host to pupate. The resulting lesion may take weeks to months to heal and may become secondarily infected. If the larvae die before leaving the skin, an abscess forms.

Semispecific myiasis is caused by flies that normally lay their eggs on decaying animal or plant matter, but it develops in a host if entry is facilitated by the presence of wounds or sores. Representatives of this group include the green-bottle flies, *Phaenicia;* blue-bottle flies, *Cochliomyia;* and black-bottle flies, *Phormia.* These flies are worldwide in distribution, and their presence is encouraged by poor sanitation. They occasionally lay their eggs on the open sores or wounds of animal and humans. Another group that causes myiasis in humans is the flesh flies, or sarcophagids. These flies have a worldwide distribution and normally breed in decomposing matter. They may deposit their larvae on foods that, if ingested, may serve as a source of infection.

Flies that produce **accidental myiasis** have no requirement for development in a host. Accidental infection may occur when eggs are deposited on oral or genitourinary openings and the resulting larvae gain entry into the intestinal or genitourinary tract. Flies that may produce accidental myiasis include *M. domestica,* the common housefly.

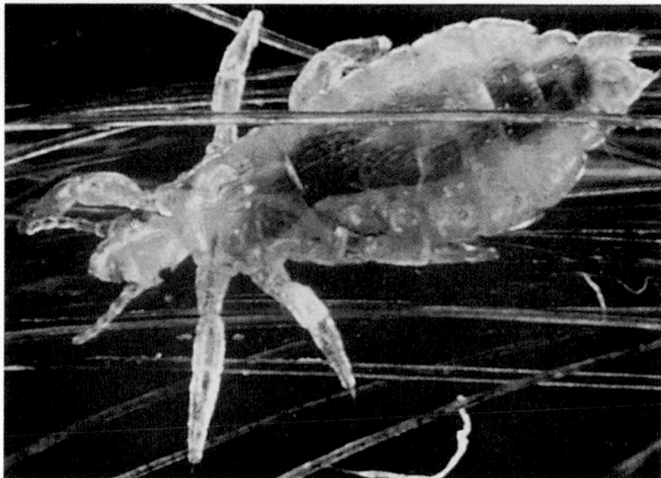

FIGURE 87–10. Body louse *(P. humanus)*. (Courtesy Oxford Scientific Films, Ltd [Dr RJ Warren]; from Peters W: *A colour atlas of arthropods in clinical medicine,* London, 1992, Wolfe.)

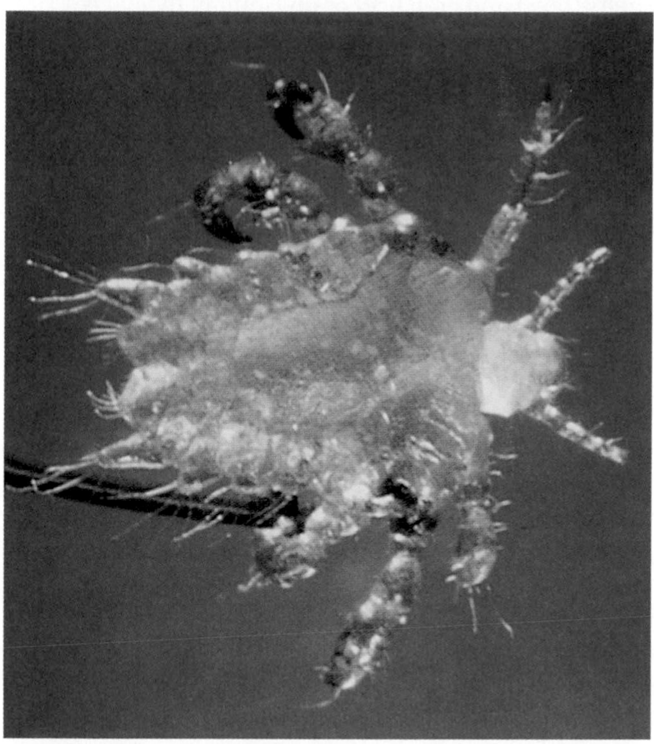

FIGURE 87–11. Crab louse *(P. pubis)*. (Courtesy Dr RV Southcott; from Peters W: *A colour atlas of arthropods in clinical medicine,* London, 1992, Wolfe.)

SUCKING LICE

Physiology and Structure

Although several species of lice *(Anoplura)* infest humans as blood-feeding parasites, only the **body louse** is important in medicine as the vector of the rickettsia of typhus and trench fevers and the vector of the spirochetes of relapsing fever (see Table 87–2). The body louse, *Pediculus humanus,* and the **head louse,** *Pediculus humanus capitis,* are elongated, wingless, flattened insects with three pairs of legs and mouthpieces adapted for piercing flesh and sucking blood (Figure 87–10). The pubic or **crab louse,** *Phthirus pubis,* has a short, crablike abdomen with clawed second and third legs (Figure 87–11).

Epidemiology

Epidemics of head lice are reported frequently in the United States, particularly among school children. The head lice inhabit the hairs of the head and are transmitted by physical contact or sharing of hairbrushes or hats. Crab lice survive on blood meals around the hairs of the pubic and perianal areas of the body. They are transmitted frequently from one person to another by sexual contact and contaminated toilet seats or clothing. Body lice are usually found on clothing. Unlike head or crab lice, they move to the body for feeding and return to the clothing after obtaining a blood meal. All of the lice inject salivary fluids into the body during the ingestion of blood, which causes varying degrees of sensitization in the human host.

Clinical Syndromes

Intense itching is the usual characteristic of infestation by lice **(pediculosis).** The patient may have pruritic, red papules around the ears, face, neck, or shoulders. Secondary infection and regional adenopathy may be present.

Diagnosis

The diagnosis is made by demonstration of the lice or eggs from a patient complaining of pruritus. Frequently, the patient has noticed the insects, and the diagnosis may be made over the telephone. The eggs, or nits, are white, round objects that may be found attached to the hair shafts (head and crab lice) or on clothing (body lice).

Treatment, Prevention, and Control

Gamma benzene hexachloride (lindane) lotion applied to the entire body and left on for 24 hours is an effective treatment for lice. Shaving the hair of affected areas is a desirable adjunct. Adult lice in clothing must be destroyed by the application of lindane or DDT powder or by boiling. Lice may survive in the environment for up to 2 weeks; thus items such as brushes, combs, and bedding must be treated with a pediculicide or by boiling.

The best strategy for primary prevention is education and practice of good hygiene habits. Secondary prevention may be practiced by a policy of routine surveillance (e.g., scalp inspections) in schools, daycare centers, military camps, and other institutions. Repellents may be necessary for people who run a high risk of exposure in crowded conditions.

FLEAS

Physiology and Structure

Fleas *(Siphonaptera)* are small, wingless insects with laterally compressed bodies and long legs adapted for jumping (Figure 87–12). Their mouthparts are adapted for sucking or "siphoning" blood from the host.

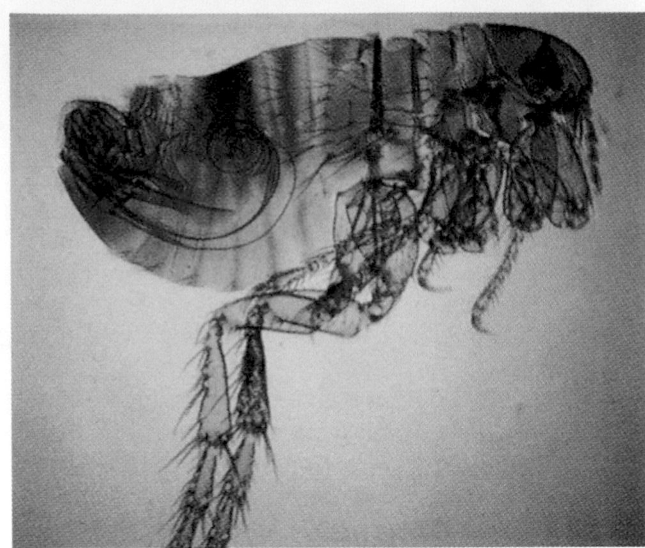

FIGURE 87–12. Flea. (From Peters W: *A colour atlas of arthropods in clinical medicine*, London, 1992, Wolfe.)

Epidemiology

Fleas are cosmopolitan in distribution. Most species are adapted to a particular host; however, they can readily feed on humans, particularly when deprived of their preferred host. Fleas are important as vectors of plague and murine typhus and as intermediate hosts for dog *(Dipylidium caninum)* and rodent (*Hymenolepis* species) tapeworms that occasionally infect humans.

In contrast to the majority of fleas that do not invade the human integument, the **chigoe flea,** *Tunga penetrans,* may cause considerable damage by actively invading the skin. The female chigoe flea burrows into the skin, often under the toenails or between the toes, where she sucks blood and lays her eggs. The chigoe flea is found in tropical and subtropical regions of America, as well as in Africa and the Far East. It is not known to transmit human pathogens.

Clinical Syndromes

As with the bites of other bloodsucking arthropods, flea bites result in pruritic, erythematous lesions of varying severity, which depends on the intensity of the infestation and the sensitivity of the bitten person. The irritation caused by the flea saliva may produce physical findings that vary from small, red welts to a diffuse, red rash. Secondary infection may be a complication.

Cutaneous invasion by the chigoe flea produces an erythematous papule that is painful and pruritic. Infested tissue can become severely inflamed and ulcerated. Secondary infection is common. In severe cases, the infestation may be complicated by tetanus or by gas gangrene, resulting in amputation.

Diagnosis

The diagnosis of flea infestation is inferred in a patient with annoying bites who is also a pet (dog or cat) owner. Examination of the patient and pet usually reveals the

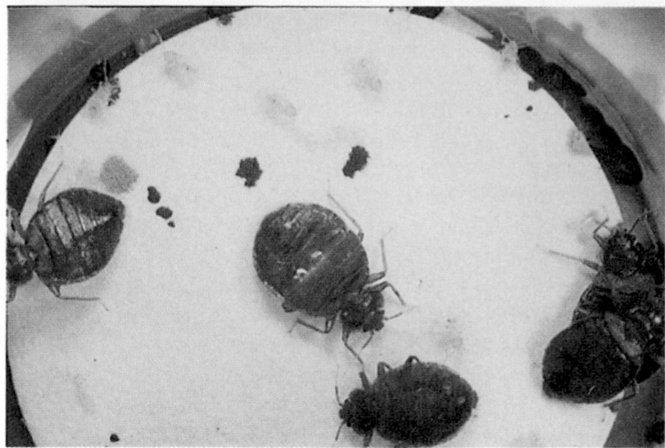

FIGURE 87–13. Bedbug *(C. lectularius).* (From Peters W: *A colour atlas of arthropods in clinical medicine,* London, 1992, Wolfe.)

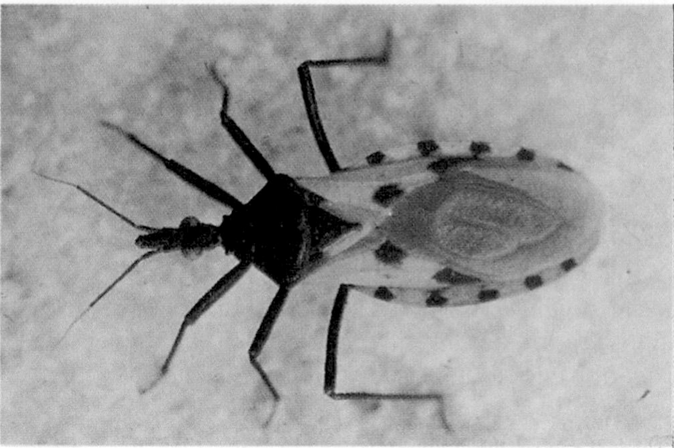

FIGURE 87–14. Triatomid bug. (Courtesy Dr D Minter; from Peters W: *A colour atlas of arthropods in clinical medicine,* London, 1992, Wolfe.

characteristic insect. Diagnosis of tungiasis is made by detecting the dark portion of the chigoe flea's abdomen as it protrudes from the skin surface in the center of an inflamed lesion.

Treatment, Prevention, and Control

Palliative treatment with antipruritics and antihistamines is indicated for most flea bites. Surgical removal of the chigoe flea is indicated.

Commercially available insecticides may control fleas at the source. Topically applied repellents can protect people against fleabites. Flea collars or powders on pets are also effective preventive measures.

BUGS

Physiology and Structure

Bugs refer specifically to two bloodsucking insects: the **bedbug** and the **triatomid bug** (Figures 87–13 and 87–14). Both bugs are characterized by a long proboscis that is folded ventrally under the body when not in use. The bedbug *(Cimex lectularius)* is a reddish-brown insect approximately 4- to 5-mm long. It has short wing pads but cannot fly. The triatomid, or **"kissing" bug,** has yellow or orange markings on the body and an elongated head. Triatomid bugs have wings and are aerial.

Epidemiology

Both bedbugs and triatomid bugs are nocturnal and feed indiscriminately on most mammals. Bedbugs are cosmopolitan in distribution, whereas triatomid bugs are limited to the Americas. Bedbugs hide during the day in cracks and crevices of wooden furniture, under loose wallpaper, in the tufts of mattresses, and in box springs. Triatomid bugs live in the cracks and crevices of walls and in thatched roofs. Bedbugs do not play a role in the transmission of human disease; however, triatomid bugs are important vectors of Chagas' disease (see Table 87–2 and Chapter 83).

Clinical Syndromes

The bites of bedbugs and triatomid bugs produce lesions that range from small, red marks to hemorrhagic bullae. Bedbugs tend to bite in linear fashion on the trunk and arms, whereas triatomid bugs bite with higher frequency on the face. The classic periorbital edema secondary to a triatomid bite is known as **Romaña's sign.** The intensity of reaction to a bite depends on the degree of sensitization of the patient. In addition to causing local lesions, bedbugs may be associated with nervous disorders and sleeplessness in children and adults.

Diagnosis

The pattern and location of bites suggests bedbugs or triatomid bugs. The detection of tiny spots of blood on bedding or the dead insects themselves is often the first sign of bedbug infestation.

Treatment, Prevention, and Control

Topical palliatives are appropriate for the relief of pruritus. Antihistamines may be indicated if dermatitis is severe. Control consists of proper hygiene and the environmental applications of insecticides.

STINGING INSECTS

Physiology and Structure

The order Hymenoptera comprises the bees, wasps, hornets, and ants. The modified ovipositor of the female, the apparatus for egg laying, serves as a stinging organ and is used for defense or to capture prey for food. Members of Hymenoptera are known for their complex social systems, castes, and elaborate hive or nest structures.

Epidemiology

Of the hymenopterans, the bees, or Apidae, live in complex social organizations, such as hives or in less-structured underground nests. Only honeybees and bumblebees are of concern to humans because of their ability to sting. The Vespidae include wasps, hornets, and yellow jackets; all are aggressive insects and a major cause of stings in humans. In the act of stinging, the aroused insect inserts the sheath to open the wound. The thrust of the stylets and injection of venom immediately follow.

One group of ants of concern in the United States is the fire ant, *Solenopsis invicta*. Fire ants are particularly common in the southeastern U.S. states. They are well camouflaged in large, hard-crusted mounds and attack when disturbed. They bite their victim with strong mandibles and then sting repeatedly.

Clinical Syndromes

An estimated 50 to 100 people die each year in the United States from reactions to stings of the hymenopterans. Severe toxic reactions such as fever and muscle cramps can be caused by as few as 10 stings. Allergic reactions are the most serious consequence, but others include pain, edema, pruritus, and a heat sensation at the site of the sting. Anaphylactic shock from bee stings has resulted in death in some instances.

Treatment, Prevention, and Control

No satisfactory treatment has been discovered for stings. If left in the wound, the sting apparatus should be removed immediately. The injection of epinephrine is sometimes necessary to counteract anaphylaxis. (Emergency kits are available by prescription for sensitive people.) For the relief of local discomfort, calamine lotion or a topical corticosteroid cream for more severe local lesions is helpful.

Although there are no effective repellents against these insects, their nests can be destroyed with any of several commercially available insecticidal compounds. General avoidance of areas inhabited by hymenopterans is advised for sensitive people.

CASE STUDY AND QUESTIONS

A 4-year-old child was brought in by her mother with a complaint of itchy hands. The child stayed at a daycare center during the day while her mother worked. The girl had intense itching and a rash on her hands and arms for approximately 2 weeks. The itching became more severe and interfered with the child's sleep. On physical examination the child appeared well nourished and cared for. The skin on her hands, wrists, and forearms appeared red and excoriated. Raised, serpiginous "tracks" were noted on the sides of her fingers, on the ventral aspects of her wrists, and in the popliteal folds. Several of the tracks were inflamed and were beginning to form pustules. The mother stated that several other children at the daycare center were experiencing a similar problem.

1. What was the likely diagnosis?
2. How would this diagnosis have been confirmed?
3. How would this child have been treated, and what advice would have been given to the mother regarding prevention?
4. Did this child require antibiotic therapy? If so, why?
5. What should have been done regarding the other children at the daycare center?

Bibliography

Binford CH, Connor DH: *Pathology of tropical and extraordinary diseases*, vol 3, Washington, 1976, Armed Forces Institute of Pathology.

Fritsche TR: Arthropods of medical importance. In Murray PR et al, editors: *Manual of clinical microbiology*, ed 8, Washington, 2003, American Society for Microbiology.

Markell EK, John DT, Krotoski WA: *Markell and Voges medical parasitology*, ed 8, Philadelphia, 1999, WB Saunders.

Najarian HH: *Textbook of medical parasitology*, Baltimore, 1967, Williams & Wilkins.

Peters W: *A colour atlas of arthropods in clinical medicine*, London, 1992, Wolfe.

Strickland GT: *Hunter's tropical medicine and emerging infectious diseases*, ed 8, Philadelphia, 2000, WB Saunders.

Van Horn KG et al: Copepods associated with a perirectal abscess and copepod pseudo-outbreaks in stools for ova and parasite examinations, *Diagn Microbiol Infect Dis* 15:561-565, 1992.

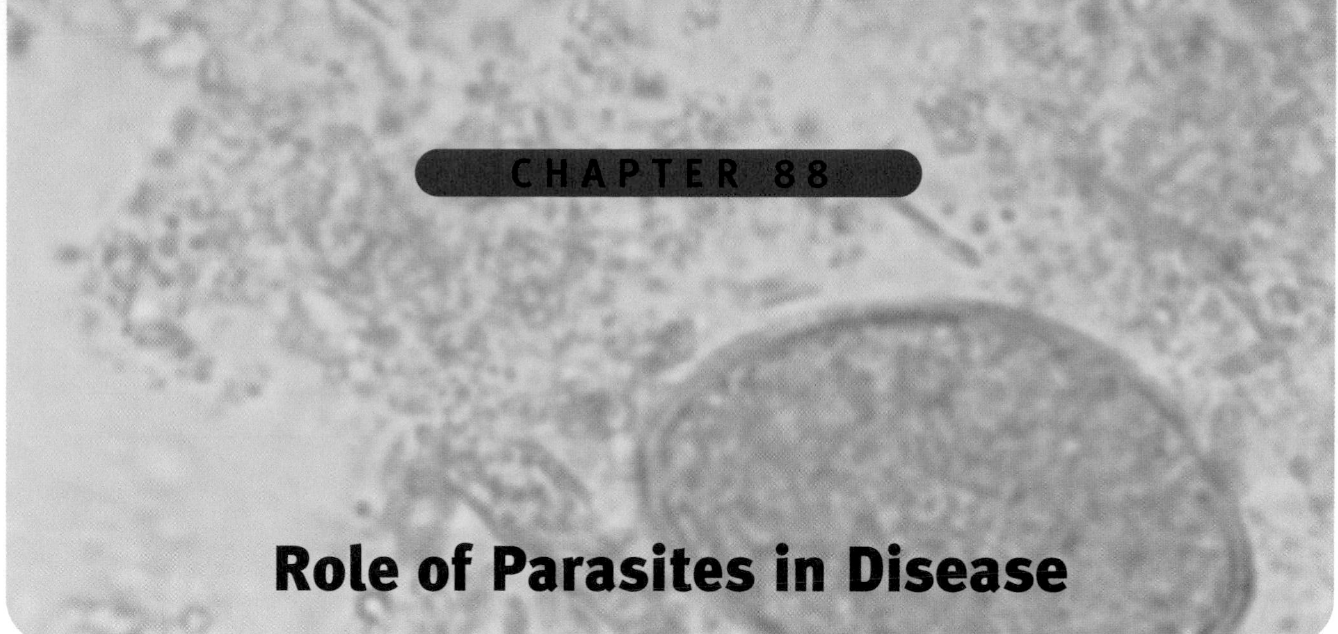

CHAPTER 88

Role of Parasites in Disease

A summary of the parasites (protozoan and helminths) most commonly associated with human disease is presented in this chapter. Although many parasites are associated with a single organ system (e.g., gastrointestinal tract) and therefore cause a disease process involving that system, some of the most dramatic manifestations of parasitic disease occur when the parasite leaves its "normal" location in the human body. Likewise, several different parasites may produce a similar disease syndrome. Given that the management of a specific parasitic infection may differ tremendously according to the etiologic agent, and that many antiparasitic treatment regimens are quite toxic, it is useful to generate a differential diagnosis that includes the most likely parasites, in order to guide both diagnostic and therapeutic efforts.

Because both the development and the prognosis of a parasitic infection often depend on factors aside from the innate virulence of the organism, one must take into account numerous factors, such as exposure history (e.g., travel to an endemic area), the potential infectious dose and/or organism burden, the use of prophylaxis (e.g., antimalarial prophylaxis), and the immunologic status of the host in determining the possibility of a parasitic infection, the meaning of any microbiologic data, and the necessity to treat and with what agent. The presentation of a given parasitic infection may be quite different in a nonimmune traveler to an endemic region versus a semi-immune resident of the same region. Likewise, the treatment and prevention strategies will be different as well.

This chapter provides a very broad listing of the various parasitic agents commonly associated with infections at specific body sites and/or specific clinical manifestations (Table 88–1). This information is meant to be used in conjunction with Table 81–1 as an aid in establishing a differential diagnosis and for selection of the most likely clinical specimens that will help establish a specific etiologic diagnosis. Other factors that may be important in determining the relative frequency with which specific parasites cause disease (e.g., travel and exposure history, specific clinical presentations) are covered in the individual chapters in this text, or in the more comprehensive infectious disease texts cited in this or other chapters.

Bibliography

Cohen J, Powderly WG, editors: *Infectious diseases*, ed 2, Philadelphia, 2004, Elsevier.

Connor DH et al, editors: *Pathology of infectious diseases*, Stamford, Conn, 1997, Appleton & Lange.

Cook G, Zumala A, editors: *Mansons tropical diseases*, ed 21, London, 2003, Elsevier Science.

Garcia LS, editor: *Diagnostic medical parasitology*, ed 4, Washington, 2001, ASM Press.

TABLE 88–1. Summary of Parasites Associated with Human Disease

System Affected and Disease	Pathogens
Blood	
Malaria	*Plasmodium* spp.
Babesiosis	*Babesia* spp.
Filariasis	*Wuchereria bancrofti, Brugia malayi, Mansonella* spp., *Loa loa*
Bone Marrow	
Leishmaniasis	*Leishmania donovani, Leishmanias tropica*
Central Nervous System	
Meningoencephalitis	*Naegleria fowleri, Trypanosoma brucei gambiense, Trypanosoma brucei rhodesiense, Trypanosoma cruzi, Toxoplasma gondii,* Microsporidia
Granulomatous encephalitis	*Acanthamoeba* spp., *Balamuthia mandrillaris*
Mass lesion Brain abscess	*T. gondii, Taenia solium, Schistosoma japonicum, Acanthamoeba* spp., *B. mandrillaris*
Eosinophilic meningitis Cerebral malaria	*Angiostrongylus cantonensis, Toxocara* spp. (Visceral larval migrans), *Plasmodium falciparum*
Cerebral paragonimiasis	*Paragonimus westermani*
Eye	
Keratitis	*Acanthamoeba* spp., Microsporidia (*Nosema* sp., *Microsporidium* spp., *Encephalitozoon hellem*), *Onchocerca volvulus*
Chorioretinitis/conjunctivitis	*T. gondii, O. volvulus, L. loa*
Ocular cysticercosis (mass lesion)	*T. solium*
Toxocariasis	*Toxocara* spp. (mimics retinoblastoma)
Intestinal Tract	
Anal pruritis	*Enterobius vermicularis*
Colitis	*Entamoeba histolytica, Balantidium coli*
Diarrhea/dysentery	*E. histolytica, Giardia lamblia (duodenalis),* Microsporidia, *Cryptosporidium parvum, Cyclospora cayetanensis, Isospora belli, Schistosoma mansoni, Strongyloides stercoralis, Trichuris trichiura*
Toxic megacolon	*Trypanosoma cruzi*
Obstruction/perforation	*Ascaris lumbricoides, Fasciolopsis buski*
Rectal prolapse	*T. trichiura*
Liver, Spleen	
Abscess	*E. histolytica, Fasciola hepatica*
Hepatitis	Microsporidia *(Encephalitozoon cuniculi, Nosema connori), T. gondii*
Biliary obstruction	*A. lumbricoides, F. hepatica, Opisthorchis (Clonorchis) sinensis*
Cirrhosis/hepatosplenomegaly	*L. donovani, L. tropica, Toxocara canis* and *T. cati* (visceral larval migrans), *S. mansoni, S. japonicum*
Mass lesions	*T. solium, Echinococcus granulosus, Echinococcus multilocularis*

TABLE 88–1. Summary of Parasites Associated with Human Disease—cont'd

Genitourinary	
Vaginitis/urethritis	*Trichomonas vaginalis, E. vermicularis*
Renal failure	*Plasmodium spp., L. donovani*
Cystitis/hematuria	*Schistosoma haematobium, P. falciparum* (blackwater fever)
Heart	
Myocarditis	Microsporidia, *T. gondii, T. cruzi*
Megacardia/complete heart block	*T. cruzi*
Lung	
Abscess	*E. histolytica, P. westermani*
Nodule/mass	*Dirofilaria immitis, E. granulosus, E. multilocularis*
Pneumonitis	*A. lumbricoides, S. stercoralis, Toxocara* spp., *P. westermani, T. gondii, Ancylostoma braziliense*
Lymphatics	
Lymphedema	*W. bancrofti, B. malayi*, other filaria
Lymphadenopathy	*T. gondii*, trypanosomes
Muscle	
Generalized myositis	*Trichinella spiralis*, Microsporidia, *Sarcocystis lindemanni, Toxocara* spp.
Myocarditis	*T. spiralis, T. cruzi*, Microsporidia, *Toxocara* spp.
Skin and Subcutaneous Tissue	
Ulcerative lesion	*Leishmania* spp., *Dracunculus medinensis*
Nodule/swellings	*O. volvulus, L. loa, T. cruzi, Acanthamoeba* spp., *Toxocara* spp.
Rash/vesicles	*T. gondii, A. braziliense*, other migrating worms, schistosomes (cercarial dermatitis)
Systemic	
General dissemination and multiple organ dysfunction	Microsporidia, *P. falciparum, T. gondii, L. donovani, T. cruzi, Toxocara* spp., *S. stercoralis, T. spiralis*
Iron deficiency, anemia	Hookworms *(Ancylostoma duodenale, Necator americanus)*
Megaloblastic anemia (Vitamin B_{12} deficiency)	*Diphyllobothrium latum*

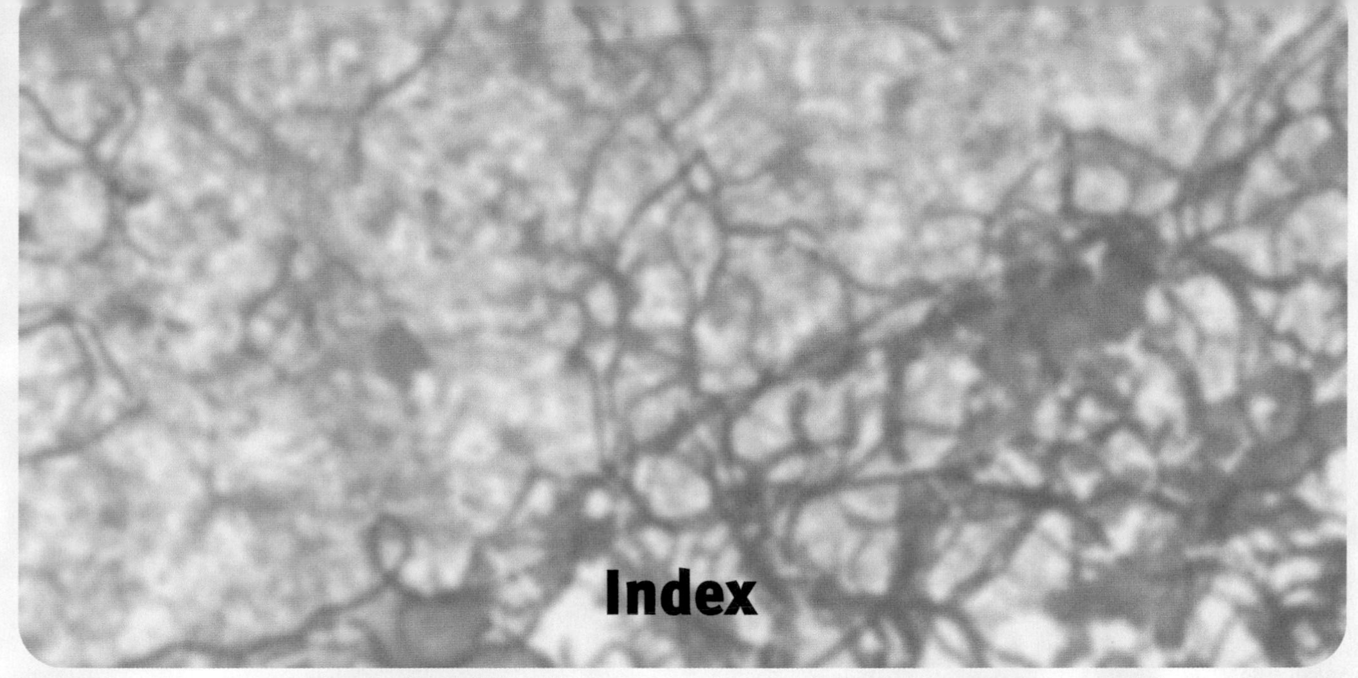

Index